NEET

EXPLORING BIOLOGY

Volume 02

Sanjay Sharma
Sudhakar Banerjee

Supported by

Mahendra Singh Rawat

arihant

ARIHANT PRAKASHAN (Series), MEERUT

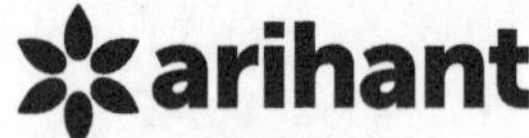

ARIHANT PRAKASHAN (Series), MEERUT

Administrative & Production Offices

Regd. Office

'Ramchhaya' 4577/15, Agarwal Road, Darya Ganj, New Delhi -110002
Tele: 011- 47630600, 43518550

Head Office

Kalindi, TP Nagar, Meerut (UP) - 250002, Tel: 0121-7156203, 7156204

Sales & Support Offices

Agra, Ahmedabad, Bengaluru, Bareilly, Chennai, Delhi, Guwahati, Hyderabad, Jaipur, Jhansi, Kolkata, Lucknow, Nagpur & Pune.

ISBN 978-93-26191-75-3

PRICE ₹735.00

PO No : TXT-XX-XXXXXXX-X-XX

Published by Arihant Publications (India) Ltd.

PRODUCTION TEAM

Publishing Manager : Keshav Mohan
Project Head : Shiva Choudhary
Project Editor : Sanubia, Kavita
Cover Designer : Bilal Hashmi
Inner Designer : Ankit Saini
Page Layouting : Deepak Bisht, Sachin, Naresh
Proof Readers : Nidhi, Nalini, Mamta

For further information about the books published by Arihant, log on to www.arihantbooks.com or e-mail at info@arihantbooks.com

Follow us on

Preface

Mastery on Biology is important for students who are planning to make their career in medicine. To get this you require an objective approach in your studies. This Objective Approach can be defined as the approach through which a student is able to master the concepts and also the skills required to tackle the questions asked in different formats in entrances such as NEET (National Eligibility cum Entrance Test).

Although the number of medical colleges imparting quality education and training has significantly increased after independence in the country but due to the simultaneous increase in the number of serious aspirants, the competition is no longer easy for a seat in a prestigious medical college today. Present changes in NEET exam Pattern has increased this challenge many fold.

Exploring Biology (Vol.1 & 2) are borne out of our experience of teaching biology to medical aspirants. The content of these books is framed to provide helps in facing present day challenges by future medicos.

The plan of the presentation of the subject matter in the books is as follows

- The whole chapter has been divided under logical topic heads to cover the whole syllabi of NEET developing the concepts in an easy going manner, taking the help of suitable examples, diagrams, flow charts, table, etc.
- Important points of the topics have been highlighted in the text under notes, some extra points regarding the topics have been given in Notes to enrich the students.
- **Check Point** Exercises given in between the text of all chapter help the readers to remain linked with the text given as they provide them an opportunity to assess themselves while studying the text.
- At the end of the theory part **Exam Points** are given in every chapter. These points are framed from last 10 years (2011-2020) questions for providing fast track revision.
- Assignments at the end of the chapters have been divided into three parts:

  Part A- 'Topical Exercises' having simple NEET level MCQs arranged in accordance with content flow of the chapter. This exercise helps in building basics about the chapter.

  Part B- 'Cumulative Exercises' has advanced level objective questions of concerned chapter. The special point of this exercise is that questions have been arranged systematically with Assertion-Reason questions in the last. This exercise helps in gaining conceptual clarity of advanced level.

  Part C- 'Medical Entrances Gallery' covering all questions asked in last 11 years' (2021-2011) in NEET & other Medical Entrances.
- The Explanation of some selected question given in different exercises have been provided.
- Appendix given in the last is an additional feature to make the text more informative.
- Multi-Coloured pictures related to important topics of chapters are given at the end of book.

At the end we would like to say that suggestions from the respected Teachers & Students for the further improvement of the book will be welcomed open heartedly.

Huge efforts have been made from our side to keep this book error free, but inspite of that if any error or whatsoever is skipped in the book then that is purely incidental, apology for the same, please write to us about that so that it can be corrected in the further edition of the book.

Sanjay Sharma
Sudhakar Banerjee

Syllabus

UNIT I Reproduction

Reproduction in organisms Reproduction, a characteristic feature of all organisms for continuation of species, Modes of reproduction–Asexual and sexual, Asexual reproduction, Modes-Binary fission, sporulation, budding, gemmule, fragmentation, vegetative propagation in plants.

Sexual reproduction in flowering plants Flower structure, Development of male and female gametophytes, Pollination-types, agencies and examples, Outbreeding devices, Pollen-Pistil interaction, Double fertilization, Post fertilization events-Development of endosperm and embryo, Development of seed and formation of fruit, Special modes-apomixis, parthenocarpy, polyembryony, Significance of seed and fruit formation.

Human Reproduction Male and female reproductive systems, Microscopic anatomy of testis and ovary, Gametogenesis-spermatogenesis and oogenesis, Menstrual cycle, Fertilisation, embryo development upto blastocyst formation, implantation, Pregnancy and placenta formation (Elementary idea), Parturition (Elementary idea), Lactation (Elementary idea).

Reproductive health Need for reproductive health and prevention of sexually transmitted diseases (STD), Birth control-Need and Methods, Contraception and Medical Termination of Pregnancy (MTP), Amniocentesis, Infertility and assisted reproductive technologies – IVF, ZIFT, GIFT (Elementary idea for general awareness).

UNIT II Genetics and Evolution

Heredity and variation Mendelian Inheritance, Deviations from Mendelism-Incomplete dominance, Co-dominance, Multiple alleles and Inheritance of blood groups, Pleiotropy, Elementary idea of polygenic inheritance, Chromosome theory of inheritance, Chromosomes and genes, Sex determination-In humans, birds, honey bee, Linkage and crossing over, Sex linked inheritance-Haemophilia, Colour blindness, Mendelian disorders in humans-Thalassemia, Chromosomal disorders in humans, Down's syndrome, Turner's and Klinefelter's syndromes.

Molecular basis of Inheritance Search for genetic material and DNA as genetic material, Structure of DNA and RNA, DNA packaging, DNA replication, Central dogma, Transcription, genetic code, translation, Gene expression and regulation-Lac Operon, Genome and human genome project, DNA finger printing.

Evolution Origin of life, Biological evolution and evidences for biological evolution from Paleontology, comparative anatomy, embryology and molecular evidence), Darwin's contribution, Modern Synthetic theory of Evolution, Mechanism of evolution-Variation (Mutation and Recombination) and Natural Selection with examples, types of natural selection, Gene flow and genetic drift, Hardy-Weinberg's principle, Adaptive Radiation, Human evolution.

UNIT III Biology and Human Welfare

Health and Disease, Pathogens, parasites causing human diseases (Malaria, Filariasis, Ascariasis, Typhoid, Pneumonia, common cold, amoebiasis, ring worm), Basic concepts of immunology-vaccines, Cancer, HIV and AIDS, Adolescence, drug and alcohol abuse.

Improvement in food production Plant breeding, tissue culture, single cell protein, Biofortification, Apiculture and Animal husbandry.

Microbes in human welfare In household food processing, industrial production, sewage treatment, energy generation and as biocontrol agents and biofertilizers.

UNIT IV Biotechnology and Its Applications

Principles and process of Biotechnology Genetic engineering (Recombinant DNA technology). Applications of Biotechnology in health and agriculture Human insulin and vaccine production, gene therapy, Genetically modified organisms-Bt crops, Transgenic Animals, Biosafety issues-Biopiracy and patents.

UNIT V Ecology and Environment

Organisms and environment Habitat and niche, Population and ecological adaptations, Population interactions-mutualism, competition, predation, parasitism, Population attributes-growth, birth rate and death rate, age distribution.

Ecosystem Patterns, components, productivity and decomposition, Energy flow, Pyramids of number, biomass, energy, Nutrient cycling (carbon and phosphorous), Ecological succession, Ecological Services-Carbon fixation, pollination, oxygen release.

Biodiversity and its conservation Concept of Biodiversity, Patterns of Biodiversity, Importance of Biodiversity, Loss of Biodiversity, Biodiversity conservation, Hotspots, endangered organisms, extinction, Red Data Book, biosphere reserves, National parks and sanctuaries.

Environmental issues Air pollution and its control, Water pollution and its control, Agrochemicals and their effects, Solid waste management, Radioactive waste management, Greenhouse effect and global warning, Ozone depletion, Deforestation, Any three case studies as success stories addressing environmental issues.

Contents

NEET
Solved Paper 2021

Scan the QR Code

CHAPTER 01

Reproduction in Organisms

The period from birth to the natural death of an organism represents its **lifespan.** It could be short as few days or long as a number of years. Lifespan cannot necessarily be correlated with the size of an organism, e.g. lifespan of mango tree is much shorter than that of peepal tree.

Irrespective of long or short lifespan of an organism, death is a certain phenomenon, i.e. no individual is immortal, except single-celled organisms like *Amoeba.* So, there must be some processes in living organisms that ensure continuity of species.

This process is reproduction. In this chapter, we will study the different modes of reproduction present in various species and the importance of this process.

Reproduction

- Every living organism passes through definite stages of life cycle. It takes birth, matures, reproduces and finally dies.
- Reproduction is thus, one of the fundamental characteristic of living organisms, through which each species ensures its continuity.
- It is a biological process through which an organism gives rise to young ones or offsprings similar to itself. It also maintains the continuous cycle of birth, growth and death.
- Reproduction performs following functions
  - (i) Maintains life on earth.
  - (ii) Enables continuity of the species, generation after generation.
  - (iii) Creates genetic variation among populations and contributes to evolutionary process.
  - (iv) Maintains populations of the young, adult and the aged persons.
- Several factors like organism's habitat, internal physiology and environmental conditions determine how an organism reproduces.
- Based on the participation of the number of organisms/parents, reproduction can be categorised into two types, i.e. **asexual** (involves only one parent) and **sexual** (involves two parents of opposite sex) reproduction.

Inside

ASEXUAL REPRODUCTION

The production of offspring by single parent without the formation or fusion of gametes is called asexual reproduction. It is also known as **agamogenesis** or **agamogeny**. In this mode of reproduction, somatic cells undergo mitosis to form a new individual (somatogenic reproduction). They do not involve meiotic divisions as the process of gamete formation is absent.

Other features of asexual reproduction are as follows

- The offspring produced in asexual reproduction are genetically similar to their parents.
- They do not show any variations due to the absence of crossing over and recombination. Such a group of morphologically and genetically similar individuals is referred to as **clone**.
- **Ramet** is the term used for a single individual of a clone.
- It occurs most commonly in unicellular, lower organisms like monerans and protists.
- It may also occur in multicellular higher plants and animals that possess relatively simple body organisations.

Modes of asexual reproduction

There can be different modes of asexual reproduction depending upon the conditions in which organism is reproducing. These modes are as follows

1. Fission

It is a mode of asexual reproduction in which the body of a mature individual divides into two or more similar and equal sized daughters.

Fission can be of two types, *viz.* binary fission or multiple fission.

Binary fission

It is the process of division of a parent cell into two daughter cells of equal size. The parent cell never dies as it continues to live in the form of daughter cells. In different organisms, binary fission occurs in following ways

- In unicellular organisms, binary fission occurs by the mitotic division of nucleus followed by cytokinesis (cytoplasmic division).
- In multicellular organisms, it is achieved by cleavage (constriction).

Types of binary fission

Depending upon the plane of division, different types of binary fission are as follows

(i) **Simple binary fission** In this type of fission, the plane of cytoplasmic division is not fixed, e.g. *Amoeba.*

The different stages in binary fission in *Amoeba* are shown in the figure below

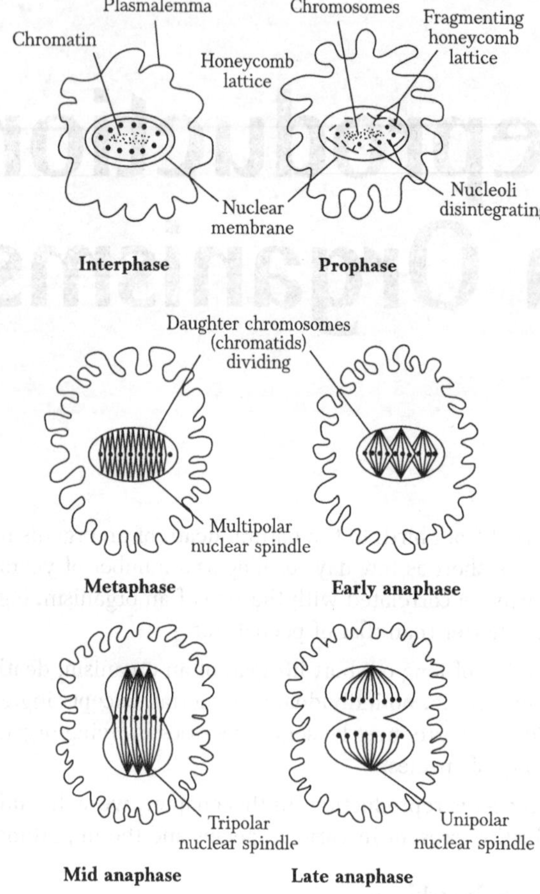

Fig. 1.1 Amoeba : Stages in binary fission

(ii) **Transverse binary fission** The plane of cytoplasmic division passes through the transverse axis of an individual, e.g. *Paramecium*, diatoms, etc.

(iii) **Longitudinal binary fission** The plane of cytoplasmic division passes through the longitudinal axis of an individual, e.g. *Euglena, Vorticella*, etc.

(iv) **Oblique binary fission** In this type of fission, plane of division is oblique, e.g. *Ceratium* and *Gonyaulax.*

Multiple fission

In this type of fission, parent cell divides several times by amitosis thus, producing several daughter cells without involving any cytokinesis. Later, each daughter nucleus gathers a small amount of cytoplasm around itself. It is a common method of reproduction in many protists, algae, protozoans and sporozoans.

Multiple fission in *Plasmodium*

In *Plasmodium*, multiple fission may occur *via* schizogony or sporogony.

The offspring produced in schizogony and sporogony are respectively, called as **merozoites** and **sporozoites**.

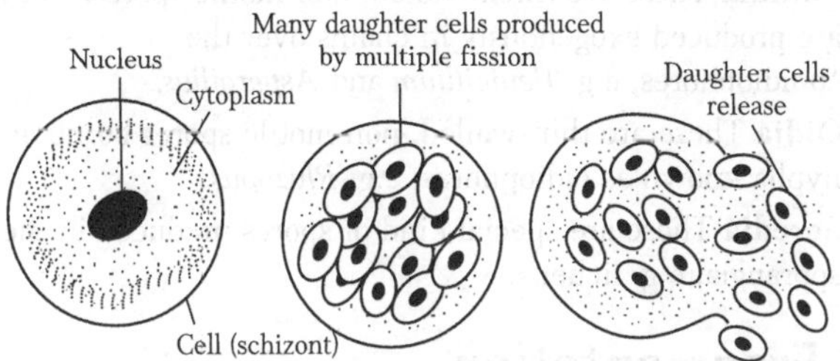

Fig. 1.2 Multiple fission in Plasmodium

Multiple fission in *Amoeba*

In *Amoeba*, multiple fission may occur with or without the formation of cyst.

(i) **Multiple fission with encystation** During unfavourable conditions, *Amoeba* develops a three-layered wall around itself to form a cyst. Inside the cyst, nucleus divides repeatedly to form several pseudopodiospores.
In favourable conditions, cyst ruptures and pseudopodiospores are liberated.

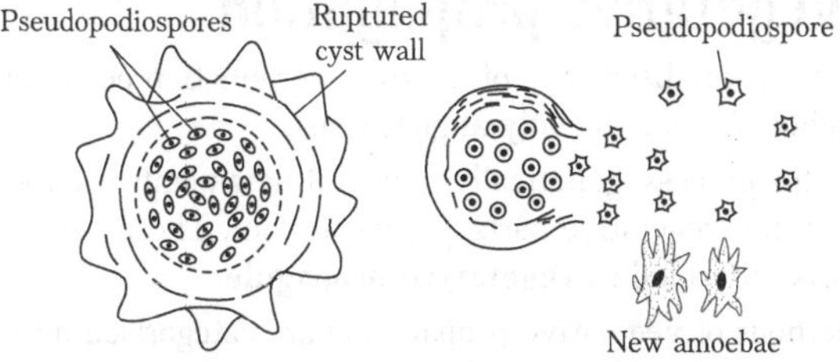

Fig. 1.3 Multiple fission with encystation

(ii) **Multiple fission without encystation** Sometimes multiple fission in *Amoeba* can also occur without encystation. This is known as **sporulation.**
In this process, after karyokinesis, spores are developed. These spores give rise to new amoebae during favourable conditions.

2. Plasmotomy

It is the division of cytoplasm in a multinucleate organism into multinucleate offspring without the involvement of nuclear division.

The daughter cells regain the same number of nuclei by further nuclear divisions, e.g. *Opalina, Pelomyxa*, etc.

3. Budding

In this process, the parent cell produces one or more protuberances called **buds** by mitosis. These buds detach from parent cell and grow into new individuals.

Budding may be of two types as follows

Exogenous budding

- During favourable conditions, a bud grows on the parent body externally (on the body surface). It shows different type of growth patterns as follows
  - Bud detaches from parent to lead a free life, e.g. *Hydra.*

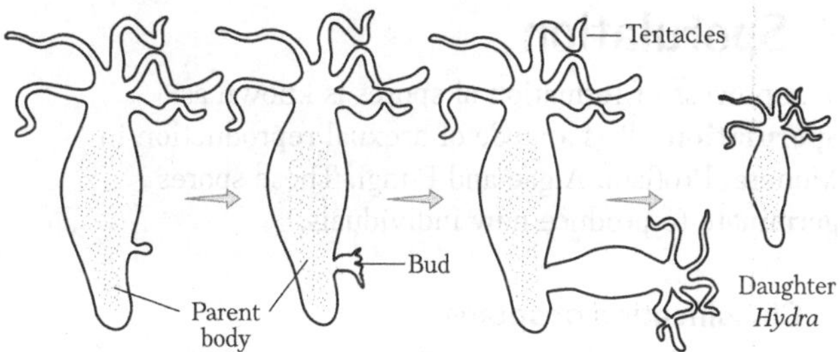

Fig. 1.4 Budding in Hydra

  - Bud remains attached to parent to form a colony, e.g. *Obelia.*
- In yeast during budding, the cell wall of the parent cell bulges out in the form of an outgrowth. The parent nucleus divides into two daughter nuclei, one of which migrates into the bud. As the bud enlarges and is fully formed, it is separated from the parent cell and grows into mature yeast.

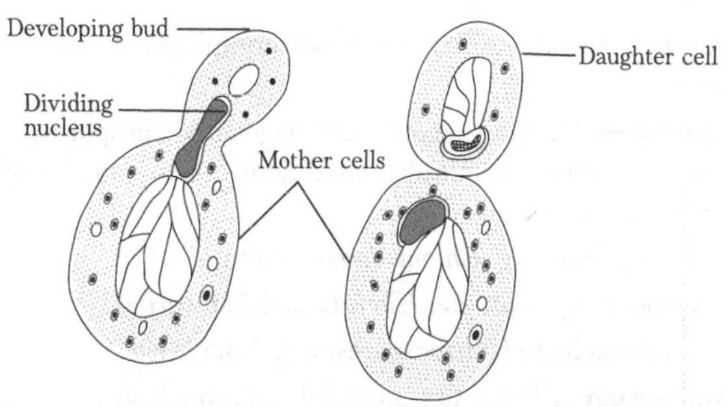

Fig. 1.5 Budding in yeast (Saccharomyces)

Endogenous budding

- In this process, the bud is formed within the parent's body. These internal buds are called **gemmules.**
- These are formed under unfavourable conditions and commonly seen in freshwater sponge, e.g. *Spongilla.*

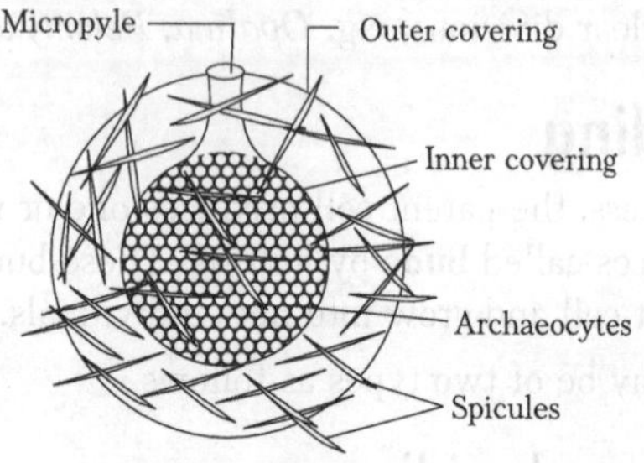

Fig. 1.6 A gemmule of sponges

- During favourable conditions, archaeocytes (totipotent cells) come out from micropyle and develop into a new complete individual.

4. Sporulation

The process of formation of spores is known as **sporulation.** It is a mode of asexual reproduction in Monera, Protista, Algae and Fungi. These spores germinate to produce new individuals.

Classification of spores

Spores are classified on the basis of structure in which these are produced, e.g. urediospore (uredium in smuts), teliospore (telium in rusts) and zygospore (zygosporangium in Zygomycetes).

Parasitic fungal spores are divided as internal spores (germinate within the host) and external spores (released by one host to infest other hosts).

Spores are also classified as

(i) **Monolete spore** A single line on the spore indicating the axis on which the mother spore was split into four spores, along a vertical axis.

(ii) **Trilete spore** All four spores share a common origin and are in contact with each other and on separation, each spore shows three lines radiating from a centre pole.

Different types of spores in various organisms are as follows

- **Zoospores** These are motile and flagellated zoospores produced during favourable conditions. These may be of following types
  - Biflagellate, e.g. *Chlamydomonas* and *Ulothrix*
  - Quadriflagellate, e.g. *Ulothrix* and *Ectocarpus*
  - Multinucleate (synzoospores) e.g. *Vaucheria*
- **Aplanospores** These are unicellular, uninucleate, non-motile and thin-walled spores produced during unfavourable conditions, e.g. *Spirogyra* and *Ulothrix.*
- **Statospores** These are thick-walled resting spores. Their wall may be smooth or variously ornamented, e.g. diatoms.
- **Neutral spores** In certain algae, the protoplast of vegetative cells directly function as spores. These spores are called as neutral spores, e.g. *Asterocystis* and *Ectocarpus.*
- **Hormospores** These are terminally located spores in blue-green algae. They are multicellular and thick-walled, e.g. *Westiella.*
- **Chlamydospores** These are thick-walled, non-motile spores, e.g. *Rhizopus, Agaricus,* etc.
- **Sporangiospores** These are non-motile spores produced inside the sporangium, e.g. *Rhizopus* and *Mucor,* etc.
- **Conidia** These are thick-walled, non-motile spores. These are produced exogenously in chains over the conidiophores, e.g. *Penicillium* and *Aspergillus.*
- **Oidia** These are thin-walled, non-motile spores borne on a hypha known as oidiophores, e.g. *Rhizopus.*
- **Soredia** These are special kind of spores produced in the sporangia, e.g. lichens.

5. Fragmentation

- It is the process of breaking down of parent individual into small pieces or fragments either accidentally or through external force.
- Each of these fragments develops into a new individual (regeneration).
- Fragmentation mainly occurs during unfavourable conditions in following organisms
  - **In plants,** it occurs commonly in algae, fungi, bryophytes and pteridophytes.
  - **Among animals,** it may occur in protists, coelenterates and many flatworms.

6. Vegetative propagation

- It is a specialised type of asexual reproduction occurring in higher plants especially angiosperms.
- In this process, genetically identical new plants are formed from the vegetative parts of parent plant. These vegetative parts are called as **vegetative propagule.**
- Methods of vegetative propagation are categorised into natural and artificial methods. These are discussed in detail below

I. Natural vegetative propagation in higher plants

This type of vegetative propagation occurs in plant naturally. A fragment of the mother plant separates and forms an independent plant under suitable conditions.

Natural propagation in higher plants may occur by the following means

(i) By roots

Tap root branches can develop adventitious buds and form new plants, e.g. guava, *Populus* and *Dalbergia*.

Similarly, fleshy adventitious roots take part in vegetative propagation, e.g. sweet potato, *Dahlia* and *Asparagus*.

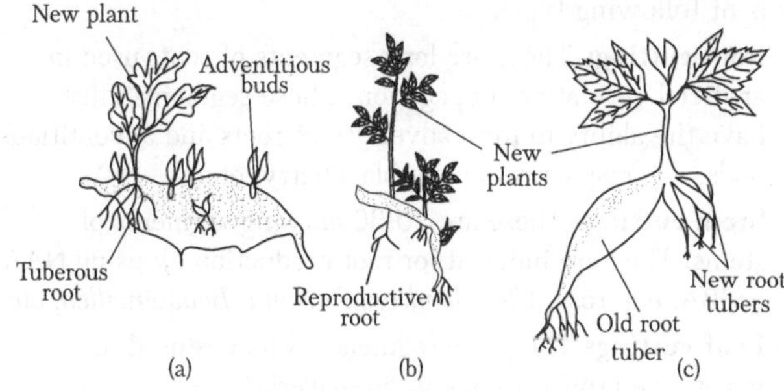

Fig. 1.7 Vegetative propagation by roots : (a) Adventitious buds growing into new shoots from tuberous root of sweet potato, (b) Young shoots arising from reproductive root of Dalbergia (Sheesham), (c) Old root tuber of Dahlia growing into new plant

(ii) By stems

In plants, vegetative propagation can also take place by stems. They modify variously to give rise to new plants in following ways

(a) **Underground stems** Various underground stems are given below

- **Tuber** is modified swollen underground stem. It bears buds on eyes or nodes. Each bud may grow into a new plant when planted, e.g. potato and artichoke.
- **Rhizome** is an underground stem having buds, nodes and internodes. Buds present on nodes give rise to new aerial shoot, e.g. banana, ginger and *Aspidium*.
- **Bulbs** are modified shoots bearing apical and axillary buds that give rise to new plants, e.g. *Narcissus*, onion and garlic.
- **Corms** bear buds that sprout to form new plants, e.g. *Crocus*, *Colocasia* and *Freesia*.

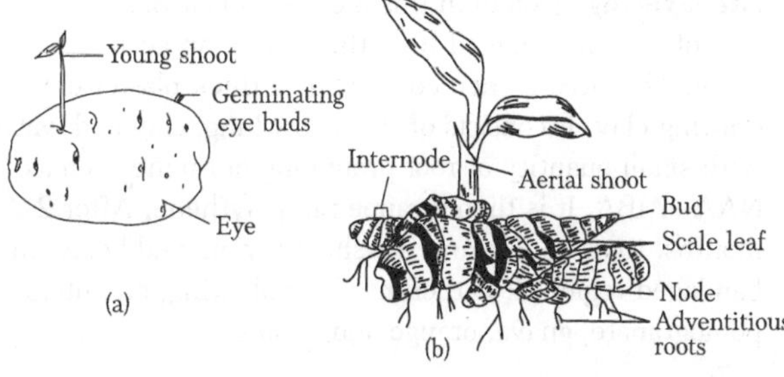

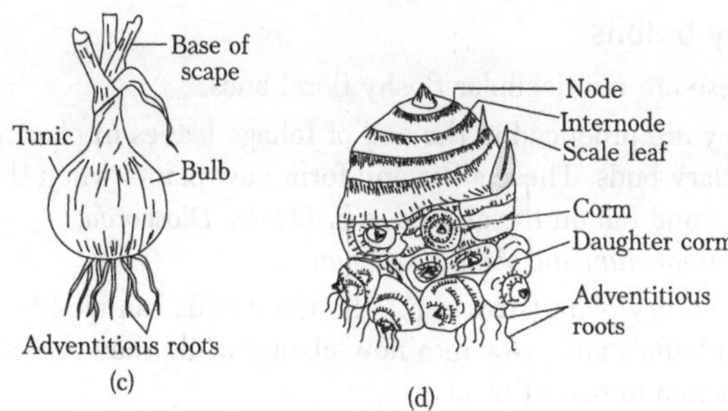

Fig. 1.8 (a) Tuber of potato, (b) Rhizome of ginger, (c) Bulb of onion, (d) Corm of Colocasia

(b) **Subaerial stems** (Creeping stems) These stems creep over the surface of soil. The various types of stems used in the development of new plants are as follows

- **Runners** are specialised narrow, green horizontal branches. They develop at the base of roots from where new crowns are formed, e.g. coriander, *Centella* and *Oxalis*.
- **Stolons** are horizontal branches that arch above the ground. They also help in vegetative propagation, e.g. strawberry, *Vallisneria*.
- **Offset** is one internode long runner found in aquatic plants. It breaks into parts and then forms new plants, e.g. *Eichhornia* (water hyacinth) and *Pistia*.
- **Suckers** arise from the base of erect shoots and grow for sometime. These detach from parent plants and then give rise to new shoots, e.g. mint and *Chrysanthemum*.

(c) **Aerial shoots** The bud bearing segments of some stems may directly give rise to new plants when fall down, e.g. sugarcane, *Opuntia* and other cacti.

(iii) By leaves

- The leaves of many plants possess adventitious buds that help in vegetative propagation, e.g. *Begonia*, *Bryophyllum*, *Saintpaulia*, etc.
- In *Begonia*, the injured leaves form new plants when they come in contact with the soil.
- However in *Bryophyllum*, marginal buds form plantlets, while they are still attached to the parent plant.

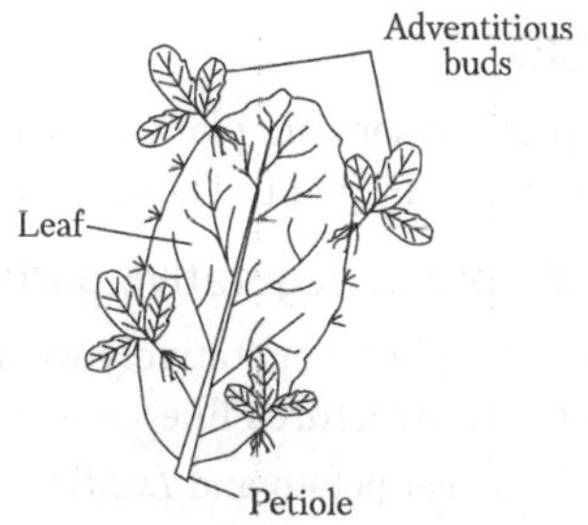

Fig. 1.9 A leaf of Bryophyllum showing formation of new plants from marginal adventitious buds

(iv) By bulbils

- These are multicellular fleshy floral buds.
- They are produced in the axil of foliage leaves in place of axillary buds. These grow and form new plants when they shed and fall on the ground, e.g. *Oxalis, Dioscorea, Chlorophytum* and *Allium sativum.*
- In century plant (*Agave* sp.), the floral buds can modify into bulbils and grow into new plants, while they are still attached to parent plant.

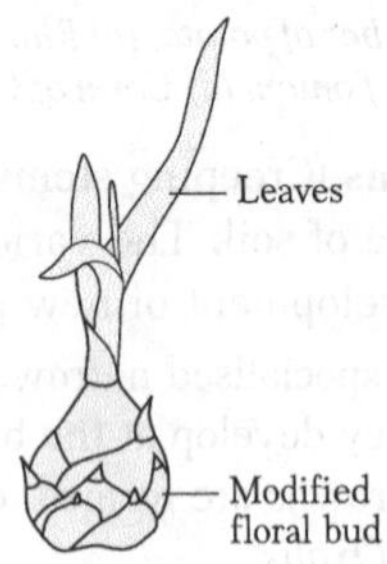

Fig. 1.10 Bulbils of Agave

(v) By turions

- These are special types of fleshy buds that develop in aquatic plants. They are swollen and contain reserve food material.
- During the spring, they form new plant for vegetative propagation, e.g. *Potamogeton* and *Utricularia.*

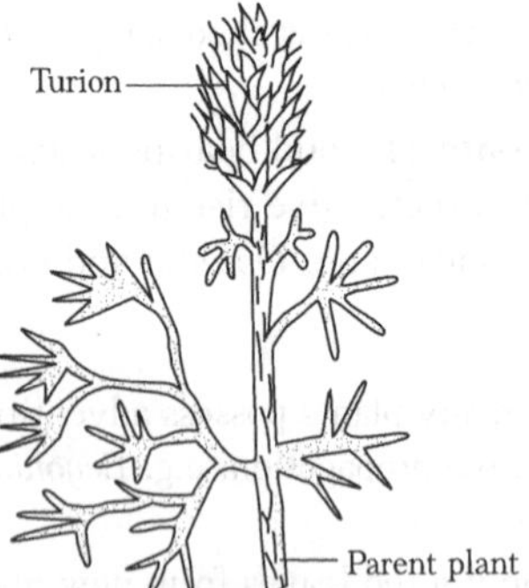

Fig 1.11 Turion of Utricularia

II. Artificial method of vegetative propagation

In this method, parts of somatic plant body are used to develop new independent plant. These are as follows

(i) By the use of special vegetative parts

Many plants are multiplied vegetatively by using their specialised vegetative structures like

- **root tubers,** e.g. sweet potato and *Dahlia*
- **corm**, e.g. *Crocus, Colocasia* and *Gladiolus*
- **bulb**, e.g. garlic and onion
- **part of rhizome**, e.g. banana and ginger
- **stem tuber,** e.g. potato
- **bulbil,** e.g. pineapple

(ii) By cuttings

When a small piece of any plant part, i.e. stem, root or leaf is used for vegetative propagation, it is called as cutting.

It is of following types

- **Root cuttings** These are long segments of roots used in artificial vegetative propagation. These segments must have the ability to form adventitious roots and adventitious buds, e.g. raspberry, lemon, blackberry, etc.
- **Stem cuttings** These are 20-30 cm long segments of stems. They are induced for root production by using NAA or IBA, e.g. rose, *Clerodendron, Duranta, Bougainvillea,* etc.
- **Leaf cuttings** These are segments of leaves used in vegetative propagation, e.g. *Sansevieria.*

(iii) By layering

In this method, adventitious roots are induced on a stem, while it is still attached to the plant. The middle part of a soft basal branch is defoliated and slightly injured. It is then pegged in the soil to develop adventitious roots.

The pegged down branch of the plant is called **layer.** Later on, this branch is separated and planted, e.g. cherry, lemon, jasmine and grapevine.

The various types of layering are as follows

- **Tip layering** In this method, only the tip of a branch is pegged down in the soil. It induces root formation followed by the growth of shoot tip, e.g. raspberry, blackberry, etc.
- **Continuous or Trench layering** In this type, a branch is pegged in horizontal position. It develops a number of vertical shoots, e.g apple and pear.
- **Serpentine layering** The basal branch is pegged at several places so as to form many plants, e.g. *Clematis.*
- **Mound layering** Shoot is pruned and its lower part is covered by soil in the form of a mound or heap. After sometime, it develops a number of shoots. Among these, the rooted ones are separated and planted, e.g. gooseberry and black currant.
- **Air layering** (gootee) In this method, about 3.5 cm ring of bark is removed from the base of an aerial shoot. This area is then covered by a thick plaster of grafting clay. It consists of hay, cowdung, clay and water with small quantity of root promoting hormone such as NAA or IBA. It is then wrapped in polythene. After 2-3 months, roots appear and the shoot is removed below the bandaged region. It is then used for planting, e.g. litchi, pomegranate, guava, orange and lemon.

Note *Plants having scattered vascular bundles like sugarcane cannot be propagated by air layering. The vascular bundles may get harmed and water and food supply is also affected in this method.*

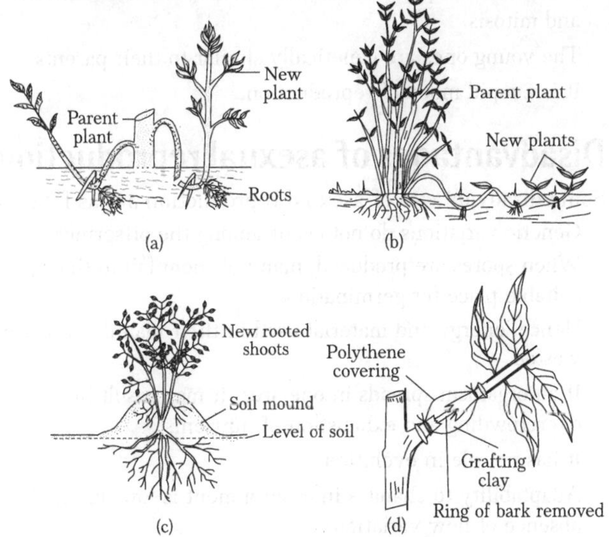

Fig. 1.12 (a) Tip layering, (b) Serpentine layering, (c) Mound layering, (d) Air layering

(iv) By grafting

- It is the most common method of artificial vegetative propagation.
- In this method, parts of two plants usually roots and shoots are joined in such a way that they grow as one plant.
- The rooted supporting portion of one plant is called as **stock**. It is joined with a twig of another plant called **scion.**
- Grafting is done between the two closely related dicotyledonous plants having vascular cambia.
- Due to joining, the cambia of these plants come in close contact. The point of contact is covered with grafting wax and bandages.
- Usually eustelic plants are used in this process, e.g. mango, rose, apple, rubber, citrus, pear, plum and peach.

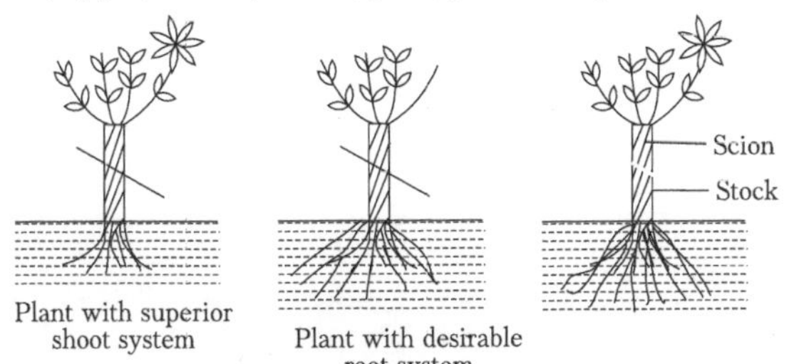

Fig 1.13 The process of grafting

- Grafting is of following four types
  (a) **Tongue or Whip grafting** Both the stock and scion are cut obliquely at about same angle.
  (b) **Wedge grafting** A V-shaped notch is made on stock and wedge-shaped cut is made on the scion.
  (c) **Crown grafting** Several scions having wedge-shaped cut are grafted on the slits at the top of stock.
  (d) **Side grafting** Single scion having wedge-shaped cut is inserted in a lateral slit of the stock.
- In case of tongue and wedge grafting, the scion and stock have almost the same diameter. In case of crown and side grafting, the stock has larger diameter than that of scion.

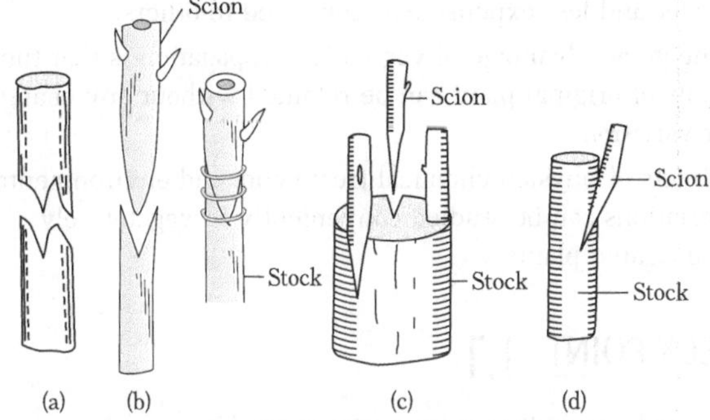

Fig 1.14 (a) Tongue grafting, (b) Wedge grafting, (c) Crown grafting, (d) Side grafting

Bud grafting

- In this method, scion is a bud with small portion of bark having intact cambium.
- This bud is inserted into a T-shaped incision made in the stock. In such a way, bud reaches up to the cambium of stock.
- The bud portion remains exposed to the air. The joint is thoroughly sealed using bandage, e.g. rose, apple, peach, etc.
- After 3-5 weeks, the bud begins to grow. As soon as the bud sprouts, the stock is cut above the level of graft, e.g. rose, apple, peach, etc.

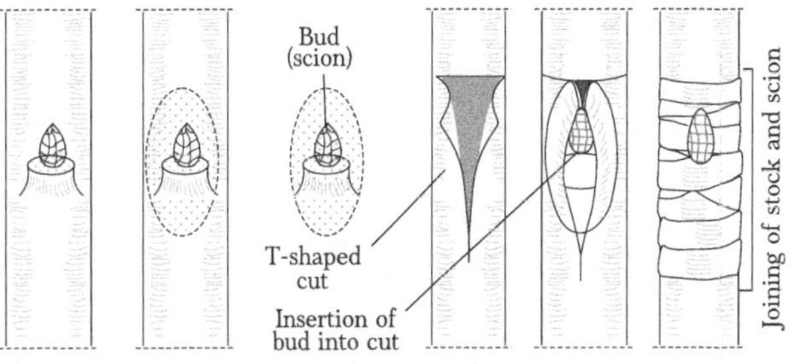

Fig 1.15 Bud grafting

Note • *Grafting can be done only in gymnosperms and dicots. It is not possible in monocot due to the absence of cambium.*
• *Grafting helps to grow the better varieties of plants with weak roots, e.g. mango, orange, etc.*

Importance of vegetative propagation

Significances of vegetative propagation are as follows

- There are some plants that lack sexual reproduction. Vegetative propagation is the only method of reproduction in those plants, e.g. banana, seedless grapes, oranges, rose, jasmine, figs, pineapple, carnation, etc.
- Plants which produce small quantities of viable seeds are mostly propagated vegetatively, e.g. *Cynodon* and *Dactylon.*
- The vegetative reproduction methods are more rapid, easier and less expensive as compared to others.
- The great advantage of vegetative propagation is that the traits of original plant can be retained without any change or variation.
- Effects of physico-chemical treatments and environmental variations can be studied conveniently in vegetatively propagated plants.

Advantages of asexual reproduction

Some advantages of asexual reproduction are listed below

- It involves simple processes of cell division like amitosis and mitosis.
- The young ones are genetically similar to their parents.
- It is a rapid mode of reproduction.

Disadvantages of asexual reproduction

Some disadvantages of asexual reproduction are as follows

- Genetic variations do not occur among the offsprings.
- When spores are produced, many of them fail to find a suitable place for germination.
  Hence, energy and material used in their manufacture are wasted.
- If an organism spreads in one area, it may result in overcrowding and exhaustion of nutrients.
- It has no role in evolution.
- Adaptability to changes in environment is low due to the absence of new variations.

CHECK POINT 1.1

1. Budding and fission are processes used by
(a) hermaphroditic organism
(b) organisms requiring new gene combinations for each generation
(c) sexually reproducing species
(d) asexually reproducing species

2. In potato, sugarcane, banana, ginger and *Dahlia*, the new plantlets invariably arise from
(a) the nodes present in the modified stems
(b) the nodes present in the modified roots
(c) the internodes present in the modified stems
(d) the margin of the leaves

3. Which pair of plants can be vegetatively propagated by leaf?
(a) *Bryophyllum* and *Saintpaulia*
(b) *Chrysanthemum* and *Agave*
(c) *Agave* and kalanchoe
(d) *Asparagus* and *Bryophyllum*

4. Vegetative propagation by stolon take place in
(a) *Eichhornia*
(b) strawberry
(c) Both (a) and (b)
(d) None of the above

5. Grafting is not possible in monocots as they
(a) lack cambium
(b) are herbaceous
(c) have conjoint open vascular bundles
(d) have parallel venation

6. One disadvantage of asexual reproduction is
(a) it does not produce variation
(b) it is complex
(c) it is a slow process
(d) None of the above

SEXUAL REPRODUCTION

It involves the formation and fusion of the male and female gametes. These gametes are produced either by same or different individuals of different sex. The gametes fuse to form a zygote which then develops to form a new organism.

Major features of sexual reproduction are as follows

- The offspring produced as a result of sexual reproduction exhibit genetic variations.
- It mainly occurs due to the involvement of meiosis and sexual fusion.
- It is a slow method of multiplication and occurs in **sexually complex organisms.**

Modes of sexual reproduction

Various modes of sexual reproduction are as follows

1. Syngamy

It is the complete and permanent fusion of male and female gametes to form the zygote. It was discovered by **Strasburger** (1884).

On the basis of structure of fusing gametes, syngamy may be of four types

(i) **Isogamy** Fusion of morphologically similar gametes, e.g. *Monocystis.*

(ii) **Anisogamy** Fusion of two dissimilar gametes, e.g. frog, rabbit and mammals.

(iii) **Oogamy** Fusion of large non-motile female gamete (egg) and small motile male gamete (antherozoid), e.g. red algae.

(iv) **Hologamy** Fusion of two organisms, which act as gametes, e.g. yeasts.

On the basis of site of occurrence, syngamy may be of two types

(i) **Exogamy** Syngamy occurs outside the body of organism in external medium (mostly water), e.g. algae, fishes, amphibians, etc.

Organisms exhibiting external fertilisation usually produce a huge number of gametes to enhance the chances of survival. This is because, their offspring are extremely vulnerable to predators.

(ii) **Endogamy** Syngamy occurs inside the body of organisms, e.g. plants like bryophytes, pteridophytes, gymnosperms, angiosperms, etc.

In order to enhance the chances of syngamy, large number of male gametes are produced in it.

2. Conjugation

- It involves the temporary union of two parents of the same species. These parents exchange their male pronuclei and then separate.
- It is somewhat like cross-fertilisation, e.g. *Paramecium*, bacteria and other ciliates.
- Conjugation is responsible for providing genetic variability even among organisms of same species.

Conjugation in Bacteria

Genetic recombination in bacteria takes place by conjugation. It was discovered by **Lederberg** and **Tatum** (1946) in *E. coli.*

The mechanism of conjugation in bacteria is as follows

- Conjugation occurs between two sexually different haploid strains of bacteria. One of them acts as donor of genes (male), while the other as recipient of genes (female).
- The donor and recipient bacteria termed as F^+ and F^-, respectively.
- The donor possesses sex factor or fertility (F) factor. It is a small genetic particle of circular DNA. Sex factor is responsible for the formation of sex pili.
- When the donor F^+ and recipient cells F^- come closer, a conjugation bridge is formed between them.
- Sex pili induces the formation of conjugation bridge.
- The F factor divides into two, out of which one remains in the donor cell and the other moves to the recipient through the conjugation bridge.
- As a result, the F^- cell now becomes F^+ cell.
- Thus, a conjugation between F^+ and F^- strains always yield F^+ progeny.

Conjugation in *Paramecium*

- It is the temporary union of two individuals (or conjugant) for the mutual exchange of their micronuclear material.
- It is the process, which occurs frequently between binary fission and is necessary for the continued vitality of species.

- The complete process of conjugation in *Paramecium* is shown in the diagram given below

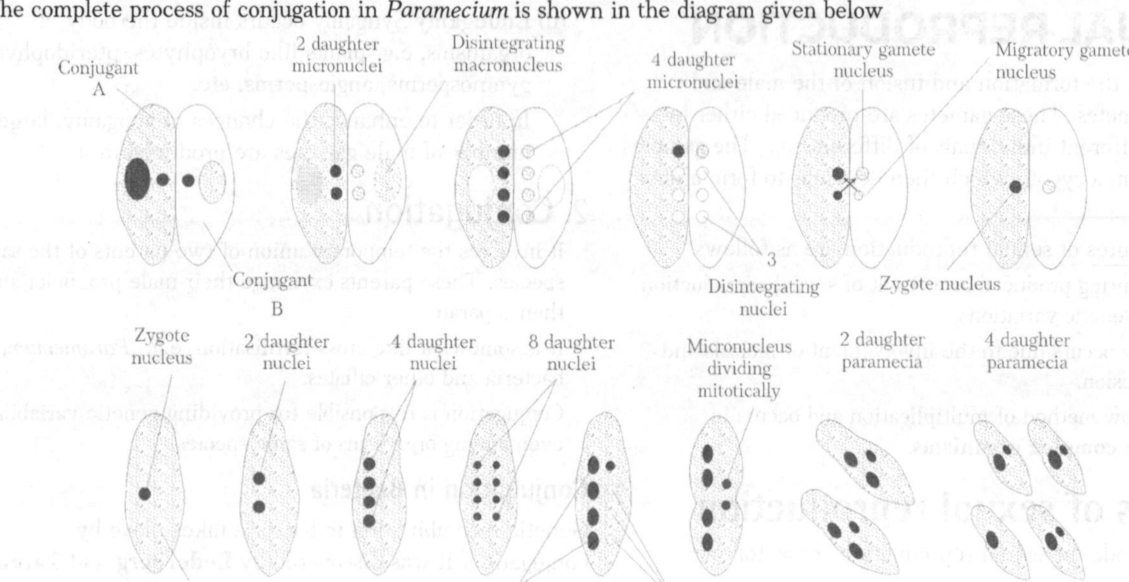

Fig. 1.16 Stages of conjugation in Paramecium

3. Sexual reproduction in lower plants

These are as follows

Sexual reproduction in algae

Depending upon the structure and behaviour of gametes, three different modes of sexual reproduction are involved in algae. These are of following types

(i) **Isogamy** or **Homogamy** It occurs in *Ulothrix, Chlamydomonas, Spirogyra, Oedogonium,* etc.
(ii) **Anisogamy** It occurs in *Chlamydomonas.*
(iii) **Oogamy** It occurs in *Chlamydomonas, Fucus, Chara, Volvox,* etc.

Sexual reproduction in fungi

It involves three processes, *viz*

- **Plasmogamy** Fusion of protoplasts of male and female cells.
- **Karyogamy** Fusion of male and female nuclei forming zygotic nucleus.
- **Meiosis** It converts diploid structure to haploid spores.

Gametes may be isogametes in lower fungi such as *Rhizopus* and *Mucor.* These gametes are labelled as plus (+) and as minus (–). They form a **zygospore** on fusion.

Sexual reproduction in different classes of fungi is explained below

- In **Oomycetes**, male gametes are produced in antheridium, while female gametes are produced in oogonium.
- In **Ascomycetes**, the sexual spores are called **ascospores**, which are formed in asci (sing. ascus) by meiosis. These asci are produced in fruiting bodies called **ascocarps**.
- In **Basidiomycetes**, haploid basidiospores are produced on the tip of the basidium. These basidiospores on germination produce monokaryotic mycelium either of plus (+) or minus (–) strain.
- In **Deuteromycetes** (fungi imperfecti), sexual reproduction is completely absent.

Note *In some fungi, sex organs are not developed and two vegetative cells fuse (somatogamy). This is mainly seen in higher fungi such as Ascomycetes and Basidiomycetes.*

Sexual reproduction in bryophytes

- Sex organs in bryophytes are formed on gametophyte. They are multicellular and are covered by multicellular sterile jackets.
- The male sex organ is **antheridium**. It encloses a mass of androcytes. These androcytes give rise to biflagellate, motile antherozoids.
- The female sex organ is the **archegonium**. It is a multicellular, flask-shaped structure having a swollen venter and elongated neck. The venter encloses the egg or oosphere.
- On maturity, the egg fuses with the antherozoid and forms a diploid zygote.

- Later the repeated cell divisions give rise to embryo, which forms a sporophytic plant.

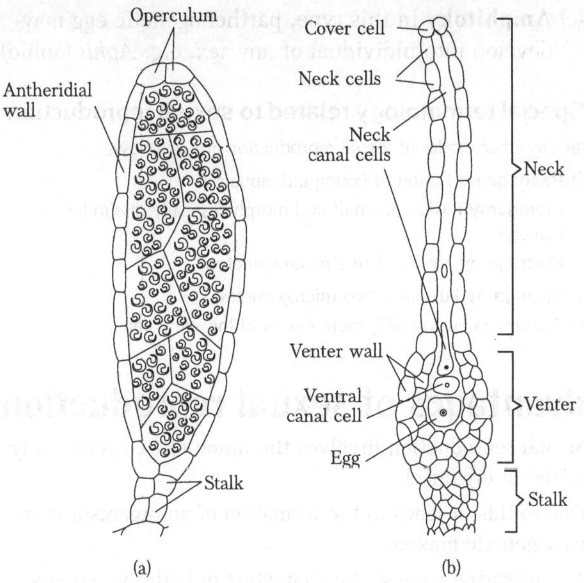

Fig. 1.17 (a) Mature antheridium ready for dehiscence, (b) A nearly mature archegonium

4. Sexual reproduction in higher plants

In higher plants, male and female gametes are produced during sexual reproduction. Characteristics of sexual reproduction in different plant group are as follows

- In **pteridophytes**, the male and female gametes are produced in sex organs called antheridia and archegonia, respectively.
- In **gymnosperms**, the male gamete is produced from microspore in antheridium, while the female gamete is produced from megaspore in archegonium.
- In **angiosperms**, the male gametes are produced inside pollen grains, whereas the female gametes are produced inside embryo sac.
- These gametes are transferred to female gamete or egg *via* the process of pollination. The fusion of gametes in all higher plants leads to the formation of zygote.
- All plants have to reach a certain stage of growth and maturity before they can reproduce sexually. This period is called **vegetative phase**. It is followed by the **reproductive** and **senescent phase.**
- In annual and biennial plants, these phases occur distinctively, but not in perennial plants.

Note
- *Bamboo species flower only once in 50-100 years.*
- *Strobilanthes kunthiana (Neelakurinji) flower once in 12 years.*

5. Sexual reproduction in lower animals

Sexual reproduction has evolved in a hierarchical pattern in animals as follows

- In protozoans, gamete formation does not occur and only the fusion of cells or nucleus occurs.
- In poriferans and coelenterates, gamete fusion occurs but specialised reproductive organs are not present.
- In coelenterates, specialised reproductive forms are seen in coelenterates (e.g. medusae).
- Well-defined reproductive organs with the capabilities of producing gametes were first evolved in Platyhelminthes.

6. Sexual reproduction in higher animals

In higher animals, **syngamy** is the main mode of reproduction. The male and female individuals are generally different. They produce male and female gametes separately. Fusion of these gametes results into the formation of zygote, which produces the young one.

In higher animals, sexual reproduction may be grouped into three distinct stages as follows

(i) **Pre-fertilisation event** It involves the formation of haploid gametes (gametogenesis) and gamete transfer.

(ii) **Fertilisation event** It invovles the fusion of gametes or syngamy. It either occurs externally or internally.

(iii) **Post-fertilisation event** It involves the events that take place after the formation of zygote till maturation.

Deviations in reproductive strategies

In plants

Deviations in reproductive strategies in plants are as follows

(i) **Parthenocarpy** It is defined as the production of fruits without fertilisation, e.g. banana, pineapple, etc.

(ii) **Polyembryony** The occurrence of more than one embryo in a seed is called polyembryony, e.g. *Citrus* etc.

(iii) **Apomixis** Generally, plants reproduce by syngamy, but sometimes involvement of usual sexual gametes do not take place. Thus, the offspring are formed due to a kind of asexual reproduction. It is known as apomixis, e.g. *Opuntia*, etc.

(iv) **Apogamy** Formation of a sporophyte directly from gametophyte without meiosis and syngamy is called as apogamy, e.g. holly fern (*Crytomium falcatum*), etc.

In animals

Though asexual and sexual reproduction are the common methods of multiplication in animals, many deviations are also observed in the reproductive strategies of animals.

These are as follows

(i) **Neoteny** The larvae of some animals fail to go through the normal metamorphosis. These result in the development of sexual maturity in the larval stage only, e.g. axolotl larva of *Necturans.*

(ii) **Paedogenesis** It is also known as reproduction by the child. It is the reproduction by immature or larval animals caused by acceleration of maturation. It occurs in very small fishes.

(iii) **Androgenesis** It is the development of an embryo with paternal (sperm) chromosomes only, accomplished by removing or destroying egg nucleus before syngamy.

(iv) **Gynogenesis** In gynogenesis, the sperm penetrates the egg and stimulates development, but soon it gets degenerated and does not take part in embryo formation. This phenomenon is called gynogenesis or **pseudogamy** or **partial fertilisation**, e.g. *Rhabditis* (roundworms) and *Dugesia* (flatworms).

In both plants and animals

Parthenogenesis It is the development of an embryo from an unfertilised egg. In this, either a spermatozoan does not penetrate the egg or the union of male and female pronuclei does not occur.

In plants, it occurs in dandelions and hawkweeds.

In animals, it occurs in rotifers, gastropods, lizards, crustaceans, etc. Male drones in honeybee are naturally produced by this process.

It is further of following types

(a) **Arrhenotoky** In this type, only males are produced by parthenogenesis, e.g. rotifers, honeybees, wasps and Turkey (bird).

(b) **Thelytoky** In this type, only females are produced by parthenogenesis, e.g. *Lacerta saxicola, Typhlina.*

(c) **Amphitoky** In this type, parthenogenetic egg may develop into individual of any sex, e.g. *Aphis* (aphid).

Special terminology related to sexual reproduction

Various other modes of sexual reproduction are as follows

(i) **Paedogamy** Fusion of young individuals.

(ii) **Merogamy** Fusion of small and morphologically dissimilar gametes.

(iii) **Macrogamy** Fusion of two macrogametes.

(iv) **Microgamy** Fusion of two microgametes.

(v) **Automixis** Fusion of gamete nuclei of the same cell.

Advantages of sexual reproduction

- Sexual reproduction involves the union of two genetically different organisms.
- Due to this, it leads to the formation of an organism with new genetic makeup.
- The offspring possess the characters of both the parents.
- Sexual reproduction results in addition of variations to the population, which ultimately contributes to evolution.

Table 1.1 Differences between asexual and sexual reproduction

Asexual reproduction	Sexual reproduction
It involves the participation of single parent.	It involves the participation of two parents.
It generally occurs without the formation of sex organs.	It usually requires the formation of sex organs.
It does not involve meiosis.	It involves meiosis, which occurs at the time of gametogenesis.
Asexual reproduction does not involve the fusion of two gametes, i.e. the zygote is not formed.	The sexual reproduction requires fertilisation to take place between two opposite gametes leading to the production of a zygote.
The offspring do not show variations and are genetically similar to the parent.	The offspring exhibit variations and are different from either of the two parents.

CHECK POINT 1.2

1. Which of the following is not true about sexual reproduction?
   (a) Gametes are diploid in humans
   (b) Sperm and ova fuse to form zygote
   (c) It introduces new gene combinations in a population
   (d) Diploid zygote divides by mitosis
2. In some algae, the two gametes are so similar in appearance that it is not possible to categorise them into male and female gametes. These gametes are called
   (a) isogametes
   (b) heterogametes
   (c) homogametes
   (d) Both (a) and (c)
3. In *Paramecium*, both autogamy and conjugation are called sexual reproduction because of
   (a) rejuvenation
   (b) gene combination
   (c) the fusion of haploid gametes
   (d) involvement of two individuals
4. Development of an organism from female gamete/egg without involving fertilisation is
   (a) adventitive embryony
   (b) polyembryony
   (c) parthenocarpy
   (d) parthenogenesis
5. Male drones in honeybee are produced by
   (a) syngamy
   (b) paedogenesis
   (c) parthenogenesis
   (d) neotany
6. Organisms belonging to pteridophytes, gymnosperms, angiosperms and most of the animal including human beings,
   (a) produce gametes by meiosis
   (b) produce gametes by mitosis
   (c) have diploid parental body
   (d) Both (a) and (c)

EXAM POINTS

- The process of reproduction ensures the continuity of life on earth. **[MHT CET 2013]**
- Reproduction in algae takes place by zoospore, in *Amoeba* by binary fission, in *Hydra* by budding, in *Penicillium* by conidia and in sponge by gemmule formation. **[Kerala CEE 2013]**
- Gemmules are asexual structure which are produced by organisms during unfavourable condition. **[JIPMER 2019]**
- Reproduction in water hyacinth occurs by offsets and in sponges by gemmule formation. **[CBSE AIPMT 2011, Kerala CEE 2011]**
- Vegetative propagule in *Agave* is termed as bulbil. **[NEET 2020]**
- Vegetative reproduction in bryophytes develops in the notches along the tip of intact leaves. **[AFMC 2012]**
- Stock and scion are used in grafting. **[WB JEE 2015]**
- In potato, banana and ginger, the plantlets arise from the internodes present in the modified stem. **[NEET 2016]**
- In ginger, vegetative propagation occurs through rhizomes. **[CBSE AIPMT 2015]**
- The correct sequence of events of sexual reproduction is Gametogenesis $\rightarrow$ Gamete transfer $\rightarrow$ Syngamy $\rightarrow$ Zygote $\rightarrow$ Cell division $\rightarrow$ Cleavage $\rightarrow$ Cell differentiation $\rightarrow$ Organogenesis. **[NEET 2019]**
- Gametogenesis is not a post-fertilisation event. **[Karnataka CET 2016]**
- The number of chromosomes in meiocyte ($2n$) of apple is 34. **[COMEDK 2015]**
- If the chromosome number in meiocyte is 34, the organism could be apple. **[Karnataka CET 2015]**
- Reproduction without actual fertilisation is called as parthenogenesis. **[JIPMER 2019]**
- Bamboo breeds only once in a lifetime. **[Kerala CEE 2015]**

Chapter Exercises

(A) Topical Exercise

Asexual Reproduction

1 There is a large diversity in the biological world and each organism has evolved its own mechanism to multiply and produce offspring. The method of reproduction depends upon
(a) habitat of organism
(b) internal physiology of organism
(c) will power
(d) Both (a) and (b)

2 There is no natural death in single-celled organisms like *Amoeba* and bacteria because **[NCERT Exemplar]**
(a) they cannot reproduce sexually
(b) they reproduce by binary fission
(c) parental body is distributed among the offspring
(d) they are microscopic

3 The following figure shows the

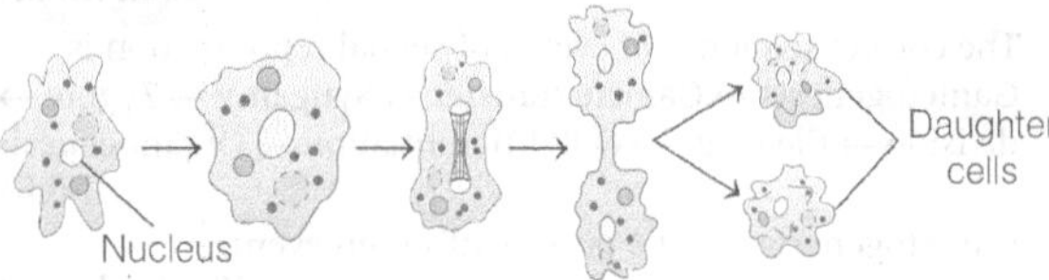

(a) Binary fission in *Amoeba*
(b) Budding in *Hydra*
(c) Equal budding in yeast
(d) Unequal budding in yeast

4 The following figure shows the

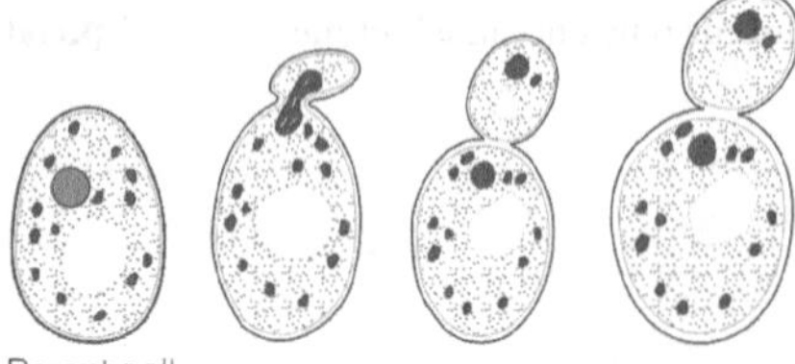

(a) Binary fission in *Amoeba* (b) Budding in *Hydra*
(c) Equal budding in yeast (d) Unequal budding in yeast

5 Which of the following is not incorrect?
(a) Clones are morphologically similar, but genetically of dissimilar
(b) The product of binary fission which are progeny of bacteria are clones
(c) The two daughter cells produced as a result of mitosis are not clones
(d) The two plasmid DNA produced as a result of replication from a parent plasmid DNA cannot be termed as gene clone

6 In *Amoeba*, under unfavourable conditions, ... *A* ... takes place but under favourable conditions, ... *B* ... occurs.

Identify *A* and *B*.

	A	***B***
(a)	sporulation	encystation
(b)	encystation	sporulation
(c)	binary fission	encystation
(d)	multiple fission	encystation

7 Match the following columns.

Column I	Column II
A. Budding	1. Breaking of multicellular animal into two or more parts
B. Multiple fission	2. Formation of gemmule
C. Gemmulation	3. An unequal division of organism in which individual arises as an out growth from the parent
D. Fragmentation	4. Division of nucleus followed by division of cytoplasm which give rise to many daughter cells

Codes

	A	B	C	D		A	B	C	D
(a)	1	2	3	4	(b)	3	4	2	1
(c)	1	3	4	2	(d)	2	4	3	1

8 Recognise the figure and find out the correct matching.

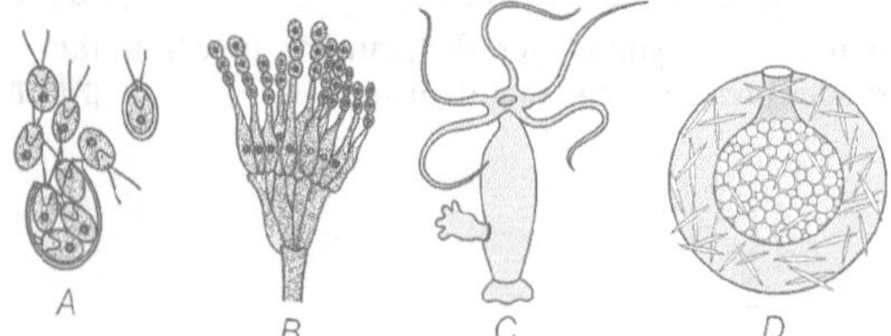

(a) *A*–Conidia, *B*–Budding, *C*–Gemmules, *D*–Zoospores
(b) A–Gemmules, *B*–Conidia, *C*–Budding, *D*–Zoospores
(c) *A*–Zoospores, *B*–Conidia, *C*–Budding, *D*–Gemmules
(d) *A*–Conidia, *B*–Gemmules, *C*–Zoospores, D–Budding

9 Match the following columns.

	Column I		Column II
A.	Binary fission	1.	Banana
B.	Budding	2.	*Paramecium*
C.	Rhizome	3.	Fungi
D.	Zoospores	4.	Yeast

Codes

	A	B	C	D		A	B	C	D
(a)	3	2	4	1	(b)	1	3	2	4
(c)	4	1	3	2	(d)	2	4	1	3

10 What is true for the structure marked *X* in the diagram given below?

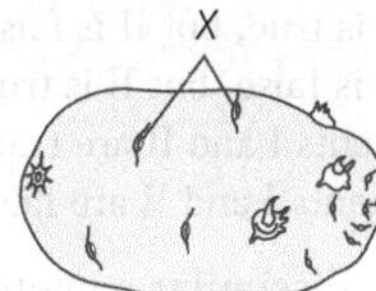

(a) *X* represents the eyes
(b) *X* represents the axillary buds
(c) *X* represents the terminal bud
(d) More than one option is correct

11 The site origin of the new plantlets in potato, ginger and banana is
(a) floral buds present on stem
(b) internodes of modified stem
(c) nodes of modified stem
(d) adventitious buds present on root

12 The vegetative propagation *via* stolons include, which of the following?
(a) Subaerial stem (b) Root
(c) Underground stem (d) None of these

13 In *Bryophyllum*, the buds that arise from the notches of margins of leaves are called
(a) apical buds (b) axillary buds
(c) adventitious buds (d) terminal buds

14 In which of the following the injured leaves form new plants when comes in contact with soil?
(a) *Begonia* (b) *Pistia*
(c) *Opuntia* (d) *Oxalis*

15 The plants which propagate through the production of turions are
(a) *Potamogeton* (b) *Utricularia*
(c) Both (a) and (b) (d) Rose

16 The swollen buds produced by aquatic plants for vegetative propagation are
(a) turions (b) layering
(c) adventitious buds (d) parenchymatous buds

17 Appearance of vegetative propagules from the nodes of plants such as sugarcane and ginger is mainly because **[NCERT Exemplar]**
(a) nodes are shorter than internodes
(b) nodes have meristematic cells
(c) nodes are located near the soil
(d) nodes have non-photosynthetic cells

18 Leaf and stem cuttings are sown
(a) vertically with morphological apical end upwards
(b) vertically with morphological basal end upwards
(c) laterally with morphological upper side upwards
(d) laterally with morphological lower side upwards

19 Recognise the figure and find out the correct matching.

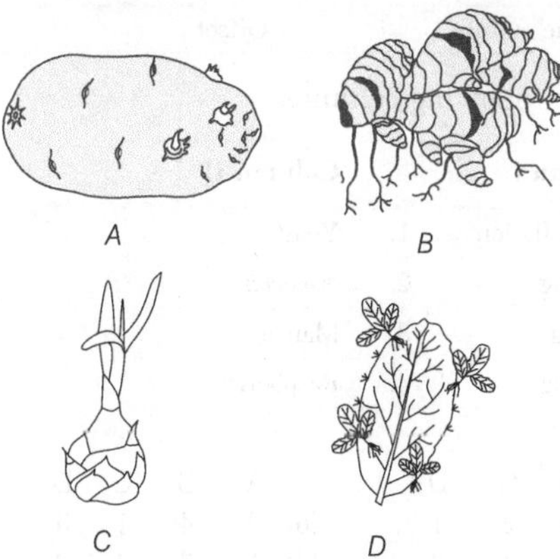

(a) *A*–Rhizome, *B*–Eyes, *C*–Leaf buds, *D*–Bulbils
(b) *A*–Eyes, *B*–Rhizome, *C*–Bulbils, *D*–Leaf buds
(c) *A*–Leaf buds, *B*–Bulbils, *C*–Rhizome, *D*–Eyes
(d) *A*–Eyes, *B*–Bulbils, C–Leaf buds, *D*–Rhizome

20 Consider the following statements.
I. The formation of rhizome, sucker, tuber, offset and bulb does not involve two parents.
II. 'Terror of Bengal' is *Eichhornia.*

Choose the correct option.
(a) Statement I is true, but II is false
(b) Statement I is false, but II is true
(c) Both statements I and II are true
(d) Both statements I and II are false

21 Stem cuttings are often treated with NAA before sowing in order to promote
(a) sprouting of buds (b) rooting
(c) layering (d) seeding

22 Girdling cannot be performed in sugarcane because its
(a) vascular bundles are scattered
(b) phloem is internal to xylem
(c) plant body is delicate
(d) inability to bear injury

23 In monocots, grafting is almost impossible because they lack
(a) vascular cambium
(b) ground tissue
(c) vascular bundle
(d) parenchymatous cells

24 Which of the following correctly depicts the natural and artificial method of vegetative propagation?

	Natural method	Artificial method
(a)	Bulb	Grafting
(b)	Rhizome	Tuber
(c)	Layering	Bulbil
(d)	Tissue culture	Offset

25 Match the following columns.

Column I	Column II
A. Binary fission	1. Yeast
B. Budding	2. *Amoeba*
C. Cutting	3. Mango
D. Grafting	4. Raspberry

Codes

	A	B	C	D		A	B	C	D
(a)	4	3	2	1	(b)	2	4	1	3
(c)	2	1	4	3	(d)	1	3	4	2

26 Both the stock and scion are cut obliquely at about same angle
(a) crown grafting
(b) side grafting
(c) whip grafting
(d) wedge grafting

Sexual Reproduction

27 Sexual reproduction results in offsprings that are not identical to the parents or among themselves because
(a) they are created as a result of fusion of male and female gametes
(b) the offspring are affected by the external environment
(c) the offsprings are affected by the internal physiology of one of the parents
(d) None of the above

28 Sexual reproduction is
(a) slow method of multiplication
(b) involves meiosis and sexual fusion
(c) fast method of multiplication
(d) Both (a) and (b)

29 Choose the correctly matched pair.
(a) Exogamy – Yeast
(b) Endogamy – Angiosperm
(c) Anisogamy – Red algae
(d) Hologamy – Fishes

30 Genetic recombination in bacteria takes place by conjugation. It was discovered by **[NCERT Exemplar]**
(a) Strasburger (b) Nawaschin
(c) Lederberg (d) JC Bose

31 Consider the following statements.
I. Conjugation occurs between two sexually different diploid strains of bacteria.
II. The donor and recipient bacteria termed as F^+ and F^-, respectively.
Choose the correct option.
(a) Statement I is true, but II is false
(b) Statement I is false, but II is true
(c) Both statements I and II are true
(d) Both statements I and II are false

32 Fusion of two dissimilar gametes is
(a) isogamy
(b) hologamy
(c) oogamy
(d) anisogamy

33 Which of the following include types of sexual reproduction in algae?
(a) Isogamy, plasmogamy, apogamy
(b) Apogamy, pseudogamy, microgamy
(c) Isogamy, anisogamy, oogamy
(d) Oogamy, somatogamy, isogamy

34 The correct sequence of sexual reproduction in fungi is
(a) Karyogamy – Meiosis – Plasmogamy
(b) Plasmogamy – Karyogamy – Meiosis
(c) Meiosis – Karyogamy – Plasmogamy
(d) Plasmogamy – Meiosis – Karyogamy

35 Choose the correctly matched pair.
(a) Oomycetes – Ascocarps
(b) Basidiomycetes – Basidiospores
(c) Ascomycetes – Mycelium
(d) Deuteromycetes – Somatogamy

36 Basidiospores on germination produce monokaryotic mycelium which is
(a) plus (+) strain only
(b) minus (–) strain only
(c) Both plus (+) and minus (–) strain
(d) Either plus (+) or minus (–) strain

37 Which one of the following statements is incorrect?
(a) Apogamy is formation of a sporophyte directly from gametophyte without meiosis and syngamy
(b) Specialised reproductive organs are present in poriferans and coelenterates
(c) No gamete formation occurs in protozoans
(d) In coelenterates, specialised reproductive forms are seen (e.g. medusa)

38 Clear-cut vegetative reproductive and senescent phase are not found in
(a) annual plants (b) perennial plants
(c) biennial plants (d) All of these

39 The sequential events in the sexual reproduction may be grouped into
(a) Two stages–gametogenesis and gamete transfer
(b) Three stages–gametogenesis and gamete transfer and fertilisation
(c) Two stages–gametogenesis and embryogenesis
(d) Three stages–pre-fertilisation, fertilisation and post-fertilisation events

40 Deviations in reproductive strategies in animals include
(a) parthenocarpy (b) gynogenesis
(c) apomixis (d) apogamy

41 Reproduction by immature or larval animals caused by acceleration of maturation is called
(a) paedogensis (b) androgenesis
(c) neoteny (d) gynogenesis

42 Drones in a colony of honeybees originate by
(a) thelytoky
(b) arrhenotoky
(c) cyclic parthenogenesis
(d) diploid parthenogenesis

43 In thelytoky type of parthenogenesis,
(a) Only males are produced parthenogenetically
(b) Only females are produced parthenogenetically
(c) Both male and females are produced parthenogenetically
(d) Parthenogenetic eggs may develop into any sex

44 Match the following columns.

Column I		Column II
A. Microgamy	1.	Fusion of young individuals
B. Paedogamy	2.	Fusion of gamete nuclei of the same cell
C. Automixis	3.	Fusion of two microgametes
D. Macrogamy	4.	Fusion of two macrogametes

Codes

	A	B	C	D		A	B	C	D
(a)	1	3	2	4	(b)	4	1	2	3
(c)	3	1	2	4	(d)	3	2	1	4

45 Advantages of sexual reproductions are
(a) formation of organism with new genetic makeup
(b) offspring possess the characters of both the parents
(c) contribute to evolution
(d) All of the above

(B) Cumulative Exercise

(Assorted Questions of the Chapter for Advanced Level Practice)

1 Examine the figures given below and select the right option out of *A-D*, in which all the four structures *A*, *B*, *C* and *D* are identified correctly.

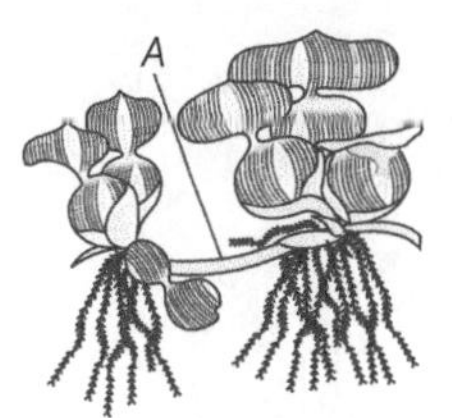

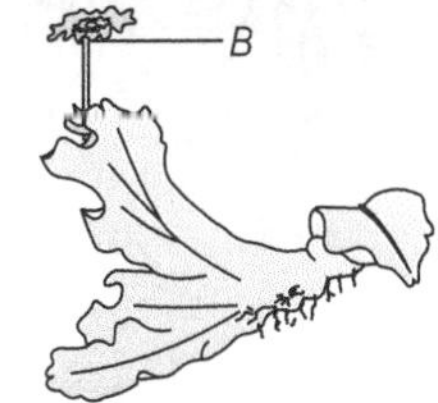

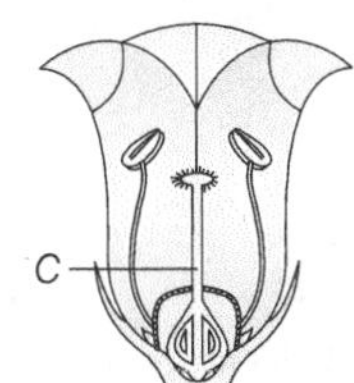

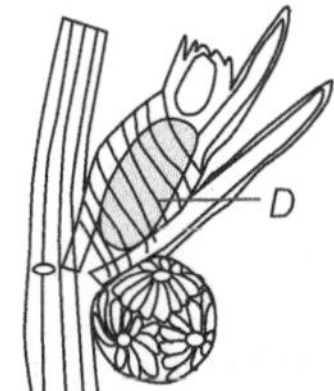

	A	*B*	*C*	*D*
(a)	Rhizome	Sporangiophore	Polar cell	Globule
(b)	Runner	Archegoniophore	Synergid	Antheridium
(c)	Offset	Antheridiophore	Carpal	Oogonium
(d)	Sucker	Seta	Megaspore mother cell	Gemma cup

2 A few statements with regard to sexual reproduction are given below. **[NCERT Exemplar]**
I. Sexual reproduction does not always require two individuals.
II. Sexual reproduction generally involves gametic fusion.
III. Meiosis never occurs during sexual reproduction.
IV. External fertilisation is a rule during sexual reproduction.

Choose the correct option.
(a) I and IV (b) I and II (c) II and III (d) III and IV

3 Match the following columns I and II and choose the correct combination from the codes given below.

Column I (Name of organisms)		Column II (Chromosome number in gametes)
A. Butterfly	1.	6
B. Housefly	2.	39
C. Dog	3.	21
D. Cat	4.	19
E. Rat	5.	190

Codes

	A	B	C	D	E		A	B	C	D	E
(a)	1	2	3	5	4	(b)	2	5	4	3	1
(c)	5	1	2	4	3	(d)	5	1	3	2	4

4 Consider the following statements with respect to reproduction in the lower living organisms.
I. Organisms like yeast and *Planaria* reproduce asexually by means of budding.
II. True regeneration is observed in *Hydra*.
III. The protonema of mosses multiply by fragmentation.
IV. In the unicellular organisms like bacteria, algae and *Amoeba*, reproduction is synonymous with growth, i.e. increase in number of cells.

Choose the correct option.
(a) I and II alone are correct
(b) II and III alone are correct
(c) I and IV alone are correct
(d) III and IV alone are correct

5 Go through the following statements.
I. Asexual reproduction occurs without the involvement of gamete formation.
II. Asexual reproduction ultimately leads to evolution.
III. Asexual reproduction occurs when the conditions are unfavourable.
IV. Asexual reproduction is a slow process.

Choose the statements correctly representing asexual reproduction.
(a) I and II (b) I and III
(c) Only I (d) II, III and IV

6 Which of the following statements, support the view that elaborate sexual reproductive process appeared much later in the organic evolution.
I. Lower groups of organisms have simpler body design.
II. Asexual reproduction is common in lower groups.
III. Asexual reproduction is common in higher groups of organisms.
IV. The high incidence of sexual reproduction in angiosperms and vertebrates.

Choose the correct option. [NCERT Exemplar]
(a) I and III (b) II and III
(c) II and IV (d) III and IV

7 Identify the organism (*X*) and the structure (*Y*) and the parts labelled as *A, B, C, D* and *E*.

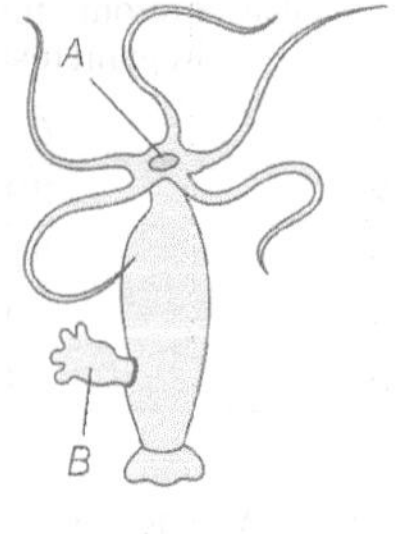

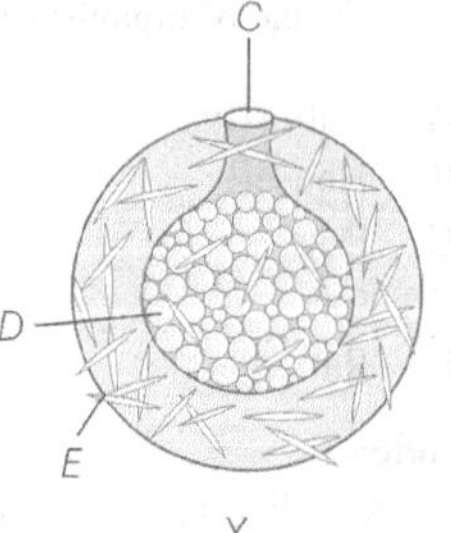

	X	A	B	Y	C	D	E
(a)	*Hydra*	Bud	Mouth	Gemmule (of sponges)	Micropyle	Archaeo-cytes	Spicules
(b)	*Obelia*	Mouth	Bud	Gemmule	Archaeocytes	Spicules	Micropyle
(c)	*Hydra*	Mouth	Bud	Gemmule (of sponges)	Micropyle	Archaeo-cytes	Spicules
(d)	*Sycon*	Mouth	Micropyle	Gemmule	Spicules	Bud	Archaeo-cytes

8 Read the following statements.
I. The vegetative phase is of same duration in different organisms.
II. Clear-cut vegetative, reproductive and senescent phases can be observed in monocarpic plants.
III. Bamboo differs from *Strobilanthes kunthiana* (Neelakurinji) in the length of juvenile phase and being monocarpic.
IV. The end of juvenile/vegetative phase in angiosperms is seen when they come to flower.
V. Sexual mode of reproduction is present in most animals.

Which of the above statement is/are incorrect?
(a) II, IV and V (b) II and III
(c) III, IV and V (d) I and III

9 Identify correctly : *A, B, C* and *D*.

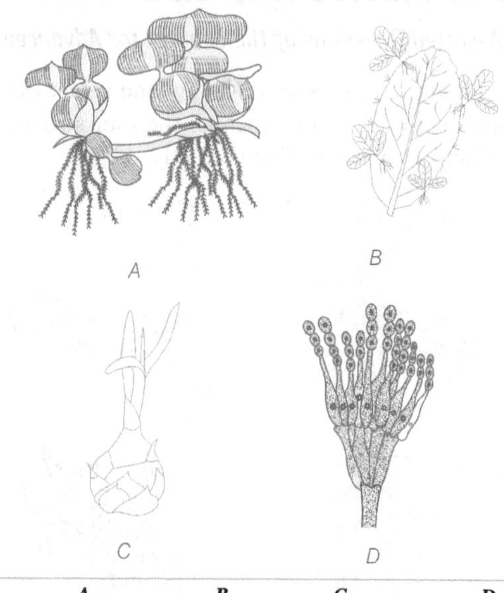

	A	B	C	D
(a)	Offset of *Eichhornia*	Leaf buds of *Bryophyllum*	Bulbil of *Agave*	*Penicillium* with conidia
(b)	Bulbil of *Agave*	Offset of *Eichhornia*	Bulbil of *Agave*	*Penicillium* with conidia
(c)	Leaf buds of *Bryophyllum*	Bulbil of *Agave*	Offset of *Eichhornia*	*Penicillium* with conidia
(d)	Offset of *Eichhornia*	Leaf buds of *Bryophyllum*	*Penicillium* with conidia	Bulbil of *Agave*

10 Given below are a few statements related to external fertilisation.

I. The male and female gametes are formed and released simultaneously.
II. Only a few gametes are released into the medium.
III. Water is the medium in a majority of organisms exhibiting external fertilisation.
IV. Offspring formed as a result of external fertilisation have better chance of survival than those formed inside an organism. **[NCERT Exemplar]**

Choose the option containing correct statements.

(a) III and IV (b) I and III
(c) II and IV (d) I and IV

11 Read the following statements and find out the incorrect statements.

I. Asexual reproduction is common among single-celled organisms, and in plants and animals with relatively complex organisations.
II. In yeast, the division is unequal and small buds are produced that remain attached initially to the parent cell which eventually gets separated and mature into new yeast organism (cells).
III. Vegetative reproduction is also a type of asexual reproduction.
IV. While in animals and other simple organisms, the term vegetative reproduction is used unambiguously, in plants, the term asexual reproduction is frequently used.
V. Water hyacinth is also called 'Terror of Bengal.'

Choose the correct option.

(a) I and IV (b) II and III
(c) I and V (d) II and IV

12 Match the following columns.

	Column I		Column II
A.	External fertilisation	1.	Human beings
B.	Internal fertilisation	2.	Algae and fishes
C.	Ovipary	3.	Bryophytes, pteridophytes and birds
D.	Vivipary	4	Reptiles and birds

Codes

	A	B	C	D		A	B	C	D
(a)	4	1	2	3	(b)	3	1	4	2
(c)	2	3	4	1	(d)	4	2	1	3

13 Fill in the blanks.

I. The ...*A*.... reproduction is the common mode of reproduction in organisms that have a relatively simple organisation like algae and fungi and they shift to ...*B*... method of reproduction just before the onset of adverse conditions.
II. Asexual (vegetative) as well as sexual modes of reproduction are exhibited by the ...*C*... .
III. Only sexual mode of reproduction is present in most of the ...*D*... .

(a) *A*–sexual, *B*–asexual, *C*–plants, *D*–animals
(b) *A*–sexual, *B*–asexual, *C*–animals, *D*–higher plants
(c) *A*–asexual, *B*–sexual, *C*–higher plants, *D*–animals
(d) *A*–asexual, *B*–sexual, *C*–animals, *D*–higher plants

14 Match the following columns I and II and choose the correct combination from the codes given below.

	Column I		Column II
A.	Coconut palm	1.	Monoecious
B.	Leech	2.	Dioecious
C.	Cockroach	3.	Seasonal breeder
D.	Frog	4.	Unisexual
E.	Date palm	5.	Bisexual

Codes

	A	B	C	D	E
(a)	1	5	2	4	3
(b)	3	1	4	2	2
(c)	5	3	2	4	2
(d)	2	1	3	5	4

15 Read the following statements.

I. *Eichhornia* is also known as 'Terror of Bengal'.
II. *Zingiber* propagates by tap roots.
III. *Bryophyllum* possesses leaf buds.
IV. Neelakurinji flower after every 50 years.

Choose the correct option containing correct statements.

(a) I and III (b) II and IV
(c) I, III and IV (d) Only I

16 Read the following statements and find out the incorrect statements.

I. In majority of organisms, male gamete is motile and female gamete is non-motile (stationary).
II. In algae and fungi, both male and female gametes are non-motile.
III. In seed plants, pollen grains are the carrier of male gametes and ovule has the egg.
IV. In dioecious plants, pollination facilitates transfer of pollen grains to the stigma.
V. In monoecious animals, since male and female gametes are formed in different individuals, the organism must evolve special mechanism for gamete transfer.

(a) II and V
(b) I and IV
(c) II and III
(d) III and V

17 Read the following statements and find out the incorrect statement.

(a) Plant, animals and fungi differ so greatly in external morphology, internal structure and physiology, when it comes to sexual mode of reproduction, they share a similar pattern
(b) In annual and biennial plants, there is a clear-cut vegetative reproductive and senescent phases, but in the perennial species, it is very difficult to clearly define these phases
(c) In animals, the juvenile phase is followed by morphological and physiological changes prior to active reproductive behaviour
(d) The females of the marsupial mammals exhibit cyclical changes in the activities of ovaries and accessory ducts as well as hormones during the reproductive phase

18 A few statements describing certain features of reproduction are given below.

I. Gametic fusion takes place.
II. Transfer of genetic material takes place.
III. Reduction division takes place.
IV. Progeny have some resemblance with parents.

Select the statements that are true for both asexual and sexual reproduction from the options. **[NCERT Exemplar]**

(a) I and II (b) II and III
(c) II and IV (d) I and III

19 Recognise the figure and find out the correct matching.

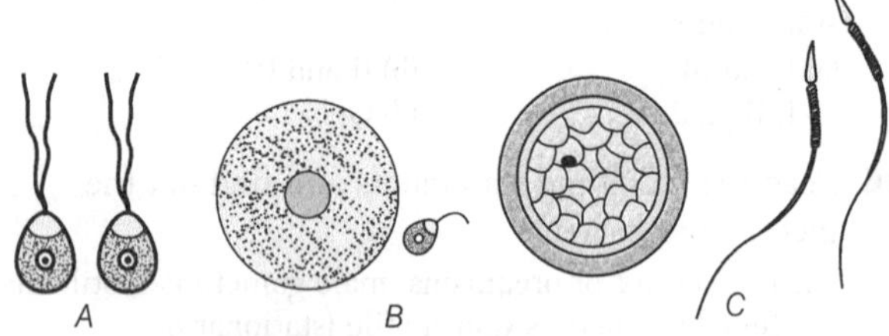

(a) *A*-Heterogametes of *Cladophora*, *B*-Heterogametes of *Homo sapiens*, *C*-Isogametes of *Fucus*
(b) *A*-Isogametes of *Fucus*, *B*-Heterogametes of *Cladophora*, *C*-Heterogametes of humans
(c) *A*-Isogametes of *Cladophora*, *B*—Heterogametes of *Home sapiens*, *C*—Heterogametes of *Fucus*
(d) *A*-Isogametes of *Cladophora*, *B*-Heterogametes of *Fucus*, *C*—Heterogametes of human beings

20 A multicellular, filamentous alga exhibits a type of sexual life cycle in which the meiotic division occurs after the formation of zygote. The adult filament of this alga has **[NCERT Exemplar]**

(a) haploid vegetative cells and diploid gametangia
(b) diploid vegetative cells and diploid gametangia
(c) diploid vegetative cells and haploid gametangia
(d) haploid vegetative cells and haploid gametangia

21 Match the following columns I and II and choose the correct combination from the codes given below.

	Column I		Column II
A.	*Drosophila*	1.	1-2 weeks
B.	Butterfly	2.	2 weeks
C.	Crow	3.	15 years
D.	Parrot	4.	60 years
E.	Tortoise	5.	140 years
F.	Crocodile	6.	100-150 years

Codes

	A	B	C	D	E	F
(a)	2	1	5	3	4	6
(b)	1	2	3	5	6	4
(c)	1	2	5	3	4	6
(d)	2	1	3	5	6	4

22 Recognise the figure and find out the correct matching.

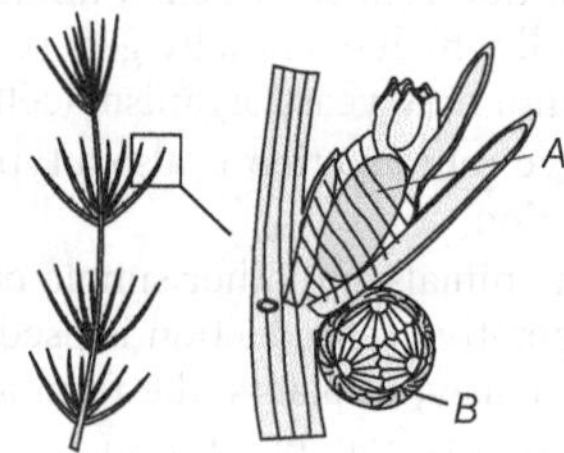

(a) *A*-Oogonium (male sex organ), *B*-Antheridium (female sex organ)
(b) *A*-Antheridium (female sex organ), *B*-Oogonium (male sex organ)
(c) *A*-Oogonium (female sex organ), *B*-Antheridium (male sex organ)
(d) *A*-Antheridium (male sex organ), *B*-Oogonium (female sex organ)

23 Which of the following situations correctly describe the similarity between an angiospermic egg and a human egg?

I. Eggs of both are formed only once in a lifetime.
II. Both the angiosperm egg and human egg are stationary.
III. Both the angiosperm egg and human egg are motile transported.
IV. Syngamy in both results in the formation of zygote.

Choose the correct option. **[NCERT Exemplar]**

(a) II and IV (b) Only IV
(c) III and IV (d) I and IV

24 Find out the incorrect statement.

I. Lifespans of organisms are necessarily correlated with their sizes.
II. The sizes of crows and parrots are not very different, but still their lifespans vary extremely.

III. A peepal tree has much shorter lifespan as compared to a mango tree.
IV. Reproduction is essential for continuity of species on the earth.

Choose the correct option.
(a) I and III
(b) I, II and III
(c) Only IV
(d) II and III

25 Select the right option in which the events (*A*, *B*, *C*, *D* and *E*) in life of general reproduction are correctly identified.

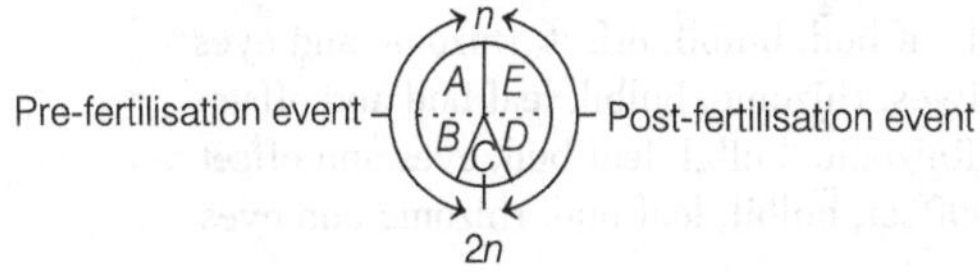

Choose the correct option.
(a) *A*-Gametogenesis, *B*-Zygote formation, *C*-Fertilisation, *D*-Gamete transfer, *E*-Embryogenesis
(b) *A*-Gametogenesis, *B*-Gamete transfer, *C*-Fertilisation, *D*-Zygote formation, *E*-Embryogenesis
(c) *A*-Gamete transfer, *B*-Gametogenesis, *C*-Fertilisation, *D*-Zygote formation, *E*-Embryogenesis
(d) *A*-Gametogenesis, *B*-Gamete transfer, *C*-Fertilisation, *D*-Embryogenesis, *E*-Zygote formation

Assertion and Reason

Direction (Q. Nos. 26–31) *In the following questions, a statement of Assertion (A) is given followed by the corresponding statement of Reason (R). Of the statements, mark the correct answer as*

(a) Both A and R are true and R is the correct explanation of A
(b) Both A and R are true, but R is not the correct explanation of A
(c) A is true, but R is false
(d) A is false, but R is true
(e) Both A and R are false

26 **Assertion** (A) An embryo is formed after some meiotic divisions by the product formed after syngamy.
Reason (R) An embryo is the first cell of sporophytic generation.

27 **Assertion** (A) Asexual reproduction requires only female animals.
Reason (R) Male animals are not capable for asexual reproduction.

28 **Assertion** (A) Bacteria divide by mitotic division.
Reason (R) Meiosis occurs in *Rhizobium.*

29 **Assertion** (A) Many plants are propagated vegetatively even though they bear seeds.
Reason (R) Potatoes multiply by tubers, apple by cutting.

30 **Assertion** (A) Asexual reproduction, is also called blastogenesis.
Reason (R) In asexual reproduction, there is no formation and fusion of gametes.

31 **Assertion** (A) Claspers of cartilaginous fishes are analogous to penis of human male.
Reason (R) Both act as copulatory organs and transfer the sperms into female.

(C) Medical Entrances' Gallery

(Collection of Questions Asked in NEET & in Various Medical Entrance Exams)

1 Vegetative propagule in *Agave* is termed as **[NEET 2020]**
(a) rhizome (b) bulbil (c) offset (d) eye

2 Choose the incorrect about gemmules. **[JIPMER 2019]**
(a) They resist desiccation
(b) They are internal buds
(c) They are asexual structure which produced by binary fission
(d) They can give rise to new organisms

3 Select the correct sequence of events. **[NEET 2019]**
(a) Gametogenesis → Gamete transfer → Syngamy → Zygote → Cell division (cleavage) → Cell differentiation → Organogenesis
(b) Gametogenesis → Gamete transfer → Syngamy → Zygote → Cell division (cleavage) → Organogenesis → Cell differentiation
(c) Gametogenesis → Syngamy → Gamete transfer → Zygote → Cell division (cleavage) → Cell differentiation → Organogenesis
(d) Gametogenesis → Gamete transfer → Syngamy → Zygote → Cell differentiation → Cell division (cleavage) → Organogenesis

4 Reproduction without actual fertilisation is called as **[JIPMER 2019]**
(a) parthenogenesis (b) parthenocarpy
(c) pseudoreproduction (d) All of these

5 Which one of the following statements is not correct? **[NEET-II 2016]**
(a) Offspring produced by the asexual reproduction are called clone
(b) Microscopic, motile asexual reproductive structures are called zoospores
(c) In potato, banana and ginger, the plantlets arise from the internodes present in the modified stem
(d) Water hyacinth, growing in the standing water, drains oxygen from water that leads to the death of fishes

6 Which one of the following generates new genetic combination leading to variation? **[NEET-II 2016]**
(a) Vegetative reproduction (b) Parthenogenesis
(c) Sexual reproduction (d) Nucellar polyembryony

7 Stock and scion are used in **[WB JEE 2015]**
(a) cutting (b) grafting
(c) layering (d) micropropagation

8 In ginger, vegetative propagation occurs through **[CBSE AIPMT 2015]**
(a) rhizome (b) offsets
(c) bulbils (d) runners

9 Which of the following pairs is not correctly matched? **[CBSE AIPMT 2015]**

Modes of reproduction		Examples
(a) Offset	–	Water hyacinth
(b) Rhizome	–	Banana
(c) Binary fission	–	*Sargassum*
(d) Conidia	–	*Penicillium*

10 Which of the following processes ensures the continuity of life on earth? **[MHT CET 2013]**
(a) Reproduction (b) Respiration
(c) Digestion (d) Growth and development

11 Match the following columns.

Column I	Column II
A. Binary fission	1. Algae
B. Zoospore	2. *Amoeba*
C. Conidium	3. *Hydra*
D. Budding	4. *Penicillium*
E. Gemmules	5. Sponge

Codes **[Kerala CEE 2013]**

	A	B	C	D	E
(a)	1	4	5	3	2
(b)	2	1	4	3	5
(c)	2	4	3	5	1
(d)	1	4	3	2	5
(e)	4	1	3	5	2

12 Which one of the following is correctly matched? **[CBSE AIPMT 2012]**
(a) Onion - Bulb (b) Ginger - Sucker
(c) *Chlamydomonas* - Conidia (d) Yeast - Zoospores

13 Vegetative reproduction in which new plants develop in the notches along the tip of intact leaves is seen in **[AFMC 2012]**
(a) *Asparagus* (b) *Agave*
(c) *Chrysanthemum* (d) *Bryophyllum*

14 Banana is vegetatively propagated by **[AMU 2012]**
(a) tubers (b) rhizomes
(c) bulbs (d) suckers

15 Find out correct order of vegetative propagules of plants like potato, ginger, *Agave*, *Bryophyllum* and water hyacinth. **[Kerala CEE 2012]**
(a) Offset, bulbil, leaf bud, rhizome and eyes
(b) Leaf bud, bulbil, offset, rhizome and eyes
(c) Eyes, rhizome, bulbil, leaf bud and offset
(d) Rhizome, bulbil, leaf bud, eyes and offset
(e) Offset, bulbil, leaf bud, rhizome and eyes

16 Match Column I with Column II and select the correct option.

Column I	Column II
A. Gemmules	1. *Agave*
B. Leaf buds	2. *Penicillium*
C. Bulbil	3. Water hyacinth
D. Offset	4. Sponges
E. Conidia	5. *Bryophyllum*

Codes **[CBSE AIPMT 2011, Kerala CEE 2011]**

	A	B	C	D	E
(a)	4	5	1	3	2
(b)	4	3	2	1	5
(c)	3	5	4	2	1
(d)	4	1	5	3	2
(e)	3	5	4	1	2

17 Which one of the following statements is incorrect for a clone? **[UP CPMT 2011]**
(a) Clones are descended from a single parent
(b) Identical twins are not clone
(c) Clone is a result of sexual reproduction
(d) Both (a) and (c)

18 Match Column I with Column II and select the correct option.

Column I (Name of the organisms)	Column II (Haploid *n* chromosome number in gamete)
A. *Ophioglossum*	1. 23
B. Rice	2. 24
C. Potato	3. 12
D. Man	4. 630

Codes **[Kerala CEE 2011]**

	A	B	C	D
(a)	1	2	3	4
(b)	2	3	4	1
(c)	3	4	2	1
(d)	4	3	2	1
(e)	4	3	1	2

ANSWERS

Check Point 1.1

1. (d)	2. (a)	3. (a)	4. (b)	5. (a)	6. (a)

Check Point 1.2

1. (a)	2. (d)	3. (c)	4. (d)	5. (c)	6. (d)

(A) Topical Exercise

1. (d)	2. (c)	3. (a)	4. (d)	5. (b)	6. (b)	7. (b)	8. (c)	9. (d)	10. (d)
11. (c)	12. (a)	13. (c)	14. (a)	15. (c)	16. (a)	17. (b)	18. (a)	19. (b)	20. (c)
21. (b)	22. (a)	23. (a)	24. (a)	25. (c)	26. (c)	27. (a)	28. (d)	29. (b)	30. (c)
31. (b)	32. (d)	33. (c)	34. (b)	35. (b)	36. (d)	37. (b)	38. (b)	39. (d)	40. (b)
41. (a)	42. (b)	43. (b)	44. (c)	45. (d)					

(B) Cumulative Exercise

1. (c)	2. (b)	3. (c)	4. (d)	5. (c)	6. (c)	7. (c)	8. (d)	9. (a)	10. (b)
11. (a)	12. (c)	13. (c)	14. (d)	15. (a)	16. (a)	17. (d)	18. (c)	19. (d)	20. (d)
21. (d)	22. (c)	23. (b)	24. (a)	25. (b)	26. (c)	27. (e)	28. (c)	29. (a)	30. (b)
31. (a)									

(C) Medical Entrances' Gallery

1. (b)	2. (c)	3. (a)	4. (a)	5. (c)	6. (c)	7. (b)	8. (a)	9. (c)	10. (a)
11. (b)	12. (a)	13. (d)	14. (b)	15. (c)	16. (a)	17. (c)	18. (d)		

Explanations

(A) Topical Exercise

31 (*b*) Statement I is false, but II is true. Incorrect statement can be corrected as

Conjugation occurs between two sexually different haploid strains of bacteria.

37 (*b*) Statement in option (c) is incorrect and can be corrected as

In poriferans and coelenterates, gamete fusion occurs, but specialised reproductive organs are not present.

42 (*b*) Based on the sex of offspring, there are four types of parthenogenesis, e.g. arrhenotoky, thelytoky, amphitoky and deuterotoky. In arrhenotoky parthenogenesis, only males or drones are produced. It occurs in honeybees, wasps, ticks, mites, etc.

43 (*b*) The production of female offspring by parthenogenesis is referred to as thelytoky, e.g. aphids.

(B) Cumulative Exercise

2 (*b*) Statements I and II are correct, while III and IV are incorrect. Incorrect statements can be corrected as

Meiosis takes place in sexual reproduction. It is not necessary in sexual reproduction, that fertilisation occurs externally. In animals like frog, fertilisation is external while in mammals, fertilisation is internal.

4 (*d*) Statements III and IV are correct, while I and II are incorrect. Incorrect statements can be corrected as

Reproduction in yeast occurs by budding while in *Planaria,* reproduction is done by regeneration.

The true regeneration is seen in *Planaria.*

5 (*c*) Statement I is correct, while statements II, III and IV are incorrect and can be corrected as

Asexual reproduction does not leads to evolution. It occurs in both favourable and unfavourable conditions. It is not slower process.

8 (*d*) Statements I and III are incorrect and can be corrected as

- The vegetative phase is different in different organisms.
- Bamboo can be monocarpic or polycarpic whereas *Strobilanthes kunthiana* is a monocarpic plant.

Rest statements are correct.

10 (*b*) Statements I and III are correct, while statements II and IV are incorrect. Incorrect statements can be corrected as

- A large number of gametes are released into the medium to increase the chances of fertilisation.
- Offspring formed as a result of internal fertilisation have better chances of survival than those formed outside an organism.

11 (*a*) Statements I and IV are incorrect and can be corrected as
- Asexual reproduction is common among unicellular organism, but in plants and animals, sexual reproduction is common. Asexual is seen under unfavourable condition.
- While in animals and other simple organisms, the term asexual reproduction is used unambiguously, in plants, the term vegetative reproduction is frequentry used.

Rest statements are correct.

16 (*a*) Statements II and V are incorrect and can be corrected as
- In algae and fungi, both male and female gametes are motile.
- In dioecious animals, male and female gametes are formed in different individuals, therefore the organism have evolve special mechanism for gamete transfer.

17 (*d*) Statement in option (d) is incorrect and can be corrected as
The female of placental mammal exhibit cyclical changes in the activities of ovaries and accessory ducts as well as hormone during the reproductive phase.

24 (*a*) Statements I and III are incorrect and can be corrected as
- Lifespans of an organism are not correlated with their sizes.
- The lifespan of peepal tree is much longer than mango tree.

Rest statements are correct.

26 (*c*) A is true, but R is false because
Syngamy involves a male gamete and an egg. It forms a diploid product, the zygote which is known as first cell of sporophytic generation, it divides by mitotic divisions and forms a multicellular structure called the embryo.

27 (*e*) Both A and R are false and can be corrected as
Asexual reproduction requires only one parental animal (either male or female), this process does not include the production and union of gametes. Due to involvement of one parent, all the offspring produced as a result of asexual reproduction are genetically identical to the parent.

28 (*c*) A is true, but R is false because
Bacteria divide by binary fission, it is a mitotic division, each bacterial cell is divided into two identical daughter cells.
Rhizobium is a nodule forming bacterium present in roots of leguminous plants. These bacteria divide by binary fission. Meiosis does not take place in bacteria because all bacteria are haploid in nature. They contain only single set of chromosomes.

29 (*a*) Both A and R true and R is the correct explanation of A.
Vegetative reproduction is asexual type of reproduction.
Potato, sugarcane, apple, etc., multiply by asexual means.

30 (*b*) Both A and R are true, but R is not the correct explanation of A.
Development of an organism forms non-reproductive units like buds, fragments, etc., is blastogenesis. In asexual reproduction, there is no formation and fusion of gametes.

31 (*a*) Both A and R true and R is the correct explanation of A.
Claspers of cartilaginous fishes (sharks) is one between the pelvic fins. Claspers are analogous to penis of human male both act as copulatory organ and transfer the sperms into female.

(C) Medical Entrances' Gallery

1 (*b*) Vegetative propagule in *Agave* is bulbil. It develops as a small bud on the axial leaf and after falling on the soil, it develops into new plants.

2 (*c*) Statement in option (c) is incorrect and can be corrected as
Gemmules are asexual structures which produced by organisms (e.g. sponges) during unfavourable condition by the process of internal budding. They resemble endospore of bacteria.
Rest of the statements are correct about gemmules.

3 (*a*) The correct sequence of events is shown by option (a), i.e. Gametogenesis (production of gametes) → Gamete transfer (movement of gamete at the site of fertilisation) → Syngamy (the fusion of gametes) → Zygote (a eukaryotic cell formed by fertilisation of gametes) → Cell division (cleavage) → Cell differentiation (i.e the process where a cell changes from one cell type to another) → Organogenesis (i.e. the process of formation of three germ layers).

4 (*a*) Reproduction without actual fertilisation is called as parthenogenesis. It is a type of reproduction in which formation of an embryo from an unfertilised egg takes place.
Parthenocarpy is the process of production of fruit without fertilisation.

5. (*c*) Statement in option (c) is not correct and can be corrected as
In potato, banana and ginger, new plantlets always arise from the nodes of the modified stem. Internodes are the area between the two nodes.
Rest of the statements are correct.

6. (*c*) The sexual reproduction brings about variation through genetic recombination. First of all, genetic recombination occurs in non-homologous chromosomes during crossing over of pachytene stage in meiotic cell division.
Secondly, the random union of gametes also contributes in forming new combinations of characters. Other options (a), (b) and (d) do not contribute in the formation of progenies with new variations.

7 (*b*) Stock and scion are used in grafting. Grafting is a horticulture technique wherein tissues from one plant are inserted into those of another, so that the two sets of vascular tissues join together.
This technique is most commonly used in asexual propagation of commercially grown plants. In this technique, one plant is selected for its roots and is called the stock or root stock.

The other plant is selected for its stems, leaves, flowers or fruits and is called the scion. The scion and stock contain the desired genes to be duplicated in future production by the stock and scion plant.

8 (*a*) In ginger, vegetative propagation occurs through rhizome. Rhizomes are stems which grow horizontally under the ground.

In ginger, the underground stems are swollen with food reserves. The terminal bud grows upward to produce the flowering shoot and the lateral buds grow out to form new plant.

9 (*c*) Option (c) in not correctly matched and can be corrected as

The plant body of *Sargassum* is a diploid sporophyte. It does not multiply asexually by means of binary fission instead, it reproduces by vegetative means, i.e. fragmentation, which is the only known method of vegetative reproduction in the free-floating species of *Sargassum.*

Rest of the options are correctly matched.

10 (*a*) Reproduction is the process of formation of new individuals of a species from the pre-existing one. It ensures the continuity of life on earth. It is meant for perpetuation of a species because the older individuals of each species undergo senescence and die.

12 (*a*) Option (a) contains the correct match. Rest of the matches are incorrect and can be corrected as

- Ginger reproduces through nodes that are present on the vegetative reproductive structure called rhizomes. Suckers are the reproductive structures through which plants like mint, *Chrysanthemum* reproduce.
- *Chlamydomonas*, a green alga reproduces through zoospores whereas conidium mode of reproduction is observed in *Penicillium.*
- Yeasts and other Ascomycetes reproduce through ascospores and Phycomycetes like *Achlya, Saprolegnia, Albugo, Phytophthora*, etc., reproduce through zoospores.

13 (*d*) *Bryophyllum* reproduces asexually through adventitious buds present at the marginal notches along the tips of intact leaves.

14 (*b*) Plants like banana, ginger, turmeric reproduce through buds present on the vegetative reproductive structures called rhizomes. Rhizomes are swollen underground stems that contain buds which lead to the formation of new shoots and become swollen due to food storage.

15 (*c*) Option (c) is the correct order of vegetative propagules of given plants.

Potato plants reproduce through nodes or eyes that are present on the vegetative reproduction structure called tubers.

Ginger plants reproduce through nodes present on rhizome, a modified stem that serves as a reproductive structure.

Agave plant reproduces through bulbils which are fleshy, modified flowering buds present on the flowering axis.

Bryophyllum reproduces through adventitious buds present on the tip of a leaf.

Water hyacinth (*Eichhornia*) reproduces through offset which breaks off to enable propagation in certain aquatic plants.

17 (*c*) Statement in option (c) is incorrect and can be corrected as

A clone is a result of asexual (not sexual) reproduction. The process of producing a clone is called cloning. All the individuals of a clone have the same genotype, which is also identical to that of the individual from which the clone was derived.

Rest of the statements are correct.

CHAPTER 02

Sexual Reproduction in Flowering Plants

All living organisms produce their progenies *via* asexual or sexual reproduction. The process of sexual reproduction is mostly seen in higher organisms such as flowering plants. **Camerarius** (1694) was the first to describe sexual reproduction in plants. This process involves the fusion of male and female gametes to form a **zygote**. The zygote in turn, gives rise to progeny after passing through various developmental processes like cleavage, differentiation, etc.

In this chapter, we will discuss all the aspects of sexual reproduction into flowering plants.

Flower

- Flowers are the main reproductive organ in angiospermic plants. They develop as a modified compressed shoots and have structures in four whorls, i.e. **sepals**, **petals**, **stamens** and **carpels.**

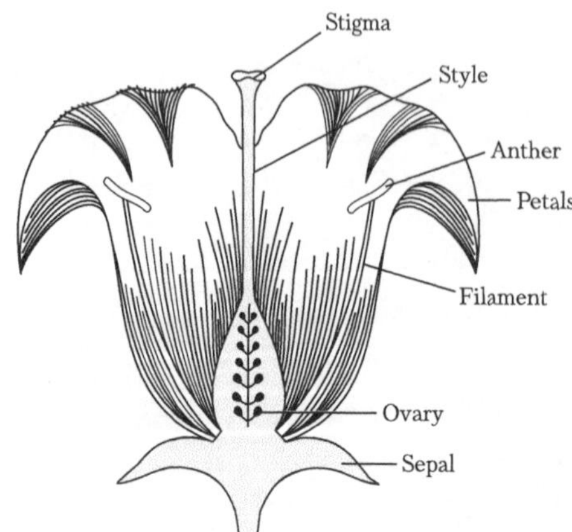

Fig. 2.1 Structure of flower

Inside

- Sepals (calyx) and petals (corolla) are of **non-essential whorls** as these are sterile in nature. Sepals are green in colour, while petals are generally brightly coloured.
- Stamens (androecium) and carpels (gynoecium) form the **essential whorls** as these constitute the fertile parts of a flower.
- Stamens and carpels contain sporangia, in which male and female gametophytes are developed.
- Male gametophytes are pollen grains, which develop inside the **microsporangia**.
- Female gametophyte is embryo sac, which develops inside **megasporangia**.

Sexual reproduction in flower

- Sexual reproduction results in the formation of a zygote through the fusion of male and female gametes. This process is known as **fertilisation**.
- Male gametes and egg cells are haploid (*n*) as these are produced through meiosis or reduction division.
- The whole process of sexual reproduction in flowering plants can be divided into the following three steps;
  1. Pre-fertilisation: Structure and events
  2. Double fertilisation
  3. Post-fertilisation: Structure and events

PRE-FERTILISATION : STRUCTURE AND EVENTS

Pre-fertilisation events occur before the fertilisation. These events are accompanied by several hormonal and structural changes which lead to the differentiation and development of floral organs of flower.

The pre-fertilisation events in plants are

1. Development of male gametophyte (microsporogenesis, microgametogenesis)
2. Development of female gametophyte (megasporogenesis, megagametogenesis)
3. Pollination
4. Pollen-pistil interaction

1. Development of male gametophyte

Pollen grains are the male gametophytes of a plant. These develop from microspores, which are formed inside the microsporangia of anthers. A typical angiospermic anther is a **bilobed** structure with each lobe having two **theca** (dithecous). These are separated by a longitudinal groove running lengthwise.

In a cross section, the anther is a four-sided (tetragonal) structure consisting of four **microsporangia** located at the corners, two in each lobe. Later, the microsporangia develop and become **pollen sacs**, which are packed with the pollen grains.

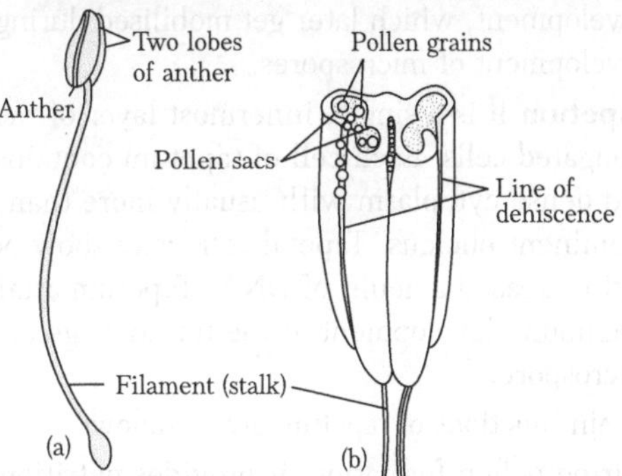

Fig. 2.2 (a) A typical stamen (b) Three-dimensional cut section of an anther

The study of pollen grain formation begins with the understanding of structure of microsporangium.

Structure of microsporangium

The wall of microsporangia consists of following four layers

(i) **Epidermis** It is a unilayer of epidermal cells, which functions as a protective covering.
The epidermis of *Arceuthobium* develops some fibrous thickenings called **exothecium.**

(ii) **Endothecium** It is present below the epidermis and is made up of radially elongated cells.
Some cells of endothecium develop fibrous thickening of α-cellulose from their inner tangential walls. These cells help in the dehiscence of anthers due to their hygroscopic nature. Fibrous bands are absent in hydrophytes, e.g. Hydrocharitaceae.
In between these cells, a few cells without thickening are also present. These thin-walled cells collectively form the **stomium** or line of dehiscence. It is the site through which pollen grains are released during anther dehiscence.

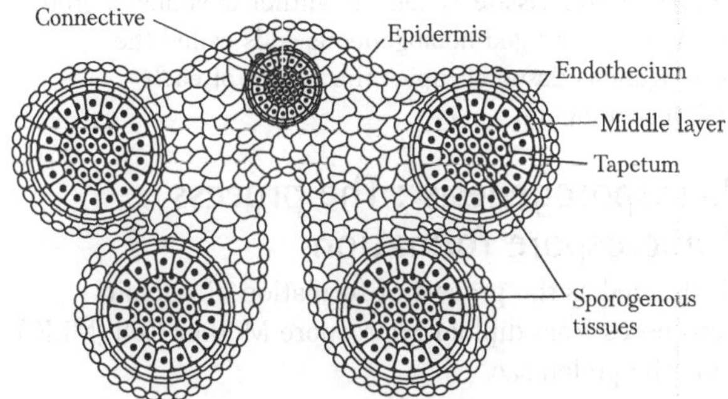

Fig. 2.3 Structure of microsporangium

(iii) **Middle layer** It consists of 2 or 3 layers of flattened and crushed parenchymatous cells. These cells store reserve food during early stages of microspore development, which later get mobilised during the development of microspores.

(iv) **Tapetum** It is a single, innermost layer of radially elongated cells. Each cell of tapetum contains a viscous and dense cytoplasm with usually more than one prominent nucleus. Tapetal cells may show polyploidy and increased amount of DNA. Tapetum attains its maximum development at the tetrad stage of microspore.

- The main functions of tapetum are as follows
  (a) During pollen formation, it provides nutrition to the pollen grains.
  (b) It produces pollenkitt material, sporopollenin, tryphine and compatibility proteins.
  (c) It secretes enzyme, e.g. callase, which degenerates the callose wall around pollen tetrad.
- On the basis of its behaviour, tapetum is of following two types
  (a) **Amoeboid** It is also named as **invasive** or **periplasmodial tapetum**. It is a primitive type of tapetum. Cells of amoeboid tapetum breakdown its radial and inner walls completely to release their protoplasmic contents in the cavity of sporangium.
  These contents later surround the developing pollen grains and provide them proper nourishment, e.g. *Arum, Typha, Mahonia, Butomus, Helianthus, Alisma, Tradescantia*, etc.
  (b) **Secretory** It is also termed as **glandular** or **parietal** tapetum and is more common type in angiosperms. Cells of secretory tapetum remain intact throughout the microspore development. It provides nourishment to developing pollen grains by secreting nutrients through its inner wall.
  These cells provide **Ubisch bodies**, which help in the ornamentation of exine as they have a chemical sporopollenin which is deposited on them.
- **Sporogenous tissue** When the anther is young, a group of compactly arranged homogeneous cells called the sporogenous tissue occupies the centre of each microsporangium.

Microsporogenesis : The process of microspore formation

It is defined as the process of formation of haploid microspores from diploid Microspore Mother Cell (MMC) inside the pollen sac.

Microsporogenesis takes place in various steps as follows

- A young anther possesses a homogeneous mass of hypodermal cells bounded by epidermis. After some time, this homogeneous mass appears like a tetra angular mass.
- Inner to this epidermis, some cells contain a prominent nucleus and abundant protoplasm, they are called **archesporial cells.** These cells undergo periclinal division (parallel to the outerwall of the epidermal cells) to form outer parietal cells and an inner sporogenous cells.
- The parietal cells divide by anticlinal and periclinal divisions to form 2-5 layered microsporangial wall. The sporogenous cells either directly function as microspore mother cells or go through some mitotic divisions and then function as **Microspore Mother Cells** (MMCs).
- Each MMC divides by meiosis and forms four haploid microspores. These microspores remain aggregated inside MMC in the form of **microspore tetrads.**
- By the end of meiosis, development of a callose wall around the microspore tetrad is seen. The individual spores are also separated from each other by callose partitions. Later, each spore starts forming its own wall, while it is still enclosed within the callose partition.
- Eventually, the microspores are set free in the anther locule by the breakdown of the callose wall.

Cell wall formation in developing pollen grains

During meiosis in MMC, two patterns of cell wall formation can be seen. These are

(a) **Successive type** In this, the cell wall is formed after meiosis-I as well as meiosis-II and thus, an **'isobilateral'** pollen tetrad is formed. It is a characteristic feature of monocots.

(b) **Simultaneous type** In this, the cell wall is formed after the completion of meiosis-II only. It gives rise to **tetrahedral** tetrad. This is found in dicots.

Other types of tetrads Many other types of tetrad have also been reported such as **decussate**, i.e. three microspores are in one phase and one in back (e.g. *Magnolia, Atriplex* and *Crocus*), **T-shaped** (e.g. *Butomopsis*) and **linear** (e.g. *Halophila*).

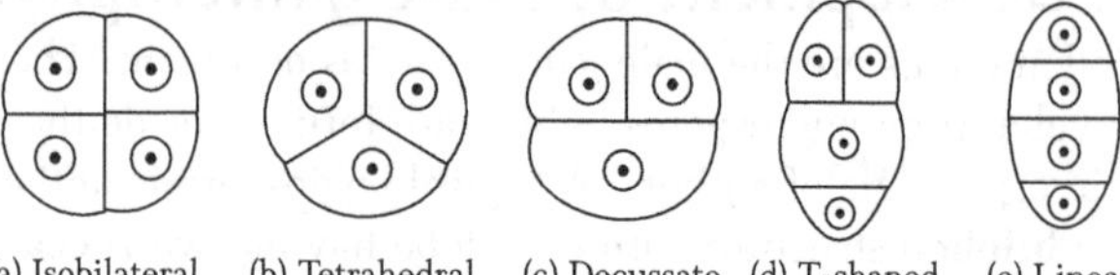

Fig. 2.4 Different types of microspore tetrads

Pollinium

In families such as Asclepiadoideae and Orchidaceae, all the microspores in a sporangium are united together to form a single structure called **pollinium**. The pollinia (pl.) of adjacent anther lobes are connected to a sticky centre or corpusculum by means of their small stalks called **caudicles**. This whole structure is called a translator apparatus.

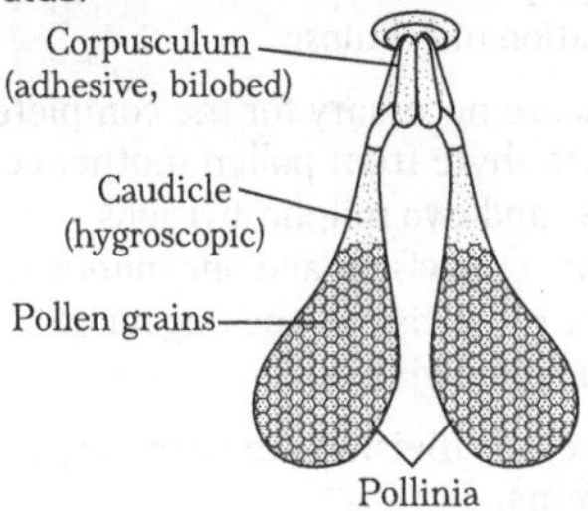

Fig. 2.5 Pollinia of Calotropis

Microgametogenesis : The process of male gamete formation

- **Microspore** is the first cell of male gametophyte. These microspores upon their release from the tetrad are called as **pollen grains.**
- They undergo mitotic division to give rise to two unequal cells.
  (i) **Vegetative cell** (the larger one) which helps in the formation of pollen tube.
  (ii) **Generative cell** (smaller one) which further divides mitotically to produce two male gametes.
- Formation of male gametes may take place after the release of pollen grains from anther. In most of the cases, anther dehiscence takes place at 2-celled stage of pollen grain.

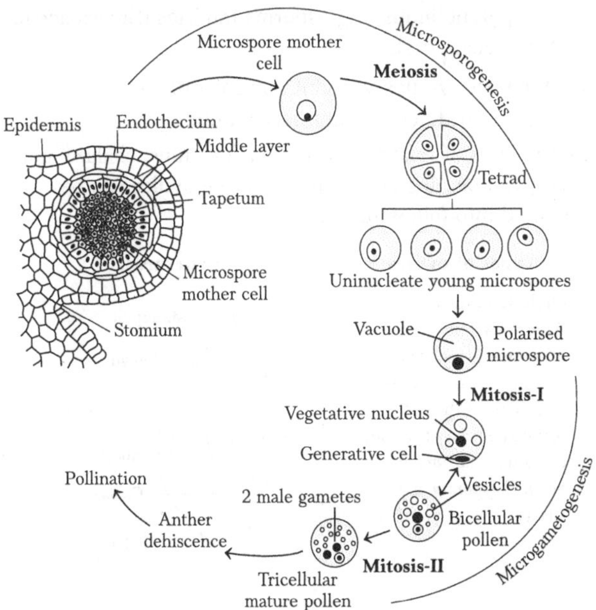

Fig. 2.6 Pollen development in flowering plants

Pollen grains : The structure

- Pollen grains are generally globular structures measuring 25-50 μm in diameter. These are either **monosiphonous** (with one pollen tube) or **polysiphonous** (with more than one pollen tube).
- The wall or covering of pollen grain is called **sporoderm.** It is made up of two layers, the outer **exine** and the inner **intine.** Both these terms, exine and intine were proposed by **Fritsch** in 1837.
- The exine is chiefly made up of **sporopollenin,** which is derived by the oxidative polymerisation of carotenoids.
- Sporopollenin is one of the most resistant biological known material. It is resistant to high temperature, acids and alkali. It cannot be degraded by any enzyme. Due to this sporopollenin, pollen grains are well preserved as microfossils.

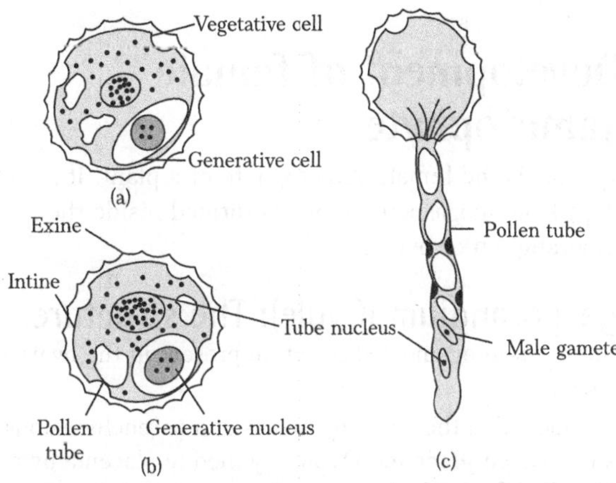

Fig 2.7 (a-b) Mature pollen grain, (c) Pollen germination

- Exine also has prominent apertures called **germ pores,** where sporopollenin is absent. Through these germ pores, pollen tubes emerge which carry male gametes in them. Exine also exhibits different patterns and designs which is of taxonomic significance.
- Intine is the inner wall which is thin and continuous and made up of **cellulose** and **pectin.**
- Cytoplasm of pollen grain is surrounded by plasma membrane. The study of pollen grains is called **polynology.**

- **Pollen allergy** Pollen grains of many species (especially anemophilous plants) cause severe allergies and bronchial afflictions in some people, often leading to chronic respiratory disorder like asthma and bronchitis, e.g. *Parthenium, Amaranthus* and *Chenopodium.*
- **Pollen products** Pollen grains are rich in nutrients, so various tablets and syrups are made out of them for consumption. These are claimed to increase the performance of athletes and race horses.
- **Pollen viability** It refers to the period in which pollen grains retain their potential to germinate. It depends on prevailing temperature, humidity and also genetic potential.
- **Pollen banks** These are centres for storage of pollens. Here, pollens are stored in liquid N_2 (–196°C) for later use in plant breeding programmes.

CHECK POINT 2.1

1. If you want to develop hybrid seeds within a bisexual flower, which of the following parts need to be removed from the same flower?
   (a) Stigma (b) Ovary
   (c) Anther (d) Oviduct
2. The anther wall consist of four wall layers where
   (a) endothecium lies inner to middle layer
   (b) tapetum lies first inner to endothecium
   (c) tapetum lies next to epidermis
   (d) middle layers lie between endothecium and tapetum
3. Ubisch bodies found in tapetal cells help in the formation of
   (a) pollenkitt and pollinia
   (b) exine
   (c) sporopollenin
   (d) intine and pollenkitt
4. Sporopollenin is derived from the
   (a) polymerisation of pectin
   (b) oxidative polymerisation of carotenoids
   (c) reductive polymerisation of carotenoids
   (d) polymerisation of cellulose
5. The processes are necessary for the complete development of male gametophyte from pollen mother cell
   (a) one meiotic and two mitotic divisions
   (b) one meiotic cell division and one mitotic cell division
   (c) two meiotic cell divisions and one mitotic cell division
   (d) two mitotic cell divisions
6. How many meiotic division are necessary to produce 100 pollen grains?
   (a) 100 (b) 25
   (c) 50 (d) 20

2. Development of female gametophyte

Embryo sac is the female gametophyte of a plant. It develops from megaspore, which is formed inside the megasporangium or ovule.

Megasporangium (Ovule): The structure

- Ovule is an integumented structure present in the ovary of a flower.
- It is attached to the ovary by means of a parenchymatous cushion called **placenta**. Ovule is joined to placenta by a stalk called **funiculus**.
- The point of attachment of the body of the ovule with the funiculus is **hilum**.
- The body of the ovule consists of a mass of parenchymatous cells called **nucellus**. It may be well-developed (crassinucellate), e.g. polypetalae or poorly developed (tenuinucellate), e.g. gamopetalae.

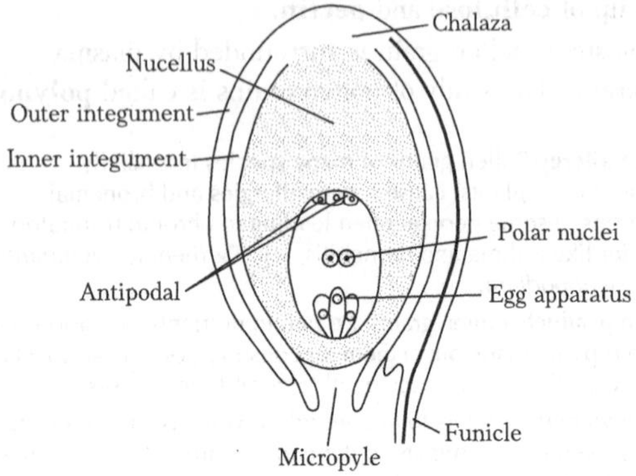

Fig. 2.8 Structure of ovule

- Embryo sac is located inside the nucellus. An ovule generally has a single embryo sac. The outermost multicellular covering of ovule is called **integument.** The integument leave a narrow pore at one end of the ovule. This pore is called **micropyle.** It represents the apical part of ovule. The basal part of ovule is called **chalaza.**

Types of ovules

- On the basis of the number of integument, ovules are of the following types
  (i) **Unitegmic** Ovules with one integument, e.g. gymnosperms and gamopetalous angiosperms families (Asteraceae, Solanaceae, etc).
  (ii) **Bitegmic** Ovules with two integuments, e.g. polypetalous angiosperms families (Brassicaceae, Malvaceae, etc).
  (iii) **Ategmic** Ovules without any integument, e.g. Loranthaceae, Santalaceae, etc.
- On the basis of relative position of funiculus, chalaza and micropyle, i.e. degree of curvature, the ovules can be classified into following six types

	Types of ovules	Structures
(i)	**Orthotropous** or **Atropous** The micropyle, chalaza and funicle are in a straight line. This is the most primitive type of ovule, e.g. *Piper nigrum*, *P. betel*, *Polygonum* and *Cycas*.	Micropyle Integuments Embryo sac Nucellus Chalaza Funiculus

Types of ovules	Structures
(ii) **Anatropous** or **Inverted** The ovule turns at 180° angle. Thus, it is an inverted ovule. Micropyle lies close to hilum or at side of hilum, e.g. found in 82% of angiospermic families.	Chalaza, Embryo sac, Raphe, Integuments, Nucellus, Hilum, Micropyle, Funicle
(iii) **Hemianatropous** The body of ovule is turned through 90° micropyle and chalaza lie in straight line. Funiculus form 90° with both micropyle and chalaza, e.g. Primulaceae and Ranunculaceae.	Integuments, Nucellus, Chalaza, Micropyle, Embryo sac, Funicle
(iv) **Campylotropous** The ovule is curved more or less at right angle to funicle. Micropylar end is bend down slightly, e.g. members of Leguminosae and Cruciferae.	Integuments, Nucellus, Embryo sac, Chalaza, Micropyle, Funicle
(v) **Amphitropous** The ovule as well as embryo sac is curved-like horse-shoe, e.g. in families-Butomaceae (*Butamus*), Rutaceae and Alismataceae (*Alisma*)	Embryo sac, Nucellus, Chalaza, Raphe, Integuments, Funicle
(vi) **Circinotropous** The ovule turns at more than 360°angle, so funicle becomes coiled around the ovule, e.g. Cactaceae (*Opuntia*), Plumbaginaceae (*Plumbago*).	Funicle, Micropyle, Embryo sac, Chalaza

Megasporogenesis: The process of megaspore formation

- A single hypodermal cell at the apex of nucellus function directly as megaspore mother cells or this cell divides periclinally to form two cells, i.e. outer parietal cell and an inner megaspore mother cell.
- The parietal cells after division form parietal tissue. The megaspore mother cell ($2n$) divides meiotically to produce a tetrad of four linear megaspores.
- Out of these four megaspores, only one megaspore is functional, while the other three degenerate.
- In majority of the angiosperms, the chalazal megaspore is functional. The functional megaspore further differentiates to form embryo sac.

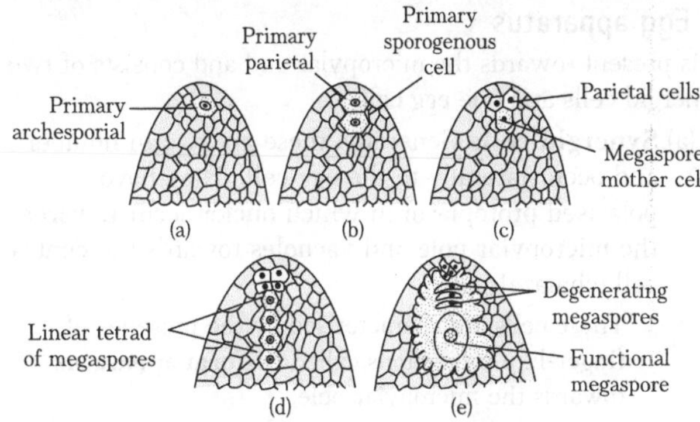

Fig 2.9 Different stages of megasporogenesis (a) to (e) showing formation of megaspore from archesporial cell (Functional hypodermal cell)

Megagametogenesis: The process of female gametophyte formation

It is the process of formation of female gametophyte (embryo sac) from megaspore. During megagametogenesis, the functional megaspore divides three times by mitotic division. As a result of this, **eight haploid nuclei** and **seven cells** are formed.

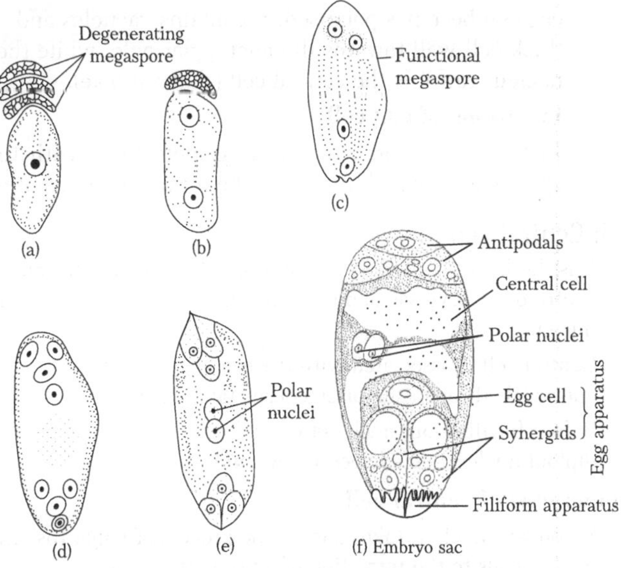

Fig. 2.10 Development of embryo sac (a-f)

Mature embryo sac : The structure

The most type of mature embryo sac in angiosperms is 7 cells and 8 nuclei in precise positions.
These are arranged in the following manner

(i) Egg apparatus

It is present towards the micropylar end and consists of two synergid cells and one egg cell.

(a) **Synergid cells** Generally, these are two in number and occur laterally to the egg cell. They have polarised protoplasm in which nuclei occur towards the micropylar pole and vacuoles towards the central cell (chalazal pole).

- These cells are characterised by the presence of finger-like projections called **filiform apparatus** towards the micropylar pole.
- The synergids degenerate before the entry of pollen tube into the embryo sac.

Functions of synergid cells

- It secretes chemotactic substances for the attraction of pollen tube during fertilisation.
- One synergid degenerate to provide a way for the entry of pollen tube into the embryo sac.
- The synergids develop haustoria and hence provide nutrition to the developing embryo sac, e.g. *Sedam, Quinchamalium, Cotula*, etc.

(b) **Egg cell** It is one in number and in general cases, it occurs between the two synergids. At maturity, the egg cell becomes polarised. It contains vacuoles and thick cell wall towards the micropylar pole, while the nucleus towards the central cell (chalazal pole).

Functions of egg cell

During fertilisation, first male gamete fuses with the egg nucleus, which results in the formation of zygote.

(ii) Central cell

- It is the largest cell of the embryo sac. It is present in the centre of embryo sac and contains (in most cases) two polar nuclei.
- Central cell is associated with the egg apparatus and antipodals through the plasmodesmatal connections.
- Before fertilisation, nuclei of central cell fuse to form a diploid nucleus called **secondary nucleus**.

Functions of central cell

- Secondary nucleus takes part in the process of triple fusion, which leads to the formation of a primary endosperm mother cell (PEM).
- It divides by mitotic divisions and forms a nutritive structure called **endosperm**, which provides nutrition to the developing embryo.

(iii) Antipodal cells

In most cases, these are three in number and occur towards the chalazal pole. Their protoplasm contains a rich amount of starch, protein, lipids, ascorbic acids, oxidases, etc.

Functions of antipodal cells

These cells limit the chalazal expression i.e. and transfer nutrients and growth hormones to developing embryo sac.

Types of embryo sac

- On the basis of number of megaspore, i.e. nuclei participating in embryo sac formation, three types of embryo sacs are recognised.
These are as follows

(i) **Monosporic embryo sac** It is derived from only one of the four megaspores. These are of two types

(a) **Polygonum type** This embryo sac is formed by the chalazal megaspore of the tetrad and is eight nucleate.

(b) **Oenothera type** This embryo sac is formed by the micropylar megaspore of the tetrad and it is four nucleate.

(ii) **Bisporic embryo sac** It is derived from two of the four megaspores. Two types of bisporic embryo sac have been recognised.

(a) **Allium type** This type develops from chalazal dyad.

(b) **Endymion type** This type develops from micropylar dyad.

(iii) **Tetrasporic embryo sac** It is derived from all the four megaspores of a tetrad.

- The following seven types of tetrasporic embryo sac have been recognised by **P Maheshwari** (1950).

(a) **Adoxa type** It has 8 nuclei, only one mitotic division occurs, e.g. *Adoxa, Sambucus, Ulmus* and *Tulipa*.

(b) **Plumbago type** This type of embryo sac is characterised by the absence of synergids and antipodals.

(c) **Penea type** It is characterised by four polar nuclei and no antipodals.

(d) **Pepromia type** It is characterised by egg apparatus which have only one synergid.

(e) **Drusa type** It is characterised by large number of antipodals.

(f) **Fritillaria type** It is characterised by triploid antipodal nuclei and tetraploid polar nucleus.

(g) **Plumbegella type** It is characterised by single triploid antipodal, no synergids and single cell egg apparatus.

CHECK POINT 2.2

1. Which one of the following pairs of plant structures has haploid number of chromosomes?
   (a) Nucellus and antipodal cells
   (b) Egg nucleus and secondary nucleus
   (c) Megaspore mother cell and antipodal cells
   (d) Egg cell and antipodal cells
2. In the angiosperm ovule, central cell of the embryo sac, prior to the entry of pollen tube, contains
   (a) a single haploid nucleus
   (b) one diploid and one haploid nucleus
   (c) two haploid polar nuclei
   (d) one diploid secondary nucleus
3. If diploid chromosome number in a flowering plants is 12, then which one of the following will have only 6? chromosomes?
   (a) Endosperm (b) Leaf cells
   (c) Cotyledons (d) Synergids
4. The hilum and micropyle lie side by side very close to each other in
   (a) anatropous ovule
   (b) campylotropous ovule
   (c) amphitropous ovule
   (d) circinotropous ovule
5. The functional megaspore undergoes
   (a) 2 meiotic divisions to form mature embryo sac
   (b) 3 mitotic divisions to form mature embryo sac
   (c) 2 mitotic divisions to form mature embryo sac
   (d) 3 meiotic divisions to form mature embryo sac
6. Four nucleated embryo sac is formed in
   (a) *Schisandra chinensis*
   (b) *Vinca rosea*
   (c) *Mirabilis*
   (d) *Commelina*

3. Pollination

It is the transfer of pollen grains from the anther of a flower to the stigma of same or other flower.

Pollination is mainly of three types

Autogamy

It involves the transfer of pollen grains from anther to the stigma of same flower. It is also known as **self- pollination.**

Autogamy is usually facilitated with the help of certain adaptations in flowers.

Some of these adaptations are as follows

(i) **Homogamy** This adaptation is seen in chasmogamous or open flowers. The anther and stigmas of these flowers are brought together by growth, bending or folding.

These mature at the same time, i.e. there is a synchrony in release of pollen and stigma maturation, e.g. *Catharanthus,* etc.

(ii) **Cleistogamy** It occurs in cleistogamous or closed flower. In such flower, the anthers and stigma lie close to each other.

Anthers do not undergo dehiscence. Germinated pollen tube pierces anther wall and enter the stigma of same flower, e.g. *Arachis hypogea*, etc.

Some plants like *Viola, Oxalis* and *Commelina* produce both types of flower, i.e. chasmogamous and cleistogamous.

(iii) **Bud pollination** Anthers and stigma ripe before the opening of the buds, hence self-pollination takes place, e.g. pea, wheat, rice, etc.

Advantages of autogamy

- It ensures fertilisation.
- Continuity of better characters can be maintained.
- Self-pollinating flowers do not waste their energy in the production of abundant pollens, colourful flowers, scent, odour, etc.
- Pollinators are not required.
- Production of large number of pollen grain is not required.

Disadvantages of autogamy

- New progenies do not show much differences from their parents.
- Adaptability to changed environment are reduced.
- Continuous selfing increases loss of vigour, which finally leads to sterility.

Geitonogamy

It involves the transfer of pollen grains from anther of a flower to the stigma of another flower of the same plant.

This pollination mainly occurs in monoecious plants.

The transfer involves an agent of pollination, hence functionally it is cross-pollination but genetically, it is similar to autogamy since the pollen grains come from the same plant, e.g. corn.

Xenogamy

It involves the transfer of pollen grains from the anther of a flower to the stigma of the genetically different flower. It is also known as **allogamy**.

Certain adaptations that facilitate xenogamy are as follows

(i) **Dichogamy** Maturation of male and female sex organs occurs at different times in a bisexual flowers. When anthers mature first, it is called **protandry**, e.g. sunflower, rose, *Impatiens* and cotton. When gynoecium matures first, it is called **protogyny**, e.g. *Vallisneria, Aristolochia* and *Scrophularia.*

(ii) **Dicliny** The presence of only one kind of essential whorl in a flower is called **dicliny** or **unisexuality**. In dioecious plants, cross-pollination is the only way of pollination, e.g. castor.

(iii) **Herkogamy** In some flowers, a mechanical barrier exists between the compatible pollen and stigma, so that self-pollination becomes impossible.

- Sometimes, a hood-like covering covers the stigma, as in *Calotropis.*
- The pollens are grouped in pollinia and remain associated to the surface till they are carried away by the insects.

(iv) **Heterostyly** In some plants, the flower may be of two or more types with regard to the length of the style and stamens. Due to this pollen from a flower cannot bring about effective pollination in flowers of its own type, e.g. *Oxalis, Lythrum, Primula.*

(v) **Self-incompatibility** In some plants, when pollen from same flower comes on the stigma, it is incapable of bringing about fertilisation. It is due to the presence of similar self-sterile genes, e.g. tobacco, potato, etc.

Types of Self-Incompatibility (SI)

SI generates and maintains genetic diversity within a species. The SI comprised of self and non-self recognition process between pollen and pistil. It is followed by selective inhibition of the development of self-pollen. These may be of two types

(i) **Sporophytic Self-Incompatibility** (SSI) Rejection of self-pollen is controlled by the genotype of the sporophytic tissue of the plant from which the pollen is derived, e.g. Brassicaceae, Asteraceae, etc.

(ii) **Gametophytic Self-Incompatibility** (GSI) Rejection of self-pollen is controlled by the genotype of male gametophyte (pollen), e.g. Solanaceae.

Sexual incompatibility may be interspecific, i.e. between the individuals of different species.

Advantages of xenogamy

- It takes place between two genetically different plants, thus offsprings formed are of new types.
- Recombination is the result of cross-pollination, which increases heterosis (increase in vigour).
- Since, two genetically different plants are involved in cross-pollination, so fertility is increased.

Disadvantages of xenogamy

- It does not ensure fertilisation.
- Cross-pollinating plants waste a lot of their energy in the formation of
  - large number of pollen grains.
  - scent or odour.
  - showy, bright-coloured petals.
- It involves different external agencies. If somehow these agencies are absent then, there will be no pollination.
- It may also lead loss of vigour.

Agencies of pollination

Various agencies helpful in cross-pollination are broadly categorised into two types, i.e. abiotic agencies and biotic agencies.

Table 2.1 Various agencies of pollination

Pollinating agencies	Processes	Agents	Examples
Abiotic agents	Anemophily	Wind	Grasses, maize and gymnosperms
	Hydrophily	Water	*Vallisneria and Hydrilla*
Biotic agents	Entomophily	Insects	Rose, poppy *and Salvia*
	Ornithophily	Birds	*Erythrena and Marcgravia*
	Cheiropterophily	Bats	*Kolabtree (Adansonia)*
	Malacophily	Snails	*Chrysanthemum and Lemma*
	Myrmecophily	Ants	

Abiotic agencies for cross-pollination

These include non-living components for pollination such as wind and water, etc.

These are given below

(i) **Anemophily** The pollination that takes place by wind is known as anemophily, e.g. *Zea mays* (maize), oaks, cotton woods, grasses, coconut, palm, date palm, *Salix, Betula, Cannabis.*

Some important features of flowers showing anemophily are as follows

- These plants have special features to assist in pollination like *Pinus* contains winged-pollen grains.
- Non-essential whorls such as calyx, corolla and bracts, bracteols are not showy.
- Flowers are devoid of scent and nectars.
- In monoecious plants, the male flowers are more in number than female flowers.
- Inflorescence is generally pendant type for swinging purpose.
- Plants grow in large groups to ensure pollination.
- In some plants, flowers appear before leaves, e.g. *Bombax*.
- Anthers are generally versatile.
- Plants produce a very large quantity of dusty pollen grains.
- Pollen grains are dry, light weight, very small-sized, non-sticky and unwettable.
- Stigma may be large and feathery (grasses) or brushy (*Typha*) and must be projected beyond the floral envelopes.

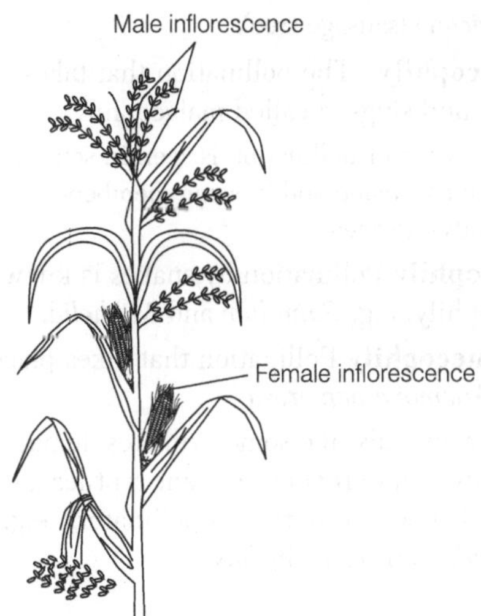

Fig 2.11 Maize : an anemophilous plant

(ii) **Hydrophily** The pollination that takes place by water is known as hydrophily.

It is of two types

- **Hypohydrophily** When pollination occurs in submerged plants, e.g. *Ceratophyllum, Najas* and *Zostera.*
- **Epihydrophily** When pollination occurs in floating hydrophytes. e.g. *Potamogeton, Vallisneria, Myriophyllum, Ruppia maritima.*

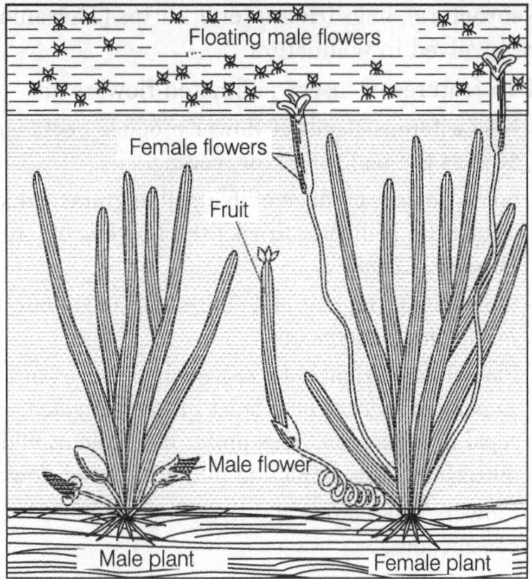

Fig 2.12 Vallisneria : a hydrophilous plant

Some specific features associated with water pollinated flowers are

- Inconspicuous and small flowers.
- Odour, nectar and colour absent in flowers.
- Flower whorls, if present are coated with wax. Stigma is unwettable, but sticky.
- Pollen grains are small, light-weighted, non-sticky and coated with wax.

Note *In Vallisneria spiralis, flowers are borne under water. Male flower gets detached from the parent plant after maturation. Female flower at the time of pollination are brought to the surface by their long stalks. As it arrives on the surface, it forms a cup-like depression to grab male flower and complete the pollination.*

Other abiotic agencies for cross-pollination

Pollination may occur *via* different mechanisms.
For example, turn pipe mechanism in *Salvia,* translator mechanism in *Calotropis,* flytrap mechanism in *Aristolochia,* trapdoor mechanism in *Ficus* and pseudocopulation mechanism in *Ophrys.*

Biotic agencies for cross-pollination

These include living agents for pollination. These are of following types

(i) **Entomophily** The pollination that takes place by insects is called entomophily. Many insects such as wasps, ants (Hymenoptera), honeybees (Diptera), moths, butterflies (Lepidoptera), grasshopper, locusts (Orthoptera), beetles (Coleoptera), dragonflies (Neuroptera), bugs (Hemiptera), thrips (Thysanioptera) are involved in pollination.

Main features of insect-pollinated flowers are

- Nectariferous glands of flower produce nectar, which attracts the pollinators for feeding.
- Some flowers produce edible pollen grains, which attract the pollinator to visit the flowers, e.g. rose, *Papaver, Clematis.*
- Flowers are fragrant and omit scent and odour, e.g. *Jasminum, Cestrum,* etc.
- Flowers are bright coloured, such as leaves in *Euphorbia pulcherrima*, bract in *Bougainvillea* and one sepal in *Mussanda.* Bees prefer blue colour, while butterflies show attraction to red coloured flowers.
- Flowers make grove and thus, become more conspicuous.
- Stigma secretes some exudates, which make stigma sticky.
- The pollen grains become sticky or develop spine around their body.

Note *Pollen/nectar robber are those insect, which consume pollen or nectar without bringing about pollination, e.g. Aquilegia spurs.*

Table 2.2 Floral features associated with pollination by different kinds of insects

Types of insects	Flower colours	Flower odours	Nectar guides
Beetles	Dull	Strong and fruity	Absent
Carrion/Dung flies	Reddish to purple-brown or greenish	Strong and foul	Absent
Bee-flies	Variable	Variable	Absent
Bees	Variable, but not solid red	Usually sweet	Present
Hawk moths	White or pale	Strong and sweet	Absent
Small moths	Variable, but not solid red	Usually sweet	Absent
Butterflies	Variable, commonly pink	Moderately strong; sweet	Present

(ii) **Ornithophily** The pollination that takes place by birds.

- Ornithophilous flowers are large-sized, brightly-coloured, odourless and they produce a large amount of mucilaginous nectar.
- *Strelitzia reginae* and *Aloe vera* are pollinated by sun birds, *Bigonia* by humming birds and *Salmelia* is by crow and mainas.

(iii) **Cheiropterophily** The pollination by bats is called cheiropterophily.

- Bat-pollinated flowers have parts, which are usually fleshy and sweet in taste, e.g. kadam, *Anthacephalus.*
- *Adonsonia digitata* pollinates the flowers of *Eidolon helvum* plant.
- *Micropteris pusillus* pollinates the flower of *Kigelia africana* (sausage tree).

(iv) **Malacophily** The pollination that takes place by snails and slugs is called malacophily.

- This type of pollination is seen in some water plants such as *Lemna* and in some members of family—Poaceae.

(v) **Ophiophily** Pollination by snakes is known as ophiophily, e.g. *Santalum* and *Michelia.*

(vi) **Myrmecophily** Pollination that takes place by ants, e.g. *Anemone nemorosa.*

(vii) Larger animals like some primates (lemur), arboreal (free-dwelling) rodent or event reptiles (gecko lizard) have also been reported as pollinators, e.g. lemur in *Ravenda* and lizard in flax.

CHECK POINT 2.3

1. Correct definition of pollination is
   (a) transfer of pollen grain from anther to stigma
   (b) germination of pollen grain
   (c) growth of pollen tube in ovule
   (d) visits of insects in flower

2. Progeny produced as a result of cross-pollination
   (a) shows high degree of variability and is evolutionary important
   (b) is sterile
   (c) has recessive character
   (d) is homozygous with phenotypic uniformity

3. Xenogamy is essentially a type of
   (a) cleistogamy
   (b) allogamy
   (c) autogamy
   (d) homogamy

4. Dichogamy which helps in cross-pollination is a floral mechanism in which of the following?
   (a) Pollen sac and stigma are at different heights
   (b) Anther and stigma mature at different times
   (c) Structure of pollen sac and stigma functions as hurdles
   (d) Pollen grain is unable to germinate on the stigma of same flowers

5. Mode of pollination in *Ruppia maritima* and *Zea mays* are
   (a) hydrophily and anemophily
   (b) entomophily and hydrophily
   (c) cheiropterophily and malacophily
   (d) anemophily and hydrophily

6. Ornithophilous flowers are
   (a) small-sized and tubular flower
   (b) large-sized and mucilaginous nectar
   (c) pollen grains are small and non-sticky
   (d) fleshy and showy

4. Pollen-pistil interaction

It is the group of events that occur from the time of pollen deposition over stigma to the time of pollen tube entry into the ovule.

The pistil has the ability to recognise the compatibility of pollen with the help of special proteins. It is a safety measure to prevent illegitimate crossing.

Precisely, these interactions are as follows

Pollen grain germination

- When stigma recognises a pollen as compatible, the pollen grain start to germinate. The compatible pollens absorb stigmatic secretions that include lipid, sugar, gum, water, etc.
- Afterwards, they germinate and produce pollen tube through one of their germ pores. This pollen tube grow and enter into the style.
- The growth and path of pollen tube through the style is also determined by specific chemicals. These chemicals are calcium, boron and isoinositol sugar.

Note *Pollen wall is boron deficient and high level of boron occurs in style and stigma of flower.*

- By the time the pollen tube cell elongates and move towards the ovule, its generative cell undergoes second mitosis (in 2-celled pollen grain) and forms two male gametes.

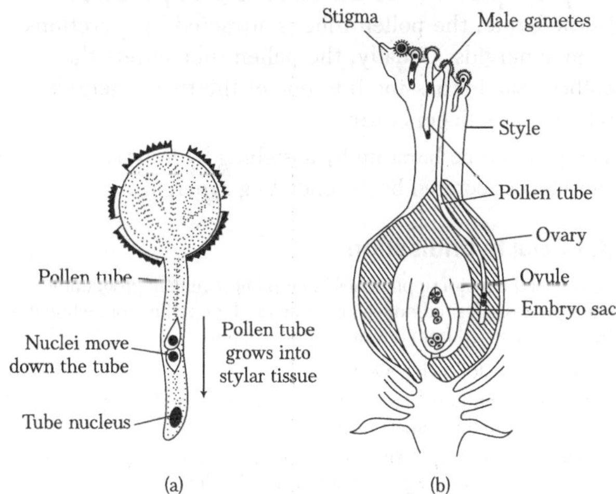

Fig 2.13 Pollen grain germination : (a) Germinated pollen grain, (b) Pollen germination on stigma

Entry of pollen tube into ovule

Pollen tube after reaching the ovary enter into ovule *via* following ways

(i) **Porogamy**, i.e. through the micropyle. It occurs in most angiosperms.

(ii) **Mesogamy**, i.e. through the integuments (e.g. *Cucurbita*) or through funiculus (e.g. *Pistacia*).

(iii) **Chalazogamy**, i.e. through the chalazal tissues, e.g. *Casuarina, Beta vulgaris, Pterocarya, Ostrya, Jaglans regia.*

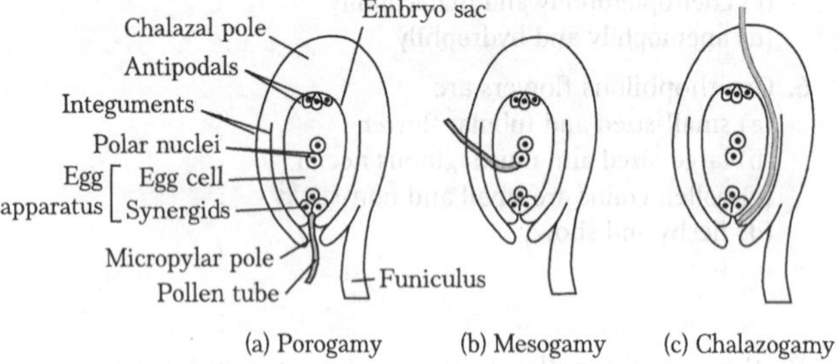

Fig 2.14 Various routes of pollen tube entry into the ovule

Entry of pollen tube into embryo sac

- In the ovule, the pollen tube is attracted by secretions from synergids. Usually, the pollen tube enters the embryo sac by passing into one of the two synergids, which starts degenerating.
- The pollen tube burst up by absorbing hydrolytic substances secreted by degenerating synergids.

Artificial hybridisation

It is one of the major approaches of crop improvement programme. In this process, desired pollen grains ae used for pollination, while the stigma is protected from unwanted pollen grains.

This is done by following two methods

(i) **Emasculation** Removal of anthers from bisexual flowers. It is done before the anthers mature.

(ii) **Bagging** Covering of emasculated flowers with a bag to prevent contamination of stigma with unwanted pollen.

DOUBLE FERTILISATION

It is the fusion of two male gametes with two different cells of the same female gametophyte to produce two different structures.

Nawaschin (1898) was the first to show that both the male gametes are involved in fertilisation in *Fritillaria* and *Lilium.*

Double fertilisation consists of two events that are as follows

(i) **Syngamy** or **Amphimixis** Fusion of the egg nucleus with one male gamete is called syngamy. This fusion results in the formation of diploid cell, the zygote.

(ii) **Triple fusion** Along with syngamy, the other male gamete moves towards the two polar nuclei located in the central cell and fuses with them to produce a triploid **Primary Endosperm Mother** (PEM) cell.

The complete process is shown in flowchart given below

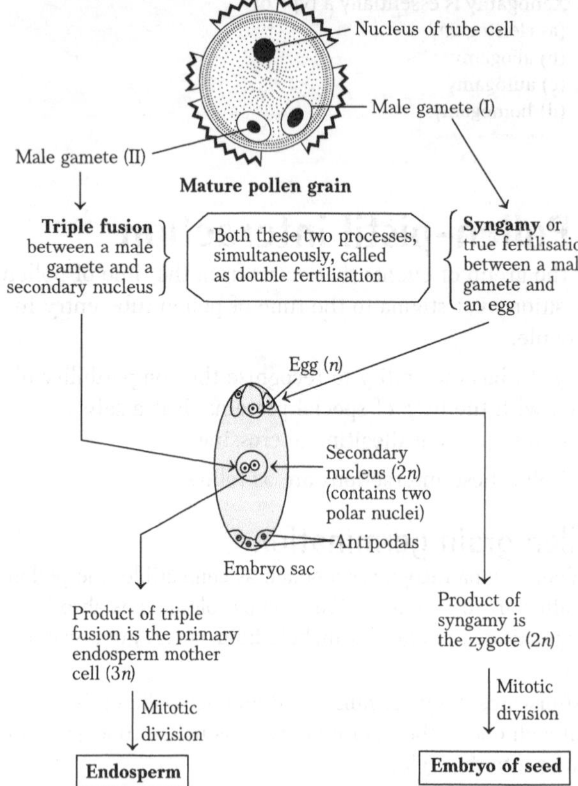

Fig. 2.15 The process of double fertilisation

Significance of double fertilisation

- The female gametophyte of angiospermic plants stop its growth at eight nucleate stage. Further growth takes place only after double fertilisation.
- The endosperm provides nutrition to the developing embryo. Thus, double fertilisation is necessary for the formation of viable seeds.
- Secondary nucleus stops its division before fertilisation. So, triple fusion induces this dormant nucleus to regain its

division power. The formation of endosperm is mainly related to its need, which arises after fertilisation, i.e. particularly for developing embryo.

Table 2.3 The changes that take place in a fertilised flower

Parts before fertilisation	Parts after fertilisation
Flower	Simple or aggregate fruit
Calyx	Fall off or remain attached as fleshy structure
Corolla	Fall off
Stamens	Fall off
Ovary wall	Pericarp of fruit
Ovary	Simple fruit
Ovule	Seed
Outer integument	Testa (tough)
Inner integument	Tegmen (delicate)
Nucellus	Perisperm
Endosperm nucleus	Endosperm
Egg cell	Embryo
Funiculus	Stalk
Antipodals	Degenerate
Synergids	Degenerate

CHECK POINT 2.4

1. Which of the following statements is correct for the pollen tube?
   (a) It shows chemotactic movement
   (b) It shows only tip growth
   (c) It is composed of three non-cellular zones
   (d) It shows rapid cytoplasmic streaming
2. A pollen tube grows down the style because
   (a) it helps in fertilisation
   (b) it takes nutrients from the style
   (c) filiform apparatus of synergids attracts the pollen tube
   (d) of chemical attraction
3. Which of the following is not true for double fertilisation?
   (a) Discovered by Nawaschin
   (b) Male gamete and secondary nucleus fused to form endosperm nucleus
   (c) Endosperm nucleus is diploid
   (d) Endosperm provides nutrition to embryo
4. Triple fusion in angiosperm is the fusion of second sperm with
   (a) antipodal cells and one synergid cell
   (b) two antipodal cells
   (c) two synergid cells
   (d) two polar nuclei

POST-FERTILISATION : STRUCTURE AND EVENTS

The major post-fertilisation events include development of endosperm and embryo, maturation of ovules into seeds and ovary into fruit. These events take place soon after the double fertilisation.

Development of embryo (Embryogeny)

- The first stage in the development of a plant zygote is a pre-determined mode of development **(embryogeny)**. It gives rise to an organised mass of cells called the **embryo** that has the potential to form a complete plant.
- Most zygotes divide only after certain amount of endosperm is formed to assure that proper nutrition is provided to the developing embryo.
- In the majority of angiosperms, the zygote (fertilised egg) divides by an asymmetric mitotic division and generates two cells with two different fates.
  (i) The smaller daughter cell with dense cytoplasm is situated towards the chalazal pole. It is called **terminal cell** or **apical cell** or **embryonal cell.**
  (ii) Another comparatively larger daughter cell situated towards the micropylar end is called **basal cell.** This cell divides transversely and gives rise to **suspensor cells.**
  The zygote gives rise to the **proembryo** and subsequently to the **globular embryo.**
- Though the seeds differ greatly, the early stages of embryo development (embryogeny) are similar upto globular stages in monocots and dicots.

Development of embryo in dicots

- In dicots, the terminal cell at chalazal end and the basal cell at micropylar end (resulted from transverse mitotic division in zygote), give rise to eight-celled octant embryo (by one transverse and two vertical divisions) and 6-10-celled filamentous suspensor, respectively.
- The cell at micropylar end of filamentous suspensor acts as **haustorium** to absorb food from endosperm. It later develops into epicotyl and plumule, whereas the suspensor cell at the chalazal end acts as **hypophysis** and generates radicle and hypocotyl.

- The suspensor cells thus, push the embryo into endosperm tissue to absorb nutrition from it. The octant developed from terminal cell soon develops into globular, then heart-shaped and mature embryo.
- A typical dicotyledonous embryo consists of an **embryonal axis** and two **cotyledons**. The portion of the embryonal axis above the level of cotyledons is the **epicotyl**, which terminates in the **plumule** or stem tip.
- The cylindrical portion below the level of cotyledons is **hypocotyl** that terminates in the **radicle** or **root tip**. The root tip is covered with a **root cap**, e.g. mango, apple, radish, rose, etc.

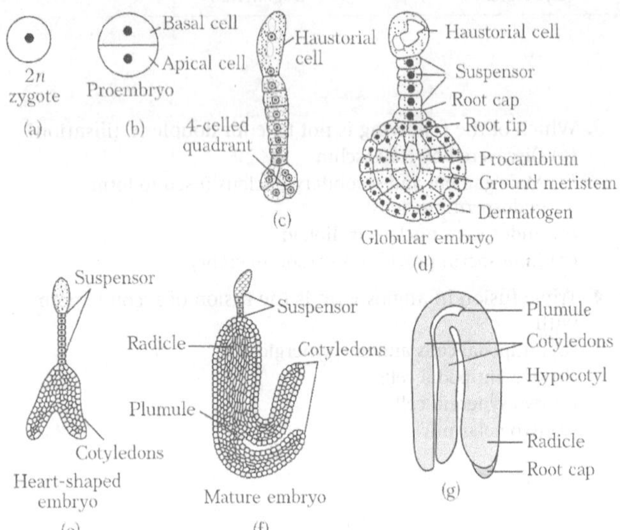

Fig. 2.16 Stages in the development of a dicot embryo

Development of embryo in monocots

- First of all zygotes divides by transverse divisions and leads to a three-celled **proembryo**. These cells are a **terminal cell** (apical cell), **basal cell** and **middle cell**.
- Larger basal cell, situated close to the micropyle, does not further divide. Instead, it enlarges in size and behaves as a **suspensor cell**.
- There are various divisions that take place in different planes in terminal cell and eventually bring about a single **cotyledon**.
- Whereas, the middle cell, by a number of vertical and transverse divisions, differentiates into **radicle, hypocotyl, plumule** and some cells of suspensor.
- Thus, the mature monocot embryo contains a laterally situated plumule and a single, terminal cotyledon.
- Embryo of monocots possesses only one cotyledon at one end (lateral) of the embryonal axis and this cotyledon is called **scutellum**.
- At the lower end, the embryonal axis has radicle and root cap enclosed in an undifferentiated sheath called **coleorhiza**. The portion of the embryonal axis above the level of attachment of scutellum is the **epicotyl**.
- The epicotyl has a shoot apex and a few leaf primordia enclosed in a hollow foliar structure called **coleoptile**, e.g. grass, banana, bamboo, palm, etc.

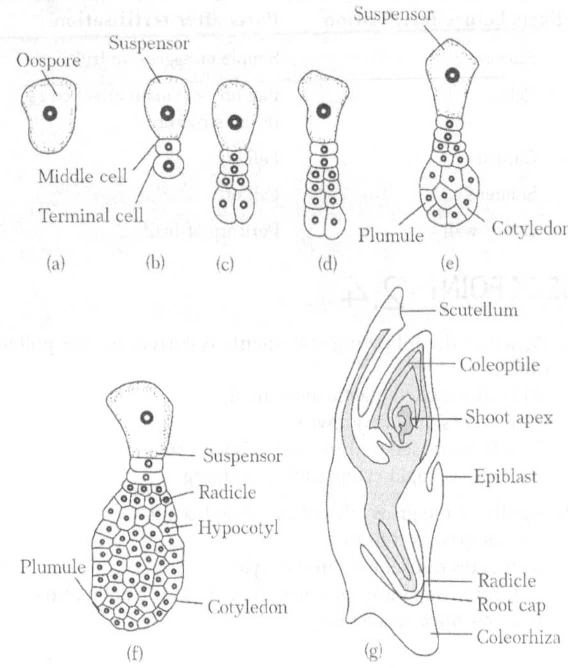

Fig. 2.17 (a-f) Stages in development of a monocot embryo, (g) A monocot embryo of a grass

Note
- ***Epiblast*** *present in monocot embryo represent secondary cotyledons.*
- *In monocot, the embryonic root is the first organ to penetrate the seed coat during seed germination.*
- ***Hypocotyl*** *is the first part of dicot embryo to appear above the ground during seed germination.*
- *Effect of pollen on endosperm is called* **xenia**.

Table 2.4 Differences between monocot embryo and dicot embryo

Characters	Monocot embryo	Dicot embryo
Number of cotyledons	One cotyledon attached to the embryonal axis.	Two cotyledons attached to an embryonal axis.
Position of plumule	Lateral	Distal
Position of cotyledons	A terminal	Lateral
Coleoptile	The envelope of plumule is called coleoptile.	Absent
Coleorhiza	This is a protective sheath of radicle.	Absent
Scutellum	A single cotyledon.	Absent
Suspensor	Comparatively small	Large

Development of endosperm

- In triple fusion, a male gamete fuses with the secondary nucleus and a triploid structure called **Primary Endosperm Mother** (PEM) cell is formed.
- It divides by mitotic division and forms a mass of nutritive cells called as endosperm.
- In Orchidaceae, Podostemaceae and Trapaceae families, endosperm is absent.
- The ploidy level of endosperm varies according to the type of embryo sac. Different embryo sacs contain different ploidy level of secondary nucleus.
- In oenothera type of embryo sac, there is haploid secondary nucleus (n). Thus, the ploidy level of endosperm is diploid ($2n$) in oenothera type embryo sac.

Internal structure of endosperm

- The endosperm is made up of isodiamorphical, triploid (in most cases) cells that store reserve food material in the form of starch, carbohydrates, proteins or fats.
- The cells of endosperm are thin-walled and do not have pits. In the presence of hemicellulose as a reserve food, the cell wall becomes thick and pitted.
- For the transfer of stored material, the plasmodesmata also occurs between the cells of endosperm.
- In cereals, the cells of the outermost layers of the endosperm become morphologically and physiologically specialised and form a layer of cells called **aleurone layer**.
- Cells of this layer contain aleurone grains, each of which is covered by a single unit membrane.
- The main components of aleurone grains are phospholipids, proteins, phytin and some carbohydrates.
- Each aleurone grain contains a globoid cavity, which is surrounded by a protein carbohydrate body. It, in turn is covered by numerous spherosomes.
- The main function of aleurone cells is the secretion of hydrolytic enzymes, protease (protein digesting enzymes) and amylase (starch digesting enzymes) in the germinating seeds.

Types of endosperm

On the basis of its development, endosperm is classified approximately into three main groups

(i) **Cellular endosperm** It is found in 25% of the angiosperm families particularly in **dicotyledons**. The primary endosperm mother cell divides by mitotic divisions and each division is followed by a cell wall formation, e.g. *Adoxa, Verbascum, Cetranthus, Scutellaria, Datura, Myostis arvensis, Impatiens, Magnolia*, etc.

(ii) **Nuclear endosperm** It is a more common type of endosperm and occurs in about 56% of the angiosperm families. In this type, PEM cell divides by free-nuclear divisions, which are not followed by the cell wall formation.

Thus, free nuclei remain in the cytoplasm of embryo sac. Later on, cell wall formation takes place from periphery to the centre (centripetal), leading to the formation of a cellular type of embryo sac, e.g. *Acer, Arachis, Gravillea, Lomatia, Phoenix, Calotropis, Primula, Citrus, Malva, Acalypha*, etc.

In coconut, Primary Endosperm Nucleus (PEN) undergoes a number of free nuclear divisions. Hence, the embryo sac gets filled with a clear fluid and this fluid is known as **coconut water**.

(iii) **Helobial endosperm** It is found in about 19% of the angiosperm families particularly in monocotyledons. It is an intermediate type between cellular and nuclear endosperms, e.g. *Asphodelus*.

Functions of endosperm

These are as follows

- Endosperm forms sufficient food for the developing embryo.
- In the absence of endosperm, the growth of embryo will be poor or suppressed and this results in the formation of non-viable seeds.
- Endosperm stores carbohydrates, fats, proteins, etc.

Note
- *Chalazal endosperm–haustorium with fingers like appendages occurs in* ***Lomatia.***
- *Only lateral endosperm–haustoria arise in* ***monochoria****.*
- *Mature endosperm with any degree of irregularity and unevenness in its surface is called* ***ruminate endosperm****, e.g. Passiflora, Myristica, etc.*
- *In* ***mosaic endosperm****, the tissue of endosperm is not homogeneous, e.g. Zea mays.*

Development of seed

- Double fertilisation in angiosperms triggers the transformation of ovule into a seed. The seeds are formed inside the fruits.
- The seeds are attached to the fruit wall by funiculus. At maturity, the funiculus abscise, leaving a scar called **hilum**. The seed has a smooth and papery seed coat.
- In some plants, such as castor bean, it has two layers, i.e. the outer layer is called **testa**, while the inner layer is called **tegmen**.
- Two cotyledons are present inside the seed coat in dicot and one cotyledon in monocot. Cotyledons are attached laterally to the **embryonal axis**.

- Depending on the presence or absence of endosperm, seeds may be
  - (i) **Endospermic** or **Albuminous seed** Endosperm is present in this seed, e.g. wheat, maize, sunflower, castor, etc.
  - (ii) **Non-endospermic** or **Exalbuminous seed** Endosperm is absent in this seed, e.g. pea, bean, groundnut, etc.

Importance of seeds

- It has reserve food for nourishing the seedling.
- Seeds are formed through sexual reproduction, thus they carry a number of variations.
- Seeds can be stored.
- Seeds have adaptive strategies to get dispersed to a new habitat and colonise the same.

Formation of fruit

It is a ripened ovary. The wall of the ovary forms the wall of the fruit, it is known as **pericarp**. Fruits that develop from the ovary are known as **true fruits**, e.g. mango, tomato, etc. Fruits that develop from other floral parts, such as thalamus along with the development of ovary wall are known as **false fruit**, e.g. apple, etc.

Importance of fruit

- These are the source of energy for animals as they use them as food.
- These also act as the source of nutrients as sugar, vitamins and minerals.
- Fruits protect the seeds from adverse environmental conditions.
- Sometimes, fruits also provide nutrition to the developing seedling.
- These also help in dispersal of seeds to new habitat, thus help the species to reach far away from the original region.

Special features arises during post-fertilisation development

During post-fertilisation, many special structures arise from various parts of the ovule. These are as follows

(i) **Caruncle** It is a fleshy, whitish structure present on micropylar end of seed. It arises due to the proliferation of cells at the tip of outer integument on the side of funiculus or all round the micropyle. It helps in seed dispersal, e.g. Euphorbiaceae.

(ii) **Aril** It is a fleshy seed appendage, which arises from the funiculus or testa or from both. Aril is regarded as the third integument because it surrounds the ovule more or less completely in the post-fertilisation stage. For example,

(a) Fruit of litchi.

(b) Dried aril of nutmeg (*Myristica fragrans*).

(c) Oily, thin-walled aril of Passifloraceae.

(d) Fimbriate aril of *Crossosoma californicum.*

(iii) **Operculum** It is a plug-like structure in micropylar part portion of the seed. It is derived from the nucellar apex, endostome, exostome or by the hilar region of the seed. It is detached during germination. It is common in monocots, but also present in some dicots.

SOME SPECIAL MECHANISMS OF REPRODUCTION

Although, seeds in general are the products of fertilisation, but a few flowering plants have evolved a special mechanism to produce seeds or to develop many embryos from a single fertilised egg. These methods are discussed below

Polyembryony

- It was first time observed in orange seeds by **Antonie van Leeuwenhoek** in 1719.
- In general, each seed bears an embryo, but sometimes there are more than one embryo in a single seed. The occurrence of more than one embryo in a seed is called polyembryony.
- On a broad basis, polyembryony is of two types
  - (i) **Spontaneous** It includes naturally occurring polyembryony.
  - (ii) **Induced** This type of polyembryony is induced experimentally.

True and false polyembryony

Ernst (1901) subdivided spontaneous polyembryony into two categories, i.e. true and false polyembryony. It is widely accepted by scientists.

(i) **True polyembryony** In this, extraembryos arise from the cells present in the same embryo sac or the cells surrounding the embryo sac, i.e. from nucellar cells or integumentary cells, e.g. *Citrus, Mangifera, Opuntia,* from synergids, e.g. *Sagittaria, Bergenia, Peltiphyllum, Argemone* and from antipodal cells, e.g. *Ulmus* or from embryo itself, e.g. *Vanda.*

EXAM POINTS

- In angiosperms, microsporogenesis and megasporogenesis involve meiosis. **[CBSE AIPMT 2015]**
- Product of sexual reproduction generally generates new genetic combination leaving to variations. **[NEET 2013]**
- Pollen grain represents the male gamete. **[UP CPMT 2012]**
- Developing pollen gets its nourishment from cells of tapetum layer. **[J&K CET 2014]**
- The isobilateral type of microspore arrangement in tetrad is present in *Zea mays*. **[AMU 2015]**
- Hardest substance in plant kingdom is sporopollenin. **[JIPMER 2019]**
- Pollen grains can be stored for several years in liquid nitrogen having temperature of −196°C. **[NEET 2018]**
- Pollen tablets are available in the market for supplementing food. **[CBSE AIPMT 2014]**
- The process of removal of anther from the flower bud before it dehisces is called as emasculation. **[AIIMS 2019]**
- Proximal end of the filament of stamen is attached to the thalamus or petal. **[NEET-I 2017]**
- Emasculation ensures cross-pollination in bisexual flower. **[RPMT 2014]**
- The ovule of an angiosperm is technically equivalent to megasporangium. **[NEET-II 2017]**
- In majority of angiosperms, reduction division occurs in the megaspore mother cells. **[NEET 2016]**
- In angiospermic plants, meiosis of megaspore mother cell generally produces linear tetrad. **[Chhattisgarh PMT 2015]**
- The body of the ovule is fused within the funicle at hilum. **[NEET 2020]**
- The embryo sac of angiosperms contains 3-celled egg apparatus, 3 antipodal cells and 2 polar nuclei. **[Haryana PMT 2014]**
- Egg in female gametophyte is accompanied by synergids. **[WB JEE 2015]**
- Transfer of pollen grains from the anther to the stigma of another flower of the different plant is known as xenogamy. **[Haryana PMT 2014]**
- Geitonogamy may require pollinators, but is genetically similar to autogamy. **[CBSE AIPMT 2015]**
- Geitonogamy involves fertilisation of a flower by the pollen form an other flower of the same plant. **[CBSE AIPMT 2014]**
- A dioecious flowering plants prevents both autogamy and geitonogamy. **[NEET 2017]**
- In papaya, both autogamy and geitonogamy are prevented. **[NEET 2019]**
- Flowers which have single ovule in the ovary and are packed into inflorescence are usually pollinated by wind. **[NEET 2017]**
- In water hyacinth and water lily, pollination takes place by insects or wind. **[NEET 2020, 16]**
- In *Vallisneria*, male flowers are carried by water currents to female flowers at the surface of water. **[NEET 2019]**
- Attractants and rewards are required for entomophily. **[NEET 2017]**
- Pollenkitt is present in entomophily. **[JIPMER 2018]**
- Nectar and pollen grains are the important floral rewards to the animal pollinators. **[CBSE AIPMT 2015]**
- Wind pollinated plants possess well exposed stamens and stigma, their flowers are small and not brightly coloured and their pollen grains are light and non-sticky. **[NEET 2020]**
- Chalazogamy is shown by *Casuarina*. **[AMU 2015]**
- Cross-pollination does not occur in cleistogamous flowers. **[MHT CET 2014]**
- Cleistogamous flowers are bisexual flowers which remain closed. **[WB JEE 2014]**
- During the process of sexual reproduction in flowering plants, double fertilisation involves fertilisation of egg cell and a central cell by two male gametes brought by same pollen tube. **[Punjab PMET 2014]**
- The endosperm in angiosperms develops from secondary nucleus. **[UP CPMT 2012]**
- Zygote is resulted by the process of syngamy. **[J&K CET 2014]**
- Filiform apparatus is characteristic feature of synergids. **[CBSE AIPMT 2015]**
- Pollen grains of many species can germinate on the stigma of a flower, but only one pollen tube of the same species grows into the style. **[NEET 2016]**
- Monosporic with three sequential mitotic division is the most common type of embryo sac. **[NEET 2019]**
- The fate of the male gamete discharged in the synergid is that, one gamete fuses with the egg and other gamete fuses with central cell nuclei. **[NEET 2019]**
- The events in post-fertilisation development in flowering plant is that zygote develops into embryo, central cell develops into endosperm and ovary develops into fruit. **[NEET 2019]**
- Embryo development other than the egg cell of haploid embryo sac from synergid and antipodals is known as apogamy. **[Chhattisgarh PMT 2015]**
- Endosperm nucleus is $3n$. **[WB JEE 2015]**
- Endosperm is present in orchids and maize, but absent in gram. **[UK PMT 2014]**
- The wheat, grain have an embryo with one large, shield-shaped cotyledon known as scutellum. **[CBSE AIPMT 2015]**
- The hilum is a scar on the seed, where funicle was attached. **[CBSE AIPMT 2015]**
- Persistent nucellus in the seed is known as perisperm. **[NEET 2019]**
- In some plants, thalamus contributes to fruit formation. Such fruits are termed as false fruits. **[NEET 2020]**
- Seed formation without fertilisation in flowering plants involves the process of apomixis. **[NEET 2016]**
- Banana is an example of parthenogenesis. **[WB JEE 2015]**

Chapter Exercises

(A) Topical Exercise

Flower and Development of Male Gametophyte

1 In a typical complete, bisexual and hypogynous flower, the arrangement of floral whorls on the thalamus from the outermost to the innermost is **[NCERT Exemplar]**

(a) calyx, corolla, androecium and gynoecium
(b) calyx, corolla, gynoecium and androecium
(c) gynoecium, androecium, corolla and calyx
(d) androecium, gynoecium, corolla and calyx

2 The male gametes of angiosperms are

(a) uniflagellate
(b) biflagellate
(c) non-motile as there is no flagellated stage in the life cycle of angiosperms
(d) None of the above

3 Wall of a pollen sac consists of

(a) endothecium and tapetum
(b) tapetum and middle layers
(c) endothecium, middle layers and tapetum
(d) epidermis, endothecium, middle layers and tapetum

4 The outermost and innermost wall layers of microsporangium in an anther are respectively

(a) endothecium and tapetum **[NCERT Exemplar]**
(b) epidermis and endodermis
(c) epidermis and middle layer
(d) epidermis and tapetum

5 Endothecium is responsible for

(a) the nourishment of anther
(b) the dehiscence of anther
(c) the formation of pollen grains
(d) None of the above

6 The given figure is an enlarged view of one microsporangium of a matured anther, identify *A*, *B* and *C*.

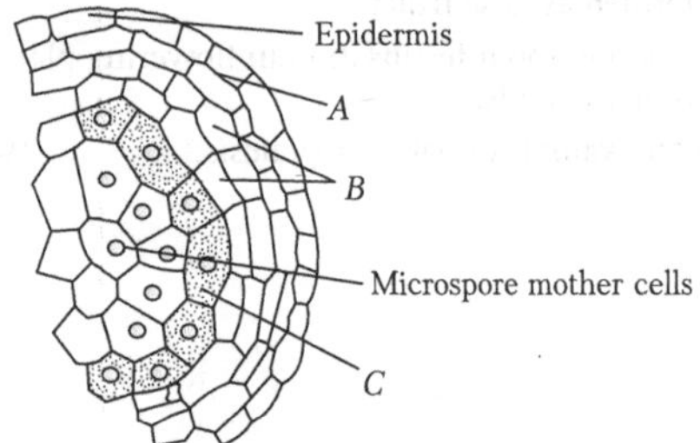

(a) *A*-Endothecium, *B*-Tapetum, *C*-Middle layer
(b) *A*-Middle layer, *B*- Endothecium, *C*-Tapetum
(c) *A*-Tapetum, *B*- Middle layer, *C*- Endothecium
(d) *A*-Endothecium, *B*- Middle layer, *C*-Tapetum

7 What is the function of tapetum in a developing anther?

(a) To draw food materials from the microspores
(b) To digest the sporocytes
(c) To supply food materials to the developing microsporocytes
(d) To give protection to the inner tissues

8 Tapetum is

(a) parietal in origin
(b) innermost wall layer of pollen sac
(c) nutritive and provides food material to pollen grains
(d) All of the above

9 What happens to tapetum on maturity?

(a) It persists
(b) It becomes sticky
(c) It is eaten up or gets degenerated
(d) It becomes fibrous

10 Middle layers of the microsporangial wall

(a) shrivel at maturity of anther
(b) persist, but remain thin-walled
(c) degenerate before maturity
(d) persist and become thickened

11 In an anther, stomium occurs

(a) at the tip
(b) in grooves of each anther lobe
(c) at the base of anther
(d) transversely on the anther

12 During formation of pollen grains, a microspore mother cell undergoes

(a) one meiotic division
(b) one mitotic division
(c) one meiotic and one mitotic division
(d) one meiotic and two mitotic divisions

13 The microsporangia develop further and become

(a) pollen grain (b) embryo sac
(c) pollen sac (d) tapetum

14 The Ubisch bodies are involved in

(a) initiating meiosis in pollen mother cell
(b) designing the external thickening of pollen
(c) providing nutrition to developing pollen
(d) no specific embryological function

15 Consider the following statements.
I. Microsporangium is generally surrounded by four wall layers-epidermis, endothecuim, middle layer and tapetum.
II. The outer three wall layers perform the function of protection and help in dehiscence of anther to release the pollen.

Choose the correct option.
(a) Statement I is true, but II is false
(b) Statement I is false, but II is true
(c) Both statements I and II are true
(d) Both statements I and II are false

16 In microsporangium, microspore tetrad are formed due to
(a) formation of callose wall
(b) formation of pectin wall
(c) formation of sporopollenin wall
(d) formation of pollenkitt

17 A typical angiospermic anther is ...*A*... where each lobe contain ...*B*... microsporangia.

	A	*B*
(a)	dithecous	two
(b)	bilobed	four
(c)	monothecous	two
(d)	single lobe	four

18 The cells of tapetum possess ...*A*... cytoplasm and generally have ...*B*... nucleus/nuclei.

	A	*B*
(a)	light	single
(b)	light	two
(c)	dense	single
(d)	dense	multiple

19 Pollen grains are generally ...*A*..., measuring about ...*B*... μm in diameter.

	A	*B*
(a)	elongated	25-50
(b)	spherical	250-1000
(c)	elongated	250-1000
(d)	spherical	25-50

20 The inner wall of the pollen grain is
(a) non-continuous (b) thick
(c) hard (d) pecto-cellulosic

21 The given figure represents some stages in microgametogenesis. Identify *A*, *B* and *C*, respectively.

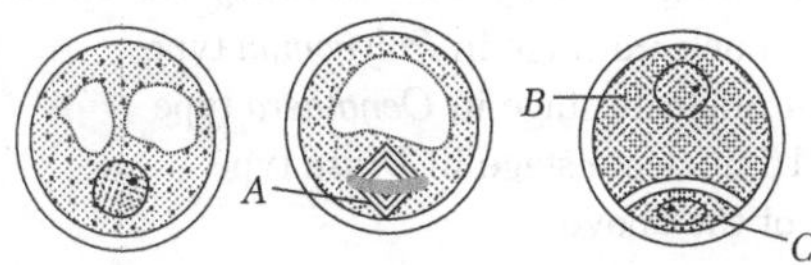

(a) *A*-Symmetric spindle, *B*-Vegetative cell, *C*-Generative cell
(b) A-Symmetric spindle, *B*-Generative cell, *C*-Vegetative cell
(c) *A*-Asymmetric spindle, *B*-Vegetative cell, *C*-Generative cell
(d) *A*-Asymmetric spindle, *B*-Generative cell, *C*-Vegetative cell

22 Which option correctly defines the property of vegetative and generative cell of a pollen grain ?

	Vegetative cell	Generative cell
(a)	Small	Big
(b)	Scanty food matter	Abundant food matter
(c)	Large with irregular-shaped nucleus	Spindle-shaped cell
(d)	Floats in the cytoplasm of generative cell	Floats in the cytoplasm of vegetative cell

23 Which of the following is secreted by tapetum?
(a) Callase enzyme (b) Compatible protein
(c) Tryphine (d) All of these

24 In given figure *A* and *B* are, respectively.

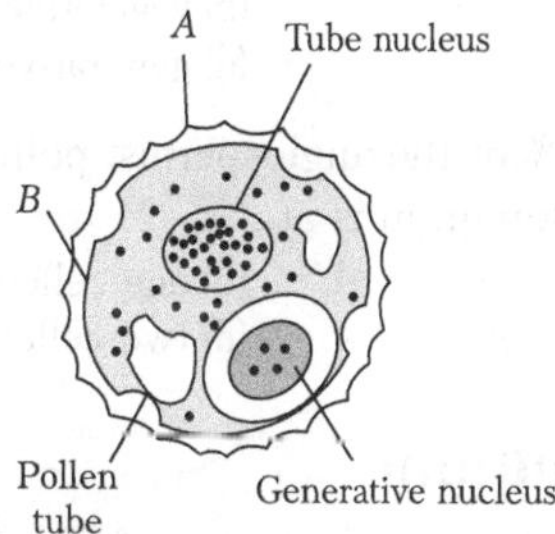

(a) Epicarp and endocarp
(b) Epidermis and endodermis
(c) Intine and exine
(d) Exine and intine

25 Pollen grain causes severe allergy and bronchial application in some people. These pollen grains belong to plants
(a) *Hibiscus*
(b) *Helianthus*
(c) *Soncus*
(d) *Parthenium*

26 The vegetative cell (tube cell) and generative cell are of unequal sizes. This is because
(a) in future, vegetative cell will undergo mitosis
(b) in future, generative cell will undergo meiosis
(c) the pollen cell produces these cells from asymmetric spindle fibres during mitosis
(d) generative cell possess more cytoplasm than vegetative cell

27 A botanist treated some pollen grains with enzymes, chemical and high temperature to break exine. After that he observed under the microscope and found that exine is still intact.

Why exine is not broken down?

(a) Because exine is cellulosic in natrue
(b) Because pollen grains are small
(c) Because exine is coated with sporopollenin
(d) None of the above

28 In some cereals like rice and wheat, pollen grains lose viability within ...*A*... but in members of Rosaceae, Leguminosae and Solanaceae, pollen viability is maintained for ...*B*... .

	A	*B*
(a)	month	year
(b)	year	month
(c)	month	30 min
(d)	30 min	month

29 The part of pollen which has prominent apertures called germ pores where sporopollenin is absent. That part is

(a) intine (b) vegetative cell
(c) exine (d) generative cell

30 In about 60% of the angiosperms, pollination occur when a pollen grain is at

(a) 3-celled stage (b) one-celled stage
(c) 4-celled stage (d) two-celled stage

Megasporangium

31 The isolation of megasporocyte from the rest of the nucellar tissue begin from

(a) micropylar region (b) chalazal region
(c) middle region (d) anywhere

32 When the body of the ovule lies at right angles to the funicle and the micropyle lies close to the later, it is termed as

(a) anatropous (b) hemianatropous
(c) campylotropous (d) amphitropous

33 *Quinchamalium chilense* is peculiar in having haustorial appendages arising from

(a) antipodals only (b) egg and synergids
(c) antipodals and synergids (d) synergids only

34 Raphe is

(a) ridge formed by union of funicle with the body of ovule
(b) distance between chalaza and micropyle
(c) distance between hilum and micropyle
(d) area between hilum and chalaza

35 Write the name of the ovule type with an example.

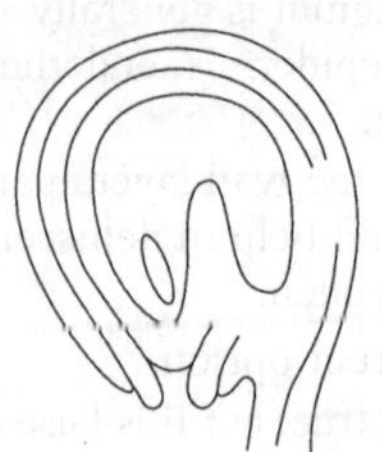

	Ovule	Example
(a)	Campylotropous	*Pisum sativum*
(b)	Anatropous	*Helianthus*
(c)	Amphitropous	*Butomaceae*
(d)	Orthotropous	*Polygonum*

36 The following figure shows the

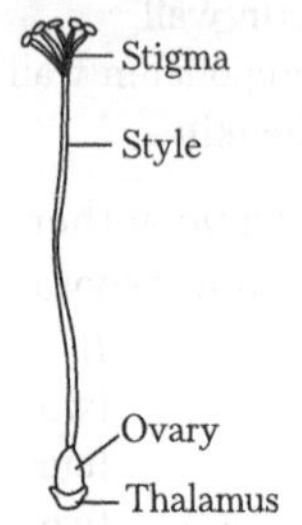

(a) Multicarpellary syncarpous pistil of *Papaver*
(b) Multicarpellary apocarpous gynoecium of *Michelia*
(c) Pentacarpellary syncarpous gynoecium of the *Hibiscus*
(d) Multicarpellary apocarpous gynoecium of the China rose

37 Consider the following statements.

I. Ovules generally differentiate a single Megaspore Mother Cell (MMC) in the chalazal region of the nucellus.
II. The MMC undergoes reduction division and produces four megaspores.

Choose the correct option.

(a) Statement I is true, but II is false
(b) Statement I is false, but II is true
(c) Both statements I and II are true
(d) Both statements I and II are false

38 Eight nucleate embryo sacs are

(a) always bisporic
(b) always tetrasporic
(c) always monosporic
(d) sometimes monosporic, sometimes bisporic and sometimes tetrasporic

39 At what stage embryo sac is ready for fertilisation?

(a) At 8 nucleate stage in *Polygonum* type
(b) At 4 nucleate stage in *Oenothera* type
(c) At 16 nucleate stage in *Drusa* type
(d) All of the above

40 In an embryo sac, the cells that degenerate after fertilisation are **[NCERT Exemplar]**
(a) synergids and primary endosperm cell
(b) synergids and antipodals
(c) antipodals and primary endosperm cell
(d) egg and antipodals

41 In a fertilised embryo sac, the haploid, diploid and triploid structures are **[NCERT Exemplar]**
(a) synergid, zygote and primary endosperm nucleus
(b) synergid, antipodal and polar nuclei
(c) antipodal, synergid and primary endosperm nucleus
(d) synergid, polar nuclei and zygote

42 Consider the following statements.
I. Mature ovules in which micropyle comes to lie close to the funiculus the ovule is anatropous.
II. When micropyle, chalaza and hilum lie in a straight line, the ovule is said to be orthotropous.
Choose the correct option.
(a) Statement I is true, but II is false
(b) Statement I is false, but II is true
(c) Both statements I and II are true
(d) Both statements I and II are false

Pollination

43 Match the following columns.

	Column I (Agents of pollination)		Column II (Technical terms)
A.	Wind	1.	Anemophily
B.	Water	2.	Hydrophily
C.	Insects	3.	Entomophily
D.	Birds	4.	Ornithophily

Codes

	A	B	C	D		A	B	C	D
(a)	1	2	3	4	(b)	1	3	2	4
(c)	4	2	3	1	(d)	3	3	4	1

44 There is only one female *Borassus* palm on an island and no male palms. There are a few male *Borassus* palms on a near by island. Birds fly frequently between these two islands. The female palm produce fruits regularly in every season. What is the agent of pollination?
(a) Water (b) Air
(c) Birds (d) None of these

45 Unisexuality of flowers prevent
(a) autogamy, but not geitonogamy
(b) Both geitonogamy and xenogamy
(c) geitonogamy, but not xenogamy
(d) autogamy and geitonogamy

46 Which type of pollination will take place in the following flower?

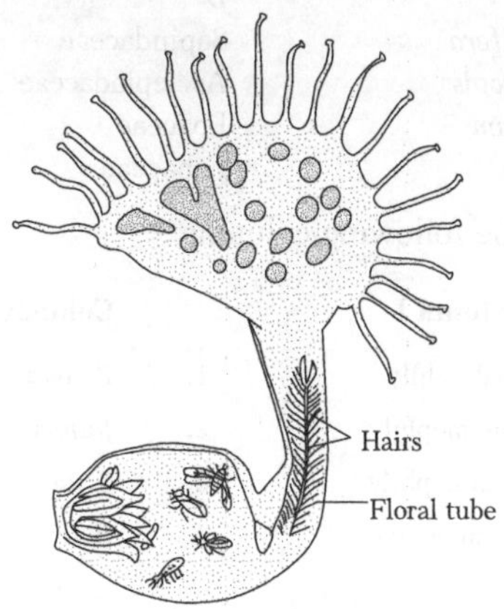

(a) Malacophily (b) Entomophily
(c) Cheiropterophily (d) Ornithophily

47 Consider the following statements.
I. Heterostyly as a contrivance for cross-pollination is found in *Primula vulgaris.*
II. Cleistogamous flower is present in *Commelina.*
Choose the correct option.
(a) Statement I is true, but II is false
(b) Statement I is false, but II is true
(c) Both statements I and II are true
(d) Both statements I and II are false

48 Match the following columns.

	Column I		Column II
A.	Zoophily	1.	Pollination by birds
B.	Ornithophily	2.	Pollination by insects
C.	Entomophily	3.	Pollination by bats
D.	Chiropterophily	4.	Pollination by animals

Codes

	A	B	C	D		A	B	C	D
(a)	3	2	1	4	(b)	1	2	3	4
(c)	4	1	2	3	(d)	4	2	1	3

49 Which of the following flowers produce assured seed set in the absence of pollinators?
(a) *Cucurbita* flower (b) Papaya flower
(c) *Oxalis* flower (d) *Hydrilla*

50 Many species of bee pollinated flowers, i.e. common dandelion have ultraviolet markings called '*A*' which help insects to locate the nectaries. Identify the *A*.
(a) Nectar
(b) Xenogamy
(c) Nectar guides
(d) Nectar violet

51 Pollinium is common in ...A... which belong to the family ...B....

	A	B
(a)	*Mangifera*	Sapindaceae
(b)	*Calotropis*	Asclepiadaceae
(c)	*Triticum*	Poaceae
(d)	*Pisum*	Fabaceae

52 Match the following columns.

	Column I		Column II
A.	Hydrophily	1.	*Zostera*
B.	Entomophily	2.	*Jasminum*
C.	Ornithophily	3.	*Triticum*
D.	Anemophily	4.	*Butea*

Codes

	A	B	C	D
(a)	4	2	1	3
(b)	4	3	1	2
(c)	1	2	3	4
(d)	1	2	4	3

53 Fill in the blanks.

I. Pollination by snakes is known as ...A... .

II. Pollination by snails is known as ...B... .

	A	B
(a)	Malcophily	Ophiophily
(b)	Ornithophily	Ophiophily
(c)	Ophiophily	Malcophily
(d)	Entomophily	Chiropterophily

54 The *Leptonycteris curasoae* bat feeds on the nectar and pollen of

(a) *Agave* and *Cactus* (b) *Oxalis* and *Catharanthus*
(c) *Viola* and *Salix* (d) All of them

55 Among abiotically pollinated sperms

(a) 9% rely on wind (b) 80% rely on water
(c) 98% rely on wind (d) 98% rely on water

56 In tape grass (*Vallisneria*),

(a) Both male and female flowers break from the plant and float on the surface of water
(b) Only the female flowers break from the plant, while the male flowers are brought to the surface by long stalks
(c) Only the male flower breaks from the plant and rise to the surface, while the female flowers are brought to the surface by long pedicels
(d) Any of the two types of flowers can break

57 Choose the correct statement from the following. **[NCERT Exemplar]**

(a) Cleistogamous flowers always exhibit autogamy
(b) Chasmogamous flowers always exhibit geitonogamy
(c) Cleistogamous flowers exhibit both autogamy and geitonogamy
(d) Chasmogamous flowers never exhibit autogamy

58 Epihydrophily occurs in

(a) *Najas* (b) *Zostera*
(c) *Vallisneria* (d) *Euphorbia*

59 Consider the following statements.

I. Self-pollination is the most economic method for plant modification.

II. Genetic stability can be maintained in the progeny through self pollination.

Choose the correct option.

(a) Statement I is true, but II is false
(b) Statement I is false, but II is true
(c) Both statements I and II are true
(d) Both statements I and II are false

60 Pollen grains of a flower fall on the stigma of another flowers of same plant. The phenomenon is

(a) genetically autogamy and ecologically geitonogamy
(b) genetically autogamy
(c) ecologically allogamy
(d) genetically allogamy and ecologically autogamy

61 Self-pollination means, pollination

(a) with different flower (b) within the ovule
(c) within the same flower (d) Both (a) and (c)

62 Given figure shows two types of primrose flowers. They occur naturally in the roughly equal numbers and differ in length of style and position of anthers. What is the advantage of such a system?

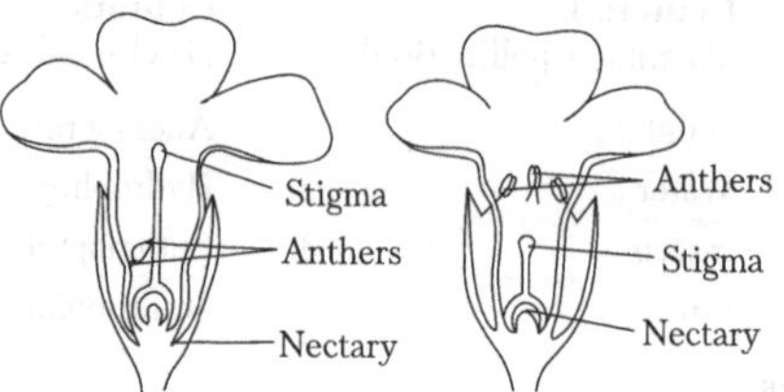

(a) It encourages inbreeding (b) It encourages outbreeding
(c) Both (a) and (b) (d) None of these

63 In which of the following cross pollination occurs?

(a) Pea (b) *Catharanthus*
(c) *Viola* (d) Rose

64 In some flowers, a mechanical barrier exists between the compatible pollen and stigma so that self-pollination becomes impossible. This situation is known as

(a) self-incompatibility (b) dictiny
(c) herkogamy (d) dichogamy

65 From among the situations given below, choose the one that prevents both autogamy and geitonogamy.

(a) Monoecious plant bearing unisexual flowers
(b) Dioecious plant bearing only male or female flowers
(c) Monoecious plant with bisexual flowers
(d) Dioecious plant with bisexual flowers

66 In sea-grasses such as *Zostera*
(a) epihydrophily occurs commonly
(b) female flowers remain submerged in water
(c) pollen grains are spherical and are carried active inside water
(d) pollen grains float on the water surface

67 Autogamy can occur in a chasmogamous flower if **[NCERT Exemplar]**
(a) pollen matures before maturity of ovule
(b) ovules matures before maturity of ovule
(c) Both pollen and ovules mature simultaneously
(d) Both anther and stigma are of equal lengths

68 The flower, in which the stamens mature first, shedding their pollens before the stigma are receptive is known as
(a) protogynous flower (b) heterostyly flower
(c) protandrous flower (d) herkogamy flower

69 Cross-pollination is preferred over self-pollination because it
(a) produces better offspring (b) forms new varieties
(c) induces parthenogenesis (d) Both (a) and (b)

70 The most exceptional feature of zoophilous flowers is
(a) scented, having nectar and mostly colourful
(b) scented, having nectar, but inconspicuous
(c) the presence of only perianth
(d) without colour and show

71 Flower with a feathery and sticky stigma, numerous light pollen, reduced petals is characteristically
(a) moth-pollinated flower (b) bird-pollinated flower
(c) bee-pollinated flower (d) wind-pollinated flower

72 A dicotyledonous plant bears flowers, but never produces fruits and seeds. The most probable cause for the above situation is **[NCERT Exemplar]**
(a) plant is dioecious and bears only pistillate flowers
(b) plant is dioecious and bears only pistillate flowers
(c) plant is monoecious
(d) plant is dioecious and bears only staminate flowers

73 The given diagram is showing hydrophily of

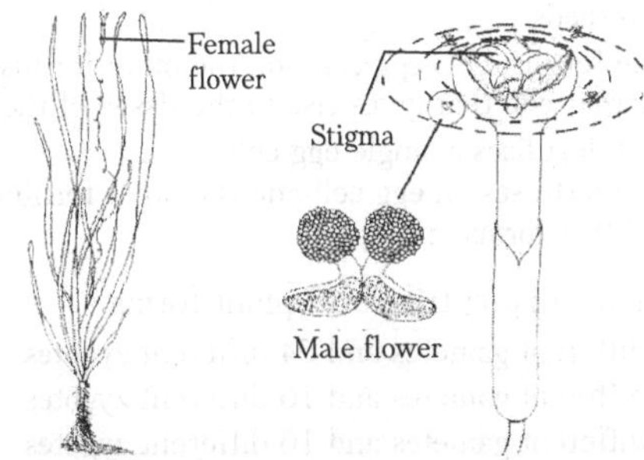

(a) *Vallisneria* (b) *Hydrilla*
(c) *Zostera* (d) Lotus

74 The below figure shows two plants of the same species. Identify the types of pollination indicated as P1, P2 and P3.

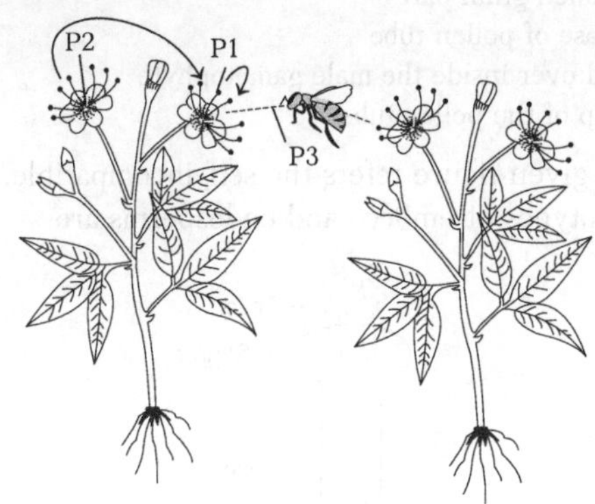

	P1	P2	P3
(a)	Autogamy	Geitonogamy	Xenogamy
(b)	Geitonogamy	Allogamy	Autogamy
(c)	Allogamy	Chasmogamy	Cleistogamy
(d)	Autogamy	Xenogamy	Geitonogamy

75 The diagram given below shows the plant of *Commelina* with two types of flowers (F_1 and F_2). The flowers are

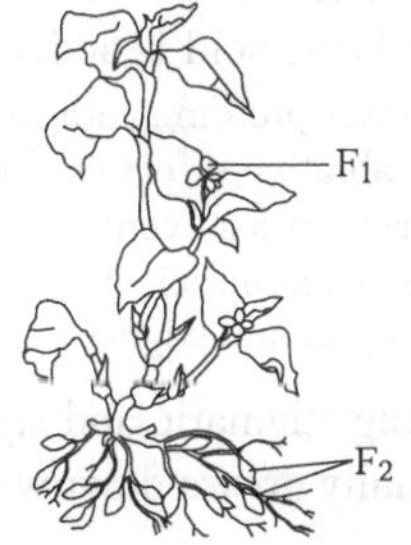

(a) F_1 - Chasmogamous, F_2 - Cleistogamous
(b) F_1 - Cryptogamous, F_2 - Ovulate
(c) F_1 - Neutral, F_2 - Staminate
(d) F_1 - Cleistogamous, F_2 - Chasmogamous

Pollen-Pistil Interaction

76 Mesogamy is
(a) fusion of male and female gametes
(b) fusion of physiologically similar and morphologically different gametes
(c) entry of pollen tube through integuments
(d) None of the above

77 What does the filiform apparatus do at the entrance into ovule?
(a) It helps in the entry of pollen tube into a synergid
(b) It prevents entry of more than one pollen tube into the embryo sac
(c) It brings about opening of the pollen tube
(d) It guides pollen tube from a synergid to egg

78 In a mature angiospermic male gametophyte, the male gametes are present in the
(a) pollen grain part
(b) base of pollen tube
(c) all over inside the male gametophyte
(d) tip of the pollen tube

79 The given figure refers the self-incompatible. Genotypes of embryo and endosperms are

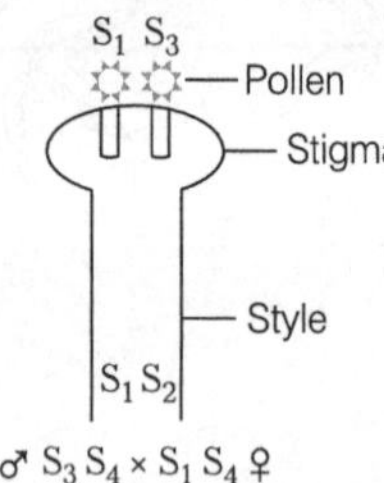

♂ $S_3 S_4 \times S_1 S_4$ ♀

	Embryo	Endosperm
(a)	S_1S_3, S_3S_4	$S_1S_1S_3$, $S_4S_4S_3$
(b)	S_1S_1	$S_1S_3S_4$
(c)	S_1S_3, S_3S_4	$S_3S_4S_4$
(d)	S_4S_4	$S_3S_4S_4$, $S_1S_1S_3$

80 Pollen grains that were easily germinate on stigma, are found to germinate *in vitro* when only 10-200 ppm of boric acid is added. This suggests that
(a) boron accelerates protein synthesis in pollen grain
(b) boron has an abrative effect on the exine
(c) boric acid serves as a solvent for sporopollenin
(d) pollen wall is boron deficient and high levels of boron occur in the styles and stigma

81 After penetrating stigmatic and stylar tissue, the pollen tube usually grows downwards towards egg because
(a) no other path to follow
(b) it grows under the control of egg nucleus
(c) attracted by dissimilar electric charge
(d) the filiform apparatus of synergids is believed to attract the pollen tube

82 The ability of the pistil to recognise the pollen followed by its acceptance or rejection is
(a) a chance factor only
(b) due to certain protein factors of petals
(c) the result of a continuous dialogue between the pistil and pollen grain
(d) is mediated physically, but not chemically

83 The growth of pollen tube into the stigma and style is
(a) intracellular and transverse
(b) intracellular and apical
(c) intercellular and transverse
(d) intercellular and apical

84 What is the role of germpore in pollen grain?
(a) Emergence of pollen tube
(b) Emergence of plumule
(c) Emergence of radicle
(d) Emergence of hypocotyl

85 Consider the following statements.
I. The events 'from pollen deposition on stigma until pollen tubes enters the ovule' are together referred to as pollen-pistil interaction.
II. Pollen-pistil interaction is mediated by chemical components of the ovule.

Choose the correct option.
(a) Statement I is true, but II is false
(b) Statement I is false, but II is true
(c) Both statements I and II are true
(d) Both statements I and II are false

86 Sporophytic self-incompatibility is observed in
(a) Solanaceae (b) Asteraceae
(c) Fabaceae (d) Liliaceae

Double Fertilisation

87 Select the incorrect statement from the following with respect to double fertilisation.
(a) Syngamy is a type of vegetative fertilisation
(b) Triple fusion is a type of vegetative fertilisation
(c) The growth of pollen tube is guided by the filiform apparatus
(d) The zygote develops into an embryo

88 Which cell of the gametophyte of a normal angiosperm (*Capsella*) is diploid at the time of fertilisation?
(a) Prothallial cell/vegetative cell
(b) Antipodal cell and synergids
(c) Secondary nucleus
(d) Generative cell

89 In angiosperms, each pollen grain produces two male cells. What do these sperms do in the fertilisation of a flower?
(a) Each one fertilises a separate egg cell to give rise to two seeds
(b) One fertilises an egg cell and the other fertilises another cell that gives rise to the tissue of the fruit
(c) Both fertilises a single egg cell
(d) One fertilises an egg cell and the other fertilises the cell that forms endosperm

90 A self-fertilising trihybrid plant forms
(a) 8 different gametes and 64 different zygotes
(b) 4 different gametes and 16 different zygotes
(c) 8 different gametes and 16 different zygotes
(d) 8 different gametes and 32 different zygotes

91 ...*A*... was the first to show that both the male gametes are invaded in fertilisation in ...*B*... .

Identify *A* and *B*.

	A	B
(a)	Nawaschin	Solanaceae
(b)	P Maheshwari	*Fritillaria*
(c)	P Maheshwari	*Kigelia*
(d)	Nawaschin	*Fritillaria*

92 There are atleast two families where the product of double fertilisation soon disintegrates and endosperm development is completely absent. These includes

(a) Orchidaceae and Podostemonaceae
(b) Asteraceae and Fabaceae
(c) Poaceae and Brassiceae
(d) All of the above

93 In monocot embryo,

(a) scutellum is absent
(b) two cotyledons found
(c) suspensor cell is 6-10 layer
(d) suspensor is single-celled

94 Identify the labelled part *A* and *B* of the following figure of fertilised embryo.

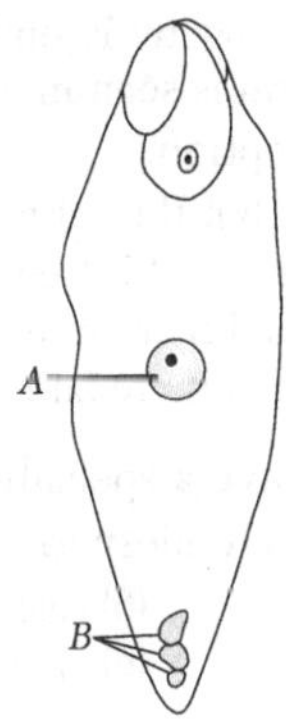

	A	B
(a)	Primary endosperm nucleus	Degenerating antipodal cells
(b)	Endosperm	Antipodal cells
(c)	Zygote	Degenerating synergids
(d)	Polar nuclei	Synergids

Post-fertilisation: Structure and Events

95 Number of chromosomes in an angiospermic plant is 14, then the number of chromosome in synergid cells will be

(a) 14 (b) 7
(c) 28 (d) 21

96 During embryo development, the lower tier of octant given rise to ...*A*... and ...*B*....

	A	*B*
(a)	plumule	cotyledon
(b)	hypocotyl	plumule
(c)	plumule	radicle
(d)	hypocotyl	radicle

97 The first mitotic division of the zygote splits the fertilised egg into a basal cell and terminal cell. This division is

(a) symmetrical (b) irregular
(c) regular (d) asymmetrical

98 The number of chromosomes in endospermic cell is 36. What will be the number of chromosomes in root tip cells?

(a) 9 (b) 18 (c) 12 (d) 24

99 Identify the incorrect statements regarding post-fertilisation development.

(a) The ovary wall develops into pericarp
(b) The outer integument of ovule develops into tegmen
(c) The fusion nucleus (triple nucleus) develops into endosperm
(d) The ovule develops into seed

100 Match the following ovular structure with post-fertilisation structure and select the correct alternative.

	Column I		Column II
A.	Ovule	1.	Endosperm
B.	Funiculus	2.	Aril
C.	Nucellus	3.	Seed
D.	Polar nuclei	4.	Perisperm

Codes

	A	B	C	D
(a)	2	3	4	1
(b)	2	3	1	4
(c)	3	2	4	1
(d)	3	2	1	4

101 Select the correct order of endosperm types.

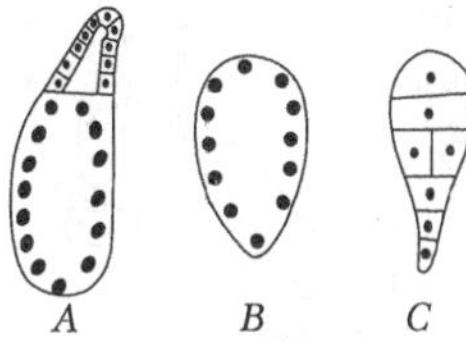

(a) *A*-Cellular, *B*-Helobial, *C*-Free nuclear
(b) *A*-Cellular, *B*-Free nuclear, *C*-Helobial
(c) *A*-Helobial, *B*-Free nuclear, *C*-Cellular
(d) *A*-Free nuclear, *B*-Cellular, *C*-Helobial

102. The given figure are shape of embryo. Identify A, B, C and D, respectively.

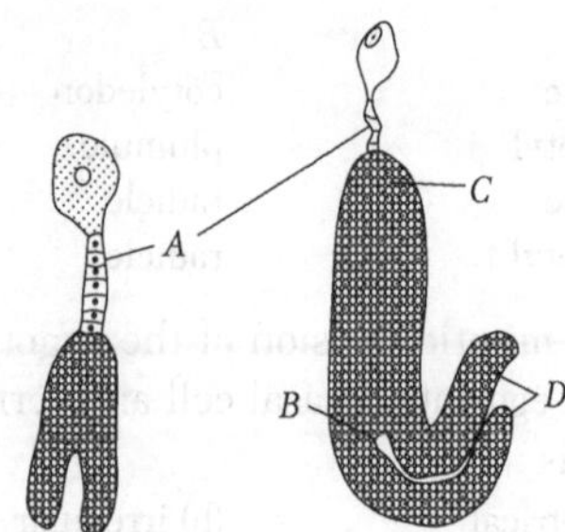

(a) Suspensor, Radicle, Plumule, Hypocotyle
(b) Suspensor, Plumule, Radicle, Cotyledons
(c) Hypophysis, Radicle, Plumule, Cotyledons
(d) Suspensor, Radicle, Plumule, Cotyledons

103 Having one cotyledon distinguishes monocot seeds from dicot seeds. What other feature is to monocot?

(a) The nutrient required for germination are stored in the endosperm
(b) The shoot apical meristem is present at the time of germination
(c) The embryonic root is the first organ to penetrate the seed coat
(d) The root apical meristem is protected by a root cap

104 Among pea, castor, groundnut, beans and coconut which of these possess non-endospermic or exalbuminous (*N*) seed and endospermic or albuminous (*E*) seeds ?

(a) *N* - Pea, groundnut, beans; *E* - Castor, coconut
(b) *N* - Pea, castor; *E* - Coconut, beans, groundnut
(c) *N* - Groundnut, beans; *E* - Pea, castor, coconut
(d) *N* - Pea, coconut; *E* - Groundnut, castor, beans

105 The given figure are related to castor seeds. Identify *A* to *D*, respectively.

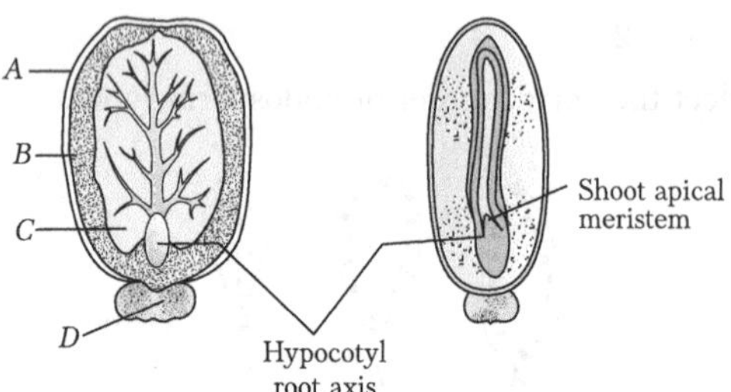

(a) *A*-Seed coat, *B*-Endosperm, *C*-Cotyledon, *D*-Caruncle
(b) *A*-Seed coat, *B*-Cotyledon, *C*-Endosperm, *D*-Caruncle
(c) *A*-Seed coat, *B*-Endosperm, *C*-Caruncle, *D*-Cotyledon
(d) *A*-Endosperm, *B*-Seed coat, *C*-Cotyledon, *D*-Caruncle

106 Which label on the diagram of a pea (shown in figure) is not correct?

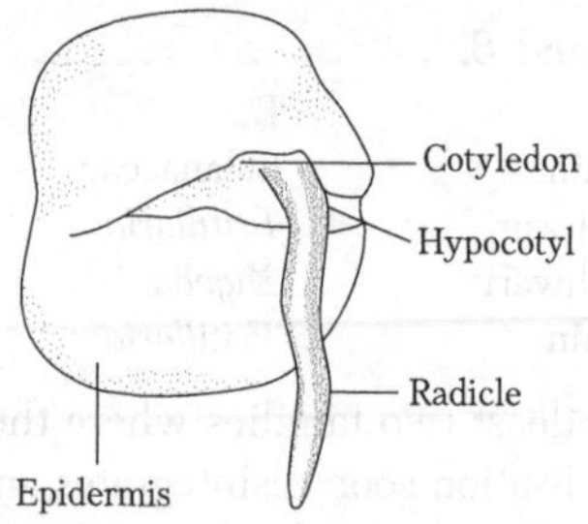

(a) Cotyledon (b) Epidermis
(c) Radicle (d) Both (a) and (c)

107 A typical dicotyledonous embryo consist of an ...*A*... axis and ...*B*... cotyledons.

	A	*B*
(a)	plumule	epicotyl
(b)	embryonal	two
(c)	embryonal	epicotyl
(d)	embryonal	plumule

108 Consider the following statements.

I. Unlike coconut, groundnut consumes endosperm completely during embryo development.
II. Though the embryogeny is similar in groundnut and coconut, perisperm is seen in coconut.

Choose the correct option.

(a) Statement I is true, but II is false
(b) Statement I is false, but II is true
(c) Both statements I and II are true
(d) Both statements I and II are false

109 Maize and wheat, have a specialised cotyledon which is pressed against the endosperm. It is known as

(a) scutellum (b) coleoptile
(c) coleorhiza (d) epicotyl

110 The sequence of development of embryo is

(a) Zygote → Basal and terminal cell → Terminal cell forms proembryo
(b) Zygote → Symmetrical division → Basal cell forms proembryo
(c) Zygote → Basal and terminal cell → Basal cell forms heart-shaped embryo
(d) Zygote → Asymmetrical division → Terminal cell forms suspensor

111 The endosperm nucleus gives rise to a number of free nuclei, which remain in the peripheral layer of embryo sac cytoplasm surrounding a large central vacuole in case of

(a) *Cocos* (b) *Capsella bursa-pastoris*
(c) datepalm (d) All of these

112 In the post-fertilisation changes within the ovule, the oospore forms the ...., while the fertilised fusion nucleus (product of triple fusion) develops the ...., respectively.
(a) endosperm, embryo
(b) embryo, endosperm
(c) nucellus, embryo
(d) embryo, nucellus

113 Which of the following workers are related as ecologist, palaeobotanist and embryologist?
(a) B. Sahni, R. Misra, P. Maheshwari
(b) R. Misra, B. Sahni, P. Maheshwari
(c) B. Sahni, P. Maheshwari, R. Misra
(d) P. Maheshwari, R. Misra, B. Sahni

114 In some organisms, karyokinesis is not followed by cytokinesis as a result of which multinucleate condition arises, leading to the formation of syncytium. The perfect example for this is
(a) appearance of a furrow in cell membrane
(b) liquid endosperm in coconut
(c) sexual reproduction
(d) fertilisation

115 Which of the following applies to the tissue indicated with the arrow in figure?

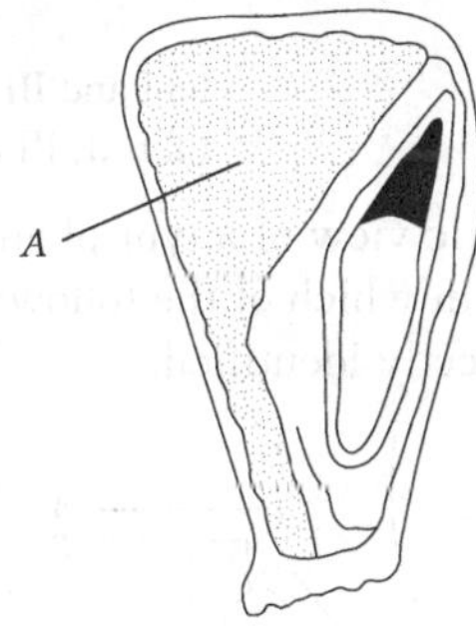

(a) It may store fat
(b) It is an endosperm
(c) It provides nutrients for the young seedlings
(d) All of the above

116 The main function of aleurone cells is the secretion of
(a) hydrolytic enzymes
(b) protease
(c) amylase
(d) All of the above

117 In the following figure.

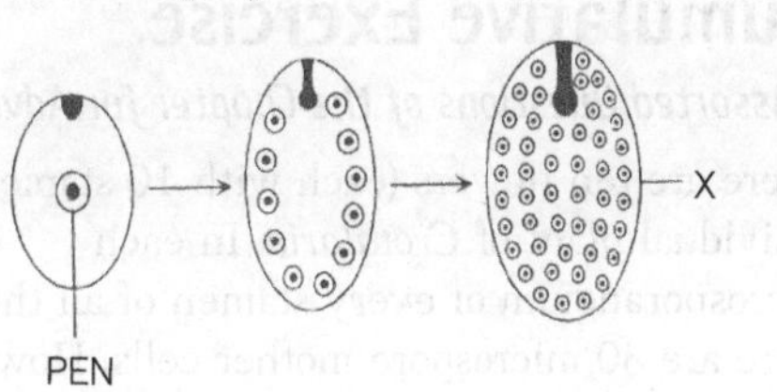

X is
(a) Ruminate endosperm (b) Nuclear endosperm
(c) Helobial endosperm (d) Cellular endosperm

118 At which stage, one can distinguish between nuclear and cellular type of endosperm?
(a) Stage following division of primary endosperm nucleus
(b) Mature stage of endosperm
(c) When embryo has started divisions
(d) At heart-shaped stage of embryo

119 Consider the following statements.
I. Helobial endosperm is intermediate between cellular and nuclear type endosperm.
II. Nuclear endosperm is the most common type of endosperm found in angiosperms.

Choose the correct option.
(a) Statement I is true, but II is false
(b) Statement I is false, but II is true
(c) Both statements I and II are true
(d) Both statements I and II are false

Special Reproductive Mechanism

120 Formation of embryo directly from nucellus and integument is
(a) adventive polyembryony (b) apospory
(c) apogamy (d) apomixis

121 In a type of apomixis known as adventive embryony, embryos develop directly from the
(a) nucellus or integuments
(b) synergids or antipodals in an embryo sac
(c) accessory embryo sacs in the ovule
(d) zygote

122 Embryogeny is a branch of embryology dealing with
(a) nutrition of embryo
(b) development of embryo
(c) formation of embryo
(d) conversion of embryo to adult plant

(B) Cumulative Exercise

(Assorted Questions of the Chapter for Advanced Level Practice)

1 There are ten flowers (each with 10 stamens) in one individual plant of *Crotalaria*. In each microsporangium of every stamen of all the flowers, there are 30 microspore mother cells. How many pollen grains are formed from that plant?

(a) 4000 (b) 10000 (c) 24000 (d) 48000

2 Read the following statements.

I. Wheat, maize, barley, castor and sunflower seeds are endospermic or albuminous.
II. Most zygotes divide only after certain amount of endosperm is formed.
III. Though the seeds differ greatly, the early stages of embryo development is similar in both monocots and dicots.
IV. The zygote divides to form proembryo and subsequently globular, heart-shaped and mature embryo.
V. Epicotyl and hypocotyl are absent in monocot seeds.

Which of the above statements are correct?

(a) I, II, III and IV (b) I, II and III
(c) I, III and V (d) III, IV and V

3 Self-incompatibility is a device for

I. ensuring cross-pollination.
II. preventing self-fertilisation.
III. ensuring self-fertilisation.
IV. genetic control for self-fertilisation.

Choose the correct statements from those given above.

(a) I, II and III (b) I, II, III and IV
(c) I, III and IV (d) I, II and IV

4 Identify the structures marked as *A*, *B*, *C* and *D* in the diagrams of dicot and monocot seeds given below.

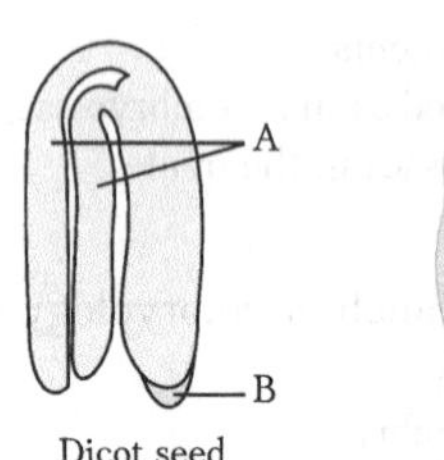

Dicot seed

(a) *A* - Cotyledons, *B* - Epiblast, *C* - Root cap, *D* - Coleoptile
(b) *A* - Cotyledons, *B* - Root cap, *C* - Epiblast, *D* - Coleorhiza
(c) *A* - Epiblast, *B* - Coleorhiza, *C* - Coleoptile, *D* - Cotyledons
(d) *A* - Cotyledons, *B* - Coleorhiza, *C* - Root cap, *D* - Epiblast

5 The diagram given below depicts an anther with pollen grains.

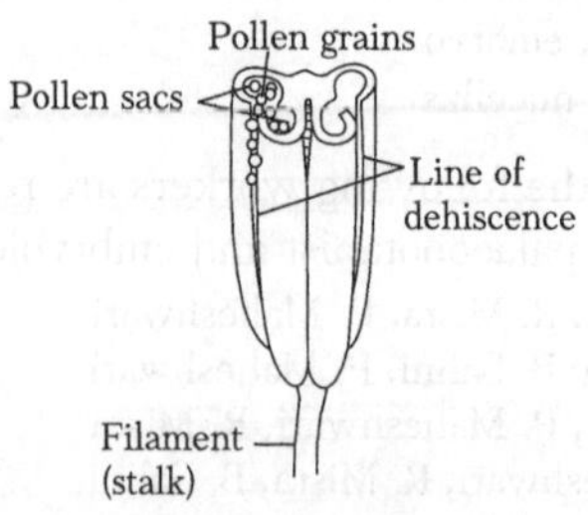

(a) Monothecous + Bisporangiate condition
(b) Dithecous + Tetrasporangiate condition
(c) Dithecous + Bisporangiate condition
(d) Monothecous + Tetrasporangiate condition

6 Which of the following statement(s) is/are correct?

I. The stigma serves as a landing platform for pollen grains.
II. Ovarian cavity is also known as ovarian locule and is present inside the ovary.
III. Placenta is located inside the ovarian cavity.
IV. The ovule is attached to the placenta by funicle.

Codes

(a) I, II and III (c) I and III
(b) I, II and IV (d) I, II, III and IV

7 A diagrammatic view of a typical anatropous ovule is given below. In which of the following option all five parts are correctly identified.

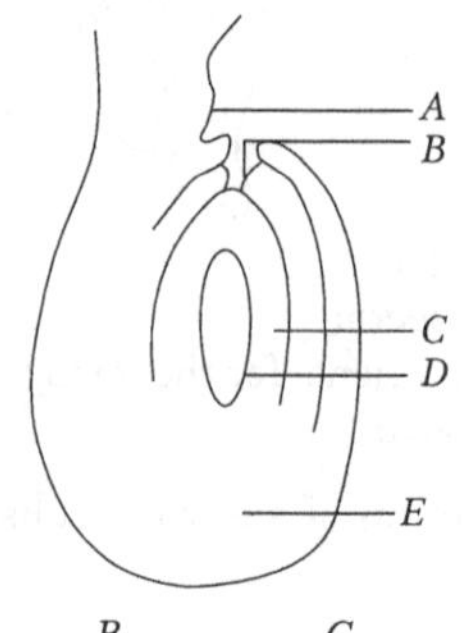

	A	*B*	*C*	*D*	*E*
(a)	Funicle	Micropyle	Female gametophyte	Embryo sac	Chalaza
(b)	Placenta	Micropyle	Egg	Embryo sac	Chalaza
(c)	Raphe	Micropyle	Egg	Embryo sac	Chalaza
(d)	Funicle	Micropyle	Nucellus	Embryo sac	Chalaza

8 Read the following statements.

I. Continued self-pollination result in inbreeding depression.
II. Wind-pollination is quite common in grasses.

III. Megasporangium is represented by the ovary in angiosperms.
IV. Cells of nucellus possess scanty food matter.
V. Embryo sac is located in the nucellus.

Which of the above statements are correct?
(a) I, II and III (b) III, IV and V
(c) I, II and V (d) I and III

9 Even after killing the generative cell with a laser beam, the pollen grain a flowering plant germinate and produce normal pollen tube because
(a) laser beam stimulates pollen germination and pollen tube growth
(b) laser beam does not the region from which pollen tube emerges
(c) the contents of the killed generative cell permit germination and pollen growth
(d) the vegetative cell has not been damaged

10 Read the following statements.
I. In a normal flower which opens and exposes the anthers and the stigma, complete autogamy is rather rare.
II. *Viola, Oxalis* and *Commelina* produce both cleistogamous as well as chasmogamous flowers.
III. Cleistogamous flowers produce assured seed set even in the absence of pollinators.
IV. Majority of the plants use abiotic agents for pollination.
V. Xenogamy does not produce any variation in the progenies after fertilisation.

Which of the following is/are correct?
(a) I, II and III (b) II, III, IV and V
(c) I, IV and V (d) V only

11 Match the following columns.

Column I	Column II
A. Place where pollen grains land.	1. Spores
B. The site, where the seeds develop.	2. Stigma
C. Reproductive cells that have exactly the same number of chromosomes as the parent plant.	3. Microspore mother cells
D. Meiotically dividing cells in the male reproductive tissues that make four microspores.	4. Ovary

Codes

	A	B	C	D
(a)	1	2	3	4
(b)	2	4	1	3
(c)	3	4	1	2
(d)	4	3	2	1

12 A total of 168 pollen grains with 14 chromosomes in each pollen grain are released from a mature microsporanguim. Mention the correct ratio of pollen mother cells, generative cells, vegetative cells and male gametes produced by the microsporangium.
(a) 1 : 1 : 1 : 4 (b) 1 : 2 : 1 : 4
(c) 1 : 4 : 4 : 8 (d) 2 : 1 : 1 : 4

13 Study the following and find correct statement(s).
I. Pollination by water is quite rare in flowering plants and is limited to about 50 genera, mostly monocotyledons.
II. Water is a regular mode of transport for the male gametes among higher plant groups.
III. Distribution of bryophytes and pteridophytes are limited because of the need of water for transport of male gametes and fertilisation.
IV. Megasporogenesis is the process of formation of megaspore.
V. Each pollen grain produces two male gametes both in gymnosperms and angiosperms.

Codes
(a) I and II (b) III, IV and V
(c) I, II and III (d) All of these

14 The given diagram is related to castor seeds. Select the incorrect statement regarding the labelled parts.

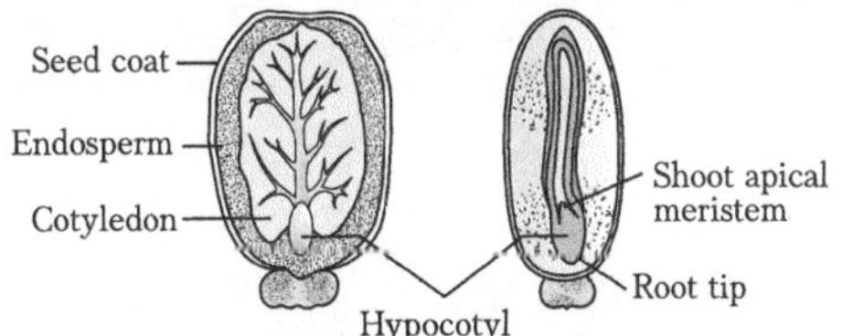

(a) Seed coat protect the seed from physical, temperature or water damage
(b) Endosperm provides nourishment to the developing embryo
(c) Castor seed has single cotyledon, i.e. monocotyledonous and is albuminous
(d) Hypocotyl terminates at its lower end in the root tip

15 Read the following statements.
I. The *Yucca* plant and the moth *Pronuba yuccasella* cannot complete their life cycles without each other.
II. In some insect species, the floral reward for pollination is the safe place to lay eggs in the flower.
III. Insect robbers consume pollens or nectar without bringing about pollination.
IV. Majority of the flowering plants produce hermaphrodite flowers.
V. Continued cross-pollination results in inbreeding depression.

Which of the above statements are correct?
(a) I, II, III and IV (b) I, II, III, IV and V
(c) I, II and III (d) I, II and V

16 Read the following statements.
I. Double fertilisation was discovered by Nawaschin in *Lilium* and *Fritillaria.*
II. The total number of nuclei involved in double fertilisation is five.
III. The central cell of embryo sac, as a result of triple fusion becomes Primary Endosperm Cell (PEC).
IV. Synergids are haploid.

Which of the above statements are correct?
(a) I, II and III
(b) II and IV
(c) III and IV
(d) I, II, III and IV

17 Choose the incorrect statement from the following.
(a) Long ribbon-like pollen grains are seen in some aquatic plants
(b) In some insect species, the floral reward for pollination is the safe place to lay eggs in the flower
(c) Autogamy is achieved within the same flower
(d) Majority of the flowering plants produce homosexual flowers

18 Identify *A, B, C* and *D* of an embryo sac.

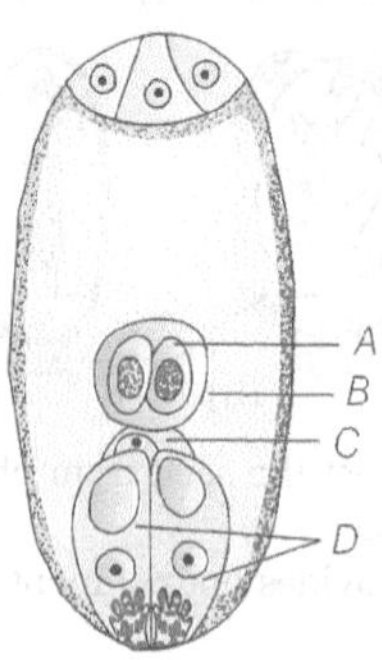

	A	*B*	*C*	*D*
(a)	Endosperm	Egg cell	Central cell	Synergids
(b)	Polar nuclei	Central cell	Synergid	Egg cell
(c)	Polar nuclei	Central cell	Egg cell	Synergid
(d)	Central cell	Polar nuclei	Forms zygote	Cooperative cell

19 What is the ploidy level of the cells of the nucellus, megaspore mother cell, megaspore and female gametophyte in an angiospermic ovule?

	Nucellus	Megaspore mother cell	Megaspore	Female gametophyte
(a)	n	$2n$	n	$2n$
(b)	n	n	$2n$	$2n$
(c)	$2n$	$2n$	n	n
(d)	$2n$	n	$2n$	n

20 Identify *A, B, C* and *D* in the diagram given below.

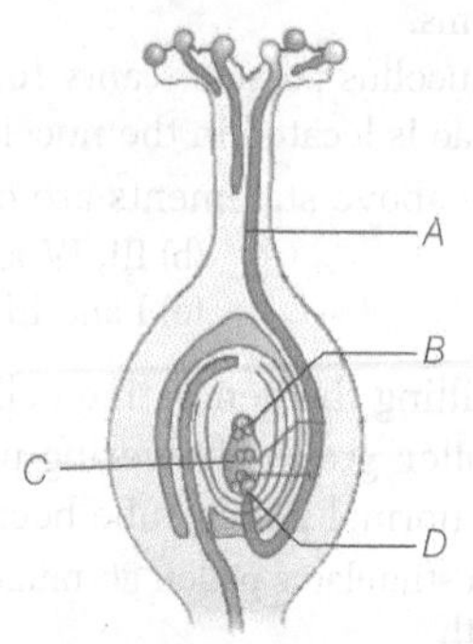

	A	*B*	*C*	*D*
(a)	Antipodals	Pollen tube	Synergids	Egg cell
(b)	Pollen tube	Antipodals	Egg cell	Synergids
(c)	Pollen tube	Synergids	Egg cell	Antipodals
(d)	Synergids	Pollen tube	Egg cell	Antipodals

21 Read the following statements with respect to embryo sac.
I. In an embryo sac, six of the eight nuclei are surrounded by cell walls and organised into cells.
II. The polar nuclei are situated just below the egg apparatus in the large central cell.
III. The egg apparatus consists of one synergid and two egg cells.
IV. A mature embryo sac possess 7-celled and 8-nucleate condition.
V. Central cell is the smallest cell of an embryo sac.

Which of the following statements are correct?
(a) I, II and IV
(b) III, IV and V
(c) III and IV
(d) IV and V

22 Arrange *A, B, C, D* and *E* in the sequence of dicot embryo development from zygote stage to mature embryo.

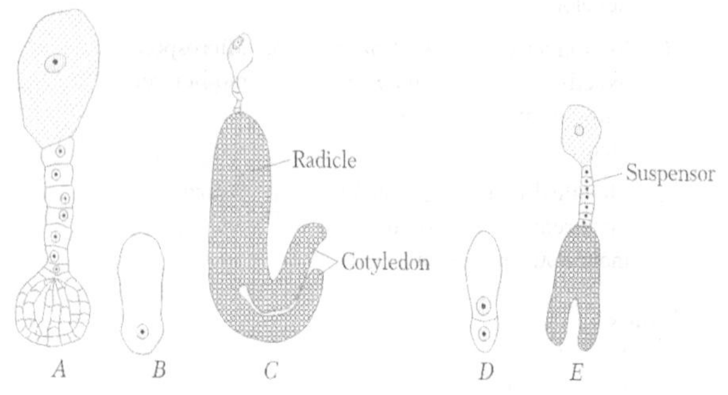

(a) $A \rightarrow C \rightarrow D \rightarrow B \rightarrow E$
(b) $C \rightarrow B \rightarrow D \rightarrow E \rightarrow A$
(c) $A \rightarrow B \rightarrow C \rightarrow E \rightarrow D$
(d) $B \rightarrow D \rightarrow A \rightarrow E \rightarrow C$

23 Read the following statements and choose the correct ones.

I. Non-essential floral organs in a flower are sepals and petals.
II. Stamens represent microsporophylls.
III. A dithecious anther consists of four microsporangia two in each lobe.
IV. The anther wall has middle layer lieing between endothecium and tapetum.

(a) I and II
(b) II and III
(c) III and IV
(d) 1, II, III and IV

24 Choose the mismatched option.

(a) Wind – *Cannabis* – Anemophily
(b) Water – *Zostera* – Hydrophily
(c) Insects – *Salvia* – Entomophily
(d) Birds – *Adansonia* – Ornithophily

25 Identify the reproductive structures of the plant shown in figure below.

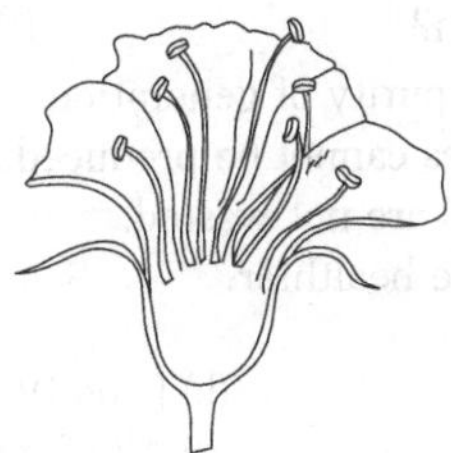

(a) *A*-Anther, *B*-Filament, *C*-Stigma, *D*-Style, *E*-Ovary
(b) *A*-Stamen, *B*-Anther, *C*-Filament, *D*-Stigma, *E*-Pistil
(c) *A*-Style, *B*-Connective, *C*-Stigma, *D*-Filament, *E*-Pistil
(d) *A*-Stigma, *B*-Filament, *C*-Style, *D*-Connective, *E*-Pistil

26 Read the following statements and choose the correct ones.

I. Emasculated flowers have to be covered with bag.
II. The suspensor helps in transferring nutrient to the embryo from endosperm.
III. In *Arceuthobium* only one microsporangia is present per anther.
IV. Tapetum completely surrounds the sporogenous tissue.

Codes

(a) I and II
(b) II and III
(c) III and IV
(d) I, II, III and IV

27 The given figure shows megasporogenesis and development of typical female gametophyte in angiosperms. Which of the following options is right in which all divisions (D_1 to D_5) and structure (S) are correctly identified?

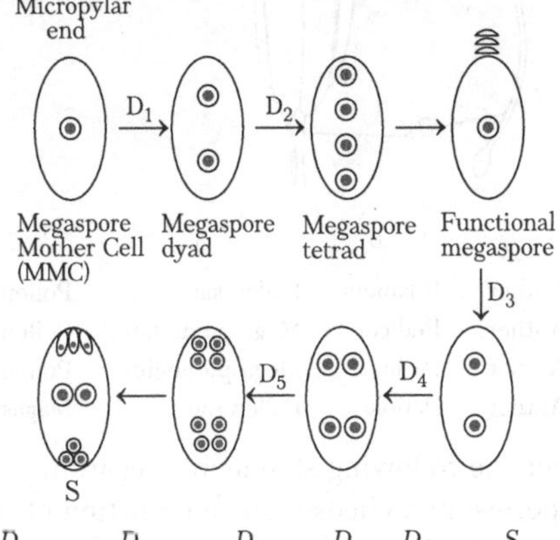

	D_1	D_2	D_3	D_4	D_5	S
(a)	Meiosis-I	Meiosis-II	Mitosis	Mitosis	Mitosis	Embryo
(b)	Meiosis-I	Meiosis-II	Mitosis	Mitosis	Mitosis	Microgametophyte
(c)	Meiosis-I	Meiosis-II	Mitosis	Mitosis	Mitosis	Embryo sac
(d)	Mitosis	Meiosis	Mitosis	Mitosis	Mitosis	Embryo sac

28 Which one of the following statements is not true?

(a) Pollen grains are released from anthers at 2-celled state
(b) Sporogenous cell directly behaves as the megaspore mother cell
(c) Megaspore divides twice to form an eight nucleate embryo sac
(d) Egg and synergids always lie near the micropylar end of ovule

29 The given figure refers to a TS of anther. Identify *A* to *E*, respectively.

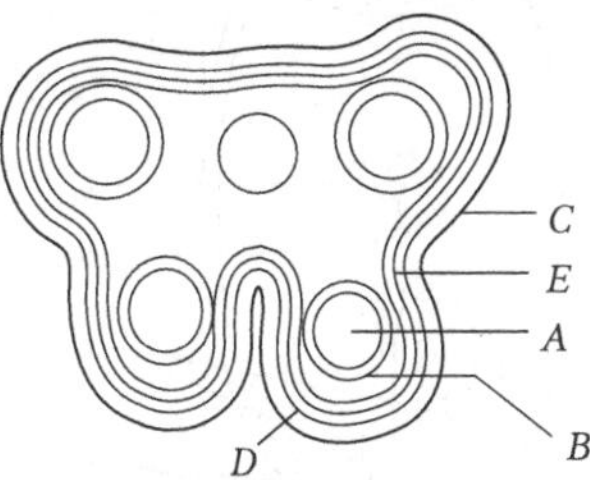

(a) *A*-Sporogenous tissue, *B*-Tapetum, *C*-Middle layer, *D*-Epidermis, *E*-Endothecium
(b) *A*-Sporogenous tissue, *B*-Epidermis, *C*-Middle layer, *D*-Tapetum, *E*-Endothecium
(c) *A*-Sporogenous tissue, *B*-Epidermis, *C*-Tapetum, *D*-Middle layer, *E*-Endothecium
(d) *A*-Sporogenous tissue, *B*-Tapetum, *C*-Epidermis, *D*-Middle layer, *E*-Endothecium

30 Identify *A*, *B*, *C* and *D* in given figure.

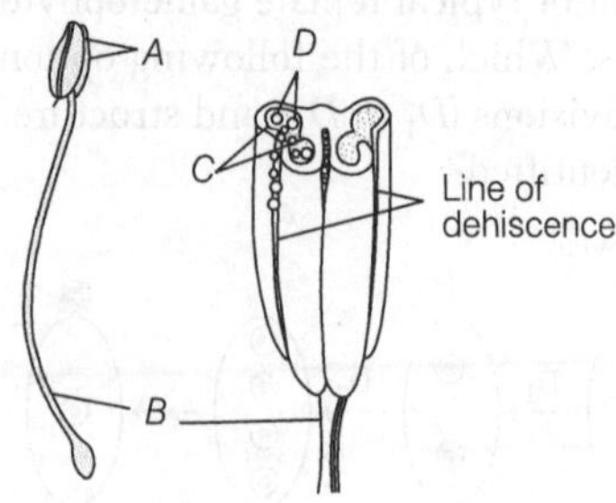

	A	*B*	*C*	*D*
(a)	Anther	Filament	Pollen sac	Pollen grains
(b)	Anther	Pedicel	Megasporangium	Pollen grains
(c)	Anther	Petiole	Megasporangium	Pollen grains
(d)	Anther	Petiole	Pollen sac	Magaspore

31 Consider the following statements regarding angiosperms and choose the combination of correct statements among these.

I. As a rule, only one pollen tube is formed from one pollen grain.
II. The protoplast of the pollen grain does not migrates at the tip of pollen tube.
III. Backward flow of cytoplasm from the tip of the pollen tube towards the microspore is prevented by the formation of callose plugs at intervals.

Codes

(a) I, II and III (b) I and III
(c) II and III (d) I and II

32 Which of the following statements is correct with respect to the given diagram?

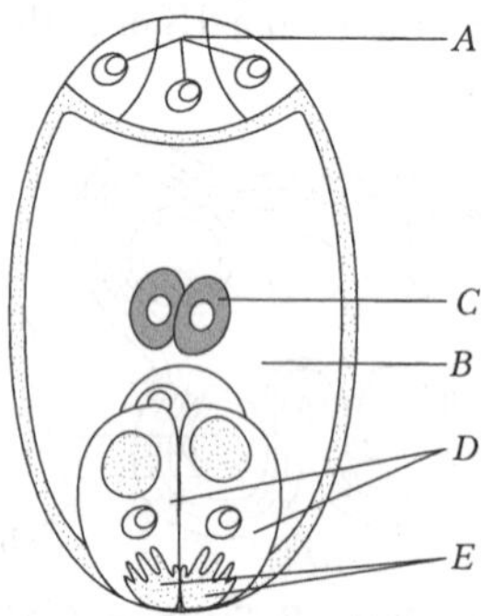

(a) *C*-Antipodal cells present at the chalazal end
(b) *E*-Filiform apparatus, which play an important role in guiding the pollen tube into synergids
(c) *B*-Synergids, which has presence of finger like projection called filiform apparatus
(d) *D*-Egg cell which fuses with male gamete to form zygote

33 Observe the four megaspores of an ovule depicted below and find out which of these (*A*, *B*, *C* and *D*) survive to form embryo sac and which of these (*A*, *B*, *C* and *D*) degenerates?

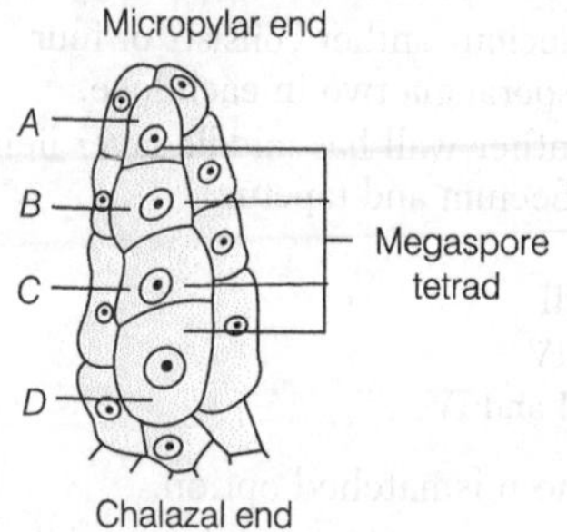

	Survives	**Degenerates**
(a)	*B*, *C*, *D*	*A*
(b)	*D*	*A*, *B*, *C*
(c)	*A*, *B*, *C*	*D*
(d)	*A*	*B*, *C*, *D*

34 Which of the following are incorrect regarding cross-pollination?

I. It maintains purity of generation.
II. New varieties cannot be produced.
III. Pollen grains are not wasted.
IV. Progenies are healthier.

Codes

(a) I and II (b) I and IV
(c) Only III (d) All of these

35 Arrange the following events in order of their occurrence.

I. Pollen tube enters *via* micropyle in the ovule.
II. Megaspore undergoes mitotic division.
III. 7-celled and 8 nucleate embryo sac formed.
IV. Three megaspores degenerate.

Codes

(a) I, II, III and IV (b) IV, II, III and I
(c) II, I, III and IV (d) IV, II, I and III

36 Match the following columns.

Column I	Column II
A. *Salvia*	1. *Pronuba*
B. *Yucca*	2. Moth
C. *Arisaema*	3. Insect
D. *Ophrys*	4. Snail

Codes

	A	B	C	D		A	B	C	D
(a)	1	2	3	4	(b)	1	3	2	4
(c)	3	1	4	2	(d)	4	2	1	3

37 Which of the following statements are correct?

I. In amphitropous ovule, curvature of ovule is more and embryo sac becomes curved like horse-shoe.

II. In anatropous ovule, the body of ovule is completely inverted.

III. In hemianatropous ovule, ovule turns at 90° angle upon the funicle.

IV. In atropous ovule, ovule is circled more or less at right angle to funicle.

Codes

(a) I and IV (b) Only IV

(c) I, II and III (d) All of these

38 Considering the genetic basis of self-incompatibility which of the following options is correct. Male plant is S_1 S_3 and female plant is S_1 S_2.

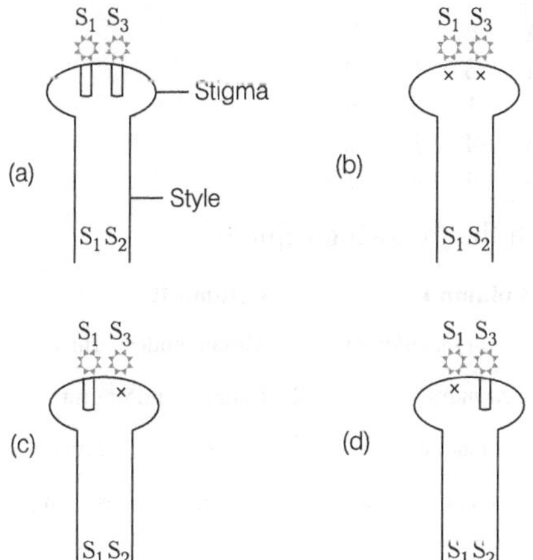

39 Choose the correct statements regarding endosperm.

I. It provides nutrition to the developing embryo.

II. It has the potentiality to form a complete plant.

III. It contains reserve food material such as fats, carbohydrates, oil, proteins, etc., in mature seeds.

IV. It continues to divide transversely and produces a thread of cells called as suspensor.

Codes

(a) II and IV (b) I and III

(c) I and II (d) III and IV

40 The given figure is associated to double fertilisation. Identify *A, B, C, D, E* and *F* respectively.

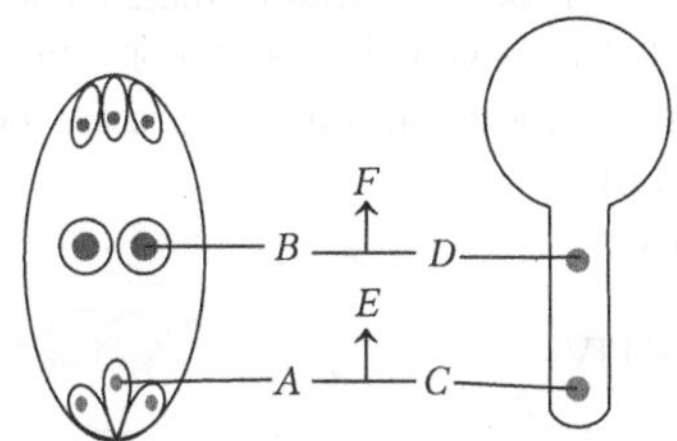

(a) Egg, Polar nuclei, Male gamete, Male gamete, Zygote and Primary Endosperm Nucleus (PEN)

(b) Egg, Male gamete, Male gamete, Polar nuclei, Primary Endosperm Nucleus (PEN) and Zygote

(c) Egg, Male gamete, Polar nuclei, Male gamete, Primary Endosperm Nucleus (PEN) and Zygote

(d) Egg, Polar nuclei, Male gamete, Male gamete, Primary Endosperm Nucleus (PEN) and Zygote

41 Read the following statements. Choose the correct statements regarding monocot embryo.

I. The envelope of plumule is called coleoptile.

II. Coleorhiza is a protective sheath of radicle.

III. Suspensor is large.

IV. Cotyledons occur laterally.

Codes

(a) Only I (b) I and II (c) III and IV (d) Only IV

42 The angiospermic endosperm, except in special cases, is a triploid ($3n$) tissue as it is a product of triple fusion involving double fertilisation. It is, thus distinct from the endosperm of gymnosperms and heterosporous pteridophytes, where the endosperm is a

(a) diploid before fertilisation

(b) simple haploid (n) tissue of the gametophyte not involving any complication like polar fusion or fertilisation

(c) polyploid formed after simple fertilisation

(d) haploid formed after fertilisation

43 In *Zea mays* 20 chromosomes are present in the cell of shoot apex. The number of chromosomes in pollen grain, nucellus, polar nucleus and aleurone layer cells will be

	Pollen grain	Nucellus	Polar nucleus	Aleurone layer
(a)	10	30	10	20
(b)	20	10	10	30
(c)	30	10	20	20
(d)	10	20	10	30

44 Study the given figure a typical dicot embryo. Select the right option in which all the labelled parts as *A*, *B* and *C* are correctly matched with their respective functions.

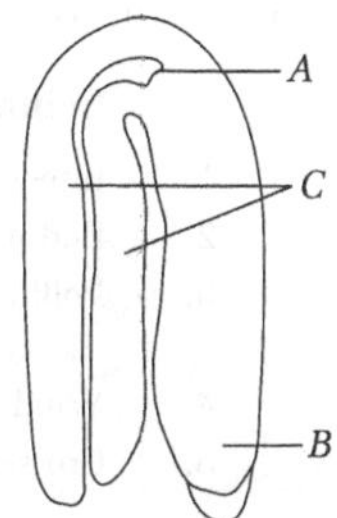

	A	B	C
(a)	Radicle, root system formation	Plumule, shoot system formation	Endosperm, food storage
(b)	Radicle, root system formation	Plumule, shoot system formation	Cotyledon, food storage
(c)	Plumule, shoot system formation	Radicle, root system formation	Cotyledon, food storage
(d)	Plumule, shoot system formation	Radicle, root system formation	Hypophysis, formation of radicle

45 Which of the following statement is incorrect regarding Ubisch bodies?

(a) These are spheroidal structures
(b) These are produced by glandular tapetum
(c) It organise the exine
(d) These are produced by amoeboid tapetum

46 Recognise the figure and find out the correct matching.

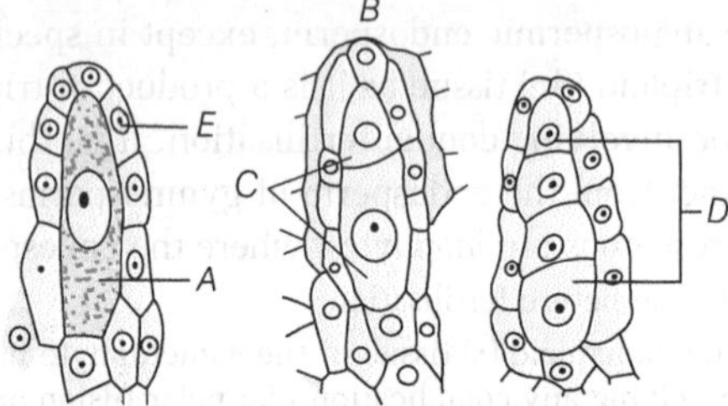

(a) *A*-Nucellus, *B*-Chalazal end, *C*-Microspore dyad, *D*-Microspore tetrad, *E*-Megaspore mother cell
(b) *A*-Megaspore mother cell, *B*-Chalazal end, *C*- Megaspore dyad, *D*-Megaspore tetrad, *E*-Nucellus
(c) *A*-Megaspore mother cell, *B*-Micropylar end, *C* - Megaspore dyad, *D*-Megaspore tetrad, *E*-Nucellus
(d) *A*-Nucellus, *B*-Micropylar end, *C*-Megaspore dyad, *D*-Megaspore tetrad, *E*-Megaspore mother cell

47 Which one of the following statements is incorrect about pollination?

(a) Anemophily occurs by wind and occurs in grasses and date palm
(b) Hydrophily occurs by water and occurs in *Zostera*, *Vallisneria* and *Ceratophyllum*
(c) Entomophily occurs by insects and occurs in rose, jasmine, *Salvia*, etc.
(d) Ornithophily occurs by birds and occurs in *Adansonia*

48 Match the entries in Column I with those of Column II and choose the correct option.

	Column I		Column II
A.	Cleistogamy	1.	Insect pollination
B.	Geitonogamy	2.	Bud pollination
C.	Entomophily	3.	Pollination between flowers in the same plant
D.	Xenogamy	4.	Wind pollination
		5.	Cross-pollination

Codes

	A	B	C	D
(a)	3	1	5	2
(b)	1	5	2	3
(c)	2	3	1	5
(d)	5	4	3	2

49 Identify the correct sequence of matches with the type of pollination and its characteristics.

	Column I		Column II
A.	Ornithophily	1.	Nocturnal flower
B.	Entomophily	2.	Light pollens
C.	Chiropterophily	3.	Funnel-shaped corolla
D.	Anemophily	4.	Pleasant fragrance and nectar

Codes

	A	B	C	D
(a)	4	3	1	2
(b)	2	1	3	4
(c)	3	4	1	2
(d)	3	4	2	1

50 Match the following columns.

	Column I		Column II
A.	*Arum maculatum*	1.	Mosaic endosperm
B.	*Zea mays*	2.	Longest endosperm
C.	*Echinocystis lobata*	3.	Highest ploidy level of endosperm
D.	*Annona squamosa*	4.	Ruminate endosperm

Codes

	A	B	C	D
(a)	4	2	1	3
(b)	2	3	1	4
(c)	4	2	3	1
(d)	3	1	2	4

51 Read the following statements.

I. Microspore tetrads possess tetraploid nucleus.
II. Sporogenous tissue occupies the centre of each microsporangium.
III. Cells of sporogenous tissue undergo meiosis.
IV. Each cell of the sporogenous tissue is a potential microspore mother cell or pollen mother cell.
V. The process of formation of male gamete in angiosperms is called megasporogenesis.

Which of the above statements are correct?

(a) I, II and III
(b) IV and V
(c) I and V
(d) II, III and IV

Assertion and Reason

Direction (Q. Nos. 52-63) *In each of the following questions, a statement of Assertion (A) is given followed by the corresponding statements of Reason (R). Of the statements, mark the correct answer as*

(a) Both A and R are true and R is the correct explanation of A
(b) Both A and R are true, but R is not the correct explanation of A
(c) A is true, but R is false
(d) A is false, but R is true
(e) Both A and R are false

52 **Assertion** (A) Pollen grains are well-preserved during fossilisation.
Reason (R) The exine of pollen grain contains sporopollenin.

53 **Assertion** (A) Pollenkitt sticks to the body of insects during pollination.
Reason (R) Pollenkitts are more common in anemophilous flowers.

54 **Assertion** (A) The cells of endothecium develop fibrous thickenings of cellulose.
Reason (R) The endothecium is hygroscopic in nature.

55 **Assertion** (A) Megaspore Mother Cell (MMC) divides mitotically and forms four megaspores.
Reason (R) Megaspore mother cells are diploid and megaspores are haploid.

56 **Assertion** (A) In hemianatropous ovule, the funiculus lies parallel to the body of ovule.
Reason (R) Here, the body of ovule is rotated by 90°C.

57 **Assertion** (A) If pollen mother cell has 42 chromosomes then pollens have only 21 chromosomes.
Reason (R) Meiosis takes place in pollen mother cells.

58 **Assertion** (A) Synergids are elongated cells that occur at the micropylar pole.
Reason (R) Synergids help in chemotropic movement of pollen tube.

59 **Assertion** (A) Helobial endosperm occurs in dicots as well as in monocot families.
Reason (R) It is the most advanced type of endosperm.

60 **Assertion** (A) An embryo is formed after some mitotic divisions.
Reason (R) An embryo is the first cell of sporophytic generation.

61 **Assertion** (A) Nuclear endosperm does not involve wall formation after each meiotic division.
Reason (R) Coconut milk is an example of cellular endosperm.

62 **Assertion** (A) Endosperm is a structure containing three complete sets of chromosomes.
Reason (R) It is formed after the fusion of secondary nucleus to a male gamete.

63 **Assertion** (A) Ovules after fertilisation develops into a fruit.
Reason (R) The angiospermic fruits contain diploid endosperm.

(C) Medical Entrances' Gallery

(Collection of Questions Asked in NEET & in Various Medical Entrance Exams)

1 In water hyacinth and water lily pollination takes place by **[NEET 2020, 2016]**
(a) water currents only
(b) wind and water
(c) insects and water
(d) insects or wind

2 The body of the ovule is fused within the funicle at **[NEET 2020]**
(a) microphyle (b) nucellus
(c) chalaza (d) hilum

3 In some plants thalamus contributes to fruit formation. Such are termed as **[NEET 2020]**
(a) false fruit
(b) aggregate fruit
(c) true fruit
(d) parthenocarpic fruit

4 Which of the following is incorrect for wind pollinated plants? **[NEET 2020]**
(a) Well exposed stamens and stigma
(b) Many ovules in each ovary
(c) Flowers are small and not brightly coloured
(d) Pollen grains are light and non-sticky

5 Which is the most common type of embryo sac in angiosperms? **[NEET 2019]**
(a) Tetrasporic with one mitotic stage of divisions
(b) Monosporic with three sequential mitotic divisions
(c) Monosporic with two sequential mitotic divisions
(d) Bisporic with two sequential mitotic divisions

6 The process of removal of anther from the flower bud before it dehisces is called as **[AIIMS 2019]**
(a) emasculation (b) bagging
(c) embryo rescue (d) budding

7 Hardest substance in plant kingdom is [JIPMER 2019]

(a) saple (b) corolla
(c) sporopollenin (d) anther

8 Find odd one out. [JIPMER 2019]

(a) Stamen (b) Stigma
(c) Style (d) Ovary

9 What type of pollination takes place in *Vallisneria*? [NEET 2019]

(a) Pollination occurs in submerged condition by water
(b) Flowers emerge above surface of water and pollination occurs by insects
(c) Flowers emerge above water surface and pollen is carried by wind
(d) Male flowers are carried by water currents to,female flowers at the surface of water

10 In which of the following, both autogamy and geitonogamy are prevented? [NEET 2019, CBSE AIPMT 2012]

(a) Wheat (b) Papaya
(c) Castor (d) Maize

11 What is the fate of the male gametes discharged in the synergid? [NEET 2019]

(a) All fuse with the egg
(b) One fuses with the egg, other (s) fuse (s) with synergid nucleus
(c) One fuses with the egg and other fuses with central cell nuclei
(d) One fuses with the egg other (s) degenerate (s) in the synergid

12 Which one of the following statements regarding post-fertilisation development in flowering plants is incorrect? [NEET 2019]

(a) Zygote develops into embryo
(b) Central cell develops into endosperm
(c) Ovules develop into embryo sac
(d) Ovary develops into fruit

13 Persistent nucellus in the seed is known as [NEET 2019]

(a) perisperm (b) hilum
(c) tegmen (d) chalaza

14 Pollen grains can be stored for several years in liquid nitrogen having temperature of [NEET 2018]

(a) −196°C (b) −80°C (c) −120°C (d) −160°C

15 Which one of the following plants shows a very close relationship with a species of moth, where none of the two can complete its life cycle without the other? [NEET 2018]

(a) Banana (b) *Yucca*
(c) *Hydrilla* (d) *Viola*

16 Pollenkitt is present in [JIPMER 2018]

(a) anemophily (b) entomophily
(c) malacophily (d) zoophily

17 Which one of the following statements is correct? [JIPMER 2017, NEET 2013]

(a) Hard outer layer of pollen is called intine
(b) Sporogenous tissue is haploid
(c) Endothelium produces the microspores
(d) Tapetum nourishes the developing pollen

18 Which one of the following statements is incorrect? [NEET-I 2017]

(a) Exine of pollen grains is made up of sporopollenin
(b) Pollen grains of many species cause severe allergies
(c) Stored pollen in liquid nitrogen can be used in the crop breeding programmes
(d) Tapetum helps in the dehiscence of anther

19 Proximal end of the filament of stamen is attached to the [NEET-I 2017]

(a) connective (b) placenta
(c) thalamus or petal (d) anther

20 The ovule of an angiosperm is technically equivalent to [NEET-II 2017, 2016]

(a) megasporangium (b) megasporophyll
(c) megaspore mother cell (d) megaspore

21 Flowers, which have single ovule in the ovary and are packed into inflorescence are usually pollinated by [NEET 2017]

(a) water (b) bee
(c) wind (d) bat

22 A dioecious flowering plant prevents both [NEET 2017]

(a) autogamy and xenogamy
(b) autogamy and geitonogamy
(c) geitonogamy and xenogamy
(d) cleistogamy and xenogamy

23 Attractants and rewards are required for [NEET 2017]

(a) anemophily (b) entomophily
(c) hydrophily (d) cleistogamy

24 **Assertion** (A) Endosperm is formed by the fusion of one male gamete and two polar nuclei.

Reason (R) In pea, the endosperm remains the part of seed as it is not completely used up during embryo development. [AIIMS 2017]

(a) Both A and R are true and R is the correct explanation of A
(b) Both A and R are true, but R is not the correct explanation of the A
(c) A is true, but R is false
(d) Both A and R are false

25 Match Column I with Column II and select the correct option using the codes given below.

Column I	Column II
A. Pistils fused together	1. Gametogenesis
B. Formation of gametes	2. Pistillate
C. Hyphae of higher ascomycetes	3. Syncarpous
D. Unisexual female flower	4. Dikaryotic

Codes [NEET-II 2016]

	A	B	C	D
(a)	4	3	2	1
(b)	2	1	4	3
(c)	1	2	4	3
(d)	3	1	4	2

26 In majority of angiosperms [NEET-II 2016]
(a) egg has a filiform apparatus
(b) there are numerous antipodal cells
(c) reduction division occurs in the megaspore mother cells
(d) a small central cell is present in the embryo sac

27 Which of the following statements is not correct? [NEET-I 2016]
(a) insects that consume pollen or nectar without bringing about pollination are called pollen nectar robbers
(b) pollen grains of many species cause severe allergies
(c) some reptiles have also been reported as pollinators in some plant species
(d) pollen grains of many species can germinate on the stigma of a flower, but only one pollen tube of the same species grows into the style

28 Seed formation without fertilisation in flowering plants involves the process of [NEET-I 2016]
(a) budding (b) somatic hybridisation
(c) apomixis (d) sporulation

29 The hilum is a scar on the [CBSE AIPMT 2015]
(a) seed, where funicle was attached
(b) fruit, where it was attached to pedicel
(c) fruit, where style was present
(d) seed, where micropyle was present

30 Which of the following may require pollinators, but is genetically similar to autogamy? [CBSE AIPMT 2015]
(a) Geitonogamy (b) Xenogamy
(c) Apogamy (d) Cleistogamy

31 Which one of the following statements is not true? [CBSE AIPMT 2015]
(a) Pollen grains are rich in nutrients and they are used in the form of tablets and syrups
(b) Pollen grains of some plants cause severe allergies and bronchial infection in some people
(c) The flower pollinated by flies and bats secrete foul odour to attract them
(d) Honey is made by bees by digesting pollen collected from flowers

32 Which of the following are the important floral rewards to the animal pollinators? [CBSE AIPMT 2015, 2011]
(a) Colour and large size of flower
(b) Nectar and pollen grain
(c) Floral fragrance and calcium crystals
(d) Protein pellicle and stigmatic exudates

33 Filiform apparatus is characteristic feature of [CBSE AIPMT 2015]
(a) generative cell (b) nucellar embryo
(c) aleurone cell (d) synergids

34 In angiosperms, microsporogenesis and megasporogenesis [CBSE AIPMT 2015]
(a) occur in anther
(b) form gametes without further divisions
(c) involve meiosis
(d) occur in ovule

35 The wheat grain has an embryo with one large, shield-shaped cotyledon known as [CBSE AIPMT 2015]
(a) epiblast (b) coleorhiza
(c) scutellum (d) coleoptile

36 Coconut water from a tender coconut is [J&K CET 2014]
(a) immature embryo
(b) free-nuclear endosperm
(c) innermost layers of the seed coat
(d) degenerated nucellus

37 Which of the following is not properly matched case of angiosperms? [Chhattisgarh PMT 2015]
(a) Exine of pollen grain - Sporopollenin
(b) Tapetum - Ubish bodies
(c) Male gametophyte of angiosperm - No prothallial cell
(d) Most common type of ovule - Orthotropous

38 Embryo development other than the egg cell of haploid embryo sac from synergid and antipodals is known as [Chhattisgarh PMT 2015]
(a) apogamy (b) apomixis
(c) amphimixis (d) isobilateral tetrad

39 In angiospermic plants, meiosis of megaspore mother cell generally produces [Chhattisgarh PMT 2015]
(a) linear tetrad (b) tetrahedral tetrad
(c) decussate tetrad (d) isobilateral tetrad

40 The isobilateral type microspores arrangement in tetrad is present in [AMU 2015]
(a) *Solanum nigrum* (b) *Zea mays*
(c) *Cassia fistula* (d) *Vigna radiate*

41 The fibrous band which develop from the cells of the anther wall layer are known as [AMU 2015]
(a) epidermis (b) endothecium
(c) middle layers (d) tapetum

42 Chalazogamy is shown by [AMU 2015]
(a) *Petunia* (b) *Cucurbita*
(c) *Pistacia* (d) *Casuarina*

43 Egg in female gametophyte is accompanied by [WB JEE 2015]
(a) antipodal cells (b) synergids
(c) definitive nucleus (d) tube nucleus

44 Endosperm nucleus is [WB JEE 2015]
(a) n (b) $2n$
(c) $3n$ (d) $4n$

45 Banana is an example of [WB JEE 2015]
(a) parthenocarpy (b) apomixis
(c) parthenogenesis (d) polyembryony

46 Geitonogamy involves [CBSE AIPMT 2014]
(a) fertilisation of a flower by the pollen from another flower of the same plant
(b) fertilisation of a flower by the pollen from the same flower
(c) fertilisation of a flower by the pollen from a flower of another plant in the same population
(d) fertilisation of a flower by the pollen from a flower of another plant belonging to a distant population

47 Pollen tablets are available in the market for [CBSE AIPMT 2014]
(a) *in vitro* fertilisation (b) breeding programmes
(c) supplementing food (d) *ex situ* conservation

48 Function of filiform apparatus is to [AIIMS 2014]
(a) recognise the suitable pollen at stigma
(b) stimulate division of generative cell
(c) produce nectar
(d) guide entry of pollen tube

49 Which one of the following statements is correct? [AFMC 2014]
(a) The seed in grasses is not endospermic
(b) Mango is a parthenocarpic fruit
(c) A proteinaceous aleurone layer is present in maize grain
(d) A sterile pistil is called a staminode

50 An angiosperm male plant with 24 chromosomes in its pollen mother cells is crossed with female plant bearing 24 chromosomes in its root cells. What would be the ploidy of embryo and endosperm, respectively formed after this cross? [MHT CET 2014]
(a) 24 and 48 (b) 24 and 24
(c) 48 and 72 (d) 24 and 36

51 Cross-pollination does not occur in [MHT CET 2014]
(a) allogamous flowers
(b) geitonogamous flowers
(c) cleistogamous flowers
(d) chasmogamous flowers

52 Select the plants pollinated by water. [Kerala CEE 2014]
I. Water hyacinth II. *Zostera*
III. *Amorphophallus* IV. *Vallisneria*
V. *Yucca*
(a) I, IV and V (b) II and V
(c) II and IV (d) II, III and IV
(e) I, II and IV

53 Which of the following feature (s) is/are common to both wind and water pollinated flowers? [Kerala CEE 2014]
I. Pollen grains are long and ribbon-like.
II. Stigma is large and feathery.
III. The flowers are not colourful.
IV. The flowers do not produce nectar.
(a) III and IV (b) II and III
(c) I and II (d) Only II
(e) Only I

54 Read the following statements and identify the correct options given below. [Kerala CEE 2014]
I. Angiosperms range in size from microscopic *Wolffia* to tall trees of *Eucalyptus.*
II. In angiosperms, the seeds are enclosed by fruits.
III. Double fertilisation is an event unique to angiosperms.
IV. In angiosperms, each cell of an embryo sac is diploid.
V. In angiosperms, the zygote develops into an endosperm.
(a) I, II and IV (b) I, II and V
(c) I, II and III (d) II, III and IV
(e) II, III and V

55 Cross-pollination through insect agent is called [WB JEE 2014; BHU 2008]
(a) anthropophily (b) malacophily
(c) entomophily (d) ornithophily

56 Cleistogamous flowers are [WB JEE 2014]
(a) bisexual flowers which remain opened
(b) bisexual flowers which remain closed
(c) open female flower
(d) open male flower

57 Emasculation ensures cross-pollination in [RPMT 2014]
(a) staminate flower
(b) bisexual flower
(c) neuter flower
(d) pistillate flower

58 Which part of the plant contains sporogenous tissue? [MP PMT 2014]
(a) Pollen (b) Microspore
(c) Young anther (d) Stamen

59 Transfer of pollen grains from the anther to the stigma of another flower of the different plant is known as **[Haryana PMT 2014]**
(a) autogamy (b) geitonogamy
(c) xenogamy (d) cleistogamy

60 The embryo sac of angiosperms contains **[Haryana PMT 2014]**
(a) 3-celled egg apparatus, 3 antipodal cells and 2 polar nuclei
(b) 2-celled egg apparatus, 3 antipodal cells and 2 polar nuclei
(c) 3-celled egg apparatus, 2 antipodal cells and 1 polar nuclei
(d) 3-celled egg apparatus, 1 antipodal cell and 2 polar nuclei

61 Zygote is resulted by the process **[J&K CET 2014]**
(a) isogamy (b) anisogamy
(c) monogamy (d) syngamy

62 Developing pollen is nourished by **[J&K CET 2014]**
(a) tapetum (b) endothecium
(c) epidermis (d) spore mother cell

63 During the process of sexual reproduction in flowering plants, double fertilisation involves **[Punjab PMET 2014]**
(a) fertilisation of egg cell by two male gametes
(b) fertilisation of egg cell and a central cell by two male gametes brought by same pollen tube
(c) fertilisation of egg cell and a central cell by two male gametes brought by different pollen tube
(d) fertilisation of two egg cells by two male gametes brought by same pollen tube

64 Endosperm, a product of double fertilisation in angiosperms is absent in the seeds of **[UK PMT 2014]**
(a) gram (b) orchids
(c) maize (d) Both (a) and (b)

65 PEN stands for **[AMU 2014]**
(a) Primary Endosperm Nucleus
(b) Poly Embryo Nourishment
(c) Primary Endosperm Nourishment
(d) Primary Embryo Nourishment

66 In which of the following plants, pollen is released before the stigma becomes receptive in the same flower? **[EAMCET 2014]**
(a) *Allium* (b) *Colchicum*
(c) *Datura* (d) *Solanum*

67 With respect to angiosperms, identify the incorrect pair from the following? **[Gujarat CET 2014]**
(a) Antipodals — $2n$
(b) Vegetative cell of male gametophyte — n
(c) Primary endosperm nucleus — $3n$
(d) Cells of nucellus of ovule — $2n$

68 In this diagram, showing the LS of an embryo of grass, identify the answer having the correct combination of alphabets with the right part. **[Gujarat CET 2014]**

D
C
F
A
B
E

(a) *A*-Root cap, *B*-Coleoptile, *C*-Scutellum, *D*-Coleorhiza, *E*-Epiblast, *F*-Shoot apex
(b) *A*-Shoot apex, *B*-Epiblast, *C*-Coleorhiza, *D*-Scutellum, *E*-Coleoptile, *F*-Radicle
(c) *A*-Epiblast, *B*-Scutellum, *C*-Coleoptile, *D*-Radicle, *E*-Coleorhiza, *F*-Shoot apex
(d) *A*-Epiblast, *B*-Radicle, *C*-Coleoptile, *D*-Scutellum, *E*-Coleorhiza, *F* Shoot apex

69 Product of sexual reproduction generally generates **[NEET 2013]**
(a) prolonged dormancy
(b) new genetic combination leaving to variation
(c) large biomass
(d) longer viability of seeds

70 Which of the following represents the male gamete? **[UP CPMT 2012]**
(a) Endosperm (b) Synergid
(c) Pollen grain (d) Antipodals

71 The endosperm in angiosperms develops from **[UP CPMT 2012]**
(a) zygote
(b) secondary nucleus
(c) chalazal polar nucleus
(d) micropylar polar nucleus

72 Even in the absence of pollinating agents, seed setting is assured in **[CBSE AIPMT 2012]**
(a) *Commelina* (b) *Zostera*
(c) *Salvia* (d) fig

73 What would be the number of chromosomes of the aleurone cells of a plant with 42 chromosomes in its root tip cells? **[CBSE AIPMT 2011]**
(a) 63 (b) 84
(c) 21 (d) 42

74 Wind pollination is common in **[CBSE AIPMT 2011]**
(a) lilies (b) grasses
(c) orchids (d) legumes

75 Nucellar polyembryony is reported in species of **[CBSE AIPMT 2011]**
(a) *Gossypium* (b) *Triticum*
(c) *Brassica* (d) *Citrus*

76 In which one of the following pollination is autogamous? **[CBSE AIPMT 2011]**
(a) Xenogamy (b) Chasmogamy
(c) Cleistogamy (d) Geitonogamy

77 Which one of the following would not lead to formation of clones? **[DUMET 2011]**
(a) Double fertilisation
(b) Apomixis
(c) Vegetative reproduction
(d) Tissue culture

78 In a flowering plant, the pollen tube first arrives in **[DUMET 2011]**
(a) egg (b) an antipodal cell
(c) a synergid (d) central cell

79 Which of the following statements is incorrect? **[DUMET 2011]**
(a) Pollen grains remain viable for several months because their outer covering is made of sporopollenin
(b) No enzyme can degrade sporopollenin
(c) Pollen grains are well-represented in fossil strata due to sporopollenin
(d) Pollen wall has cavities containing proteins

80 Long, ribbon-like pollen grains are seen in some **[DUMET 2011]**
(a) aquatic plants
(b) wind pollinated grasses
(c) gymnosperms
(d) bird pollinated flowers

81 If the number of chromosomes in egg cell is 8, then what is the number of chromosomes in endosperm ? **[UP CPMT 2011]**
(a) 24 (b) 8
(c) 16 (d) 12

82 Ruminate endosperm is found in the seeds of family **[UP CPMT 2011]**
(a) Compositae (b) Cruciferae
(c) Euphorbiaceae (d) Annonaceae

83 Pericarp is formed of **[OJEE 2011]**
(a) endosperm (b) ovary wall
(c) tapetum (d) epidermis

84 Find out the odd one. **[OJEE 2011]**
(a) Micropyle
(b) Embryo sac
(c) Nucellus
(d) Pollen grain

85 The ovule is attached to the placenta of ovary wall by **[OJEE 2011]**
(a) raphae (b) micropyle
(c) funicle (d) hilum

86 Entry of pollen tube with two male gametes and tube nucleus through micropyle, is **[OJEE 2011; BHU 2009]**
(a) mesogamy (b) porogamy
(c) chalazogamy (d) None of these

87 Ovule integument gets transformed into **[WB JEE 2011]**
(a) seed (b) fruit wall
(c) seed coat (d) cotyledons

88 The ovule in which the funicle, chalaza and micropyle lie in one vertical plane, is called **[J&K CET 2011]**
(a) campylotropous (b) amphitropous
(c) orthotropous (d) anatropous

89 Testa of a seed is produced from **[J&K CET 2011]**
(a) ovary wall
(b) hilum
(c) outer integument of ovule
(d) funicle

90 Cleistogamous flower is found in **[J&K CET 2011]**
(a) Tobacco (b) *Viola*
(c) *Mirabilis* (d) None of these

91 The following is the diagram of TS of anther. Identify the parts labelled as *A*, *B* and *C*. **[KCET 2011]**

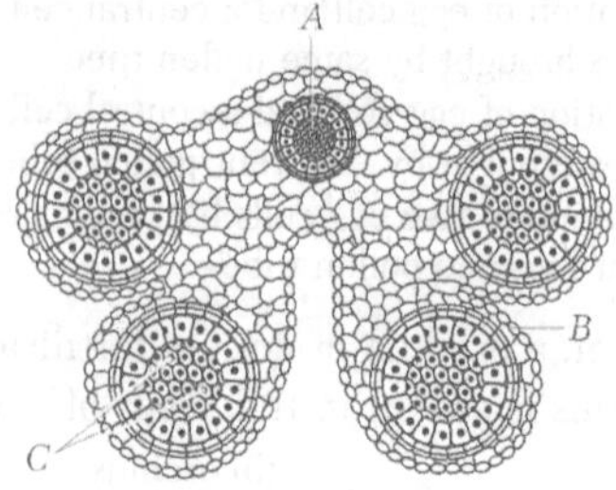

(a) *A*-Connective, *B*-Endothecium, *C*-Pollen grain
(b) *A*-Endothecium, *B*-Connective, *C*-Pollen grain
(c) *A*-Pollen grain, *B*-Connective, *C*-Endothecium
(d) *A*-Endothecium, *B*-Pollen grain, *C*-Connective

92 Study the following statements and choose the correct option. **[Kerala CEE 2011]**
I. Tapetum nourishes the developing pollen grains.
II. Hilum represents the junction between ovule and funicle.
III. In aquatic plants such as water hyacinth and water lily, pollination is by water.
IV. The primary endosperm nucleus is triploid.
(a) I and II are correct, but III and IV are incorrect
(b) I, II and IV are correct, but III is incorrect
(c) II, III and IV are correct, but I is incorrect
(d) I and IV are correct, but II and III are incorrect
(e) II and IV are correct, but I and III are incorrect

ANSWERS

Check Point 2.1

1. (c) 2. (d) 3. (b) 4. (b) 5. (a) 6. (b)

Check Point 2.2

1. (d) 2. (c) 3. (d) 4. (a) 5. (b) 6. (a)

Check Point 2.3

1. (a) 2. (a) 3. (b) 4. (b) 5. (a) 6. (b)

Check Point 2.4

1. (a) 2. (c) 3. (c) 4. (d)

Check Point 2.5

1. (b) 2. (c) 3. (b) 4. (c) 5. (b) 6. (c) 7. (d)

(A) Topical Exercise

1. (a) 2. (c) 3. (d) 4. (d) 5. (b) 6. (d) 7. (c) 8. (d) 9. (c) 10. (c)
11. (b) 12. (a) 13. (c) 14. (b) 15. (c) 16. (a) 17. (a) 18. (d) 19. (d) 20. (d)
21. (c) 22. (c) 23. (d) 24. (d) 25. (d) 26. (c) 27. (c) 28. (d) 29. (c) 30. (d)
31. (b) 32. (b) 33. (c) 34. (a) 35. (c) 36. (c) 37. (b) 38. (d) 39. (d) 40. (b)
41. (a) 42. (c) 43. (a) 44. (b) 45. (a) 46. (b) 47. (c) 48. (c) 49. (c) 50. (c)
51. (b) 52. (d) 53. (c) 54. (a) 55. (c) 56. (c) 57. (a) 58. (c) 59. (c) 60. (a)
61. (c) 62. (b) 63. (d) 64. (c) 65. (b) 66. (b) 67. (c) 68. (c) 69. (b) 70. (a)
71. (d) 72. (d) 73. (a) 74. (a) 75. (a) 76. (c) 77. (a) 78. (b) 79. (a) 80. (d)
81. (d) 82. (c) 83. (b) 84. (a) 85. (a) 86. (b) 87. (a) 88. (c) 89. (d) 90. (a)
91. (d) 92. (a) 93. (d) 94. (a) 95. (b) 96. (d) 97. (d) 98. (d) 99. (b) 100. (c)
101. (c) 102. (b) 103. (c) 104. (a) 105. (a) 106. (a) 107. (b) 108. (a) 109. (a) 110. (a)
111. (d) 112. (b) 113. (b) 114. (b) 115. (d) 116. (d) 117. (b) 118. (a) 119. (c) 120. (a)
121. (a) 122. (b)

(B) Cumulative Exercise

1. (d) 2. (a) 3. (d) 4. (b) 5. (b) 6. (d) 7. (d) 8. (c) 9. (d) 10. (a)
11. (b) 12. (c) 13. (b) 14. (c) 15. (a) 16. (d) 17. (d) 18. (c) 19. (c) 20. (b)
21. (a) 22. (d) 23. (d) 24. (d) 25. (a) 26. (d) 27. (c) 28. (c) 29. (d) 30. (a)
31. (b) 32. (b) 33. (b) 34. (a) 35. (b) 36. (c) 37. (c) 38. (d) 39. (b) 40. (a)
41. (b) 42. (b) 43. (d) 44. (c) 45. (d) 46. (c) 47. (d) 48. (c) 49. (c) 50. (d)
51. (d) 52. (a) 53. (c) 54. (a) 55. (d) 56. (a) 57. (a) 58. (b) 59. (e) 60. (c)
61. (c) 62. (a) 63. (e)

(C) Medical Entrances' Gallery

1. (d) 2. (d) 3. (a) 4. (b) 5. (b) 6. (a) 7. (c) 8. (a) 9. (d) 10. (b)
11. (c) 12. (c) 13. (a) 14. (a) 15. (b) 16. (b) 17. (d) 18. (d) 19. (c) 20. (a)
21. (c) 22. (b) 23. (b) 24. (c) 25. (d) 26. (c) 27. (d) 28. (c) 29. (a) 30. (a)
31. (d) 32. (b) 33. (d) 34. (c) 35. (c) 36. (b) 37. (d) 38. (a) 39. (a) 40. (b)
41. (b) 42. (d) 43. (b) 44. (c) 45. (a) 46. (a) 47. (c) 48. (d) 49. (c) 50. (d)
51. (c) 52. (c) 53. (a) 54. (c) 55. (c) 56. (b) 57. (b) 58. (c) 59. (c) 60. (a)
61. (d) 62. (a) 63. (b) 64. (a) 65. (a) 66. (a) 67. (a) 68. (d) 69. (b) 70. (c)
71. (b) 72. (a) 73. (a) 74. (b) 75. (d) 76. (c) 77. (a) 78. (c) 79. (d) 80. (a)
81. (a) 82. (d) 83. (b) 84. (d) 85. (c) 86. (b) 87. (c) 88. (c) 89. (c) 90. (b)
91. (a) 92. (b)

Explanations

(A) Topical Exercise

37 (*b*) Statement I is false, but II is true because
Ovules generally differentiate a single megaspore mother cell in the micropylar region of the nucellus.

85 (*a*) Statement I is true, but II is false and it can be corrected as
The pollen-pistil interaction is mediated by chemical components of the pollen.

87 (*a*) Statement in option (a) is incorrect and can be corrected as
Syngamy is a type of generative fertilisation.

95 (*b*) Synergids are haploid (*n*). If the plant has 14 chromosomes, synergids will have 7 chromosomes.

99 (*b*) Statement in option (b) is incorrect and can be corrected as
The outer integument of ovule develops into testa.

108 (*a*) Statement I is true, but II is false and it can be corrected as
Perisperm is present in castor, not in coconut.

(B) Cumulative Exercise

1 (*d*) Option (d) is correct.
There are 10 flowers (each with 10 stamens). So, total of 100 stamens are there.
Now each stamen consist of four microsporangia.
So, $= 100 \times 4 = 400$ microsporangia are present in 10 flowers.
Each microsporangium has 30 microspore mother cells. So, 400 microsporangia will have
$= 400 \times 30 = 12000$ microspore mother cell
Now, each microspore mother cell give rise to tetrad pollen grain by meiosis. So,
$= 12000 \times 4 = 48000$
$\therefore$ Total 48000 pollen grains will be formed from the plant of *Crotalaria*.

2 (*a*) All statements are correct except statement V and it can be corrected as Epicotyl and hypocotyl are present in monocot seeds.

8 (*c*) Statements I, II and V are correct. Other statements are incorrect and can be corrected as
- Megasporangium is represented by ovule.
- Nucellus have abundant reserve food materials.

10 (*a*) Statements I, II and III are correct. Other statements are incorrect and can be corrected as
- Majority of plants use biotic agents for pollination.
- Xenogamy is cross-pollination, thus is responsible for producing variation in progeny.

12 (*c*) Option (c) is correct.
Pollen mother cell undergo meiotic division to produce 4 pollen grains.
So, for generation of 168 pollen grains, 168/4 = 42 pollen mother cells undergo meiotic division.
Each pollen grain undergo mitotic division to give two unequal cells, i.e. one larger vegetative cells and one smaller generative cell.
So, total number of vegetative cells will be -168
and total number of generative cells will be - 168.
Now, each generative cell further produce two male gametes by another mitotic division.
So, 168 generative cell will produce 336 male gametes.
Now, the ratio of pollen mother cells, generative cells, vegetative cells and male gametes produced by the microsporangium will be
$= 42 : 168 : 168 : 336$
Or $1 : 4 : 4 : 8$

13 (*b*) Statements III, IV and V are correct. Other statements are incorrect and can be corrected as
- Pollination by water is quite rare in flowering plants and is limited to about 30 genera, mostly monocotyledons, e.g. *Vallisneria*.
- Water is a regular mode of transport for male gametes among lower plant groups like algae, bryophytes, etc.

14 (*c*) The statement in option (c) is incorrect and can be corrected as
Castor seed is dicotyledonous, i.e. with two cotyledons and is albuminous, i.e. having residual endosperm.
Rest of the statements are correct.

15 (*a*) Statements I, II, III and IV are correct. Statement V is incorrect and can be corrected as
Continued self-pollination results in inbreeding depression.

17 (*d*) Statement in option (d) is incorrect and can be corrected as
Majority of flowering plants produce bisexual flowers.

21 (*a*) Statements I, II and IV are correct. Other statements are incorrect and can be corrected as
- The egg apparatus consists of two synergid and one egg cell.
- Central cell is the largest cell of an embryo sac.

24 (*d*) The mismatched option is (d). It can be corrected as
Adansonia is pollinated by bats (cheiropterophily).

28 (*c*) Statement in option (c) is not true and can be corrected as
Megaspore divides three times mitotically to form an eight nucleate embryo sac.

31 (*b*) Statements I and III are correct while II is incorrect and can be corrected as
The cytoplasm of the pollen grain containing the male gametes flows towards the tip of the pollen tube.

34 (*a*) Statements I and II are incorrect and can be corrected as
- Cross-pollination does not maintains purity of generation as it produces variation.
- Cross-pollination produces new varieties.

37 (*c*) Statements I, II and III are correct while IV is incorrect and it can be corrected as
In atropous ovule, the body of the ovule is erect or straight. The hilum, chalaza and micropyle lie in a straight line, e.g. *Polygonum*.

39 (*b*) Statements I and III are correct about endosperm. Other statements are incorrect and can be corrected as
- Endosperm cells cannot form complete plant, instead it is a nourishment providing cell.
- Suspensor cells are not formed form endosperm. They are formed from embryo cells.

41 (*b*) Statements I and II are correct for monocot embryo. Other statements are incorrect and can be corrected as
- Suspensor is small.
- Cotyledon is terminal in position.

45 (*d*) Statement (d) is incorrect and it can be corrected as Ubisch bodies are produced only by glandular tapetum not by amoeboid tapetum.

47 (*d*) Statement in option (d) is incorrect and can be corrected as Ornithophily occurs by birds but *Adansonia* is pollinated by bats not birds.

51 (*d*) Statements II, III and IV are correct. Other statements are incorrect and can be corrected as
- Microspore tetrads possess haploid nucleus.
- The process of formation of male gamete in angiosperms is called microsporogenesis.

52 (*a*) Both A and R are true and R is the correct explanation of A.
Sporopollenin is found in the exine of pollen grains. It is resistant to microbial and chemical decomposition, that is why, pollen grains are well-preserved during fossilisation.

53 (*c*) A is true, but R is false because
Pollenkitt occurs over the cell wall of pollen grains of insect-pollinating flowers. Pollenkitt is an oily layer, it provides stickiness, specific odour to pollen grains. Thus, it helps in insect pollination, i.e. entomophily.

54 (*a*) Both A and R are true and R is the correct explanation of A.
Anther wall of mature anther consists of epidermis (outermost layer), followed by endothecium then one to three middle layers and an innermost tapetum layer. The cells of endothecium are radially elongated and at maturity develop, fibrous thickenings of cellulose and thus hygroscopic in nature. Endothecium attains its maximum development when the anther is ready for dehiscence. This hygroscopic nature of endothecial cells helps in the dehiscence of anther.

55 (*d*) A is false, but R is true because
Megaspore Mother Cells (MMCs) are diploid mother cells of megaspores. Each MMC divides by a meiosis division and forms four haploid megaspores.

56 (*a*) Both A and R are true and R is the correct explanation of A.
When the funiculus lies at right angle (90°) to the body of ovule and the chalazal and micropylar ends are in straight line then the ovule is called **hemianatropous**.

57 (*a*) Both A and R are true and R is the correct explanation of A.
Pollen Mother Cells (PMCs) are diploid structures. These divide by meiotic division and form pollen tetrad (haploid).

58 (*b*) Both A and R are true, but R is not the correct explanation of A.
Synergids are found at the micropylar pole and their position is lateral to an egg. During pollen germination, synergids release some chemicals, which attract the pollen tube towards the embryo sac, such type of attraction is known as chemotropism.

59 (*e*) Both A and R are false. These can be corrected as Helobial type of endosperm occurs in 19% families of monocots. It is an intermediate type of endosperm.

60 (*c*) A is true, but R is false
Syngamy involves a male gamete and an egg. It forms a diploid product, the zygote, which is known as first cell of sporophytic generation. It divides by some mitotic divisions and forms a multicellular structure called the embryo.

61 (*c*) A is true, but R is false because
Nuclear type of endosperm is formed after free nuclear divisions in primary endosperm mother cell. Here, each mitotic divisions does not follow wall formation.
Hence, many nuclei are formed, which remain together in a mass of protoplasm of the embryo sac. Coconut milk is an example of liquid endosperm which is made up of nuclear endosperm.

62 (*a*) Both A and R are true and R is the correct explanation of A.
Endosperm contains three sets of chromosomes (it is a triploid structure), two sets come from a diploid secondary nucleus and one from a male gamete.

63 (*e*) Both A and R are false. These can be corrected as Ovules after fertilisation develop into seeds that may or may not bear triploid endosperm.

(C) Medical Entrances' Gallery

1 (*d*) In water hyacinth and water lily the flowers emerge above the level of water and are thus pollinated by insects or winds. Water lily and water hyacinth are in the water, but their stem part which is above the thalamus is not in water. The pollen grains are in the upper part of thalamus, so pollination cannot be done by water. That is why, it is done by insect or wind.

2 (*d*) The attachment point of funicle and body of ovule is known as hilum. It is the point where ovule attaches to the base. It is generally present as an eye of the seed as it is present as scar.

3 (*a*) A fruit in which floral parts other than ovary like thalamus, base of sepals, petal, etc., fuse with pericarp and contribute in fruit formation is called false fruit or pseudocarp. Apple, mulberry and strawberry are false fruits.

4 (*b*) Option (b) is incorrect because
Wind pollinated plants have single ovule in each ovary. In case of wind pollination or anemophily, many pollens are produced because anemophily is highly wasteful and is a non-directional process.
These pollens are also light-weighed, small, dusty and dry. To catch the wind borne pollens stigma is exposed and hairy. Flowers are small and inconspicous, colourless and nectarless.

5 (*b*) The most common type of female gametophyte (embryo sac) in angiosperms is the monosporic embryo sac in which the embryo sac develops from a single functional megaspore (n), while the other three megaspores degenerate. The functional megaspore undergoes three sequential mitotic divisions and gives rise to 8-nucleate and 7-celled mature embryo sac.

6 (*a*) The process of removal of anther from flower bud before it dehisces is called as emasculation. In bagging, emasculated flower is covered with a bag of suitable size to prevent contamination of its stigma with unwanted pollen.

7 (*c*) Sporopollenin is the hardest substance in plant kingdom. It is the major constituent of outer layer (exine) of pollen grains. It is the most resistant organic material that can withstand high temperature as well as strong acids and alkali. No enzyme is known which can degrade it.

8 (*a*) Stamen is the odd one out among other options. Stamen represents the male reproductive part of a flower, whereas, stigma, style and ovary are the parts of a carpel or pistil which represents the female reproductive part of flower.

9 (*d*) *Vallisneria* is a water pollinated plant. In *Vallisneria*, the female flowers reach the surface of water by the long stalk and the male flowers or pollen grains are released onto the surface of water. They are carried passively by water currents to female flowers at the surface of water.

10 (*b*) Autogamy and geitonogamy, i.e. self-pollnation either in the same flower and in different flowers of same plant, both are prevented in papaya plant. In papaya, male and female flowers are present on different plants that in each plant is either male or female (dioecy).

11 (*c*) Out of the male gametes discharged in the synergid, one fuses with the egg and other fuses with central cell nuclei. The fusion between male gamete and egg is called syngamy or true fertilisation which forms zygote ($2n$). The fusion between male gamete and central cell nuclei is called triple fusion and it results in the formation of a triploid primary endosperm nucleus ($3n$).

12 (*c*) The statement-'ovules develop into embryo sac' is incorrect. Correct information about the statement is as follows

During post-fertilisation event, ovule develops into seed. On the other hand, embryo sac is a multicellular structure which is derived from the megaspore. Rest statements regarding post-fertilisation development in flowering plants are correct.

13 (*a*) Persistent nucellus in the seed is known as perisperm.

The albuminous seeds usually retain a part of endosperm as it is not completely used up during embryo development.

But in some seeds, remnants of nucellus are also persistent, e.g. black pepper and beet.

14 (*a*) Pollen grains can be stored for several years in liquid nitrogen having a temperature of $-196°$ C (cryopreservation). These pollen grains can be later used in plant breeding programmes.

15 (*b*) *Yucca gloriosa* has developed in obligate symbiotic relationship with *Pronuba yuccasella* moth. Both of them cannot complete their life cycle without each other. The moth deposits its egg in the locule of the ovary and the flower, in turn, gets pollinated by the moth. The larvae of the moth come out of the eggs as the seed start developing.

16 (*b*) Pollenkitt is present in entomophily. It is a yellowish, sticky and oily covering on the surface of pollen grains. Its major function is to make the pollen stick to the bugs. Thus, it helps in the pollination.

17 (*d*) Statement in option (d) is correct. Tapetum is the innermost nutritive structure of anther wall which nourishes the developing pollen grain. Other incorrect statements can be corrected as

Hard outer layer of pollen is called exine. Sporogenous tissue is diploid. Microsporangia produce the microspores.

18 (*d*) Statement in option (d) is incorrect and can be corrected as Tapetum is the inner layer of microsporangium (anther), which provides nourishment to developing pollen grain after meiotic cell division.

19 (*c*) A typical stamen consists of anther and filament. The proximal end of filament is attached to thalamus or petal of the flower whereas distal end to the anther.

20 (*a*) Ovule of an angiosperm is equivalent to megasporangium which consists of 2 synergids, 1 egg cell, 3 antipodal cells and a secondary nucleus.

21 (*c*) The flowers with packed inflorescence and single ovule in the ovary are wind pollinated. These flowers have pollen grains produced in large numbers, which are light weighted, sometimes winged, e.g. cereals and grasses.

22 (*b*) Dioecious flowering plants prevent both autogamy and geitonogamy because they contain unisexual flower. In dioecious condition, male and female flowers occur on different plants.

However, autogamy takes place in bisexual flowers and geitonogamy takes place between different flowers of the same plant.

23 (*b*) Attractants and rewards are required for entomophily (insect pollination). Flowers have nectar glands and are highly fragrant to attract insects for effective pollination. To sustain animal visits, flowers provide them rewards also, i.e. nectar and pollen grains.

24 (*c*) A is true, but R is false because

Endosperm is a nutritive tissue present in the seeds. It provides nutrition to the developing embryo. It develops from fusion of one male gamete and two polar nuclei. In pea (dicot) seed, there is no residual endosperm as it is completely consumed during embryo devlopemnt. These types of seeds are called non-endospermic seeds.

27 (*d*) Statement in option (d) is not correct and can be corrected as

Pollen grains of different species are incompatible, so when they fall on stigma only the pollen of the same species germinate and can form pollen tube which grows and finally dispatches male gamete to embryo sac.

31 (*d*) Statement in option (d) is not correct and can be corrected as

Honey is made by bees from nectar and pollens. Bees collect pollen and nectar in the spring when most flowers and plants are in bloom. They collect them in their stomach for about an hour, the nectar mixes with the proteins and enzymes produced by bees, which convert it to honey.

37 (*d*) Option (d) is incorrectly matched pair. It can be corrected as

Most common type of ovule is anatropus ovule.

49 (*c*) Statement in option (c) is correct. A proteinaceous aleurone protein layer is present in maize grain which start to develop approximately 10-15 days after pollination. Other statements are incorrect and can be corrected as

- Seed in grasses is endospermic.
- Banana (not mango) is a parthenocarpic fruit.
- Sterile pistil is called pistillode.

50 (*d*) 24 and 36 are the ploidy of embryo and endosperm, respectively. The male plant has 24 chromosomes in its pollen mother cells, i.e. $2n = 24$ or $n = 12$. The root cells of female plant bear 24 chromosomes, i.e. $n = 24$ or $n = 12$. An embryo ($2n$) is formed from fusion of egg (n) and male nuclei (n), i.e. $2n = 24$. An endosperm is formed after triple fusion of central cell ($2n$) and male nuclei (n), i.e. $3n = 36$.

54 (*c*) Statements I, II and III are correct. Angiosperms range in size from microscopic *Wolffia* to tall trees of *Eucalyptus*. The seeds are enclosed by fruits in angiosperms and double fertilisation is an event unique to them.

Rest statements are incorrect and can be corrected as
In angiosperms, each cell of an embryo sac is haploid and zygote develops into an embryo (not endosperm).

67 (*a*) Option (a) represents incorrectly matched pair. It can be corrected as

Antipodals cells are haploid (n) in nature.

73 (*a*) The outermost cell layer of the endosperm ($3n$) of seed is called **aleurone layer**. Since, the cells of aleurone layer are triploid, the number of chromosomes would be 63, as root tip cells ($2n$) has 42 chromosomes.

75 (*d*) Occurrence of more than one embryo in a seed is referred as polyembryony. In many *Citrus* and mango varieties, some of the nucellar cells surrounding the embryo sac start dividing, protrude into the embryo sac and develop into the embryos. In such species, each ovule contains many embryos (nucellar polyembryony).

76 (*c*) Bisexual flowers which remain always closed are called cleistogamous and such condition of flowers is called cleistogamy. In such flowers, the anthers and stigma lie close to each other. When anthers dehisce in the flowers buds, pollen grains come in contact with stigma to effect pollination. Thus, cleistogamous flowers are invariably autogamous.

77 (*a*) Clone is an individual obtained from single parent through apomixis, vegetative reproduction and tissue culture. The process of fusion of two male gametes in a single embryo sac is called **double fertilisation**. It is found in sexual reproduction of angiosperms only and discovered by Nawaschin (1898).

78 (*c*) The typical embryo sac (*Polygonum* type) is 7-celled, 8-nucleate (two synergids, one egg, three antipodal and one central cell). The synergids are also known as helpers. They help in distribution of nutrients in embryo sac with the help of filiform apparatus and also help in attracting pollen tube towards egg cell.

79 (*d*) Statement in option (d) is incorrect and can be corrected as Pollen wall comprises of two principal layers, the inner intine and outer exine. The intine is pectocellulosic in nature. A special feature of intine is the presence of beads, ribbons or plates of enzymatic proteins particularly in vicinity of germ pores. The exine is composed of sporopollenin which is derived from carotenoids by oxidative polymerisation. It is resistant to physical and biological decomposition. Due to this, pollen walls are often preserved for long periods in fossil deposits.

80 (*a*) In most water pollinated plants, the pollen grains are long and ribbon-like and are protected from wetting by mucilagenous covering.

81 (*a*) Egg cell is haploid, whereas endosperm is triploid as it is formed by the fusion of one male gamete with two polar nuclei. Therefore, the number of chromosomes in endosperm will be $8 \times 3 = 24$.

82 (*d*) Mature endosperm with any degree of irregularity and unevenness in its surface contour is called **ruminate endosperm**. It is known to occur in about 32 families of angiosperms. In family-Annonaceae, the ruminate endosperm is found.

83 (*b*) With the development of seed, the tissue of ovary wall is also stimulated to grow. It produces pericarp.

84 (*d*) Pollen grain is male reproductive part of angiospermic plant while embryo sac, micropyle and nucellus are female reproductive parts.

85 (*c*) Ovule is the integumented indehiscent megasporangium, which develops as a small outgrowth from the tissue of placenta. It is attached to placenta by a stalk called **funiculus**.

86 (*b*) The pollen tube containing male gametes enters the ovule in majority of cases through micropyle by a process termed as porogamy.

87 (*c*) Some post-fertilisation changes are

Ovule	– Seed
Ovary	– Fruit
Outer integument	– Testa (outer seed coat)
Inner integument	– Tegmen (inner seed coat)

88 (*c*) The ovule in which the funicle, chalaza and micropyle lie on the vertical plane is called **orthotropous** (Gk. *orthos* - straight; *trope* - turned). In this type, the body of ovule is straight. Hilum and chalaza occur nearly. It is also called **atropous** or **erect ovule**, e.g. Piperaceae, Polygoniaceae, Urticaceae, etc. It is the most primitive and simplest type of ovule in angiosperms.

89 (*c*) The outer seed coat (testa) of a seed is produced from outer integument of ovule. The inner integument forms tegmen (inner seed coat). Ovary wall forms pericarp (fruit wall).

90 (*b*) Bisexual flowers which do not open at all are called **cleistogamous**. In such flowers, anthers and stigma lie close to each other. *Viola* (common pansy) has both cleistogamous and chasmogamous flowers. Chasmogamous flowers remain open with exposed anthers and stigma.

92 (*b*) All statements are correct except III. Incorrect statement can be corrected as

In majority of aquatic plants such as water hyacinth and water lily, the flower emerge above the level of water and are pollinated by insects or wind as in most of the land plants.

CHAPTER 03

Human Reproduction

Humans are sexually reproducing viviparous (i.e. give birth to young ones) organisms. They are also unisexual, i.e. male and female sexes are separate and each sex has reproductive organs (gonads), reproductive ducts and accessory structures. There are remarkable differences between the reproductive events in males and females.

Human beings show prominent sexual dimorphism, the male and female differ from each other by a number of primary and secondary sex characteristics. **Primary sex characters** are those which are present in both males and females since birth like external genitalia.

Whereas, **secondary sex characters** appear after puberty and include a number of traits like presence of thick facial hairs, low pitch voice, etc., in males and well-developed mammary glands, high pitch voice, etc., in females.

Reproductive organs are also divided into the following types

(i) **Primary sex organs** These produce gametes and sex hormones.

(ii) **Secondary sex organs** These do not produce gametes or sex hormones but play an important role during reproduction.

In this chapter, we will study about the different reproductive systems in male and female and also the various events of human reproduction.

Inside

MALE REPRODUCTIVE SYSTEM

It is found in the pelvic region of body. It consists of a pair of testes, accessory ducts, glands and external genitalia. The structures present in this system are either paired or unpaired.

The diagram showing detailed internal structure of male reproductive system is given below

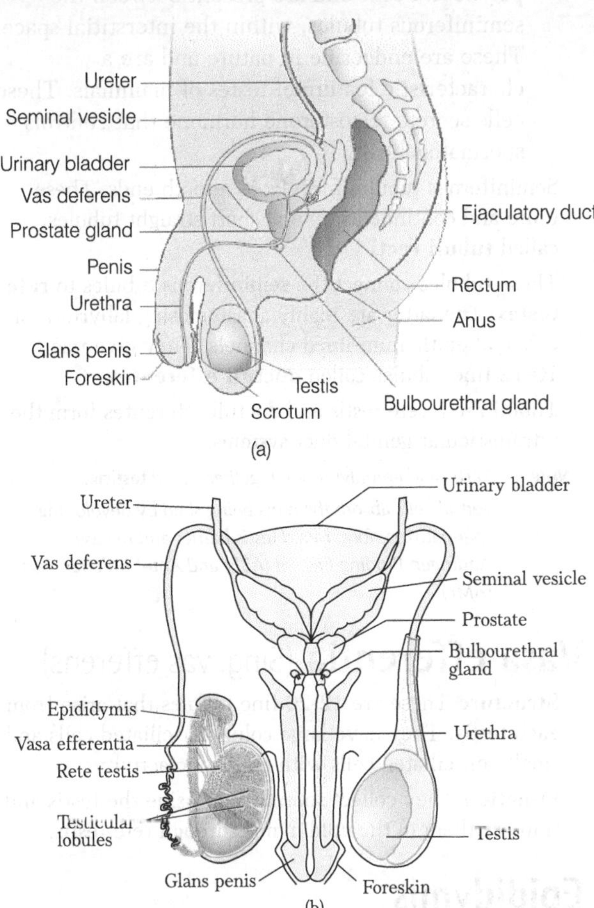

Fig. 3.1 (a) Diagrammatic sectional view of male pelvis showing reproductive system, (b) Front view of male reproductive system

Before discussing the structural details of male reproductive system, let us study the secondary sexual characters that appear during puberty.

Table 3.1 Development of secondary sexual characteristics in boys at puberty

Characteristics	Ages of first appearance	Hormonal stimulations
Sperm production by testes	10-14 yrs	Testosterone, FSH and growth hormone
Pubic hair	10-15 yrs	Testosterone
Body growth	10-16 yrs	Testosterone, growth hormone
Growth of penis	11-15 yrs	Testosterone
Voice change	Sametime as growth of penis	Testosterone
Facial and axillary (under arm) hair	About 2 yrs after the appearance of pubic hair	Testosterone
Exocrine gland or sweat glands and sebaceous glands; acne (from blocked sebaceous glands)	About the same time as facial and axillary hair growth	Testosterone

The major structures of male reproductive systems are discussed below

Scrotal sac (Scrotum)

- In human males, testes are situated outside the abdominal or pelvic cavity in a darkly pigmented sac of skin called the scrotal sac or scrotum.
- It acts as a thermoregulator to keep the testicular temperature 2-3°C lower than the normal internal body temperature. This is the optimum temperature necessary for sperm production (spermatogenesis).

Testes

- These are the primary male gonads in man.
- Each testis is oval in shape, with a length of about 4-5 cm, width of 2-3 cm and 3 cm thick.
- Testes develop in the abdominal cavity during early foetal life. They descend in the scrotum during the seventh month of foetal development.
- The passage through which testes descend is called **inguinal canal**. The spermatic cord which passes through this canal connects the testis with abdominal cavity.
- Testes are positioned by the **cremaster** muscles and **Dartos** muscles of the scrotal sac. At low temperature, these muscles contract to move the testes close to the abdomen and *vice-versa.*

Note
- *Cremaster muscle and connective tissues surround all structures passing through inguinal canal including spermatic cord.*
- *If testes fail to descend, this condition is called **cryptorchidism,** it leads to sterility. Inflammation of testis is called **orchitis**.*
- *Gubernaculum is a fibrous cord that extends from caudal end of testis to scrotal wall. It helps to keep testis in position.*

Coverings

The testis is surrounded by three protective coverings known as **tunicae**. These are as follows

(i) **Tunica vaginalis** It is the outer covering of testes.

(ii) **Tunica albuginea** It is a white fibrous capsule. It forms partitions (septa) through its interior surface to divide the testis into lobules.

(iii) **Tunica vasculosa** It contains a network of capillaries which are supported by delicate connective tissue.

Seminiferous tubules

- Each testis has about 250 compartments called **testicular lobules.**
- Each lobule contains one to three highly coiled seminiferous tubules, where the sperms are produced.
- The tubules of ductuli efferentes combine to form the ductus epididymis.

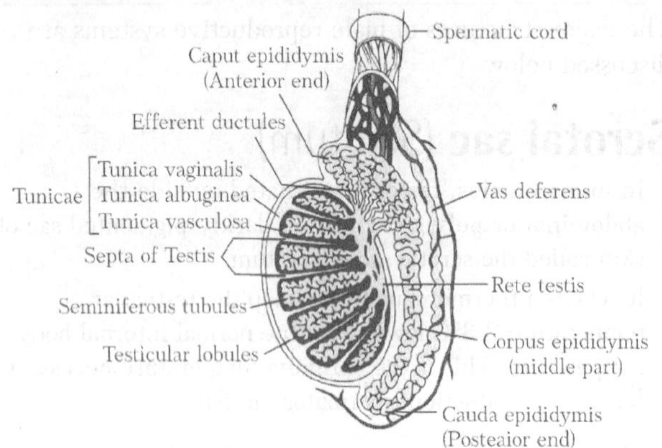

Fig. 3.2 LS of testis showing various parts

- The stratified epithelium of seminiferous tubule is made up of three types of cells
  (i) **Sertoli cells** (Supporting cells) These are also called **sustentacular cells** or **nurse cells**. They are elongated and pyramidal, which partially envelope the spermatogenic cells. These cells provide nourishment to developing germ cells and also secrete a glycoprotein hormone called **inhibin.** It is involved in the negative feedback control of sperm production by checking FSH activity.
  (ii) **Spermatogenic cells** These cells line the space between the basal lamina and the lumen of the tubule. These cells divide several times and differentiate to produce spermatozoa.

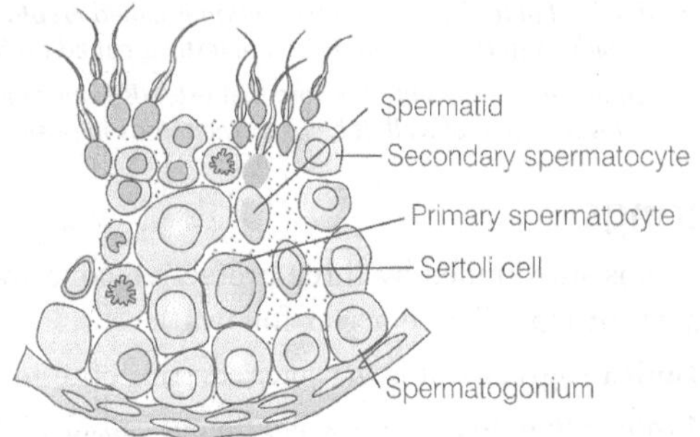

Fig. 3.3 Diagrammatic sectional view of a seminiferous tubule (enlarged)

  (iii) **Leydig cells** (Interstitial cells) They are group of polyhedral cells and are present between the seminiferous tubules, within the interstitial space. These are endocrine in nature and are a characteristic feature of testes of mammals. These cells secrete testosterone hormone that controls spermatogenesis.
- Seminiferous tubules form loops at both ends. These unite and continue as several short straight tubules, called **tubuli recti**.
- These tubules connect the seminiferous tubules to **rete testes.** The latter are highly anastomosing labyrinth of cuboidal epithelium-lined channels. They give rise to 10-12 fine tubules called **ductuli efferentes.**
- Tubuli recti, rete testis and ductuli efferentes form the intratesticular genital duct systems.

Note
- *Testis and epididymis are together called **testicle**.*
- *Sertoli cells absorb the parts being shed by developing spermatozoa, form blood testis barrier and release Androgen Binding Protein (ABP) and Anti-Mullerian Factor (AMF).*

Vasa efferentia (Sing. vas efferens)

- **Structure** These are 12-20 fine tubules that arise from each testis. They have large columnar ciliated cells and small non-ciliated cells with endocytic activity.
- **Function** They collect sperm from inside the testis and transfer them to the epididymis through rete testis.

Epididymis

- **Structure** The epididymis is a coiled tube, which consists of three parts. The anterior end called **caput epididymis,** middle part **corpus epididymis** the posterior end is **cauda epididymis.** It is lined by pseudostratified columnar epithelium.
- **Function** It stores the sperm temporarily. It also produces essential chemicals required for the nourishment and maturation of sperms.

Vasa deferentia (Sing. vas deferens)

- **Structure** Vas deferens is also called **ductus deferens** or **sperm duct.** It arises from cauda epididymis, ascends to abdomen, passes over the urinary bladder. It receives the duct from seminal vesicle behind the urinary bladder and form ejaculatory duct.
- **Function** It is a straight tube, which carries sperm to the urethra. Most of the sperms are stored in vas deferens.

Ejaculatory ducts

- **Structure** These are short, straight muscular tubes. These are formed by the union of vas deferens and duct of seminal vesicle.
- **Function** The two ejaculatory ducts pass through prostate and open into urethra to release sperms into it.

Urethra

- **Structure** It comprises of three regions
  - A short proximal prostatic urethra surrounded by **prostate gland.**
  - A very short middle **membranous urethra.**
  - A long distal **penile urethra** or **spongy urethra** that passes through penis to its external opening called **urethral meatus.**
- **Function** It carries urine from the bladder as well as, sperms from the vasa deferentia to penis. Thus, it is known as **urinogenital system** as it provides a common pathway for the flow of both urine and semen.

Penis

- It is the external genitalia in males. It is suspended from pubic region in front of scrotum.
- **Structure** It is vascular, spongy containing erectile tissue and a pensile organ.
- **External structure** Erect penis on an average is about 15 cm long. It has glans penis at the tip. It is covered with a loose fold of skin called **prepuce** or **foreskin.** Margin of glans penis is known as **corona.**
- **Internal structure** The interior of penis consists of three cylindrical cords made up of spongy and erectile (cavernous) tissue.
- Two of these cords are thick and lie parallel on the left and right side. These are called **corpora cavernosa.**
- These become superio-posterior, when penis is erect.
- The third cord smaller cord is **corpus urethral** or spongiosum. It remains inferio-anterior in position in erect penis. It is called so, because urethra runs from this cord.
- The pineal mass is covered by a dense connective tissue, called **tunica albuginea.**
- The extended part of corpus spongiosum is enlarged and form a bulged structure called **glans penis.** Its surface is formed of thin smooth hairless skin. This loose skin folds over and is retractile on glans penis. It is called **prepuce** or **foreskin.** At the tip of glans, urethral opening or meatus is present.
- **Tyson's gland** or **preputial gland** present in the skin of penis neck secrete a white sebaceous substance called **smegma.**
- The diagram showing TS penis is given below

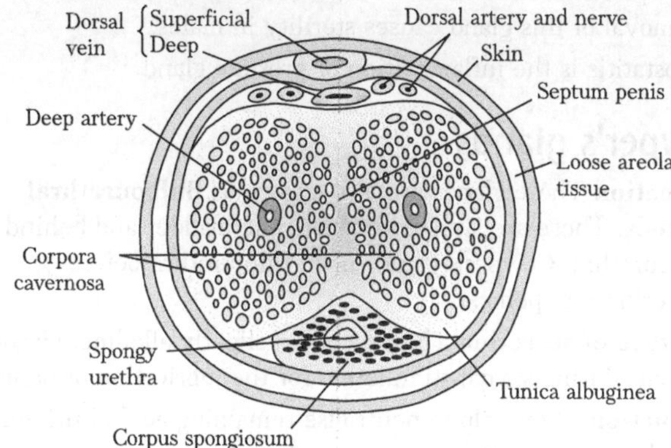

Fig. 3.4 TS of penis

- **Function** During sexual arousal, erectile tissue fills with blood. It causing the penis to become hard and erect to facilitate copulation and transmit sperms into vagina of the female. Therefore, it is also called **copulatory organ.**

Male accessory glands

The male accessory glands include paired seminal vesicles, a prostate gland and paired bulbourethral glands. The secretion of these glands constitutes the seminal plasma. It is rich in fructose, calcium and certain enzymes. These glands are discussed in detail below

Seminal vesicles

- **Location** These are paired, tubular glands present below urinary bladder.
- **Nature of secretion** They secrete alkaline nutritive seminal fluid which constitutes the main part of ejaculate.
  Seminal fluid contains fructose, citrate, inositol, prostaglandins and several proteins.
  They maintain viability and motility of sperms.
- **Function** Fructose, which is present in seminal fluid, is not produced anywhere else in the body. Its presence in the female's genital tract confirms sexual intercourse and also provides a forensic test in case of rape.

Prostate gland

- **Location** It is a single, large gland consisting of 30-40 tubuloalveolar glands. It is situated around the first part of the urethra. It contains prostatic utricle and acini and is covered by a capsule.
- **Nature of secretion** It secretes a slightly acidic (pH~6.5) milky fluid. It contains calcium, citrate ion, phosphate ion, a proteolytic enzymes (prefibrinolysin, fibrinolysin and fibrinogenase) and other enzymes like acid phosphatase, amylase, pepsinogen, etc.

- **Function** Secretion of prostate gland nourishes and activates the spermatozoa to swim. It is essential for sperm motility. Removal of this gland causes sterility in males.
- Prostatitis is the inflammation of prostate gland.

Cowper's glands

- **Location** These glands are also known as **Bulbourethral glands.** These are situated beneath the bladder and behind the urethra. Cowper's glands open into urethra before entering into penis.
- **Nature of secretion** They secrete a slightly alkaline, viscous mucus during sexual stimulation for the lubrication of penis.
- **Function** They help to neutralise remaining acid of urine in urethra during coitus.
- Secretion of Cowper's gland carries some spermatozoa released before ejaculation. This is one of the reasons for high failure rate of withdrawl method of birth control.

Semen

- It is ejaculated during the male sexual act.
- **Composition** It is composed of the fluid and sperms from the vas deferens (about 10% of the total), fluid from the seminal vesicles (almost 60 %) and prostate gland (about 30%). It also contains small amount of mucus from Bulbourethral gland.
- **Volume** The average volume of semen in an ejaculation is 2.5-5 mL, with a sperm count of 200 to 300 million sperms.
- **pH** The average pH of the semen is about 7.5 (alkaline).
- **Lifespan** The lifespan of sperm after ejaculation is 24-48 hrs. Longevity of sperms can be increased by preserving them at temperature below –100°C (cryopreservation).

Table 3.2 Organs of male reproductive system in a nutshell

Types	Organs	Paired/ Unpaired	Descriptions and locations	Functions
Glands	Testes	Paired	Primary sex organs, posterior to the penis within the scrotum.	Produce spermatozoa (gametes) and testosterone (male sex hormone).
	Seminal vesicle	Paired	Club-shaped glands posterior to the prostate, attached to the ejaculatory ducts.	Secretes alkaline fluid containing nutrients, like fructose and prostaglandins.
	Cowper's gland	Paired	Pea-sized glands inferior to the prostate, empty into the membranous urethra.	Secretes fluid that lubricates urethra and end of penis.
	Prostate gland	Unpaired	Walnut-sized gland at the base of the urinary bladder, surrounding the prostatic urethra.	Secretes alkaline fluid that helps neutralise acidic environment of the vagina, enhances motility of spermatozoa.
Ducts	Epididymis	Paired	Mass of tubules attached to the posterior surface of the testes.	Site of sperm maturation, store spermatozoa.
	Vas deferens	Paired	Ducts extending from the epididymis to the ejaculatory ducts.	Store spermatozoa, transport spermatozoa during ejaculation.
	Ejaculatory duct	Paired	Short ducts between the ductus deferentia and the prostatic urethra.	Receive spermatozoa and additives to produce seminal fluid.
Supporting structures	Scrotum	Unpaired	Pouch of skin, posterior to the penis.	Encloses and protects testes.
	Penis	Unpaired	Pendant organ, anterior to the scrotum and attached to the pubis.	Convey urine and seminal fluid to outside of body, organ of coitus.

CHECK POINT 3.1

1. Which of the following is the endocrine structure of testes?
   (a) Interstitial cells or cells of Leydig
   (b) Inguinal canal
   (c) Spermatic cord
   (d) Epidermis
2. The vasa efferentia leave the testis and open into
   (a) epididymis located along the posterior surface of each testis
   (b) epididymis located along the anterior surface of each testis
   (c) rete testis
   (d) testicular lobules
3. If for some reason, the vasa efferentia in the human reproductive system get blocked, the gametes will not be transported from
   (a) vagina to uterus
   (b) testis to epididymis
   (c) epididymis to vas deferens
   (d) ovary to uterus
4. The elastic tissue connecting the cauda epididymis to the scrotal sac is
   (a) gubernaculum
   (b) tendinous cord
   (c) scrotal ligament
   (d) caput epididymis
5. Seminal plasma in human is rich in
   (a) fructose, calcium, certain enzymes
   (b) fructose and calcium, but has no enzymes
   (c) glucose and certain enzymes, but has no calcium
   (d) fructose and certain enzymes, but poor in calcium
6. Choose the odd one out.
   (a) Epididymis
   (b) Vas deferens
   (c) Seminal vesicle
   (d) Ejaculatory duct

FEMALE REPRODUCTIVE SYSTEM

It consists of a pair of ovaries, oviducts, uterus, cervix, vagina and external genitalia in pelvic region. All these structures are found in either paired and unpaired condition. A detailed diagram showing all the major structures of female reproductive system is given below

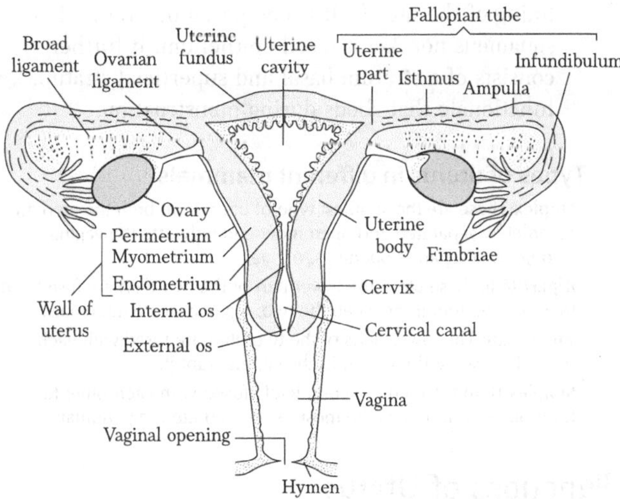

Fig. 3.5 Female reproductive system (representation)

The secondary sexual characters in females appear during puberty.

Table 3.3 Development of secondary sexual characteristics in girls at puberty

Characteristics	Ages of first appearance	Hormonal stimulations
Appearance of breast buds	8-13 yrs	Oestrogen, progesterone, growth hormone, thyroxine, insulin and cortisol
Pubic hair	8-14 yrs	Adrenal androgens
Menarche (first menstrual flow)	10-16 yrs	Oestrogen and progesterone
Axillary (under arm) hair	About 2 yrs after the appearance of pubic hair.	Adrenal androgens
Exocrine glands or sweat glands and sebaceous glands, acne (from blocked sebaceous glands)	About the same time as axillary hair growth.	Adrenal androgens

The main structures of female reproductive system are discussed in detail below

Ovaries

- These are the primary sex organs of a woman.
- Each ovary is almond-shaped structure of about 3 cm diameter.
- They are located near kidneys. These remain attached to abdominal wall by a ligament called **mesovarium.**
- Free surface of ovaries is covered by germinal epithelium. It is composed of cubical cells. This epithelium is continuous with mesothelium called **peritoneum.**
- The germinal epithelium encloses ovarian stroma. It is divided into two regions as follows
  (i) The outer cortex which is covered by **tunica albuginea** (dense connective tissue).
  It contains sac-like masses called **ovarian follicles** and remains of ovum called **corpus luteum.**
  (ii) The inner medulla which consists of loose connective tissue, elastic fibres, blood vessels and smooth muscle fibres.

Fallopian tubes

- Fallopian tubes or **Oviducts** or **Mullerian ducts** are two tubes (about 10 cm long) lying on either sides of uterus near kidney. Its lumen is lined by ciliated epithelium. Each Fallopian tube is suspended by mesosalpinx.
- The wall of oviduct is made up of three layers, outermost serosa, middle muscular layer and the innermost mucous membrane.
- Oviducts are differentiated into following parts
  (i) **Infundibulum** is the funnel-shaped part, which lies near to oviduct. Its edges possess finger-like projections called **fimbriae.** These help in the collection of ovum after ovulation.
  Infundibulum opens into abdominal cavity by an aperture called **ostium.**
  (ii) The infundibulum leads to a wider part of oviduct called **ampulla.**
  (iii) **Isthmus** is the last part having a narrow, thick -walled, ciliated lumen.
  (iv) **Uterine part** is the inner, narrow part which opens in the uterus.

Function of Fallopian tubes

- These tubes are involved in the conduction of the ovum or zygote towards the uterus by peristalsis and ciliary action.
- It also acts as the site of fertilisation (fertilisation occurs at the junction of ampulla and isthmus).

Uterus

- The uterus (or **womb** or **hystera**) is a single, pear-shaped, hollow, muscular structure.
- It is present within the pelvis between the bladder and rectum. It is suspended by a mesentery, i.e. mesometrium.
- It consists of following parts
  (i) **Fundus** It is the dome-shaped part present above the opening of Fallopian tubes.
  (ii) **Corpus** (body) The tapered central region of the uterus is its body. Its interior portion forms the uterine cavity.
  (iii) **Cervix** The lower narrow portion which protrudes into the vagina is cervix. It communicates with the body of uterus by an aperture called **internal os** and with vagina by **external os.** It is formed of the most powerful sphincter muscle in the body. The interior of cervix is called **cervical canal.**

Wall of the uterus

It is composed of three layers

(i) **Perimetrium** It is the thin outer covering or peritoneal layer.

(ii) **Myometrium** It is thick membranous layer composed of smooth muscle layers. These are thickest in the fundus and thinnest in the cervix.

(iii) **Endometrium** It is the inner highly vascular mucosal lining of the uterus. It is composed of stratified squamous non-keratinised epithelium. It further consists of a stratum basal and superficial stratum functionale that sheds during menstruation.

Types of uterus in different mammals

- **Duplex** These are the simplest type of uteri. In it, both the uteri are completely separated and open independently into the vagina through two separate openings, e.g. rat.
- **Bipartite** In these uteri, the lower part of the two uteri are fused and there is a septum in between the two, e.g. carnivore mammals.
- **Bicornuate** The lower parts of the two uteri are fused with each other, but the partition wall is absent, e.g. rabbit.
- **Simplex** Both the uteri are completely fused with each-other to form one structure, it is the most developed uteri, e.g. human.

Functions of Uterus

Uterus acts as the site of foetal growth during pregnancy. It also takes part in placenta formation and helps in pushing the baby out during parturition.

Vagina

- This is a muscular tube that is 8-10 cm long and contains elastic walls. It extends backward in front of rectum and anal canal from cervix to vestibule. The vagina opens to the exterior by an aperture called **vaginal orifice.**

- The opening of vagina is covered partially by a membrane called **hymen**. During the first coitus, the hymen is often torn. In some cases, it persists even after the coitus. However, it can be broken by a sudden fold, fall or during some vigorous physical activities.
- **Linings of vagina** It consists of a mucosa, a muscular layer and an adventitia. The mucosal layer is raised into transverse ridges called **vaginal rugae** and it contains few glands. The acidic mucus that is present in the vagina comes primarily from the glands within the uterus.
- **pH** The pH of the vagina is acidic (about 4.0) due to the presence of certain bacteria (e.g. *Lactobacillus*). It brings about fermentation and produces acid, so as to inhibit the growth of other microorganisms.
- **Function** It acts as copulation canal as it receives the sperms from penis during copulation. It also acts as a birth canal along with cervix during parturition.

External genitalia

Various structures of external genitalia are as follows

(i) **Vulva** It is external genital structure of the female reproductive system.

(ii) **Mons pubis** It is the most anterior structure of vulva. It is also called **mons Veneris**. It remains covered by pubic hair.

(iii) **Skin folds** The two longitudinal folds of skin, called the **labia majora** (labia means lips) form the boundary of vulva. It is homologous to male's scrotum. Labia majora covers two additional folds of skin called the **labia minora**. Labia majora and labia minora protect the vaginal and urethral openings. The labia minora also covers the openings of several tiny ducts that produce a mucus like secretion during sexual intercourse.

(iv) **Fourchette** Labia minora fuse posteriorly to form a membranous fold called fourchette.

(v) **Perineum** The area between fourchette and anus is called perineum.

(vi) **Clitoris** It is a tiny erectile finger-like structure. It lies at the upper junction of the two labia minora above urethral opening. It is homologous to penis.

Female accessory glands

The detailed description of female accessory glands is given below

Vestibular glands

They are similar to Cowper's gland in males. These are of following two types

(i) **Lesser vestibular glands** or **Paraurethral** or **Skene's glands** These are present around the urethral and vaginal orifice. They secrete mucus.

(ii) **Greater vestibular glands or Bartholin's glands** These are present on either side of vaginal orifice. They secrete alkaline secretion. These help in vestibular lubrication and neutralizing the urinary acidity.

Mammary glands

- There are two mammary or milk producing glands found in each normal female.
- These are present over the pectoralis major muscle on front wall of thorax.
- These start developing under the influence of oestrogen and progesterone during puberty.

External structure

Each mammary gland has a median nipple, surrounded by a pigmented area, called the **areola**. Various sebaceous glands are present on the surface of areola called **areolar glands**.

Internal structure

Mammary glands consist of three types of tissues. Three types of tissues are as follows

(i) **Glandular tissue** comprises of about 15-20 mammary lobes in each breast. From each lobe, excretory lactiferous ducts emerge which carry milk from one of the lobes to exterior.

(ii) **Fibrous tissue** supports alveoli and ducts.

(iii) **Adipose tissue** determines the size of breasts.

The diagram showing all the associated structures of mammary gland is given below

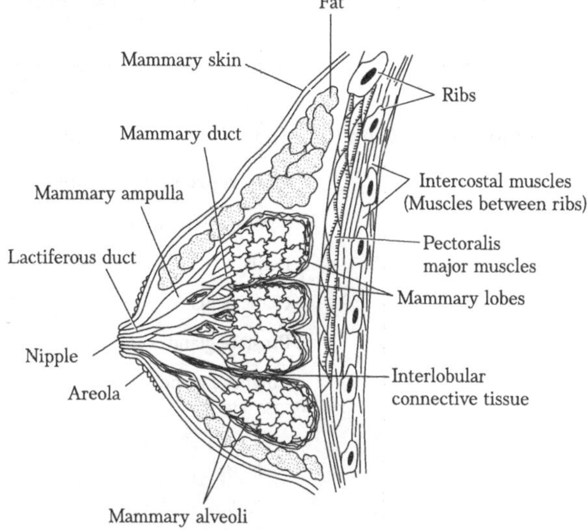

Fig 3.6 Sectional view of mammary gland

Function

- The mammary glands are modified sweat glands. The production of milk in these glands is stimulated by the hormone **prolactin.** It is secreted by the anterior part of pituitary gland.
- The ejection of milk into the ducts of mammary glands is stimulated by oxytocin hormone. The latter is secreted by the posterior part of pituitary gland.
- The path of milk ejection is as follows
Mammary alveolus → Mammary duct → Ampulla → Lactiferous duct → Nipple

Composition of milk

Milk secreted by mammary gland contains casein (milk protein), lactose (milk sugar), fat droplets, water, mineral salts (sodium, calcium, potassium, phosphorus, etc.) and vitamins. Milk from mammary gland is poor in iron content and vitamin-C.

Table 3.4 Organs of female reproductive system in a nutshell

Types	Organs	Paired/ Unpaired	Descriptions and locations	Functions
Glands	Ovaries	Paired	Primary sex organ, upper pelvic cavity on both lateral sides of uterus.	Production of ova (gametes) and female sex hormones, oestrogen and progesterone.
	Vestibular glands	Paired	Subcutaneous within the wall of the vaginal opening.	Secrete lubricating fluid into the vestibule and vaginal opening during coitus.
	Mammary glands	Paired	Composed of lobes within the breasts.	Produce and secrete milk for nourishment of an infant.
Ducts	Fallopian tube	Paired	Open-ended tubes that extend from the ovaries to the uterus.	Convey ova toward uterus, site of fertilisation, convey developing blastocyst to uterus.
Supporting-structures	Uterus	Unpaired	Hollow-shaped like an inverted pear, maintained in position within the pelvic cavity by muscles and ligaments.	Site of implantation, sustains life of embryo and foetus during pregnancy, plays active role in parturition.
	Vagina	Unpaired	Hollow, positioned between the urinary bladder and urethra anteriorly and the rectum posteriorly.	Conveys uterine secretion to outside of body, receives erect penis and semen during coitus, passage way for foetus during parturition.
	Labia majora	Unpaired	Two longitudinal folds of skin that extend from the mons pubis to the perineum; separated longitudinally by the pudendal cleft.	Form margins to enclose and protect other external reproductive organs.
	Labia minora	Unpaired	Two longitudinal folds of skin medial to the labia majora; separated longitudinally by the vaginal vestibule.	Form margins of vestibule, protect openings of vagina and urethra.
	Clitoris	Unpaired	Rounded projection at the upper part of the pudendal cleft, sheathed by a prepuce.	Provides feeling of pleasure during sexual stimulation.

The homology between the organs/structures of male and female reproductive system are tabulate below

Male reproductive system	Female reproductive system
Scrotum/Scrotal sac	Labia majora
Penis	Clitoris
Glans penis	Glans clitoris
Prostate gland	Paraurethral/Skene's gland
Cowper's gland	Bartholin's gland

CHECK POINT 3.2

1. The structure which attaches the ovaries with the dorsal wall is known as
   (a) Wolffian body (b) mesovarium
   (c) mesorchium (d) fimbricated body
2. The characteristic of human uterus is
   (a) paired with well separated oviducts
   (b) single large chamber with posterior part of oviduct fused to it anteriorly
   (c) paired with partially fused oviduct
   (d) a single large chamber with completely fused oviducts
3. The female external genitalia do not include
   (a) labia majora, labia minora, mons pubis and hymen
   (b) hymen, clitoris and mons
   (c) labia majora and labia minora only
   (d) vagina and cervix
4. In female, Bartholin's gland opens into the
   (a) vestibule and releases a lubricating fluid in the vagina
   (b) uterus and releases lubricating fluid during the birth of young ones
   (c) urinary bladdar and assists in release of urine
   (d) Fallopian tube and releases a secretion which makes sperm motile
5. The glandular tissue of each breast is divided into .... containing clusters of cells called alveoli.
   (a) 2-3 mammary lobes
   (b) 15-20 mammary ducts
   (c) 2-3 mammary ducts
   (d) 15-20 mammary lobes
6. Choose the incorrectly matched pair.
   (a) Vestibular gland – Unpaired (b) Uterus – Unpaired
   (c) Ovaries – Paired (d) Fallopian tube – Paired

GAMETOGENESIS

- It is the process of formation of haploid gametes from undifferentiated, diploid germ cells in the gonads of both males and females.
- The production of male gametes or sperms is called **spermatogenesis.** The production of female gametes or ova is called **oogenesis.**
- These processes involve meiotic division due to which haploid gametes are formed.
- Both spermatozoa and ova originate from Primordial Germ Cells (PGCs). These cells are **extragonadal** in **origin.**
- They originate from **extraembryonic mesoderm** during early embryonic development. They migrate to yolk sac endoderm and ultimately to the gonads of developing embryo, where they undergo further development.

Spermatogenesis

It is the process of formation of spermatozoa. This process begins with the Primordial Germ Cells (PGCs) present in the outer wall of seminiferous tubules.

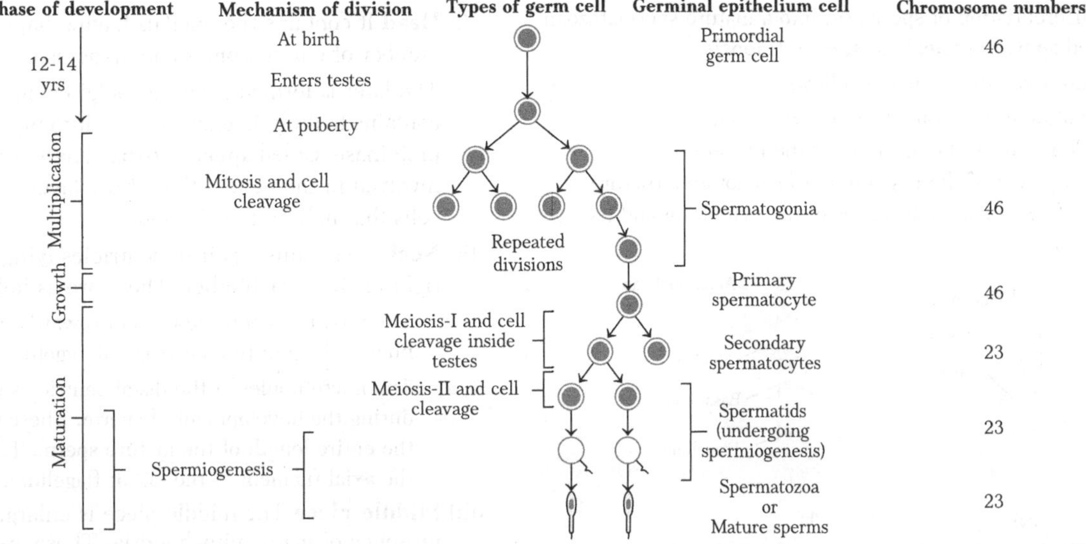

Fig. 3.7 Process of spermatogenesis

Spermatogenesis is completed in two major steps

A. Spermatocytogenesis

It includes multiplication phase, growth phase and maturation phase.

(i) **Multiplication phase** The spermatogonial cells are small cells. They divide several times by mitosis to produce a large number of cells called **spermatogonia.** Some of them continue as stem cells for spermatogenic lineage and called as **type A spermatogonia.** Rest of the spermatogonia differentiate into progenitor cells to form primary spermatocytes and called as **type B spermatogonia.**

(ii) **Growth phase** Type B spermatogonia take nourishment from germinal cells to double up their volume. This growth requires synthetic activities that are required for the initiation of meiosis. This ultimately forms the **primary spermatocytes.** These cells are large and diploid ($2n$). Thus, they possess 44 + XY (total 46) chromosomes.

(iii) **Maturation phase** This phase is also called meiotic and it includes following events

(a) **Meiosis-I** The primary spermatocytes undergo the first meiotic division. It leads to the formation of daughter cells which are smaller and termed as **secondary spermatocytes.** They are haploid (n) and contain 22 + X or 22 + Y (total 23) chromosomes.

(b) **Meiosis-II** The secondary spermatocytes undergo meiosis-II and produce the **spermatids.**
In this way, from each type B spermatogonium, 4 haploid spermatids are produced.

B. Spermiogenesis

- The differentiation of spermatid into a mature spermatozoan is called **spermiogenesis** or **spermateleosis.**
- It includes various events as follows
  - Formation of acrosome from Golgi complex
  - Condensation and elongation of the nucleus
  - Development of the flagellum as locomotory structure
  - Loss of redundant substances of the cytoplasm and its organelles.

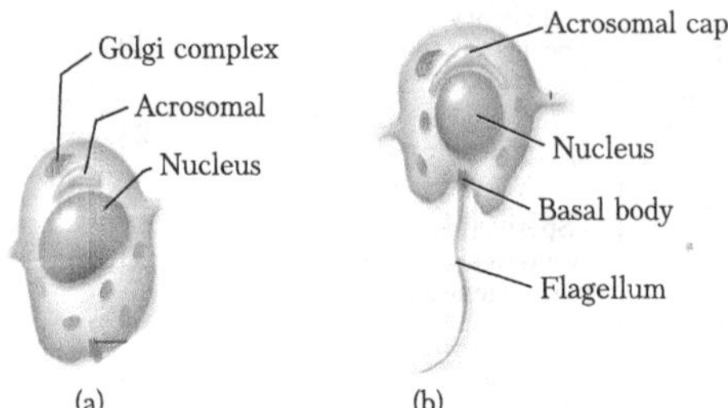

Fig. 3.8 (a) Appearance of acrosomal, (b) Development of acrosomal cap and flagellum

- The continuation of reduction in cytoplasm levels and development of flagellum results in the formation of mature spermatozoa as shown below

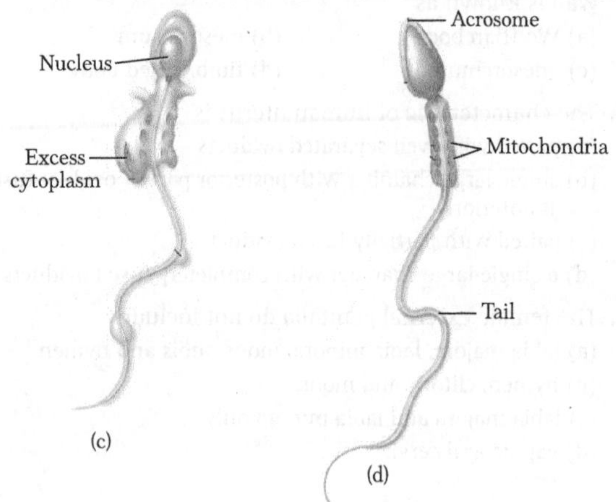

Fig. 3.9 (c) Shedding of excess cytoplasm, (d) Mature sperm

- **Spermiation** After spermiogenesis, sperm heads become embedded in Sertoli cells. These are finally released from the seminiferous tubule by the process called spermiation.

Sperm

The human sperm was first seen by **Antonie van Leeuwenhoek** in 1677. A mature spermatozoan or sperm cell is a microscopic, tadpole-shaped cell of about 2-5 μm in diameter and 60 μm long. It consists of an oval head,
a cylindrical body (neck and body piece) and an elongated tail. All these structures are discussed in delail below

(i) **Head** It contains the nucleus having haploid number of chromosomes and an acrosome.
The later is formed from the Golgi complex. It contains hydrolytic enzymes (hyaluronidase and proteinase) called **sperm lysins.** These are involved in the penetration of the layers of sperm cells that help in fertilisation.

(ii) **Neck** It contains a pair of centrioles lying at the right angle to each other. These are as follows

- The proximal centriole present towards the nucleus help in first cleavage of zygote.
- The microtubules of the distal centrioles elongate during the development of sperm. These run along the entire length of the mature sperm. They form the axial filament of the tail or flagellum.

(iii) **Middle piece** The middle piece is enlarged by the presence of many mitochondria. These are a arranged in spiral turns around the axial filament called **mitochondrial spiral.** Mitochondria carryout aerobic respiration and produce ATP as a source of energy. It is used in the movement of sperm tail. Thus, it allows the sperms to swim at the rate of about 1-4 mm per min.

(iv) **Tail** It is several time longer than the head and is composed of cytoplasm. Axial filament or axoneme occurs through out it. Basal granule of tail is distal centriole.

It has two parts as follows

- The main piece has a covering of cytoplasm, while
- The end piece consists of naked filament alone and lacks cytoplasm.

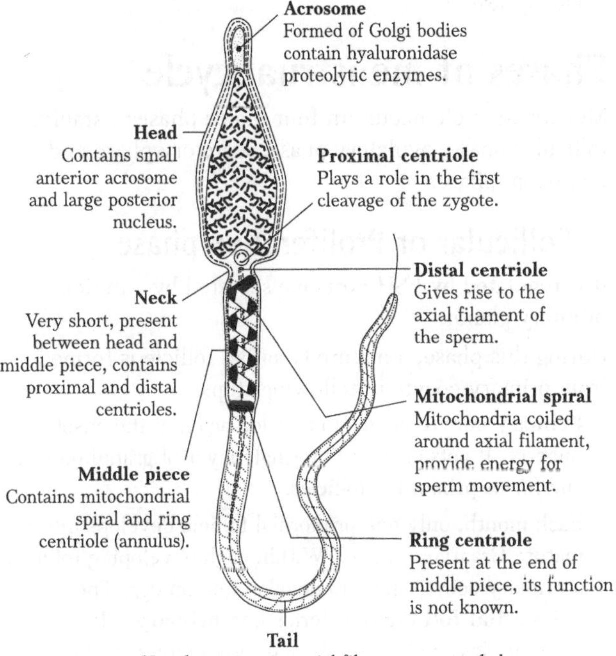

Fig. 3.10 Human sperm

The human male ejaculates about 200-300 million sperms during a coitus. Out of these, 60% should have normal shape and 40% should show vigorous motility for normal fertility.

Hormonal control of spermatogenesis

- Spermatogenesis is controlled by various hormones. It starts at puberty due to increase in **Gonadotropin Releasing Hormone** (GnRH) by hypothalamus.
- It acts on anterior pituitary, which stimulates the production of two gonadotropins, **Luteinizing Hormone** (LH or ICSH) and **Follicle Stimulating Hormone** (FSH).
- Luteinizing Hormone (LH) acts on Leydig cells. It helps in the synthesis and secretion of androgens to stimulate spermatogenesis.
- Follicle Stimulating Hormone (FSH) acts on Sertoli cells. The latter secretes inhibin, required for suppressing FSH synthesis. FSH also stimulates spermiogenesis.

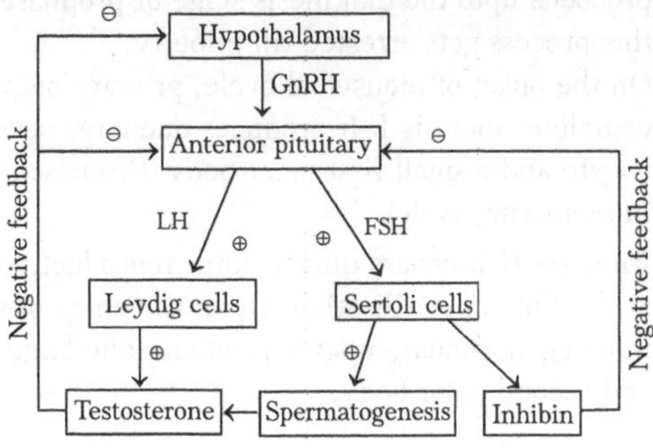

Fig. 3.11 Hormonal control of male reproductive system

Note
- *In positive feedback loop, hormones released by one gland, stimulate the other which further lead to significant changes.*
- *In negative feedback loop, product of a process inhibits its own production.*

Oogenesis

The process of formation of a mature female gamete is called oogenesis. This process begins in foetal life and it lasts upto adult reproductive life as shown in the diagram below

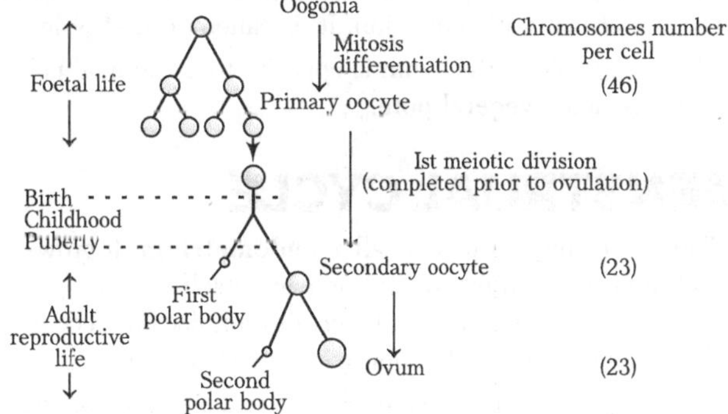

Fig. 3.12 Schematic representation of oogenesis in human female

Oogenesis comprises of three phases, *viz.* multiplication phase, growth phase and maturation phase. All these three phases occur during the foetal life only. However, the completion of maturation phase occur after puberty and during adult reproductive life.

(i) **Multiplication phase** Primordial germ cells divide mitotically to form oogonia. These undergo mitosis and form primary oocyte.

(ii) **Growth phase** Primary oocytes undergo growth. It is a prolonged and slow process. During this period, primary oocytes secrete zona pellucida outside its plasma membrane. Other processes like increase in reserve food material, nucleus size, mitochondria number, etc., also occur during this phase.

(iii) **Maturation phase** Two meiotic divisions, *viz.* meiosis-I and meiosis-II occur during this phase.

- **Meiosis-I** Primary oocyte undergoes meiosis-I. It proceeds upto the diakinesis stage of prophase-I and this process gets arrested till puberty.
  On the onset of menstrual cycle, primary oocyte completes meiosis-I. It produces one large secondary oocyte and a small first polar body (Discussed in detail in menstrual cycle).
- **Meiosis-II** It occurs during adult reproductive life, at the time of fertilisation. Upon the entry of sperm into egg, secondary oocyte produces one large ovum and second polar body.

Ovum

- Human egg or ovum is non-cledoic (without shell) and alecithal (yolk is absent).
- It is a microscopic structure with about 0.1-0.13 mm or 100-130 μm diameter. It is formed as a result of oogenesis.
- The ovum possesses three coverings, *viz.* inner plasma membrane, middle glycoprotein layer called zona pellucida and the outer cellular layer, corona radiata.
- Fertilizin is a compatibility receptor proteins found in zona pellucida.
- Human egg has two poles. The uppermost pole of an egg is the site of maturation division. It is called **animal pole.**
- The lower pole of the ovum is opposite to the animal pole and it is called **vegetal pole.**

MENSTRUAL CYCLE

- The inner lining of uterus called **endometrium.** It grows and thickens each month and prepares itself for the implantation of an embryo. If fertilisation does not occur, the endometrium sheds along with menstrual flow.
- This monthly event of development and shedding of the functional layer of the uterus is called the **menstrual phase.**
- The monthly maturation of an egg and its release is called the **ovarian cycle.** A typical menstrual cycle completes in an average of about 28 days.
- Cyclic mensturation is an indicator of normal reproductive phase and extends between menarche and menopause.

Menarche

- The release of the first menstrual flow is called **menarche.**
- It marks the beginning of a female's reproductive life. It is one of the most obvious signals of the onset of puberty.
- Menarche usually occurs between the age of 11-14 yrs. The ovaries are stimulated by the gonadotropins released from the anterior pituitary gland.

Menopause

It is the condition in which menstrual cycle stops naturally. The average age of menopause in woman is 45-50 yrs.

Various features of menopause are as follows

- In menopause, the size of ovaries gets decreased.
- Graafian follicle gets replaced by fibrous tissue.
- Ova, corpora lutea and internal secretions of the ovary are not further formed.
- The uterus and vagina become atrophic.
- Woman does not remain reproductively active after menopause.

Phases of menstrual cycle

Menstrual cycle occurs in four major phases namely, follicular phase, ovulatory phase, secretory phase and menstrual phase.

1. Follicular or Proliferative phase

It is regulated by FSH hormone secreted by anterior pituitary gland.

During this phase, a mature Graafian follicle is formed from primary oocyte in following steps

- **Primary oocyte** begins to develop again at the onset of puberty. It gets enclosed by single layer of granulosa cells and forms primordial follicles.
- Each month, only one primordial follicle develops into a mature Graafian follicle. Within each developing follicle, a primary oocyte starts to develop into an egg. The **primordial follicle** transforms into **primary follicle** as the granulosa cells multiply and form many layers of cells around the primary oocyte.
- The cells from the stroma of the ovary form further layers of granulosa cell and the theca around primary follicle to form **secondary follicles.**
- The outer part of the theca contains blood vessels and merges with the stroma. The inner part of the theca secretes female sex hormones.
- Secondary follicle transforms into a **tertiary follicle.** It is characterised by a fluid-filled space called **antrum.**
- Oestrogen further stimulates the growth of follicle. It eventually becomes a mature follicle, known as **Graafian follicle** or **mature follicle.** It is about 1 cm in diameter.
- Graafian follicle secretes oestradiol which stimulates the proliferation of endometrium and the enlargement of uterine glands.

Note • *Initial steps of oogenesis occur **prior to birth** in **25 weeks old foetus.***

- *The maturing oocytes adhere to wall of follicle through a stalk, cumulus oophorus formed by granulosa cells.*
- *About 2 million primordial follicles are present in the ovary before birth. But during reproductive life, only about 450 eggs are released from ovaries. Rest of these eggs undergo follicular attresia.*

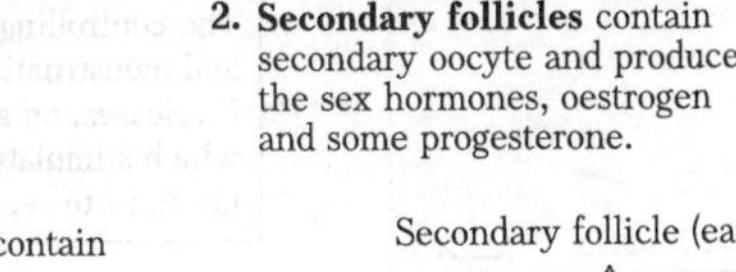

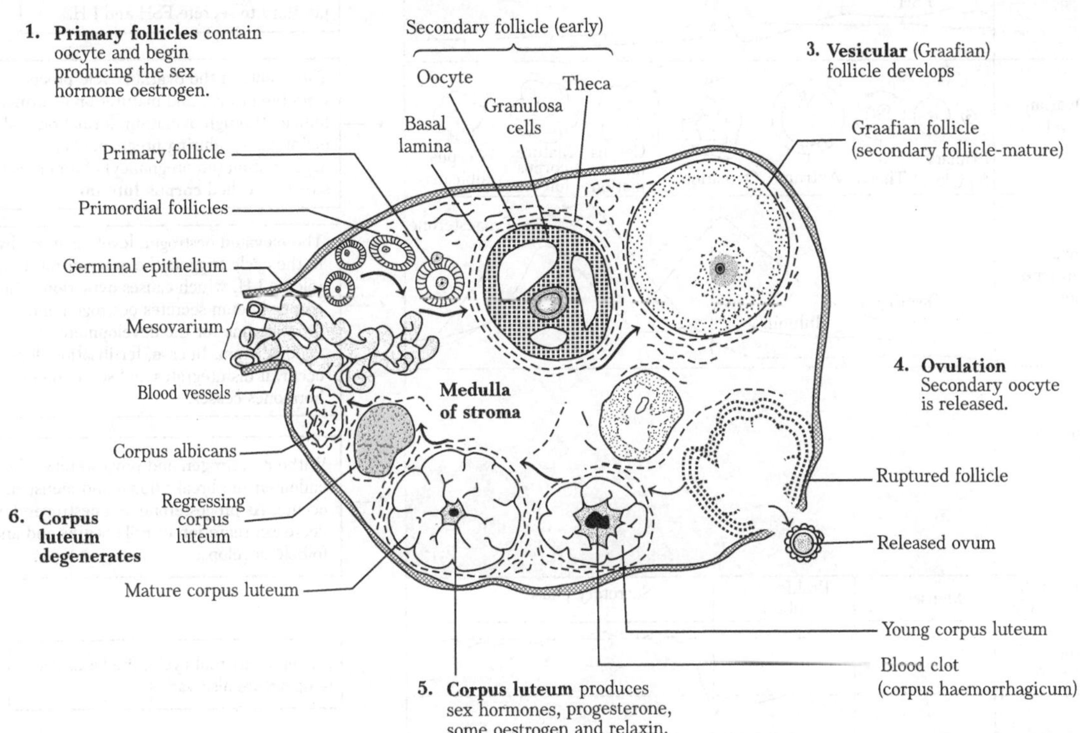

Fig. 3.13 Different stages of follicle development

2. Ovulatory phase

During this phase, Graafian follicle gets ruptured to release the secondary oocyte or ovum. This event occurs due to increased secretion of LH (LH surge) from anterior pituitary on the 14th day of cycle.

3. Secretory phase or Luteal phase

This phase of menstrual cycle is marked by the presence of corpus luteum (yellow body).

The fate of corpus luteum depends upon the presence or absence of fertilisation.

(i) During pregnancy, this yellow body secretes hormone, i.e. **human Chorionic Gonadotropin** (hCG) and **progesterone**. These hormones help to keep endometrium intact and prepare it for implantation of fertilised ovum.

(ii) In the absence of pregnancy, it regresses to form corpus albicans and menstruation start (menstrual phase).

Corpus luteum secretes oestrogen and progesterone. As a result, endometrium remains intact and the release of FSH and LH is inhibited. This prevents the development of new follicles. This phase lasts for 14 days.

4. Menstrual phase

It occurs due to the breakdown of endometrium lining of uterus and blood vessels. Menstrual blood contains fibrinolytic enzyme due to which the blood in menses do not clot. It lasts for 3-4 days.

The correlation of menstrual cycle with hormonal control at its various phase is described in the diagram given below

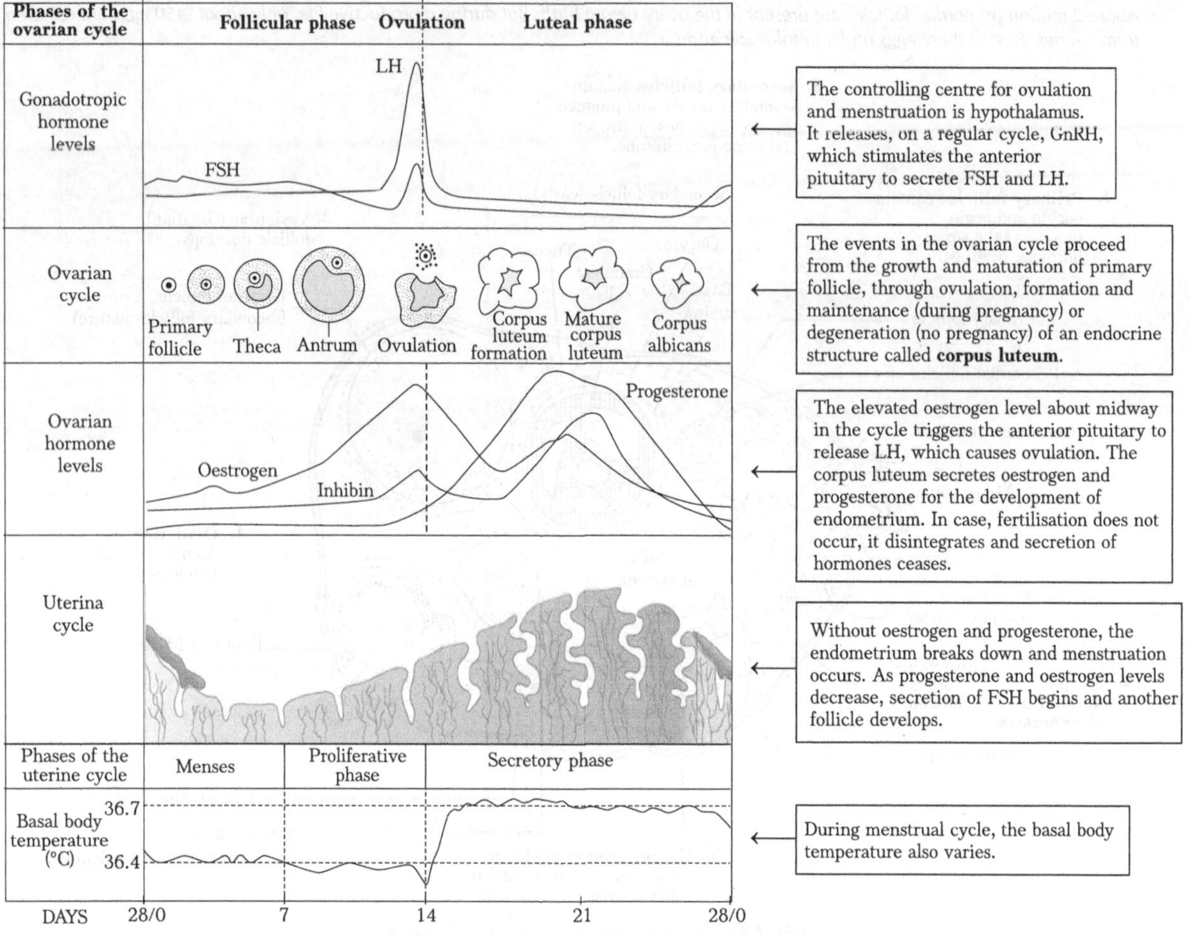

Fig. 3.14 *Menstrual cycle in a normal female*

Table 3.5 Various phases of the menstrual cycle

Phases of cycle		Hormonal changes		Tissue changes	
Ovarian	**Endometrial**	**Pituitary**	**Ovary**	**Ovarian**	**Endometrial**
Follicular (1-4 days)	Menstrual	Low secretion of FSH and LH	Oestradiol and progesterone remain low	Primary follicles grow	Outer two-thirds of endometrium shed off, accompanying bleeding
Follicular (5-13 days)	Proliferative	FSH slightly higher than LH secretion in early follicular phase	Oestradiol secretion rises (due to FSH stimulation of follicles)	Follicles grow, Graafian follicle develops (due to FSH stimulation)	Increases in the thickness of endometrium, spiral arteries develop (due to oestradiol stimulation)
Ovulatory (14 days)	Proliferative	LH surge and increased FSH stimulated by positive feedback from oestradiol	Oestradiol secretion falls	Graafian follicle ruptures and secondary oocyte is extruded into uterine tube	No change
Luteal (15-28 days)	Secretory	LH and FSH decrease (due to negative feedback from steroids)	Progesterone and oestrogen secretion increase, then fall	Development of corpus luteum (due to LH stimulation), regression of corpus luteum	Glandular development in endometrium (due to progesterone stimulation)

Hormonal control of oogenesis

The menstrual cycle is under the control of various hormones are as follows

- The hypothalamus secretes GnRH. It stimulates the anterior lobe of pituitary gland to secrete LH and FSH.
- FSH stimulates the growth of ovarian follicles. It also helps in the development of secondary oocyte.
- FSH also stimulates oestrogen formation.
- LH stimulates the corpus luteum to secrete progesterone. The latter inhibits the production of GnRH. It ultimately inhibits the secretion of FSH, LH and progesterone.

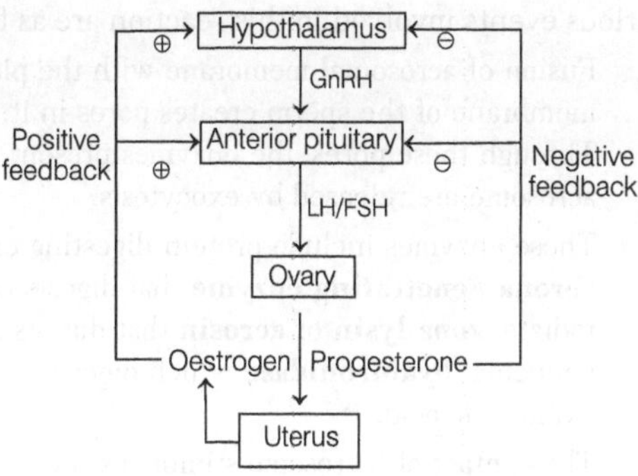

Fig. 3.15 Hormonal control of oogenesis

CHECK POINT 3.3

1. In spermatogenesis, a primary spermatocyte produces four similar sperms while in oogenesis, a primary oocyte forms
   (a) four similar ova
   (b) three large ova and one polar body
   (c) two large ova and two polar bodies
   (d) one large ova and 2-3 polar bodies
2. Spermiogenesis changes
   (a) spermatogonium to primary spermatocytes
   (b) primary spermatocytes to secondary spermatocytes
   (c) secondary spermatocytes to spermatids
   (d) spermatids to sperm
3. The second maturation division of the mammalian ovum occurs
   (a) in the Graafian follicle following first maturation division
   (b) shortly after ovulation before the ovum makes entry into Fallopian tube
   (c) until ovum is penetrated by sperm
   (d) until nucleus of sperm has fused with ovum
4. Which one of the following is the most likely the root cause, why menstruation is not taking place in human female having regular menstrual cycle?
   (a) Maintenance of hypertrophical endometrium living
   (b) Maintenance of high concentration of sex hormone in blood
   (c) Retention of well-developed corpus luteum
   (d) Fertilisation of ovum
5. Ovulation in the human female normally takes place during the menstrual cycle
   (a) at the mid secretory phase
   (b) just before the end of the secretory phase
   (c) at the beginning of the proliferative phase
   (d) at the end of proliferative phase
6. Inhibition of uterine contraction ceases and the bleeding and cramps of menstruation begin due to
   (a) increase in level of progesterone
   (b) decrease in level of progesterone
   (c) increase in level of LH
   (d) decrease in level of FSH

FERTILISATION

It involves the union of ovum and sperm to form a diploid zygote. During fertilisation, the sperm cell enters the cytoplasm of the much larger egg cell. Within 12 hrs, the nuclear membrane of the ovum disappears. The haploid chromosome in the ovum fuses with that of sperm cell. Thus, a fertilised egg or zygote is formed. It contains the diploid number of chromosomes, i.e. 46.

Steps of fertilisation process

Various steps of fertilisation are as follows

(i) **Insemination** Male discharges semen in female's vagina, close to the cervix. The sperm swims and prostaglandins of semen help in the movement of sperm or spermatozoa in the female genital tract.

Fertilisation can occur only when both ovum and sperms are transported simultaneously to the ampullary-isthmic junction. This is why, not all copulations lead to fertilisation and pregnancy.

(ii) **Capacitation** In this process, the spermatozoa acquire the capacity to fertilise the eggs. It involves

- Dilution of inhibitory factors of semen.
- Removal of cholesterol vesicles that cover sperm head and acrosome.
- Increase in the permeability of acrosome covering for Ca^{2+} **ions** and their entry into the sperm.

(iii) **Penetration of sperm** It is a chemical mechanism and involves the following reactions

(a) **Acrosome reaction** The interaction of sperm with the zona pellucida of ovum triggers an acrosomal reaction.

Various events involved in this reaction are as follows

- Fusion of acrosomal membrane with the plasma membrane of the sperm creates pores in it. Through these pores, the enzymes present in acrosome are released by exocytosis.
- These enzymes include protein-digesting enzyme, **corona penetrating enzyme** that digests corona radiata, **zona lysin** or **acrosin** that digests zona pellucida, **hyaluronidase** which digests hyaluronic acid.
- The contact of acrosome stimulates the development of an outgrowth in oocyte called **fertilisation cone** or **cone of reception.**

(b) **Fertilizin-antifertilizin reaction** The compatability reaction between sperm and surface of the ovum occurs by special fertilizin and antifertilizin reaction. **Fertilizin** is a glycoprotein or acid mucopolysaccharide present on the surface layer of the egg. **Antifertilizin** is present on the surface layer of the cytoplasm of spermatozoa.
These reactions result in the agglutination of the spermatozoa by egg. They lead to the adhesion of the spermatozoa to the egg membranes or egg surface.

(c) **Cortical and zona reaction** The stepwise processes that occur during this reaction are as follows

- As the sperm head comes in contact with the fertilisation cone, it causes opening of Na^+ channels.
- It causes depolarisation of ovum (fast block to check polyspermy) and Ca^{+2} moves into the egg.
- Sperm and egg membrane get dissolved.
- Male pronucleus and proximal centriole of sperm enter egg's cytoplasm.
- Ca^{+2} influx causes extrusion of cortical granules (cortical reaction).

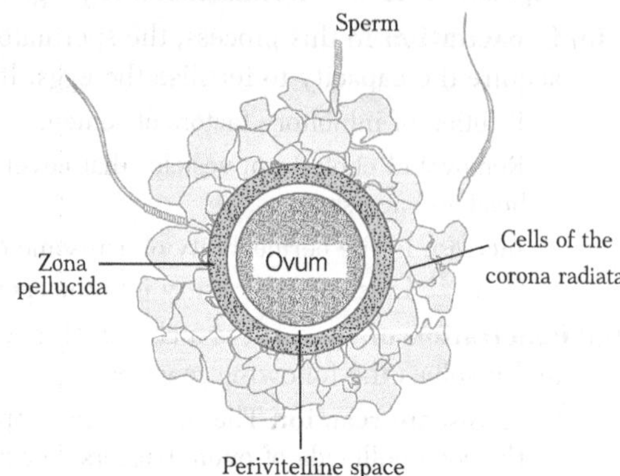

Fig. 3.16 Ovum surrounded by few sperms

- Zona pellucida becomes impervious to second sperm by destroying sperm receptors (zona reaction). It acts as the slow block to check polyspermy.
- The entry of sperm causes the breakdown of **Metaphase Promating Factor** (MPF) and turn on **Anaphase Promoting Complex** (APC).
- It further induces completion of second meiotic division of secondary oocyte.
- This division forms a second polar body and a haploid ovum (ootid). Soon, the haploid nucleus of sperm and that of ovum fuse together to form a diploid zygote.

EMBRYONIC DEVELOPMENT OR EMBRYOGENESIS

It is the development of embryo from fertilised egg and its subsequent development into a young organism. It includes cleavage, blastulation, implantation, gastrulation and organogenesis.

Cleavage

It starts after 30-36 hrs of fertilisation. It involves following events

- The zygote moves through the isthmus of oviduct towards the uterus. Meanwhile, it divides mitotically *via* a process called cleavage into two smaller cells (also called blastomeres).
- Second cleavage occurs about 40 hrs after fertilisation. It produces four cells, followed by a third cleavage which occurs after 50-60 hrs of fertilisation.
- This leads to the formation of a ball of a solid mass of cells called a **morula** (Latin-*mulberry*).

Laws related to cleavage

(i) **Sach's law** (1877) Cells divide into equal daughter cells. Each new division plane tends to intersect the preceding plane at right angles. It helps to maintain the spheroidal shape of blastomeres.

(ii) **Hertwig's law** (1881) The nucleus and achromatic figures occupy the centre of 'protoplasmic density' of the egg or blastomeres in which it lies. The axis of mitotic spindle occupies the longest axis of the protoplasmic mass in which it lies. The division therefore, tends to cut this axis transversely.

(iii) **Balfour's law** (1885) The rate of cleavage is inversely proportional to the amount of yolk or deutoplasm.

(iv) **Pfulger's law** The mitotic spindle always elongates in the direction of least resistance.

Various types, patterns and planes of cleavage are discussed in the table below

Table 3.6 Types, patterns and planes of cleavage

Types	Patterns	Planes
Holoblastic The cleavage furrow extends completely through entire length of egg and divides it into equal parts. It is of two types (a) **Equal** Blastomeres are of equal sized, e.g. placental mammals. (b) **Unequal** Blastomeres are of variable size, e.g. amphibians.	**Radial** It involves successive cleavage planes through the egg at right angles, e.g. *Synapta paracentrotus* **Biradial** The first three planes of division are not at right angle to each other, e.g. Ctenophora.	**Meridional plane** When the cleavage furrow bisects animal and vegetal pole.
Meroblastic The yolk remains undivided as cleavage furrow restricts to germinal disc. It is divided into two types (a) **Discoidal cleavage** It restricted to disc-shaped cytoplasm, e.g. reptiles and birds. (b) **Superficial cleavage** It is restricted to cytoplasm, e.g. insects.	**Spiral** It involves the arrangement of the blastomeres of each upper tier over the cell junctions of lower tier, so that they move spirally around pole to pole axis, e.g. nematodes.	**Vertical plane** When cleavage furrow passes through animal to vegetal pole but not through median plane.
	Determinate The fate of blastomeres is predetermined. This is also called **mosaic development**, e.g. molluscs, nematode.	**Equatorial plane** When cleavage furrow passes through equator.
	Indeterminate The fate of blastomeres is not predetermined. This is also called **regulative development**, e.g. echinoderms, chordates.	**Latitudinal or Transverse or Horizontal plane** When cleavage furrow passes horizontally on either side of equator.

Morula

- It is a solid ball of cells, having 16-32 blastomeres. Morula undergoes compaction and possesses two type of cells
  - The outer/peripheral cells are smaller/flat with tight junction.
  - The inner cell mass is slightly large, rounded and with gap junction.
- Morula descends slowly towards the uterus in 4-6 days and corona radiata detaches during this period.

Blastulation or Blastocyst formation

As the morula enters the uterus, it obtains rich supply of nutrients from endometrium. The fate of different cells formed in morula is as follows

- The outer peripheral cells enlarge to form **trophoblast** or **trophoectoderm**. Trophoblast cells secrete a fluid into the interior creating a cavity called **blastocoel**.
- The **inner cell mass** comes to lie on one side as embryonal knob. Cells of trophoblasts in contact with the inner cell mass are called **cells of Rauber**. Thus, morula is converted to blastula, which is called **blastocyst in mammals**.
- Further changes in blastocyst occur in following manner
  - Due to the pressure of growing blastocyst, a slit is produced in zona pellucida from which growing blastocysts comes out.
  - At times, it gets broken into two parts which give rise to **identical twins** or **monozygotic twins**.
  - The area of embryonal knob represents animal pole.
  - Soon embryonal knob shows rearrangement to form embryonal disc.
  - Cells of trophoblast layer divide periclinally. They give rise to two layers, *viz.* outer syncytiotrophoblast and inner cytotrophoblast.
  - The two layers later form chorion, amnion and foetal part of placenta.

Types of blastula in animals

- **Coeloblastula** A hollow blastula in which blastocoel is surrounded by either single layered (e.g. echinoderms, amphioxus) or many layered blastoderms (e.g. frog).
- **Amphiblastula** It is a type of coeloblastula surrounded by two types of cells., *viz.* upper micromeres and lower macromeres, e.g. frog.
- **Stereoblastula** Solid blastula with no blastocoel, e.g. coelenterates, annelids and molluscs.
- **Discoblastula** The blastula is multilayered flat disc at the animal pole lying on the top of well-developed yolk. It is found in reptiles, birds, prototherians and fishes.
- **Blastocyst** In this, the blastula possesses two types of cells, i.e.
  - an outer epithelium like layer of trophoblast or nutritive cells;
  - an inner mass of formative cells collectively called **embryonal knob**. It is found in mammals.
- **Superficial blastula or Periblastula** In this, the blastocoel is filled with yolk and is surrounded by a peripheral layer of cells. It is found in insects.

The diagram showing foetal development in early weeks of pregnancy is given below

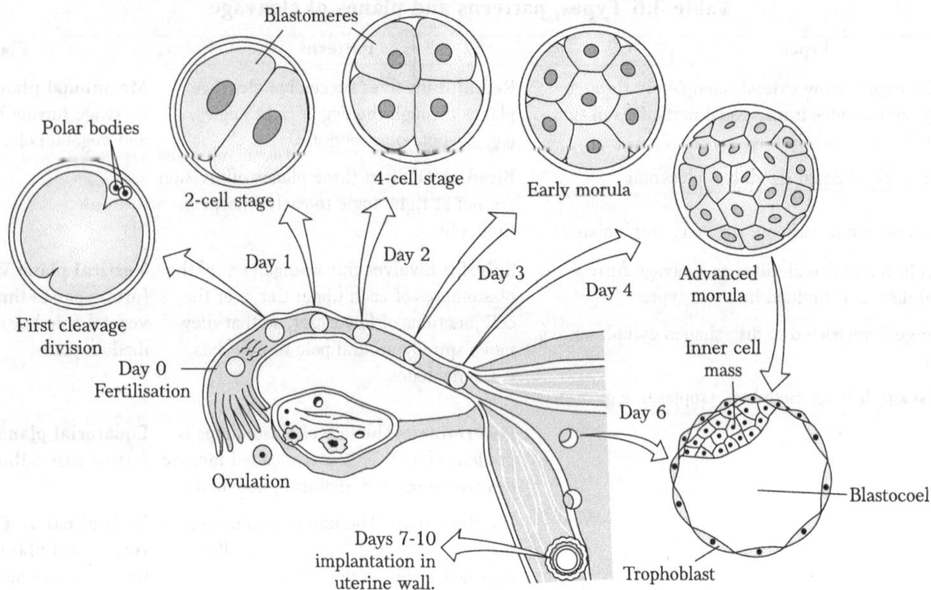

Fig. 3.17 Foetal development during the first and second weeks

Implantation

- The embedding of blastocyst in the endometrium is called implantation.
- The side containing the inner mass is positioned against the uterine wall.
- The trophoblast cells produce lytic enzymes that erode endometrial lining. It allows the blastocyst to penetrate into the thick endometrium.
- They also give rise to finger-like outgrowth called **villi**. These villi help in the fixation and absorption of nutrients.
- Implantation causes nutrient enrichment, enlargement of cells and formation of uterine part of placenta called **decidua** (*L. deciduos*-falling off).
- Decidua has three regions, which are as follows
  - (i) **Decidua basalis** This part of decidua underlies the chorionic villi and overlying the myometrium.
  - (ii) **Decidua capsularis** It lies between embryo and lumen of uterus.
  - (iii) **Decidua parietalis** This part of decidua lines the uterus at places other than the site of attachment of embryo.
- Trophoblast covering secretes a hormone called **human Chorionic Gonadotropin** (hCG).
- **Significance of hCG** Detection of hCG in the urine is the basis of **pregnancy/Gravidex test.** hCG maintains the corpus luteum beyond its normal lifetime.

Gastrulation

- It is the process of the embryonic development during which cell movements establish the three primary germinal layers. These are ectoderm, mesoderm and endoderm.
- During gastrulation, the cells move to occupy their definite position. The product of gastrulation is called **gastrula.**
- Archenteron is the cavity which occurs inside the gastrula. It forms the future alimentary canal. It opens to the outside through blastopore which later on gets closed down.
- The cell movements that occur during gastrulation are called **morphogenetic movements,** since they lead to initiation of morphogenesis.

Note *Fate mapping can be done in polar blastula or early gastrula. It was first tried by SPECT (1919) and first done by **W. Vogt** (1929).*

Types of gastrular movement or Morphogenetic movement

Following types of gastrular movements are found in different animals.

(i) **Epiboly** It involves the morphogenetic movement of prospective ectodermal (micromeres) blastomeres antero-posteriorly. It envelops the presumptive endodermal and mesodermal blastomeres. It is found in telolecithal egg of frog.

(ii) **Emboly** It involves inward movement of prospective endodermal and chorda-mesodermal blastomeres from the surface of blastula.

Emboly occurs through following methods

- **Invagination** It involves insinking of endodermal cells in the blastocoel to form archenteron. It is found in amphioxus.
- **Involution** It involves the rolling of the chorda-mesodermal blastomeres inside the ectodermal cells over the lips of blastopore. It is also found during the gastrulation in frog.
- **Ingression or Polyinvagination** In this, individual blastomeres migrate into the blastocoel in two ways
  - From only vegetal pole (called **unipolar ingression**, e.g. *Obelia*).
  - From all sides (called **multipolar ingression**, e.g. *Hydra*) to form a solid gastrula called **stereogastrula**.
- **Delamination** It involves splitting off the blastoderm into two layers by the appearance of grooves. It results in the formation of hypoblast. It is found in birds.

Formation of primary germinal layers

The cells of the inner cell mass or embryonal knob get rearranged to form a **flat embryonic** or **germinal disc.** The latter differentiate into two layers

(i) **Outer epiblast of larger columnar cells**

- Epiblast forms both ectoderm and mesoderm of the embryo.
- It laterally divides to produce ectoderm.
- Epiblast cells proliferate to form first cellular elevation called **primitive streak.**
- The cells continue to proliferate and pass out in between epiblast and hypoblast.
- They form the third germinal layer called **mesoderm** (intraembryonic mesoderm).

(ii) **Inner hypoblast of smaller cuboidal cells**

- Hypoblast functions as embryonic endoderm.
- It is the first germinal layer to differentiate and grow on the sides to forms a covering of blastocoel.
- Meanwhile, embryonic endoderm forms a tube of its own. The tubular structure is the gut tract of the embryo.

The fate of different germ layers is shown in the line diagram below

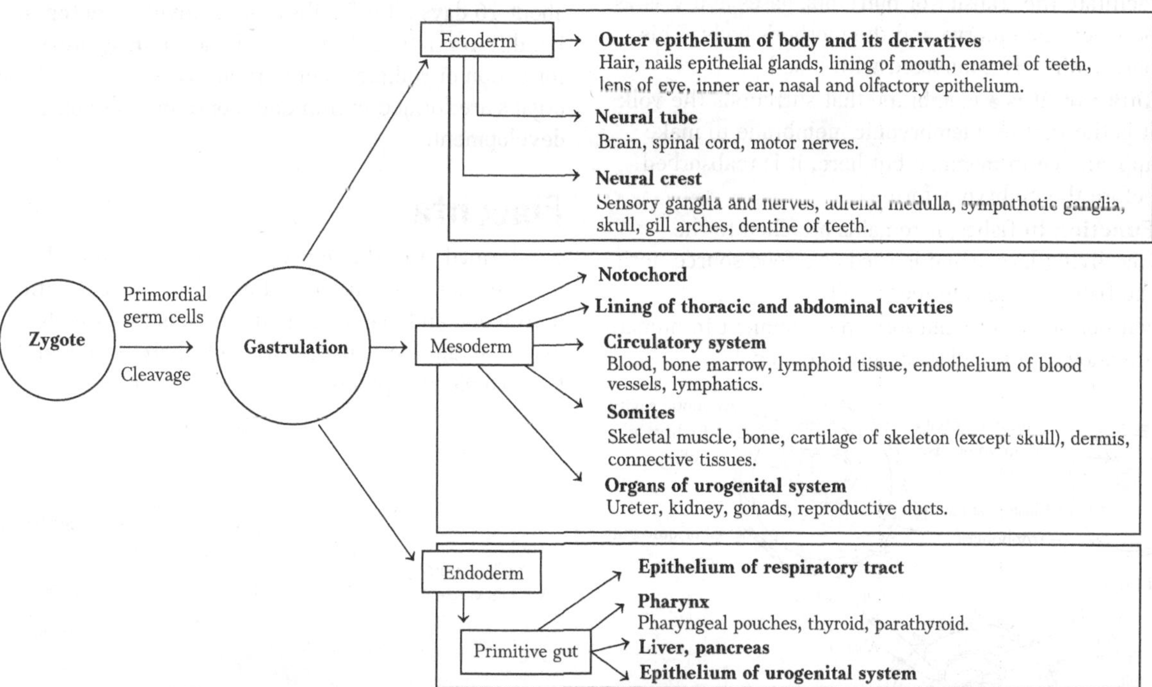

Fig. 3.18 *Derivatives of the primary germ layers in mammals*

Foetal membranes

These are also called **extraembryonic membranes** because these are not a part of the embryo body.

These membranes play some role in the life support of pre-embryo, the embryo and the foetus. These membranes are formed from the trophoblast. The space present between ectoderm and trophoblast is called the amniotic cavity. It is filled with the amniotic fluid.

The four foetal membranes are as follows

(i) **Amnion** It is a thin, fluid (amniotic fluid) filled sac that fully encloses the embryo.
Function It helps to protect the embryo from shocks and adhesion.

(ii) **Allantois** It is a tiny sausage-shaped pouch which arises from the gut of the embryo near the yolk sac.
Function In human, it supplies the blood vessels to the placenta. But in reptiles, birds and egg laying mammals, it helps in the exchange of oxygen and carbon dioxide.

(iii) **Chorion** It lies just beneath the egg shell. It completely encloses the developing embryo and extraembryonic tissues.
Function The chorion is highly specialised to facilitate the transfer of nutrients, gases and wastes between the embryo and the mother's body. This part is directly connected with blood.

(iv) **Yolk sac** It is a membrane that surrounds the yolk. It is the first extraembryonic membrane to make appearance in mammal but here, it is reabsorbed before the embryo is formed.
Function In fishes, it remains attached to the free-living larvae and is used as a food source until the fish can begin to feed itself.
Various stages of embryonic development in humans are shown in the diagram given below

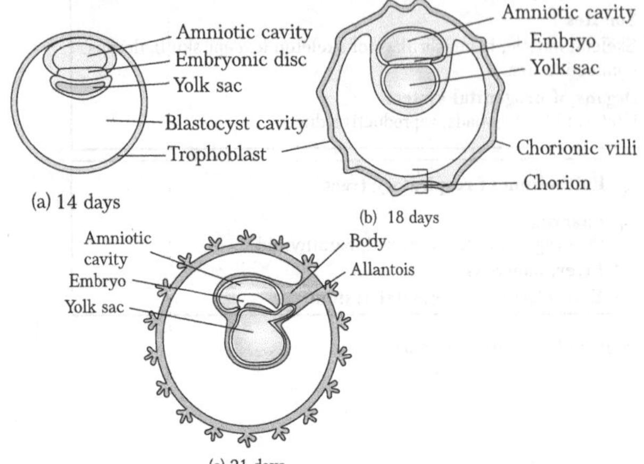

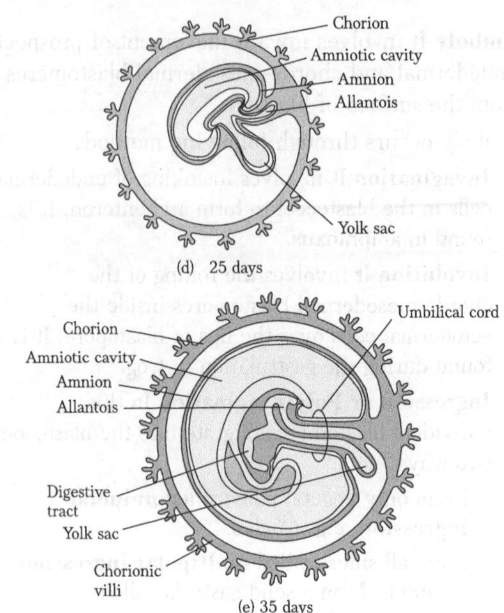

Fig. 3.19 Human embryonic development

Organogenesis

It is the process of development and differentiation of organs and tissues in the embryo. Organogenesis begins about 16 days after fertilisation. It involves **notogenesis,** i.e. differentiation of notochord and **neurogenesis**, i.e. formation of rudiments of nervous system. Most of the organs are formed within one month of embryonic development.

Placenta

It is formed after the implantation of embryo in the uterine wall. This structure formed by the association of both foetal and maternal tissue. It constitutes both maternal and foetal parts, although there is no blending of the two blood supplies.

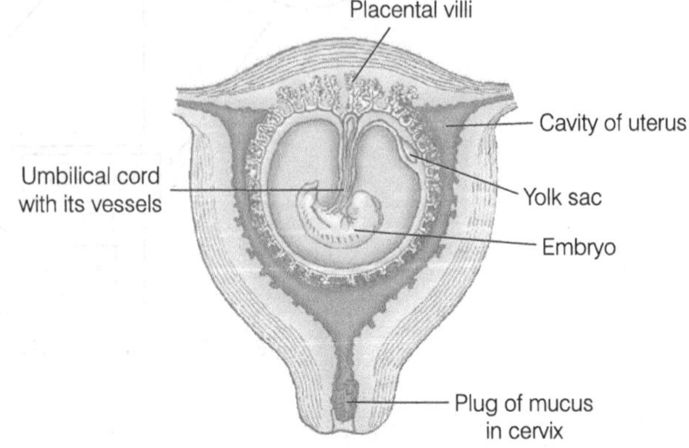

Fig. 3.20 The human foetus within the uterus

Structure

Placenta consists of two parts, (i) **foetal part**, the chorion and (ii) **maternal part**, the decidua basalis.

The human placenta is referred as **chorioallantoic placenta** because chorion and allantois take part in its formation. It also consists of uterine epithelium, uterine connective tissue and endothelium of maternal blood vessels.

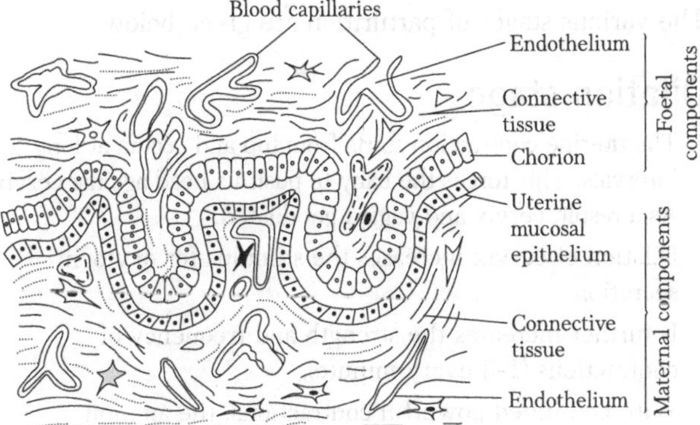

Fig. 3.21 Structure of typical placenta

Types of placenta

1. On the basis of structure, placenta are of following types
   (i) **Epitheliochorial** Placenta with all six barriers between foetal and maternal blood, e.g. horse and ass.
   (ii) **Syndesmochorial** Uterine epithelium breaks down, only five barriers left, e.g. cow, buffalo, sheep, goat and camel.
   (iii) **Endotheliochorial** Uterine epithelium and connective tissue gets eroded, only four barriers left, e.g. tiger, lion, cat and dog.
   (iv) **Haemochorial** Placenta with only three barriers, the maternal part of placenta gets eroded, e.g. human, ape and lemurs.
   (v) **Haemoendothelial** All barriers, except for the endothelium of the foetal part of placenta gets eroded, e.g. rat and rabbit.
2. On the basis of the nature of uterine wall after parturition, the placenta may be categorised as follows
   (i) **Non-deciduous** No part of uterine portion of placenta is broken off, e.g. horse and ass.
   (ii) **Deciduous** A portion of uterine tissue called decidua is detached and passed out at birth, e.g. most of the mammals.
   (iii) **Contra deciduous** Even the foetal part of placenta is retained and gets absorbed to provide nourishment, e.g. *Talpa* and *Perameles.*
3. On the basis of distribution of villi on the surface, placenta are categorised into six types
   (i) **Diffuse placenta** Villi distributed uniformly all over the surface, e.g. horse and pig.
   (ii) **Cotyledonary** Villi form tufts which fit into the corresponding caruncles, in the uterine part of placenta, e.g. cow, buffalo and sheep.
   (iii) **Intermediate** Villi occur singly as well as in tufts, e.g. camel and giraffe.
   (iv) **Zonary** Villi arranged in two transverse bands, e.g. tiger, lion, cat, dog and elephant.
   (v) **Discoidal** Villi are confined to a disc-like area, e.g. rat, rabbit and bat.
   (vi) **Metadiscoidal** Villi are initially distributed uniformly all over the surface. Later on, villi get confined to a disc-like area fitting into a corresponding depression on the uterine wall. In this, the placenta diffuses at first, but later on becomes discoidal, e.g. human beings and apes.

Functions of placenta

- It transports nutrients from maternal blood stream into the foetus.
- It helps in exchange of gases between mother and foetus, elimination of nitrogenous discharge and other wastes from foetus.
- Placenta acts as an endocrine gland and synthesises large quantities of proteins and some hormones. These include human Chorionic Gonadotropin (hCG), chorionic thyrotropin, chorionic corticotropin, chorionic somatomammotropin, oestrogens and progesterone.
- It secretes relaxin hormone that facilitates parturition by softening the connective tissue of the pubic symphysis for easy childbirth.

Note *Placenta and umbilical cord are rich sources of stem cells. These cells can be stored and preserved through placenta banking.*

Teratogens

During the first trimester of pregnancy, the basic structure of the baby is formed. During this period, the developing baby, called **foetus** is very sensitive to viral infection of the mother, e.g. measles or exposure to certain chemicals such as drugs, alcohols, etc., These may cause malformations in the developing embryo. Such agents are called teratogens (monster forming agents). They cause miscarriage or abortion in the first trimester. By three months, all the systems of the baby have been formed, at least in a rudimentary way. From then on, the development of the foetus is primarily a matter of growth and minor structural modifications.

Pregnancy or Gestation period

The time period during which the embryo remains in the uterus, i.e. the time from conception to the day of parturition (birth of a baby) is known as gestation period. In human, this period is about 280 days (9 month + 10 days).

Table 3.7 Average gestation period in some mammals

Mammals	Gestation periods	Mammals	Gestation periods
Elephant	620 days	Human	280 days
Rhinoceros	560 days	Lion	106 days
Giraffe	450 days	Panther	93 days
Camel	395 days	Dog	50-60 days
Horse	330 days	Rat	20 days
Cow	280 days		

PARTURITION

The act of giving birth to a baby is called parturition. Progesterone is called **pregnancy hormone** because it is required continually during entire period of gestation or pregnancy.

The mechanism of parturition is explained in stepwise manner below

- Parturition is induced by a complex neuroendocrine mechanism.
- The signals for parturition originate from the fully developed foetus and the placenta.
- It induces mild uterine contractions called **foetal-ejection reflex.**
- The simulatory reflex between the uterine contraction and oxytocin secretion result in stronger contraction. It results in the expulsion of the baby. The most common method by which a baby comes out during parturition is left anterior oblique. In this position, the head comes out first during vaginal birth.

Stages of parturition

The various stages of parturition are given below

Dilation stage

- The uterine contraction starts from top and occurs at long intervals. This forces the baby to push its head against cervix. As a result, cervix and vagina get dilated.
- Dilation of cervix increases the stimulus for oxytocin secretion.
- It further increases the strength and frequency of contractions (1-3 every minute).
- With continued powerful contractions, the amnion ruptures and the amniotic fluid flows out through the vagina.

Expulsion stage

- With further increase in the intensity of uterine and abdominal contraction, the baby comes out through cervix and vagina. It may take 20-60 min.
- Umbilical cord is cut after the expulsion of newborn. Within 10-15 min after delivery, the placenta and the remains of the umbilical cord are expelled out. It is called after birth.

The summary of pregnancy in humans in different weeks is given in the table below

Table 3.8 Summary of human pregnancy from fertilisation to birth of the baby

Week 1	Week 2	Week 3
Fertilisation, cleavage to form a blastocyst (4-5 days after fertilisation), implantation (6-9 days after fertilisation).	The three basic layers of the embryo developed are, ectoderm, mesoderm and endoderm. No research allowed on human embryos beyond this stage.	Woman does not mensurate. This may be the first sign that she is pregnant. Beginnings of the backbone, neural tube develops, the beginning of the brain and spinal cord (first organs). Embryo about 2 mm long.
Week 4	**Week 5**	**Week 6**
Heart, blood vessels, blood and gut start forming. Umbilical cord developing. Embryo about 5 mm long.	Brain developing. 'Limb buds', small swellings forms, which are the beginnings of the arms and legs. Heart is a large tube and starts to beat, pumping blood. This can be seen on an ultrasound scan. Embryo about 8 mm long.	Eyes and ears start to form.

Week 7	Week 12	Week 20
All major internal organs developing. Face forming. Eyes have some colour. Mouth and tongue. Beginnings of hands and feet. Foetus is 17 mm long.	Foetus fully formed, with all organs, muscles, bones, toes and fingers. Sex organs well-developed. Foetus is moving. For the rest of the gestation period, it is mainly growing in size. Foetus is 56 mm long from head to bottom. Legal limit for abortion in most circumstances.	Hair beginning to grow, including eyebrows and eyelashes. Fingerprints developed. Finger nails and toe nails growing. Firm hand grip. Between 16 and 20 weeks baby usually felt moving for the first time. Baby is 160 mm long from head to bottom.
Week 24	**Week 26**	**Week 28**
Eyelids open.	Baby has a good chance of survival if born prematurely.	Baby moving vigorously. Responds to touch and loud noises. Swallowing amniotic fluid and urinating.
Week 30	**40 weeks** (9 months)	
Baby usually lying head down, ready for birth. Baby is 240 mm from head to bottom.	Birth	

LACTATION

The production and release of milk from the mammary glands of mother after the birth of baby is called lactation. The first milk which comes out from the mother's mammary glands just after childbirth is known as **colostrum.**

Colostrum is rich in proteins and energy but the fat content is almost negligible . It also contains antibodies that provide passive immunity to the newborn infant. Milk synthesis is stimulated by pituitary hormone, prolactin.

Milk contains inhibitory peptides which accumulate and inhibit milk production, if the breasts are not fully emptied.

CHECK POINT 3.4

1. Sperm of animal species *A* cannot fertilise ovum of species *B* because
   (a) fertilizin of *A* and antifertilizin of *B* are not
   (b) antifertilizin of *A* and fertilizin of *B* are not compatible
   (c) fertilizin of *A* and *B* are not compatible
   (d) antifertilizin of *A* and *B* are not compatible
2. What is true about cleavage in the fertilised egg in humans?
   (a) It is meroblastic
   (b) It starts while the egg is in Fallopian tube
   (c) It is identical to the normal mitosis
   (d) It starts when the egg reaches in uterus
3. Embryologists can presume the future organs of the embryo in
   (a) blastula (b) gastrulation
   (c) 32-celled stage (d) 64-celled stage
4. The 'cells of Rauber' are
   (a) secretory cells of endometrium in uterus
   (b) inner mass of blastocoel
   (c) outer cells of trophoblast in contact with uterine wall
   (d) cells of trophoblast, in contact with inner cell mass of blastocyst
5. After gastrulation, the roof of archenteron is formed by
   (a) neural plate
   (b) mesoderm
   (c) ectoderm
   (d) chorda-mesoderm
6. The foetal membrane which is the source of first blood corpuscle to enter the circulation of embryo is called
   (a) amnion (b) chorion
   (c) trophoblast (d) yolk sac

EXAM POINTS

- The testes of humans are situated outside the abdominal cavity inside a pouch called scrotum to maintain the scrotal temperature lower than the internal body temperature. **[CBSE AIPMT 2011]**
- LH acts on Sertoli cells and stimulates the process of spermiogenesis. **[Karnataka CET 2015]**
- The correct sequence for transport of sperm cells in male reproductive system is Seminiferous tubule → Rete testis → Vasa efferentia → Epididymis → Vas deferens → Ejaculatory duct → Urethra → Urethral meatus. **[NEET 2019, 2016]**
- In spermiogenesis, spermatozoa are formed while in spermiation, spermatozoa are released from Sertoli cells into the cavity of seminiferous tubule. **[NEET 2018]**
- Spermatogonia during gametogenesis is normally diploid. **[CBSE AIPMT 2015]**
- Number of chromosomes present in spermatogonium is 46. **[JIPMER 2019]**
- Number of chromosomes present in secondary spermatocyte is 23. **[JIPMER 2019]**
- The correct sequence of sperm formation is Spermatogonia → Spermatocytes → Spermatid → Spermatozoa. **[NEET 2013]**
- The main function of the fimbrae of the Fallopian tube in female is to help in the collection of the ovum. **[Kerala CEE 2011]**
- Fertilisation in human is practically feasible only if the ovum and sperms are transported simultaneously to ampullary-isthmic junction of the Fallopian tube. **[NEET 2016]**
- Extrusion of second polar body from egg nucleus occurs after the entry of sperm, but before fertilisation. **[NEET 2019]**
- Graafian follicle of ovary in mammals acts as an endocrine gland after ovulation. **[AIIMS 2017]**
- Level of LH is maximum at the time of ovulation. **[JIPMER 2019]**
- Menstrual flow occurs due to lack of progesterone. **[NEET 2013, BHU 2012]**
- During menstrual cycle, the cyclic changes take place in endometrium. **[Karnataka CET 2015]**
- Corpus luteum releases progesterone. **[DUMET 2011]**
- The secretion of corpus luteum prepares the inner wall of uterus for implantation. **[UP CPMT 2012]**
- Formation of corpus luteum is induced by LH. **[JIPMER 2018]**
- The secretory phase in the human menstrual cycle is also called as luteal phase and it lasts for about 13 days. **[JIPMER 2017]**
- No new follicles develop in the luteal phase of the menstrual cycle because both FSH and LH level are low. **[NEET 2019]**
- Capacitation refers to changes in the sperm before fertilisation. **[CBSE AIPMT 2015]**
- Capacitation of sperm occurs in female reproductive tract. **[NEET 2017]**
- In humans, cleavage divisions are slow and synchronous. **[DUMET 2011]**
- Gastrulation is the process where the cell moves to occupy their definite position. **[UP CPMT 2011]**
- Gastrulation involves the formation of three germ layers. **[JIPMER 2019]**
- The amnion of mammalian embryo is derived from ectoderm and mesoderm. **[NEET 2018]**
- Structure analogous to the placenta in mammals is chorion. **[JIPMER 2019]**
- Hormones secreted by the placenta to maintain pregnancy are hCG, hPL, progesterone, oestrogen. **[NEET 2018]**
- Changes in GnRH pulse frequency in females is controlled by circulating levels of oestrogen and progesterone. **[NEET-I 2016]**
- Signal for parturition originates from both placenta as well as fully developed foetus. **[CBSE AIPMT 2012]**
- Oxytocin hormone is responsible for both the milk ejection reflex and the foetal-ejection reflex. **[NEET 2019]**
- Colostrum, the yellowish fluid secreted by mother during the initial days of lactation is very essential to impart the immunity to the infants because it contains immunoglobin-A. **[NEET 2019]**

Chapter Exercises

(A) Topical Exercise

Male Reproductive System

1 In humans, the testes are located in
(a) abdominal cavity (b) thoracic cavity
(c) extra-abdominal cavity (d) pericardial cavity

2 Temperature in scrotum necessary for sperm formation should be
(a) 2°C above the body temperature
(b) 2°C below the body temperature
(c) 7°C above the body temperature
(d) 7°C below the body temperature

3 The role of Leydig cells of testis is
(a) to provide nourishment to sperms
(b) synthesis of testosterone hormone
(c) to provide motility to sperm
(d) to bring about maturation of sperms

4 The seminiferous tubules open into ...*A*... through ...*B*... .

	A	*B*
(a)	vasa efferentia	epididymis
(b)	testicular tubules	epididymis
(c)	vasa efferentia	rete testis
(d)	rete testis	vasa efferentia

5. The regions just outside the seminiferous tubules contain
(a) small blood vessels, but lack interstitial cells
(b) cells which secrete testosterone
(c) cells which get stimulated by LH of pituitary gland
(d) Both (b) and (c)

6. In which of the following structures, sperms undergo maturation?
(a) Epididymis
(b) Seminiferous tubules
(c) Vasa efferentia
(d) Rete testis

7 Consider the following statements.
I. Vasa efferentia connect the testis with epididymis.
II. They have large columnar ciliated cells and small non-ciliated cells.
Choose the correct option.
(a) Statement I is true, but II is false
(b) Statement I is false, but II is true
(c) Both statements I and II are true
(d) Both statements I and II are false

8 Which of the following options is/are correct about male reproductive system?
(a) The head of epididymis is called caput epididymis
(b) Epididymis and seminal vesicle are paired structures
(c) Both (a) and (b)
(d) The head of epididymis is called output epididymis

9 Consider the following statements.
I. Vas deferens receives a duct from the seminal vesicle and opens into urethra as ejaculatory duct.
II. It stores and transports sperms.
Choose the correct option.
(a) Statement I is true, but II is false
(b) Statement I is false, but II is true
(c) Both statements I and II are true
(d) Both statements I and II are false

10 Glands of male reproductive system are
(a) prostate and seminal vesicles
(b) prostate, Bartholin's glands and corpus luteum
(c) vestibular gland and Bartholin's glands
(d) prostate, Cowper's glands and seminal vesicles

11 Consider the following statements.
I. Prostate secretions inactivate sperm.
II. In most mammals, testis is located in the scrotal sac.
Choose the correct option.
(a) Statement I is true, but II is false
(b) Statement I is false, but II is true
(c) Both statements I and II are true
(d) Both statements I and II are false

12 Which of the following is a part of mammalian male reproductive system?
(a) Vas deferens (b) Cowper's gland
(c) Both (a) and (b) (d) Fallopian tube

13 The parts of male urethra are
(a) corpora cavernosa, ventral corpus spongiosum
(b) prostatic, membranous and penile
(c) seminal vesicles, prostate and Cowper's gland
(d) prostate, Bulbourethral and Cowper's gland

14 Match the following columns.

	Column I		Column II
A.	Male reproductive organ	1.	Semen
B.	Site of sperm maturation and storage	2.	Seminiferous tubules
C.	Unit of testis	3.	Testis
D.	Substance containing sperm and other secretions	4.	Epididymis

Codes

	A	B	C	D		A	B	C	D
(a)	3	1	2	4	(b)	1	2	3	4
(c)	3	4	2	1	(d)	4	3	1	2

15 Gubernaculum cords is a contractile structure that
(a) pulls down the testis during breeding season into the scrotal sac
(b) allows daily migration of the testis from the abdominal cavity into the scrotum
(c) facilitates ejaculation of spermatozoa from the testis
(d) keeps the testis in position

16 In man, the sperms released from the testis take the following route to reach the ureter.
(a) Vasa efferentia → Bidder's canal → Uriniferous tubules → Nephrostome
(b) Vasa efferentia → Epididymis → Vas deferens → Urethra
(c) Vasa efferentia → Bidder's canal → Nephrostome
(d) Vasa efferentia → Collecting tubules → Bidder's canal

17 Which of these pairs is mismatched?
(a) Interstitial cells – Testosterone
(b) Seminiferous tubules – Sperm production
(c) Vasa deferentia – Seminal fluid production
(d) Urethra – Conducts sperm

18 Cryptorchidism is the condition in man when
(a) there are two testes in each scrotum
(b) testes do not descent into the scrotum
(c) testes enlarge in the scrotum
(d) testes degenerate in the scrotum

19 Orchidectomy is
(a) surgical removal of testes
(b) surgical removal of ovaries
(c) inflammation of testes
(d) non-descent of testes in scrotum

Female Reproductive System

20 Identify the parts as *A*, *B*, *C* and *D* in the given diagram.

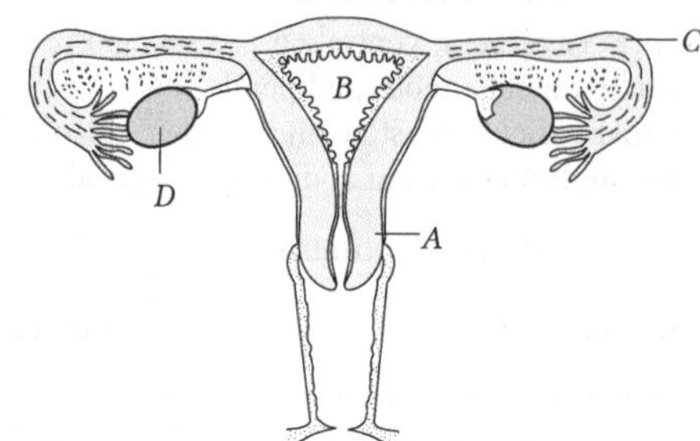

(a) *A*-Oviduct, *B*-Uterus, *C*-Oviduct, *D*-Ovary
(b) *A*-Cervix, *B*-Uterus, *C*-Ovary, *D*-Tumour
(c) *A*-Uterus, *B*-Uterine cavity, *C*-Oviducal funnel, *D*-Ovary
(d) *A*-Cervix, *B*-Uterine cavity, *C*-Fallopian tube, *D*-Ovary

21 Which of the following statements is incorrect?
(a) Each ovary is about 2-4 cm in length and is connected to the pelvic wall and uterus by ligaments
(b) Each ovary is covered by a thin epithelium which encloses the ovarian stroma
(c) Ovaries do not produce any steroid hormones
(d) The stroma of ovary is divided into a peripheral cortex and an inner medulla

22 The part of Fallopian tube near uterus is called ...*A*... and near the ovary is called ...*B*... .

	A	*B*
(a)	Uterus	Isthmus
(b)	Cervical canal	Isthmus
(c)	Isthmus	Ampulla
(d)	Isthmus	Infundibulum

23 Match the following columns.

	Column I		Column II
A.	Oviduct	1.	Narrow lumen
B.	Isthmus	2.	Womb
C.	Uterus	3.	Fallopian tube
D.	Infundibulum	4.	Funnel-shaped

Codes

	A	B	C	D
(a)	1	4	3	2
(b)	2	1	3	4
(c)	3	1	2	4
(d)	4	2	1	3

24 Which of the following statements is false for uterus?
(a) It is also called womb and its shape is like an inverted pear
(b) It is supported by ligaments attached to the pelvic wall
(c) It opens into oviducts through cervix whose cavity is called cervical canal
(d) It is bounded by three layers, outer perimetrium, middle myometrium and inner endometrium

25 Match the following columns.

	Column I (Layers of uterus)		Column I (Features)
A.	Perimetrium	1.	Inner glandular layer of uterus
B.	Endometrium	2.	External thin membrane of uterus
C.	Myometrium	3.	Middle thick membrane of uterus

Codes

	A	B	C		A	B	C
(a)	2	1	3	(b)	1	2	3
(c)	3	2	1	(d)	3	1	2

26 Bartholin's glands of female correspond to which glands in male?
(a) Cowper's glands
(b) Inguinal glands
(c) Rectal glands
(d) Prostate glands

27 Bartholin's glands are situated
(a) on either side of vagina in human
(b) on either side of vas deferens in human
(c) on the sides of the head of some amphibians
(d) at the reduced tail end of birds

28 Consider the following statements.
I. Vulva consists of the external genital organs of a woman.
II. The vulva includes mons pubis, labia majora, labia minora, clitoris and hymen.
Choose the correct option.
(a) Statement I is true, but II is false
(b) Statement I is false, but II is true
(c) Both statements I and II are true
(d) Both statements I and II are false

29 Find out the correct pathway of milk flow in the breast.
I. Mammary duct
II. Lactiferous duct
III. Mammary tubules
IV. Alveoli lumen
V. Mammary ampulla
(a) IV $\rightarrow$ III $\rightarrow$ V $\rightarrow$ I $\rightarrow$ II
(b) III $\rightarrow$ I $\rightarrow$ IV $\rightarrow$ II $\rightarrow$ V
(c) IV $\rightarrow$ III $\rightarrow$ I $\rightarrow$ V $\rightarrow$ II
(d) IV $\rightarrow$ III $\rightarrow$ II $\rightarrow$ I $\rightarrow$ V

Gametogenesis

30 Which one is not associated with gametogenesis?
(a) Formation of ova
(b) Formation of spermatids
(c) Release of ova
(d) Change of spermatid to spermatozoa

31 Primordial germ cells are present in the
(a) seminiferous tubules (b) epididymis
(c) seminal vesicles (d) prostate glands

32 Which one is correct?
(a) Meiosis-I occurs in primary spermatocyte
(b) Meiosis-I occurs in secondary spermatocyte
(c) Meiosis-I takes place in spermatids
(d) Meiosis-II occurs in spermatids

33 In human, at the end of the first meiotic division, the male germ cells differentiate into the
(a) primary spermatocytes (b) secondary spermatocytes
(c) spermatids (d) spermatogonia

34 The number of sperm(s) formed from one secondary spermatocyte is ...*A*... whereas the number of ovum/ova formed from one secondary oocyte is ...*B*...

	A	*B*		*A*	*B*
(a)	2	1	(b)	3	1
(c)	1	2	(d)	4	1

35 The acrosome of sperm is formed from
(a) centrosome of spermatid
(b) nucleus of spermatid
(c) Golgi complex of spermatid
(d) mitochondria of spermatid

36 Consider the following statements.
I. Human sperm cells move by means of a flagellum.
II. Centrioles of sperm control the movement of tail.
Choose the correct option.
(a) Statement I is true, but II is false
(b) Statement I is false, but II is true
(c) Both statements I and II are true
(d) Both statements I and II are false

37 Consider the following statements.
I. The head of sperm contains material which helps in sex-determination in foetus.
II. The function of mitochondria in sperm is to provide energy for the movement of sperm.
Choose the correct option.
(a) Statement I is true, but II is false
(b) Statement I is false, but II is true
(c) Both statements I and II are true
(d) Both statements I and II are false

38 A cross-section at the midpoint of the middle piece of a human sperm shows
(a) centriole, mitochondria and 9 + 2 arrangement of microtubules
(b) centriole and mitochondria
(c) mitochondria and 9 + 2 arrangement of microtubules
(d) 9 + 2 arrangement of microtubules only

39 In oogenesis, when a diploid cell in the ovary undergoes meiosis, how many ova results?
(a) 1 (b) 2 (c) 3 (d) 4

40 Which of the following statements is not correct for oogonia?
(a) They are million gamete mother cells
(b) They are formed within each foetal ovary
(c) They are formed throughout the life of female
(d) They start division and get arrested at prophase-I of meiotic division

41 Polar bodies formed during the formation of oocytes are
(a) smaller cells formed due to unequal meiosis of oocyte
(b) structures which bud off during oogenesis
(c) structures formed during spermatogenesis
(d) daughter cells formed after mitosis

42 What is the advantage of unequal cell division (meiosis) during the formation of ovum?
(a) Mature ovum retains most of the cytoplasm
(b) Retention of more cytoplasm in ovum provides it with ample nutrients during development
(c) Retention of more cytoplasm in ovum allow it to survive for long duration
(d) more than one option is correct

43 Human females possess 44+XX chromosomes. The secondary oocyte shall have
(a) 44 + XX (b) 22 + XX
(c) 22 (d) 44

Menstrual Cycle

44 Stages in menstrual cycle are
(a) recovery and proliferative phase only
(b) proliferative and secretory phase only
(c) proliferative, secretory and menstrual phase
(d) recovery, secretory and phase of menstrual flow

45 Match the following columns.

	Column I		Column II
A.	Menstrual phase	1.	Day 15-28
B.	Luteal phase	2.	Day 1-5
C.	Ovulation	3.	Day 1-13
D.	Follicular phase	4.	Day 14

Codes

	A	B	C	D		A	B	C	D
(a)	2	4	1	3	(b)	2	1	4	3
(c)	1	3	2	4	(d)	2	1	3	4

46 Choose the incorrect statement for the hormones *A*, *B*, *C* and *D* is graph shown. These hormones include oestrogen, Luteinizing hormone, progesterone and follicle stimulating hormone.

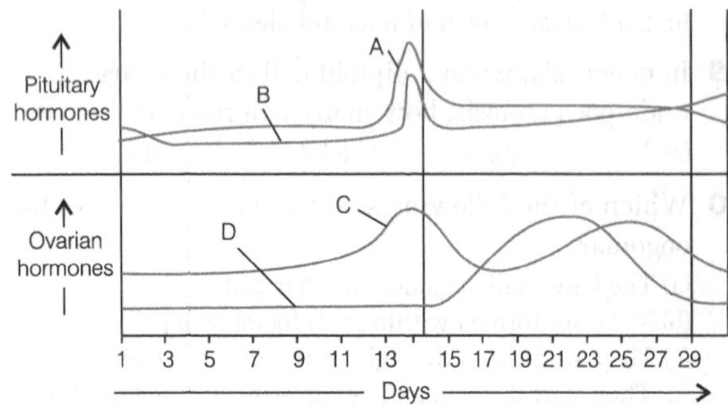

(a) At menopause, there is a rise in the urinary excretion of *B*
(b) *D* is secreted by corpus luteum
(c) *B* stimulates the secretion of *C*
(d) *A* which is steroidal hormone causes ovulation

47 Correct sequence of hormone secretion from beginning of menstruation is
(a) FSH → Progesterone → Oestrogen
(b) Oestrogen → FSH → Progesterone
(c) FSH → Oestrogen → Progesterone
(d) Progesterone → FSH → Oestrogen

48 Consider the following statements.
I. One ovum is released (ovulation) during the middle of each menstrual cycle.
II. Menstruation is repeated at an average interval of about 28 days.

Choose the correct option.
(a) Statement I is true, but II is false
(b) Statement I is false, but II is true
(c) Both statements I and II are true
(d) Both statements I and II are false

49 Consider the following statements.
I. The menstrual phase is followed by the follicular phase.
II. The changes in the ovary and uterus during menstrual cycle are induced by the changes in the levels of ovarian hormones only.

Choose the correct option.
(a) Statement I is true, but II is false
(b) Statement I is false, but II is true
(c) Both statements I and II are true
(d) Both statements I and II are false

50 Yellow corpus luteum occurs in mammals in
(a) heart to initiate heartbeat
(b) skin to function as pain receptor
(c) brain and connects cerebral hemispheres
(d) ovary for the secretion of progesterone

51 Follicle Stimulating Hormone (FSH)
(a) is secreted by females, but not males
(b) stimulates the seminiferous tubules to produce sperm
(c) secretion is controlled by Gonadotropic Releasing Hormone (GnRH)
(d) Both (b) and (c)

52 Which of the following is correct for a typical menstrual cycle?
(a) Endometrium regenerates between 5th-10th day
(b) Rise in the level of progesterone occur after 15th day
(c) Both (a) and (b)
(d) Rise in the level of oestrogen in the first 5 days

53 Consider the following statements.
I. Both LH and FSH attain a peak level in the middle of cycle, i.e. about 24th day.
II. Rapid secretion of LH leading to its maximum level during the mid-cycle called 'LH-surge' induces rupture of Graafian follicle and thereby, ovulation.

Choose the correct option.
(a) Statement I is true, but II is false
(b) Statement I is false, but II is true
(c) Both statements I and II are true
(d) Both statements I and II are false

54 Which one of the following events is correctly matched with the time period in a normal menstrual cycle?
(a) Release of egg : 5th day
(b) Endometrium regenerates : 5-10 days
(c) Endometrium secretes nutrients for implantation 11-18 days
(d) Rise in progesterone level : 1 - 15 days

55 If pregnancy does not occur, the corpus luteum will disintegrate and turn into
(a) corpus albicans
(b) corpus allatum
(c) corpus callosum
(d) corpus cavernosum

56 Which one of the following is the correct matching of the events occurring during menstrual cycle?

(a)	Ovulation	–	LH and FSH attain peak level and sharp fall in the secretion of progesterone
(b)	Proliferative	–	Rapid regeneration of myometrium and maturation of Graafian follicle
(c)	Development of corpus luteum	–	Secretory phase and increased secretion of progesterone
(d)	Menstruation	–	Breakdown of myometrium and ovum not fertilised

Fertilisation, Embryonic Development and Implantation

57 Fertilisation is depicted by the condition
(a) $n \rightarrow 2n$
(b) $2n \rightarrow 3n$
(c) $2n \rightarrow 4n$
(d) $4n \rightarrow 8n$

58 Fertilisation is the fusion of
(a) diploid spermatozoan with diploid ovum to form diploid zygote
(b) haploid spermatozoan with diploid ovum to form diploid zygote
(c) diploid spermatozoan with haploid ovum to form diploid zygote
(d) haploid spermatozoan with haploid ovum to form diploid zygote

59 Which of the following statements is incorrect?
(a) Fertilisation occurs in Fallopian tube
(b) Fertilisation is mechanical events
(c) Cleavage produces morula
(d) None of the above

60 The initial step in the activation of ovum during the process of fertilisation is the
(a) penetration of sperm in the egg
(b) fertilizin-antifertilizin reaction
(c) formation of the fertilisation cone
(d) formation of fertilisation membrane

61 During fertilisation, a sperm comes in contact with the zona pellucida layer of the ovum and induces changes in the membrane that block the entry of ...*A*... . The secretions of the ...*B*... help the sperm to enter into the cytoplasm of ovum.

	A	*B*
(a)	eggs	zona pellucida
(b)	eggs	acrosome
(c)	additional sperms	acrosome
(d)	additional sperms	zona pellucida

62 Capacitation of sperm in mammals involves
(a) sperm size change
(b) acrosome reaction
(c) nuclear chromatin change
(d) mitochondrial alignment

63 Arrange the events of fertilisation sequentially.
I. Acrosomal reaction
II. Karyogamy
III. Entry of sperm into egg cytoplasm
IV. Completion of meiosis-II in ovum
V. Zygote formation

Choose the correct option.
(a) I $\rightarrow$ II $\rightarrow$ III $\rightarrow$ V $\rightarrow$ IV
(b) II $\rightarrow$ I $\rightarrow$ III $\rightarrow$ V $\rightarrow$ IV
(c) I $\rightarrow$ III $\rightarrow$ II $\rightarrow$ IV $\rightarrow$ V
(d) I $\rightarrow$ III $\rightarrow$ IV $\rightarrow$ II $\rightarrow$ V

64 The second maturation division of the mammalian ovum occurs
(a) in the Graafian follicle following the first maturation division
(b) shortly after ovulation before the ovum makes entry into the Fallopian tube
(c) until after the ovum has been penetrated by a sperm
(d) until the nucleus of the sperm has fused with that of the ovum

65 If a sperm enters an ovum, the entry of other sperms is prevented by the
(a) formation of fertilisation membrane
(b) formation of vitelline membrane
(c) Both (a) and (b)
(d) secretion of endolysin by sperms

66 The function of hyaluronidase in fertilisation is
(a) to form cone of reception in egg
(b) to puncture the vitelline membrane of egg
(c) to inactivate the neighbouring sperms
(d) None of the above

67 A change in ova after sperm penetration is
(a) formation of first polar body
(b) meiosis-I start
(c) meiosis-II start
(d) formation of second polar body

68 Match the following columns.

	Column I		Column I
A.	Acrosin	1.	Dissolves corona radiata
B.	Corona penetrating enzyme	2.	Dissolves cementing material between the corona radiata cells
C.	Hyaluronidase	3.	Digests zona pellucida

Codes

	A	B	C		A	B	C
(a)	3	2	1	(b)	1	2	3
(c)	2	1	3	(d)	3	1	2

69 Animals which possess cleidoic eggs exhibit
(a) external fertilisation and internal development
(b) internal fertilisation and internal development
(c) internal fertilisation and external development
(d) external fertilisation and external development

70 Cleavage differs from mitosis because in cleavage,
(a) there is no growth phase
(b) consumption of oxygen increases
(c) nucleo cytoplasmic ratio increases
(d) All of the above

71 Which one of the following statements with regard to embryonic development in human is correct?
(a) Cleavage divisions bring about considerable increase in the mass of protoplasm
(b) In the second cleavage division, one of the two blastomeres usually divides a little sooner than the second
(c) With more cleavage divisions, the resultant blastomeres become larger and larger
(d) Cleavage division results in a hollow ball of cells called morula

72 Consider the following statements.
I. Cleavage starts while the egg is still in the Fallopian tube.
II. The resultant daughter cells of cleavage are blastomere.

Choose the correct option.
(a) Statement I is true, but II is false
(b) Statement I is false, but II is true
(c) Both statements I and II are true
(d) Both statements I and II are false

73 Implantation of the blastocyst occurs
(a) just prior to conception
(b) one week after fertilisation
(c) at one month's gestation
(d) just prior to birth

74 Study and identify the given structure represents

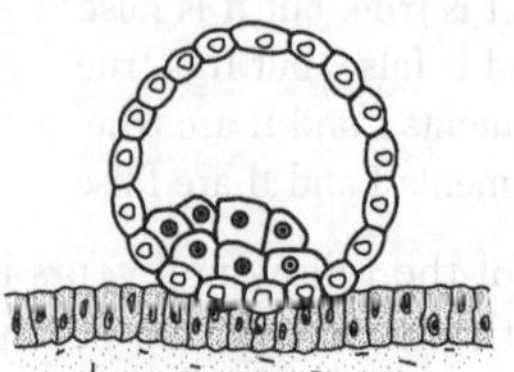

(a) morula (b) zygote (c) blastocyst (d) gastrula

75 Consider the following statements.
I. Zona pellucida remains intact throughout the cleavage divisions.
II. Cleavage results in a solid ball of cells called morula with eight to sixteen cells.

Choose the correct option.
(a) Statement I is true, but II is false
(b) Statement I is false, but II is true
(c) Both statements I and II are true
(d) Both statements I and II are false

76 Arrange the events of embryo formation sequentially.
I. Blastocyst II. Mature embryo
III. Morula IV. Zygotic cleavage
V. Blastomere

Choose the correct option.
(a) IV → III → I → V → II
(b) V → II → I → III → IV
(c) IV → III → V → I → II
(d) IV → V → III → I → II

77 Study the chart given below.

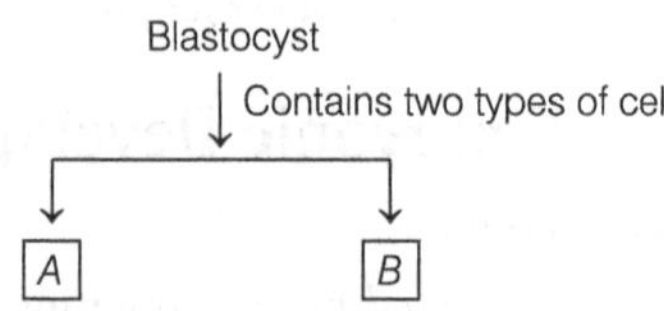

Select the option that correctly identify *A* and *B*.
(a) *A*-Trophoblast, *B*-Inner cell mass
(b) *A*-Placenta, *B*-Embryoblast
(c) *A*-Placenta, *B*-Trophoblast
(d) None of the above

Gastrulation and Organogenesis

78 Consider the following statements.
I. Gastrulation is the early phase in the embryonic development during which the blastula is reorganised into multilayered gastrula.
II. Cavity of gastrula is archenteron.

Choose the correct option.
(a) Statement I is true, but II is false
(b) Statement I is false, but II is true
(c) Both statements I and II are true
(d) Both statements I and II are false

79 Termination of gastrulation is marked by
(a) obliteration of archenteron
(b) closure of neural tube
(c) obliteration of blastocoel
(d) None of the above

80 Primary germ layers are
(a) trophoblast, ectoderm, mesoderm and endoderm
(b) endoderm, trophoectoderm and trophomesoderm
(c) trophomesoderm and trophoectoderm
(d) ectoderm, mesoderm and endoderm

81 Match the following columns with respect to germ layers.

	Column I		Column I
A.	Ectoderm	1.	Muscles, skeleton, heart, kidney, gonads
B.	Mesoderm	2.	Nervous system, skin
C.	Endoderm	3.	Respiratory organs and midgut

Codes

	A	B	C		A	B	C
(a)	1	2	3	(b)	2	1	3
(c)	3	2	1	(d)	2	3	1

82 Which of these pairs is mismatched?
(a) Brain – Ectoderm
(b) Gut – Endoderm
(c) Bone – Mesoderm
(d) Lens – Endoderm

83 Mesoderm proliferates from
(a) trophoblast
(b) cephalic end of embryonic disc
(c) caudal end of embryonic disc
(d) ectoderm of embryonic disc

84 Presumptive ectoderm is that
(a) layer which presumably is ectoderm
(b) layer which may or may not develop into ectoderm
(c) area around the margin of the blastopore which rolls into the interior of the embryo, thus forming the lining of primitive gut
(d) None of the above

85 All of the following structure are ectodermal except one, which is mesodermal. Identify that structure
(a) epithelium of retina (b) optic nerve
(c) eye lens (d) ciliary body

86 Identify the correctly matched pair/pairs of the germ layers and their derivatives.
I. Ectoderm – Epidermis
II. Endoderm – Pineal gland
III. Mesoderm – Muscles
IV. Mesoderm – Cartilage
V. Endoderm – Enamel of teeth

Choose the option containing the correctly matched pairs.
(a) I and IV (b) I and II
(c) I, III and IV (d) I, II, III and V

87 Vitellogenesis is the process of formation of
(a) vitelline membrane around the developing egg cells
(b) yolk sac membrane around the yolk mass during the development of reptiles and birds
(c) yolk and its deposition within the growing oocyte of amphibians
(d) archenteron around the egg cells

88 Arrange the foetal membrane from outside to inside
I. Amnion II. Allantois
III. Chorion

Codes
(a) III → II → I (b) III → I → II
(c) II → I → III (d) I → II → III

89 Identify the correct statement(s) for placenta.
(a) It facilitates the supply of O_2 and nutrients to embryo
(b) It is connected to embryo through umbilical cord
(c) It removes CO_2 and excretory material produced by embryo
(d) All of the above

90 In human, the placenta develops from the chorion. This indicates that human development
(a) resembles that of the chick
(b) is associated with extraembryonic membranes
(c) cannot be compared to the development of lower animals
(d) Both (a) and (b)

91 The first movement of the foetus and appearance of hair on the head are usually observed during which month of pregnancy?
(a) 3rd month (b) 9th month
(c) 2nd month (d) 5th month

Parturition and Lactation

92 Why are contractions necessary during birth?
(a) So that the mother will know that the baby is about to arrive
(b) Vagina will expand to accept the baby
(c) Ovaries will know when to resume oocyte production
(d) Cervix will expand to let the baby through

93 The foetal-ejection reflex in human females is induced by
(a) fully developed foetus and placenta
(b) release of oxytocin from the anterior pituitary
(c) amniotic fluid
(d) Luteinizing hormone

94 Name *A*, *B* and *C* hormones in the given figure.

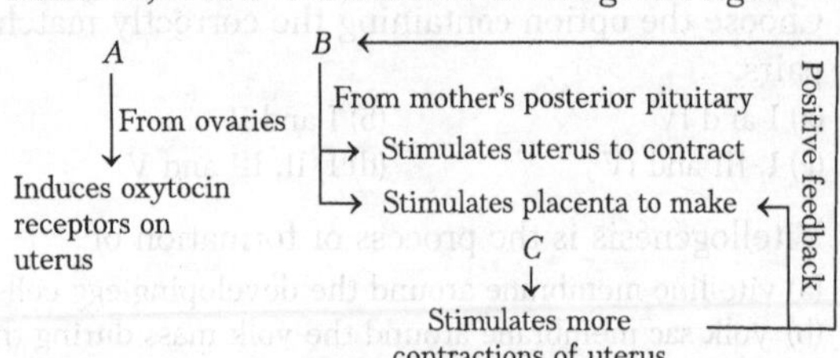

(a) *A*–Prostaglandin, *B*–Oxytocin, *C*–Oestrogen
(b) *A*–Oestrogen, *B*–Oxytocin, *C*–Prostaglandin
(c) *A*–Oestrogen, *B*–Prostaglandin, *C*–Oxytocin
(d) *A*–Prostaglandin, *B*–Oestrogen, *C*–Oxytocin

95 Identify the correct sequence in which the various stages of parturition take place.
(a) Shedding of placenta → Dilation of cervix → Delivery of the baby
(b) Dilation of the cervix → Shedding of placenta → Delivery of the baby
(c) Dilation of the cervix → Delivery of the baby → Shedding of placenta
(d) None of the above

96 The fluid released from the vagina just prior to childbirth is the
(a) baby's accumulated urine
(b) amniotic fluid
(c) mother's plasma form the umbilical cord
(d) baby's plasma from its foetal circulation

97 The female hormone that causes an increased in blood vessels in the uterus and development of milk glands in the breast is
(a) Luteinizing hormone
(b) follicle-stimulating hormone
(c) oestrogen
(d) progesterone

98 Consider the following statements.
I. Generally, a woman does not conceive during lactation period.
II. The hormone prolactin initiates and maintains lactation in a woman.

Choose the correct option.
(a) Statement I is true, but II is false
(b) Statement I is false, but II is true
(c) Both statements I and II are true
(d) Both statements I and II are false

99 Colostrum is important for newly born because
(a) it contains essential antigen
(b) it contains essential antibodies
(c) Both (a) and (b)
(d) it has more iron than ordinary milk

100 Match the following columns.

Column I	Column II
A. Parturition	1. Milk production
B. Lactation	2. Initial milk with several antibodies, healthy protein and less fat
C. Colostrum	3. Foetus delivery
D. Oxytocin	4. Uterine contraction

Codes

	A	B	C	D
(a)	4	1	2	3
(b)	2	4	1	3
(c)	3	2	4	1
(d)	3	1	2	4

101 What is 'after birth' referred to?
(a) amniotic fluid passing out
(b) expulsion of baby
(c) expulsion of placenta, umbilical cord and foetus membrane
(d) secretion of hormone relaxin

102 Consider the following statements.
I. Gestation period in human is about 280 days.
II. The lungs of infant expand and breating begins after the expulsion of baby from mother's body.

Choose the correct option.
(a) Statement I is true, but II is false
(b) Statement I is false, but II is true
(c) Both statements I and II are true
(d) Both statements I and II are false

(B) Cumulative Exercise

(Assorted Questions of the Chapter for Advanced Level Practice)

1 Consider the following statements.

I. Low pitched voice and apparent larynx are secondary sexual characters in females.
II. Acrosome does not have nucleus.
III. Acrosome of sperm contains sperm lysins.
IV. Spirally arranged mitochondria are found in the mid-piece of sperm.

Choose the option with containing correct statements.

(a) I and IV (b) III and IV (c) I and II (d) II and III

2 Correct sequence in development is

(a) fertilisation → zygote → cleavage → morula → blastula → gastrula
(b) fertilisation → zygote → blastula → morula → cleavage → gastrula
(c) fertilisation → cleavage → morula → zygote → blastula → gastrula
(d) cleavage → zygote → fertilisation → morula → blastula → gastrula

3 Choose the correct combination of labelling the hormonal control of female reproductive system.

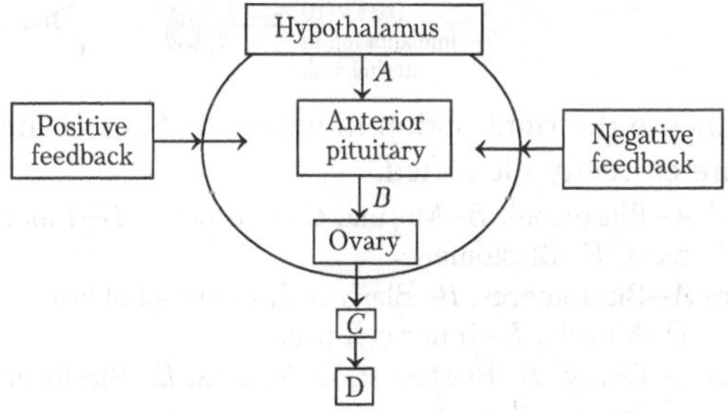

(a) *A*-GnRH, *B*-TSH, *C*-LTH, *D*-Uterus
(b) *A*-GnRH, *B*-LH/FSH, *C*-Oestrogen or Progesterone, *D*-Uterus
(c) *A*-GnRH, *B*-STH, *C*-LH, *D*-Uterus
(d) *A*-GnRH, *B*-ACTH, *C*-LH, *D*-Uterus

4 The given figure belongs to human sperm. Identify *A*, *B* and *C*, respectively.

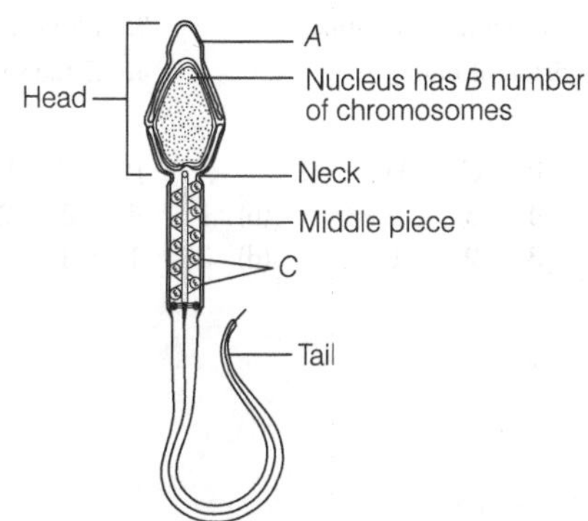

(a) *A*–Acrosome, *B*–23, *C*–Spirillum
(b) *A*–Lysosome, *B*–23, *C*–Mitochondria
(c) *A*–Acrosome, *B*–23, *C*–Mitochondria
(d) *A*–Acrosome, *B*–46, *C*–Mitochondria

5 Consider the following statements.

I. Oogenesis is initiated during the embryonic development stage.
II. At puberty, only 60,000-80,000 primary follicles are left in each ovary.
III. The primary follicles gets surrounded with many layers of granulosa cells to form secondary follicles.
IV. Changing of sanitary napkins or pads after every 4-5 hours is necessary for maintaining menstrual hygiene.

Choose the correct option.

(a) I and II
(b) I, II, III and IV
(c) I and III
(d) None of the above

6 The following diagram refers the changes taking place during the human menstruation cycle.

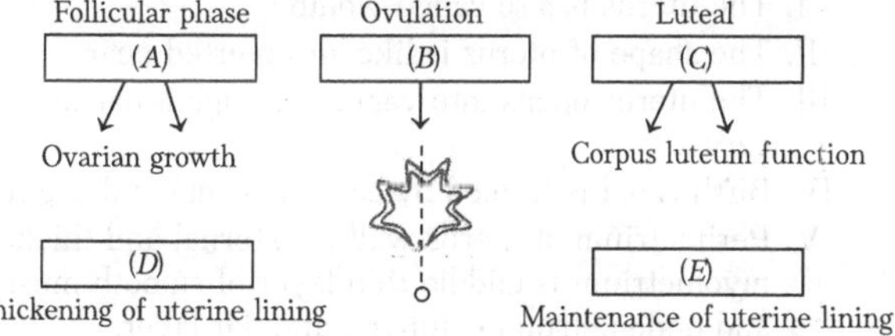

In each of the boxes shown in the diagram fill the name of the hormone controlling the stage in the human menstrual cycle.

(a) *A*–FSH, *B*–LH, *C*–LH, *D*–Progesterone, *E*–Oestrogen
(b) *A*–FSH, *B*–LH, *C*–FSH, *D*–Oestrogen, *E*–Progesterone
(c) *A*–LH, *B*–FSH, *C*–LH, *D*–Oestrogen, *E*–Progesterone
(d) *A*–FSH, *B*–LH, *C*–Progesterone, *D*–Oestrogen, *E*–Progesterone

7 Given below is a diagrammatic sketch of a portion of human male reproductive system. Select the correct set of names of the parts labelled *A*, *B*, *C* and *D*.

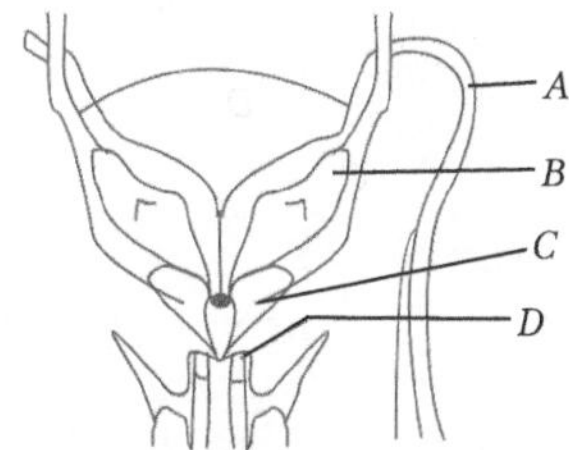

	A	B	C	D
(a)	Ureter	Prostate	Seminal vesicle	Bulbourethral gland
(b)	Vas deferens	Seminal vesicle	Prostate	Bulbourethral gland
(c)	Vas deferens	Seminal vesicle	Bulbourethral gland	Prostate
(d)	Ureter	Seminal vesicle	Prostate	Bulbourethral gland

8 Which is the correctly matched pair among the following?

I.	Colostrum	–	Secretion found in seminal fluid
II.	Areola	–	Pigmented circular area around the nipple
III.	Sexual intercourse	–	Coitus
IV.	Bartholin's gland	–	Erectile body in female homologous to glans penis of male

Codes

(a) II and III (b) III and IV
(c) I and IV (d) II and IV

9 Consider the following statements.

I. The uterus is also called womb.
II. The shape of uterus is like an inverted pear.
III. The uterus opens into vagina through a narrow cervix.
IV. Birth canal is formed by cervical canal and vagina.
V. Perimetrium of uterus wall is external and thick, myometrium is middle thin layer of smooth muscles and endometrium is inner glandular layer.

Choose the correct option.

(a) I, II and III (b) I, II, III and IV
(c) IV and V (d) I and V

10 Identify the parts labelled (*A* to *G*) in the given figure of male reproductive system from the list I to X.

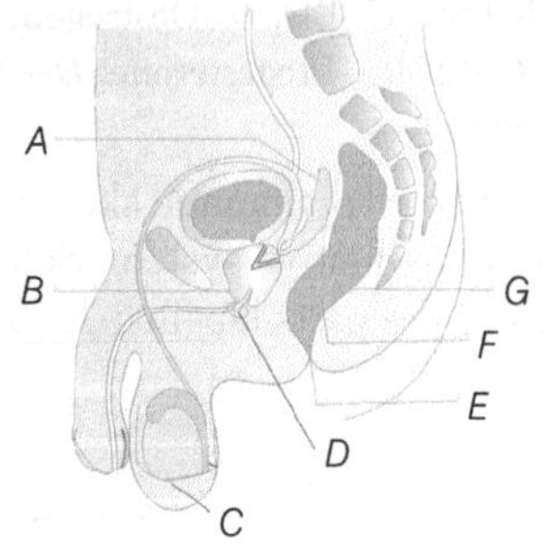

I. Fundus II. Uriniferous tubules
III. Seminiferous tubules IV. Seminal vesicle
V. Prostate VI. Ejaculatory duct
VII. Rectum VIII. Anus
IX. Bulbourethral gland
X. Scrotum

(a) *A* - IV, *B* - V, *C* - X, *D* - IX, *E* - VIII, *F* - VII, *G* - VI
(b) *A* - X, *B* - IX, *C* - VIII, *D* - IV, *E* - III, *F* - II, *G* - I
(c) *A* - IV, *B* - V, *C* - I, *D* - III, *E* - IX, *F* - X, *G* - II
(d) *A* - V, *B* - III, *C* - I, *D* - II, *E* - IV, *F* - VI, *G* - VIII

11 Label the given figure which illustrates fertilisation followed by cleavage and the early stages of embryonic development.

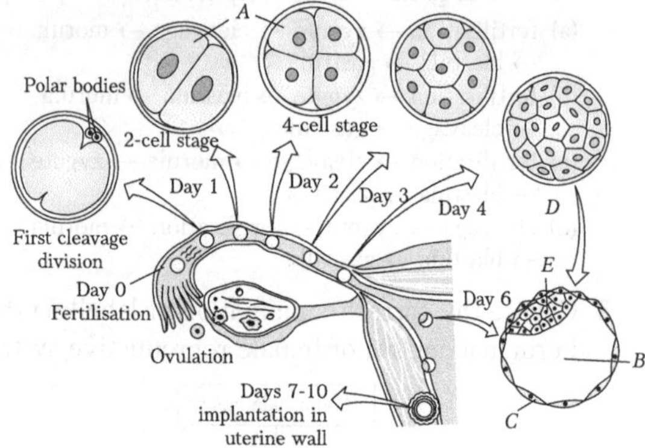

Choose the right option in which *A, B, C, D* and *E* are correctly identified.

(a) *A*–Blastocoel, *B*–Morula, *C*–Blastocyst, *D*–Inner cell mass, *E*–Blastomeres
(b) *A*–Blastomeres, *B*–Blastocoel, *C*–Trophoblast, *D*–Morula, *E*–Inner cell mass
(c) *A*–Ovary, *B*–Blastocyst, *C*–Morula, *D*–Blastocoel, *E*–Inner cell mass
(d) *A*–Ovary, *B*–Blastocyst, *C*–Gastrula, *D*–Inner cell mass, *E*–Trophoblast

12 Match the following columns.

Column I	Column II
A. A hollow ball of cells	1. Cleavage
B. Outer germ layer	2. Blastula
C. Cavity within a blastula	3. Blastocoel
D. Division of embryo	4. Ectoderm

Codes

	A	B	C	D		A	B	C	D
(a)	2	4	3	1	(b)	1	4	3	2
(c)	4	3	2	1	(d)	3	1	4	2

13 The figure given below is an incomplete chart showing influence of hormones on gametogenesis in males. Examine the chart carefully and select the appropriate words for the blanks *A*, *B*, *C* and *D*.

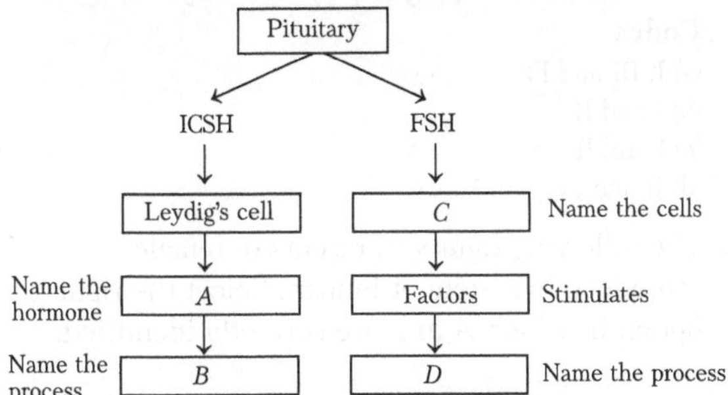

(a) *A*–Testosterone, *B*–Spermatogenesis, *C*–Sertoli cells, *D*–Spermiogenesis
(b) *A*–Testosterone, *B*–Spermiogenesis, *C*–Sertoli cells *D*–Spermatogenesis
(c) *A*–Testosterone, *B*–Spermatogenesis, *C*–Testis, *D*–Spermiogenesis
(d) *A*–LH, *B*–Spermatogenesis, *C*–Sertoli cells, *D*–Spermiogenesis

14 Given below are four statements (I-IV) regarding embryonic development in humans.

I. Cleavage divisions bring about considerable increase in the mass of protoplasm.
II. With more cleavage divisions, the resultant blastomeres become smaller and smaller.
III. The blastomeres in the blastocyst are arranged into two layers, i.e. trophoblast and endometrium.
IV. Cleavage divisions result in a solid ball of cells called morula.

Which of the above two statements are correct?
(a) I and III (b) II and IV
(c) I and II (d) III and IV

15 Match the following columns.

Column I	Column II
A. The process of start of menstrual cycle in the life of a human female	1. Capacitation
B. The process of maturation of sperms	2. Luteal phase
C. The process of transformation of ruptured Graafian follicle into corpus luteum	3. Spermiogenesis
D. The process of activation of sperms in female reproductive system after their ejaculation into it	4. Menarche

Codes

	A	B	C	D		A	B	C	D
(a)	4	3	2	1	(b)	1	2	3	4
(c)	2	1	3	4	(d)	3	1	2	4

16 The following figure refers to LS of testis showing various parts. In which option all the six parts *A*, *B*, *C*, *D*, *E* and *F* are correctly identified

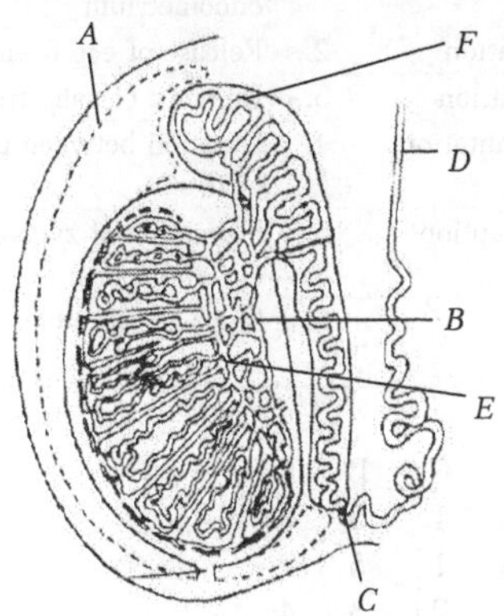

(a) *A*–Tunica vaginalis, *B*–Rete testis, *C*–Caput epididymis, *D*–Mediastinum testis, *E*–Vas deferens, *F*–Cauda epididymis
(b) *A*–Tunica vaginalis, *B*–Rete testis, *C*–Cauda epididymis, *D*–Vas deferens, *E*–Mediastinum testis, *F*–Caput epididymis
(c) *A*–Tunica vaginalis, *B*–Rete testis, *C*–Cauda epididymis, *D*–Mediastinum testis, *E*–Vas deferens, *F*–Caput epididymis
(d) *A*–Tunica vaginalis, *B*–Rete testis, *C*–Caput epididymis, *D*–Vas deferens, *E*–Mediastinum testis, *F*–Cauda epididymis

17 In the diagram of section of Graafian follicle, different parts are indicated by alphabets, choose the answer in which these alphabets have been correctly matched with the parts they indicate.

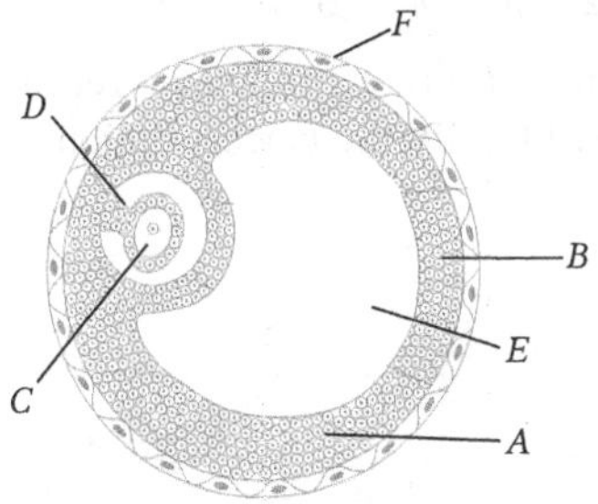

(a) *A*–Theca externa, *B*–Theca interna, *C*–Ovum, *D*–Cumulus oophorus, *E*–Antrum, *F*–Membrana granulosa
(b) *A*–Membrana granulosa, *B*–Theca externa, *C*–Ovum, *D*–Cumulus oophorus, *E*–Antrum, *F*–Theca interna
(c) *A*–Membrana granulosa, *B*–Theca interna, *C*–Ovum, *D*–Cumulus oophorus, *E*–Antrum, *F*–Theca externa
(d) *A*–Theca externa, *B*–Theca interna, *C*–Ovum, *D*–Membrana granulosa, *E*–Antrum, *F*–Cumulus oophorus

18 Match the following columns.

	Column I		Column II
A.	Parturition	1.	Attachment of zygote to endometrium
B.	Gestation	2.	Release of egg from Graafian follicle
C.	Ovulation	3.	Delivery of baby from uterus
D.	Implantation	4.	Duration between pregnancy and birth
E.	Conception	5.	Formation of zygote by fusion of the egg end sperm
		6.	Stoppage of ovulation and menstruation

Codes

	A	B	C	D	E
(a)	2	4	1	5	3
(b)	4	3	1	5	2
(c)	5	1	2	3	4
(d)	3	4	2	1	5

19 Match the following columns.

	Column I		Column II
A.	Hyaluronidase	1.	Acrosomal reaction
B.	Corpus luteum	2.	Morphogenetic movements
C.	Gastrulation	3.	Progesterone
D.	Capacitation	4.	Mammary gland
E.	Colostrum	5.	Sperm activation

Codes

	A	B	C	D	E
(a)	5	2	4	1	3
(b)	1	3	2	5	4
(c)	3	2	5	4	1
(d)	1	2	3	4	5

20 The given figure refers to female reproductive system of human. Identify the correct option.

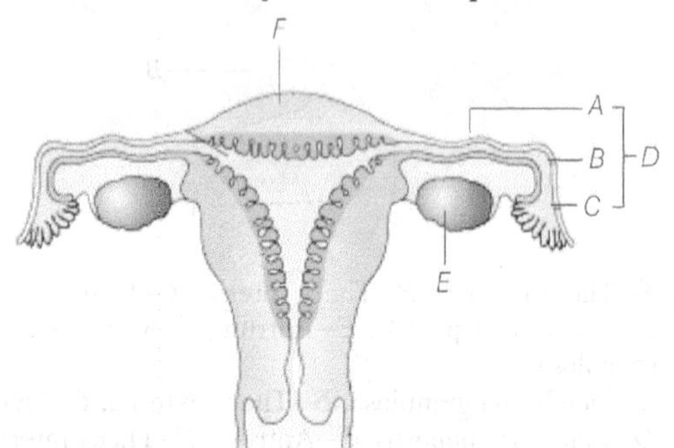

(a) *A*-Isthmus—wider part of oviduct
(b) *C*-Ampulla—narrow part of oviduct
(c) *F*-Ovrary—primary sex organ of a woman
(d) *C*-Infundibulum—helps in collection of ovum after ovulation

21 Menstrual cycle is controlled by
I. androgens from Leydig cells.
II. FSH and LH of pituitary.
III. oxytoxin hormone.
IV. oestrogen and progesterone of ovary.

Codes
(a) I, III and IV
(b) I and II
(c) I and III
(d) II and IV

22 The following figure represents to female reproductive system of human. Select the right option in which *A* to *E* are correctly identified.

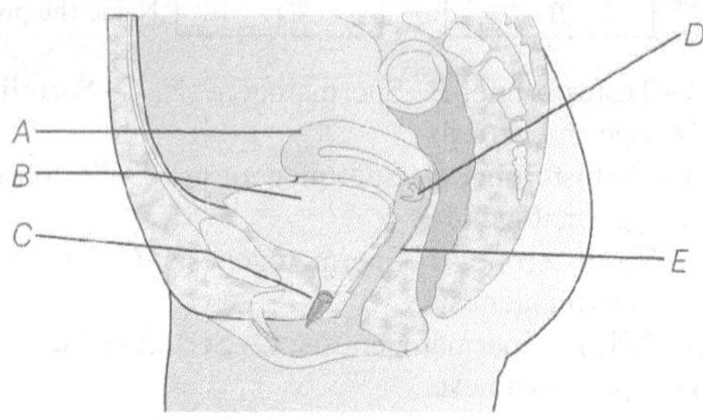

(a) *A*–Uterus, *B*–Urinary bladder, *C*–Urethra, *D*–Cervix, *E*–Vagina
(b) *A*–Urethra, *B*–Urinary bladder, *C*–Uterus, *D*–Cervix, *E*–Vagina
(c) *A*–Uterus, *B*–Urinary bladder, *C*–Urethra, *D*–Vagina, *E*–Cervix
(d) *A*–Urethra, *B*–Urinary bladder, *C*–Uterus, *D*–Cervix, *E*–Vagina

23 The given diagram shows to ovum surrounded by few sperms. Identify all the alphabets correctly.

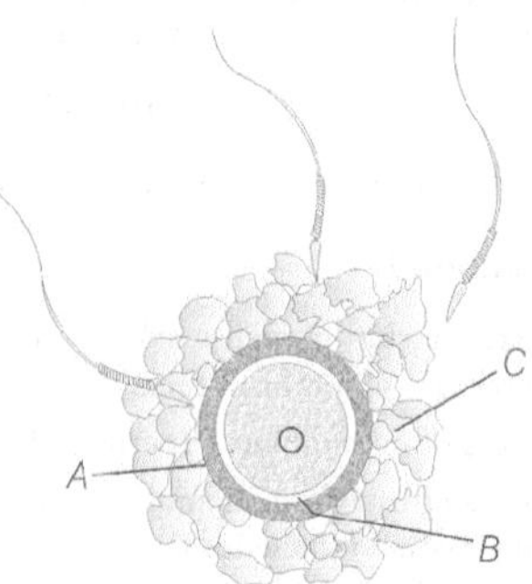

(a) *A* - Oolemma, *B* - Perivitelline space, *C* - Corona radiata
(b) *A* - Zona pellucida, *B* - Perivitelline space, *C* - Corona radiata
(c) *A* - Zona pellucida, *B* - Vitelline membrane, *C* - Corona radiata
(d) *A* - Zona pellucida, *B* - Perivitelline space, *C* - Corona reticulata

24 Match the following columns.

	Column I		Column II		Column III
1.	Interstitial cells	A.	Cortex of ovary	I.	Follicular fluid
2.	Sertoli cells	B.	Ovarian follicle	II.	Progesterone
3.	Granulosa cells	C.	Testes	III.	Attachment of sperm bundle
4.	Cells of corpus luteum	D.	Seminiferous tubules	IV.	Testosterone

(a) 2-A-III, 1-C-IV, 3-B-I, 4-D-II
(b) 1-C-IV, 2-D-III, 3-B-I, 4-A-II
(c) 1-D-III, 2-A-IV, 3-B-I, 4-C-II
(d) 2-D-III, I-C-IV, 3-A-II, 4-B-I

25 Identify the stages labelled as *A*, *B*, *C* and *D* in the schematic diagram of spermatogenesis.

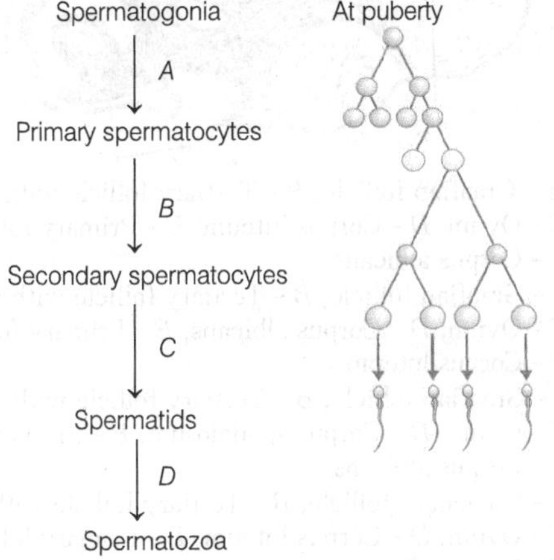

	A	B	C	D
(a)	Mitosis and differentiation	Meiosis-I	Meiosis-II	Differentiation
(b)	Mitosis	Meiosis-I	Meiosis-II	Mitosis
(c)	Meiosis-I	Meiosis-I	Mitosis	Differentiation
(d)	Mitosis and differentiation	Mitosis	Meiosis-I	Meiosis-II

26 Identify the parts *A*, *B*, *C*, *D*, *E* and *F* in the diagrammatic view of male reproductive system.

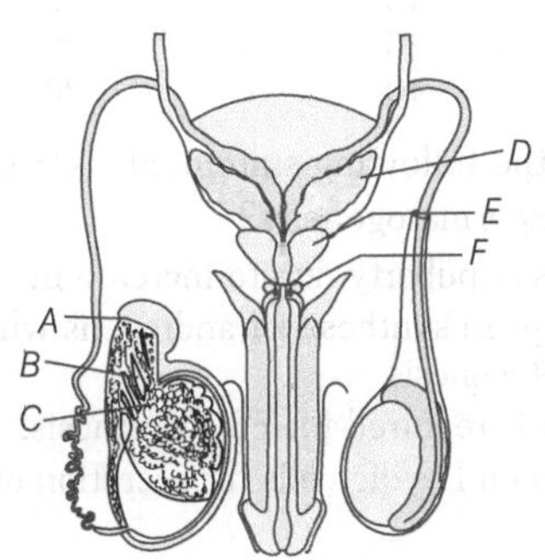

	A	B	C	D	E	F
(a)	Epididymis	Rete testis	Vasa efferentia	Seminal vesicle	Prostate gland	Bulbourethral gland
(b)	Vasa efferentia	Epididymis	Rete testes	Seminal vesicle	Prostate gland	Bulbourethral gland
(c)	Rete testis	Vasa efferentia	Epididymis	Seminal vesicle	Prostate gland	Bulbourethral gland
(d)	Epididymis	Vasa efferentia	Rete testis	Seminal vesicle	Prostate gland	Bulbourethral gland

27 Identify *A*, *B*, *C* and *D* in the diagrammatic sectional view of seminiferous tubule.

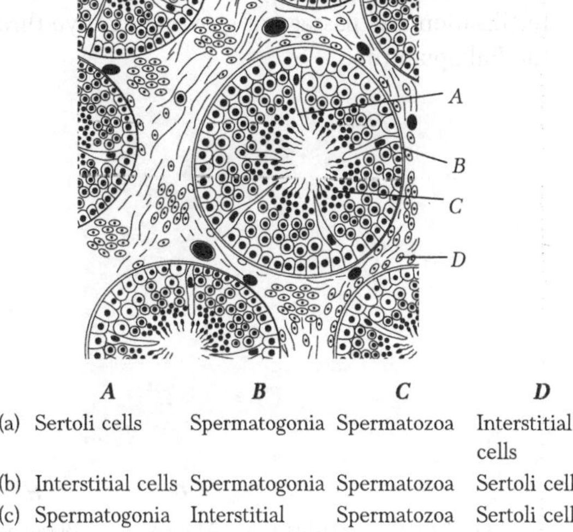

	A	B	C	D
(a)	Sertoli cells	Spermatogonia	Spermatozoa	Interstitial cells
(b)	Interstitial cells	Spermatogonia	Spermatozoa	Sertoli cells
(c)	Spermatogonia	Interstitial cells	Spermatozoa	Sertoli cells
(d)	Spermatozoa	Spermatogonia	Interstitial cells	Sertoli cells

28 Identify the hormones (*W*, *X*, *Y*, *Z*) and the structures (*A*, *B*) labelled in the diagram.

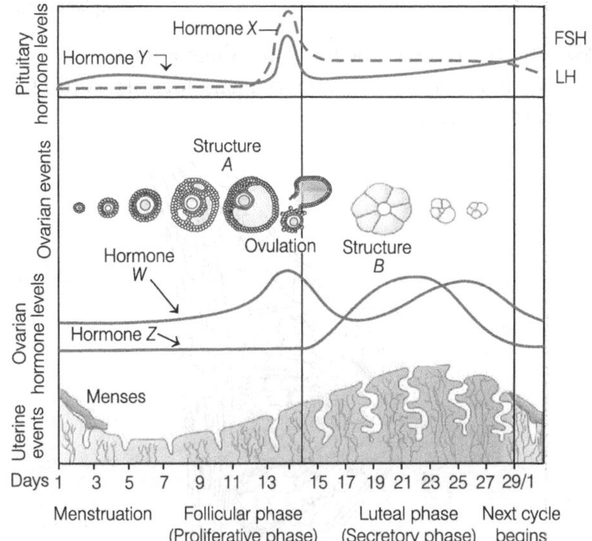

	Hormones X	Hormones Y	Structures A	Structures B	Hormones W	Hormones Z
(a)	FSH	LH	Mature follicle	Corpus luteum	Oestrogen	Progesterone
(b)	LH	FSH	Mature follicle	Corpus luteum	Progesterone	Oestrogen
(c)	FSH	LH	Mature follicle	Regressing corpus luteum	Progesterone	Oestrogen
(d)	LH	FSH	Mature follicle	Corpus luteum	Oestrogen	Progesterone

29 Identify *B, E G* and *H* in the diagram showing fertilisation and passage of growing embryo through the Fallopian tube.

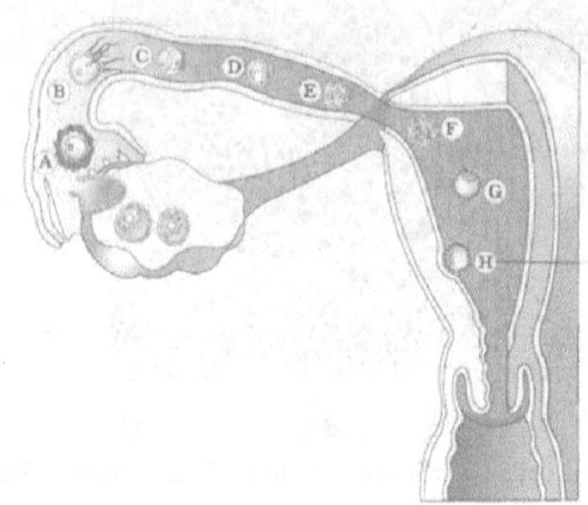

	B	*E*	*G*	*H*
(a)	Ovulation	Fertilisation	Morula	Blastocyst
(b)	Blastocyst implantation	Fertilisation	Morula	Ovulation
(c)	Fertilisation	Morula	Blastocyst	Blastocyst implantation
(d)	Morula	Blastocyst	Fertilisation	Blastocyst implantation

30 The figure given below is the diagrammatic sectional view of mammary gland identify *A* to *D*, respectively.

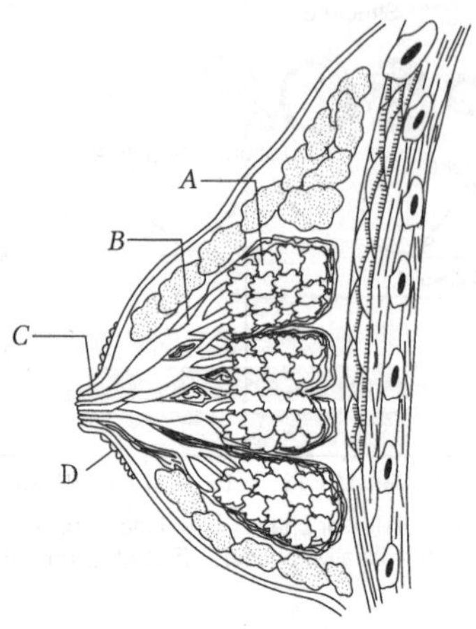

(a) *A* - Alveolus, *B* - Mammary duct, *C* - Lactiferous duct, *D* - Lactogenic spot
(b) *A* - Alveolus, *B* - Lactiferous duct, *C* - Mammary duct, *D* - Areola
(c) *A* - Alveolus, *B* - Mammary duct, *C* - Lactiferous duct, *D* - Areola
(d) *A* - Gland, *B* - Mammary duct, *C* - Lactiferous duct, *D* - Areola

31 The figure shows a section of human ovary. Select the option which gives the correct identification of *A* to *F*.

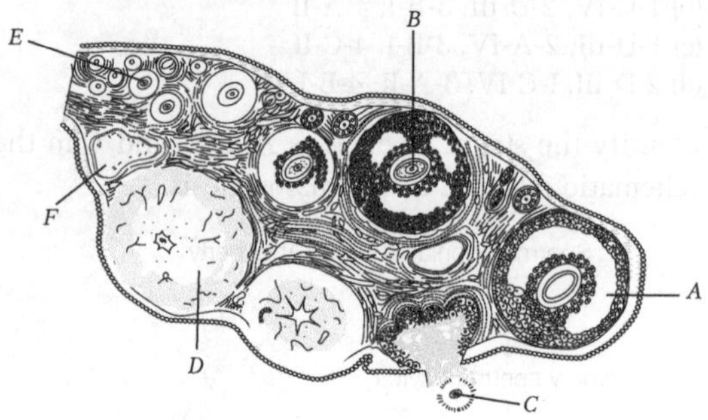

(a) *A* - Graafian follicle, *B* - Tertiary follicle with antrum, *C* - Ovum, *D* - Corpus luteum, *E* - Primary follicle, *F* - Corpus albicans
(b) *A* - Graafian follicle, *B* - Tertiary follicle with antrum, *C* - Ovum, *D* - Corpus albicans, *E* - Primary follicle, *F* - Corpus luteum
(c) *A* - Graafian follicle, *B* - Tertiary follicle with antrum, *C* - Ovum, *D* - Corpus spongiosum, *E* - Primary follicle, *F* - Corpus albicans
(d) *A* - Secondary follicle, *B* - Tertiary follicle with antrum, *C* - Ovum, *D* - Corpus luteum, *E* - Primary follicle, *F* - Corpus albicans

32 Identify *A, B, C, D* and *E* in the table provided.

Cell type	Ploidy	DNA content
Oogonium	*A*	2*n* or 4C
Primary oocyte	2*n*	*B*
Secondary oocyte	C	*D*
Ovum	*n*	*E*

	A	*B*	*C*	*D*	*E*
(a)	2*n*	2C	*n*	2C	1C
(b)	4*n*	4C	*n*	2C	1C
(c)	*n*	2C	*n*	2C	1C
(d)	2*n*	4C	*n*	2C	1C

33 Which of the following statements is/are false regarding spermatogenesis?

I. It starts at puberty due to increase in GnRH.
II. LH helps in synthesis of androgens which stimulates spermatogenesis.
III. Inhibin is required for FSH synthesis.
IV. LH acts on Leydig cells for secretion of androgens.

Codes

(a) Only IV (b) I and II (c) Only III (d) II and IV

34 Some important events in the human females reproductive cycle are given below. Arrange the events in a proper sequence.

I. Secretion of FSH
II. Growth of corpus luteum
III. Growth of the follicle and oogenesis
IV. Ovulation
V. Sudden increase in the levels of LH

(a) III → I → IV → II → V (b) I → III → V → IV → II
(c) I → IV → III → V → II (d) II → I → III → IV → V

35 Which of the following is true about mammalian placenta?

I. It acts as endocrine gland.
II. It secretes relaxin hormone which prevents parturition.
III. It secretes chorionic gonadotropin.
IV. It helps in mixing of foetal and maternal blood.

Codes

(a) I, II and IV (b) I, IV and III
(c) II, III and IV (d) I, II and III

36 The events of the menstrual cycle are represented below. Select the right option in which the level of FSH, LH and progesterone are mentioned correctly.

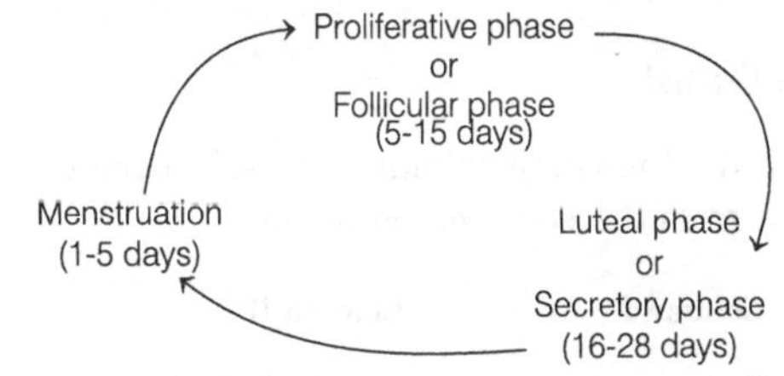

	13th - 14th day			21st - 23rd day		
	FSH	LH	Progesterone	FSH	LH	Progesterone
(a)	High	High	Low	Low	Low	High
(b)	High	High	High	Low	Low	Low
(c)	Low	Low	Low	High	High	High
(d)	Low	Low	High	High	Low	Low

37 Identify the hormones *W*, *X*, *Y* and *Z* for the hormonal control of female reproductive system.

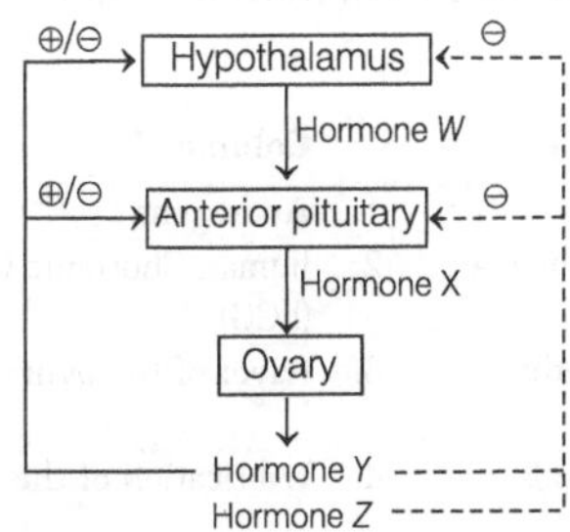

	W	*X*	*Y*	*Z*
(a)	GnRH	FSH/LH	Progesterone	Oestrogen
(b)	GnRH	FSH/LH	Oestrogen	Progesterone
(c)	FSH/LH	GnRH	Oestrogen	Progesterone
(d)	FSH/LH	GnRH	Progesterone	Oestrogen

38 Which of the following is correct for *A*, *B*, *C* and *D*.

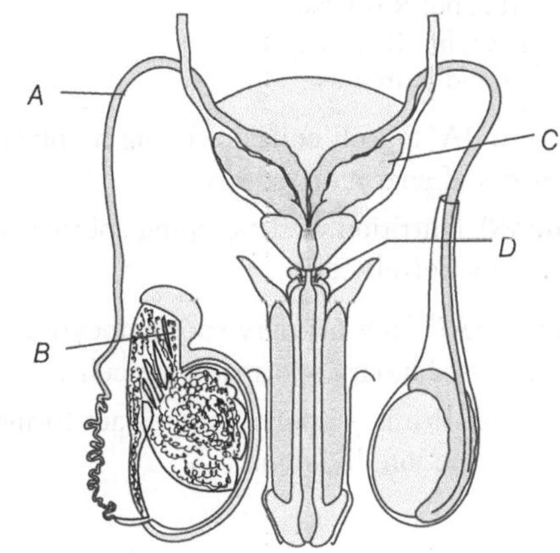

	A	*B*	*C*	*D*
(a)	Carries sperm	Stores sperm permanently	Secretes a fluid that lubricates ureter	Secretes a fluid that ultimately becomes semen
(b)	Carries Sertoli cells	Stores sperm	Carries urine	Stores sperm
(c)	Carries sperm	Stores sperm	Secretes a fluid that ultimately becomes semen	Secretes a fluid that lubricates distal urethra
(d)	Carries sperm	Stores sperm permanently	Secretes a fluid that lubricates distal urethra	Secretes a fluid that ultimately becomes semen

39 Match the following columns.

	Column I		Column II
A.	Endometrium	1.	Zona pellucida
B.	Clitoris	2.	Alveoli
C.	Mammary gland	3.	Erectile organ
D.	Secondary oocyte	4.	Womb

Codes

	A	B	C	D		A	B	C	D
(a)	4	3	1	2	(b)	2	4	1	3
(c)	3	1	4	2	(d)	4	3	2	1

Assertion and Reason

Direction (Q. Nos. 40-46) *In each of followed the following questions, a statement of Assertion (A) is given followed by the corresponding statements of Reason (R). Of the statements, mark the correct answer as*

(a) Both A and R are true and R is the correct explanation of A
(b) Both A and R are true, but R is not the correct explanation of A
(c) A is true, but R is false
(d) A is false, but R is true
(e) Both A and R are false

40 **Assertion** (A) Sertoli cells are being involved in the process of spermatogenesis.
Reason (R) Nutrition of developing sperms is provided by Sertoli cells.

41 **Assertion** (A) Each primary spermatocyte cell gives rise to four secondary spermatocyte cells.
Reason (R) Primary spermatocytes are formed through reduction division.

42 **Assertion** (A) Scrotum is a pouch in which testes are held.
Reason (R) A pocketed sac of the abdominal cavity or pelvic cavity holds testes.

43 **Assertion** (A) Generally, sperm cells are larger than egg cells.
Reason (R) Spermatozoa consist of acrosome and mitochondria.

44 **Assertion** (A) First meiotic division in primary oocytes results in the formation of two equal sized cells.
Reason (R) Both of these cells are equally functional.

45 **Assertion** (A) Only a single functional female gamete is formed from each primary oocyte cell.
Reason (R) Meiosis in each primary oocyte gives rise to only one cell which functions as ovum.

46 **Assertion** (A) A chemical substance fertilizin is present in eggs.
Reason (R) It helps in maturation of embryo after fertilisation.

(C) Medical Entrances' Gallery

(Collection of Questions Asked in NEET & in Various Medical Entrance Exams)

1 In human beings, at the end of 12 weeks (first trimester) of pregnancy, the following is observed. **[NEET 2020]**
(a) Eyelids and eyelashes are formed
(b) Most of the major organ systems are formed
(c) The head is covered with fine hair
(d) Movement of the foetus

2 Which of the following hormone levels will cause release of ovum (ovulation) from the Graafian follicle? **[NEET 2020]**
(a) High concentration of progesterone
(b) Low concentration of LH
(c) Low concentration of FSH
(d) High concentration of oestrogen

3 Meiotic division of the secondary oocyte completed **[NEET 2020]**
(a) at the time of copulation
(b) after zygote formation
(c) at the time of fusion of a sperm with an ovum
(d) prior to ovulation

4 Select the correct option of haploid cells from the following groups. **[NEET 2020]**
(a) Primary oocyte, secondary oocyte, spermatid
(b) Secondary spermatocyte, first polar body, ovum
(c) Spermatogonia, primary spermatocyte, spermatid
(d) Primary spermatocyte, secondary spermatocyte, second polar body

5 Match the following columns and select the correct option from the codes given below.

Column I		Column II
A. Ovary	1.	Human chorionic gonadotropin
B. Placenta	2.	Oestrogen and progesterone
C. Corpus luteum	3.	Androgens
D. Leydig cells	4.	Progesterone only

Codes **[NEET 2020]**

	A	B	C	D
(a)	4	3	2	1
(b)	1	2	3	4
(c)	1	3	2	4
(d)	2	1	4	3

6 Match the following columns and select the correct option.

Column I		Column II
A. Placenta	1.	Androgens
B. Zona pellucida	2.	human Chorionic Gonadotropin (hCG)
C. Bulbourethral glands	3.	Layer of the ovum
D. Leydig cells	4.	Lubrication of the penis

[NEET 2020]

Codes

	A	B	C	D
(a)	1	4	2	3
(b)	3	2	4	1
(c)	2	3	4	1
(d)	4	3	1	2

7 Choose the correct option.

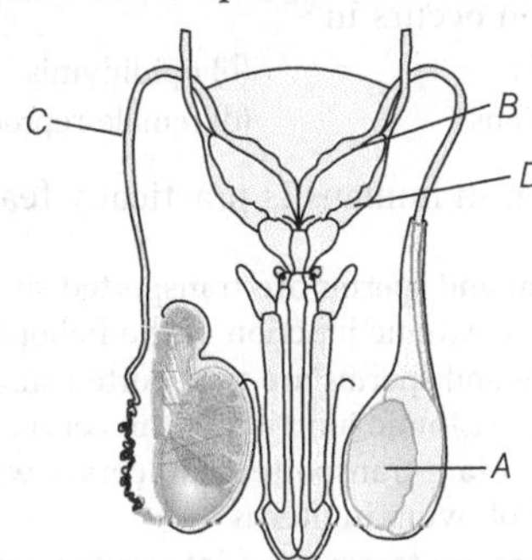

[AIIMS 2019]

(a) *A*-Testis - Possesses 3-4 testicular lobule
(b) *B*-Seminal vesicle - Storage of sperm
(c) *C*-Vas deferens - Helps in sperm transfer
(d) *D*-Prostate gland - Secretes seminal fluid

8 Select the correct sequence for transport of sperm cells in male reproductive system. **[EAMCET 2015, NEET 2019]**

(a) Seminiferous tubules → Rete testis → Vasa efferentia → Epididymis → Vas deferens → Ejaculatory duct → Urethra → Urethral meatus
(b) Seminiferous tubules → Vasa efferentia → Epididymis → Inguinal canal → Urethra
(c) Testis → Epididymis → Vasa efferentia → Vas deferens → Ejaculatory duct → Inguinal canal → Urethra → Urethral meatus
(d) Testis → Epididymis → Vasa efferentia → Rete testis → Inguinal canal → Urethra

9 Extrusion of second polar body from egg nucleus occurs **[NEET 2019]**

(a) after fertilisation
(b) before the entry of sperm into ovum
(c) simultaneously with first cleavage
(d) after the entry of sperm, but before fertilisation

10 Which of the following hormones is responsible for both the milk ejection reflex and the foetal-ejection reflex? **[EAMCET 2015, NEET 2019]**

(a) Oestrogen (b) Prolactin
(c) Oxytocin (d) Relaxin

11 Colostrum, the yellowish fluid, secreted by mother during the initial days of lactation is very essential to impart immunity to the newborn infants because it contains **[NEET 2019]**

(a) monocytes (b) macrophages
(c) immunoglobulin-A (d) natural killer cells

12 Gastrulation means **[JIPMER 2019]**

(a) conversion of blastula into morula
(b) formation of 3 germ layers
(c) a phase in which organogenesis takes place
(d) a phase characterised by inner cell mass

13 Structure analogous to the placenta in mammals. **[JIPMER 2019]**

(a) Chorion (b) Amnion (c) Yolk sac (d) Allantois

14 No new follicles develop in the luteal phase of the menstrual cycle because **[NEET 2019]**

(a) follicles do not remain in the ovary after ovulation
(b) FSH levels are high in the luteal phase
(c) LH levels are high in the luteal phase
(d) Both FSH and LH levels are low in the luteal phase

15 Number of chromosomes present in secondary spermatocyte is **[JIPMER 2019]**

(a) 22 (b) 23 (c) 24 (d) 25

16 Level of LH is maximum **[JIPMER 2019]**

(a) just before ovulation
(b) just after ovulation
(c) at the time of ovulation
(d) during menstrual bleeding phase

17 Number of chromosomes present in spermatogonium is **[JIPMER 2019]**

(a) 46 (b) 23 (c) 48 (d) 43

18 Which one of the labelled parts utilises fructose as a source of energy? **[JIPMER 2019]**

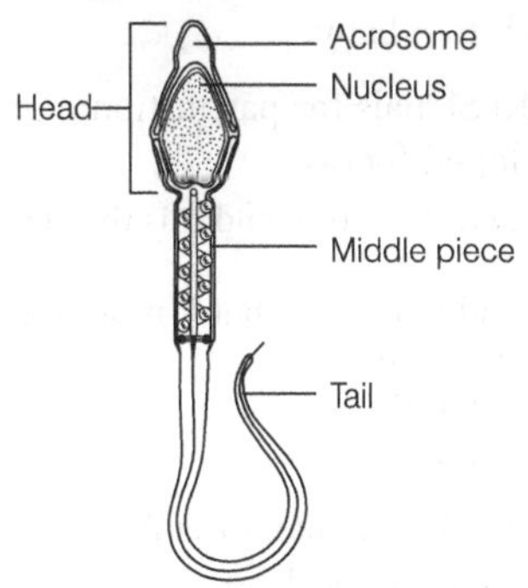

(a) Head (b) Tail
(c) Acrosome (d) Middle piece

19 The difference between spermiogenesis and spermiation is **[NEET 2018]**

(a) in spermiogenesis, spermatozoa from Sertoli cells are released into the cavity of seminiferous tubules, while in spermiation, spermatozoa are formed
(b) in spermiogenesis, spermatozoa are formed while in spermiation, spermatids are formed
(c) in spermiogenesis, spermatids are formed while in spermiation, spermatozoa are formed
(d) in spermiogenesis, spermatozoa are formed, while in spermiation, spermatozoa are released from Sertoli cells into the cavity of seminiferous tubules

20 Match the items given in Column I with those in Column II and select the correct option given below.

Column I	Column II
A. Proliferative phase	1. Breakdown of endometrial lining
B. Secretory phase	2. Follicular phase
C. Menstruation	3. Luteal phase

Codes [NEET 2018]

	A	B	C		A	B	C
(a)	2	3	1	(b)	1	3	2
(c)	3	2	1	(d)	3	1	2

21 Formation of corpus luteum is induced by [JIPMER 2018]
(a) LH (b) oestrogen
(c) FSH (d) progesterone

22 What is incorrect about inhibin? [JIPMER 2018]
(a) It is a lipoprotein
(b) Decreases FSH secretion
(c) Molecular weight is between 10k-30k Dalton
(d) Secreted by Sertoli cells

23 Hormones secreted by the placenta to maintain pregnancy are [NEET 2018]
(a) hCG, hPL, progesterone, oestrogen
(b) hCG, hPL, oestrogen, relaxin, oxytocin
(c) hCG, hPL, progesterone, prolactin
(d) hCG, progesterone, oestrogens, glucocorticoids

24 **Assertion** (A) In females, parturition is the act of giving birth to a baby.

Reason (R) Signals for parturition originate from a fully developed foetus. [AIIMS 2018]
(a) Both A and R are true and R is the correct explanation of A
(b) Both A and R are true, but R is not the correct explanation of A
(c) A is true, but R is false
(d) Both A and R are false

25 The amnion of mammalian embryo is derived from
(a) mesoderm and trophoblast [NEET 2018]
(b) endoderm and mesoderm
(c) ectoderm and mesoderm
(d) ectoderm and endoderm

26 The correct sequence is [JIPMER 2018]
(a) Zygote → Cleavage → Morula → Blastula → Gastrula
(b) Cleavage → Zygote → Morula → Blastula → Gastrula
(c) Zygote → Morula → Blastula → Cleavage → Gastrula
(d) Zygote → Blastula → Morula → Cleavage → Gastrula

27 Which part of ovary in mammals acts as an endocrine gland after ovulation? [AIIMS 2017]
(a) Graafian follicle (b) Vitelline membrane
(c) Germinal epithelium (d) Chorion

28 The secretory phase in the human menstrual cycle is also called as [JIPMER 2017]
(a) luteal phase and lasts for about 6 days
(b) follicular phase lasting for about 6 days
(c) luteal phase and lasts for about 13 days
(d) follicular phase and lasts for about 13 days

29 Capacitation occurs in [NEET 2017]
(a) rete testis (b) epididymis
(c) vas deferens (d) female reproductive tract

30 Fertilisation in humans is practically feasible only if [NEET-I 2016]
(a) the ovum and sperms are transported simultaneously to ampullary-isthmic junction of the Fallopian tube
(b) the ovum and sperms are transported simultaneously to ampullary-isthmic junction of the cervix
(c) the sperms are transported into cervix within 48 hrs of released of ovum in uterus
(d) the sperms are transported into vagina just after the release of ovum in Fallopian tube

31 Select the incorrect statement. [NEET-I 2016]
(a) LH and FSH triggers ovulation in ovary
(b) LH and FSH decrease gradually during the follicular phase
(c) LH triggers secretion of androgens from the Leydig cells
(d) FSH stimulates the Sertoli cells which help in spermiogenesis

32 Identify the correct statement on inhibin. [NEET-I 2016]
(a) It is produced by granulosa cells in ovary and inhibits the secretion of FSH
(b) It is produced by granulosa cells in ovary and inhibits the secretion of LH
(c) It is produced by nurse cells in testes and inhibits the secretion of LH
(d) It inhibits the secretion of LH, FSH and prolactin

33 Which of the following depicts the correct pathway of transport of sperms? [NEET-II 2016]
(a) Rete testis → Efferent ductules → Epididymis → Vas deferens
(b) Rete testis → Epididymis→ Efferent ductules → Vas deferens
(c) Rete testis → Vas deferens → Efferent ductules → Epididymis
(d) Efferent ductules → Rete testis → Vas deferens → Epididymis

34 Match the following columns.

Column I	Column II
A. Mons pubis	1. Embryo formation
B. Antrum	2. Sperm
C. Trophoectoderm	3. Female external genitalia
D. Nebenkern	4. Graafian follicle

[NEET-II 2016]

Codes

	A	B	C	D
(a)	3	4	2	1
(b)	3	4	1	2
(b)	3	1	4	2
(d)	1	4	3	2

35 Several hormones like hCG, hPL, oestrogen, progesterone are produced by **[NEET-II 2016]**
(a) ovary (b) placenta
(c) Fallopian tube (d) pituitary

36 The hormone which acts on Sertoli cells and stimulates the process of spermiogenesis is **[Karnataka CET 2015, Manipal 2012]**
(a) GnRH (b) androgen
(c) FSH (d) LH

37 During menstrual cycle, the cyclical changes takes place in **[Karnataka CET 2015]**
(a) perimetrium
(b) endometrium
(c) corpus luteum
(d) myometrium

38 Which one of the following is not function of placenta? **[NEET 2013]**
(a) It secretes oestrogen
(b) It facilitates removal of carbon dioxide and waste material from embryo
(c) It secretes oxytocin during parturition
(d) It facilitates supply of oxygen and nutrients to embryo

39 What is the correct sequence of sperm formation? **[NEET 2013]**
(a) Spermatogonia, Spermatocyte, Spermatozoa, Spermatid
(b) Spermatogonia, Spermatozoa, Spermatocyte, Spermatid
(c) Spermatogonia, Spermatocyte, Spermatid, Spermatozoa
(d) Spermatid, Spermatocyte, Spermatogonia, Spermatozoa

40 Menstrual flow occurs due to lack of **[NEET 2013, BHU 2012]**
(a) FSH (b) oxytocin
(c) vasopressin (d) progesterone

41 Secretion from which of the following structures is preparing inner wall of uterus for implantation? **[UP CPMT 2012]**
(a) Ovary
(b) Pituitary gland
(c) Corpus luteum
(d) Ovarian follicle

42 Withdrawal of which of the following hormones is the immediate cause of menstruation? **[UP CPMT 2012]**
(a) Oestrogen (b) FSH
(c) FSH-RH (d) Progesterone

43 Which one of the following statements is false in respect of viability of mammalian sperm? **[CBSE AIPMT 2012]**
(a) Sperm is viable for only up to 24 hrs
(b) Survival of sperm depends on the pH of the medium and is more active in alkaline medium
(c) Viability of sperm is determined by its motility
(d) Sperms must be concentrated in a thick suspension

44 Signals for parturition originate from **[CBSE AIPMT 2012]**
(a) Both placenta as well as fully developed foetus
(b) oxytocin released from maternal pituitary
(c) placenta only
(d) fully developed foetus only

45 In a normal pregnant woman, the amount of total gonadotropin activity was assessed. The result expected was **[CBSE AIPMT 2012]**
(a) high level of circulation FSH and LH in the uterus to stimulate implantation of the embryo
(b) high level of circulating hCG to stimulate endometrial thickening
(c) high levels of FSH and LH in uterus to stimulate endometrial thickening
(d) high level of circulating hCG to stimulate oestrogen and progesterone synthesis

46 Which of the following hormones is not a secretory product of human placenta? **[Manipal 2012]**
(a) Human chorionic gonadotropin
(b) Prolactin
(c) Oestrogen
(d) Progesterone

47 The figure given below depicts a diagrammatic sectional view of the female reproductive system of humans. Which one set of three parts out of *A*-*F* have been correctly identified? **[CBSE AIPMT 2011]**

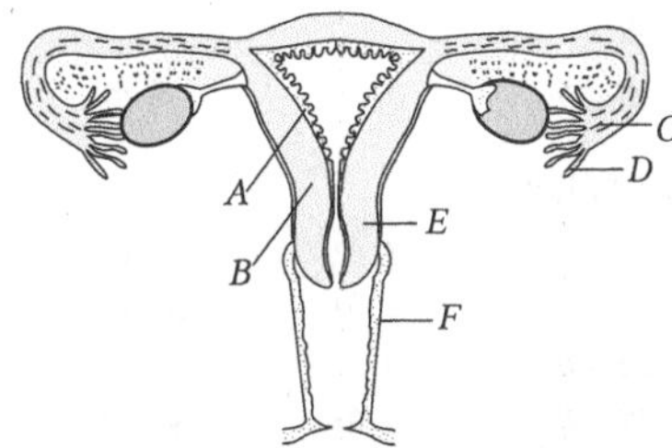

(a) *C*-Infundibulum, *D*-Fimbriae, *E*-Cervix
(b) *D*-Oviducal funnel, *E*-Uterus, *F*-Cervix
(c) *A*-Perimetrium, *B*-Myometrium, *C*-Fallopian tube
(d) *B*-Endometrium, *C*-Infundibulum, *D*-Fimbriae

48 The testes in humans are situated outside the abdominal cavity inside a pouch called scrotum. The purpose served is for **[CBSE AIPMT 2011]**
(a) escaping any possible compression by the visceral organs
(b) providing more space for the growth of epididymis
(c) providing a secondary sexual feature for exhibiting the male sex
(d) maintaining the scrotal temperature lower than the internal body temperature

49 The main function of the fimbriae of the Fallopian tube in females is to **[Kerala CEE 2011]**
(a) release to ovum from the Graafian follicle
(b) make necessary changes in the endometrium for implantation
(c) help in the development of corpus luteum
(d) help in the collection of the ovum after ovulation
(e) help in the development of ovary

50 At the time of implantation, the human embryo is called **[RPMT 2011]**
(a) embryo (b) blastocyst (c) zygote (d) foetus

51 Which of the following organs is devoid of glands? **[DUMET 2011]**
(a) Uterus (b) Vagina
(c) Vulva (d) Oviduct

52 Corpus luteum releases **[DUMET 2011]**
(a) oestrogen (b) progesterone
(c) androgen (d) Both (a) and (b)

53 Primary spermatocyte differs form spermatogonium in **[DUMET 2011]**
(a) number of chromosomes
(b) size and volume
(c) DNA content
(d) size of chromosomes

54 In human, cleavage/divisions are **[DUMET 2011]**
(a) slow and synchronous (b) fast and synchronous
(c) slow and asynchronous (d) fast and asynchronous

55 The number of autosomes in human primary spermatocyte is **[DUMET 2011]**
(a) 46 (b) 44 (c) 23 (d) 22

56 Sperm acrosome is derived from **[J&K CET 2011]**
(a) Golgi bodies (b) endoplasmic reticulum
(c) lysosome (d) mesosome

57 In human beings, normally in which one of the following parts, does the sperm fertilise the ovum? **[MHT CET 2011]**
(a) Cervix (b) Fallopian tube
(c) Lower part of uterus (d) Upper part of uterus

58 The best definition of the process of gastrulation is that it is a process where the **[UP CPMT 2011]**
(a) single layered blastula becomes two-layered
(b) archenteron is formed
(c) zygote gets converted into larva
(d) cells move to occupy their definite position

ANSWERS

Check Point 3.1

1. (a)	2. (a)	3. (b)	4. (a)	5. (b)	6. (c)

Check Point 3.2

1. (b)	2. (b)	3. (d)	4. (a)	5. (d)	6. (a)

Check Point 3.3

1. (d)	2. (d)	3. (c)	4. (d)	5. (d)	6. (b)

Check Point 3.4

1. (b)	2. (b)	3. (a)	4. (d)	5. (d)	6. (d)

(A) Topical Exercise

1. (c)	2. (b)	3. (b)	4. (c)	5. (d)	6. (a)	7. (c)	8. (c)	9. (c)	10. (d)
11. (b)	12. (c)	13. (b)	14. (c)	15. (d)	16. (b)	17. (c)	18. (b)	19. (a)	20. (d)
21. (c)	22. (d)	23. (c)	24. (c)	25. (a)	26. (a)	27. (a)	28. (c)	29. (c)	30. (c)
31. (a)	32. (a)	33. (b)	34. (a)	35. (c)	36. (c)	37. (c)	38. (c)	39. (a)	40. (c)
41. (a)	42. (d)	43. (b)	44. (c)	45. (b)	46. (d)	47. (c)	48. (c)	49. (a)	50. (d)
51. (d)	52. (c)	53. (b)	54. (b)	55. (a)	56. (c)	57. (a)	58. (d)	59. (b)	60. (b)
61. (c)	62. (b)	63. (d)	64. (c)	65. (a)	66. (b)	67. (d)	68. (d)	69. (c)	70. (d)
71. (c)	72. (c)	73. (b)	74. (c)	75. (c)	76. (d)	77. (a)	78. (c)	79. (a)	80. (d)
81. (b)	82. (d)	83. (c)	84. (c)	85. (d)	86. (c)	87. (c)	88. (b)	89. (d)	90. (b)
91. (d)	92. (d)	93. (a)	94. (b)	95. (c)	96. (b)	97. (d)	98. (c)	99. (b)	100. (d)
101. (c)	102. (c)								

(B) Cumulative Exercise

1. (b)	2. (a)	3. (b)	4. (c)	5. (b)	6. (d)	7. (b)	8. (a)	9. (b)	10. (a)
11. (b)	12. (a)	13. (a)	14. (b)	15. (a)	16. (b)	17. (c)	18. (d)	19. (b)	20. (d)
21. (d)	22. (a)	23. (b)	24. (b)	25. (a)	26. (d)	27. (a)	28. (d)	29. (c)	30. (c)
31. (a)	32. (a)	33. (c)	34. (b)	35. (b)	36. (a)	37. (b)	38. (c)	39. (d)	40. (a)
41. (e)	42. (b)	43. (d)	44. (e)	45. (a)	46. (c)				

(C) Medical Entrances' Gallery

1. (b)	2. (d)	3. (c)	4. (b)	5. (d)	6. (c)	7. (c)	8. (a)	9. (d)	10. (c)
11. (c)	12. (b)	13. (a)	14. (d)	15. (b)	16. (c)	17. (a)	18. (d)	19. (d)	20. (a)
21. (a)	22. (a)	23. (a)	24. (b)	25. (c)	26. (a)	27. (a)	28. (c)	29. (d)	30. (a)
31. (b)	32. (a)	33. (a)	34. (b)	35. (b)	36. (c)	37. (b)	38. (c)	39. (c)	40. (d)
41. (c)	42. (d)	43. (a)	44. (a)	45. (d)	46. (b)	47. (a)	48. (d)	49. (d)	50. (b)
51. (d)	52. (b)	53. (a)	54. (a)	55. (b)	56. (a)	57. (b)	58. (d)		

Explanations

(A) Topical Exercise

11 (*b*) Statement I is false, but II is true. Incorrect statement can be corrected as

Prostate secretions activate the sperms.

17 (*c*) Pair in option (c) is incorrect and can be corrected as

Vasa deferentia help in the conduction of sperms from testis to penis. They have no role in seminal fluid production.

Rest options are correctly matched pairs.

21 (*c*) Statement in option (c) is incorrect and can be corrected as

Ovaries produce steroid hormones like oestradiol, progesterone, etc.

24 (*c*) Statement in option (c) is incorrect and can be corrected as

Uterus opens into the vagina through cervix.

38 (*c*) The middle piece of human sperm contains mitochondria coiled around the axial bundles of microtubules. The latter possesses 9 +2 arrangement.

40 (*c*) Statement in option (c) is incorrect and can be corrected as

Oogonia are formed during the foetal life only.

No new oogonia are formed after the birth of females.

46 (*d*) Statement in option (d) is incorrect for hormone A and can be corrected as

Here, A represents Luteinizing Hormone (LH). It is a peptide hormone and increased amount of this hormone causes ovulation.

49 (*a*) Statement I is true, but II is false. Incorrect statement can be corrected as

The changes in the ovary and uterus during menstrual cycle are induced by the ovarian hormones and anterior pituitary hormones.

59 (*b*) Satement in option (b) is incorrect and can be corrected as

Fertilisation is a physio-chemical event that involves movement and entry of sperm into ovum through various chemical reactions.

82 (*d*) Option (d) is mismatched and can be correctly matched as

Lens of human eye is ectodermal in origin.

(B) Cumulative Exercise

1 (*b*) Statements III and IV are correct.

Statements I and II are incorrect and can be corrected as

Low pitched voice and apparent larynx are secondary sexual characters in males.

Acrosome contains nucleus having haploid set of chromosomes.

8 (*a*) II and III are correctly matched pairs while I and II are incorrect. Incorrectly matched pairs can be corrected as

- Colostrum is the first milk which comes out from the mother's mammary gland just after childbirth.
- Bartholin's gland in female is homologous to cowper's gland in male.

9 (*b*) All the given statements are correct except V.

Incorrect statement can be corrected as

Perimetrium is thin outer covering and myometrium is thick middle layer.

14 (*b*) Statements II and IV are correct wheresas I and III are incorrect. Incorrect statements can be corrected as

Cleavage divisions do not increase the protoplasm content in blastomeres.

In blastocyst, blastomers are arranged as trophoblast and inner cell mass.

33 (*c*) Statement III is false and can be corrected as

Inhibin is secreted when FSH from anterior pituitary acts upon Sertoli cells. It inhibits FSH synthesis in negative feedback loop.

35 (*b*) All statements are true about mammalian placenta except II. Incorrect statement can be corrected as

Relaxin is secreted by ovary and placenta at the end of gestation period because it aids in parturition.

16-celled stage. It develops into blastula, which is the 64-celled stage. It contains a fluid-filled cavity called blastocoel. It ultimately leads to the stage called gastrula, a multilayered structure, which is then followed by organogenesis.

27 (*a*) Following ovulation, Graafian follicle bursts to release the ovum, after which granulosa and interstitial cells together form a mass of large, conical cells called corpus luteum. It acts as an endocrine gland because it secretes progesterone hormone for the maintenance of pregnancy.

28 (*c*) The secretory or luteal phase of human menstrual cycle is called the second phase of human menstrual cycle and it lasts for about 13 days.

Here, the LH is secreted by anterior lobe of pituitary leading to LH surge and subsequently ovulation.

29 (*d*) Capacitation is a pre-fertilisation process, where the spermatozoa acquire the capacity to fertilise the eggs (i.e. maturation). It occurs in the female reproductive tract.

Capacitation involves following changes

- Dilution of inhibitory factors of semen.
- Removal of cholesterol vesicles covering sperm head and acrosome.
- Increase in the permeability of acrosome.

38 (*c*) Option (c) is not function of placenta.

The placenta facilitates the supply of oxygen and nutrients to the embryo and also removal of carbon dioxide and excretory/waste materials produced by the embryo. The placenta is connected to the embryo through a cord, which helps in the transport of substances to and from the embryo. Placenta also acts as an endocrine tissue and produces several hormones like human Chorionic Gonadotropin (hCG), human Placental Lactogen (hPL), oestrogens, progestogens, etc.

40 (*d*) Decreased level of progesterone results in the menstrual flow. During this phase, uterine endometrium, epithelial glands and connective tissues are broken.

43 (*a*) Option (a) is false and can be corrected as

Sperms are viable for up to 24-48 hrs, whereas the human ovum is viable for only up to 24 hrs.

44 (*a*) Parturition is induced by complex neuroendocrine mechanism. These signals originate from fully developed foetus and placenta which induces mild uterine contraction called foetal ejection reflex. This reflex triggers the release of oxytocin from the maternal pituitary and acts on uterine muscles. It causes more contractions, which inturn secretes more oxytocin.

45 (*d*) In a normal pregnant woman, the level of human Chorionic Gonadotropin (hCG), oestrogen and progesterone are high. This is because the placenta (develops in pregnant women) acts as endocrine gland resulting in synthesis and secretion of these hormones.

52 (*b*) The ruptured follicle of ovary after ovulation gives rise to corpus luteum, which is the source for the secretion of progesterone. This hormone is responsible for growth and maintenance of foetus. Oestrogen is produced by theca interna cells of Graafian follicles.

53 (*a*) Undifferentiated primordial germ cells undergo mitotic division to produce spermatogonia. Each spermatogonium grows to a larger primary spermatocyte by obtaining nutrients from the nursing cells. The DNA content remains the same ($2n$) in both spermatogonia and primary spermatocyte.

54 (*a*) Cleavage in human is simple holoblastic, slow and synchronous. Cleavage in mammals ovum takes place during its passage through the Fallopian tube to the uterus. The resultant cells of cleavage are called blastomeres.

CHAPTER 04

Reproductive Health

According to the World Health Organisation (WHO), reproductive health means total well-being in physical, emotional, behavioural and social aspects of reproduction.

It deals with the reproductive processes, functions and systems at all stages of life. Reproductive health is a crucial part and a central feature of human health and development. Its ultimate purpose is the enhancement of life and personal relations. Thus, it is not merely the absence of reproductive diseases or infirmity.

In this chapter, we will deal with various aspects of reproductive health including human population, its explosion and control measures. We will also discuss about STDs, infertility and assisted reproductive technologies.

REPRODUCTIVE HEALTH : PROBLEMS AND STRATEGIES

India is amongst the pioneer countries of the world to initiate plans and programmes for attaining reproductive health as a social goal. The basic problems of reproductive health that are addressed in these programmes are as follows

- During adolescent stage, the reproductive organs are not completely developed. So, if marriages happen at early stage and the female gets pregnant, the development of the body stops, thus leading to various health issues.
- Lack of proper care and nutrition of the pregnant mother can lead to mortality of both mother and child.
- Lack of education about reproductive health and hygiene.
- Frequent pregnancies during adolescent stage.
- Lack of awareness about various family planning strategies and birth control measures.

A programme was initiated in 1951 to combat these problems and it was called **family planning programme**. Since then, it has been periodically assessed and improved. Some, additional programmes covering wider reproduction-related areas are currently in operation under the popular **'Reproductive and Child Healthcare** (RCH) **Programmes'**. This programme was launched throughout the country on 15th October, 1997.

Inside

The aspects that are taken care of in RCH programmes are as follows

(i) **Sex education** Introduction of sex education in schools should be encouraged to provide right information to the young generation. This would discourage children from believing in myths and having misconceptions about sex related aspects.

(ii) **Awareness about reproduction and STDs** Proper information about reproductive organs, adolescence and related changes, safe and hygienic sexual practices, Sexually Transmitted Diseases (STDs), AIDS, etc., would help the individuals in adolescent age group to lead a reproductively healthy life.

(iii) **Knowledge of birth control devices and pregnancy** The fertile couples and those in marriageable age group should be educated about available birth control options, care of pregnant mother, postnatal care of the mother and child, importance of breastfeeding, equal opportunities of male and female child, etc.

(iv) **Prevention of sex abuse and related crimes** Awareness of problems due to uncontrolled population growth, social evils like sex abuse and sex related crimes, etc., needs to be created. It would enable people to think and take up necessary steps to prevent these crimes and thereby, buildup a socially responsible and healthy society.

(v) **Development of new techniques** Implementation of better techniques and new strategies from time to time are required to provide more efficient care and assistance to people.

The development of these techniques requires strong infrastructural facilities, professional expertise and material support.

These efforts are essential to provide medical assistance and care to people in reproduction related problems like pregnancy, delivery, STDs, abortions, contraception, menstrual problems and infertility, etc.

(vi) **Prevention of female foeticide** Strict ban on amniocentesis is implemented to legally control the increased incidences of female foeticides.

(vii) **Child immunisation** It has a major role in RCH programmes. Vaccines are given to people of different age groups to combat different diseases.

(viii) **Research on reproduction-related areas** It should be encouraged and supported by the governmental and non-governmental agencies to find out newer methods and/or to improve the existing ones.

POPULATION EXPLOSION AND BIRTH CONTROL

The total number of individuals of a species living in an area form a population. The scientific study of all aspects of human population is called **demography**.

Population explosion

A sudden and rapid increase in population in a relatively shorter time period is known as population explosion.

In recent time, the world population which was around 6.102 billion in 2000 rocketed to about 7.2 billion in 2011. A similar trend of population explosion was observed in India too, due to improved medical facilities and quality of life.

Causes of population explosion

The main causes of population explosion are as follows

- Decrease in death rate
- Increase in average lifespan
- Decline in Maternal Mortality Rate (MMR) and Infant Mortality Rate (IMR)
- Increase in number of people in reproducible age group
- Better medical facilities
- Control of insect vectors that cause fatal diseases and epidemics
- Better sanitation
- Proper care of newborn children and their mothers

Census gives us information about the population of a country.

An account of census from 1991 to 2011 is tabulated below

Table 4.1 Details of India's population of 1991, 2001 and 2011

Data	1991 Census	2001 Census	2011 Census
1. Population			
Total	843,930,861	1,027,015,247	1,210,193,422
Males	437,597,929	531,277,078	623,724,248
Females	406,332,932	495,738,169	586,469,174
2. Decennial population growth			
Absolute	160,601,764	183,084,386	201,047,089
Percentage	23.50%	21.34%	17.7%
3. Annual population growth rate			
	2.35%	2.13%	1.77%

Data	1991 Census	2001 Census	2011 Census
4. Population density per square kilometre (maximum in Paschim Banga)			
	267	312.5	382
5. Sex ratio			
	929 females per 1000 males	933 females per 1000 males	943 females per 1000 males
6. Literacy rate			
Total	52.11%	65.28%	74.04%
Males	63.86%	76.40%	82.14%
Females	39.42%	54.16%	65.46%

Note • *The annual average population growth rate in India was about 2.1% per year during the period of 1965 to 1970 which has now dropped to 1.77%. The present doubling time of population in India is still 33 years.*

• *The population of India is projected close to 1.38 billion or 138 crore in 2020.*

Population growth rate

It is indicated by two factors, i.e.

- **Annual average growth rate** The annual growth rate of population in per cent is equal to $\frac{P_2 - P_1}{P_1 \times N} \times 100$,

  where, P_1 is the population size at the time of previous census, P_2 is the population size during present census and N is the number of years between the two census.
- **Doubling time** It is the number of years required for a population to double.

Demographic cycle

During technological and social development of a country, the population passes through five phases. These are as follows

- **High stationary** Both birth and death rates are high and population remains stationary.
- **Early expanding** Death rate falls, but birth rate continues to be high.
- **Late expanding** Both birth and death rates fall.
- **Low stationary** Both birth and death rates are low, but still birth rate is more than death rate.
- **Declining** It is temporary and shows birth rate to be lower than death rate, so that population tends to fall.

Effects of population explosion

Population explosion has become major problem because of its following effects

- Socioeconomic problems due to shortage of space, food, unemployment, poverty, educational and medical facilities.
- Energy crisis due to greater demands of oil and electricity.
- Rapid ecodegradation due to deforestation and pollution.

Therefore, the government has been forced to take up serious measures to check this population growth rate.

Control of population

The various methods that can be adopted in order to check overpopulation are as follows

- People, especially adolescents should be educated about the advantages to smaller families.
- Raising the marriageable age of females to 18 yrs and that of males to 21 yrs.
- Incentives are being offered to couples with small families.
- Utilisation of birth control measures which can check birth rate.

Birth control

The process used to prevent conception or pregnancy without interfering with the reproductive health of individuals is called birth control.

The methods or devices used to limit the number of offsprings are called **birth control methods** or **contraceptives.**

An ideal contraceptive should be comfortable, i.e. easy to use, safe, easily available and effective with no side effects. Most of the birth control methods act by blocking the transport of sperm to ova, ovulation or implantation.

Methods of birth control

The various methods of birth control are listed in the table given below

Table 4.2 Methods of contraception or birth control

Methods	Basis of actions	Note on uses	Approximate failure rates	Relative advantages	Relative disadvantages
1. **Natural methods** (NFP stands for Natural Method of Family Planning)					
Rhythm method or **abstinence**	Avoid sexual intercourse around the time of ovulation, i.e. total abstinence from day 10-17 of menstrual cycle.	—	20%	Natural and acceptable	High failure rate, even higher if periods are irregular. Requires good knowledge of body and good record-keeping. Requires period of abstinence.
Temperature method	There is a rise in temperature by 1° F during/at ovulation and avoiding sexual intercourse at that time could help in birth control.	—	Upto 20%	Can increase reliability of rhythm method	Same as above
Coitus interruptus (withdrawal method)	Penis is withdrawn from vagina before ejaculation, so as to prevent insemination.	—	20%	Accepted by Roman Catholic church	High failure rate. Requires self-discipline. Penis may leak some sperm before ejaculation (Pre-ejaculation)
Lactational amenorrhea	During lactation, high level of prolactin prevents the menstrual cycle by inhibiting the secretion of gonadotropins, LH and FSH. Hence, ovulation does not occur.	—	Less just after childbirth	No efforts required	Effective only up to a period of 4-6 months. (After parturition)
2. **Barrier methods**					
Condom	A thin, strong rubber sheath, prevents sperm from entering the vagina.	Placed over erect penis just before sexual intercourse, e.g. Nirodh (the common brand provided by the family welfare services).	10-12% with experienced use.	Cheap, easy and convenient to use. Easily obtained, gives protection against sexually transmitted diseases such as HIV, etc.	Not as reliable as the pill, Relies on male will, may tear or slip off.
Fem-shield (Femidom)	Female equivalent of the condom, a thin rubber or polyurethral tube with one closed end. It fits inside vagina and an open end have two fixable rings, one on each end, to keep it in place.	Inserted before intercourse and removed any time later.	Relatively new so no data. Probably simil ar to condom.	Help of male partner and erection of penis is not required. Also protects against STD.	• Difficult to insert • Can break or leak • Expensive than male condom

Methods	Basis of actions	Note on uses	Approximate failure rates	Relative advantages	Relative disadvantages
Diaphragm, cervical cap and vaults	These are tubular rubber sheath with flexible metal or spring ring at the margin (**diaphragm**) or rubber nipple (**cervical cap**) fitted inside and over the cervix, respectively. **Vault** is a rubber dome, which fits over the vaginal vault or cervix. These prevent entry of sperm into the uterus. Used with a spermicidal cream or jelly (a spermicide is a chemical which kills sperms).	Inserted before intercourse and must be left in place at least 6 hours after the intercourse.	3-15%	It can be inserted at any time before sex. However, extra spermicide must be used to increase effectiveness.	Suggestion of doctor is required for proper size selection. Training is required to fit. Occasionally causes abdominal pain. It should not be left for more than 30 hours as it may cause toxic shock syndrome. Examination required after every 6 months that cap is of right size.
3. **Chemical methods**					
Spermicides	Chemical which kills sperm, e.g. lactic acid, boric acid, zinc sulphate in the form of creams (e.g. delfen), jellies (e.g. perceptin) and foam tablets (e.g. chlorimin-T).	Placed in vagina to cover lining of vagina and cervix. Effective for about 1 hour.	10-25%	Can be quite effective when used along with condom or diaphragm.	High failure rate if used on its own.
Sponge	Polyurethane sponge impregnated with spermicide (e.g. non-oxynol 9). Fits over cervix and is disposable.	Fitted up to 24 hours before intercourse. Leave in place for least 6 hours after intercourse.	10-25%	One size fits all and no fitting required.	High failure rate
4. **Injectable contraceptives**					
Hormone injections (depo-provera)	Progesterone derivative injections that either suppress or prevent ovulation, e.g. Depot Medroxy Progesterone Acetate (DMPA) and NorEthisterone Enanthate (NETEN). Cyclofem and Mesigyna are combined injectable contraceptives containing progestin and oestradiol.	Given once every 1-3 months		Convenient and highly effective.	No serious side effects, occasionally there is menstrual bleeding.
5. **Oral contraceptives**					
Pills	Contains either progestin alone (e.g. minipill) or combination of hormones oestrogen and progesterone (e.g. Mala-D). Oestrogen prevents development of eggs and ovulation by inhibiting secretion of FSH. Progesterone inhibits LH production; acts on cervical mucus to prevent penetration of sperm. They can also prevent the blastocyst implantation by alternation in endometrium, e.g. Mala-D, Mala-L.	One pill taken orally each day during first 3 weeks of cycle. After 4 weeks, menstruation starts and the pill is taken again.	1%	Very reliable (almost 100% if properly used). Woman has control.	Short-term side effects, may include nausea, fluid retention and weight gain. Long-term side effects, not fully understood, but high risk of blood clotting may occur in some women. Not recommended for older women.
Saheli (non-steroidal pill)	It is a non-hormonal pill that contains centchroman. It acts by inhibiting oestrogen activity. This alters uterus lining and thus, prevent implantation. It was developed by Central Drug Research Institute (CDRI), Lucknow.	It is taken once a week.	1%	Non-steroidal, less side effects	

Methods	Basis of actions	Note on uses	Approximate failure rates	Relative advantages	Relative disadvantages
Minipill or **Progestin Only Pill** (POP)	Contains progestin, a synthetic progesterone only. Ovulation may occur, but cervical mucus is thickened, preventing entry of sperms.	Must be taken within 3 hours of same time every day, but newer generation have the relaxations of 12 hours.	2%	Very reliable. Lower dose of hormones than pill. Therefore, less risk to older women.	Bleeding between periods. May cause headache.
Morning after pill or **Emergency contraceptives**	Contains RU486, an antiprogesterone. They prevent implantation, e.g. i-pill, PILL-72 and unwanted 72.	They are taken within 3 days (72 hours) of sexual intercourse.		Highly effective	For use only in emergencies. Long term effects not known.
6. **IUD** (Intrauterine Device) or **Coil** Increase spermphagocytosis and prevent fertilisation and implantation					
1st generation (non- medicated, e.g. Lippes loops, rings).		These are inserted in uterus, to make it unfit for sperm.	3%	Can be left in place for long periods (up to 10 years). Suitable for women who have had children (easier to fit in larger uterus).	May cause bleeding and discomfort. IUD may come out. Other complications include tubual pregnancy, perforation of uterus.
2nd generation (copper devices) e.g. Cu T-200, Multiload, Cu T-375, Cu 7.	The copper ions suppress the motility and fertilisation capacity of sperm.				
3rd generation (hormonal devices) e.g. Progestasert and Levonorgestrel IUD, e.g. LNG-20.	These make the uterus unsuitable for implantation and the cervix hostile to sperms.				
7. **Implants**					
	Hormone containing devices implanted subdermally for providing long term contraception, e.g. Norplant (progestin only device), Implanon (3-keto-desogestrel)	Inserted under the skin inside upper arm or forearm through a small incision.	Less than 1%	Effective for 5-3 yrs.	May cause discomfort.
8. **Abortion** (discussed later in this chapter as MTP)					
	Premature voluntary termination of pregnancy by surgical intervention.	Upto 20 weeks		A measure of last resort.	Risk of infertility and other complications. Emotionally difficult and ethically wrong.
9. **Sterilisation** (surgical methods)					
Vasectomy	Vas deferens are cut and tied.		Less than 1%	Very reliable. No side effects. Simple.	Very difficult to reverse. Need to use alternative method upto 2-3 months after vasectomy.
Tubectomy	Both oviducts are cut and tied (now laparoscopic methods are used).		Less than 1%	Very reliable.	Even more difficult to reverse than vasectomy.

Medical Termination of Pregnancy (MTP)

- Voluntary or Intentional termination of pregnancy before full term is called **Medical Termination of Pregnancy** (MTP) or **Induced Abortion.**
- It is the termination or removal of embryo from the uterus by using pharmacological or surgical methods.
- MTP is considered relatively safe during the first trimester, i.e. upto 12 weeks of pregnancy, but can be performed upto 20 weeks.
- Government of India legalised MTP under 'Medical Termination of Pregnancy Act, 1971' with some strict conditions to avoid its misuse. The act has been amended in 2002.
- About 45-50 million, MTPs are performed in a year all over the world. It accounts to 1/5th of the total number of conceived pregnancies in a year.

Significance of MTP

- MTP has a significant role in decreasing the population though it is not meant for that purpose.
- MTPs are essential in certain cases where continuation of the pregnancy could be harmful to the mother, foetus or both.

Disadvantages of MTP

- A majority of the MTPs are performed illegally by unqualified persons. It is not only unsafe, but could be fatal too.
- MTP is often misused to abort female foetus.
- MTP has raised many emotional, ethical, religious and social issues.

Amniocentesis

It is also referred to as Amniotic Fluid Test (AFT). It is a medical procedure used in prenatal diagnosis of **chromosomal abnormalities** and **foetal infections**. In this process, a small amount of amniotic fluid containing foetal cells is extracted from the amnion or amniotic sac surrounding a developing foetus. The foetal DNA is then examined for genetic abnormalities. Using this process, the sex of a child can also be determined, hence this procedure has some legal restrictions.

Misuse of amniocentesis

Unfortunately, it is being misused to know the sex of unborn baby followed by medical termination of foetus, in case its female. Determination of sex by amniocentesis has been banned in India.

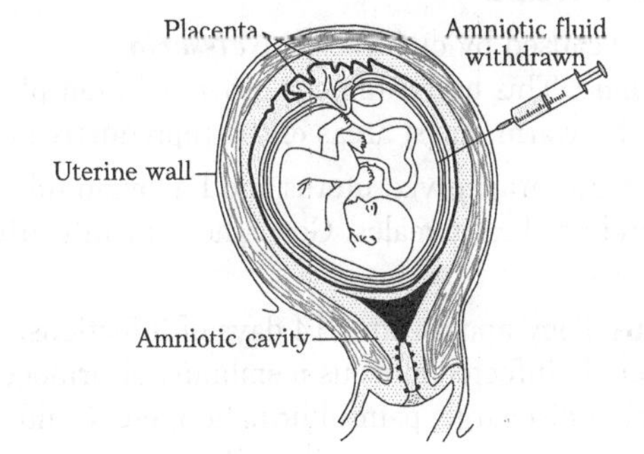

Fig. 4.1 Amniocentesis

CHECK POINT 4.1

1. Increased IMR and decreased MMR in a population will
   (a) cause rapid increase in growth rate
   (b) result in decline in growth rate
   (c) not cause significant change in growth rate
   (d) result in an explosive population
2. A stable population is one which has got
   (a) no growth of population in the last decade
   (b) constant rate of growth of population in last decade
   (c) slow growth of population in last decade
   (d) growth of 20% in excess than the last decade
3. Which of the following birth control measure can be considered as the safest?
   (a) The rhythm method
   (b) The use of withdrawl method
   (c) Terminalisation of unwanted pregnancy
   (d) Sterilisation technique
4. Which of the following is not a barrier method of birth control?
   (a) Vault (b) Implant
   (c) Diaphragm (d) Fem-shield
5. Use of which of the following contraceptive device has increased in recent years due to its additional benefit of protecting the user from contracting STDs?
   (a) Diaphragms and cervical cap
   (b) IUDs
   (c) Condoms
   (d) Contraceptive pills
6. Choose the odd one out.
   (a) Vasectomy
   (b) Contraceptive pills
   (c) Amniocentesis
   (d) Implanon

SEXUALLY TRANSMITTED DISEASES (STDs)

Diseases or Infections, which are transmitted through sexual intercourse with infected person are collectively called **Sexually Transmitted Diseases** (STDs) or **Veneral Diseases** (VD) or **Reproductive Tract Infections** (RTIs).

These diseases if not cured in time, can lead to complications, which include Pelvic Inflammatory Diseases (PIDs), abortions, still births, ectopic pregnancies, infertility or even cancer of the reproductive tract.

The common sexually transmitted diseases are as follows

1. Gonorrhoea

Cause It is caused by diplococcus ***Neisseria gonorrhoeae***. This bacterium can grow and multiply easily in the warm, moist areas of the reproductive tract.

It includes urethra, cervix, uterus and Fallopian tubes in women and urethra in males. Gonorrhoea mainly affects women.

Symptoms They appear after 14 days of infections. These include infected mucous membrane of urinogenital tract, genital discharge, painful urination, etc. Children born to infected mother naturally suffer eye infection.

2. Syphilis

Cause It is caused by a bacterium named ***Treponema pallidum*** that can grow and multiply easily in the warm, moist areas of the reproductive tract.

Symptoms Sores and lessions in genital tract, painful urination, small painless sore or chancre at the point of sexual contact (first stage), skin rash, joint and muscle ache, swollen lymph gland, etc. (second stage).

3. Chlamydiasis

Cause It is a common STD caused by a bacterium named ***Chlamydia trachomatis***.

Symptoms It can damage female reproductive organs. Chlamydia infection may even cause infertility in women.

4. Trichomoniasis

Cause It is also a very common STD caused by a protozoan parasite called ***Trichomonas vaginalis***.

Symptoms Most commonly infected parts of women body in this disease include vulva, vagina and urethra. Thus, it causes vaginal itching, discharge, urethritis, etc.

5. Chancroid

Cause It is caused by Gram negative bacilli ***Haemophilus ducrei***. The incubation period is of about 3-5 days.

Symptoms The initial lesion at the site of inoculation breaks down to form a painful, soft ulcer with a necrotic base.

6. Genital warts

Cause These are infectious diseases caused by viruses like **Human Papilloma Virus** (HPV). Patients with a history of genital warts may be at increased risk for cervical, vaginal, anal, vulvar and penile cancers.

Symptoms Hard outgrowth with horny surface over the skin and mucosal surface of external genitalia and perianal area.

7. Genital herpes

Cause It is a sexually transmitted disease caused by the **Herpes Simplex Viruses-type** 1 (HSV-1) or **type** 2 (HSV-2). Most genital herpes are caused by HSV-2.

Symptoms Painful genital blisters on and around penis in males; vaginal discharge, blisters, fever, itching, etc., in females.

8. Hepatitis-B

Cause It is caused by **Hepatitis-B Virus** (HBV) which is transmitted through sexual contact, blood transfusion, etc.

Symptoms Yellowing of skin, persistant low-grade fever, jaundice, dark urine, light-coloured stools, cirrhosis, etc.

Note *Hepatitis-B is diagnosed by Australian antigen test or Hepatitis-B surface antigen test (HBSAg).*

9. AIDS

(Acquired Immuno Deficiency Syndrome)

Cause It is caused by **Human Immunodeficiency Virus** (HIV). This virus is pathogenic to human beings as it damages the immune system of the human body.

Symptoms Fever, lethargy, pharyngitis, weight loss, nausea, headache, rashes, weakened immune system, etc.

Transmission AIDS along with hepatitis-B can also be transmitted by sharing of injection needles, surgical instruments, etc., with infected persons, transfusion of blood or from an infected mother to the foetus too.

The first case of AIDS was reported from California in 1981 (US). HIV was first isolated by **Montagnier *et al.*** (1983) of the **Pasteur Institute of Paris**. In India, first case of AIDS was detected in Chennai. More details about AIDS are discussed in chapter Human Health and Diseases.

Generalised symptoms of STDs

The initial symptoms of most of the sexually transmitted diseases mentioned above are minor.

These include

- Itching (irritation inside the penis), burning sensations after urination or ejaculation, fluid discharge, mild pain and swellings, etc., in the genital region.
- Infected females may often be asymptomatic, hence may remain undetected for long.
- In women, the most commonly infected part of the body is the lower genital tract (vulva, vagina or urethra) and in men, the most commonly infected body part is the inside of the penis (urethra).
- Discharge from penis in a gonorrhoea infected person is yellow, white or green in colour.
- Absence or less significant symptoms in the early stages of infection and the social stigma attached to the STDs, prevent the infected person from undergoing timely detection and proper treatment.
- Except for hepatitis-B, genital herpes and HIV infections, other STDs are completely curable, if detected early and treated properly.
- **Age group vulnerable to STDs** All persons are vulnerable to these infections. However, their incidences are reported to be very high among persons in the age group of 15-24 years, i.e. the adolescent age group. Therefore, one should be very alert and disciplined, so that STDs cannot ruin their health and happiness.

Preventive measures (Prophylaxis) of STDs

Prevention or early detection and cure of sexually transmitted diseases are given prime consideration under the reproductive healthcare programmes.

Prevention of sexually transmitted diseases can be done by the simple practices given below

- Avoid sex with unknown partners/multiple partners.
- Always use condoms during coitus.
- Use of sterilised needles and syringes during immunisation, blood transfusion, etc.
- Education about the sexually transmitted diseases should be given to the people.
- Any genital symptoms such as discharge or burning sensation during urination or unusual sore or rash are alert signals of STD and one should see a doctor immediately.
- Screening of blood donors should be mandatory.

INFERTILITY

- It refers to the failure to achieve a clinical pregnancy even after 12 months or more of regular unprotected sexual intercourse. It is different from sterility, which means the complete inability to conceive. Thus, infertility is often termed as **relative sterility.**
- The reasons for infertility could be many, such as physical, congenital diseases, drugs, immunological or even psychological.
- Infertility can be of two types
  - (i) **Primary infertility** It is found in patients, who have never conceived.
  - (ii) **Secondary infertility** It is found in patients, who were able to conceive at least once previously.
- Infertility is caused by defects found in males, females or in both of them.

Infertility in males

Normal fertile male may ejaculate 2.5-5 mL semen with a sperm count of over 200-300 million per ejaculation. Any defect in the sperm count, sperm structure, sperm motility of seminal fluid may cause infertility in males.

The main reasons of infertility in males are given below

- Low sperm count in males, i.e. **oligospermia**.
- Absence of sperm in semen, i.e. **azoospermia**.
- Low sperm motility, i.e. **asthenozoospermia**.
- Defective sperm morphology, i.e. **tetrazoospermia**.
- Failure of testes to descend into scrotum, i.e. **cryptorchidism**.
- Blocked vas deferentia and vasa efferentia.
- High temperature of scrotum, i.e. **hyperthermia**.
- Infections such as orchitis (inflammation of testis) brochiectasis and chlamydiasis, etc.
- Alcoholism, use of cytotoxic drugs, radiations and antidepressant suppress spermatogenesis.
- Gonadotropin deficiency, Klinefelter's syndrome, etc.
- Low fructose content, high prostaglandin content, high viscosity and low volume of ejaculate lead to male infertility.

Infertility in females

A fertile woman is the one who regularly ovulates, passes the egg down the reproductive tract, develops conditions for smooth passage of sperms and implantation of fertilised egg.

The main reasons of infertility in females are listed below

- Irregular menstrual cycle
- Polycystic Ovarian Disease (PCOD)
- Inadequate growth and functioning of corpus luteum
- Blockage of Fallopian tube
- Vaginal and cervical infections
- Non-canalisation of uterus
- Hypothalamic and pituitary dysfunction may cause **anovulation** (non-ovulation) and **oligo-ovulation** (deficient ovulation).
- Fibroid uterus
- Defective vaginal growth
- The ovum is not liberated, but remains trapped inside the follicle due to hyperprolactinaemia.

Note
- *A woman who has never conceived in 20 years is said to be **nulliparous**.*
- *Total fertility rate is average number of children born to a woman and replacement fertility rate is number of offsprings produced by a couple to replace themselves.*

ASSISTED REPRODUCTIVE TECHNOLOGY (ART)

It refers to techniques or procedures adopted for the correction of infertility in males and females.

These procedures are usually paired with more conventional therapies such as fertility drugs, to increase success rates.

A brief account of various ARTs is given below

1. *In vitro* Fertilisation (IVF)

The term '*in vitro*' is used to refer any biological procedure that is performed outside the organism's body.

In this technique, egg cells are fertilised by sperms outside the woman's womb in a test tube. It is a major treatment for infertility when other methods of achieving conception have failed.

The major steps of IVF are as follows

- The process involves hormonally controlled ovulatory process, removal of ova (eggs) from the woman's ovaries by transvaginal oocyte retrieval technique and then letting the sperms fertilise them in a fluid medium.
- Once fertilisation has occurred, the embryo is allowed to develop for 3-5 days.
- It is then transferred to the patient's uterus.
- A general term for babies conceived due to IVF is test tube babies. **Dr. Patrick Steptoe** and **Dr. Robert Edwards** reported first successful test tube baby, **Louise Joy Brown** on July 25, 1978 England. In India, the first test tube baby was born on August 6, 1986 at KEM Hospital, Mumbai. She was named **Kumari Harsha**. The doctor was **Indira Hinduja**.

2. Intra Cytoplasmic Sperm Injection (ICSI)

This is the technique to assist fertilisation of an egg. In this, one sperm is injected into the cytoplasm of an egg with a microscopic needle to allow fertilisation with that sperm only. ICSI is different from IVF because in IVF, many sperms are positioned close to the egg in a test tube. Once fertilisation occurs, the resulting embryo is placed inside the uterus as done in IVF.

3. Intra Uterine Insemination (IUI)

In this technique, a woman is first given a small amount of ovarian stimulation to maximise the maturity of the egg and the lining of the uterus. This is followed by the intrauterine insemination of the best of the sperm from a man's ejaculate. It is suitable for couples with unexplained infertility or minor semen problems provided the woman's Fallopian tubes are normal.

4. Artificial Donor Insemination (ADI)

This is a treatment in which donated sperm is inseminated into woman's uterus. It is suitable for couples where the partner has no sperm in the reproductive tract.

It is also suitable, if the man carries a genetic disease. The first reported birth from this technique was in 1984.

5. Oocyte Donation Procedure (ODP)

This is a treatment for women who are no longer producing their own eggs. It involves an oocyte donor (who can be known to the couple) going through an IVF treatment cycle. The donor's eggs are fertilised with the partner's sperm and the embryos are transferred into the uterus of his partner.

6. Gamete Intra Fallopian Transfer (GIFT)

In this technique, eggs are removed from the woman and placed in one of the Fallopian tubes, along with the sperm. Thus, fertilisation takes place inside the woman's body only. Therefore, it is considered *in vivo* fertilisation as gametes fuses inside the body. This technique is suitable for couples where the Fallopian tubes are healthy and the sperm can produce adequate fertilisation rates.

7. Zygote Intra Fallopian Transfer (ZIFT)

In this process, the pre-embryos (zygotes upto 8 cells) rather than gametes are transferred into the oviducts. The advantage of ZIFT over IVF is that the embryo enters the uterus after 24 hrs in ZIFT.

8. Intra Uterine Transfer (IUT)

When the zygote with more than 8 blastomeres stage is placed into uterus, it is termed as **Intrauterine Transfer** (IUT). It can be performed either in genetical mother or surrogate mother, i.e. a woman who substitutes the real mother to nurse the embryo.

9. Testicular Sperm Extraction (TSE)

It is a surgical technique to collect sperm from the testis or epididymis of a man who has blockage in his sperm ducts passage, due to which he is unable to ejaculate. Collection is usually done by needle aspiration of a small biopsy of the testes.

10. Pre-implantation Genetic Diagnosis (PGD)

This is a technique used when one or both partner's carry a serious genetic disease. It combines the techniques of IVF and ICSI. When the embryo is 3 days old, its one or two cells are removed.

These cells are examined to see if the embryo is at risk of having a genetic condition. Only those embryos that are not affected are transferred.

CHECK POINT 4.2

1. The sexually transmitted disease that can affect both the male and female genitals and may damage the eyes of babies born of infected mother is
   (a) AIDS (b) gonorrhoea (c) syphilis (d) hepatitis
2. Genital warts are due to sexually transmitted disease spread by
   (a) Herpes virus (b) Papillomavirus
   (c) Hepatitis-A (d) *Trichomonas*
3. In women, this sexually transmitted disease can result in infertility.
   (a) Human Papilloma Virus (HPV)
   (b) Pelvic inflammatory disease
   (c) Genital herpes
   (d) None of the above
4. ART does not include
   (a) zygote extra Fallopian transfer
   (b) *in vitro* fertilisation and embryo transfer
   (c) artificial insemination
   (d) gamete intra Fallopian transfer
5. Choose the incorrect option with respect to ART.
   (a) ZIFT is Zygote Intra Fallopian Transfer
   (b) Zygote is transferred into Fallopian tube after IVF
   (c) Early embryo of upto 8 blastomeres can be transferred to Fallopian tube
   (d) Embryo with more than 8 blastomeres are transferred to Fallopian tube

EXAM POINTS

- The study of human population is called demography. **[HPMT 2010]**
- Lactational amenorrhea, pills, emergency contraceptives are the contraceptive methods that involve a role of hormone. **[NEET 2019]**
- The contraceptive 'Saheli' blocks oestrogen receptors in the uterus, preventing eggs from getting implanted. **[NEET 2018]**
- Saheli was developed at CDRI, Lucknow. **[UK PMT 2014]**
- Progestasert is an IUD, which makes the uterus unsuitable and cervix hostile to the sperms as they are hormone releasing IUDs. **[KCET 2015]**
- Progestasert, LNG-20 are the hormone releasing intrauterine devices. **[NEET 2019, 16]**
- The function of copper ions in copper releasing IUDs is to suppress sperm motility and fertilising capacity of sperms. **[NEET 2017]**
- Vasectomy is used to block the passage of sperm from testes to penis. **[MHT CET 2014]**
- After tubectomy, Fallopian tube of female reproductive system is blocked. **[UK CET 2020, 15]**
- Purpose of tubectomy is to prevent embryonic development. **[BCECE 2012]**
- MTPs are considered safe during the first trimester of pregnancy. **[UK PMT 2014]**
- Amniocentesis can be used for the detection of cleft palate. **[NEET 2016]**
- AIDS and hepatitis-B are sexually transmitted diseases do not specifically affect reproductive organs. **[NEET 2019]**
- Gonorrhoea, syphilis, genital herpes are sexually transmitted diseases. **[NEET 2018, 2020]**
- Embryo with more than 16 blastomeres formed due to *in vitro* fertilisation is transferred into uterus. **[NEET 2016]**
- Assisted reproductive technology does not include zygote extra Fallopian transfer. **[KCET 2015]**
- In IVF, zygote is transferred into the Fallopian tube. **[CBSE AIPMT 2014]**
- In Intrauterine insemination, donor semen is artificially introduced into the uterus. **[J&K CET 2014]**
- GIFT stands for Gamete Intra Fallopian Transfer. **[GCET 2015]**

Chapter Exercises

(A) Topical Exercise

Reproductive Health and Population Explosion

1 The term 'Health' is defined in many ways. The most accurate definition of the health would be
(a) health is the state of body and mind in a balanced condition
(b) health is the reflection of a smiling face
(c) health is a state of complete physical, mental and social well-being
(d) health is the symbol of economic prosperity

2 The term reproductive health refers to
(a) sound mind in sound body
(b) creating awareness about reproductive organs
(c) normal functioning of reproductive organs
(d) Both (b) and (c)

3 Problems associated with reproductive health are
(a) myths and misconceptions about sex
(b) increased STD and sex crime
(c) lack of knowledge about the options of birth control devices
(d) All of the above

4 NRHM mainly emphesises on
(a) rural economic development
(b) to provide health care to rural population
(c) prevent migration of rural population
(d) to provide sex education to rural population

5 In India, population is tremendously increasing from last 30 years as a result of
(a) long lifespan of many individuals and of high birth rate
(b) short lifespan and low birth rate
(c) long lifespan and low birth rate
(d) short lifespan and high birth rate

6 The population generally stabilises
(a) around the carrying capacity
(b) below the carrying capacity
(c) above the carrying capacity
(d) irrespective of the carrying capacity

7 Consider the following statements.
I. The term demography was coined by Guillard.
II. The present doubling time of Indian population is 33 years.
Choose the correct option.
(a) Statement I is true, but II is false
(b) Statement I is false, but II is true
(c) Both statements I and II are true
(d) Both statements I and II are false

8 Population explosion in India is mainly due to
(a) climate change (b) increased birth rate
(c) lack of education (d) Both (b) and (c)

9 Which factor contributed most to rapid rise in human population?
(a) Decrease in infant mortality
(b) Polygamy
(c) Decrease in the death rate of old people
(d) Increase in birth rate

10 Which of the following is not a response of an animal population to high density?
(a) Starvation (b) Emigration
(c) Cannibalism (d) Increased natality rate

11 If the rate of addition of new members increases with respect to the individual lost of the same population, then the graph obtained has
(a) declined growth
(b) exponential growth
(c) zero population growth
(d) None of the above

12 In India, human population has higher number of younger age group because of
(a) long lifespan and low birth rate
(b) short lifespan and high birth rate
(c) short lifespan and low birth rate
(d) birth rate is equal to death rate

13 A population is said to achieve demographic transition, if
(a) birth rate is equal to death rate
(b) emigration is equal to immigration if population is same in both places
(c) doubling time is 33 years
(d) Both (a) and (b)

14 In a demographic cycle, when overall births and deaths rates are low, but birth rate is still more than death rate is
(a) low stationary (b) exponential stage
(c) early growth stage (d) acceleration stage

Birth Control

15 What is true for natural methods of contraception?
(a) They increase phagocytosis of sperms
(b) They employ barriers to prevent fertilisation
(c) They are natural ways of avoiding chances of fertilisation
(d) They are surgical methods

16 In the rhythm method of birth control, the couple refrains from intercourse
(a) one day before and after ovulation
(b) two days before and after ovulation
(c) seven days before and after ovulation
(d) on the day of ovulation

17 Which of the following is/are natural method of birth control? **[NCERT Exemplar]**
I. Abstinence
II. Rhythm method
III. Temperature method
IV. IUD
Codes
(a) Only I (b) Only III
(c) I, II and III (d) None of these

18 Coitus interruption method of birth control involves
(a) avoiding intercourse
(b) withdrawl of penis from vagina before male ejaculates
(c) application of cream in vagina before coitus
(d) use of foam during coitus

19 In lactational amenorrhea, high level of prolactin helps to
(a) inhibit the release of gonadotropins
(b) inhibit the release of oestrogen and progesterone
(c) stimulate the release of FSH and LH
(d) stimulate the release of oestrogen and progesterone

20 Which of the following method of contraception is effective only up to a maximum period of 6 months, following parturition?
(a) Coitus interruptus
(b) Lactational amenorrhea
(c) Periodic abstinence
(d) Condoms

21 Condoms are one of the most popular contraceptives because of the following reasons.
(a) These are effective barriers for insemination
(b) They do not interfere with coital act
(c) These help in reducing the risk of STDs
(d) All of the above

22 Consider the following statements.
I. Diaphragm acts as a chemical barrier for sperm entry.
II. Diaphragm is placed to cover the cervical region.
Choose the correct option.
(a) Statement I is true, but II is false
(b) Statement I is false, but II is true
(c) Both statements I and II are true
(d) Both statements I and II are false

23 Castration cannot be taken as a contraceptive device, because
(a) deficiency of testosterone hormone will deprive a person of sexual drive, desire and/or the sexual act
(b) it inhibits gamete transport
(c) this technique is highly effective, but its reversibility is poor
(d) All of the above

24 Choose the odd one out.
(a) Cyclofem (b) Mesigyma
(c) DMPA (d) Delfen

25 Consider the following statements with respect to contraceptive pills.
I. They inhibit ovulation and implantation.
II. They alter the quality of cervical mucus to prevent or retard the entry of sperms.
Choose the correct option.
(a) Statement I is true, but II is false
(b) Statement I is false, but II is true
(c) Both statements I and II are true
(d) Both statements I and II are false

26 The pills mostly used for birth control contains
I. oestrogen II. progesterone
III. prolactin IV. cholecystokinin
Codes **[NCERT Exemplar]**
(a) I and II (b) II and IV
(c) Only I (d) Only II

27 Progestin in the contraceptive pill
(a) inhibits Luteinizing hormone
(b) inhibits oestrogen
(c) checks attachment of zygote to endometrium
(d) All of the above

28 Oral contraceptives check ovulation by inhibiting the secretion of
(a) follicle stimulating hormone
(b) Luteinizing hormone
(c) progesterone
(d) Both (a) and (b)

29 Mark the incorrectly matched pair.
(a) Minipill – Contains oestrogen and progestin
(b) Morning pill – Contains RU 486
(c) Implant – Effective for 3-5 years
(d) Multiload – Placed in uterus

30 The pill Saheli is taken
(a) weekly (b) monthly
(c) daily (d) once in 3 months

31 RU486 (Mifepristone) is
(a) a steroid having affinity for progesterone hormone receptor
(b) a contraceptive pill taken daily
(c) morning after pill
(d) Both (a) and (c)

32 Emergency contraceptives are effective if used within
(a) 72 hrs of coitus (b) 72 hrs of ovulation
(c) 72 hrs of menstruation (d) 72 hrs of implantation

33 The pill Mala-D is taken
(a) daily for 3 weeks (b) twice in a day
(c) twice in a week (d) None of these

34 The contraceptives which are implanted include
(a) progestin (b) minipill
(c) copper-T (d) Both (a) and (c)

35 Which of the following statements is correct?
(a) Hormone releasing IUD make uterus unsuitable for implantation
(b) IUDs are ideal contraceptives for females who want to delay pregnancy
(c) IUD is the most widely accepted method of contraception in India
(d) All of the above

36 Consider the following statements.
I. IUDs increase phagocytosis reaction in the uterus.
II. IUDs once inserted, need not to be replaced.
Choose the correct option.
(a) Statement I is true, but II is false
(b) Statement I is false, but II is true
(c) Both statements I and II are true
(d) Both statements I and II are false

37 The copper ions of IUDs
(a) suppress the motility and fertilisation capacity of sperms
(b) make the vagina unsuitable for implantation
(c) increase sperms fertilising capacity
(d) prevent ovulation

38 Find out the incorrect statement for IUD.
(a) They can be self-inserted
(b) They are inserted by expert nurses/doctors
(c) They may be non-medicated IUDs, copper releasing IUDs or hormone releasing IUDs
(d) They are intrauterine devices

39 'Norplant' is the new form of birth control and it
(a) allows ovulation but does not allow fertilisation
(b) makes the cervical mucus thin to prevent sperm entry into the uterus
(c) has progestin as the active ingredient
(d) is effective for a maximum of 1 year

40 Match the following columns.

Column I (Names of IUDs)	Column II (Examples of IUDs)
A. Non-medicated IUD	1. Progestasert and LNG-20
B. Copper releasing IUD	2. Lippes loop
C. Hormone releasing IUD	3. Cu-T, Cu-7 and Multiload-375

Codes

	A	B	C
(a)	3	2	1
(b)	1	2	3
(c)	2	3	1
(d)	2	1	3

41 The leproscopy procedure is used in
(a) removal of uterus
(b) cutting and ligation of oviducts
(c) fitting of copper-T
(d) removal of ovaries

42 The correct surgical procedure as a contraceptive method is **[NCERT Exemplar]**
(a) ovariectomy
(b) hysterectomy
(c) vasectomy
(d) castration

43 Vasectomy has no effect on the sexual life of male because
(a) he can still ejaculate and has normal secretion of sex hormones in blood
(b) vasectomy affects the hormonal secretion, but the person can ejaculate semen with normal number of sperms
(c) he cannot ejaculate, but the hormone levels are normal
(d) vasectomy does not affect the sexual desire but can cause impotency

44 What is the figure given below showing in particular?

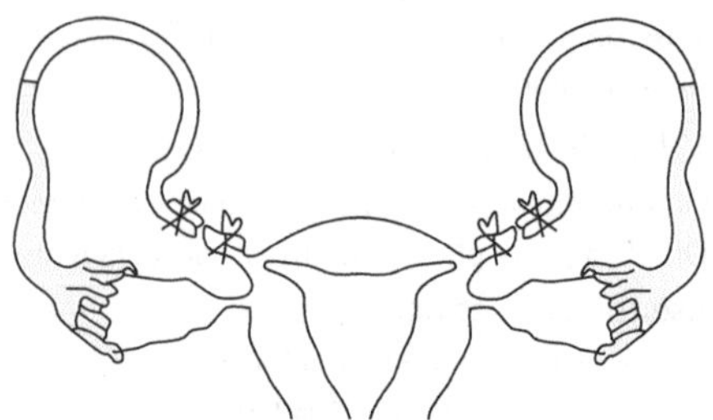

(a) Ovarian cancer
(b) Uterine cancer
(c) Tubectomy
(d) Vasectomy

45 Given below are the four methods and their modes of action in achieving contraception. Select their correct matching from the four options that follows.

	Column I (Birth control measures)		Column II (Modes of action)
A.	Pill	1.	Prevents sperms reaching cervix
B.	Condom	2.	Prevents implantation
C.	Vasectomy	3.	Prevents ovulation
D.	Copper-T	4.	Semen contains no sperms

Codes

	A	B	C	D
(a)	3	4	1	2
(b)	2	3	1	4
(c)	3	1	4	2
(d)	4	1	2	3

46 Match the contraceptive methods given under Column I with their examples given under Column II.

	Column I		Column II
A.	Chemical	1.	Tubectomy and vasectomy
B.	IUD	2.	Copper-T and loop
C.	Barriers	3.	Condom and cervical cap
D.	Sterilisation	4.	Spermicidal jelly and foam

Codes

	A	B	C	D
(a)	4	2	3	1
(b)	4	1	2	3
(c)	1	3	2	4
(d)	1	2	3	4

47 The success of birth control programmes in controlling population growth is dependent on
(a) use of contraceptives
(b) tubectomy
(c) vasectomy
(d) acceptability of the above by the people

48 Which of the following methods is used during abortion?
(a) Vacuum aspiration
(b) infusion of a saline solution/antiseptics
(c) Scraping
(d) All of the above

49 Which of the following statements is correct?
(a) MTP has a significant role in decreasing the population
(b) Government of India legalised MTP in 1977 with some strict conditions
(c) MTP is relatively safe during the first trimester
(d) All of the above

50 In which of the following conditions, MTP is performed legally?
I. To get rid of unwanted pregnancy due to casual unprotective intercourse.
II. To get rid of unwanted pregnancy due to failure of the contraceptive used during coitus or rapes.
III. Where the continuation of the pregnancy could be harmful or even fatal to the mother or to foetus or both.
IV. To get rid of pregnancy as the foetus is found to be female.
(a) I and II
(b) II and III
(c) I, II and III
(d) I, II, III and IV

51 Amniocentesis technique is commonly used for the determination of
I. sex
II. condition of the foetus
III. child heartbeat rate
IV. None of the above
Codes **[NCERT Exemplar]**
(a) Only I (b) I and II
(c) Only III (d) I, II, III and IV

52 All the following are use of aminocentesis, but one is misuse.
Which one is misuse?
(a) The centres for genetic counselling offer amniocentesis on request to women for chromosome analysis
(b) This technique has been developed for detecting foetal abnormalities by analysing chromosomal defect
(c) It is used to study metabolic defect of foetus
(d) It is done of examine the sex of foetus, leading to female foeticide

53 The term infanticide refers to
(a) a condition of dwarfism
(b) killing of live foetus before birth
(c) killing of baby after birth
(d) premature birth of the baby

Sexually Transmitted Disease

54 Consider the following statements.
I. STDs lead to the minor complications like itching, fluid discharge, slight pain, swellings.
II. STDs lead to the cancer of the reproductive tract.
Choose the correct option.
(a) Statement I is true, but II is false
(b) Statement I is false, but II is true
(c) Both statements I and II are true
(d) Both statements I and II are false

55 Which of the following statements is incorrect regarding gonorrhoea?
(a) It is caused by diplococcus bacterium
(b) The bacterium passess through sexual contact
(c) It is caused by herpes simplex virus
(d) All of the above

56 Which of the following cannot be taken as the symptom of a female suffering from gonorrhoea?
(a) Inflammation of urethra with painful urination
(b) Discharge of pus from vagina
(c) Inflammation of uterine tubes
(d) Peritonitis or inflammation of the peritoneum

57 Which of the following is an important detection technique for syphilis?
(a) Gram staining of the discharge
(b) Nucleic acid hybridisation, PCR
(c) Antibody detection, e.g. VDRL
(d) Microscopic examination of culture

58 Which one of the following correctly matches a sexually transmitted disease with its pathogen?
(a) Urethritis – *Bacillus anthracis*
(b) Soft sore – *Bacillus brevis*
(c) Syphilis – *Treponema pallidum*
(d) Gonorrhoea – *Entamoeba histolytica*

59 Which of the following symptoms can be related to the tertiary stage of syphilis?
(a) Appearance of painless open sore
(b) Skin rash, fever
(c) Joint aches
(d) Signs of organ degeneration

60 The most common site of infection in case of *Chlamydia* in female is
(a) cervix
(b) urethra
(c) uterine tubes
(d) bladder

61 Match the following columns.

	Column I (STDs)		Column II (Causal agents)
A.	Chlamydiasis	1.	*Chlamydia trachomatis*
B.	Chancroid	2.	*Haemophilus ducreyi*
C.	Trichomoniasis	3.	*Trichomonas vaginalis*
D.	Genital herpes	4.	Herpes simplex virus

Codes

	A	B	C	D
(a)	1	3	2	4
(b)	4	1	3	2
(c)	1	2	3	4
(d)	1	2	4	3

62 Which of the following statements about hepatitis-B is incorrect?
(a) It is one of the examples of STD
(b) It is spread primarily by sexual contact, even by contaminated syringes and blood transfusion
(c) It is 42 nm enveloped virus containing *ss*RNA as the genetic material
(d) Recombivax HB vaccine is available to prevent hepatitis-B infection

63 Consider the following statements.
I. HBV causes yellowing of skin and cirrhosis.
II. HBV is diagnosed by HBSAg and ELISA.
Choose the correct option.
(a) Statement I is true, but II is false
(b) Statement I is false, but II is true
(c) Both statements I and II are true
(d) Both statements I and II are false

64 From the sexually transmitted diseases mentioned below, identify the one which does not specifically affect the sex organs. **[NCERT Exemplar]**
(a) Syphilis
(b) AIDS
(c) Gonorrhoea
(d) Genital warts

65 Match Column I with Column II and select the correct option from the codes given below.

	Column I (Diseases)		Column II (Diagnostic tests)
A.	Syphilis	1.	PCR test
B.	Genital herpes	2.	VDRL test
C.	AIDS	3.	Urine test
D.	Gonorrhoea	4.	ELISA

Codes

	A	B	C	D
(a)	1	2	3	4
(b)	2	1	4	3
(c)	4	3	2	1
(d)	3	4	1	2

Infertility and ART

66 Which of the following is the most appropriate statement of infertility?
(a) Couple is unable to produce children in spite of unprotected sexual cohabitation
(b) Infertility is defined as the inability to produce a viable offspring and is always due to defects/abnormalities in the female partner
(c) Infertility is due to immature sex organs
(d) All of the above

67 The term oligospermia refers to
(a) low sperm motility
(b) absence of sperm in semen
(c) low sperm count
(d) defective sperm morphology

68 Replacement level fertility rate is
(a) average number of children a women is likely to have
(b) number of children a couple must bear to replace themselves
(c) average number of children in a family
(d) number of surviving children in the family

69 Total Fertility Rate (TFR) is
(a) average number of children born by a woman
(b) number of children a couple must bear to replace themselves
(c) average number of children in a family
(d) number of surviving children in a family

70 The first case of IVF-ET technique success was reported by
(a) Louis Joy Brown and Banting Best
(b) Partrick Steptoe and Robert Edwards
(c) Robert Steptoe and Gilbert Brown
(d) Baylis and Starling Taylor

71 The technique used for retrieving the egg from the patient while performing IVF is known as
(a) transvaginal oocyte retrieval technique
(b) transuterine oocyte retrieval technique
(c) transovarian oocyte retrieval technique
(d) None of the above

72 *In vitro* fertilisation is a technique where
(a) zygote is taken from the oviduct cultured and then implanted
(b) ovum is taken out, then fertilised and implanted
(c) sperm and ovum are fused and zygote grown in a test tube
(d) ovum and sperm are fertilised internally and grown in test tube

73 Choose the correct statement regarding the ZIFT procedure. **[NCERT Exemplar]**
(a) Ova collected from a female donor are transferred to the Fallopian tube to facilitate zygote formation
(b) Zygote is collected from a female donor and transferred to the Fallopian tube
(c) Zygote is collected from a female donor and transferred to the uterus
(d) Ova collected from a female donor and transferred to the uterus

74 Which method is used for the implantation of a blastocyst with more than 8 cells?
(a) Intrauterine transfer
(b) Interuterine transfer
(c) Zygote intra-Fallopian transfer
(d) Zygote inter Fallopian transfer

75 Which method can be used for carrying out *in vivo* fertilisation in a sterile female?
(a) ZIFT (b) AT (c) GIFT (d) IUT

(B) Cumulative Exercise

(Assorted Questions of the Chapter for Advanced Level Practice)

1 Mark the incorrect statement.
(a) According to 2011 census, our population growth rate is 1.7%
(b) Marriageable age for male and female is 18 and 21 years, respectively
(c) An ideal contraceptive should be reversible
(d) The problem of infertility in India lies most often in female partner

2 Which of the following given statements are not correct?
I. A statutory ban has been implemented on amniocentesis because of its regular misuse.
II. Surgical methods are also called sterilisation as they block the release of gametes into secretions.
III. All sexually transmitted diseases are completely curable.
IV. MTPs are relatively safe upto 20 weeks of pregnancy.
(a) I and III (b) III and IV
(c) II and III (d) I and II

3 Match the following columns.

	Column I		Column II
A.	Gonorrhoea	1.	HSV 1 and HSV 2 viruses
B.	Syphilis	2.	HIV virus
C.	Chlamydia	3.	*Treponema pallidum*
D.	AIDS	4.	*Neisseria gonorrhoeae*
E.	Herpes	5.	*Chlamydia trachomatis*

Codes

	A	B	C	D	E
(a)	4	3	2	1	5
(b)	4	3	5	2	1
(c)	3	5	1	2	4
(d)	1	2	4	3	5

4 Which of the following have been found to be very effective as emergency contraceptives as they can be used to avoid possible pregnancy due to rape if given within 72 hrs?

I. Administration of antiprogestogens.
II. Progestin-oestrogen combination.
III. IUDs
IV. Condoms

Codes

(a) Only IV (b) I and II
(c) I, II and III (d) I, II, III and IV

5 Match the following columns.

	Column I	Column II
A.	Government of India legalised MTP in	1. 1951
B.	Family planning introduced in India	2. 1971
C.	Nirodh	3. Barrier contraceptive
D.	Mala-D and Mala-N	4. Hormonal contraceptive

Codes

	A	B	C	D
(a)	1	2	3	4
(b)	2	1	3	4
(c)	4	3	2	1
(d)	1	4	3	2

6 Consider the statements given below regarding contraception and answer as directed thereafter.

I. Medical Termination of Pregnancy (MTP) during first trimester is generally safe.
II. Generally, the chances of conception are nil until mother breastfeeds the infant up to two years.
III. Intrauterine devices such as copper-T are effective contraceptives.
IV. Contraception pills may be taken up to 1 week after coitus to prevent conception.

Which two of the above statements are correct?

(a) I and III (b) I and II
(c) II and III (d) III and IV

7 Which of the following statements is correct with reference to a test tube baby?

(a) Fertilisation of egg is completed outside the body; the fertilised egg is then placed in the womb of the mother where gestation is completed
(b) Fertilisation of egg is completed in the female genital tract. It is then taken out and grown in a large test tube
(c) A prematurely born baby is reared in an incubator
(d) Fertilisation of egg and growth of embryo is completed in a large test tube

8 In India, population crossed one billion mark in May 2000. The probable reasons for this are decline in

I. Maternal Mortality Rate (MMR)
II. Infant Mortality Rate (IMR)
III. Number of people in reproducible age
IV. Medical facilities

(a) I and II only (b) I, II and III
(c) I, II and IV (d) I, II, III and IV

9 Which of the following can be complications resulting from STDs without timely detection and treatment?

I. Pelvic Inflammatory Disease (PID)
II. Still births
III. Infertility or even cancer of reproductive tract
IV. Ectopic pregnancies

Codes

(a) I and II (b) I, II and III
(c) Only I (d) I, II, III and IV

10 Match the following columns.

	Column I (Contraceptive methods)		Column II (Categories)
A.	Periodic abstinence	1.	Natural methods
B.	Vasectomy	2.	Barrier methods
C.	Coitus interruptus	3.	Surgical methods
D.	IUDs		
E.	Lactational amenorrhea		
F.	Cervical caps		

Codes

	A	B	C	D	E	F
(a)	1	1	2	3	2	3
(b)	1	3	2	1	3	2
(c)	2	1	2	1	3	3
(d)	1	3	1	2	1	2

11 Mark the incorrect statements.

I. Castration is a method of contraception.
II. MTPs have a significant role in decreasing the size of population, so it is legal.
III. Amniocentesis for sex-determination is banned in our country.
IV. Nearly 45 to 50 million, MTPs are performed in a year all over the world.

(a) I and II
(b) III and IV
(c) I, II and III
(d) I, II, III and IV

12 Sterilisation techniques are generally full proof methods of contraception with least side effects. Yet, this is the last option for the couples because

I. it is almost irreversible.
II. their is misconception that it reduces sexual urge.
III. it is a surgical procedure.
IV. it lacks sufficient facilities in many parts of the developing country.

Choose the correct option

(a) I and III
(b) II and III
(c) II and IV
(d) I, II, III and IV

13 Which of the following graphs is the correct representation of the level of progesterone in a female who has been using Mala-D as a method of birth control?

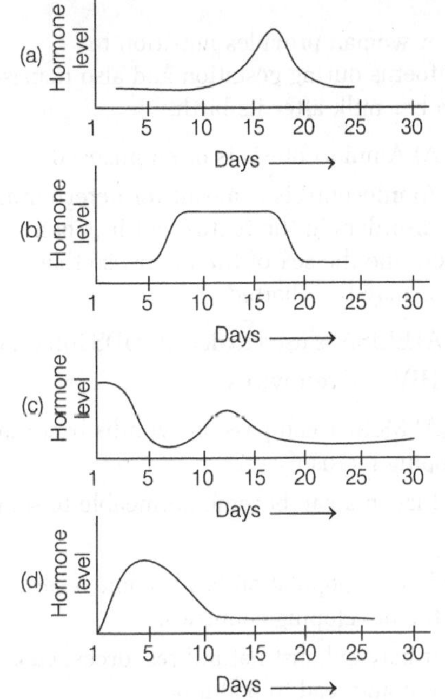

14 Match the following columns.

Column I	Column II
A. IUD	1. Intra Uterine Device
B. Spermicide	2. *In vitro* fertilisation
C. Temperature method	3. Kills the sperms
D. IVF	4. Natural birth control method

Codes

	A	B	C	D		A	B	C	D
(a)	1	3	4	2	(b)	2	1	3	4
(c)	4	3	1	2	(d)	3	2	1	4

15 The following figure shows the uterine tubes of four women (P, Q, R and S).

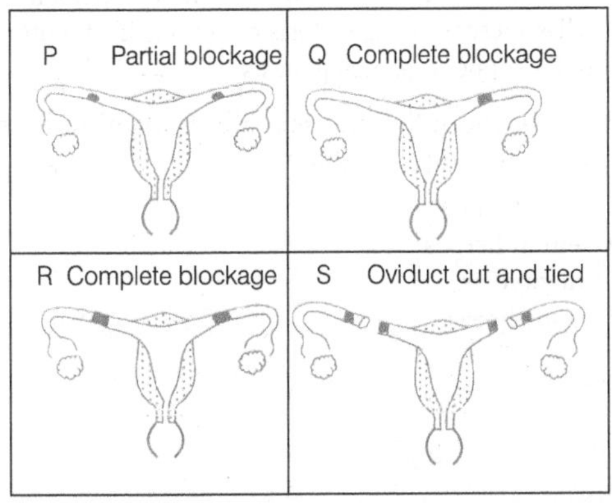

Out of them fertilisation is impossible in which two women at present?

(a) P and Q (b) Q and R
(c) R and S (d) S and P

16 Following statements are given regarding MTP.

I. MTPs are generally advised during first trimester.
II. MTPs are used as contraceptive method.
III. MTPs are always done surgically.
IV. MTPs require the assistance of qualified medical personnel.

Choose the option containing correct statements.

(a) I and III (b) II and III
(c) I and IV (d) I and II

17 Match the following figures with the related method of birth control

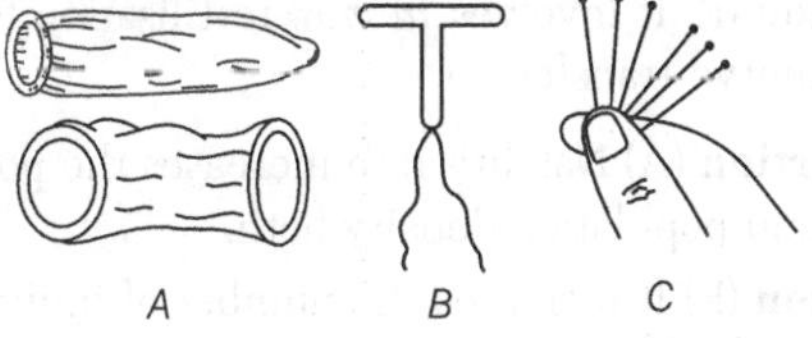

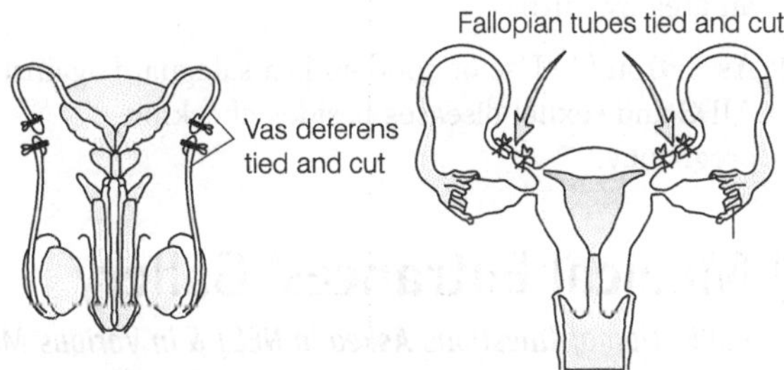

1. Tubectomy 2. Vasectomy
3. Implants 4. Condoms
5. Copper-T 6. Cervical caps

Codes

	A	B	C	D	E
(a)	6	5	4	1	2
(b)	4	5	3	2	1
(c)	3	5	4	1	2
(d)	6	5	3	2	1

Assertion and Reason

Direction (Q. Nos. 18–26) *In the following questions, a statement of Assertion (A) is given followed by the corresponding statement of Reason (R). Of the statements, mark the correct answer as*

(a) Both A and R are true and R is the correct explanation of A
(b) Both A and R are true, but R is not the correct explanation of A
(c) A is true, but R is false
(d) A is false, but R is true
(e) Both A and R are false

18 Assertion (A) The technique shown in the given figure is frequently used in prenatal disease treatment.

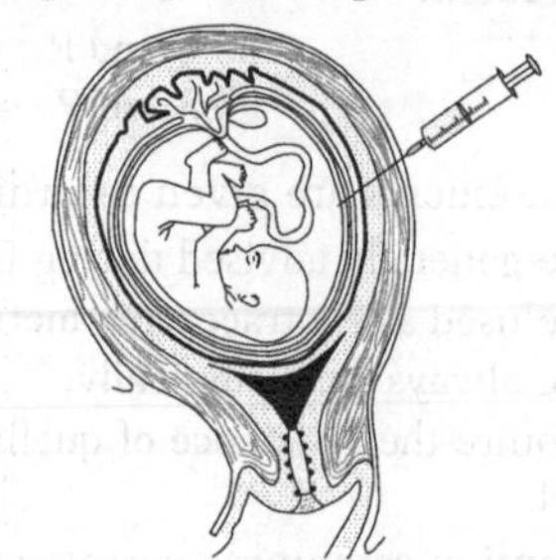

Reason (R) This technique cannot be used for sex-determination of child.

19 Assertion (A) Test tube baby has raised several legal problems.

Reason (R) It involves *in vitro* fertilisation followed by embryo transfer.

20 Assertion (A) Natality rate increases the population size and population density both.

Reason (R) It increases the number of individuals in an area by births.

21 Assertion (A) Use of condom is a safeguard against AIDS and sexual diseases besides checking pregnancy.

Reason (R) Certain contraceptives are planted under the skin of the upper arm to prevent pregnancy.

22 Assertion (A) Biologically, woman is superior to man.

Reason (R) A woman provides nutrition to developing foetus during gestation and also nourishes the baby on her milk after its birth.

23 Assertion (A) Amniocentesis is often misused.

Reason (R) Amniocentesis is meant for determining the genetic disorders in the foetus, but it is being used to determine the sex of the foetus, so that female foetus may the aborted.

24 Assertion (A) ELISA is used to detect AIDS infection.

Reason (R) HIV is a retrovirus.

25 Assertion (A) Mother can pass on syphilis bacteria to their developing foetus.

Reason (R) Placenta can become permeable to some pathogens.

26 Assertion (A) Overpopulation has become a serious problem in the developing countries.

Reason (R) It may exhaust natural resources, cause unemployment and lead to pollution.

(C) Medical Entrances' Gallery

(Collection of Questions Asked in NEET & in Various Medical Entrance Exams)

1 Select the option including all sexually transmitted diseases. **[NEET 2020]**

(a) Gonorrhoea, malaria, genital herpes
(b) AIDS, malaria, filaria
(c) Cancer, AIDS, syphilis
(d) Gonorrhoea, syphilis, genital herpes

2 Which of the following STDs are not curable? **[NEET 2020]**

(a) Genital herpes, hepatitis-B, HIV infection
(b) Chlamydiasis, Syphilis, genital warts
(c) HIV, gonorrhoea, trichomoniasis
(d) Gonorrhoea, trichomoniasis, hepatitis-B

3 Which of the following contraceptive methods do involve a role of hormone? **[NEET 2019]**

(a) Barrier method, lactational amenorrhea, pills
(b) Cu-T, pills, emergency contraceptives
(c) Pills, emergency contraceptives, barrier methods
(d) Lactational amenorrhea, pills, emergency contraceptives

4 Select the hormone releasing intrauterine devices. **[NEET 2019, NEET-II 2016]**

(a) Multiload-375, Progestasert
(b) Progestasert, LNG-20
(c) Lippes loop, Multiload-375
(d) Vaults, LNG-20

5 Which of the following is a correct statement? **[NEET 2019]**

(a) IUDs once inserted need not to be replaced
(b) IUDs are generally inserted by the user herself
(c) IUDs increase phagocytosis of sperms in the uterus
(d) IUDs suppress gametogenesis

6 Which of the following sexually transmitted diseases is not completely curable? **[NEET 2019]**

(a) Genital warts
(b) Genital herpes
(c) Chlamydiasis
(d) Gonorrhoea

7 Which of the following sexually transmitted diseases do not specifically affect reproductive organs? **[NEET 2019]**
(a) Genital warts and hepatitis-B
(b) Syphilis and genital herpes
(c) AIDS and hepatitis-B
(d) Chlamydiasis and AIDS

8 The contraceptive 'Saheli' **[NEET 2018]**
(a) is an IUD
(b) increases the concentration of oestrogen and prevents ovulation in females
(c) blocks oestrogen receptors in the uterus, preventing eggs from getting implanted
(d) is a post-coital contraceptive

9 The function of copper ions in copper releasing IUDs is **[NEET 2017, CBSE AIPMT 2017]**
(a) they suppress sperm motility and fertilising capacity of sperms
(b) they inhibit gametogenesis
(c) they make uterus unsuitable for implantation
(d) they inhibit ovulation

10 In case of a couple, where the male is having a very low sperm count, which technique will be suitable for fertilisation? **[NEET 2017, MHT CET 2017]**
(a) Intrauterine transfer
(b) Gamete intracytoplasmic Fallopian transfer
(c) Artificial insemination
(d) Intracytoplasmic sperm injection

11 Match the following sexually transmitted diseases (Column-I) with their causative agents (Column II) and select the corect option.

	Column I		Column II
A.	Gonorrhoea	1.	HIV
B.	Syphilis	2.	*Neisseria*
C.	Genital warts	3.	*Treponema*
D.	AIDS	4.	Human Papilloma Virus

Codes **[NEET 2017]**

	A	B	C	D
(a)	2	3	4	1
(b)	3	4	1	2
(c)	4	2	3	1
(d)	4	3	2	1

12 Which of the following is incorrect regarding vasectomy? **[NEET-II 2016]**
(a) No sperm occurs in seminal fluid
(b) No sperm occurs in epididymis
(c) Vas deferentia are cut and tied
(d) Irreversible sterility

13 Embryo with more than 16 blastomeres formed due to *in vitro* fertilisation is transferred into **[NEET-II 2016]**
(a) uterus (b) Fallopian tube
(c) fimbriae (d) cervix

14 Which of the following approaches does not give the defined action of contraceptive? **[NEET-I 2016]**
(a) Intrauterine devices – Increase phagocytosis of sperms suppress sperm motility and fertilising capacity of sperms
(b) Hormonal contraceptives – Prevent/retard entry of sperms, prevent ovulation and fertilisation
(c) Vasectomy – Prevents spermatogenesis
(d) Barrier methods – Prevent fertilisation

15 In context of amniocentesis, which of the following statements is incorrect? **[NEET-I 2016]**
(a) It is used for prenatal sex-determination
(b) It can be used for detection of Down's syndrome
(c) It can be used for detection of cleft palate
(d) It is usually done when a woman is between 14-16 weeks pregnant

16 Progestasert is an IUD, which makes the uterus unsuitable and cervix hostile to the sperms as they are **[Karnataka CET 2015]**
(a) hormone releasing IUDs (b) copper releasing IUDs
(c) ideal contraceptive (d) non-medicated IUDs

17 Match the following columns I, II with III.

Column I	Column II	Column III
A. Trichomoniasis	1. *Herpes simplex*	(i) Pain in lower abdomen
B. Syphilis	2. *Neisseria gonorrhoeae*	(ii) Inflammation and itching in and around vagina
C. Gonorrhoea	3. *Treponema pallidum*	(iii) Patchy hair loss
D. Genital herpes	4. *Trichomonas vaginalis*	(iv) Feeling of uneasiness

Codes **[Gujarat CET 2015]**

	A	B	C	D
(a)	1-(iii)	2-(ii)	4-(iv)	3-(i)
(b)	4-(ii)	1-(iii)	2-(i)	3-(iv)
(c)	4-(i)	1-(iv)	2-(ii)	3-(iii)
(d)	4-(ii)	3-(iii)	2-(i)	1-(iv)

18 Which of the following is not a sexually transmitted disease? **[Gujarat CET 2015]**
(a) Syphilis
(b) Acquired Immuno Deficiency Syndrome (AIDS)
(c) Trichomoniasis
(d) Encephalitis

19 A childless couple can be assisted to have a child through a technique called GIFT. The full form of this technique is **[Gujarat CET 2015]**

(a) Gamete Inseminated Fallopian Transfer
(b) Gamete Intra Fallopian Transfer
(c) Gamete Internal Fertilisation and Transfer
(d) Germ Cell Internal Fallopian Transfer

20 Amniocentesis can diagnose which of the following defects?

I. Trisomy
II. Neural tube defects
III. Infection
IV. Lung maturity

Codes **[Chhattisgarh PMT 2015]**

(a) I, II and III (b) I, II and IV
(c) II, III and IV (d) I, II, III and IV

21 After tubectomy, which part of female reproductive system remains blocked? **[Uttarakhand CET 2015]**

(a) Cervix
(b) Uterine cavity
(c) Ovary
(d) Fallopian tube

22 Tubectomy is a method of sterilisation in which **[CBSE AIPMT 2014]**

(a) small part of the Fallopian tube is removed or tied up
(b) ovaries are removed surgically
(c) small part of vas deferens is removed or tied up
(d) uterus is removed surgically

23 Assisted reproductive technology, IVF involves transfer of **[CBSE AIPMT 2014]**

(a) ovum into the Fallopian tube
(b) zygote into the Fallopian tube
(c) zygote into the uterus
(d) embryo with 16 blastomeres into the Fallopian tube

24 The technique used to block the passage of sperm in male is **[MHT CET 2014]**

(a) tubectomy (b) vasectomy
(c) coitus interruptus (d) rhythm method

25 Which of the following statements is incorrect? **[WB JEE 2014]**

(a) Test tube baby grows inside test tube
(b) Test tube baby grows within mother's womb
(c) Test tube baby grows within surrogate mother's womb
(d) Test tube baby grows following uterine fertilisation

26 In which technique, the donor semen is artificially introduced into the uterus? **[J&K CET 2014]**

(a) Intravaginal insemination
(b) Intrauterine insemination
(c) Intracytoplasmic sperm injection
(d) Gamete intra Fallopian transfer

27 IUDs which are used by females **[KCET 2014]**

(a) act as spermicidal jellies
(b) block the entry of sperms into vagina
(c) are implanted under the skin and they release progestogen and oestrogen
(d) release copper ions in the uterus that increase phagocytosis of sperms

28 Oral contraceptive pills for females developed at CDRI, Lucknow is **[UK PMT 2014]**

(a) Mala-D (b) Cortisol
(c) Saheli (d) None of these

29 MTPs are considered relatively safe during the **[UK PMT 2014; CBSE AIPMT 2010]**

(a) first trimester
(b) second trimester
(c) third trimester
(d) None of the above

30 In which 'Assisted Reproductive Technology' (ART), 'test tube baby' procedure is applied? **[EAMCET 2014]**

(a) Gamete Intra Fallopian Transfer (GIFT)
(b) Intra Cytoplasmic Sperm Injection (ICSI)
(c) *In Vitro* Fertilisation and Embryo Transfer (IVF-ET)
(d) Zygote Intra Fallopian Transfer (ZIFT)

31 One of the legal methods of birth control is **[NEET 2013]**

(a) by abstaining from coitus from day 10-17 of the menstrual cycle
(b) by having coitus at the time of day break
(c) by a premature ejaculation during coitus
(d) abortion by taking an appropriate medicine

32 Artificial insemination means **[NEET 2013]**

(a) transfer of sperms of husband to a test tube containing ova
(b) artificial introduction of sperms of a healthy donor into the vagina
(c) introduction of sperms of a healthy donor directly into the ovary
(d) transfer of sperms of a healthy donor to a test tube containing ova

33 The test tube baby programme employs which one of the following techniques? **[CBSE AIPMT 2012]**

(a) Intra Cytoplasmic Sperm Injection (ICSI)
(b) Intra Uterine Insemination (IUI)
(c) Gamete Intra Fallopian Transfer (GIFT)
(d) Zygote Intra Fallopian Transfer (ZIFT)

34 Purpose of tubectomy is to prevent **[BCECE 2012]**

(a) fertilisation
(b) coitus
(c) egg formation
(d) embryonic development

35 One of the group includes all sexually transmitted diseases. **[AMU 2012]**

(a) AIDS, syphilis, cholera
(b) HIV, malaria, trichomoniasis
(c) Gonorrhoea, hepatits-B, chlamydiasis
(d) Hepatitis-B, haemophilia, AIDS

36 It is a disease which mainly affects mucous membrane of urinogenital tract. In males, burning feeling on passing urine, after a yellow discharge occurs, that is accompanied by fever, headache and feeling of illness. **[AMU 2012]**

(a) Syphilis (b) Gonorrhoea
(c) AIDS (d) None of these

37 The most important factor which determined the increase in human population in India during the 20th century was **[DUMET 2011]**

(a) natality (b) mortality
(c) immigration (d) emigration

38 Study of human population is **[HPMT 2010]**

(a) demography (b) chronology
(c) population science (d) None of these

39 AIDS stands for **[AFMC 2010]**

(a) Acquired Immuno Deficiency Syndrome
(b) Access Immuno Deficiency Syndrome
(c) Actual Immuno Deficiency Syndrome
(d) Apparent Deficiency Syndrome

ANSWERS

Check Point 4.1

1. (c)	2. (b)	3. (d)	4. (b)	5. (c)	6. (c)

Check Point 4.2

1. (b)	2. (b)	3. (b)	4. (a)	5. (d)

(A) Topical Exercise

1. (c)	2. (d)	3. (d)	4. (b)	5. (a)	6. (a)	7. (c)	8. (d)	9. (a)	10. (d)
11. (b)	12. (b)	13. (d)	14. (a)	15. (c)	16. (c)	17. (c)	18. (b)	19. (a)	20. (b)
21. (d)	22. (b)	23. (a)	24. (d)	25. (c)	26. (a)	27. (a)	28. (d)	29. (a)	30. (a)
31. (d)	32. (a)	33. (a)	34. (c)	35. (d)	36. (a)	37. (a)	38. (a)	39. (c)	40. (c)
41. (b)	42. (c)	43. (a)	44. (c)	45. (c)	46. (a)	47. (d)	48. (d)	49. (d)	50. (c)
51. (b)	52. (d)	53. (b)	54. (c)	55. (c)	56. (a)	57. (c)	58. (c)	59. (d)	60. (a)
61. (c)	62. (c)	63. (c)	64. (b)	65. (b)	66. (a)	67. (c)	68. (b)	69. (a)	70. (b)
71. (a)	72. (b)	73. (b)	74. (a)	75. (c)					

(B) Cumulative Exercise

1. (d)	2. (b)	3. (b)	4. (b)	5. (b)	6. (a)	7. (a)	8. (c)	9. (d)	10. (d)
11. (a)	12. (d)	13. (b)	14. (a)	15. (c)	16. (c)	17. (b)	18. (e)	19. (b)	20. (a)
21. (b)	22. (a)	23. (a)	24. (b)	25. (a)	26. (a)				

(C) Medical Entrances' Gallery

1. (d)	2. (a)	3. (d)	4. (b)	5. (c)	6. (b)	7. (c)	8. (c)	9. (a)	10. (c)
11. (a)	12. (a)	13. (a)	14. (c)	15. (c)	16. (a)	17. (d)	18. (d)	19. (b)	20. (d)
21. (d)	22. (a)	23. (b)	24. (b)	25. (d)	26. (b)	27. (d)	28. (c)	29. (a)	30. (c)
31. (a)	32. (b)	33. (b)	34. (a)	35. (c)	36. (b)	37. (a)	38. (a)	39. (a)	

Explanations

(A) Topical Exercise

4 (*b*) NRHM stands for National Rural Health Mission. This programme was launched on 12th April, 2005 to provide affordable, quality health care to rural population.

19 (*a*) In lactational amenorrhea, high level of prolactin inhibits the release of gonadotropins, LH and FSH. Due to this, ovulation is suppressed and thus chances of conception are negligible.

22 (*b*) Statement I is false, but II is true. Incorrect statement can be corrected as

Diaphragm acts as a physical barrier for sperm entry. It is used by females to cover cervical region during coitus.

24 (*d*) Option (d) is odd one out because

Delfen is a spermicidal cream whereas other three are injectable contraceptives.

26 (*a*) Birth control pills either contain progesterone alone or a combination of oestrogen and progesterone. Prolactin and cholecystokinin are not used in it as these hormones are not associated with female's reproductive cycle.

29 (*a*) Option (a) shows incorrectly matched pair and can be corrected as

Minipill contains progestin, a synthetic progesterone only.

36 (*a*) Statement I is true, but II is false. Incorrect statement can be corrected as

IUDs are needed to be replaced after 3-5 years.

38 (*a*) Statement in option (a) is incorrect. It can be corrected as

IUDs cannot be self-inserted, but require the help of trained medical practioner.

50 (*c*) Statements I, II, III are correct, but IV is incorrect. Incorrect statement can be corrected as

MTP is illegal to get rid of female foetuses.

55 (*c*) Statement in option (c) is incorrect and can be corrected as

Gonorrhoea is caused by *Neisseria gonorrhoeae.*

57 (*c*) Syphilis is diagnosed by clinical symptoms, microscopic examination and antibody detection, e.g. VDRL (Venereal Disease Research Laboratory).

62 (*c*) Statement in option (c) is incorrect and can be corrected as

The genetic material of hepatitis-B virus is double-stranded (*ds*) DNA.

(B) Cumulative Exercise

1 (*d*) Statement in option (d) is incorrect and can be corrected as

The problem of infertility in India or elsewhere in world could be associated with male, female or both.

2 (*b*) Statements III and IV are not correct. They can be corrected as

- Sexually transmitted diseases are completely curable except hepatitis-B, genital herpes and HIV infections.
- MTPs are relatively safe upto 12 weeks of pregnancy.

6 (*a*) Statements I and III are correct, while II and IV are incorrect. Incorrect statements can be corrected as

In breastfeeding mother, conception does not occur upto 6 months.

Contraceptive pills are taken within 72 hours after coitus.

7 (*a*) In test tube baby or *in vitro* fertilisation technique, the ovum is fertilised with the sperm outside the body of a woman providing the ovum with the same environmental conditions as it would have got inside the uterus. The zygote formed is grown inside a culture and when embryo is formed, it is implanted into the uterus.

11 (*a*) Statements I and II are incorrect. These can be corrected as

Castration is not a method of contraception.

MTP is considered illegal if it is carried out due to irrelevant purposes, other than risk pregnancy.

13 (*b*) The woman that has been using Mala-D would not ovulate as the level of progesterone remain high throughout 21 days.

18 (*e*) Both A and R are false and can be corrected as

The technique shown in figures is amniocentesis. It is a foetal sex-determination and disorder test based on chromosomal pattern in the amniotic fluid surrounding the developing foetus. This technique is banned in India at present due to its role in increased female foeticides.

19 (*b*) Both A and R are true, but R is not the correct explanation of A.

In very rare cases, a surrogate mother may have to be used to bring up *in vitro* fertilised ovum to maturity. Though biological realisation of a test tube baby is a remarkable achievement, it has raised several ethical and legal problems like the right over the child.

The technique of *in vitro* fertilisation followed by the embryo-transfer in the uterus of the normal female to start the development and finally leading to normal birth, is called test tube baby.

20 (*a*) Both A and R are true and R is the correct explanation of A.

Natality is generally expressed as number of births per 1,000 individuals of a population per year. Crude birth rate is the number births per 1,300 persons in the middle of a given year, i.e. on july 07. It increases the population size (total number of individuals of a population) and population density.

21 (*b*) Both A and R are true, but R is not the correct explanation of A.

Use of condom is a simple, but effective method and has no side effect. It checks pregnancy by preventing deposition of semen in the vagina. Condom should be used regularly and put on before starting coital activity, otherwise sperm containing lubricating fluid may be left in the vagina. Condom is also a safeguard against infection of AIDS and sexual diseases (STDs).

Certain contraceptives, such as progestin, minipill or progestogen in combination with oestrogen are also used by the females as injections or implants under the skin of the upper arm.

22 (*a*) Both A and R are true and R is the correct explanation of A.

Woman plays an important role in the continuity of the family and human race. She provides nutrition to the foetus in her womb for about nine months (280 days) through placenta. Even after birth, she nourishes the infant on her milk. Hence, biologically woman is superior to man.

23 (*a*) Both A and R are true and R is the correct explanation of A.

Amniocentesis is a prenatal diagnostic technique to determine the genetic disorders such as Down's syndrome, Turner's syndrome and Klinefelter's syndrome, etc. Since, the cells withdrawn with needle from the amniotic fluid are examined for chromosomal abnormalities. So, some people illegally use this technique for determining the sex of unborn child.

24 (*b*) Both A and R are true, but R is not the correct explanation of A.

HIV (Human Immunodeficiency Virus) is one of the large group of immunodeficiency viruses. It is a causative agent of AIDS (Acquired Immunodeficiency Syndrome). ELISA, (Enzymc Linked Immuno Sorbent Assay) is used to test HIV infections. Western blot test is another widely used confirmatory test for HIV infection.

25 (*a*) Both A and R are true and R is the correct explanation of A.

At the time of childbirth during withdrawn of placenta, the parasite of syphilis enters the newborn baby through the placental blood. This is called congenital syphilis. This occurs because the blood of mother enters the foetus through the placenta.

26 (*a*) Both A and R are true and R is the correct explanation of A.

The overpopulation can exhaust natural resources and create severe competition.
It causes socioeconomic problems due to shortage of space, food and educational and medical facilities and due to unemployment and poverty. It also causes pollution due to rapid ecodegradation.

(C) Medical Entrances' Gallery

1 (*d*) Gonorrhoea, syphilis, genital herpes are sexually transmitted diseases.

Gonorrhoea is caused by a bacterium *Nesseria gonorrhoeae.* It is a Sexually Transmitted Disease (STD) that can infect both men and women. It can cause infections in the genitals, rectum and throat.

Syphilis is caused by a bacterium *Treponoma pallidum.* It starts as painless sore typically on the genitals, rectum or mouth.

Genital herpes is caused by virus Type II herpes simplex virus. It causes herpetic sores which are painful bilsters (fluid-filled bumps) that can break open and ooze fluid.

2 (*a*) Except for hepatitis-B, genital herpes and HIV infections, other sexually transmitted diseases are completely curable if deteted early and treated properly.

3 (*d*) Lactational amenorrhea, pills and emergency contraceptives provide contraception due to the role of hormones.

- In lactational amenorrhea, high prolactin level during active lactation period decreases the gonadotropin level in the blood.
- Pills usually contain progesterone or progesterone-oestrogen combinations, which prevent ovulation.
- Emergency contraceptives also contain progesterone and oestradiol preparation.
- Whereas barrier method represents a physical method of contraception and copper-T (Cu-T) acts by releasing copper and not any hormone.

4 (*b*) Progestasert and LNG-20 are hormone releasing Intrauterine Devices (IUDs). These devices release small quantity of hormones which makes the uterus unsuitable for implantation and the cervix hostile to the sperms.

Whereas, Multiload-375 is copper releasing IUD, Lippes loop is non-medicated IUD and vaults are the barrier type of contraceptive devices.

5 (*c*) Statement in option (c) is correct.

Rest of the statements are incorrect and can be corrected as

- IUDs can be replaced as these are a reversible contraception method.
- IUDs are inserted by doctors or expert nurses in the uterus through vagina.
- IUDs do not affect gametogenesis.

6 (*b*) Genital herpes is sexually transmitted disease, which is not completely curable. It is caused by herpes simplex virus. Treatment is available for herpes symptoms, but the virus remains in the body and becomes active again. Whereas, genital warts, chlamydiasis and gonorrhoea are completely curable diseases.

7 (*c*) AIDS and hepatitis-B are sexually transmitted diseases, which do not specifically affect reproductive organs. AIDS affects the overall immune system of the individual and hepatitis B affects the liver. These are called STDs, because these spread through unsafe or unprotected sex.

8 (*c*) The contraceptive pill 'Saheli' is developed by CDRI, Lucknow. It blocks oestrogen receptors in the uterus, preventing eggs from getting implanted by altering the lining of uterus. It is once a week pill that contains a non-steroidal preparation, Centchroman with high contraceptive value.

9 (*a*) The copper releasing IUDs primarily work by disrupting sperm motility and damaging the sperm by increasing their phagocytosis. Copper acts as a spermicide and suppresses the fertilising ability of sperms. Whereas, hormone releasing IUDs alter the endometrial (uterus) lining, preventing implantation.

10 (*c*) Artificial insemination, a type of Assisted Reproductive Technology (ART) is suitable for this case.

In this method, the semen is collected either from husband or a healthy donor and then artificially introduced into the vagina or into the uterus of the female. It is commonly used in cases, where male partners are unable to inseminate the female due to very low sperm counts in the ejaculate.

12 (*a*) Statement in option (a) is incorrect regarding vasectomy and can be corrected as

Epididymis is an accessory duct present in the male reproductive system.

Rest other statements are correct regarding vasectomy.

Sperms produced by testes are sent here by vasa efferentia and are temporarily stored here. These sperms do not reach seminal vesicle when vas deferens are cut and tied in vasectomy.

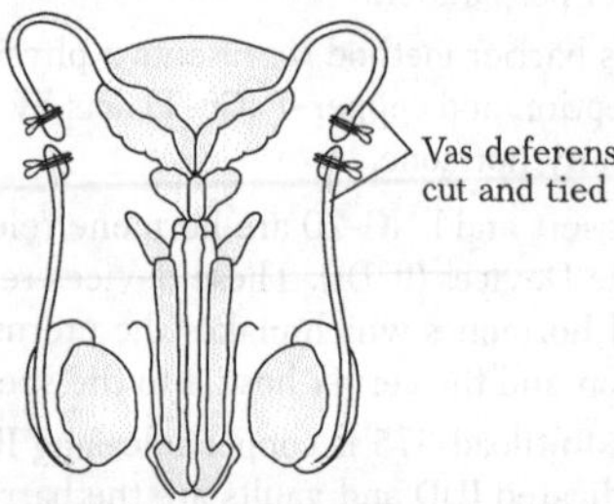

13 (*a*) Embryo with more than 16 blastomeres formed due to *in vitro* fertilisation is transferred into the uterus to complete its further development.
Intra Uterine Transfer or IUT is an assisted reproductive technology to solve the infertility problems.

In this process, embryo is implanted in the uterus where its further development occurs. On completion of gestation, the mother gives birth to a normal child.

14 (*c*) Option (c) does not give the defined action of contraceptive and can be corrected as
In vasectomy, a small part of the vas deferens is removed or tied up through a small incision on the scrotum in males. Vasectomy blocks the gamete transport and does not affect spermatogenesis.

15 (*c*) Statement in option (c) is incorrect and can be corrected as
Cleft palate is a developmental abnormality which may occur in the developing foetus and so, it can be detected by sonography, not by amniocentesis.
Amniocentesis is often misused for foetal sex-determination test, so it is banned in India.

20 (*d*) Amniocentesis is an invasive, diagnostic prenatal test. It involves taking sample of amniotic fluid in order to examine foetal cells found in this fluid. The amniotic fluid extracted contains cells from the amnion and foetal skin, lungs and urinary tract. Amniocentesis is used to detect genetic defects (e.g. trisomy), lung maturity, foetal infection, neural tube defects (by checking acetylcholinesterase and alpha-fetoprotein level), etc.

26 (*b*) Intra Uterine Insemination (IUI) is the technique in which semen is collected either from the husband or a healthy donor and then artificially introduced into the uterus of the female.

35 (*c*) Gonorrhoea, hepatitis-B and chlamydiasis are sexually transmitted diseases. Whereas, cholera is transmitted through unhygienic water or food, malaria is transmitted by mosquito and haemophilia is a genetic disorder.

36 (*b*) Gonorrhoea mainly affects mucous membrane of urinogenital tract in males. The symptoms include burning sensation on passing urine, fever, headache and feeling of illness.

37 (*a*) Population growth can be determined by the number of individuals added to the population.
The addition of individuals may take place through natality (by birth) or through immigration (i.e. entry of individual from outside). The human population of India increased in 20th century due to increased in natality rate.

38 (*a*) The scientific study of vital and social statistics, such as births, deaths, diseases, etc., of human or any other population is called demography. In brief, demography is the study of factors that affect the growth and decline of population.

CHAPTER 05

Growth, Regeneration and Ageing

Growth is a vital feature of all living organisms. It enables multicellular organisms to attain their full shape and size. In animals, considerable growth occurs during late embryonic or foetal period, which continues even after birth until the attainment of adulthood.

Regeneration and regular replacement of worn out cells with the new cells occur in all stages of life. The process of growth and regeneration diminish with ageing and ultimately ends with death.

In this chapter, we will study about various aspects of growth, regeneration and ageing.

GROWTH

Growth in living beings can be defined as 'the irreversible increase in overall size and weight of an organism due to the synthesis of new protoplasm'.

Forms of growth

In living organisms, growth can occur in two following forms

(i) **Intussusception** It is internal type of growth. In this form, the surface area of cell increases *via* deposition of new particles that are synthesised by the existing body cells.

(ii) **Apposition** It is external type of growth. In this form, the surface area of cell increases *via* deposition of any external material that is not the constituent of the cell.

Non-living things like mountains, sand mounds and snow also grow by apposition, if increase in body mass is the criterion. However, this growth occurs by the accumulation of material on the surface only.

Inside

Features of growth

At the cellular level, growth involves following features

- Increase in size of cells due to the synthesis of protoplasmic structures (**hypertrophy**).
- Increase in the number of cells by cell division (**hyperplasia**).
- Increase in the amount of apoplasmatic structures like fibres, matrix, etc.

Different cells may grow differently in humans.
For example,

- Eye lens cells grow by multiplication.
- Cardiac and skeletal muscle cells grow by an increase in volume.
- Neurons (nerve cells) grow by extension and growth of their axons and dendrites.
- Cartilage and bone cells grow by the secretion of extracellular matrix.

Pattern of growth

On the basis of changes in the body proportions, there are two types of growth patterns.

(i) **Isometric growth** It is a type of growth in which all the parts grow at the same rate and same time. Thus, there is no change in the form and body proportion, e.g. fish, locust and grasshopper.

(ii) **Allometric growth** It is a type of growth, in which different organs grow at different rates and at different times. Thus, the external form and body proportions change with the stages of growth, e.g. mammals.

Types of growth

The different types of growth seen in the bodies of living organisms are as follows

(i) **Auxetic growth** It is the growth due to increase in size of cells (not number), e.g. nematodes, rotifers and tunicates (early chordates).

(ii) **Multiplicative growth** It is the growth of body due to increase in the number of cells, e.g. embryonic development of higher vertebrates.

(iii) **Accretionary growth** It is the growth in which undifferentiated reserve cells get differentiated to perform specific functions, e.g. formation of erythrocytes from erythropoietic tissue, replacement of worn out cells of skin, secretion of extracellular matrix by chondrocytes and bone osteocytes.

Growth curve

- It is a graphic representation of growth against time. The **sigmoid curve** or **S-shaped growth curve** is the characteristic growth curve of all higher animals including humans.
- In the initial phase, the curve rises at a very slow rate (lag phase).
- In the middle part, the curve rises steeply indicating very fast rate of growth (acceleration phase).
- Finally, in the last part, rate of growth again slows down till the curve becomes horizontal (Plateau phase).
- It signifies that no further growth is taking place and the individual is simply maintaining itself.
- Hence, animals show differential growth rate.

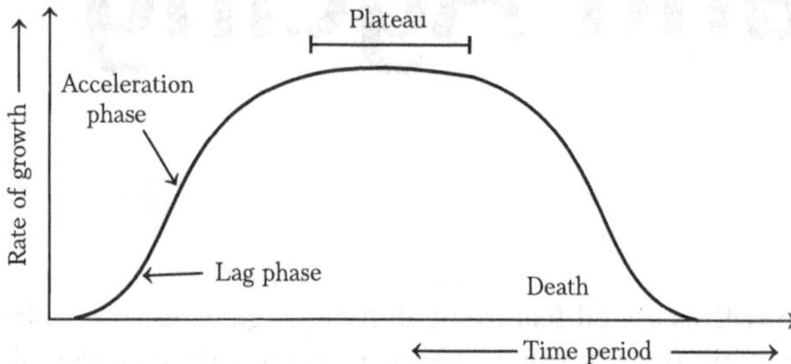

Fig. 5.1 Growth curve

An absolute growth rate curve shows how much the rate of growth changes with time, whereas relative growth rate curve takes into account the existing size.

Life expectancy and lifespan

- Life expectancy is the number of years an individual can expect to live, which is based on average lifespan.
- Lifespan is defined as the age at which half the population still survives. It is the characteristic of a population.
- The maximum lifespan of human has been estimated to be about 121 yrs. This is based on the fact that a man in Japan, Shigechiyo Izumi, reached the age of 120 yrs, 237 days in 1986.
- In general, the rate of mortality of human has gone down and the lifespan has increased. It is approximately 56 in India, whereas in the USA, it is 78.

Positive and negative growth

(i) **Positive growth** occurs when synthesis (anabolism) of materials exceeds the breakdown (catabolism) of materials. In some cases, continuous positive growth is found, e.g. monocotyledonous leaves, many non-vertebrates, fish and certain reptiles. In such cases, growth curve may continue to rise slightly until the organism dies.

(ii) **Negative growth** occurs when catabolism exceeds anabolism. It is found during germination of seeds.

Germination of seeds includes a period of negative growth, which becomes positive when seedlings start photosynthesise and make their own food. In certain cnidarians, the growth curve gets flattened thus, indicating zero growth.

Growth in humans

Human body undergoes following pre-birth phases of growth

1. Cellular growth

- Unicellular organisms grow only through the cell growth. In multicellular organisms, growth is the sum total of growth shown by their cells.
- The steps involved in cellular growth initiate with cell division followed by cell enlargement and cell differentiation, finally leading to maturation.
- Cell growth occurs during post-mitotic phase and interphase.

2. Embryonic growth

- In humans, early embryonic developmental stages constitute transitional growth.
- During cleavage and blastula formation, the cells exhibit little growth.
- During gastrulation (early embryonic state), rudiments of primary organs develop, but they are in their prefunctional state.
- With further development, the rudimentary organs grow, differentiate and become functional.
- Overall growth of the foetus occurs mainly in the period after the basic morphological plane is established, i.e. at the onset of fourth month.

3. Post-embryonic growth

Animals do not show any uniformity in the rate of growth. They grow at different rates at different periods of life.

For example, human embryo is about 150 μm at the time of implantation. It does not grow much in the first 2 months. But after 4 months, embryo grows 10 cm/month and during first year, 2 cm/month, after the age of 22-23 the growth stops.

Control of growth

Growth depends on growth factors and hormones.

The various growth factors involved in the control of growth in human body are discussed in table below

Table 5.1 Growth factors of mammalian cells

Growth factors	Ranges of specificity	Effects
Epidermal Growth Factor (EGF)	Broad	Stimulates cell proliferation in many tissues, plays key role in regulating embryonic development.
Erythropoietin (EPO)	Narrow	Required for proliferation of red blood cell precursors and their maturation into erythrocytes (red blood cells).
Fibroblast Growth Factor (FGF)	Broad	Initiates proliferation of many cell types, inhibits maturation of many types of stem cells, acts as a signal in embryonic development.
Insulin-like Growth Factor (IGF)	Broad	Stimulates metabolism of many cell types, potentiates the effects of other growth factors in promoting cell proliferation.
Interleukin-2	Narrow	Triggers the division of activated T-lymphocytes during the immune response.
Mitosis Promoting Factor (MPF)	Broad	Regulates entrance of the cell cycle into the M-phase.
Nerve Growth Factor (NGF)	Narrow	Stimulates the growth of neuron during neural development.
Platelet-Derived Growth Factor (PDGF)	Broad	Promotes the proliferation of many connective tissues.
Transforming Growth Factor- β (TGF-β)	Broad	Inhibits the responses of many cell types, often plays an important role in cell differentiation.

Hormonal control of growth

There are some hormones which play an important role in the growth of human body. These hormones are as follows

- Thymosin hormone assists GH (Growth Hormone) for early slow growth from birth to puberty period.
- During puberty (14-18 yrs of age), the rate of growth increases. It is due to increased secretion of thyroxine hormone and growth hormone. These are secreted from thyroid gland and anterior lobe of pituitary gland, respectively.
- During puberty, the secretion of sex hormones, i.e. testosterone in the male and oestrogens and progesterone in the female begins. This leads to the development of secondary sex organs and characters.

CHECK POINT 5.1

1. Hypertrophy is said to occur when
   (a) an organ or tissue is forced to cease functioning and decrease in size
   (b) a hollow organ undergoes growth in which the over all size and volume is enlarged
   (c) there is generalised reduction in the size of body tissues
   (d) All of the above

2. Among the following animals, isometric growth is seen in
   (a) teleosts and arthropods (b) arthropods and molluscs
   (c) birds and mammals (d) amphibians and mammals

3. This cannot be called accretionary growth.
   (a) Replacement of worn out cells of skin
   (b) Red blood formation from erythropoietin tissue
   (c) Embryonic development in higher vertebrates
   (d) Chondrocytes and osteocytes secreting extracellular matrix

4. Growth curve indicates
   (a) percentage increase in muscle mass
   (b) a growth parameter at various intervals
   (c) absolute growth
   (d) None of the above

5. Growth occurs when
   (a) anabolism is higher than catabolism
   (b) catabolism is higher than anabolism
   (c) Both anabolism and catabolism are equal
   (d) None of the above

6. Human foetus is under rapid growth and development during pregnancy. Out of the different time duration, the maximum growth in foetus occurs at the age of
   (a) 8 months (b) 6 months
   (c) 4 months (d) 2 months

REGENERATION

It is the capacity of the body to produce the lost parts by proliferation of cells. Regeneration leads to the healing of wounds, replacing of worn out cells and even the formation of a complete individual.

Types of regeneration

There are mainly two types of regeneration. These are as follows

1. Reparative regeneration

- It is regeneration to allow repair of certain damaged cells of the body.
- It is quite common in both invertebrate and vertebrate groups, e.g. earthworms, amphibians, salamanders and axolotl larvae.
- Reparative regeneration also involves **compensatory hypertrophy**, i.e. growth of a part that is removed or damaged, e.g. liver in mammals has the extensive power of reparative regeneration.

2. Restorative regeneration

- It is the restoration or replacement of a lost body part. In this process, even a complete organism can be formed from a fragment of body, e.g. *Hydra, Planaria* and sponges.
- Restorative regeneration decreases with the increase in complexity of organisation of animals.
- It involves dedifferentiation of cells, mitotic divisions, cell movements, autotomy, etc.

Autotomy is the voluntary casting off a part of the body when an animal is attacked. For example,

- Crabs break of their leg on approaching the enemy.
- Lizards throw off their tail.
- Holothurian (echinoderm) throw off their internal viscera (respiratory tree).
- Startish can regenerate the whole arm.

Mechanism of regeneration

TH Morgan recognised two primary mechanisms of regeneration. These are as follows

(i) **Morphallaxis** (Morphallactic regeneration) It involves reconstitution of the body from small fragments. In this, the reorientation and reorganisation of the existing body cells occur. Thus, the regenerated animal is smaller than the original one after the completion of the process, e.g. *Hydra*.

(ii) **Epimorphosis** (Epimorphic regeneration) It takes place by the proliferation of new cells from the surface of the wound. For example,
   - Regeneration of arm in starfish, tail in lizard, etc.
   - In case of crustacean, if antenna is cut, it may be replaced by an eye or *vice-versa.* This is called **heteromorphosis.**
   - In regeneration of mammalian liver or kidney, the cells divide, but do not form an undifferentiated mass of cells or tissues. These produce cells similar to themselves and maintain their differentiated function. This intermediate type of regeneration is called **compensatory regeneration.**

Examples of regeneration

Regeneration occurs in the organisms of almost each class. Some examples of regeneration in different animal groups are given below

- **Protozoans** Ciliates like *Stentor*, *Blepharisma* and *Spirostomum* require only cell cortex for regeneration. About 1/100th part of body of *Acetabularia* can regenerate the entire body.
- **Poriferans** They possess remarkable power of regeneration. Any part of the body cut off or injured is readily repaired. Small pieces of sponges (containing amoebocytes) can grow into complete individual.
- **Coelenterates** *Hydra* has excellent power of regeneration that was discovered by **Trembley**. He cut the body into sections and the lost part was regenerated with exact polarity.
    - In the hydroids, interstitial cells are totipotent and responsible for complete regeneration.
    - In *Hydra,* regeneration will be faster if it is cut off from tentacles.
    - The hypostome (oral end) in *Hydra* can also regenerate again and again. This is called **repetitive regeneration** that has made it virtually immortal.
- **Planarians** (Platyhelminthes) They have stock of undifferentiated cells called **neoblasts**, which are omnipotent.
    - They may regenerate the cut portions, lost parts and even the whole body.
    - *Planaria* shows **super regeneration**, i.e. the development of cells or organ in a number that is more than required.
- **Annelids** Sealing of the wounds by neoblast cells.
- **Molluscs** Regeneration is poor in gastropods. Eye stalk with eye may be regenerated. Cephalopods may regenerate their arms.
- **Nematodes** Regeneration is poor, only closure of superficial wound is observed.
- **Arthropods** Limited renewal of lost appendages as in certain crustaceans and spider takes place by regeneration.
- **Echinoderms** Starfishes, brittle stars and sea lilies can regenerate arms and parts of disc.
- **Fishes** Regeneration is restricted to fish fins.
- **Amphibians** Limb regeneration occurs.
- **Reptiles** Lizards regenerate their tails by the process of autotomy.
- **Birds** Parts of beak can be regenerated, otherwise regenerative ability is poor.
- **Mammals** Extremely poor regenerative capacity, few marsupials can regenerate part of the limbs and liver.

AGEING

- It may be defined as the progressive deterioration in structure and function of the cells, tissues and organs of an organism with the advancing age.
- The branch of biology that deals with the study of the process of ageing in humans is called **Gerontology.**
- The process of ageing may also occur in plants as senescence. In plants, it includes necrosis and apoptosis.
- In **necrosis**, injured cell swells and bursts thus, releasing its contents, on the other hand, in **apoptosis,** programmed cell death occurs wherein cells shrivel and shrink.

The process of ageing is always accompanied by certain changes.

Changes with ageing

In humans, ageing leads to changes in morphological, physiological and cellular forms. These changes are as follows

Morphological changes

Various morphological changes due to ageing are given below

- Thin, shrivelled and stooping body
- Dry and wrinkled skin
- Brittle bones

Physiological changes

Changes in physiology of body due to ageing are given below

(i) **Heart** It grows slightly larger with age. Cardiac output stays nearly the same as the heart pumps more efficiently.

(ii) **Lungs** Reduced oxygen uptake, maximum breathing (vital) capacity may decline up to 40% between the ages of 20 and 70.

Maximal oxygen consumption during exercise declines in men up to 10% with each decade of adult life and in women up to 7.5%.

(iii) **Brain** With age, the brain loses some cells (neurons) while others become damaged.

However, it adapts by increasing the number of cell synapses and by regrowing the dendrites and axons.

(iv) **Kidneys** These gradually become less efficient in extracting wastes from the blood. Reduced blood supply leads to reduced urine output.

(v) **Body fat** The body does not lose fat with age, but redistributes it from just under the skin to deeper parts of the body.

(vi) **Muscles** Without exercise, estimated muscle mass declines 22% in women and 23% in men between the ages of 30 and 70.

(vii) **Sight** Difficulty in focusing nearby objects may begin in forties. From fifties, there is increased susceptibility to glare, greater difficulty in seeing at low levels of illumination and more difficulty in detecting moving targets.

The ability to distinguish fine details may begin declining in the seventies.

(viii) **Hearing** It becomes more difficult to hear higher frequencies with age. It declines more quickly in men than in women.

Cellular changes

Various cellular changes due to ageing are given below

- Increased number of chromosomal aberrations in the liver cells.
- The increased defects in the DNA structure produce greater amount of defective proteins in the body cells.
- Increased accumulation of pigments in body cells especially in the brain tissue and muscles.
- Decreased power of multiplication in cells, though it differs in various tissues.
- Activity of many enzymes, e.g. glucose-6-phosphate dehydrogenase, lactate dehydrogenase and acetylcholinesterase is reduced.

Causes of ageing

There are various theories regarding the causes of ageing. These theories of ageing mainly fall into two groups, i.e. programmed theories and damage or error theories.

1. Programmed theories

These theories stress upon the role of internal biological clock within an organism. Programmed theories have various subcategories, which are given below

(i) **Endocrine theory** This theory states that the biological clock acts through the hormones to control the pace of ageing.

For example, during ageing, level of growth hormone declines to about half that of adults.

Thus, following changes occurs

- Fall in sex hormone.
- Fall in oestrogen causes weakening of bones, frailty and disability.
- Decrease in the level of melatonin, thymosin and Dehydroepiandrosterone (DHEA).

(ii) **Programmed senescence theory** Ageing is the result of sequential switching on and off of certain genes.

- Studies of immune system reveal that B or T-lymphocytes having the receptors for self-antigens undergo programmed cell death or apoptosis.
- This mechanism eliminates about 90% of all the B-cells made in bone marrow. A parallel process occurs with T-cells in the thymus.
- Programmed cell death in humans mainly occurs due to the antagonistic action of *bax* and *bcl*-2 gene. *bax* gene promotes ageing, whereas *bcl*-2 prevents ageing.

(iii) **Immunity theory** It states that the size of thymus decreases with the progress in ageing. It increases the vulnerability to disease.

2. Damage or Error theories

These theories stress upon the external or environmental factors that cause ageing. These have following subcategories

(i) **Living theory** It states that ageing is a byproduct of metabolism. The greater an organism's rate of oxygen basal metabolism, the shorter is its lifespan.

(ii) **Free radical theory** According to this theory, due to the damage caused by highly reactive free oxygen radical, the cells and organs stop functioning.

These free radicals are found to be involved in degenerative disorders, including cancer, atherosclerosis, cataracts and neurodegeneration.

(iii) **Cross linking theory** This theory highlights that an accumulation of cross-linking proteins damages cells and tissues which slow down the body processes and results in ageing.

For example, glucose combines with protein *via* glycosylation resulting in cross-linking.

This can alter their biological role and may cause some of the deterioration associated with ageing.

(iv) **Wear and tear theory** According to this theory, the cells and tissues have vital parts that wear out and bring up ageing. Due to the normal wear and tear of cells, DNA gets damaged.

- This damage leads to malfunctioning of genes, proteins, cells and deterioration of tissues and organs, e.g. telomerase enzyme degradation causes ageing.
- Thus, DNA damage and repair is somewhat, a part of the ageing process.

Death

- A biological phenomenon which results in irreversible breakdown of the body functions is known as death. It results from the failure of either of heart or nervous system.
- Although, death is often related with age, it is not known if the process of ageing itself is a disease or a natural process of the organism.
- Scientists are trying to distinguish between changes, which are associated with normal ageing and those associated with external or internal pathological effects.

CHECK POINT 5.2

1. What will you call if the cells of liver and kidney divide, but do not form undifferentiated tissue?
   (a) Compensatory hypertrophy
   (b) Morphallaxis
   (c) Epimorphosis
   (d) Compensatory regeneration
2. To demonstrate the fastest regeneration capacity in *Hydra*, the scientist show cut its
   (a) basal disc region (b) middle body
   (c) tentacles (d) bud
3. Apoptosis is programmed cell death, but certain cells cannot be destroyed by apoptosis. These are
   (a) immune cells
   (b) cells with damaged DNA
   (c) cancer cells
   (d) cells infected with virus
4. A 68-years old woman suddenly lost conscious. Upon awaking 1 hour later, she could not speak. 2 months later, CT scan showed, cystic lesion in her brain. What is the most likely pathological change occurred in the brain?
   (a) Apoptosis
   (b) Necrosis
   (c) Senescence
   (d) Tumours
5. Genes in the somatic cells of the body undergoes mutation with the passage of time. Such mutations cause senescence. It is related with
   (a) hormonal theory
   (b) programmed senescence theory
   (c) error or damage theories
   (d) immunological theories

EXAM POINTS

- The process of growth is maximum during log phase. **[NEET 2020]**
- Due to fragmentation in *Planaria*, each part develops the remaining body parts and becomes a complete animal. Differentiated tissue present in each broken part of *Planaria* undergoes dedifferentiation and then differentiation for regeneration. **[Gujarat CET 2011]**
- Lowest regeneration power is found in brain cells. **[UP CPMT 2011]**
- Morphallaxis is regeneration of two transversely cut equal pieces of one *Hydra* into two small *Hydra*. **[UP CPMT 2011]**
- In epimorphosis, the cut or injured part of the organism is repaired, e.g. lizard repairs its cut tail. **[UP CPMT 2011]**

Chapter Exercises

(A) Topical Exercise

Growth

1 Neurons grow by
(a) multiplication
(b) increase in volume
(c) extension of axons and dendrites
(d) Both (a) and (b)

2 Isometric growth is found in
(a) fish (b) locust
(c) grasshopper (d) All of these

3 Find the odd one out with respect to the pattern of growth.
(a) Humans (b) *Pteropus* (c) *Chelone* (d) Whale

4 Auxetic growth is
(a) increase in cell volume only
(b) increase in cell number only
(c) increase in fatty tissue
(d) increase in intercellular material

5 Consider the following statements.
I. Growth due to mitotic multiplication of reserve cells occurring in specific location of the body is accretionary growth.
II. The kind of growth in which undifferentiated reserve cells get differentiated is accretionary growth.

Choose the correct option.
(a) Statement I is true, but II is false
(b) Statement I is false, but II is true
(c) Both statements I and II are true
(d) Both statements I and II are false

6 Post-embryonic growth is
(a) accretionary (b) auxetic
(c) multiplicative (d) All of these

7 Choose the incorrect statement for growth.
(a) Growth is an important property of life
(b) Multiplicative growth is found in embryo
(c) Early embryonic development stages constitute transitional growth
(d) In animals, growth rate is uniform

8 The growth curve is
(a) uniform and sigmoid
(b) non-uniform and straight
(c) uniform and straight
(d) non-uniform and sigmoid

9 The nearest approach to pure exponential growth is found in
(a) rod-shaped bacteria
(b) multicellular organisms
(c) larvae of insects in which complete metamorphosis
(d) All of the above

10 Which of the following correctly signifies the phases found in a sigmoid curve?
(a) Lag phase, plateau, acceleration
(b) Plateau, acceleration, lag phase
(c) Log phase, plateau, exponential phase
(d) Lag phase, acceleration, plateau

11 Choose the incorrect match pair.
(a) Hypertrophy–Increase in cell size due to synthesis of protoplasmic structures
(b) Hyperplasia–Increase in cell number
(c) Negative growth–Formation of leaves
(d) Positive growth–Embryo formation

12 Select the correct statement.
(a) Average lifespan of man is longer than that of woman
(b) Average lifespan of woman is longer than that of man
(c) Average lifespan in both sexes is same
(d) None of the above

13 With the increase in age, which of the following organ in mice, dog and man exhibits increase in chromosomal aberrations?
(a) Liver (b) Brain
(c) Kidney (d) Gonads

14 In human beings, which part shows the minimum increase in weight from birth to adulthood?
(a) Muscles (b) Skeleton
(c) Fat (d) Brain

15 In human beings, which part shows the maximum increase in weight from birth to adulthood?
(a) Brain (b) Fat
(c) Muscles (d) Skeleton

16 Adult females tend to have less weight than adult males due to lesser development of
(a) muscles (b) skeleton
(c) Both (a) and (b) (d) fat

17 Human body regularly looses cells in the region of
(a) skin surface
(b) lining layer of gut
(c) red blood cells
(d) All of the above

18 Which of the following factors triggers the division of activated T-lymphocytes?
(a) Epidermal growth factor
(b) Erythropoietin
(c) Interleukin-2
(d) Both (a) and (c)

19 Which of the following growth factor promotes the proliferation of many connective tissues?
(a) Interleukin-2
(b) Insulin like growth factors
(c) Epidermal growth factors
(d) Platelet-derived growth factors

20 Consider the following statements.
I. Growth in the first 10-13 yrs of age is controlled by thyroxine.
II. Growth at the end of the childhood and during puberty is controlled by thyroxine and GH.
Choose the correct option.
(a) Statement I is true, but II is false
(b) Statement I is false, but II is true
(c) Both statements I and II are true
(d) Both statements I and II are false

Regeneration

21 Healing of cuts and wounds are examples of
(a) proliferation (b) differentiation
(c) regeneration (d) degeneration

22 Regeneration of liver is
(a) metamorphosis (b) reparative regeneration
(c) epimorphosis (d) morphogenesis

23 Which of the following is found in animals with higher and complex organisation?
(a) Restorative regenerations
(b) Reparative regeneration
(c) Both (a) and (b)
(d) None of the above

24 Restorative regeneration decreases with
(a) increase in complexity of organisation
(b) decrease in organisational complexity
(c) development of hormones
(d) development of nerves

25 The voluntary casting off a part of the body when an animal is attacked is known as
(a) autotomy (b) autogamy
(c) amputation (d) regeneration

26 Autotomy is recorded in
(a) legs in crabs
(b) tail of lizards
(c) viscera in holothurian echinoderms
(d) All of the above

27 Morphallaxis is
(a) reconstruction of the whole body
(b) growth of lost limb
(c) healing of injury
(d) regeneration with the help of blastema

28 Morphallaxis is reported in
(a) poriferans
(b) coelenterates and flatworms
(c) nemerteans and some ascidians
(d) All of the above

29 Accumulation of cells and formation of a bud at the site of amputation is
(a) morphallaxis (b) epimorphosis
(c) repair (d) compensatory regeneration

30 Regeneration of a limb or tail is an example of
(a) compensatory hypertrophy
(b) epimorphosis
(c) morphallaxis
(d) autotomy

31 If one kidney of a man is lost, the other kidney enlarges to take over the function of the missing kidney and is called
(a) restorative regeneration
(b) reparative regeneration
(c) autotomy
(d) compensatory regeneration

32 Consider the following statements.
I. The process of regeneration was first discovered in *Hydra*.
II. The mechanism of regeneration in *Hydra* was discovered by Trembley.
Choose the correct option.
(a) Statement I is true, but II is false
(b) Statement I is false, but II is true
(c) Both statements I and II are true
(d) Both statements I and II are false

33 Choose the incorrect statement.
(a) In lizards, regeneration occurs in tail
(b) In birds, regeneration occurs in beak
(c) In fish, regeneration occurs in fins
(d) In tadpoles, regeneration occurs in jaws and eyes

34 Consider the following statements.
I. Crustaceans, insects and spiders are able to regenerate their legs.
II. Salamander is capable to regenerate its limbs, external gills and tail.
Choose the correct option.
(a) Statement I is true, but II is false
(b) Statement I is false, but II is true
(c) Both statements I and II are true
(d) Both statements I and II are false

Ageing and Death

35 Ageing is characterised by
(a) decline in metabolic activity
(b) increased metabolic activity
(c) increased anabolism
(d) decrease number of free radicals

36 Ageing of leaves is called
(a) senescence
(b) necrosis
(c) photoperiodism
(d) vernalisation

37 Gerontology is the branch of science that deals with
(a) sexual reproduction
(b) ageing
(c) embryo development
(d) regeneration

38 Which of the following is an immortal being not subjected to ageing?
(a) *Periplaneta* (b) Starfish
(c) *Hydra* (d) All of these

39 Which of the following is a morphological change occurring during ageing?
(a) Brittle bone
(b) Stooping body
(c) Wrinkled skin
(d) All of the above

40 Possible cause of brittle bones with ageing may be
(a) decrease amount of DHEA in body
(b) excess of calcium in body
(c) increased amount of oestrogen in body
(d) None of the above

41 Which of the following theory falls under the category of programmed theories of ageing?
(a) Cross linking theory (b) Living theory
(c) Free radical theory (d) Endocrine theory

42 Consider the following statements.
I. According to programmed senescence theory, *bax*-1 gene prevents ageing.
II. Free radicals are involved in causing neurodegradation.
Choose the correct option.
(a) Statement I is true, but II is false
(b) Statement I is false, but II is true
(c) Both statements I and II are true
(d) Both statements I and II are false

43 Accumulation of .... in the skin causes premature ageing of the skin in women.
(a) phosphorus (b) collagen
(c) calcium (d) magnesium

44 With increasing age, secretion of which of the following reduces to almost half?
(a) GTH (b) Melatonin
(c) hGH (d) Oestrogen

45 Fall in oestrogen during ageing may cause
(a) thinning of bones (b) frailty
(c) disability (d) All of these

46 In many mammals, even humans, ageing can be due to
(a) malnutrition and stress
(b) interaction between hereditary factors and the environment
(c) adverse alterations in the environment
(d) All of the above

47 Wear and tear theory of ageing is given by
(a) TH Morgan
(b) E Darwin
(c) August Weismann
(d) Sutton

48 A biological phenomenon which results in irreversible breakdown of the body functions is
(a) ageing (b) apoptosis
(c) regeneration (d) death

(B) Cumulative Exercise

(Assorted Questions of the Chapter for Advanced Level Practice)

1 Read the following statements.

I. In auxetic growth, the volume of body is increased.
II. Auxetic growth occurs without any division and increases in the number of cells.
III. Accretionary growth in post-embryonic period of organism's life is due to increase in number of cells.
IV. The pre-natal growth of higher vertebrates is an example of accretionary growth.

Choose the correct option containing correct statements.

(a) I and II (b) III and IV (c) Only III (d) I, II and IV

2 Which of the following statements correctly defines growth?

I. Increases in size of cells.
II. Increases in the number of cells.
III. Increases in the amount of apoplasmatic structures.
IV. Decreases in amount of living material.

Codes

(a) Only I (b) I and II
(c) I, II and III (d) I, II, III and IV

3 Match the following columns.

Column I	Column II
A. Morphallaxis	1. Deterioration in the structure and function of the body cells, tissues and organs of an animal.
B. Epimorphosis	2. Replacement or reconstruction of lost parts.
C. Autotomy	3. Proliferation of the new tissue cells from the surface of wound.
D. Regeneration	4. Reconstruction of the whole body from a small fragment.
E. Senescence	5. Voluntary casting off a part of the body when an animal is attached.

Codes

	A	B	C	D	E
(a)	3	5	4	1	2
(b)	1	2	4	5	3
(c)	4	2	5	3	1
(d)	1	3	4	5	2

4 Consider the following match pairs.

I. Coelenterates – Lost part regenerated with exact polarity
II. Molluscs – Sealing of wounds by neoblast cells
III. Nematodes – Only closure of superficial wound
IV. Arthropods – Regenerate parts of disc

Choose the correct option containing incorrectly match pairs.

(a) Only I (b) Only III (c) II and IV (d) I and III

5 Read the given statements regarding changes occurring in organisms during ageing.

I. Heart rate decreases slightly with age.
II. The brain loses some cells (neurons) and others become damaged.
III. Enzyme aldolase becomes more effective.
IV. Collagen becomes less permeable, rigid and insoluble.

Which of the following changes occur in human beings?

(a) Only I (b) I and IV (c) II and IV (d) I and III

6 Match the following columns.

Column I	Column II
A. Earthworms	1. Limbs, tails, external gills, jaws, intestine, etc.
B. Mollusca	2. Few body segments
C. Salamander and axolotl	3. Liver
D. Mammals	4. Part of eye, eye-stalk, head, foot, etc.

Codes

	A	B	C	D		A	B	C	D
(a)	2	4	3	1	(b)	1	2	4	3
(c)	2	4	1	3	(d)	4	3	2	1

7 Which of the following cases are of epimorphosis?

I. Formation of sperms from small clumps of cells.
II. Regeneration of tail in a lizard.
III. Replacement of severed arm in starfish.
IV. Replacement of limb in salamander.

Codes

(a) I and II (b) II and IV
(c) I, II and III (d) II, III and IV

Assertion and Reason

Direction (Q. Nos. 8-18) *In each of the following questions, a statement of Assertion (A) is given followed by the corresponding statement of Reason (R). Of the statements, mark the correct answer as*

(a) Both A and R are true and R is the correct explanation of A
(b) Both A and R are true, but R is not the correct explanation of A
(c) A is true, but R is false
(d) A is false, but R is true
(e) Both A and R are false

8 **Assertion** (A) Growth involves the synthesis of protoplasmic materials.

Reason (R) During growth, catabolic activities are faster than anabolic activities.

9 **Assertion** (A) Coelenterates and flatworms show morphallactic regeneration.

Reason (R) In both of these, a body fragment can develop into complete organism.

10 **Assertion** (A) Growth curve of higher animals is sigmoid.

Reason (R) Absolute growth is the difference between initial and final weight/size of an organism.

11 **Assertion** (A) Growth of different body parts is differential.

Reason (R) During human growth, muscles show minimum growth, while brain shows maximum growth.

12 **Assertion** (A) In ageing, power of intake of useful materials and expelling of harmful materials out of the cells both decrease.

Reason (R) With age, collagen protein of connective tissue becomes less flexible, less permeable and insoluble.

13 **Assertion** (A) Death is an essential and inescapable biological phenomenon.

Reason (R) Death maintains ecological homeostasis and justifies the need of reproduction.

14 **Assertion** (A) A regenerated tail of wall lizard shows heteromorphosis.

Reason (R) Newly formed tail is different from original tail in being without vertebrae.

15 **Assertion** (A) Brain of man shows compensatory hypertrophy.

Reason (R) It grows larger than its normal size when a part is lost.

16 **Assertion** (A) Regeneration blastema is a bud-like structure formed during regeneration of limb in salamander.

Reason (R) Formation of regeneration blastema involves dedifferentiation.

17 **Assertion** (A) Old age is not an illness. It is a continuation of life with decrease capacity for adaptation.

Reason (R) Cessation of mitosis is normal genetically programmed event.

18 **Assertion** (A) Senescence is the time when age associated defects are manifested.

Reason (R) Certain genes may be undergoing sequential switching on and off during one's life.

(C) Medical Entrances' Gallery

(Collection of Questions Asked in NEET & in Various Medical Entrance Exams)

1 The process of growth is maximum during **[NEET 2020]**

(a) lag phase (b) senescence
(c) dormancy (d) log phase

2 Which is the correct example of the type of regeneration out of the two major types? **[UP CPMT 2011]**

(a) Morphallaxis – Regeneration of two transversely cut equal pieces of one *Hydra* into two small *Hydra*

(b) Epimorphosis – Replacement of old and dead erythrocytes by the new ones

(c) Morphallaxis – Healing of wound in the skin

(d) Epimorphosis – Regeneration of crushed and filtered out pieces of *Planaria* into as many new planarian

3 Lowest regeneration power is found in **[UP CPMT 2011]**

(a) *Amoeba* (b) sponges
(c) coelenterates (d) brain cells

4 **Assertion** (A) Due to fragmentation in *Planaria*, each part develops the remaining body parts and becomes a complete animal.

Reason (R) Differentiated tissue present in each broken part of *Planaria* undergoes dedifferentiation and then differentiation for regeneration. **[Gujarat CET 2011]**

(a) Both A and R are true and R is the correct explanation of A
(b) Both A and R are true, but R is not the correct explanation of A
(c) A is true, but R is false
(d) Both A and R are false

ANSWERS

CHECK POINT 5.1

1. (b) 2. (a) 3. (c) 4. (b) 5. (a) 6. (c)

CHECK POINT 5.2

1. (d) 2. (c) 3. (c) 4. (b) 5. (c)

(A) Topical Exercise

1. (c) 2. (d) 3. (c) 4. (a) 5. (c) 6. (c) 7. (d) 8. (d) 9. (c) 10. (d)
11. (c) 12. (b) 13. (a) 14. (d) 15. (c) 16. (c) 17. (d) 18. (c) 19. (d) 20. (c)
21. (c) 22. (b) 23. (b) 24. (a) 25. (a) 26. (d) 27. (a) 28. (d) 29. (b) 30. (b)
31. (d) 32. (c) 33. (d) 34. (c) 35. (a) 36. (a) 37. (b) 38. (c) 39. (d) 40. (b)
41. (d) 42. (b) 43. (b) 44. (c) 45. (d) 46. (d) 47. (c) 48. (d)

(B) Cumulative Exercise

1. (a) 2. (c) 3. (c) 4. (c) 5. (b) 6. (c) 7. (d) 8. (c) 9. (a) 10. (b)
11. (c) 12. (a) 13. (a) 14. (u) 15. (e) 16. (b) 17. (c) 18. (a)

(C) Medical Entrances' Gallery

1. (d) 2. (a) 3. (d) 4. (a)

Explanations

(A) Topical Exercise

3 (*c*) Humans, *Pteropus* and whale show allometric growth while *Chelone* shows isometric growth. Hence, option (c) is correct.

7 (*d*) Statement in option (d) is incorrect and can be corrected as
In animals, growth rate is non-uniform.
Rest statements are correct for growth.

11 (*c*) Option (c) is incorrect match pair and can be corrected as
Negative growth is seen in germination of seeds.
Rest options are correct match pairs.

33 (*d*) Statement in option (d) is incorrect and can be corrected as
In tadpoles, regeneration occurs in limbs.
Rest statements are correct.

42 (*b*) Statement I is false, but II is true. Incorrect statement can be corrected as
According to programmed senescence theory, *bax* gene promotes ageing.

(B) Cumulative Exercise

1 (*a*) Statements I and II are correct whereas III and IV are incorrect. Incorrect statements can be corrected as

- Accretionary growth in post-embryonic period of organism's life is not due to increase in number of cells. It is growth in undifferentiated reserve cells when they get differentiated to perform specific function.
- Formation of erythrocytes from erythropoietic tissue is an example of accretionary growth (not pre-natal growth in higher vertebrates).

2 (*c*) All statements correctly define growth except IV. Incorrect statement can be corrected as
Growth causes increase in amount of living material.

4 (*c*) Matched pairs in II and III are incorrect and can be corrected as

- Sealing of wounds by neoblast cells occurs in annelids.
- Echinoderms regenerate parts of disc.

Rest others are correct matched pairs.

5 (*b*) Statements I and IV are correct regarding human ageing. Statements II and III are incorrect and can be corrected as

- Heart rate remains same with age.
- Enzyme aldolase becomes less effective.

7 (*d*) Epimorphosis replaces a lost organ of the body for proliferating new cells from the surface of the wound on injured part, e.g. regeneration of tail in lizard, replacement of arm in starfish and limb in salamander.
Thus, option (d) is correct.

8 (*c*) A is true, but R is false because
Growth may be defined as 'the increase in size and weight of an organism due to synthesis of new protoplasmic' materials. Growth occurs when the anabolic activities exceed the catabolic activities.

9 (*a*) Both A and R are true and R is the correct explanation of A.
If *Hydra* (coelenterates) is cut transversely into two or more parts. Then, these parts can grow into complete organism of smaller size similarly *Planaria* (flatworm) can also develop into a complete animal though it has smaller size than the parental animal by morphallactic regeneration as in *Hydra*.

10 (*b*) Both A and R are true, but R is not the correct explanation of A.

Growth curve is the graphic representation of the growth of a living organism. Growth curve of higher animals, including man, is S-shaped and is called sigmoid growth curve. The difference between the initial and final weight (or size) of an individual in a given period of time is called absolute growth.

11 (*c*) A is true, but R is false because

The growth rate is not uniform, but it is different at different period of life. So, the growth is differential. In human beings, the muscles show maximum growth, i.e. from 0.8 kg in newly born body to 30 kg in adult, while brain shows minimum growth, i.e. from 0.4 kg in newly born body to 1 kg in adult, from birth to adulthood.

12 (*a*) Both A and R are true and R is the correct explanation of A.

Collagen forms about 40% of total protein contents of the body in young age-groups. It is permeable, flexible and soluble, so there is easy exchange of materials between the cell cytoplasm and interstitial fluid through the semipermeable cell membrane. But with advancing age, the collagen protein becomes less flexible, less permeable and insoluble.
Due to these changes, there is a decreased inflow of nutritive substances and oxygen into the cells and also decreased loss of nitrogenous wastes and CO_2 from the body cells. This causes decreased efficiency of body cells and induces ageing.

13 (*a*) Both A and R are true and R is the correct explanation of A.

Death is an essential and inescapable biological phenomenon, which helps in maintaining ecological balance or homeostasis in nature. It prevents overcrowding of the members of a specific species and justifies the continuity of life on earth.

14 (*a*) Both A and R are true and R is the correct explanation of A.

Wall lizard can regenerate its lost tail when severed in autotomy, but the regenerated tail differs from the original one in shape. It is mainly due to lack of vertebrae and the type of scales covering it. This is known as heteromorphosis.

15 (*e*) Both A and R are false and can be corrected as

Maximum reparative regeneration is found in the liver of mammals. If a part of liver is surgically removed, then the cells of the remaining part undergo repeated mitotic divisions and original volume of the liver is maintained.
Similarly, if one kidney of man is lost, the other kidney enlarges to take over the function of the missing kidney and is called compensatory regeneration. It is not found in brain.

16 (*b*) Both A and R are true, but R is not the correct explanation of A.

Formation of a conical bulge called regeneration blastema or bud, below the newly formed epidermal cover so that the epidermis starts bulging during the regeneration of limb of salamander. A number of evidences have supported that the mitotically proliferating cells in a regenerating limb are derived by a regressive process called transformation or dedifferentiation of specialised or fully differentiated cells of the skin, muscles, bones, etc.

17 (*c*) A is true, but R is false.

Old age is not the age of illness. It includes progressive deterioration of the structure and functions of cells, tissue, organs and organ systems. With the increasing age, the efficiency of heart decreases and consequently, the blood going to the brain and kidney, is reduced to 80% and 42%, respectively. Arthritis, weak eyesight, less secretion of digestive juices, etc., are some degenerative diseases.
Cessation of mitosis is not a genetically programmed event.

18 (*a*) Both A and R are true and R is the correct explanation of A.

Senescence is the process of ageing which involves the progressive deterioration in activity of cells, tissues, organs, etc.

Ageing may be due to the gradual accumulation of somatic mutations or very late expressions of genes, not subject to strong selections. It is genetically controlled programme regulated by the regulatory genes.

(C) Medical Entrances' Gallery

1 (*d*) The process of growth is maximum during log phase (exponential phase) because during log phase, the growth rate of the cells gradually increases, at a maximum rate.

In exponential growth, the initial growth is slow (lag phase) and thereafter it increases rapidly.

2 (*a*) Option (a) is the correct example of the type of regeneration out of the two major types. Rest options are incorrect and can be corrected as

- Morphallaxis involves the reconstruction of whole body from small fragment by reorganising the existing cells, e.g. regeneration of *Hydra* from its piece.
- In epimorphosis, the cut or injured part of the organism is repaired, e.g. lizard repairs its cut tail.

3 (*d*) Regeneration is defined as replacement, repair or restoration of the lost or damaged structures or reconstitution of the whole body from a small fragment of it during post-embryonic life of an organism. Brain cells have lowest power of regeneration due to highly specific differentiation.

4 (*a*) Both A and R are true and R is the correct explanation of A.

Regeneration is the capacity of the body to produce the lost part by proliferation of cells. Planarians have remarkable power of regeneration.

The differentiated tissue in each broken part of *Planaria* undergoes dedifferentiation and then differentiation to become complete animal.

CHAPTER 06

Mendelian Basis of Inheritance

We all know, reproduction in living organisms is done to facilitate continuity of life. The progeny produced, often resemble their parents in most of the characteristics. This transmission of characters from parents to their offsprings is called **heredity** and the process by which characters pass from one generation to the next is called **inheritance**. However, all characteristics of offsprings are not similar to their parents. Some of them show **variations** or **differences** also. These variations infact signify their own characteristics.

The study of heredity and variations is called **genetics**. This term was proposed by **William Bateson** (1905). The basic principles of genetics were discovered by **Gregor Johann Mendel** (1822-84). That is why, he is also known as the **'Father of Genetics'**.

Branches of genetics

Scientists often divide genetics into following three main branches

(i) **Transmission genetics** It is also called as **classical genetics**. It involves the transmission of genetic material from one generation to the other. It is further subdivided into Mendelian genetics, Morganian genetics (i.e. recombination in all kinds of organisms), non-Mendelian genetics and mutations.

(ii) **Molecular and biochemical genetics** It involves the study of structural and functional aspects of genes at a molecular level.

(iii) **Population and biometrical genetics** It involves the study of behaviour and effects of genes in various biological populations.

As initial working on genetics was done by Mendel, so, the genetics can be categorised into Pre-Mendelian, Mendelian and Post-Mendelian eras of working.

Inside

PRE-MENDELIAN CONCEPTS OF INHERITANCE

Before the ideas of Mendel were accepted, there were many philosophers, thinkers and workers who gave various theories to explain heredity or inheritance. These theories are called Pre-Mendelian concept of heredity. Some of these are given below

(i) **Moist vapour theory—Pythagoras** (580-500 BC) proposed that various body parts emit certain vapour, which gets aggregated to form a new individual.

(ii) **Fluid theory—Empedocles** (504-433 BC) thought that every part of the body produces a fluid. This fluid then mixes up to form an offspring. Any defect in this fluid results in the formation of defective organs.

(iii) **Preformation theory** This was given by **Swammerdam** (1679) and was advocated by **Malpighi** (1673). They believed that the miniature form of an individual is already present in the sperm or egg called **'homonculus'**. Fertilisation is required to stimulate its growth.

(iv) **Particulate theory—Maupertvuis** (1689-1759) proposed that various parts of the body produce minute particles for reproduction. An individual is formed when the particles from male and female unite.

(v) **Theory of pangenesis—Darwin** (1868) proposed that each body part produces a gemmule or pangene. These pangenes carry parental traits as well as variations. Their aggregation results to form gamete. On fusion, these give rise to a new individual.

Pre-Mendelian experiments

Among the workers who performed experiments before Mendel, the most important name is **J Kolreuter** (1733-1806). He was a German botanist who worked on tobacco plant.

Other persons who worked on hybridisation before Mendel, include **Bartner** (1772-1850), **Naudin** (1815-1899), **Koght** (1799) and **Goss** (1824). But none of these workers were able to rationalise and explain the results with a sure degree of repetitions.

It is better to explore certain facts related to Gregor Johann Mendel and related genetic terms before moving to Mendelian inheritance.

Gregor Johann Mendel

Gregor Johann Mendel was an Australian Monk (Brunn, Austria, Czech Republic). He was born in 1822 in the Central European village of Heinzendorf. In 1843, he was admitted to the Augustinian Monastery of St. Thomas in Bruno.

Work

- Mendel worked on *Pisum sativum* (garden pea) for 7 years between 1856 and 1863.
- The results of his experiments were presented in 1865 before the local Natural History Society of Brunn.
- He published his paper '*Experiments on Plant Hybridisation*' in the proceedings of Natural Science Society of Brunn in the year 1866.

Results

- Although his work was widely available after 1866, the scientific community was not ready to appreciate Mendel's great contribution until the turn of century.
- He died in 1884 due to kidney disorder without getting any recognition for his work.

Rediscovery of Mendel's work

- Mendel's work was rediscovered in the year 1900 after a time span of about 34 years.
- **Hugo de Vries** of Netherland, **Karl Correns** of Germany and **Erich von Tschermak** of Austria were the three independent contributors of Mendelian facts rediscovery.
- Following facts are considered as the major reasons for the lapse of these 34 years.
  - Communication was difficult, so Mendel's work could not be widely published.
  - His concept of stable, unblending and discrete units or factors for various traits did not find acceptance from the contemporaries.
  - He could not provide any physical proof for the existence of factors.
  - His approach of using mathematical and statistical tools to explain biological phenomenon was new and unacceptable.
  - Mendel's paper were republished in the 'journal Flora' in 1901.

Reasons for Mendel's success

The reasons of Mendel's success are stated under following headings

1. Method of working

- Focus on one character at a time
- Used true breeding pea lines
- Avoided cross-pollination by undesirable pollen
- Kept accurate records of results obtained

2. Selection of pea plant

Mendel used garden pea for his experiment because it has following advantages

- Many distinct alternative traits (clear contrasting characters).
- Produces large number of seeds.
- Short lifespan.
- Predominantly self-pollinating, i.e. true breeding.
- Cross-pollination produces fertile hybrids.

3. Mendel's crossing method

Crossing method of Mendel is summerised in following steps

- Mendel conducted artificial pollination or cross-pollination experiments using several true breeding pea lines. He used dwarf plant as female parent.
- Since pea is self fertilising plant, the anthers should be removed before maturity for cross-pollination. The process of removal of anther is called **emasculation.**
- He then took pollen from tall plant, i.e. male parent and dusted on the stigma of dwarf plant, i.e. female parent.
- The cross-pollinated flowers of female parent were then covered with small bags to prevent contamination. The process of covering with bags is called **Bagging**.
- The process of identification of particular gene responsible for a particular biological process is called **genetic dissection.** Mendel is regarded as a first genetic surgeon.

Genetic terms

A list of important terms used to study genetics are given below

1. **Gene** (unit factor) It is considered as the determinant of a characteristics pertaining to a particular organism. Mendel used the word unit factors or pair factors for the units that control various traits.

   Thus, a gene is a unit of inheritance. It is a piece of DNA that carries the information needed to make a specific protein. The term 'Gene' was given by **Johannsen.**
2. **Character,** i.e. the feature or characteristic of an individual like height, colour, shape, etc.
3. **Trait** It is an inherited character, i.e. the feature, which is normally inherited and has its detectable variant too. For example, in pea plant tall and dwarf are traits of a character, i.e. height.
4. **Gene locus** It is the particular position of a gene on a chromosome. Various alleles of a gene occupy the same locus on similar or homologous chromosomes.
5. **Alleles or Allelomorphs** It is the alternate forms or varieties of genes in a particular gene pair that occupies same locus (position) on homologous pair of chromosome. This term was given by **Bateson.**
6. **Homozygous** When a gene pair (allele) in an organism contains two identical genes which control similar trait of a character, then the organism is considered as homozygous for that particular trait.
7. **Heterozygous** When a gene pair (allele) contains two different genes which control different traits of a character in an organism, then the organism is considered as heterozygous for that particular trait.
8. **Dominant allele** An allele which expresses itself phenotypically whether present in homozygous or in heterozygous conditions.
9. **Recessive allele** An allele which expresses itself phenotypically when present in homozygous condition, but remains suppressed in heterozygous conditions.
10. **Genotype** It is the complete genetic constitution of an individual.
11. **Phenotype** It is the physical appearance of an individual. It is the result of genotype and environmental interactions.
12. **Gamete** A mature reproductive cell, which is specialised for amphimixis (fusion) with other similar type of cell is called gamete.
13. **Hybrid** The literary meaning of this word is mixture. In genetics, we define it as an offspring, which is obtained from a cross between two genetically different parents.
14. **F_1-generation** First filial (*filial*—offspring) generation, i.e. the generation of hybrids, which are obtained from a cross between two genetically different parents.
15. **F_2-generation** Second filial generation, i.e. individuals normally obtained after self-crossing the individuals of F_1-generation.
16. **Cross** Mating between two individuals, leading to the fusion of gametes and resulting in offsprings or progenies. The crosses may be
    (i) **Monohybrid cross,** i.e. when only one pair of contrasting character is considered.
    (ii) **Dihybrid cross,** i.e. when two pairs of contrasting characters are considered (similarly trihybrid and so on).

(iii) **Reciprocal cross** is the cross that could be made either way or independent of the sex of parents.

(iv) **Back cross**, i.e. the cross of the hybrids of F_1-generation with either of its parents. Thus, there can be two possibilities.

(a) F_1 hybrid to be crossed with homozygous dominant parent (outcross)

(b) F_1 hybrid to be crossed with homozygous recessive parent (test cross)

(v) **Test cross** is a back cross between F_1 hybrid and its homozygous recessive parent. It is called test cross because it helps to find, whether the given dominant phenotype is homozygous or heterozygous. The test cross always results in 1:1 phenotypic ratio.

17. **Punnett square** It is a grid devised by a British geneticist **RC Punnett** (1927). It is used to determine the various genotypes and phenotypes resulting from the combination of all possible gametes.

Genetic symbols

According to the **classical method of symbolisation** used by Mendel, the dominant character is expressed in a capital alphabet and recessive character is expressed in a small alphabet.

For example, tall is dominant character for height, its first letter in capital form (T) represents tallness (dominant) and in small form (t) represents dwarfness (recessive).

In modern genetical literature, **wild type symbolism** is normally used. In this, the phenotype which is of much more common occurrence in a population is called wild type and is represented by (+) symbol.

On the other hand, the phenotype which is of rare occurrence is called **mutant type**. It is represented by a capital or small letter depending upon whether mutant is dominant or recessive.

Case I If the mutant gene is recessive, then its symbol will be a small alphabet, which is the initial letter of trait itself. Its wild type is symbolised as either same letter superscript with (+) sign, suppose W for wings or simply by the (+) sign only.

Case II On the other hand, if the mutant trait is dominant, then its wild type is symbolised by its initial alphabet in capital and mutant type by same alphabet along with (+) sign in superscript or only (+) sign.

CHECK POINT 6.1

1. Transmission of genetic material from one generation to the other is called

(a) population genetics (b) classical genetics
(c) biometrical genetics (d) biochemical genetics

2. All allelomorphic pair implies

(a) a pair of contrasting traits
(b) a pair of non-contrasting characters
(c) any two characters
(d) sex-linked characters

3. A heterozygous parent produces

(a) one kind of gamete
(b) two kinds of gametes each having two alleles
(c) two kinds of gametes each having one allele in equal proportion
(d) two kinds of gametes

4. An allele is dominant if it expresses itself

(a) both in homozygous and heterozygous state
(b) only in homozygous conditions
(c) neither in homozygous nor in heterozygous condition
(d) only in heterozygous conditions

5. Phenotype of an organism is the result of

(a) mutation and linkage
(b) cytoplasmic effects and nutrition
(c) environmental changes and sexual dimorphism
(d) genotype and environmental interactions

6. The genotype of a plant showing the dominant phenotype can be determined by

(a) test cross (b) dihybrid cross
(c) pedigree analysis (d) back cross

MENDELIAN INHERITANCE

The study of experiments of Mendel and his conclusion in combined form is called Mendelian inheritance.

Mendel's hybridisation experiments

- Mendel used hybridisation technique to conduct his experiments.
- **Hybridisation** is the crossing of two different individuals to produce an offspring which will have character of both parents.
- He crossed parents with contrasting traits. Firstly, he made monohybrid cross followed by dihybrid cross and finally trihybrid cross. In the experiments, the F_1 hybrids were self-crossed to give rise to F_2-generations.
- Mendel selected 14 true breeding pea lines for his experiments.
- A **true breeding line** is the one that shows stable trait's inheritance and expression for several generation on undergoing continuous self-pollination. These true breeding lines were taken as pairs which were similar except for a contrasting trait.
- Thus, Mendel selected **14 contrasting traits** for **7 characters** in pea (*Pisum sativum*) for his experiments. It is now known that these 7 characters are located on only **4 chromosomes** of pea plant.

Monohybrid cross

It is a cross which involves single pair of contrasting traits of a character. All the contrasting traits used by Mendel and his results are given in the table below

Table: 6.1 Results of seven characters with their contrasting traits used by Mendel in his monohybrid crosses

Characters	Contrasting traits	Dominant/ Recessive	F_1 results	F_2 results	F_2 ratio
Shape of the seeds	Round × Wrinkled	Round/Wrinkled	All round	5474 round 1850 wrinkled	2.96:1
Colour of the seeds	Yellow × Green	Yellow/Green	All yellow	6022 yellow 2001 green	3.01:1
Shape of the pods	Full × Constricted	Full/Constricted	All full	882 full 299 constricted	2.95:1
Colour of the pods	Green × Yellow	Green/Yellow	All green	428 green 152 yellow	2.82:1
Colour of the flowers	Violet × White	Violet/White	All violet	705 violet 224 white	3.15:1
Position of the pods	Axial × Terminal	Axial/Terminal	All axial	651 axial 207 terminal	3.14:1
Height of the stem	Tall × Dwarf	Tall/Dwarf	All tall	787 tall 277 dwarf	2.84:1

Results

- When a cross is made between pure tall and pure dwarf plant in F_1-generation, all plants will be tall.
- When F_1-plants are self-pollinated, then in F_2-generation, both tall and dwarf plants are found in approximate ratio of 3:1. This cross is shown in the **figure (6.1)**.
- Mendel in his experiments used the first letter of dominant traits to express the contrasting trait, e.g. 'T' and 't' to represent tall and dwarf traits, respectively. However, modern scientist use first letter of recessive trait, e.g. 'D' instead of 'T' and 'd' instead of 't'.
- For convenience sake, we are using modern terminology here while in rest of the chapter, we will be using Mendel's terminology throughout.
- The dwarf plants of F_2-generation on self-pollination, produce dwarf plants generation after generation.
- On the other hand among tall plants, only 1/3 rd show this character generation after generation (pureline) and rest 2/3rd produce tall and dwarf in 3:1 ratio again (F_3-generation).

Mathematical interpretation

In mathematical terms, the result can be rewritten as follows

- 1/4th of the random fertilisation lead to DD, 1/2 lead to Dd and 1/4th to dd genotype.
- The 1/4 : 1/2 : 1/4 ratio of DD : Dd : dd is mathematically condensable to form the binomial expression $(ax + by)^2$ that has the gametes bearing D or d in equal frequency of 1/2. Terms 'a' and 'b' in above expression represents frequency, while 'x' and 'y' represent genes controlling different traits of same character.

- The expression is expanded as

$$\left(\frac{1}{2}D + \frac{1}{2}d\right)^2 = \frac{1}{4}DD + \frac{1}{2}Dd + \frac{1}{4}dd \text{ or } 1 : 2 : 1$$

Mendel also carried out reciprocal crosses and obtained the same result.

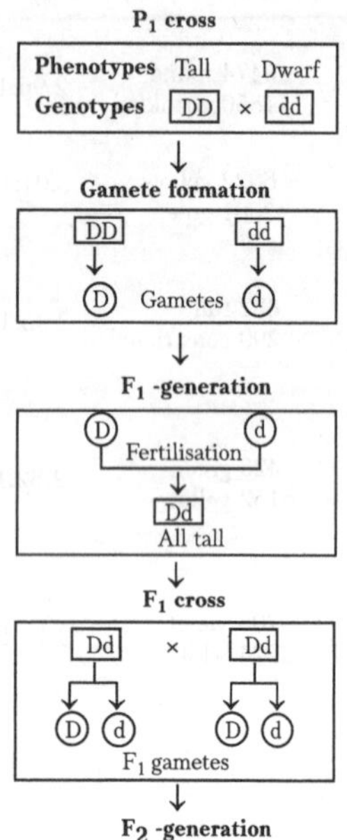

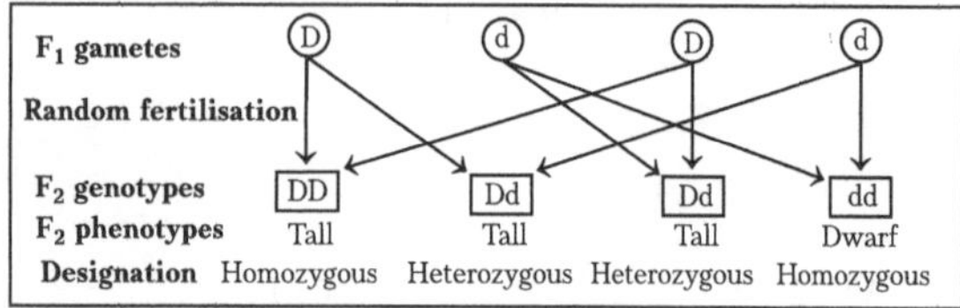

Phenotypic ratio Tall : Dwarf = 3 : 1

Genotypic ratio DD : Dd : dd = 1 : 2 : 1

Fig. 6.1 *The monohybrid cross between tall and dwarf*

Reciprocal cross

- In such crosses, the parent that provides male gamete in one cross, provides female gamete in the second experiment and *vice-versa.*
- The result of reciprocal crosses proves that both gametes produce the same effect and it does not matter which parent provides male and which one provides female gamete.

Mendel's postulates based on monohybrid cross

On the basis of his experimental crosses, Mendel formulated four postulates. Out of these, three postulates were based on monohybrid cross or one-gene interaction and the last postulate was based on dihybrid cross or two genes interaction.

(i) **Postulate on factors of genetics** It states that characters are controlled by a pair of unit factors. Two such factors are now called **alleles** or **allelomorphic pair.**

(ii) **Postulate on dominance and recessivesness** If two dissimilar unit factors are present in an individual, then only one of them expresses itself. This is known as the **dominant factor,** while the second which does not express at all is known as the **recessive factor.**

(iii) **Postulate on segregation** It states that any two contrasting alleles responsible for contrasting traits present in an individual do not get mixed. These get separated or segregated from each other at the time of gamete formation by F_1 hybrid.

(iv) **Postulate on independent assortment** It states that in a hybrid, segregation of one pair of trait is independent to the other similar one. **Karl Correns** later changed the term. Mendel's postulates to Mendel's laws of inheritance in 1901.

Mendel's laws of inheritance

1. Law of dominance

- It states that when two contrasting alleles for a character come together in an organism, then only one of them expresses itself completely and shows visible effect. This allele is called **dominant** and the other allele of the pair which does not express and remains hidden is called **recessive.**
- For example, in the monohybrid cross, when dwarf plant is crossed with tall plant, the F_1-generation have all tall plants. This shows that allele for tallness is dominant.
- Besides pea plant, the law of dominance has also been observed in different characters of many plants. For example,

(i) **Sunflower** (branching) Branched habit is dominant over unbranched habit.

(ii) **Cotton** (colour of lint) Coloured lint is dominant over white lint.

(iii) **Maize** (type of kernel) Round starchy kernal is dominant over wrinkled sugary kernel.

(iv) **Snapdragon** (colour of flower) Red-coloured flowers are dominant over non-red flowers.

(v) **Wheat** (rust susceptibility) Susceptibility to rust is dominant over immunity to rust.

- The law of dominance is applicable well to animals also. Examine the following cross of homozygous black Guinea pig with homozygous white Guinea pig. The cross clears the dominance of black colour on white one.

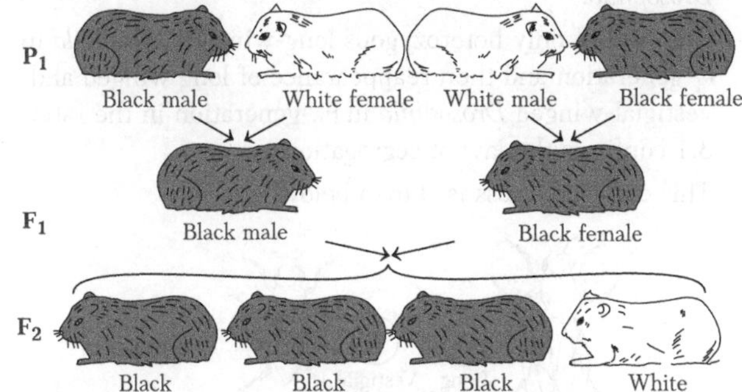

Fig. 6.2 A cross between black and white Guinea pigs

The dominant and recessive traits in some other animals are as follows

1. **Cat**	(a) Coat colour	- Tabby colour coat is dominant over black or blue colour coat.
	(b) Length of hair	- Short hairs are dominant over long hairs (Angora).
2. **Cattle**	(a) Colour of face	- White face colour is dominant over coloured face.
	(b) Horn	- Polled or hornless are dominant over horned cattle.
3. **Dog**	(a) Coat colour	- Grey colour is dominant over black colour.
	(b) Tail	- Stumpy tail is dominant over normal tail.
4. ***Drosophila***	(a) Eye colour	- Red colour is dominant over white.
	(b) Wings	- Flat and yellow wings are dominant over curled and white.
	(c) Body colour	- Grey body colour is dominant over white.
5. **Salamander**	Dark body colour	- Dark body colour is dominant over light.

Dominant and recessive characters in humans are as follows

Normal	Abnormal
Curly hairs are dominant over straight ones.	Absence of body hairs is dominant over their presence.
Dark hairs are dominant over light ones.	Presence of short, webbed and extra digits is dominant over normal ones.
Dark skin colour is dominant over light one.	Free ear lobes are dominant over attached ear lobes.
Normal (brown or pigmented) skin is dominant over skin without pigment.	Presence of glaucoma is dominant over its absence.
Brown iris (eye) colour is dominant over blue colour.	Taste bitter to PTC is dominant over tasteless to PTC.

Deviation from law of dominance

The law of dominance is not applicable universally. After Mendel, several cases were recorded by scientists where a clear cut deviation from law of dominance was seen. These are discussed below

(i) Incomplete dominance (1 : 2 : 1)

When F_1 hybrids exhibit a mixture or blending of characters of two parents, the case is considered as incomplete or blending inheritance. It simply means that the two genes of allelomorphic pair are not related as dominant or recessive, but each of them express itself partially. For example,

(a) Inheritance of flower colour in the 4 O' clock plant (*Mirabilis jalapa*) and snapdragon (*Antirrhinum majus*). When plants with red flower (homozygous RR) are crossed with plants having white flower (homozygous rr), the heterozygous F_1 hybrid (Rr) bear pink flowers. When these pink flowers are self-pollinated, they develop red (RR), pink (Rr) and white (rr) flowers in the ratio 1:2:1, respectively. The cross is shown below

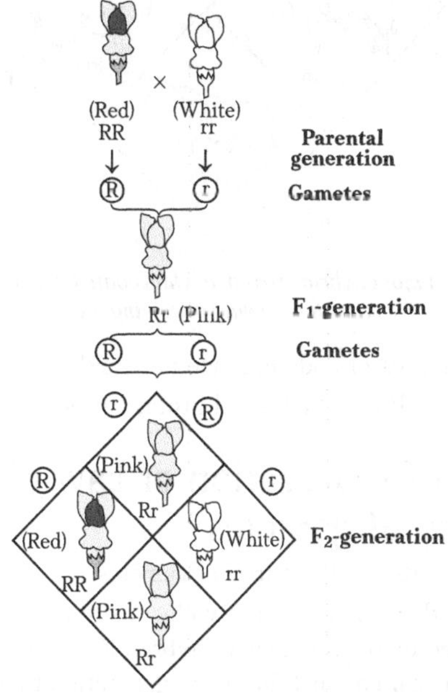

Fig. 6.3 The inheritance of flower colour in the snapdragon

(b) In case of animals, when a homozygous fowl with black feathers is crossed with a homozygous fowl having splashed white feathers, the F_1 hybrids are found to contain blue feathers.

(ii) Codominance (1 : 2 : 1)

Here, both alleles of a pair express themselves fully in F_1 hybrid. It is contrary to the situation seen in incomplete dominance, where traits express themselves only partially.

Coat colour in cattle is an example of codominance. When a cattle with red coat is crossed with the cattle having white coat, the F_1 hybrid possesses roan appearance. In roan appearance, the red and white hair occur in patches, but no hair have intermediate colour of red and white. The ratio of codominance is **1:2:1**. The cross is shown below

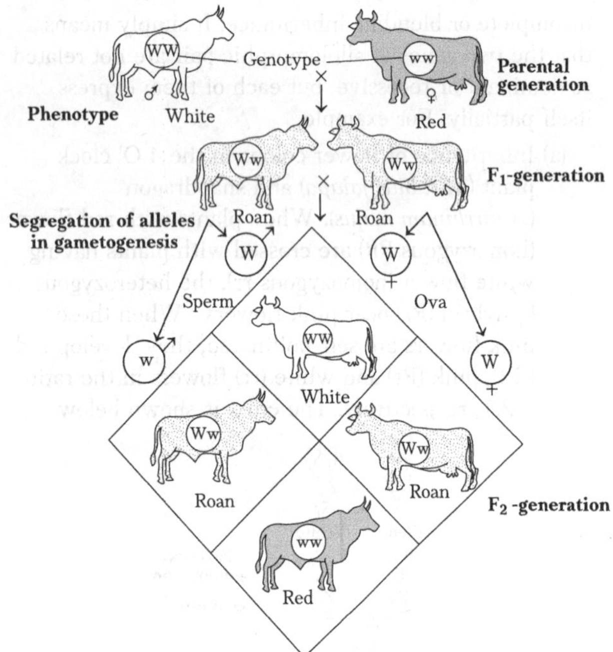

Fig. 6.4 A monohybrid cross in a white coated and a red coated cattle showing codominance

Other examples of codominance are sickle-cell anaemia (Hb^A Hb^S), AB and MN blood group antigens in human.

2. Law of segregation or Law of purity of gametes

- This law ensures the purity of gametes.
- It is based on the fact that two factors of a character do not get mixed up (blending) in F_1 hybrid. Rather both the traits are seen again as such in the F_2-generation though one of these was not seen at the F_1-generation.
- Actually, during gamete or spore formation, traits of a pair separate or segregate from each other, so that a gamete carries only one trait of a character. It means gametes are always pure for a particular trait.
- This law is universally applicable.
- In plants, this law can be explained by Mendel's monohybrid cross, taking tall and dwarf plants as two contrasting traits.
- In animals, this law was experimentally proved by TH Morgan in *Drosophila.*
- Morgan crossed a long winged dominant homozygous *Drosophila* with a vestigial-winged recessive homozygous *Drosophila.*
- Presence of only heterozygous long-winged *Drosophila* in F_1-generation and then reappearance of long winged and vestigial-winged *Drosophila* in F_2-generation in the ratio 3:1 confirms the law of segregation.
- This complete cross is shown below

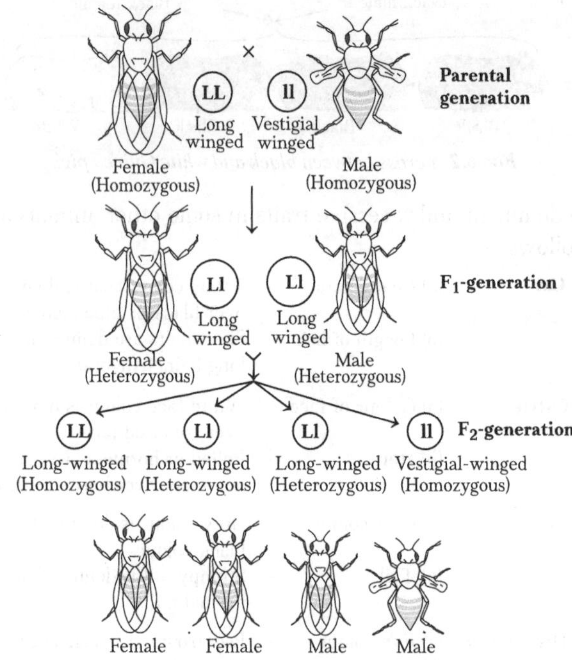

Fig. 6.5 Cross between long-winged and vestigial-winged Drosophila

Dihybrid cross

- When two or more than two characters are taken into consideration within a cross, it is called as **polyhybrid cross**, e.g. dihybrid cross, trihybrid cross, etc. A **dihybrid cross** is a cross involving two pairs of contrasting characters.
- For examples, when a cross is made between plants having yellow round and wrinkled green seeds (both pureline homozygous), only yellow round seeds are seen in F_1-generation.
- In F_2-generation, four types of combinations are observed. Two of these combinations are similar to the parental combinations and other two are new combinations. These are **round green** and **wrinkled yellow**.
- The ratio of four combinations in F_2-generation comes out to be 9 (round, yellow) : 3 (round, green) : 3 (wrinkled, yellow) : 1 (wrinkled, green).

- This ratio is called **phenotypic dihybrid ratio.** The phenotypic ratio of **dihybrid test cross** is 1:1:1:1. The cross can be seen as shown in the figure below

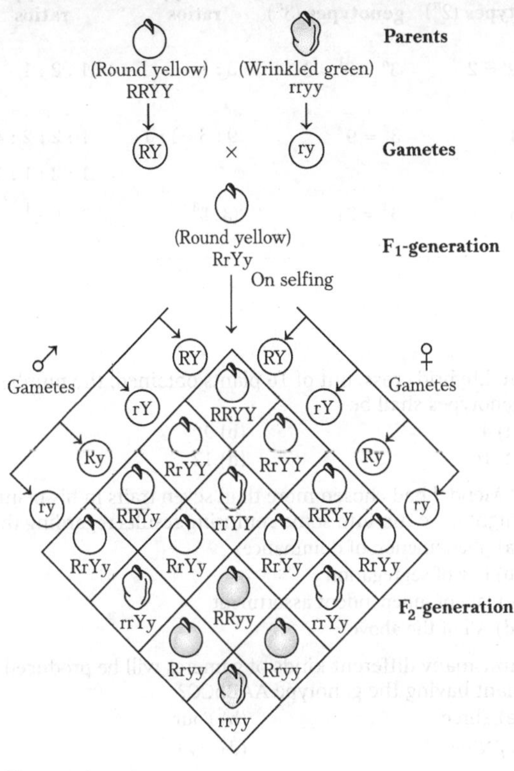

Phenotypic ratio

Round yellow : Round green : Wrinkled yellow : Wrinkled green
9 : 3 : 3 : 1

Genotypic ratio

1 : 2 : 2 : 4 : 1 : 2 : 1 : 2 : 1

***Fig 6.6** Dihybrid cross between the two parents differed in two pairs of contrasting traits, i.e. seed colour and shape*

3. Law of independent assortment

- This law states that when two pairs of traits are combined in a hybrid, segregation of one pair of trait is independent of the other pair of trait.
- For example, in the above dihybrid cross, the presence of new combinations, i.e. round-green and wrinkled-yellow suggests that the genes for shape of seed and colour of seed are assorted independently.
- The results (9:3:3:1) indicate that yellow and green seeds appear in the ratio of 9+3:3+1=3:1.
- Similarly, the round and wrinkled seeds appear in the ratio of 9+3:3+1=3:1.
- This indicates that each of the two pairs of alternative characters, i.e. yellow-green seed colour is inherited independent of the round-wrinkled characters of the seed. This could be possible only when at the time of gamete formation, the factor (gene) for yellow colour entered the gametes independent of the factor of shape of seed.

Condition for independent assortment

- Law of independent assortment was, in fact, an effort of Mendel to find out how different characters would behave in relation to each other during inheritance.
- This law fails to have a universal applicability. Cytological studies have revealed that only those factors or genes assort independently during meiosis, which are located on different homologous pair of chromosomes. But if the genes of different character occupy different locus on same homologous pair, they will pass to the same gamete. Thus, law of independent assortment does not apply to such cases.

Trihybrid inheritance (Trihybrid cross)

- It is the cross involving three pairs of contrasting characters in it. When a cross is made between pea plants having tall stem, yellow seed colour with round seeds (TTYYRR) and short stem, green seed colour with wrinkled seeds (ttyyrr), all F_1 hybrids are tall with yellow, round seeds (TtYyRr). These are called trihybrids.
- On selfing the trihybrids, F_2 phenotypic ratio is 27 : 9 : 9 : 9 : 3 : 3 : 3 : 1. The ratio for a trihybrid test cross is 1 : 1 : 1 : 1 : 1 : 1 : 1 : 1.

Fork line method

Gamete formation for polyhybrid cross (trihybrid onwards) can be easily done with the help of fork line method as shown below, e.g. gamete formation for the trihybrid cross can be worked in following way

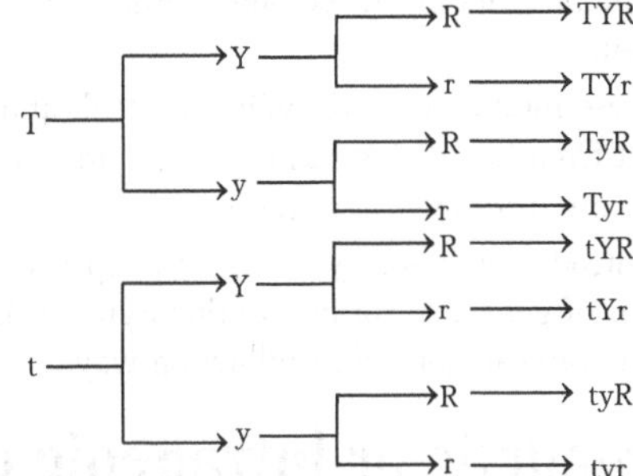

Table 6.2 Summarised account of Mendel's experiments

Numbers of traits hybrid (n)	Experiments	Types of gametes (2^n)	Numbers of zygotes/offsprings (gametes)	Numbers of phenotypes (2^n)	Numbers of genotypes (3^n)	Phenotypic ratios	Genotypic ratios
1.	Monohybrid cross (Aa × Aa)	$2^n = 2^1 = 2$	$2^2 = 4$	$2^n = 2^1 = 2$	$3^n = 3^1 = 3$	3 : 1	1 : 2 : 1
2.	Dihybrid cross (AaBb × AaBb)	$2^2 = 4$	$4^2 = 16$	$2^2 = 4$	$3^2 = 9$	9 : 3 : 3 : 1	1 : 2 : 2 : 4 : 2 1 : 2 : 1 : 1
3.	Trihybrid cross AaBbCc × AaBbCc	$2^3 = 8$	$8^2 = 64$	$2^3 = 8$	$3^3 = 27$	$(3:1)^3$	$(1:2:1)^3$

CHECK POINT 6.2

1. In Mendel's experiment, nature of seed coat, flower colour, position of flower, pod colour, stem height, etc., are referred to as
(a) alleles (b) genotypes
(c) phenotypes (d) characters

2. Percentage of heterozygous individuals obtained from selfing of any Rr individuals is
(a) 100% (b) 75% (c) 50% (d) 25%

3. The proportion of the plants that Mendel found on self-pollination of F_1 plants, was
(a) 1/4th tall and 3/4th dwarf
(b) 1/4th dwarf and 3/4th tall
(c) 1/4th dwarf, 1/2nd hybrid and 1/4th tall
(d) 1/2nd dwarf, 1/2nd hybrid and 1/4th tall

4. In dihybrid cross, out of 16 plants obtained, the number of genotypes shall be
(a) 4 (b) 9
(c) 16 (d) 12

5. If Mendel had chosen more than seven traits in his plants, he might have run into some confusing results regarding the
(a) phenomenon of dominance
(b) law of segregation
(c) law of independent assortment
(d) All of the above

6. How many different kinds of gametes will be produced by a plant having the genotype AABbCC?
(a) Three (b) Four
(c) Nine (d) Two

POST-MENDELIAN INHERITANCE (GENE INTERACTIONS)

- Genes usually function or express themselves singly or individually. But many cases were seen by geneticists where two genes of the same allelic pair or genes of two or more different allelic pairs influence one another. This is called **gene interaction.**
- Each of these interactions are typical in itself and ratio obtained is different from Mendelian ratios, i.e. 3:1 for monohybrid, 9:3:3:1 for dihybrid in F_2-generation.
- **Bateson** introduced factor hypothesis to explain these interactions of genes. According to this hypothesis, these interactions can categorised in following ways

1. Inter-allelic or Intragenic gene interactions

- These are genetic interactions between the alleles of a single gene.
- Under inter-allelic gene interaction, we study the cases of incomplete dominance, codominance, multiple allelism and pleiotropic genes.
- Out of these, incomplete dominance and codominance have already been discussed.

Multiple allelism

- When multiple forms of a gene occupy the same gene locus in a given pair of homologous chromosomes, they are said to constitute a series of multiple alleles.
- A classical example of multiple alleles is found in the ABO blood group system of humans.
- Inheritance of A, B, AB and O blood types in man was discovered by the German mathematician **Felix Bernstein** in 1925.
- Other examples of multiple alleles are coat colour in *Drosophila* and self-incompatibility in tobacco. We will study more about multiple allelism in next chapter.

Pleiotropic gene (Lethal genes)

- The term 'pleiotropy' is derived from the Greek words *Pleio*-many and *tropic*-affecting.
- Thus, a pleiotropic gene is the single gene which produces many or multiple unrelated phenotypes.

- A good example of pleiotropic genes are lethal genes. These genes are known to control the manifestation of some phenotypic trait along with affecting the viability of organism.
- Lethal gene may be dominant, partial dominant or recessive. The monohybrid ratio of lethal gene is 3:0 or 2:1.
- Examples of dominant lethals include
  - yellow lethal in mice
  - creeper lethal in chickens
  - bulldog calves in cattle
  - Sickle-cell anaemia in man.

The recessive lethals are expressed only when they are in homozygous state and their examples include

- Tay Sach's lethals in man
- hydrocephaly in mouse

2. Non-allelic or Intergenic gene interactions

These are the interactions between genes located at different loci on the same or on different chromosomes for controlling a single phenotype to produce a different expression. These interactions have following specific phenomena.

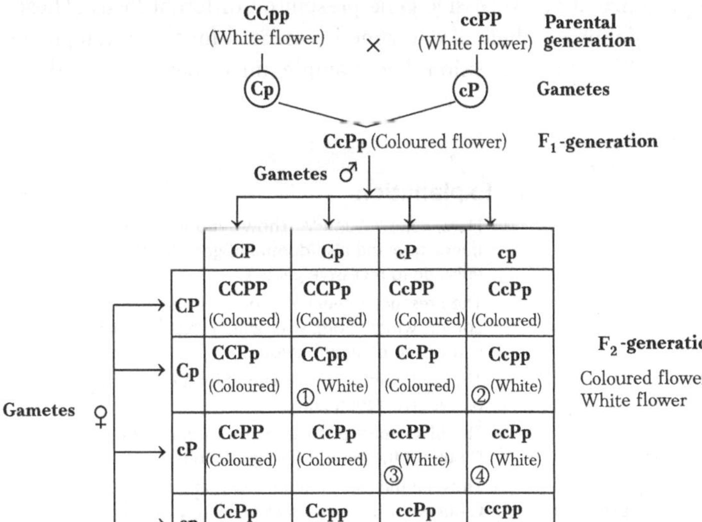

Fig. 6.7 The results of an experiment to show the operation of complementary genes in the production of flower colour in sweet pea (Lathyrus)

Epistasis

In this interaction, one gene complement, masks, inhibits or suppresses the expression of the other gene. Here, the gene that produces the effect on the other gene is called **epistatic gene.** Whereas the gene whose expression is suppressed is called **hypostatic gene/ masked gene.**

Following types of epistasis are reported so far

(i) **Complementary genes** (9 : 7) These are two pairs of non-allelic dominant genes, which interact to produce only one phenotypic trait, but neither of them if present alone produces the trait in the absence of other. For the development of dominant character, the presence of both of the genes is necessary.

For example, the flower colour in *Lathyrus odoratus*, i.e. sweet pea. In this, the two non-allelic complementary genes C and P are required to synthesise anthocyanin pigment responsible for the production of coloured flowers. This phenomenon was first seen by **Bateson.**

The inheritance of both the genes is shown in the cross given below

Explanation

- Actually, gene C produces an enzyme that catalyses the formation of colourless chromogen for the **formation of anthocyanin** pigment.
- The gene P, on the other hand, controls the formation of another enzyme, which catalyses the transformation of chromogen into anthocyanin.
- Thus, both the genes are **complementary**. It only one of them is present, the result is colourless or white flowers.
- In the cross, the ratio **9 : 7** is called the **complementary ratio.**
- Another examples of complementary genes include maize, where purple colour of flower depends upon three dominant genes for its appearance, i.e. A, C and R. Absence of any of these produces white seeds.
- In man, **deaf mutism** is complementary gene dependent. It depends upon two dominant genes, i.e. A and B. The presence of both of them is responsible for normal hearing and speech.

(ii) **Dominant epistasis or Inhibiting genes** (12 : 3 : 1) When a dominant gene does not allow the expression of other non-allelic gene, it is called dominant epistasis, e.g. inheritance of coat colour in dogs.

Their inheritance is shown in the cross given below

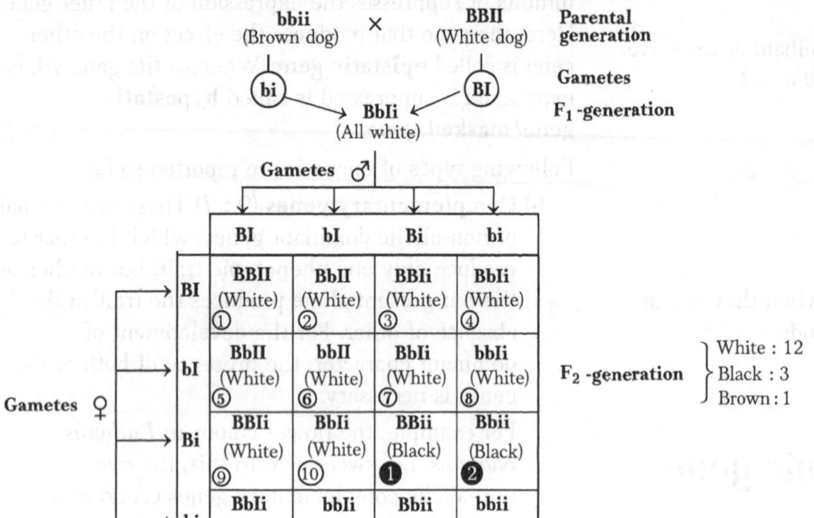

Fig. 6.8 Interaction of inhibiting genes in dog for coat colour showing dominant epistasis

Explanation

- In dogs, white coat colour appears to be dominant. It develops due to a gene I, which prevents the formation of pigment responsible for colour of coat. The hypostatic gene B produces black coat, while its counterpart b produces brown colour only when gene I is homozygous recessive.
- Thus all those cases, where I is present, are white in colour. Similarly, all those cases with at least one B but absence of I are black, while the case in which both B and I are absent produces brown individual.
- The dominant epistasis ratio is 12 : 3 : 1.
- Another example of dominant epistasis is fruit colour in *Cucurbita pepo*.

(iii) **Recessive epistasis or Supplementary gene** (9 : 3 : 4) It is seen when out of the two pairs of genes, the recessive epistatic gene masks the activity of dominant gene on the other gene locus. In other words, we can say that a dominant gene expresses itself only in the presence of one recessive gene present on different locus. These are also called supplementary genes because here the dominant allele of one gene is essential for the development of the concerned phenotype, while the other gene modifies the expression. For example, mice coat colour with agouti (greyish), black and white varieties.

The inheritance of mice coat colour is shown below

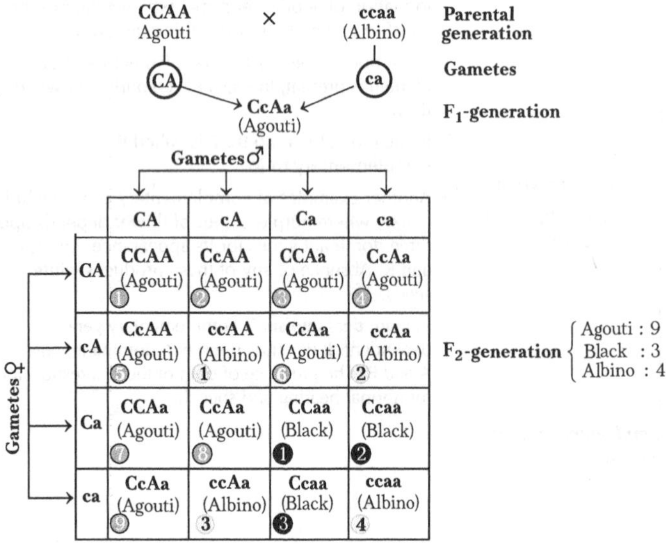

Fig. 6.9 Interaction of supplementary genes in mice for coat colour

Explanation

- Here, gene 'C' and 'A' show supplementary interaction and also dominant gene 'A' is epistatic to recessive gene 'C'.
- The presence of gene C produces black colour, which along with gene A results in the expression of agouti colour.
- Thus, all combinations with at least one C and one A give agouti colour.
- The black mice possess factor for black colour C but not the gene A for agouti colour.
- Thus, all the combinations with at least one C but without A produces black individuals.
- If gene for black colour is absent, agouti is unable to express itself, hence, albinos are seen.
- Thus in all combinations, where C is absent in the presence or absence of A, the individuals are albinos.
- The ratio of this interaction is **9 : 3 : 4**.

(iv) **Duplicate genes** (15 : 1) In this interaction, dominant alleles of two gene loci produce same or nearly same phenotype whether inherited together or separately. Hence, either of the gene is able to produce the character. For example, fruit shape in Shepherd's purse (*Capsella bursa pastoris*). Their inheritance is shown in the cross given below

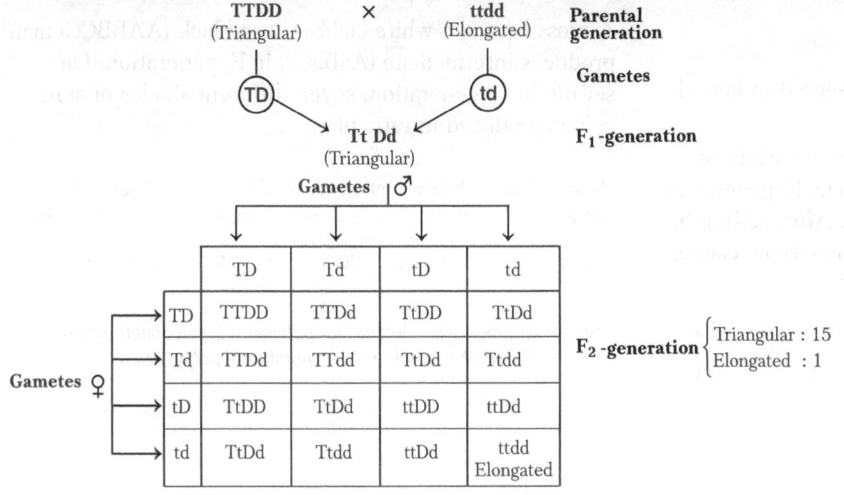

	TD	Td	tD	td
TD	TTDD	TTDd	TtDD	TtDd
Td	TTDd	TTdd	TtDd	Ttdd
tD	TtDD	TtDd	ttDD	ttDd
td	TtDd	Ttdd	ttDd	ttdd Elongated

Fig. 6.10 Interaction of duplicating genes in Shepherd's purse for seed pods

Explanation

- This inheritance was studied by **Shull**, who found two types of seed capsule in plant
  (a) Triangular
  (b) Elongated or Top-shaped
- It is clear from the cross itself that the triangular shape is the dominant factor and both of the genes either present singly or collectively produce this dominant trait.
- Out of 16 individual of F_2-generation, this trait is not seen in one individual only, which is homozygous recessive for both the genes. The duplicate genes are also called **pseudoalleles**.
- Its ratio of this interaction is 15 : 1.

(v) **Collaborator genes** (9 : 3 : 3 : 1) These are two gene pairs present on separate locus but interact to produce a totally new trait or phenotype that neither of the genes alone could produce. For example, inheritance of combs in poultry. Inheritance of collaborator genes is shown in the cross given below

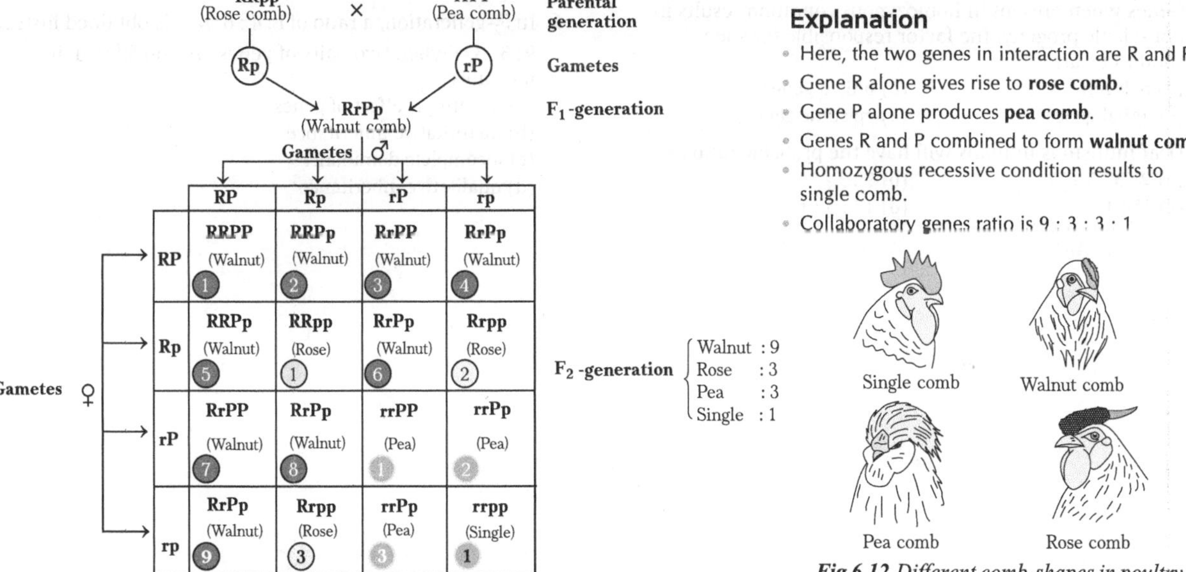

	RP	Rp	rP	rp
RP	RRPP (Walnut) 1	RRPp (Walnut) 2	RrPP (Walnut) 3	RrPp (Walnut) 4
Rp	RRPp (Walnut) 5	RRpp (Rose) 1	RrPp (Walnut) 6	Rrpp (Rose) 2
rP	RrPP (Walnut) 7	RrPp (Walnut) 8	rrPP (Pea) 1	rrPp (Pea) 2
rp	RrPp (Walnut) 9	Rrpp (Rose) 3	rrPp (Pea) 3	rrpp (Single) 1

Fig. 6.11 Inheritance of rose and pea comb in poultry

Explanation

- Here, the two genes in interaction are R and P.
- Gene R alone gives rise to **rose comb.**
- Gene P alone produces **pea comb.**
- Genes R and P combined to form **walnut comb.**
- Homozygous recessive condition results to single comb.
- Collaboratory genes ratio is 9 : 3 : 3 : 1

Fig 6.12 Different comb-shapes in poultry

Polygenic inheritance

- It is also called **quantitative inheritance.**
- In this inheritance, the trait is controlled by one or more genes, where the dominant alleles give cumulative effect. Thus, each dominant allele expresses a part or unit of a trait. The full trait being shown only when all the dominant alleles are present.

The genes responsible for polygenic inheritance are called **polygenes** or **multiple** or **cumulative genes,** e.g. skin colour in human, kernel colour in wheat, corolla length in tobacco, etc.

Examples with Ratio

(i) Polygenic inheritance was first observed in kernel colour of wheat.

H. Nilsson Ehle crossed red kerneled variety of wheat with white kernel variety. The F_1-generation had intermediate coloured kernels. After selfing in the F_2-generation, five different phenotypic classes were appeared in the ratio of

Extreme red	:	Deep red	:	Intermediate red	:	Light red	:	White
1	:	4	:	6	:	4	:	1

(ii) Similarly in human, skin colour is determined by three pairs of genes. These genes present on different loci. Each of the dominant gene is responsible for human skin colour.

A cross between white (aabbcc) and black (AABBCC) man produces intermediate (AaBbCc) in F_1-generation. On selfing in F_2-generation, seven different shades of skin colour produced in ratio of

Very dark	:	Dark	:	Fairly dark	:	Intermediate	:	Fairly light	:	Light	:	Very light
1	:	6	:	15	:	20	:	15	:	6	:	1

Note *Number of phenotypes for polygenes is calculated by the formula 2n + 1 where 'n' is number of polygenes.*

CHECK POINT 6.3

1. Sometimes, there are more than two alleles for a given chromosome locus, in this case, a trait is controlled by
(a) codominance
(b) pseudodominance
(c) incomplete dominance
(d) multiple alleles

2. Genes when present in homozygous condition results in non-viable progeny, the factor responsible for such conditions are
(a) polygenes (b) linked genes
(c) lethal genes (d) epistatic genes

3. Deaf mutism is humans will have the probable ratio as
(a) 9 : 3 : 3 1 (b) 9 : 7
(c) 15 : 1 (d) 12 : 3 : 1

4. The dihybrid ratio 9:3:4 comes in case/s of
(a) recessive epistasis (b) supplementary gene ratio
(c) Both (a) and (b) (d) dominant epistasis

5. The ratio 15 : 1 comes for
(a) multiple alleles (b) codominant alleles
(c) pseudoalleles (d) None of these

6. In F_2-generation, a ratio of 1 : 4 : 6 : 4 : 1 is obtained instead of 9 : 3 : 3 : 1 when two pairs of genes are considered, it indicates
(a) pleiotropic effect of genes
(b) quantitative inheritance
(c) incomplete dominance
(d) qualitative inheritance

EXAM POINTS

- The number of contrasting characters studied by Mendel for his experiments was seven. **[NEET 2020]**
- The period of Mendel's hybridisation experiments is 1856-1863, i.e. 7 years. **[NEET 2017]**
- Mendel selected 14 true-breeding pea plant varieties in pairs, which were similar except for one character with contrasting traits. **[NEET 2020]**
- A true breeding plant is homozygous and produces offspring of its own kind. **[NEET 2016]**
- Mendel called the genes by the term factors. **[AMU 2015]**
- Alleles are different molecular forms of a gene. **[CBSE AIPMT 2015]**
- Dominance is seen in a heterozygous organism only one allele expresses itself. **[NEET 2016]**
- If a genotype consists of different alleles, it is heterozygous. **[AMU 2015]**
- Punnett square was developed by a British scientist. **[NEET 2018]**
- Punnett square is the graphical representation to calculate possible genotype of offspring. **[Kerala CEE 2014]**
- Reciprocal cross yields identical result. It means, sex has no influence on the dominance of traits. **[KCET 2013]**
- Aa × aa is a type of test cross. **[WB JEE 2011]**
- In a test cross, F_1 is crossed with homozygous recessive parent. **[UP CPMT 2013]**
- The production of gametes by the parents, the formation of zygotes, the F_1 and F_2 plants can be understood using Punnett square. **[NEET 2019]**
- The number of gametes are calculated by the formula 2^n, where n = number of heterozygotes. **[WB JEE 2015]**
- Inheritance in snapdragon (*Antirrhinum*) plant is incomplete dominance. **[NEET 2019]**
- Codominance means both alleles express equally. **[NEET 2016, AIIMS 2019]**
- MN blood group shows codominance. **[BCECE 2012]**
- In codominance, both alleles of a gene have the ability to express independently in heterozygotes. **[CBSE AIPMT 2015]**
- In codominance, F_1-generation resembles both parents. **[NEET 2013]**
- ABO blood grouping shows codominance. **[NEET 2018]**
- Inheritance of blood groups in human shows dominance, codominance and multiple allele. **[NEET 2018]**
- Multiple allelism observed in ABO blood group. **[Kerala CEE 2014]**
- ABO blood grouping is inherited by single gene with more than two alleles. **[WB JEE 2015]**
- I^A and I^B alleles of ABO blood group gene, I produces sugar but third allele, I^C does not produce any sugar. **[KCET 2015]**
- A person will have only two of the three alleles of ABO blood groups, i.e. I^A, I^B and I^0. **[NEET 2020]**
- Pleiotropy is when a single gene influence many characters. **[NEET 2016]**
- Pleiotropic gene is one gene which shows multiple phenotypic expression. **[AIIMS 2019]**
- The best example for pleiotropy is phenylketonuria. **[NEET 2020]**
- Fruit colour in squash is an example of dominant epistasis. **[CBSE AIPMT 2014]**
- Epistasis is non-allelic gene inheritance. **[AIIMS 2019]**
- In polygenic inheritance, many genes govern a single character. **[NEET 2016]**
- Skin colour in man is example of polygenic inheritance. **[EAMCET 2014]**

Chapter Exercises

(A) Topical Exercise

Pre-Mendelian and Mendelian Inheritance

1 Genetics is
(a) genes + alleles (b) heredity + variation
(c) DNA + RNA (d) dominant + recessive

2 The term genetics was given by
(a) Bateson (b) Morgan
(c) Mendel (d) Johansan

3 Which of the following does not come under transmission genetics?
(a) Molecular genetics (b) Mendelian genetics
(c) Morganian genetics (d) Non-Mendelian genetics

4 The miniature form of individuals discussed in preformation theory are
(a) sperms (b) pangenes
(c) homunculus (d) gemmules

5 The work of Mendel was published in 1866 before the Natural Science Society of Brunn in a paper named
(a) hybridisation on pea plant
(b) inheritance pattern in pea plant
(c) experiments on plant hybridisation
(d) Mendelian experiments on pea plant

6 Mendel was the first biologist
(a) to study the mechanism of inheritance
(b) to discover that chromosomes are responsible for inheritance
(c) to use statistical methods in analysing his results
(d) All of the above

7 How did Mendel's studies in genetics differ from earlier studies of breeding and inheritance?
(a) Mendel worked with plants; earlier studies used animals
(b) Mendel was able to explain the 'blending' hypothesis
(c) Mendel's work was more quantitative
(d) Mendel worked with wild species, not the domesticated ones

8 In 1900 AD, three biologists independently discovered Mendel's principles. They are
(a) de Vries, Correns and Tschermak
(b) Sutton, Morgan and Bridges
(c) Avery, McLeod and McCarty
(d) Bateson, Punnett and Bridges

9 One reason for Mendel's success was that he
(a) repeated his experiments many times
(b) used carefully controlled experiments
(c) used plants with easily observable traits
(d) All of the above

10 Mendel started his experiments with pure strains of peas. A pure strain was developed by removing all
(a) ovules (b) anthers
(c) stigma (d) weak plants

11 Why was Mendel fairly certain that he had a pure-bred variety when he collected seeds from a pea plant?
(a) The flower is self-pollinating in these plants
(b) Peas bear a large number of offspring
(c) Because the varieties are so distinctive
(d) He maintained extremely accurate records

12 Who coined the term gene
(a) Johannsen (b) Bateson
(c) Morgan (d) Correns

13 When a gene pair contains two different genes controlling different traits of a character, it is
(a) homozygous (b) heterozygous
(c) monozygous (d) None of these

14 An organism with two copies of the same allele is
(a) homozygous for that trait
(b) homologous for the allele
(c) heterozygous for that trait
(d) heterologous for the allele

15 Phenotype is
(a) the genetic makeup of an individual
(b) the same for parent and offspring
(c) the account of physiological activities
(d) the appearance of an individual

16 A wild type is
(a) the phenotype found most commonly in nature
(b) the dominant allele
(c) designated by a small letter if it is recessive or a capital letter if it is dominant
(d) All of the above

17 When a monohybrid is crossed with a recessive parent, the cross is described as a
(a) test cross (b) monohybrid cross
(c) dihybrid cross (d) None of these

18 The graphical representation to calculate the probability of all possible genotypes of offspring in a genetic cross is called
(a) pedigree analysis (b) karyotype
(c) Punnett square (d) chromosome map

Mendel's Hybridisation Experiments

19 A true breeding line is one that
(a) having undergone continuous self-pollination
(b) shows the stable trait inheritance
(c) shows expression for several generation
(d) All of the above

20 Which statement describes the work of Gregor Mendel?
(a) He developed some basic principles of heredity without having knowledge of chromosomes
(b) He developed the microscope for the study of genes in pea plants
(c) He explained the principle of dominance on the basis of the gene chromosome theory
(d) He used his knowledge of gene mutations to explain the appearance of new traits in organisms

21 Mendel studied seven contrasting characters for his breeding experiments with *Pisum sativum*, which one of the following characters he did not use?
(a) Pod shape (b) Leaf shape
(c) Plant height (d) Pod colour

22 Genes controlling the seven pea characters studied by Mendel are now known to be located on how many different chromosomes?
(a) Five (b) Four (c) Seven (d) Six

23 Mendel's law is still true because it takes place in
(a) sexually reproducing plants
(b) asexually reproducing plants
(c) Both (a) and (b)
(d) apomictic reproducing plants

24 What phenotypes are possible from the cross, between round seeded plant and wrinkled seeded plants if both the parents are homozygous?
(a) All round
(b) Round and wrinkled
(c) All wrinkled
(d) Slightly wrinkled

25 What would be the parent's genotypes if both were heterozygous for flower colour (purple-W, white-w)?
(a) ww and ww
(b) Ww and Ww
(c) WW and WW
(d) WW and ww

26 In a monohybrid cross, when F_1 is crossed with homozygous dominant parent then which type of offsprings will obtain?
(a) Dominant : Recessive, 3 : 1
(b) Only recessive
(c) Dominant : Recessive, 1 : 1
(d) No recessive

27 When looking at the inheritance of a single characteristic, Mendel found that a cross between two true breeding peas (between purple and white, for example) always yielded a .... in the F_2-generation.
(a) 1 : 1 phenotypic ratio
(b) 3 : 1 genotypic ratio
(c) 1 : 2 : 1 phenotypic ratio
(d) 3 : 1 phenotypic ratio

28 If an organism with the genotype Ww is crossed with a Ww organism, what would be the proportion of offsprings that would be heterozygous?
(a) 1/4 (b) 1/2
(c) 3/4 (d) All would be heterozygous

29 In addition to pea, Mendel had carried out hybridisation experiments in another plant also, where he could not establish the findings he had previously obtained on pea plants. This plant was
(a) bean (b) maize
(c) *Hieracium* (d) None of these

30 Which of the following statements is/are correct for Mendel's law of dominance?
(a) Characters are controlled by factors
(b) Factors occur in pairs
(c) In a dissimilar pair of factors, one member of the pair dominates the other
(d) All of the above

31 The law of dominance is used to explain
(a) the expression of only one of the parental characters in a monohybrid cross in the F_1
(b) the expression of both the parental characters in a monohybrid cross in the F_2
(c) the proportion of 3 : 1 obtained at the F_2
(d) All of the above

32 Which of the following statements is correct, when we use alphabetical symbols for each gene?
(a) Capital letter is used for the trait expressed at the F_1 stage and small alphabet for the other trait
(b) Small letter is used for the trait expressed at the F_1 stage and capital alphabet for the other trait
(c) Both capital and small letters are used for the both F_1 stage and other
(d) Either (a) or (b)

33 When a particular characteristic of an individual, e.g. petal colour, shows variation among the offspring produced after the individual is selfed, it is said to be

(a) pure-breeding (b) true-breeding
(c) homozygous (d) heterozygous

34 When two individuals, heterozygous for the same genes, are bred together, they produce

(a) only dominant phenotypes, all of the same genotypes
(b) only recessive phenotypes
(c) only dominant phenotypes of different genotypes
(d) both recessive and dominant phenotypes. The latter being of two genotypes

35 A 1 : 1 phenotypic ratio in a test cross indicates that

(a) the alleles are dominant
(b) one parent must have been homozygous recessive
(c) the dominant phenotype parent was a heterozygote
(d) the alleles segregated independently

36 How many different kinds of female gametes are produced by the F_1 offsprings from a cross between a pure strain of plants with yellow peas and a pure strain of plants with green peas?

(a) One (b) Two (c) Four (d) Eight

37 If a cross is made between AA and aa, the nature of F_1 progeny will be

(a) genotypically AA, phenotypically a
(b) genotypically Aa, phenotypically a
(c) genotypically Aa, phenotypically A
(d) genotypically aa, phenotypically A

38 In squirrels, the gene for grey fur (G) is dominant over the gene for black fur (g). If 50% of a large litter of squirrels are grey, the parental cross that produced this litter was most likely

(a) GG × Gg (b) Gg × gg (c) GG × GG (d) gg × gg

39 In a certain species of mouse, grey fur (G) is dominant over cream-coloured fur (g). If a homozygous grey mouse is crossed with a cream-coloured mouse, the genotype of the F_1-generation will most likely be

(a) 100% Gg
(b) 25% GG, 50% Gg and 25% gg
(c) 50% GG and 50% gg
(d) 75% Gg and 25% gg

40 The F_2-generation of a cross

(a) has a phenotypic ratio of 3 : 1
(b) is the result of the self-fertilisation or crossing of F_1 individuals
(c) can be used to determine the genotype of individuals with the dominant phenotype
(d) has a phenotypic ratio that equals its genotypic ratio

41 The crossing of a homozygous tall plant with a dwarf in F_2 would yield plants in the ratio of

(a) all homozygous dwarf
(b) all heterozygous tall
(c) one homozygous tall, one homozygous dwarf and two heterozygous tall
(d) two tall and two dwarf

42 Mendel crossed a pure white-flowered recessive pea plant with a dominant pure red-flowered plant. The first generation of hybrids from the cross should show

(a) 50% white-flowered plants and 50% red-flowered plants
(b) all red-flowered plants
(c) 75% red-flowered plants and 25% white-flowered plants
(d) all white-flowered plants

43 Choose the incorrect pair regarding the dominant characters in given organisms.

	Organisms		Dominant characters
(a)	Salamander	–	Dark body colour
(b)	Cat	–	Angora hair
(c)	Human	–	Curly hair
(d)	None of the above		

44 An embryo resulting from the mating of two albino rabbits is transplanted into the uterus of a brown rabbit. The phenotype of this transplant will most probably be

(a) all brown
(b) all white
(c) brown with white spots
(d) white with brown spots

45 If heterozygous round seeded pea plants are self-pollinated, the offsprings will be

(a) 75% round (b) 50% heterozygous
(c) 25% wrinkled (d) All of these

46 A cross between two tall plants resulted in offspring having few dwarf plants. What would be the genotype of both the parents? **[NCERT Exemplar]**

(a) TT and Tt (b) Tt and Tt
(c) TT and TT (d) Tt and tt

47 Assume that in mice, B = black fur, b = brown fur. If a heterozygous black mouse mates with a homozygous brown mouse, what per cent of their offspring will have black fur?

(a) 25% (b) 50%
(c) 75% (d) 100%

48 When two hybrids are crossed, the percentage of recessive population is

(a) 25% (b) 100%
(c) 50% (d) 75%

49 Choose the incorrect statement.
(a) Tabby colour is dominant over black in cats
(b) Stumpy tail is dominant over normal tail in dogs
(c) Horned cattle is dominant over hornless
(d) None of the above

50 Which of the following pair is incorrect?
(a) Presence of webbed digit in humans – Recessive
(b) Presence of glaucoma in humans – Dominant
(c) Attached ear lobes – Recessive
(d) Brown iris colour – Dominant

51 Which of the following pea plants will always be white flowered?
(a) CcPp (b) CCPP (c) ccPP (d) CCpP

52 The validity of the F_1 hybrid is determined by
(a) breeding together brothers and sisters of the F_1-generation
(b) back crossing one or more of the F_1 individuals
(c) test crossing one or more of the F_1 individuals
(d) producing large progeny

53 Which of the following statement is correct?
(a) Each back cross is a test cross
(b) Each test cross is a back cross
(c) Both tests have the same meaning
(d) Disappearance of similar characters in a test cross is called a back cross

54 Imagine that in a pea plant, the factors for controlling seed coat colour and shape of seeds are present on the same chromosomes are very close together. Performing dihybrid experiments with these characters Mendel would not have been able to arrive at the idea of
(a) independent assortment (b) dominance
(c) incomplete dominance (d) segregation

55 Inheritance of flower colour is an example of incomplete dominance, which is seen in
(a) *Antirrhinum* (b) *Pisum*
(c) *Solanum* (d) *Hibiscus*

56 1 : 2 : 1 phenotypic and genotypic ratio is found in
(a) complementary genes (b) blending inheritance
(c) multiple alleles (d) pseudoalleles

57 In Guinea pigs, black fur (B) is dominant over white fur (b) and rough fur (R) is dominant over smooth fur (r). A cross between two Guinea pigs hybrid for both traits (BbRr × BbRr) produces some offsprings that have rough, black fur and some that have smooth, black fur. The genotypes of these offsprings illustrate the genetic concept of
(a) intermediate inheritance (b) multiple alleles
(c) independent assortment (d) codominance

58 A monohybrid cross between two plants, one having 24 cm long internodes, produces F_1 hybrids all having 18 cm long internodes. This is a case of
(a) recessive dominance (b) multiple allelism
(c) complete dominance (d) incomplete dominance

59 In case of incomplete dominance, F_2-generation has
(a) genotypic ratio equals to phenotypic ratio
(b) genotypic ratio is 3 : 1
(c) phenotypic ratio is 3 : 1
(d) None of the above

60 If fur colour in mice is caused by the following genes : B = black and b = brown, choose the genotype for the organism, which will have brown fur?
(a) BB (b) bB (c) bb (d) Either (a) or (b)

61 *Mirabilis*, a homozygous plant with red flowers, if crossed with another homozygous plant with white flowers, produces pink-flowered progeny.
(a) This is an example of a test cross
(b) It would be expected that the pinks would not breed true
(c) This shows that the genes blend in F_1
(d) This proves that colour has a genetic basis

62 Which one of the following cannot be explained on the basis of Mendel's law of dominance?
(a) The discrete unit controlling a particular character is called a factor
(b) Out of one pair of factors one is dominant and the other is recessive
(c) Alleles do not show any blending and both the characters recover as such in F_2-generation
(d) Factors occur in pairs

63 A brown mouse is mated with a white mouse. All of their offsprings are brown. If two of these brown offsprings are mated, what fraction of their offspring will be white?
(a) 1/4 (b) 1/2
(c) 1/6 (d) None of these

64 The independent assortment of two pairs of genes located on non-homologous chromosomes occur as a result of the random orientation of chromosomes during
(a) telophase of the first meiotic division
(b) the brief interphase between the two meiotic divisions
(c) prophase of the second meiotic division
(d) metaphase of the first meiotic division

65 Person having genotype $I^a I^b$ would show the blood group as AB. This is because of **[NCERT Exemplar]**
(a) pleiotropy (b) codominance
(c) segregation (d) incomplete dominance

66 If red short horn cows are mated with white short horn bulls, the coat of the resulting calves carry both red and white hair, giving a red horn. This is a case of
(a) incomplete dominance
(b) codominance
(c) epistasis
(d) complete dominance

67 Choose the best statement that explains Mendel's law of segregation.
(a) Dominant and recessive traits are transmitted independently from one generation to the next so that neither trait has any influence on the inheritance of the other
(b) Inheritance of one gene is not influenced by the inheritance of another and genes assort independently in successive generations
(c) One allele of a gene is dominant over the other
(d) One gene masks the effect of the other and is not transmitted independently from one generation to another

68 A plant is heterozygous and is designated Bb. It produces two kinds of gametes, B or b. The probability of gamete B fertilising either B or b is
(a) 1/2 (b) 0/2 (c) 1/1 (d) 1/4

69 How many different kinds of gametes can an organism of genotypes A/a; B/B; C/c produce?
(a) 3 (b) 4 (c) 9 (d) 16

70 In Mendel's experiments, there are two alleles of the gene that causes pea shape–R (round) and r (wrinkled) and two alleles of the gene that causes plant height–T (tall) and t (short). How many different kinds of eggs are produced by a short plant with wrinkled peas?
(a) One (b) Two
(c) Four (d) Eight

71 From a single ear of corn, a farmer planted 200 kernels which produced 140 tall and 40 dwarf plants. The genotypes of these offsprings are most likely
(a) TT, Tt and tt (b) TT and tt
(c) TT and Tt (d) tt and tt

72 How many genetically different kinds of gametes will an individual with genotype AAbb produce?
(a) One (b) Two (c) Three (d) Four

73 Which one of the following individuals can produce sixteen different gametes?
(a) Aa, Bb, Cc, Dd
(b) Aa, Bb, cc, DD, Ee, Ff
(c) Aa, Bb, Cc, dd, EE, FF
(d) Aa, Bb, Cc, DD, Ee, Ff

74 A hybrid black coated Guinea pig produces 2 million sperm cells. Approximately, what number of its sperm cells contain the recessive gene for white colour?
(a) 1.0 million (b) 2.0 million
(c) 2.25 million (d) 3.5 million

75 Mendel's principle of segregation was based on the separation of alleles in the garden pea during
(a) pollination (b) embryonic development
(c) seed formation (d) gamete formation

76 When two heterozygous tall plants are crossed, some short plants appear in the offspring. The appearance of these short plants illustrates
(a) segregation and recombination
(b) intermediate inheritance
(c) crossing over and differentiation
(d) codominant inheritance

77 In raccoons, a dark face mask is dominant over a bleached face mask. Several crosses were made between raccoons that were heterozygous for dark face mask and that were homozygous for bleached face mask. What percentage of the offspring would be expected to have a dark face mask?
(a) 0% (b) 50%
(c) 75% (d) 100%

78 In a certain variety of chicken, the genes for black feather colour and the genes for white feather colour are codominant. This variety of chicken will most likely have
(a) three possible phenotypes for feather colour
(b) only two genotypes for feather colour
(c) white feather colour only
(d) black feather colour only

79 Which of the following statements is correct for Mendel's law of independent assortment?
(a) When two pairs of traits are combined in a hybrid, segregation of one pair of characters is independent of the other pair of characters
(b) When two pairs of trait are combined in a hybrid, segregation of one pair of character is dependent of the other pair of characters
(c) When two pairs of trait are segregated, the character of one pair is dependent on the character of the other pair
(d) When two pairs of trait are segregated, the characters of the both pairs are independent

80 In a dihybrid cross, if you get 9 : 3 : 3 : 1 ratio it denotes that **[NCERT Exemplar]**
(a) the alleles of two genes are interacting with each other
(b) it is a multigenic inheritance
(c) it is a case of multiple allelism
(d) the alleles of two genes are segregating independently

81 What will be the result of a cross between TtGG and ttGG?
(a) One TtGG and one ttGG
(b) Three TtGg and one ttgg
(c) Two TtGg, one TTGG and one ttGG
(d) Nine TtGG, three TTGG, three TtGg and one ttgg

82 Genes A and B are necessary for normal hearing. A deaf man marries a deaf woman and all their children have normal hearing. The genotype of the parents are
(a) AAbb and AAbb
(b) Aabb and aaBb
(c) AAbb and aaBB
(d) aaBB and aaBb

83 In the Punnett square given below, the genotype of the female parent (?) must be

		Male gametes			
Female gametes	?	AB	Ab	aB	ab
		AaBB	AaBb	aaBB	aaBb

(a) AaBb (b) aaBB
(c) aaBb (d) AaBB

84 In the F_2 progeny of a dihybrid cross, the expected genotypic proportion of individuals homozygous for both the dominant character will be
(a) 1/16 (b) 3/16
(c) 9/16 (d) 12/16

85 A human male produces sperms with the genotypes AB, Ab, aB and ab pertaining to two diallelic characters in equal proportions. What is the corresponding genotype of this person?
(a) AaBb (b) AaBB
(c) AABb (d) AABB

86 In pea plants, yellow seeds are dominant to green. If a heterozygous yellow seeded plant is crossed with a green seeded plant, what ratio of yellow and green seeded plants would you expect in F_1-generation?
(a) 50 : 50 (b) 9 : 1 (c) 1 : 3 (d) 3 : 1

87 If AAbb × aaBB, then phenotypic ratio of its progeny (F_2-generation) will be
(a) 9 : 3 : 3 : 1 (b) 1 : 2 : 1
(c) 1 : 1 : 1 : 1 (d) 4 : 1

88 When heterozygous red (dominant) flower is crossed with white flower, the ratio of the progeny will be
(a) 350→ red : 350→ white
(b) 450→ red : 250→ white
(c) 380→ red : 320→ white
(d) None of the above

89 A dihybrid test cross-yielding a result of 1:1:1:1 ratio is indicative of
(a) four different types of gametes produced by the F_1-dihybrid
(b) homozygous condition of the F_1-hybrid
(c) four different types of F_1-generation hybrid
(d) four different types of gametes produced by the P_1-parent

90 In order to find out the different types of gametes produced by a pea plant having the genotype AaBb. It should be crossed to a plant with the genotype
(a) aaBB (b) AaBb (c) AABB (d) aabb

91 In the F_2-generation of a Mendelian dihybrid cross, the number of phenotypes and genotypes are
(a) phenotype-4; genotype-16 **[NCERT Exemplar]**
(b) phenotype-9; genotype-4
(c) phenotype-4; genotype-8
(d) phenotype-4; genotype-9

92 In an experiment with homozygous pea plants, the round yellow seeded plants were crossed with the plants producing wrinkled green seeds. What will be the phenotypic ratio of the progeny?
(a) All round yellow
(b) 1 round yellow, 1 round green, 3 wrinkled green
(c) 1 round yellow, 1 round green, 1 wrinkled yellow, 1 wrinkled green
(d) Data are insufficient

93 Two true breeding varieties of garden peas are crossed. One parent had red, axial flowers and the other had white, terminal flowers. All F_1 individuals had red, axial flowers. If 100 F_2 offsprings were counted, how many of them would you expect to have red, axial flowers?
(a) 6 (b) 25 (c) 19 (d) 56

94 If the P or parental generation was pure strain with green peas crossed with a pure strain with yellow peas and their offsprings (the F_1-generation) were self-pollinated, then the F_2-generation would be
(a) all plants with green peas
(b) all plants with yellow peas
(c) half plants with green peas and half plants with yellow peas
(d) 3/4 plants with yellow peas and 1/4 plants with green peas

95 Some dogs bark, while tailing; others are silent. The barker gene is dominant, the silent gene is recessive. The gene for normal tail is dominant over the gene for screw (curly) tail. A barker dog with a normal tail which is heterozygous for both characteristics is mated with another dog of the same genotype. What

fraction of their offspring will be barkers with the screw tails?
(a) 3/4 (b) 9/16
(c) 3/16 (d) 1/4

96 Two heterozygous tall pea plants with purple flowers are crossed. The probability that one of their offspring will have white flowers is 1/4. The probability that one of their offspring will be short is 1/4. What is the probability that one of their offspring will be short with white flowers?
(a) Zero (b) 1/16
(c) 1/8 (d) 1/4

97 Kernel colour in corn is a trait determined by two alleles. The dominant allele (P) produces a purple colour and the recessive allele (p) produces a yellow colour. The diagram given below shows an ear of corn produced by crossing between two corn plants. The shaded kernels are purple and the unshaded ones are yellow.

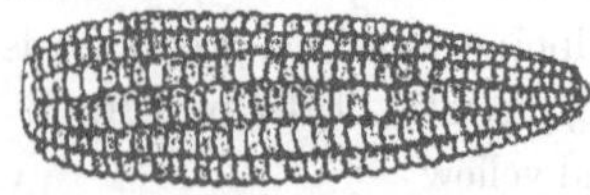

The yellow kernels can be best described as
(a) homozygous dominant
(b) hybrid
(c) heterozygous
(d) homozygous recessive

98 In pigeons, checkered pattern is dominant over plain pattern and red colour is dominant over brown. A checkered brown female mated with a plain red male produced two checkered red, two plain red and one checkered brown offspring. What are the probable genotypes of the parents?
(a) CCRR and ccrr
(b) CcRr and CRrr
(c) CcRr and ccRR
(d) Ccrr and ccRr

99 Pea plants that were heterozygous for both height and colour of seed coat (TtYy) were crossed with pea plants that were homozygous recessive for both traits (ttyy). The offsprings from this cross included tall plants with green seeds, tall plants with yellow seeds, short plants with green seeds and short plants with yellow seeds. This cross best illustrates
(a) gene mutation
(b) independent assortment of chromosomes
(c) environmental influence on heredity
(d) intermediate inheritance

100 In a given plant, red colour (R) of fruit is dominant over white fruit (r) and tallness (T) is dominant over dwarfness (t). If a plant with genotype RRTt is crossed with a plant over genotype rrtt, what will be the percentage of tall plants with red fruits in the next generation?
(a) 100% (b) 25% (c) 50% (d) 75%

101 If the cell of an organism is heterozygous for two pairs of genes represented by Aa, Bb which undergoes meiosis, then the possible genotypic combination of gametes will be
(a) AB, aB, Ab, ab (b) AB, ab
(c) Aa, Bb (d) None of these

102 Two genes 'A' and 'B' are linked in a dihybrid cross involving these two genes, the F_1 heterozygote is crossed with homozygous recessive parental type (aabb). What would be the ratio of offspring in the next generation? **[NCERT Exemplar]**
(a) 1 : 1 : 1 : 1 (b) 9 : 3 : 3 : 1
(c) 3 : 1 (d) 1 : 2 : 1

103 Mendel's law of independent assortment holds good for genes situated on the **[NCERT Exemplar]**
(a) non-homologous chromosomes
(b) homologous chromosomes
(c) extranuclear genetic element
(d) same chromosome

104 It is said that Mendel proposed that the factor controlling any character is discrete and independent. This proposition was based on the
(a) results of F_3-generation of a cross **[NCERT Exemplar]**
(b) observations that the offspring of a cross made between the plants having two contrasting characters show only one character without any blending
(c) self-pollination of F_1 offsprings
(d) cross-pollination of parental generations

105 Which phase of meiosis is most directly related to the law of independent assortment?
(a) Anaphase-II (b) Prophase-II
(c) Metaphase-I (d) Metaphase-II

106 The principle of independent assortment of characters is proved by the
(a) appearance of tall and dwarf plants in F_2 population
(b) appearance of tall and dwarf in the ratio 3 : 1 and also the appearance of smooth and wrinkled seeded plant in the ratio 3 : 1
(c) appearance of smooth and wrinkled seed plants in the F_2 population
(d) observation that F_1 progeny is tall

107 All of the offsprings produced in a cross involving a brown mink and a silver-blue mink are brown. When these brown mink offsprings were crossed with each other, the ratio of brown to silver blue was 3:1. The results of these crosses are best explained by

(a) independent assortment and crossing over
(b) codominance, segregation and recombination
(c) dominance, segregation and recombination
(d) recombination and intermediate inheritance

108 Using the results of his experiments with pea plant crosses, Gregor Mendel discovered the

(a) principles of dominance, segregation and independent assortment
(b) intermediate inheritance and gene linkage
(c) pea plants develop mutations after exposure to radiation
(d) DNA is involved in the inheritance of dominant traits

109 If Mendel had studied 8 traits using pea plant with 14 chromosomes, he would

(a) not have proposed that chromosomes are carriers of hereditary factor
(b) not have discovered the law of independent assortment
(c) have not discovered sex linkage
(d) have discovered polygenic inheritance

110 In Mendel's garden peas, the tall allele (D) is dominant over the dwarf allele (d) and the green pod allele is dominant (Y) over the yellow pod allele (y). What is the genotype of a heterozygous tall, homozygous green pod pea plant?

(a) DdYy (b) DDYY (c) DdYY (d) DDYy

111 When a pure strain of tall plants with round peas is crossed with a pure strain of short plants with wrinkled peas, what proportion of the F_1-generation will be short with wrinkled peas?

(a) Zero (b) 1/16 (c) 1/2 (d) 9/16

112 When a pure strain of tall plants with round peas is crossed with a pure strain of short plants with wrinkled peas, how many different kinds of gametes can their offsprings (F_1-generation) produce?

(a) One (b) Two (c) Four (d) Eight

113 The important assumption is made by Mendel and substantiated by the discovery of meiosis is/are the

(a) law of segregation
(b) law of independent assortment
(c) Both (a) and (b)
(d) constant number of chromosomes in members of the same species, which is maintained by the formation of gametes and the act of fertilisation

114 Which two processes are best represented by the diagram shown below?

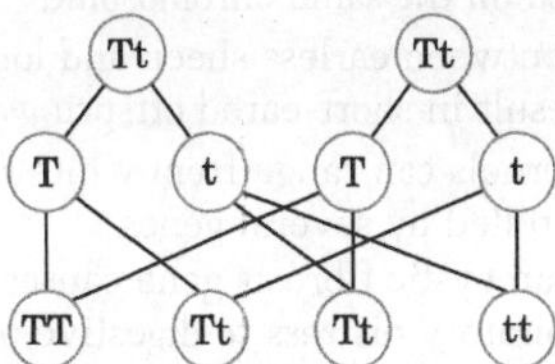

(a) Recombination and codominance
(b) Segregation and recombination
(c) Segregation and intermediate inheritance
(d) Codominance and gene linkage

115 A plant of F_1-generation has genotypes 'AABbCC'. On selfing of this plant, the phenotypic ratio in F_2-generation will be

(a) 3 : 1
(b) 1 : 1
(c) 9 : 3 : 3 : 1
(d) 27 : 9 : 9 : 9 : 3 : 3 : 3 : 1

Gene Interaction

116 Which of the following is not a non-allelic gene interaction?

(a) Epistasis
(b) Duplicate gene
(c) Incomplete dominance
(d) Complementary gene

117 Self-incompatibility in tobacco is an example of

(a) pleiotropic gene
(b) complementary genes
(c) multiple allelism
(d) epistasis

118 Mother and father of a person with 'O' blood group have 'A' and 'B' blood group, respectively. What would be the genotype of both mother and father? **[NCERT Exemplar]**

(a) Mother is homozygous for 'A' blood group and father is heterozygous for 'B'
(b) Mother is heterozygous for 'A' blood group and father is homozygous for 'B'
(c) Both mother and father are heterozygous for 'A' and 'B' blood group, respectively
(d) Both mother and father are homozygous for 'A' and 'B' blood group, respectively

119 Pleiotropy occurs when a gene has

(a) a complementary gene elsewhere
(b) a small effect on one trait
(c) reversible effects on the phenotype, depending on age
(d) many effects on the phenotype

120 Which of the following illustrates pleiotropy?
(a) In fruit flies, the genes for scarlet eyes and hairy body are located on the same chromosome
(b) Matings between earless sheep and long-eared sheep always result in short-eared offspring
(c) Wheat kernels can range from white to red in colour, a trait controlled by several genes
(d) The human cystic fibrosis gene causes many symptoms, from respiratory distress to digestive problems

121 The process that involves intergenic suppression or the masking effect, which one gene locus has upon the expression of another is called
(a) epistasis (b) dominance
(c) incomplete dominance (d) recessive

122 In *Cucurbita pepo*, 'W' gene is epistatic over 'Y and y' (responsible for the appearance of yellow and green coloured fruits respectively) while 'w' gene is ineffective. The ratio of the fruits of different colours in the progeny of the cross WwYy × WwYy is
(a) 9 white : 7 yellow : no green
(b) 3 white : 4 yellow : 1 green
(c) 12 white : 3 yellow : 1 green
(d) 2 white : 1 yellow : 1 green

123 In *Cucurbita pepo*, gene for white fruit colour (W) is epistatic over yellow (Y) which is dominant over green (y). It produces white flowers. What will be the ratio of fruits colour in the cross WwYy × wwYy ?
(a) 9 white : 7 yellow
(b) 4 white : 3 green : 1 yellow
(c) 12 white : 3 yellow : 3 green
(d) 6 white : 1 yellow : 1 green

124 Mating between black rats of identical genotype produced offspring - 14 creamy, 47 black and 19 albino. What epistatic ratio is expected and what type of epistasis is operative?
(a) 1 : 2 : 1, incomplete dominance
(b) 9 : 3 : 4, recessive epistasis
(c) 12 : 3 : 1, dominant epistasis
(d) None of the above

125 Consider the following statements.
I. Mice coat colour is an example of recessive epistasis.
II. The coat colour of mice will be black when CCaa.
Choose the correct option.
(a) Statement I is true, but II is false
(b) Statement I is false, but II is true
(c) Both statements I and II are true
(d) Both statements I and II are false

126 Find the correct match.
(a) Duplicate genes – Multiple allele
(b) Complementary gene – ABO blood group
(c) Recessive epistasis genes – Flower colour in *Lathyrus odoratus*
(d) Duplicate genes – Fruit shape in Shepherd's purse

127 The modified dihybrid ratio of duplicate genes is
(a) 9 : 6 : 1
(b) 13 : 3
(c) 15 : 1
(d) 12 : 3 : 4

128 In poultry birds, the inheritance of combs is controlled by
(a) duplicate genes
(b) collaborator gene
(c) complementary gene
(d) Both (a) and (b)

129 Consider the following statements.
I. Two non-allelic genes produce the new phenotype when present together, but fail to do so independently. It is called complementary gene.
II. Complementary genes were demonstrated by Bateson in *Lathyrus odoratus.*
Choose the correct option.
(a) Statement I is true, but II is false
(b) Statement I is false, but II is true
(c) Both statements I and II are true
(d) Both statements I and II are false

130 Which of the following gene controls the formation of enzyme which catalyses transformation of chromogen into anthocyanin?
(a) Gene P (b) Gene I
(c) Gene C (d) Gene B

131 When a wheat variety of red kernel is crossed with white kerneled wheat, the F_2 ratio would be
(a) 1 : 10 : 4 : 1
(b) 9 : 7
(c) 1 : 2 : 4 : 2 : 4 : 2 : 1
(d) 1 : 4 : 6 : 4 : 1

132 Which of the following statements is incorrect?
(a) TtRr represents the genotype of dihybrid condition
(b) Epistatic gene masks the expression of non-allelic dominant gene
(c) 9 : 3 : 4 phenotypic ratio is an instance of recessive epistasis
(d) Eye colour in humans is an example of codominance

(B) Cumulative Exercise

(Assorted Questions of the Chapter for Advanced Level Practice)

1 Which of the following statements are correct?

I. Expressivity of a gene is defined as the ability to express itself uniformly in all the individuals with same genotype.

II. When one gene masks, inhibits or suppresses the expression of other, the phenomenon is called epistasis.

III. Gene penetrance is the ability of gene to express itself in an individual that carries it.

IV. Inhibiting genes interact in such a way that one dominant gene produces its effect irrespective of the presence or absence of other.

Codes

(a) I, II and III (b) II and IV
(c) III and IV (d) II and III

2 Which of the following statements are correct?

I. Hybrid breakdown refers to condition when offsprings are physiologically inferior to F_1- generation.

II. The collaborator genes are also called pseudoalleles.

III. Complementary genes mask the expression of other gene.

Codes

(a) I, II and III (b) II and III
(c) I and III (d) Only I

3 In his experiments, Mendel obtained wrinkled pea. The wrinkling was due to deposition of sugar instead of starch. This happened due to the

(a) amylase enzyme
(b) invertase enzyme
(c) diastase enzyme
(d) absence of starch-branching enzyme

4 Match the following columns.

Column I		Column II
A. Pleiotropy	1	Heterozygote is intermediate between homozygous phenotypes
B. Epistasis	2	Cross that involves two different gene pairs
C. Dihybrid cross	3	One gene influences the expression of other gene
D. Incomplete dominance	4	Two or more genes with additive effect on phenotype

Codes

	A	B	C	D
(a)	4	3	2	1
(b)	1	2	3	4
(c)	3	1	4	2
(d)	2	4	1	3

5 Match the following columns.

Column I	Column II
A. An organism that has two identical alleles for a given characteristic	1. Law of segregation
B. An organism that has one copy of each allele for a given characteristic	2. Rule of multiplication
C. Principle that describes the probability of a given outcome when that outcome can happen in two or more ways	3. Rule of addition
D. Principle that describes the probability of any two or more events happening together	4. Heterozygous
E. The observations that genetic elements separate when gametes are formed	5. Homozygous

Codes

	A	B	C	D	E
(a)	1	5	2	3	4
(b)	5	4	3	2	1
(c)	4	2	3	5	1
(d)	3	1	2	5	4

6 According to Mendel's law of purity of gametes,

I. in F_1 hybrid, the dominant and recessive characters though remain together for long time but do not contaminate or mix with each other.

II. the inheritance of one character is always independent to the inheritance of other character within the same individual.

III. the gamete formed contains the factor, which determines single trait pertaining to a particular character.

IV. two genes of allelomorphic pair are not related as dominant or recessive but each of them express itself partially.

Choose the correct option containing statements.

(a) I and II (b) III and IV
(c) I and IV (d) II and III

7. Match the following columns.

Column I		Column II
A. Monohybrid cross	1.	T and t
B. Test cross	2.	TT
C. Alleles	3.	Tt × Tt
D. Homozygous tall	4.	tt
	5.	Tt × tt

Codes

	A	B	C	D		A	B	C	D
(a)	3	5	1	2	(b)	5	3	2	4
(c)	3	4	1	2	(d)	3	1	5	2

31 In pea plants, round seed is dominant over wrinkled seed. A plant heterozygous for round seeds was crossed with a plant with wrinkled seeds, which one of the following progenies agrees with expected result?
(a) 99 round and 300 wrinkled
(b) 301 round and 100 wrinkled
(c) 305 round and 301 wrinkled
(d) 200 round and 100 wrinkled

32 In man, brown eyes (B) are dominant over blue (b) and dark hair (D) dominant over red hair (d). A man with brown eyes and red hair marries a woman with blue eyes and dark hair. They got two children; one resembling the man and other the woman, genotypes of the man and woman were
(a) BBdd, bbDD (b) Bbdd, bbDd
(c) BBdd, bbDd (d) Bbdd, bbDD

33 Resistance to a fungus in pea plants is conferred by gene 'H', which is completely recessive to its allele 'h' for susceptibility. If a resistant female plant is crossed with a homozygous susceptible male, what would be the order of genotype in pistillate parent, staminate parent, male gametes and egg?
(a) Hh, HH, H, h (b) hh, Hh, h, h
(c) hh, HH, H, h (d) Hh, HH, h, H

34 A purple flowered plant is cross-pollinated with a yellow flowered plant of the same species. The F_1 plants are all yellow-flowered. If a yellow-flowered F_1 plant is cross-pollinated with a purple-flowered plant, what percentage of the offsprings do you expect to have purple flowers?
(a) 75% (b) 50% (c) 25% (d) 100%

35 The mating of a red fruit bearing tomato plant with yellow fruit bearing plants yielded 173 plants. Out of these, 84 bore red fruits, while 89 bore yellow fruits. The genotypes of the parents are most likely
(a) RR, rr (b) RR, Rr
(c) Rr, rr (d) rr, rr

36 Three yellow round pea seeds labelled A, B, C were taken and grown into plants. The plants were crossed to a plant grown from a green wrinkled pea.
100 seeds issuing from each cross were sorted into phenotypic classes as follows
I. A : 100 yellow round
II. B : 51 yellow round, 49 green round
III. C : 24 yellow round, 26 yellow wrinkled, 25 green round, 24 green wrinkled
The genotype of plant C would be
(a) YYRR (b) YyRr
(c) YyRR (d) YYRr

37 Mendel crossed plants with red and white flowers. In the F_1, only red flowered plants were found. Two F_1 plants were crossed and in F_2-generation, 2950 red and 1050 white flowered plants were obtained. It is reasonable, he concluded that
(a) mutation had occurred
(b) the genes for white flower is incompletely dominant
(c) the probability of white flowered plant is 1/4
(d) no reason can be attributed

38 Mendel studied inheritance for seven pairs of characters in pea. For a study of independent assortment, seven characters can be arranged in 21 possible pairs. If you are told that in one of these of 21 pairs, independent assortment was not observed in repeated later studies, what would be your reaction?
(a) It is impossible
(b) All the later workers must have committed mistakes
(c) Mendel might not have studied cell with 21 combinations
(d) Mendel's principle of independent assortment may be wrong

39 In pea plant, the genes for tallness (T) and for green pod colour (G) are dominant and present on separate chromosomes. Its recessive alleles are t and g. What would be the genotype of female gamete of TtGg and of male gamete of TTgg?
(a) TG, Tg, tG, tg female and Tg male
(b) Female TT, TG, Tg and tg and male Tg
(c) Female TT and Tg and male Tg
(d) Female TT and TG and male Tg

40 Choose the best explanation for the mechanism of inheritance, keeping in mind Mendel's laws of segregation and independent assortment.
(a) A characteristic is inherited 'in combination' with others
(b) The presence of one characteristic (e.g. colour) modifies the inheritance of the other (e.g. shape)
(c) A characteristic (say shape) is inherited independent of the influence of others (e.g. colour)
(d) Rare combinations of characters are always due to mutations, which are inherited by the progeny

41 Two black Guinea pigs are mated together on several occasions. Their offsprings are invariably black. However, when their black offsprings are mated with white Guinea pigs, half the matings result in litters containing black babies only and the other half equal numbers of black and white babies. If colour is determined by a single pair of alleles, the genotypes of the two parents are
(a) homozygous dominant and heterozygous recessive
(b) homozygous dominant and homozygous recessive
(c) Both homozygous dominant
(d) Both heterozygous

42 When a pure strain of tall plants (T/T) with round peas (R/R) is crossed with a pure strain of short plants (t/t) with wrinkled peas (r/r), a F_1-generation is produced. When these F_1 plants self-pollinate, how many genotypes (with regard to the genes for height and pea shape) are produced in the F_2-generation?
(a) 4 (b) 6 (c) 9 (d) 16

43 When a pure strain of tall plants (T/T) with round peas (R/R) is crossed with a pure strain of short plants (t/t) with wrinkled peas (r/r), a F_1-generation is produced. The alleles for short and wrinkled are recessive to those for tall and round, respectively. When these F_1 plants self-pollinate, what proportion of the F_2-generation is short with wrinkled peas?
(a) Zero (b) 1/16 (c) 1/2 (d) 9/16

44 In watermelon, the allele for green colour (G) is dominant over the allele for striped colour (g) and the allele for short shape (S) is dominant over the allele for long shape (s). When long, striped watermelons are crossed with watermelons heterozygous for both traits, what proportion of the offspring are striped and short?
(a) 0 (b) 1/4
(c) 1/2 (d) 9/16

45 One pure strain of pea plants developed by Mendel had yellow peas and another strain had green peas. All the offsprings from crosses between these two parental (P) strains of plants had yellow peas. In these plants, the allele for yellow pea colour is
(a) recessive to the allele for green colour
(b) dominant over the allele for green colour
(c) epistatic over other alleles
(d) expressed only in gametes

46 If an animal's coat colour depends on two separate gene pairs, in which the pair A codes for the pigment protein and the pair B codes for the control mechanism that turns on pigment production, then a cross between two albinos (no pigments), one with defects at locus A and the other with defects at locus B will produce offsprings that are all
(a) albinos
(b) streaked, in which pigmented areas are mixed with unpigmented areas
(c) pink-eyed and blind
(d) normally pigmented

47 Normal maize has starchy seeds which remain smooth when dry. A mutant form has sugary seeds, which go wrinkled when dry. When a mutant was crossed with a normal plant, an F_1 was produced which has smooth seeds. What would be the relative ratios of the different seed types, if the F_1 was allowed to self
(a) 1 smooth : 3 sugary (b) 3 smooth : 1 sugary
(c) 1 smooth : 1 sugary (d) All sugary

48 A black female is test crossed, producing 6 black offsprings. The probability that a black heterozygous female would this by chance alone is approximately
(a) 50% (b) 25%
(c) 1% (d) cannot be determined

49 Short hair is due to a dominant gene L and long hair to its recessive allele l (in rabbit). A cross between a short-haired female and a long haired male produces a litter of 1 long haired and 7 short haired bunnies. What are the genotypes of the parents?
(a) LL (male) × ll (female) (b) ll (male) × LL (female)
(c) Ll (female) × ll (male) (d) Ll (male) × ll (female)

50 Why were pea plants more suitable than dogs for Mendel's experiment?
(a) There were no pedigree records of dogs
(b) Pea plants can be self-fertilised
(c) All pea plants have $2n$ number of chromosomes
(d) Dogs have different colour

51 In Mendel's crosses beginning with two pure strains of pea plants, one with yellow peas (Y/Y) and the other with green peas (y/y), the test cross was done between F_2 offspring with yellow peas and a pure strain of plants with the genotype
(a) Y/Y (b) y/y (c) Y/y (d) YG

52 The allele for black hair colour (B) is dominant over the allele for white hair colour (b) in Guinea pigs. A test cross between a black male and a white female produced a litter of five black and one white Guinea pigs. The genotype of the father is
(a) unknown, due to the small sample size
(b) B/B
(c) B/b
(d) b/b

Assertion and Reason

Direction (Q. Nos. 53-57) *In each of the following questions, a statement of Assertion (A) is given followed by corresponding statement of Reason (R). Of the statements, mark the correct answer as*

(a) Both A and R are true and R is the correct explanation of A
(b) Both A and R are true, but R is not the correct explanation of A
(c) A is true, but R is false
(d) A is false, but R is true
(e) Both A and R are false

53 **Assertion** (A) In a monohybrid cross, we study two characters.
Reason (R) In a monohybrid cross, alleles exhibit dominant recessive relationship.

54 **Assertion** (A) The genetic complement of an organism is called genotype.
Reason (R) Genotype is the type of hereditary properties of an organism.

55 **Assertion** (A) Mendel worked on garden pea (*Pisum sativum*).
Reason (R) Garden pea belongs to family-Malvaceae.

56 **Assertion** (A) Mendel was successful in knowing the process of inheritance.
Reason (R) He considered a single character at one time.

57 **Assertion** (A) Test cross is used to determine as unknown genotype within one breeding generation.
Reason (R) It is a cross between F_1 hybrid and dominant parent.

(C) Medical Entrances' Gallery

(Collection of Questions Asked in NEET & in Various Medical Entrance Exams)

1 Identify the incorrect statement with reference to the gene 'I' that controls ABO blood groups. **[NEET 2020]**
(a) A person will have only two of the three alleles
(b) When I^A and I^B are present together, they express same type of sugar
(c) Allele 'I' does not produce any sugar
(d) The gene (I) has three alleles

2 How many true breeding pea plant varieties did Mendel select as pairs, which were similar except in one character with contrasting traits? **[NEET 2020]**
(a) 2 (b) 14 (c) 8 (d) 4

3 The number of contrasting characters studied by Mendel for his experiments was **[NEET 2020, CBSE AIPMT 2015]**
(a) 14 (b) 4 (c) 2 (d) 7

4 The best example for pleiotropy is **[NEET 2020]**
(a) skin colour
(b) phenylketonuria
(c) colour blindness
(d) ABO blood group

5 Match the following columns and choose the correct option from the codes given below.

Column I	Column II
A. Pleiotropic gene	1. Both alleles express equally
B. Codominance	2. Change in nucleotides
C. Epistasis	3. One gene shows multiple phenotypic expression
D. Mutation	4. Non-allelic gene inheritance

Codes **[AIIMS 2019]**

	A	B	C	D		A	B	C	D
(a)	1	2	3	4	(b)	2	3	4	1
(c)	3	1	4	2	(d)	1	3	4	2

6 The production of gametes by the parents, the formation of zygotes, the F_1 and F_2 plants, can be understood using **[NEET 2019]**
(a) pie diagram (b) a pyramid diagram
(c) Punnett square (d) Venn diagram

7 In *Antirrhinum* (snapdragon), a red flower was crossed with a white flower and in F_1-generation, pink flowers were obtained. When pink flowers were selfed, the F_2-generation showed white, red and pink flowers.
Choose the incorrect statement from the following. **[NEET 2019]**
(a) Pink colour in F_1 is due to incomplete dominance
(b) Ratio of F_2 is $\frac{1}{4}$ (Red) : $\frac{2}{4}$ (Pink) : $\frac{1}{4}$ (White)
(c) Law of segregation does not apply in this experiment
(d) This experiment does not follow the principle of dominance

8 Which one of the following pairs is incorrectly matched? **[NEET 2018]**
(a) XO type sex-determination - Grasshopper
(b) ABO blood grouping - Codominance
(c) Starch synthesis in pea - Multiple alleles
(d) TH Morgan - Linkage

9 Select the correct statement. **[NEET 2018]**
(a) Spliceosomes take part in translation
(b) Punnett square was developed by a British scientist
(c) Franklin Stahl coined the term 'linkage'
(d) Transduction was discovered by S Altman

10 Which of the following characteristics represents 'inheritance of blood groups' in humans?
1. Dominance 2. Codominance
3. Multiple allele 4. Incomplete dominance
5. Polygenic inheritance **[NEET 2018]**

Choose the correct option.
(a) 2, 4 and 5 (b) 1, 2 and 3
(c) 2, 3 and 5 (d) 1, 3 and 5

11 AB blood group shows [NEET 2018]
(a) codominance (b) incomplete dominance
(c) polygenic inheritance (d) pleiotropy

12 In pea plants, green pod colour is dominant over yellow pods. 1000 seeds taken from a pea plant on germination produces 760 green pod and 240 yellow pod plants. The parental genotype and phenotype of the seed plant are [AIIMS 2017]
(a) heterozygous and yellow (b) heterozygous and green
(c) homozygous and yellow (d) homozygous and green

13 Which one from those given below is the period of Mendel's hybridisation experiments? [NEET 2017]
(a) 1856-1863 (b) 1840-1850
(c) 1857-1869 (d) 1870-1877

14 The genotypes of a husband and wife are and i. Among the blood types of their children, how many different genotypes and phenotypes are possible? [NEET 2017]
(a) 3 genotypes, 3 phenotypes
(b) 3 genotypes, 4 phenotypes
(c) 4 genotypes, 3 phenotypes
(d) 4 genotypes, 4 phenotypes

15 If two people with AB blood group marry and have sufficiently large number of children, these children could be classified as A blood group, AB blood group and B blood group in 1 : 2 : 1 ratio.
Modern technique of protein electrophoresis reveals the presence of both A and B type proteins in AB blood group individuals. This is an example of [JIPMER 2017]
(a) codominance (b) incomplete dominance
(c) partial dominance (d) complete dominance

16 A true breeding plant is [NEET-II 2016]
(a) one that is able to breed on its own
(b) produced due to cross-pollination among unrelated plants
(c) homozygous and produces offspring of its own kind
(d) always homozygous recessive in its genetic constitution

17 A tall true breeding garden pea plant is crossed with a dwarf true breeding garden pea plant. When the F_1 plants were selfed the resulting genotypes were in the ratio of [NEET-I 2016]
(a) 1 : 2 : 1 :: Tall heterozygous : Tall homozygous : Dwarf
(b) 3 : 1 :: Tall : Dwarf
(c) 3 : 1 :: Dwarf : Tall
(d) 1 : 2 : 1 :: Tall homozygous : Tall heterozygous : Dwarf

18 Match the terms in Column I with their description in Column II and choose the correct option.

Column I	Column II
A. Dominance	1. Many genes govern a single character
B. Codominance	2. In a heterozygous organism, only one allele expresses itself
C. Pleiotropy	3. In a heterozygous organism, both alleles express themselves fully
D. Polygenic inheritance	4. A single gene influences many characters

Codes [NEET-I 2016]

	A	B	C	D		A	B	C	D
(a)	2	3	4	1	(b)	4	1	2	3
(c)	4	3	1	2	(d)	2	1	4	3

19 A pure pea plant with round seeds having large starch grains is crossed with another pure pea plant with wrinkled seeds having small starch grains. The F_1 heterozygotes formed are self-pollinated. What is the phenotypic ratio of plants with round seeds and intermediate starch grains to plants with wrinkled seeds and larger starch grains expected in the F_2-generation? [EAMCET 2016]
(a) 3 : 4 (b) 6 : 1 (c) 5 : 6 (d) 2 : 3

20 A gene showing codominance has [CBSE AIPMT 2015]
(a) one allele dominant on the other
(b) alleles tightly linked on the same chromosome
(c) alleles that are recessive to each other
(d) both alleles independently expressed in the heterozygote

21 Alleles are [CBSE AIPMT 2015]
(a) different phenotype
(b) true breeding homozygotes
(c) different molecular forms of a gene
(d) heterozygotes

22 Arrange the following in decreasing order based on the result obtained in the F_2 progeny of a dihybrid cross.
I. Total number of parental genotypes
II. Total number of recombinant genotypes
III. Total phenotypes
IV. Total genotypes [EAMCET 2015]
Codes
(a) III, II, IV and I (b) I, III, IV and II
(c) IV, I, III and II (d) IV, II, III and I

23 A male rabbit of genotype AABBDDEE is crossed with a female rabbit of genotype aabbddee, to produce F_1 hybrid offspring. How many genetically different gametes can be produced by this F_1 hybrid? [WB JEE 2015]
(a) 4 (b) 8 (c) 16 (d) 32

24 Which of the followings is/are correct for the inheritance of genes involved in human 'ABO' blood grouping? **[WB JEE 2015]**
(a) It is inherited by complete dominant allele
(b) It is inherited by complete recessive allele
(c) Both (a) and (b)
(d) It is inherited by single gene with more than two alleles

25 During the experiments, Mendel called genes by the term **[AMU 2015, UK PMT 2014]**
(a) traits (b) characters (c) factors (d) qulities

26 If a genotype consists of different types of alleles, it is called **[AMU 2015]**
(a) homozygous (b) heterozygous
(c) monoallelic (d) uniallelic

27 The alternative form of gene is called **[AMU 2015]**
(a) dominant (b) recessive character
(c) alternative genes (d) allele

28 Identify the incorrect statement. **[Karnataka CET 2015]**
(a) Alleles b and c also produce sugar
(b) Alleles I^A and I^B produce sugars
(c) When I^B and b or I are present only I^B is expressed
(d) Both I^A and I^B are present together and they express because of codominance

29 A character which is expressed in a hybrid is called **[J&K CET 2015]**
(a) dominant (b) recessive
(c) codominant (d) epistatic

30 In Mendel's experiments with garden pea, round seed-shape (RR) was dominant over wrinkled seed (rr), yellow cotyledon (YY) was dominant over green cotyledon (yy). What are the expected phenotypes in the F_2-generation of the cross RRYY × rryy? **[J&K CET 2015]**
(a) Only wrinkled seeds with green cotyledons
(b) Only wrinkled seeds with yellow cotyledons
(c) Only round seeds with green cotyledons
(d) Round seeds with yellow cotyledons, round seeds with green cotyledons, wrinkled seeds with yellow cotyledons and wrinkled seeds with green cotyledons

31 Fruit colour in squash is an example of **[CBSE AIPMT 2014]**
(a) recessive epistasis (b) dominant epistasis
(c) complementary genes (d) inhibitory genes

32 Which of the following cross will give recessive progeny in F_1-generation? **[MHT CET 2014]**
(a) TT × tt (b) Tt × tt
(c) tt × tt (d) TT × TT

33 Multiple allelism is observed in **[Kerala CEE 2014]**
(a) flower colour in snapdragon
(b) pod colour in *Pisum sativum*
(c) haemophilia in human
(d) sex-determination in birds
(e) ABO blood types

34 The graphical representation to calculate the probability of all possible genotypes of offspring in a genetic cross was developed by **[Kerala CEE 2014]**
(a) Gregor Johann Mendel (b) Kornberg
(c) Har Gobind Khorana (d) George Gamow
(e) Reginald C Punnett

35 In a plant species, flower colour yellow is dominant over white and fruit shape round is dominant over elongated. Crossing was performed between two pure lines, i.e. one having yellow-flower and round-fruit and another with white-flower and elongated-fruit. About 20 plants survived in F_1 progeny. Plants of F_1 were allowed to self-fertilise and about 960 plants survived in F_2. If the traits follow Mendelian inheritance, the number of plants that would have yellow-flower and round-fruit in F_1 and F_2 are respectively. **[WB JEE 2014]**
(a) 20, 960 (b) 20, 540
(c) 10, 180 (d) 10, 60

36 Mendel conducted hybridisation experiments on garden peas for **[J&K CET 2014]**
(a) 7 years (b) 6 years (c) 5 years (d) 4 years

37 Two plants one with black flower and other with white coloured flower were crossed in an experiment. In next generation, grey coloured flowers were obtained, the reason for the result is **[J&K CET 2014]**
(a) incomplete dominance (b) pseudodominance
(c) codominance (d) None of these

38 Some genomic representation of skin colour are given below.
I. AAbbCC II. AAbbcc
III. AABBCC IV. aabbcc
Which of the option is correct for showing the darkness of colour of the skin in decreasing order? **[UK PMT 2014]**
(a) III → II → I → IV (b) I → IV → II → III
(c) III → I → II → IV (d) I → III → II → IV

39 Skin colour in man is an example of **[EAMCET 2014]**
(a) sex-linked inheritance (b) multiple allelism
(c) pleiotropy (d) polygenic inheritance

40 A cross between two tall garden pea plants produced all tall plants. The possible genotypes of the parents are **[EAMCET 2014]**

I. TT, TT II. TT, Tt
III. Tt, tt IV. Tt, Tt

The correct answer is
(a) III and IV (b) I and IV (c) I and II (d) II and III

41 Tall (T) is completely dominant over dwarf (t). Red flower colour (R) is incompletely dominant over white (r), the heterozygote being pink. Plant having genotype of TtRr is self-pollinated. What would be the proportion of plants with dwarf and pink characters in its progeny? **[EAMCET 2014]**

(a) $\frac{2}{16}$ (b) $\frac{1}{16}$
(c) $\frac{9}{16}$ (d) $\frac{3}{16}$

42 In garden pea, round shape of seeds is dominant over wrinkled shape. A pea plant heterozygous for round shape of seed is selfed and 1600 seeds produced during the cross are subsequently germinated. How many seedlings would have the parental phenotype? **[Karnataka CET 2014]**

(a) 1600 (b) 800 (c) 400 (d) 1200

43 Which Mendelian idea is depicted by a cross in which the F_1-generation resembles both the parents? **[NEET 2013]**

(a) Law of dominance
(b) Inheritance of one gene
(c) Codominance
(d) Incomplete dominance

44 When two hybrids rrTt and Rrtt are crossed, the phenotype ratio of offspring would be **[UP CPMT 2013]**

(a) 3:1 (b) 9:3:3:1
(c) 1:1 (d) 1:1:1:1

45 Test cross is when **[UP CPMT 2013; WB JEE 2010]**

(a) F_1 crossed with heterozygous parents
(b) F_2 crossed with homozygous recessive parents
(c) F_1 crossed with homozygous recessive parents
(d) F_1 crossed with homozygous parents

46 In a typical Mendelian cross, which is a dihybrid cross, one parent is homozygous for both dominant traits and another parent is homozygous for both recessive traits. In the F_2-generation, both parental combinations and recombinations appear. The phenotypic ratio of parental combinations to recombinations is **[Karnataka CET 2013]**

(a) 10:6 (b) 12:4
(c) 9:7 (d) 15:1

47 Mendel found that the reciprocal crosses yielded identical results. From that it was concluded **[Karnataka CET 2013]**

(a) there is no dominance of any trait
(b) sex has no influence on the dominance of traits
(c) there is independent assortment of traits
(d) sex plays a role in deciding the dominance of a trait

48 F_2-generation in a Mendelian cross showed that both genotypic and phenotypic ratios are same as 1:2:1. It represents a case of **[CBSE AIPMT 2012]**

(a) codominance
(b) dihybrid cross
(c) monohybrid cross with complete dominance
(d) monohybrid cross with incomplete dominance

49 In a dihybrid cross, where two parents differ in two pairs of contrasting traits like seed colour yellow (YY) and seed colour green (yy) with seed shape round (RR) and seed shape wrinkled (rr), the number of green coloured seeds (yy) among sixteen products of F_2-generation will be **[AMU 2012]**

(a) 2 (b) 4 (c) 6 (d) 8

50 Mating of an organism to a double recessive in order to determine whether it is homozygous or heterozygous for a character under consideration, is called **[JCECE 2012, Odisha JEE 2010, AIIMS 2008]**

(a) reciprocal cross (b) test cross
(c) dihybrid cross (d) back cross

51 Which of the following is best suited for codominance? **[BCECE 2012]**

(a) Flower colour in snapdragon
(b) MN blood group in human
(c) Both (a) and (c)
(d) Skin colour in human

52 A common test to find the genotype of hybrid is **[Manipal 2012]**

(a) crossing of one F_2 progeny with male parent
(b) crossing of one F_2 progeny with female parent
(c) studying the sexual behaviour of F_1 progenies
(d) crossing of one F_1 progeny with recessive parent

53 Mendel's principle of segregation means that the germ cells always receive **[AFMC 2012]**

(a) one pair of alleles (b) one quarter of genes
(c) one of the paired alleles (d) any pair of alleles

54 When two unrelated individuals or lines are crossed, the performance of F_1 hybrid is often superior to both its parents. This phenomenon is called **[CBSE AIPMT 2011]**

(a) transformation (b) splicing
(c) metamorphosis (d) heterosis

55 If two pea plants having red (dominant) coloured flowers with unknown genotypes are crossed, 75% of the flowers are red and 25% are white. The genotypic constitution of the parents having red coloured flowers will be **[DUMET 2011]**

(a) Both homozygous
(b) One homozygous and other heterozygous
(c) Both heterozygous
(d) Both hemizygous

56 A polygenic trait is controlled by 3 genes A, B and C. In a cross AaBbCc × AaBbCc, the phenotypic ratio of the offsprings was observed as 1: 6 : x : 20 : x : 6 :1. What is the possible value of x? **[DUMET 2011]**

(a) 3 (b) 9 (c) 15 (d) 25

57 The F_1-generation has all tall and F_2 ratio 3 : 1, it proves **[Odisha JEE 2011]**

(a) law of dominance (b) incomplete assortment
(c) law of segregation (d) linkage

58 Multiple phenotype is seen in **[Odisha JEE 2011]**

(a) pleiotropy (b) incomplete dominance
(c) multiple allelism (d) polygenic inheritance

59 If a cross between two individuals produces offsprings with 50% dominant character (A) and 50% recessive character (a), then the genotypes of parents are **[WB JEE 2011]**

(a) Aa × Aa (b) Aa × aa (c) AA × aa (d) AA × Aa

60 Allelism refers to **[J&K CET 2011]**

(a) genic interactions controlling a character
(b) multiple genes controlling a character
(c) expression of many characters by a single gene
(d) alternative forms of a gene at a given locus

61 Mendelian principles are not applicable in case of

(a) sex-linked alleles **[J&K CET 2011]**
(b) asexually reproducing forms
(c) sexually interbreeding forms
(d) diploid homozygous forms

62 Genotypic and phenotypic ratio in monohybrid cross remains the same in case of **[J&K CET 2011]**

(a) sex-linked genes
(b) pseudoallelic genes
(c) intermediate inheritance
(d) dominant and recessive genes

63 Mendel was successful in discovering the principles of inheritance as **[J&K CET 2011]**

(a) he took pea plants for his experiments
(b) he did not encounter linkage between the genes for the characters he considered
(c) he had an in-depth knowledge on hybridisation
(d) he was a famous mathematician

64 Independent assortment means **[Odisha JEE 2011]**

(a) separation of parental characters
(b) segregation of parental characters
(c) recombination of parental characters
(d) non-separation of parental characters

65 In Mendelian dihybrid cross, when heterozygous Round Yellow are self-crossed, Round Green offsprings are represented by the genotype **[Kerala CEE 2011]**

(a) RrYy, RrYY and RRYy
(b) Rryy, RRyy and rryy
(c) rrYy and rrYY
(d) Rryy and RRyy
(e) RrYy, rryy and Rryy

ANSWERS

Check Point 6.1

1. (b)	2. (a)	3. (c)	4. (a)	5. (d)	6. (a)

Check Point 6.2

1. (b)	2. (c)	3. (c)	4. (b)	5. (c)	6. (d)

Check Point 6.3

1. (d)	2. (c)	3. (b)	4. (c)	5. (c)	6. (b)

(A) Topical Exercise

1. (b)	2. (a)	3. (a)	4. (c)	5. (c)	6. (d)	7. (c)	8. (a)	9. (d)	10. (b)
11. (a)	12. (a)	13. (b)	14. (a)	15. (d)	16. (a)	17. (a)	18. (c)	19. (d)	20. (a)
21. (b)	22. (b)	23. (a)	24. (a)	25. (b)	26. (d)	27. (d)	28. (b)	29. (c)	30. (d)
31. (d)	32. (a)	33. (d)	34. (d)	35. (c)	36. (b)	37. (c)	38. (b)	39. (a)	40. (b)
41. (c)	42. (b)	43. (b)	44. (b)	45. (d)	46. (b)	47. (b)	48. (a)	49. (c)	50. (a)
51. (c)	52. (c)	53. (b)	54. (a)	55. (a)	56. (b)	57. (c)	58. (d)	59. (a)	60. (c)
61. (c)	62. (c)	63. (a)	64. (d)	65. (b)	66. (b)	67. (a)	68. (d)	69. (b)	70. (a)
71. (a)	72. (a)	73. (b)	74. (a)	75. (d)	76. (a)	77. (b)	78. (a)	79. (a)	80. (d)
81. (a)	82. (c)	83. (b)	84. (a)	85. (a)	86. (a)	87. (a)	88. (a)	89. (a)	90. (d)
91. (a)	92. (a)	93. (d)	94. (d)	95. (c)	96. (b)	97. (d)	98. (d)	99. (b)	100. (c)
101. (a)	102. (a)	103. (b)	104. (b)	105. (c)	106. (b)	107. (c)	108. (a)	109. (b)	110. (c)
111. (a)	112. (c)	113. (c)	114. (b)	115. (a)	116. (c)	117. (c)	118. (c)	119. (d)	120. (d)
121. (a)	122. (c)	123. (b)	124. (b)	125. (c)	126. (d)	127. (c)	128. (b)	129. (c)	130. (a)
131. (d)	132. (d)								

(B) Cumulative Exercise

1. (a)	2. (d)	3. (d)	4. (a)	5. (b)	6. (a)	7. (a)	8. (c)	9. (d)	10. (a)
11. (d)	12. (b)	13. (a)	14. (c)	15. (b)	16. (b)	17. (c)	18. (d)	19. (c)	20. (d)
21. (d)	22. (d)	23. (a)	24. (b)	25. (c)	26. (b)	27. (c)	28. (a)	29. (b)	30. (c)
31. (c)	32. (b)	33. (c)	34. (b)	35. (c)	36. (b)	37. (c)	38. (c)	39. (a)	40. (c)
41. (a)	42. (d)	43. (b)	44. (b)	45. (b)	46. (a)	47. (b)	48. (a)	49. (c)	50. (b)
51. (b)	52. (c)	53. (d)	54. (b)	55. (c)	56. (a)	57. (c)			

(C) Medical Entrances' Gallery

1. (b)	2. (b)	3. (d)	4. (b)	5. (c)	6. (c)	7. (c)	8. (c)	9. (b)	10. (b)
11. (a)	12. (b)	13. (a)	14. (c)	15. (a)	16. (c)	17. (d)	18. (a)	19. (b)	20. (d)
21. (c)	22. (c)	23. (c)	24. (d)	25. (c)	26. (b)	27. (d)	28. (a)	29. (a)	30. (d)
31. (b)	32. (c)	33. (e)	34. (e)	35. (b)	36. (a)	37. (a)	38. (c)	39. (d)	40. (c)
41. (a)	42. (d)	43. (c)	44. (d)	45. (c)	46. (a)	47. (b)	48. (d)	49. (b)	50. (b)
51. (b)	52. (d)	53. (c)	54. (d)	55. (c)	56. (c)	57. (c)	58. (a)	59. (b)	60. (d)
61. (b)	62. (c)	63. (b)	64. (c)	65. (d)					

Explanations

(A) Topical Exercise

43 (*b*) Option (b) is incorrect pair and can be corrected as

In cat, angora (long) hair is recessive trait whereas short hair is a dominant trait.

Rest options are correct pair regarding the dominant character.

44 (*b*) The term albino signifies white rabbit only. Since, both parents are albino, the resulting progeny would be albino or white only. Colour of surrogate rabbit would not affect the progeny inheritance.

49 (*c*) Statement in option (c) is incorrect and can be corrected as

Hornless cattle is dominant over horned cattle.

Rest statements are correct.

50 (*a*) Option (a) is incorrect pair and can be corrected as

Presence of webbed digits in human is an abnormal trait. However, it is a dominant trait over the normal digits

Rest options are correct pairs.

68 (*d*) The probability of gamete B to fuse with B or b are mutually exclusive events.

According to product rule of probability,

- Probability of B to fuse with B is $B\ (\frac{1}{2}) \times B\ (\frac{1}{2}) = BB\ (\frac{1}{4})$
- Probability of B to fuse with b is $B\ (\frac{1}{2}) \times b\ (\frac{1}{2}) = Bb\ (\frac{1}{4})$

71 (*a*) Mature corn plants produce ears that contain hundreds of seeds. Each seeds is formed by fertilisation and it has both alleles for height, i.e. T and t.

So, offspring produced by crossing Tt and Tt will have genotypes TT, Tt and tt.

Out of these, 140 are tall (TT and Tt) and 40 are dwarf (tt).

72 (*a*) Number of gametes = 2^n

Where, n = Number of heterozygotes

In AAbb, $n = 0$

Thus, $2^0 = 1$ (Any number raised to the power zero is one).

88 (*a*) When heterozygous red flower (Rr) is crossed with white flower (rr), red and white flowers will be produced in equal ratio.

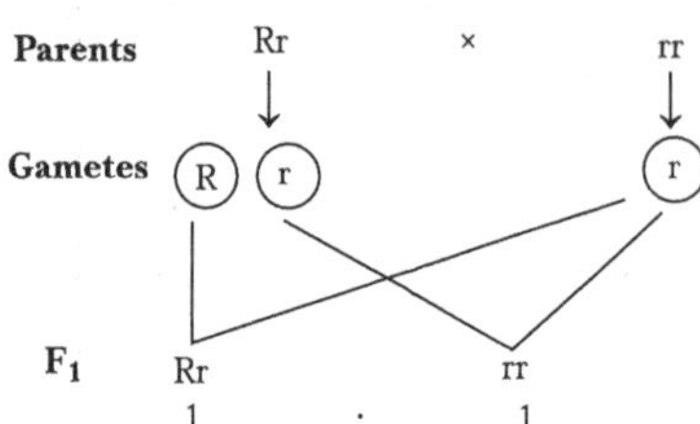

Thus, option (a) is correct.

93 (*d*) Since, the F_1 progeny had red, axial flower, it indicates a dihybrid cross.

Thus, the F_2-generation would have 9 : 3 : 3 : 1 ratio.

The frequency of dominant red, axial trait would be 9/16.

The total number of offsprings are 100.

Thus, $\left(\frac{9}{16}\right) \times 100 = 56.25 \sim 56$

100 (*c*)

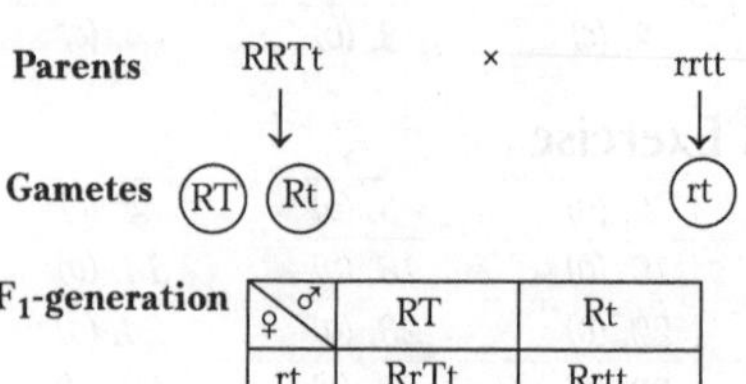

F_1-generation

♀ \ ♂	RT	Rt
rt	RrTt	Rrtt

Thus, 50% plants would have tall height and red fruit.

111 (*a*)

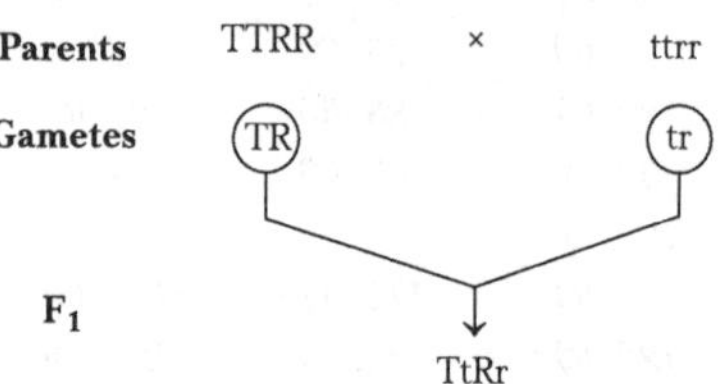

Thus, the proportion of dwarf plant with wrinkled seed is zero.

115 (*a*) The genotype of F_1-generation is AABbCC. Number of gametes produced by it = $2^n = 2^1 = 2$

Hence, there will be two gametes, ABC and AbC.

On selfing, the phenotype of F_2 would be 3 : 1.

♀ \ ♂	ABC	AbC
ABC	AABBCC	AABbCC
AbC	AABbCC	AAbbCC

123 (*b*) A cross between WwYy (white) and wwYy (yellow) would produce 8 white, 6 yellow and 2 green progenies.

Thus, the ratio is 4 : 3 : 1.

♀ \ ♂	wY	wy	wY	wy
WY	WwYY (White)	WwYy (White)	WwYY (White)	WwYy (White)
Wy	WwYy (White)	Wwyy (White)	WwYy (White)	Wwyy (White)
wY	wwYY (Yellow)	wwYy (Yellow)	wwYY (Yellow)	wwYy (Yellow)
wy	wwYy (Yellow)	wwyy (Green)	wwYy (Yellow)	wwyy (Green)

132 (*d*) Statement in option (d) is incorrect and can be corrected as

Eye colour in humans is an example of polygenic inheritance. This trait is influenced by about 16 different genes.

Rest statements are correct.

(B) Cumulative Exercise

1 (*a*) Statements I, II, III are correct, whereas IV is incorrect.
Incorrect statement can be corrected as
Inhibiting genes prevent the expression of another gene.

2 (*d*) Only statement I is correct whereas II and III are incorrect.
Incorrect statements can be corrected as
- Sometimes duplicate genes are referred to as pseudoalleles.
- Epistatic alleles mask the expression of other gene.

11 (*d*) Option (d) represents incorrect matched pair and can be corrected as
Incomplete dominance was reported by Karl Correns.
Rest options represent correct match pairs.

15 (*b*) Statement in option (b) is false and can be corrected as
In cats, tortoise-shell is a sex-linked trait and it is restricted to females only. Thus, male-tortoise shell kittens cannot be produced.
Rest statements are true.

20 (*d*) Statement in option (d) is correct.
A cross between black hybrid and pure brown mouse would produce equal proportion of black and brown progenies regardless of their sex.

26 (*b*) Cross between Aa and aa would generate progenies in the ratio of 1:1 because it is a test cross.
The approximate values are being represented by option (b) thus it is correct.

35 (*c*) Since, the mating yielded both dominant and recessive traits in 1:1 ratio, one of the parent should be heterozygous (Rr), while the other should be homozygous (rr) recessive
Thus, option (c) is correct.

44 (*b*) When ssgg (long striped) watermelon is crossed with heterozygous (SsGg) watermelon, four progenies would be produced in 1:1:1:1 ratio as it is a test cross.
The progenies would be
Gg Bb – Green short
Gg bb – Green long
gg Bb – Striped short
gg bb – Striped long
Thus, option (b) is correct

53 (*d*) A is false, but R is true. A can be corrected as
In monohybrid cross, single character each controlled by a single pair of genes or alleles are considered. In F_2-generation, monohybrid cross shows 3:1 ratio between dominant character and recessive character.

54 (*b*) Both A and R are true, but R is not the correct explanation of A.
Genotype is the hereditary properties of an organism and genetic complement of an organism.

55 (*c*) A is true, but R is false, because
Mendel worked on garden pea (*Pisum sativum*) as plant material for his experiments because of their following advantages such as
Well defined characters, bisexual flowers, predominantly self-fertilisation, easy hybritisation.
Pea is a leguminous crop which belong to family-Fabaceae.

56 (*a*) Both A and R are true and R is the correct explanation of A.
Although hybridisation experiments were conducted earlier by workers like Knight (1799), Goss (1824) and J Kolreuter, but they considered the individual as a whole complex of characters. Mendel's success was mainly based on the fact that he considered a single character at one time.

57 (*c*) A is true, but R is false. R can be corrected as
Test cross is a cross between F_1 hybrid individual and its recessive parent. By crossing an organism having an unknown genotype with a homozygous recessive organism, it is possible to determine an unknown genotype within one breeding generation.

(C) Medical Entrances' Gallery

1 (*b*) Statement in option (b) represents incorrect statement with reference to the gene 'I' that controls ABO blood group and can be corrected as
I^A and I^B are completely dominant over I^0, When I^A and I^B are present together, they both express their own sugar and thus behave as codominant alleles.
Rest statements are correct.

2 (*b*) Mendel (father of genetics) selected 14 true-breeding pea plant varieties, in pairs, which were similar except for one character with contrasting traits. A true breeding line refers to the plant that has undergone continuous self-pollination and showed stable trait inheritance and expression for several generations.

3 (*d*) Mendel conducted breeding experiments on garden pea by selecting 7 pairs of contrasting characters. Luckily all these characters were related as dominant and recessive and none of them showed linkage.

4 (*b*) The best example for pleiotropy is phenylketonuria which occurs in humans. In pleiotropy, a single gene can exhibit multiple phenotypic expressions. This gene is called pleiotropic gene. In phenylketonuria, a single gene mutation that codes for enzyme phenylalanine hydroxylase is seen
This manifests itself through phenotypic expression characterised by mental retardation and a reduction in hair and skin pigmentation.

6 (*c*) The production of gametes by the parents, the formation of zygotes and the F_1 and F_2 plants can be understood from a diagram called Punnett square. It was developed by a British geneticist, Reginald C Punnett. It is a graphical representation to calculate the probability of all possible genotypes of offspring in a genetic cross.

7 (*c*) Statement in option (c) that 'law of segregation does not apply in this experiment' is incorrect and can be corrected as
The law of segregation applies universally. The reappearance of parental (red and white) flowers in the F_2-generation also confirms, that law of segregation applies in this experiment.
Rest of the statements are correct.

8 (*c*) In the given pairs, option (c) is incorrectly matched and can be corrected as
Starch synthesis in pea is an example of pleiotropy. A pleiotropic gene is a single gene which produces many or multiple unrelated phenotypes.
Rest of the pairs are correctly matched.

9 (*b*) Statement in option (b) is correct.
Punnett square is a checker board used to show the result of a cross between two organisms. The checker board was devised by a British geneticist, Reginald Punnett (1927). It depicts both the genotype and the phenotype of the progeny.
Other statements are incorrect and can be corrected

- Spliceosome is formed during post-transcriptional changes in eukaryotes.
- Franklin Stahl with Matthew Meselson proved the semiconservative replication of DNA.
- Transduction is a method of sexual reproduction in bacteria. It was discovered by Zinder and his teacher Lederberg (1952) in *Salmonella typhimurium*.

10 (*b*) Dominance, codominance and multiple alleles are the characteristics that represent 'inheritance of blood groups' in humans. ABO blood groups are determined by the gene I. There are multiple (three) alleles, I^A, I^B and i of this gene. Alleles I^A and I^B are dominant over i. However, when I^A and I^B alleles are present together, they show codominance. Therefore, option (b) is correct.

11 (*a*) In humans, AB blood group shows codominance. Here, allele I^A for A-type blood is codominant with allele I^B for B-type blood. In heterozygotes, I^AI^B expresses the characteristics of both A and B antigens, i.e. I^AI^B possesses RBCs that carry both A and B antigens at their surface.

12 (*b*) Since, the ratio of 760 green pod and 240 yellow pod plants is 3:1, it is evident that the parent plant is a heterozygous dominant (green). This is in accordance with the law of dominance. This law states that when homozygous parents for contrasting traits are crossed then the F_1 hybrid progeny expresses the dominant trait.

13 (*a*) Mendel was a great mathematician and an Austrian Monk. He became interested in genetics and conducted experiments in pea plant (*Pisum sativum*). He hybridised the contrasting characters of the plant and conducted his experiments between 1856-1863. His experimental data was published in 1865.

14 (*c*) A cross between two individuals, one with AB blood group (I^AI^B) and the other with A blood group (I^Ai) will produce four genotypes and three phenotypes.

♀ \ ♂	I^A	I^B
I^A	I^AI^A	I^AI^B
i	I^A i	I^B i

Offspring

Genotypes : 4(I^AI^A, I^AI^B, I^A i, I^B i)

Phenotypes : 3 (A, B, AB)

15 (*a*) AB blood group is characterised by the presence of both antigens A and B, i.e. I^A and I^B over the surface of RBCs. Here, both alleles A and B are able to express themselves. This is called as codominance,

17 (*d*) **Parents** TT (Tall) × tt (Dwarf)

F_1-generation Tt (Heterozygous tall)

On selfing

Pollen → / Egg ↓	T	t
T	TT (Tall)	Tt (Tall)
t	Tt (Tall)	tt (Dwarf)

F_2-generation

Phenotypic ratio = 3 : 1 [Tall : Dwarf]

Genotypic ratio = 1 : 2 : 1

[Tall homozygous : Tall heterozygous : Dwarf]

19 (*b*)

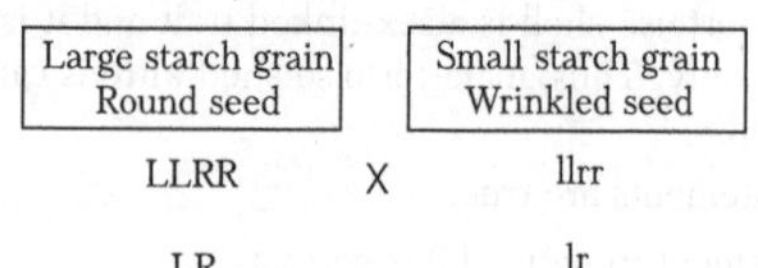

Ll Rr (F_1-generation)

After self crossing of F_2-generation, results obtained are

Gametes	LR	Lr	lR	lr
LR	LLRR	LLRr	LlRR	LlRr
Lr	LLRr	LLrr	LlRr	Llrr
lR	LlRR	LlRr	llRR	llRr
lr	LlRr	Llrr	llRr	llrr

Wrinkled and larger starch grains = 1

Round and intermediate starch grains = 6

So, ratio will be 6 : 1

Size of starch grains characters show incomplete dominance.

22 (*c*)

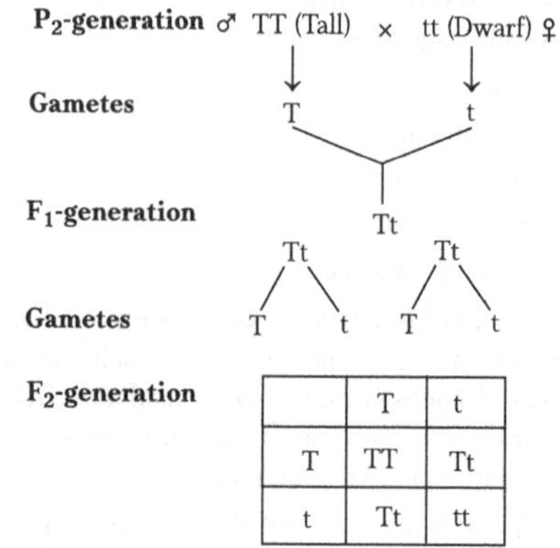

Phenotypic ratio = 3 : 1 } of **F_2-generation**
Genotypic ratio = 1 : 2 : 1 }
Parental generation ratio of genotypes (including both generations) = 1 : 1 : 1
Recombination genotypes = 1
Therefore, option (c) is correct.

23 (c)

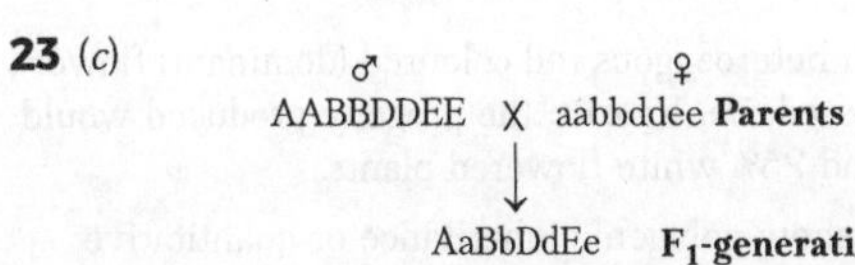

Types of gametes formed = 2^n(n = number of heterozygous genes)

$\therefore \quad 2^4 = 2 \times 2 \times 2 \times 2 = 16$ gametes

24 (d) Human blood type is determined by codominant alleles. It is inherited by single gene (present on autosome chromosome) with more than two alleles.

Since, there are three different alleles, these are a total of different genotypes at the human ABO genetic locus.

Genes	Blood group
I^AI^A	Blood group-A
I^AI^B	Blood group-AB
I^Ai	Blood group-A
I^BI^B	Blood group-B
I^Bi	Blood group-B
ii	Blood group-O

32 (c) Out of the crosses given in the option, the appropriate option is the cross between both homozygous recessive parents, i.e. tt × tt. As only parents having recessiveness can have recessive, F_1 progeny.

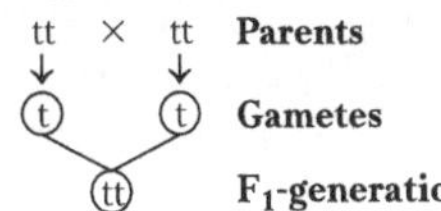

35 (b) (Yellow round flower, fruit) × (White elongated flower, fruit)
YYRR yyrr

F_1-generation
(20 plants survived)

YyRr
(Yellow round flower, fruit) Selfing

F_2-generation Yellow rounded : Yellow elongated : White rounded : White elongated
9 : 3 : 3 : 1

Now, out of total 960 species survived in F_2-generation, the number of plants that would have yellow flower and round fruit in F_2-generation will be $\frac{9 \text{ (round yellow)}}{16 \text{ (total progeny)}} \times 960$

(Total survived) = 540 plants

Thus, in F_1 and F_2-generation, total yellow colour, round fruit plants survived will be 20,540.

38 (c) According to the given question,

The ratio of darkness in decreasing order will be

AABBCC (III) ⟶ AAbbCC (I) ⟶
(All alleles are dominant and most dark) (Two alleles are dominant and less dark)

AAbbcc (II) ⟶ aabbcc (IV)
(Only one allele is dominant over other two so, it will be little less darker than previous) (Homozygous recessive, no allele will be able to express itself so, it will be least darker)

Thus, option (c) is correct.

40 (c) Since, F_1 has all tall plants, the possible genotypes of parents can be TT, TT or TT, Tt.

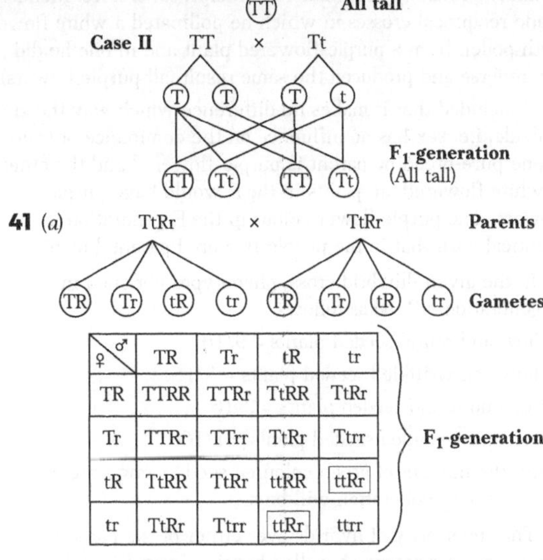

Plants with dwarf and pink characters (ttRr) are 2/16.

42 (d) Round shape in pea plant is dominant (R) over wrinkled (r). If pea plant in heterozygous state is self-crossed, following results would obtain.

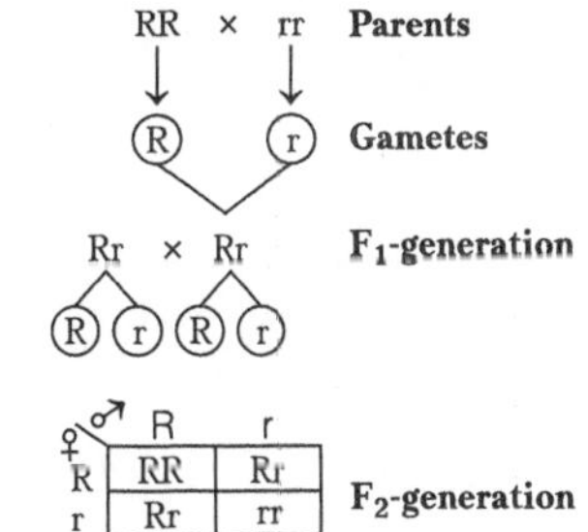

Phenotype 3 : 1(Round : Wrinkled)

If total 1600 seeds produced during the cross were subsequently germinated. The seeds that would have the parental phenotype will be $\left(\frac{3}{4} \times 1600 = 1200\right)$.

44 (d) All the offsprings have different phenotypes.

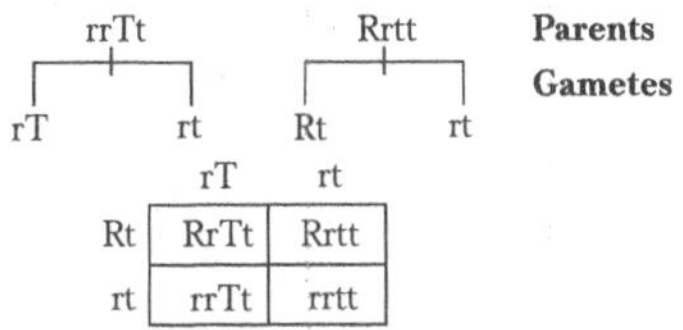

Therefore, the phenotypic ratio obtained by crossing rrTt and Rrtt is 1:1:1:1.

46 (a) A cross of round yellow seeds (both dominant and green wrinkled seeds (both recessive) plants produced 9 : 3 : 3 : 1 ratio of plants (phenotypic) in F_2-generation. The ratio of parental to recombinant is 10 : 6 here because 9 and 1 are parental type whereas 3 and 3 are recombinant type.

47 (*b*) In most plants, any cross can be made in two ways, depending on which phenotype is used as male or female. For example,

Phenotype A (female) × Phenotype B (male) and Phenotype B (female) × Phenotype A (male) are reciprocal crosses. Mendel made reciprocal crosses in which he pollinated a white flower with pollen from a purple-flowered plant and in one he did the reverse and produced the same result (all purple flowers).

He concluded that it makes no difference which way the cross is made, i.e. sex has no influence on the dominance of traits. If one pure-breeding parent is purple-flowered and the other is white flowered, all plants in the F_1 would have purple flowers. The purple flower colour in the F_1-generation is identical with that in the purple-flowered parental plants.

49 (*b*) In the given dihybrid cross, phenotypes obtained in F_2-generation will be as follows

Yellow and round seeded plants = 9/16

Yellow and wrinkled seeded plants = 3/16

Green and round seeded plants = 3/16

Green and wrinkled seeded plants = 1/16

Thus, the number of green coloured seed among sixteen products of F_2-generation will be 4.

54 (*d*) The superiority of hybrids over either of the parents (dominant or recessive) is called hybrid vigour (G Shull). Heterosis is equivalent of hybrid vigour.

55 (*c*) When both heterozygous red coloured (dominant) flower plants are crossed, i.e. Rr × Rr, the progeny produced would be 75% red and 25% white flowered plants.

56 (*c*) Polygenes show polygenic inheritance or quantitative inheritance. As genes are present on different chromosomes they segregate independently during meiosis.

$$\text{Types of gametes} = 2^n$$

$$\text{Number of individuals in } F_2 = (\text{Types of gametes})^2 = (2^n)^2$$

n = Number of heterozygous genes present

$$= (2^3)^2 = 8^2 = 64 \text{ individuals}$$

$$1 + 6 + 2x + 20 + 6 + 1 = 64$$

$$2x = 64 - 34$$

$$x = \frac{30}{2} = 15$$

59 (*b*) A cross between homozygous recessive (aa) and heterozygous plant (Aa) is called test cross. It gives 1:1 ratio in monohybrid and 1:1:1:1 ratio in dihybrid cross.

61 (*b*) Mendelian principles are not based asexually reproducing forms because gametes are not formed in them.

65 (*d*) Heterozygous round yellow has the genotype RrYy. On selfing, round green offsprings are produced and are represented by RRyy and Rryy genotypes only (R= Round; yy = Green).

CHAPTER 07

Chromosomal Basis of Inheritance

The machinery of inheritance lies in the nucleus as chromosomes, i.e. they form the basis of inheritance. The transmission of chromosomes occurs through male and female gametes.

In this chapter, we will discuss various topics related to inheritance, beginning with the chromosomal theory of inheritance.

Inside

CHROMOSOMAL THEORY OF INHERITANCE

Wilhelm Roux in 1833 stated that the chromosomes within the nucleus are involved in the hereditary process. Later on, **T Boveri** and **WS Sutton** studied the behaviour of chromosomes in 1902. They noted a close similarity between thc behaviour of chromosomes and that of Mendelian factors (genes). Based on their observations, they proposed the 'Chromosomal Theory of Inheritance'.

The factual details of this theory are given below

- This theory identified chromosomes as the genetic material responsible for Mendelian inheritance.
- Mendelian factors are located at specific loci on these chromosomes. They segregate and assort independently during meiosis and then pass on to the next generation.

Further, the chromosomal theory was confirmed when **TH Morgan** gave his theory of the gene as a discrete unit of chromosome.

Parallelism between chromosomes and genes

Based on chromosomal theory, a parallelism can be drawn between the chromosomes and genes as given below

1. Each species possesses a specific and characteristic number of chromosomes in its cells. In diploid cells (having two sets of chromosomes), these chromosomes are found in pairs. These pairs are called **homologous pairs** and resemble in morphology as well as in genetic content.

Out of the two sets of homologous pair, one set belongs to paternal side and the other set belongs to maternal side. Genes on the other hand, also exist in **allelomorphic pairs**, which are equally contributed by two parents.

2. Each chromosome is a distinct double-stranded structure consisting of two sister chromatids.
   (i) **During mitosis**, the two sister chromatids get separated into two daughter nuclei. Thus, both the alleles of a gene find place in two different daughter nuclei.
   (ii) **During meiosis**, two chromosomes of a homologous pair are separated and pass on to daughter nuclei. Similarly, the alleles of a gene also get separated (just like mitosis).
   Hence, each haploid cell or gamete contains only one chromosome of a type and only one of the two alleles of a trait.
3. During fertilisation, when two haploid gametes fuse, the paired condition of chromosome and alleles is restored.

Interpretation of Mendelian laws

On the basis of chromosomal theory of inheritance and parallelism between chromosomes and genes, we can easily explain the principle of segregation and independent assortment as follows

(i) With the separation of members of homologous chromosomes, the alleles of a gene also segregate and go to different gametes. This explains the principle of segregation.

(ii) When gametes belonging to two different homologous pairs fuse, a new allelic pair is formed. This explains the principle of independent assortment.

Experimental proof of chromosomal theory

- In 1916, a student of **Morgan** named **C Bridges** gave the experimental proof of chromosomal theory through his **non-disjunction experiment**. This **non-disjunction** refers to the occasional failure of two X-chromosomes to get separated from each other during gametogenesis.
- In this experiment, a cross was made between white-eyed females and red-eyed males of *Drosophila*. This cross resulted in F_1 flies possessing red-eyed females and white-eyed males.
- He noted that one in about every 2000 F_1 flies was an exception, i.e. either a white-eyed female or a red-eyed male.
- Bridges showed that these rare offsprings result from non-disjunction. This leads to the formation of some eggs with two X-chromosomes and others with none.
- The complete cross is given below

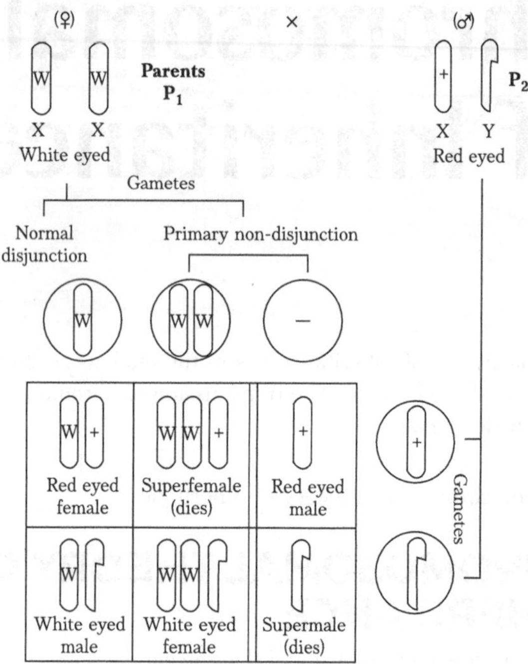

Fig. 7.1 Non-disjunction experiment of Bridges

- Usually animals with no X-chromosome are not detected because embryos that lack an X-chromosome are not viable. Similarly, most progeny with three X-chromosomes die early during development.
- Thus from the above cross, it can be interpreted that proper segregation of homologous chromosomes and the genes present on them is a pre-requisite for the viability of organisms. Any variation in the process leads to the formation of exceptional offsprings.

Evidences of chromosomal theory

Other processes of inheritance, which can be explained on the basis of chromosomal theory are as follows

1. Determination of sex
2. Crossing over
3. Linkage
4. Linkage maps
5. Different allelic phenomena like isoallele, pseudoallele and multiple allele
6. Mutation

DETERMINATION OF SEX

- The first definite evidence of chromosomal theory came from sex-determination. The sex behaves as a Mendelian character and its inheritance follows the law of segregation. Mostly the mechanisms of determination and differentiation of sexes are under the genetic control.
- Biologically, sex is an aggregate of morphological, physiological and behavioural qualities that differentiate males from females. This separation of two types of sexes is called as **gonochorism**.
- In plants, male and female do not differ morphologically except in floral characters, hence gonochorism is a rare phenomenon in them.

Sex-determination in animals

The various mechanisms of sex-determination in animals are discussed below

1. Chromosomal theory of sex-determination

- This theory was worked out by **EB Wilson** and **Stevens** (1902-1905). According to this theory, the male (♂) and female (♀) individuals normally differ in their chromosomal constitution.
- Following two types of chromosomes are present in these individuals.
  (i) **Sex chromosomes** or **Allosomes**, i.e. chromosomes responsible for the determination of sex, e.g. X and Y-chromosomes.
  (ii) **Autosomes**, i.e. chromosomes having no relation with the sex and contain genes which determine the somatic characters.

Note
- *The X-chromosome was first observed by German biologist **Henking** in 1891, during his studies on spermatogenesis in male bug. He called it **X-body**.*
- *Y-chromosome was discovered by **Stevens** in 1902.*

Parent types and systems

- On the basis of their constitution of sex chromosome, parents can be of following two types
  (i) **Homogametic** (homomorphic gametes), i.e. with similar gametes.
  (ii) **Heterogametic** (heteromorphic gametes), i.e. with different gametes.
- Among these, the heterogametic parent plays crucial role in determination of sex. Thus on this basis, we have following two types of systems among diploid organisms.
  - System having heterogametic males.
  - System having heterogametic females.

Sex-determination involving heterogametic males

The various mechanisms of sex-determination involving heterogametic male are as follows

(i) XX-XY pattern

- This is the most common method of sex-determination. It is found in mammals like humans and certain insects like *Drosophila*.
- In this pattern, the female possesses two homomorphic X-chromosomes (i.e. XX) and being homogametic, produces only one kind of eggs, i.e. their all eggs have one X-chromosome each.
- The male on the other hand are heteromorphic and possesses one X and one Y-chromosome (i. e. XY) and thus, produces two kinds of sperms. Half of these sperms consists of X-chromosome, while the other half consists of Y-chromosome.
- The sex of embryo depends upon the kind of sperm that fertilises the egg. A female individual is produced if egg is fertilised with a sperm having X-chromosome and a male is produced if the egg is fertilised with Y-chromosome bearing sperm.
- A complete cross of this sex-determination is given below

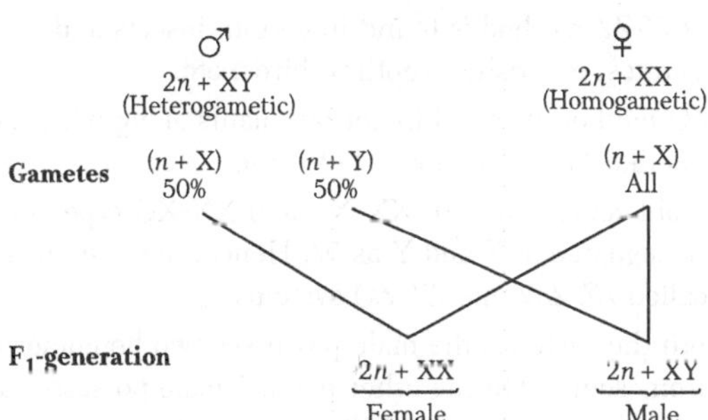

Fig. 7.2 XX-XY pattern of sex-determination

Note *The Y-chromosome supports the male sex as it has the genes for secondary sexual characters. Most of the part of it is present as heterochromatic region.*

(ii) XX-XO pattern

- This pattern is found in certain insects, especially those of class—Hemiptera (true bugs) and order—Orthoptera, e.g. grasshopper.
- In this pattern, the female has two X-chromosomes (called XX), while male has only one X-chromosome (called XO).
- The Y-chromosome is completely absent. Thus, the presence of unpaired X-chromosome determines the masculine sex.
- The female produces only one type of eggs and male produces two types of sperms, i.e. 50% with one X-chromosome and 50% without any sex chromosome.

- The sex of offspring depends upon the type of sperm, which fertilises the egg as shown below

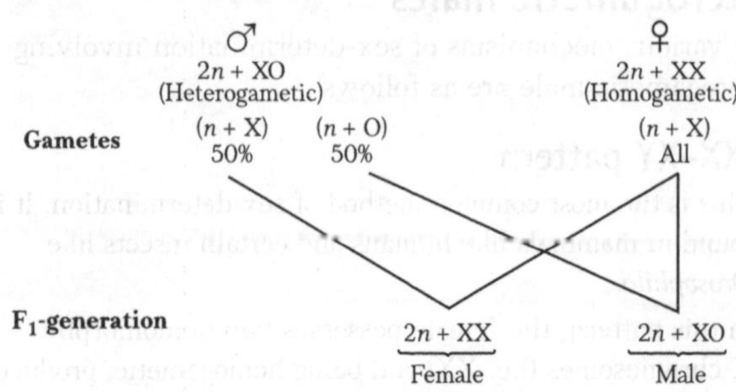

Fig. 7.3 XX-XO pattern of sex-determination

Note *Although in the XX-XX and XX-XO methods, it is the type of sperm, which plays major role. The sex is ascertained on the basis of the presence or absence of paired X-chromosome. If the X-chromosome is paired, result is seen as female and if it is unpaired, the result is seen as a male.*

Sex-determination involving heterogametic female

Sex determining patterns based on this system are as follows

ZZ-ZW and ZZ-ZO pattern

- The ZW-ZZ method is found in certain insects and vertebrates, e.g. fishes, reptiles, birds, etc.
- ZZ-ZO method is found in certain plants along with some insects like *Fumea* (a moth), butterflies, etc.
- To avoid confusion with XX-XY and XX-XO type here, X is designated as Z and Y as W. Hence, the systems here are called ZZ-ZW and ZZ-ZO systems.
- In both the systems, the male possesses two homomorphic Z-chromosomes. On the other hand, female possesses a single Z-chromosome in ZZ-ZO system and a Z-chromosome supported by the W-chromosome in ZZ-ZW systems.
- Thus, the female produces two types of gametes, i.e. 50% with Z-chromosome and rest 50% either with W-chromosome or without Z-chromosome.
- The mechanism sex-determination in both the systems is same. The paired Z results in male, while single Z or Z with W defines the female.

The chromosomal mechanism discussed above are not always correct. It was **Patterson** who reported that sometimes in *Drosophila*, the Y-chromosome is heterochromatic and plays a insignificant role in sex-determination. He gave the theory of genic balance.

2. Genic balance mechanism

- It has been observed that an organism generally have inherent potentialities for both the sexes and each individual is intermediate between male and female sexes.
- In *Drosophila*, it is the ratio between the X-chromosome and autosome, which determines the sex. These observations were based upon various experiments carried on *Drosophila* triploids.

Bridges experiment of genic balance

According to **CB Bridges** in *Drosophila*,

- **X-chromosome** is responsible for female characteristics.
- **Y-chromosome** is responsible for male characteristics.
- **Autosome** is necessary for the fertility of sex, but not responsible for any sex-determination.
- A single X-chromosome in a diploid organism produces male sex and XX combination within a diploid organism produces females.
- In his experiments, bridges crossed a triploid female (3A+ XXX) with a diploid male (2A+ XY) are obtained intersexes, supermales and superfemales as shown in the result below

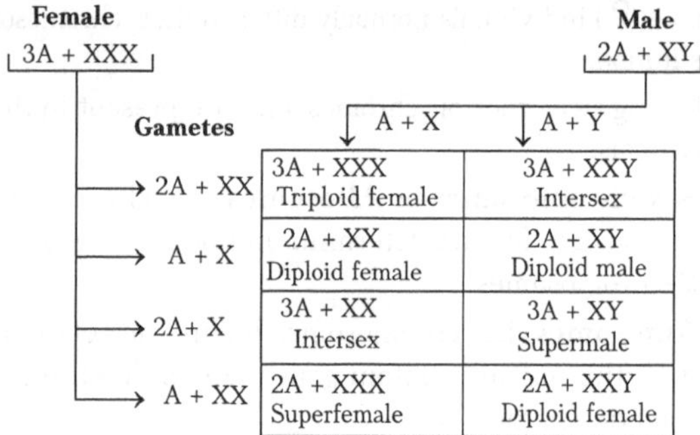
Female: 3A + XXX; Male: 2A + XY

Gametes	A + X	A + Y
2A + XX	3A + XXX Triploid female	3A + XXY Intersex
A + X	2A + XX Diploid female	2A + XY Diploid male
2A+ X	3A + XX Intersex	3A + XY Supermale
A + XX	2A + XXX Superfemale	2A + XXY Diploid female

Fig 7.4 Genic balance in Drosophila

- The presence of triploid intersexes in the above experiment is a proof that autosomes also carry genes for sex-determination.
- The interpretation of results was based on the following ratio between number of X-chromosomes and set of autosomes (A)
  (i) 1.0-female
  (ii) 0.5-male
  (iii) More than 1-superfemale
  (iv) Less than 0.5-supermale
  (v) Between 0.5 to 1-intersex

- Thus according to him, it is the delicate balance between the X-chromosomes and autosomes which is responsible for sex-determination.
- This theory is very helpful in predicting the sex of individuals that arise from non-disjunction of X-chromosome during meiosis in female.

Gynandromorphs

- In *Drosophila*, occasionally flies are obtained with one half of body having male characteristics and another half having female characteristics, as shown below

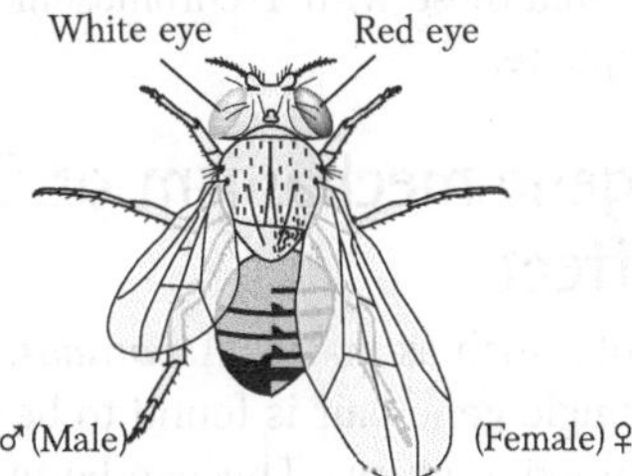

Fig. 7.5 Gynandromorph of Drosophila, in which right half is male while the left half is female

- Such flies with both the male and female characters are known as **gynandromorphs** or **sex mosaic**.
- These are formed when there is formation of two blastomeres with unequal number of X-chromosomes during first zygotic division.
- The blastomere with $2n$ + X-chromosome forms the male half and the blastomere with $2n$ + XX-chromosome forms the female half.
- The occurrence of gynandromorphs clearly indicates that the number of X-chromosome determines the sex of individual and it is due non-disjunction of X-chromosomes during first (mitotic) division of zygote.
- In *Drosophila*, another possibility is also visible. The fly may be a male or female with patches of tissue of other sex on it, is called **gynander**.

3. Haplo-diploidy mechanism

- Another mechanism of sex-determination is male haploidy or haplodiploidy or **arrhenotoky**.
- This mechanism is particularly common in hymenopteran insects, e.g. honeybee, wasp, ants, etc.
- All these insects have one thing in common, i.e. they show parthenogenesis.
- So in these insects, following three types of individuals are seen.
  (i) **Diploid queen** These are fully functional females developed from fertilised eggs.
  (ii) **Diploid workers** These are underdeveloped or sexually non-functional females developed from fertilised eggs.
    - In actual, the fertilised egg gives rise to the females only. Out of these, the female which fed on Royal jelly (a specialised food) becomes queen and rest develop into **workers.**
    - The workers perform specific function of protection of colony, while queen is involved in egg production.
    - The workers are unable to perform fertilisation and egg laying. The organs of oviposition in workers are modified into sting apparatus.
  (iii) **Haploid males or Drones** Functional males are developed parthenogenetically from haploid eggs.
    - These males are short-lived and normally die after fertilisation.
    - Since, males develop parthenogenetically, we can say that in this mechanism parthenogenesis plays a major role in the determination of sex. The sex chromosomes have no significance here.
    - In certain extreme cases, males are altogether absent and females are produced by parthenogenesis. These females are always diploid, e.g. *Lacerta sexicola.*

Special haplodiploidy in parasitic wasp (Bracon hebetor)

- In *Habrobracon juglandis* (a parasitic wasp, also called *Bracon hebetor*), the initial sex-determination mechanism is similar to wasps and bees.
- In them, unfertilised eggs develop into males and fertilised eggs develop into females.
- The difference lies in the fact that some fertilised eggs also develop into males. This is due to the presence of a number of alleles promoting maleness and femaleness, e.g. X_A, X_B, X_C and X_D, etc.
- The diploid males have homozygous condition of these alleles, while diploid females have heterozygous condition.

4. Hormonal control of sex-determination

Apart from above written mechanisms of genetic control, hormonal and environmental factors are also involved in determining the sex. The sex-determination theories (chromosomal theory and genic balance) are applicable to lower animals but in higher vertebrates, hormones, especially the gonadal hormones may considerably alter the sexual characters. For example,

- In fowl, if the ovary from a genetic female is removed (intentionally or accidentally), it results into the development of male comb along with male plumage and in extreme cases, testes will also appear (findings of crene).
- The above case of sex reversal can be explained by assuming that as soon as the ovary was removed or destroyed, the production of ovarian hormones were stopped. After some time, the dormant testes present as rudiments in almost all the female birds start functioning.
- This leads to the production of male hormones which help in the development of secondary sexual characters and sperm formation in extreme cases.
- Cases of such sex reversal are also observed in some fishes, amphibians, birds and even in mammals. In mammals, such cases are reported as free martins by **FrLillie**.

5. Environmental control of sex-determination

- **F Baltzor** first observed that sex-determination in a marine worm, *Bonellia viridis* is controlled by environmental factors. In *Bonellia*, usually all the larvae are genetically and cytologically similar.
- If the larva settles near the proboscis of an adult female, it develops into the male individual. If the larva settles in mud, it develops into a female.
- In **turtles**, a temperature below 28°C produces more males, above 33°C produces more females and between 28-33°C produces males and females in equal proportion.

Sex-determination in plants

Most flowering plants are monoecious, hence they are without sex chromosomes. The well-known examples of dioecious plants are usually under the direct control of single gene locus.

The mechanism of sex-determination in plants is given below

1. Sex chromosome mechanism

- Chromosomal activity has been reported in many plant species, like *Melandrium album, Coccinia indica* and *Vallisneria spiralis,* etc.
- In *Coccinia* and *Melandrium,* XX-XY type of mechanism is seen. The male plant have XY combination, while female plant have XX combination.
- The sex chromosome mechanism of sex-determination is observed in certain monoploid bryophytes like *Sphaerocarpus.* In these plants also, XX female and XY male is seen. It means that the sporophyte containing XY combination produces two types of meiospores, some with X and other with Y-chromosome.
- The meiospores with X-chromosome form female gametophyte and those with Y-chromosome produces male gametophyte.

2. Single gene mechanism or Single gene effect

In certain plants, such as maize, *Asparagus, Neurospora,* yeast, etc., a single gene pair is found to be responsible for the determination of sex. This can be understood with the help of following example of *Asparagus.*

- *Asparagus* is a dioecious plant in which female flowers bear rudimentary anthers and male flowers bear rudimentary pistils. However, it may be seen that the male flowers sometimes set the seed.
- In one such case, when seeds obtained from a rare male flower were raised into plants and allowed to self-fertilise, the male and female plants of next generation were found to be present in the ratio of 3:1.
- Hence in this case, maleness is dominant over femaleness and the rare male plant is heterozygous as shown below

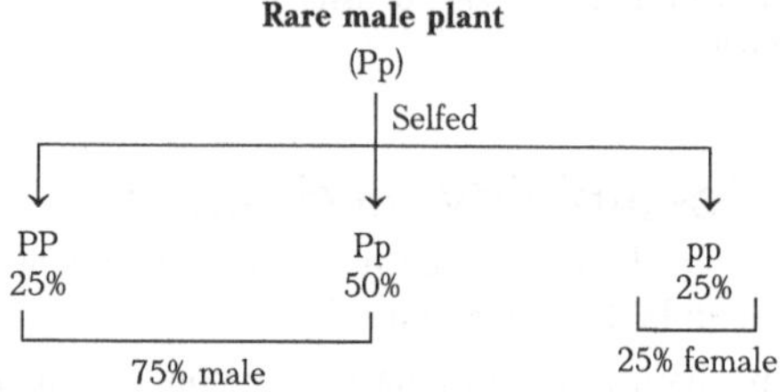

***Fig. 7.6** Single gene effect*

- Similarly, when these male plants were raised and used to pollinate female flowers, only 2/3rd of them show segregation, suggesting the control of sex by a single gene pair.

CHECK POINT 7.1

1. Sutton and Boveri argued that the pairing and separation of a pair of chromosomes would lead to
   (a) the segregation of a pair of factors they carried
   (b) the segregation of the characters
   (c) recombination of the factors they carried
   (d) Both (b) and (c)

2. In bugs, cockroach and roundworms, the male possesses
   (a) one chromosome less than the female
   (b) two similar sex-chromosomes
   (c) one chromosome different from rest
   (d) a Y-chromosome

3. Sex-determination ratio in an organism is given by $\frac{X}{A} = 1.5$, then organism will be
   (a) male (b) female
   (c) superfemale (d) intersex

4. In *Drosophila*, a male or female with the patches of other sex is called
   (a) Bracon hebetor
   (b) Gynandromorph
   (c) Gynander
   (d) free martin

5. The sex-determination mechanism which is associated with parthenogenesis is
   (a) genic balance mechanism
   (b) sex chromosome
   (c) haplodiploidy
   (d) Environmental control

6. Plant showing single gene mechanism of sex-determination are dioecious. In then which of the following gene effect will show female plant?
   (a) PP (b) Pp (c) pp (d) All of these

CROSSING OVER

- It is the process of interchanging the segments between non-sister chromatids of homologous chromosomes. The chromatin resulting from such interchanges of chromosomal parts are called **crossovers.**
- Crossing over produces new combinations (recombinants) of genes. It occurs in pachytene stage of prophase of cell division. During the process, homologous chromosomes are at 4 stranded stage. The 2:2:2:2 arrangement of ascospores in ascus of *Neurospora* proves that crossing over occurs at 4 strand stage.
- Crossing over may even lead to the separation of linked genes.

Types of crossing over

The crossing over can be of following types

1. Somatic or Mitotic crossing over

- This crossing over occurs in somatic cells of an organism during mitotic cell division and thus, has no genetic significance. It is the process of very rare occurrence.
- Somatic crossing over was first reported by **Curt Stern** in somatic cells of *Drosophila* for bristles and hair. Later on, **G Pontecarvo** described it in fungus, *Aspergillus nodulans.*
- The somatic crossover produces patches of crossover tissue between the normal cells, i.e. mosaic appearance. A mosaic of even one cell has been recognised in *Drosophila* for bristles and hair.

2. Germinal or Meiotic crossing over

It occurs in germ cells or germinal cells during meiosis, i.e. during gametogenesis. Germinal crossing over is of universal occurrence and is of great genetic significance. Usually, it is of following three types

(i) **Single crossing over,** i.e. the condition in which crossing over is seen only at one point within a homologous pair. As a result of single crossing over, only one chiasma is formed.

(ii) **Double crossing over,** i.e. the condition in which crossing over takes place at two points within the same homologous pair. This leads to the formation of two chiasma (reciprocal or complementary).

(iii) **Multiple crossing over,** i.e. the condition in which crossing over takes place at more than two points within the same homologous pair. It results in the formation of many chiasma.

Mechanism of crossing over

It involves the following steps

Synapsis

First of all, pairing of homologous chromosomes takes place during zygotene stage of prophase-I. This process is called synapsis. The resultant paired chromosomes are called **bivalents.**

Duplication of chromosomes

- This is followed by chromosome duplication in which each homologous chromosome of bivalent, splits longitudinally to form two identical sister chromatids.
- These are held together by an unsplitted centromere. Now, each bivalent contains four arms with two chromatids. At this stage, it is referred to as **tetrad.**

Crossing over by breakage and union

- After tetrad formation, crossing over occurs during which two non-sister chromatids exchange their segments. After exchange, the chromosomal parts start repelling each other except at the point of contact. As a result, cross-shaped or X-shaped structures called **chiasmata** are formed.
- The number of chiasmata depends upon the length of chromosome and the type of crossover.
- The formation of chiasmata between any two gene loci has a characteristic probability, i.e. the more apart the two genes are located, the greater probability of chiasmata formation they have.

Enzymes in Crossing over

Stern and Hotta (1969) have described that the breakage of chromatids is brought about by a nuclear enzyme endonuclease. The fusion of broken segments takes place due to the action of another enzyme ligase. Thus, these two enzymes help in the exchange of segments during crossing over.

Terminalisation

- After chiasmata formation, the chromosomes start separating progressively from each other, beginning at centromere and moving towards the chiasma.
- In this process, the chiasma itself move in a zipper-like fashion towards the ends of tetrads. This zipper movement of chiasma is called **terminalisation** and it results into complete separation of homologous pairs.
- All the steps are shown in following figure

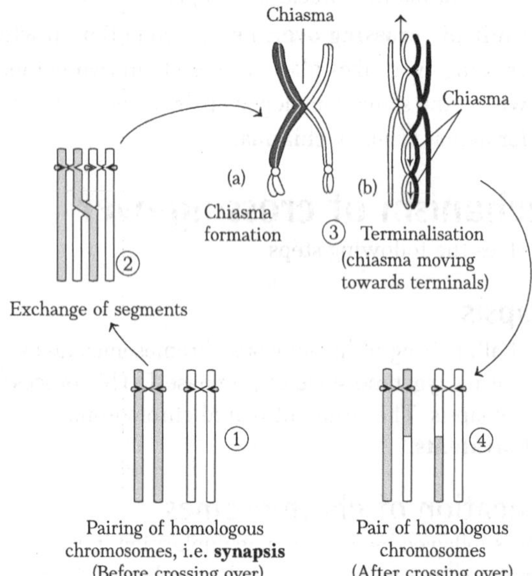

Fig 7.7 Crossing over

Factors affecting crossing over

Many factors affect the frequency of crossing over. These are

- **Distance** The frequency of crossing over of genes is directly proportional to the distance between them in the chromosome. This statement is called **Morgan** and **Sturtevant's hypothesis.** The more distance between two genes, the greater opportunity they have for crossing over and *vice-versa.*
- **Age** Crossing over frequency generally decreases with increasing age.
- **X-rays** Exposure to X-rays increases the frequency of crossing over.
- **Sex** Crossing over has not been reported in male fruitfly. Male mammals have less frequent crossing over than their female counterparts.
- **Temperature** Variations in temperature increase the frequency of crossing over.
- **Location** The genes which are located near the ends and centromere, the frequency of crossing over is very much reduced.
- **Interference** One crossover lessens the chance of another crossing over to occur near it.

LINKAGE

- In most organisms, the number of genes per individual far exceed the number of chromosomal pairs. It means that each chromosome bears many genes. These genes are usually arranged in linear fashion over the chromosome and do not show independent assortment.
- The phenomenon of genic inheritance in which genes of a particular chromosome show the tendency to inherit together is known as **linkage.**
- The genes showing linkage are known as **linked genes.** Such genes retain their parental combination even in the offsprings.
- The strength of linkage between any two genes is inversely proportional to the distance between the two genes.

Linkage groups

- All the linked genes located on a single chromosome constitute a linkage group. The total number of linkage groups in an organism are always equal to the haploid number of chromosomal number of that species.

- All the genes of a chromosome have their identical allelomorphs on the homologous chromosomes, therefore linkage group of a homologous pair of chromosome is considered one. For example, *Drosophila melanogaster* has four linkage groups. Similarly, 23 linkage groups are present in man, seven in sweet pea, etc.

Mechanism of linkage

The mechanism of linkage was explained by **TH Morgan** and **Castle** in 1911 in chromosome theory of linkage. However, its existence was predicted even before by different workers.

First suggestion about this tendency was given by **Sutton** in 1903, but he was lacking in experimental verifications of his thoughts. Afterwards, **Bateson** and **Punnett** in 1906, suggested the existence of linkage in their coupling and repulsion experiment.

Coupling and repulsion experiment

Bateson in 1905 performed a cross in *Lathyrus odoratus* (sweat pea) where he observed a deviation from Mendel's law of independent assortment.

In this experiment, following two cases were discussed

Case I

- Plants of sweet pea having blue flowers and long pollen (**BBLL**) were crossed with red flowers and round pollen (**bbll**).
- The F_1 individuals thus obtained had long pollen and blue flowers with genetic constitution BbLl. These were then test crossed.
- Normally, if independent assortment takes place, the expected ratio in a test cross is 1:1:1:1. But here, the ratio obtained in test cross was 7:1:1:7. Bateson called it **gametic coupling**.
- This complete cross is shown below

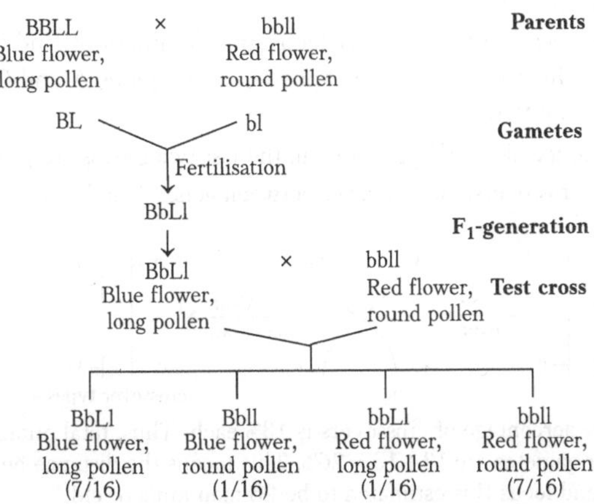

Fig.7.8 Cross showing the coupling experiment

- The ratio obtained by Bateson was due to the fact that during coupling, the two dominant or recessive genes that come from same parents tend to remain together.

Case 2

- Similar results were observed when the plants with genetic constitution **BBll** (i.e. blue flower round pollen) were crossed with plants of genetic constitution **bbLL** (i.e. red flower long pollen).
- The F_1 hybrid had plants with BbLL (i.e. blue flower long pollen). The F_1 test cross resulted in1:7:7:1 instead of expected 1:1:1:1. Bateson called this deviation as **gametic repulsion**. This complete cross is shown below

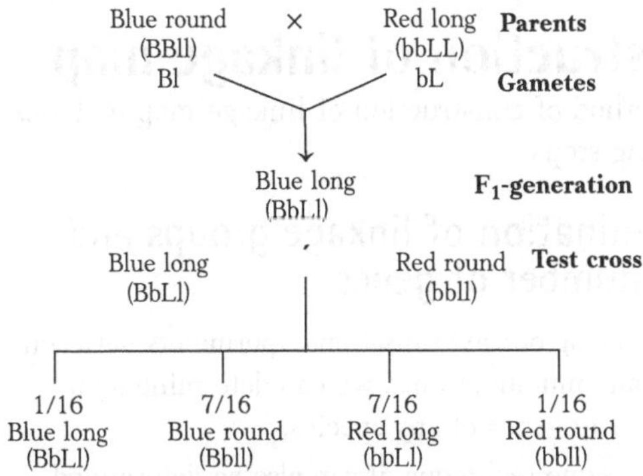

Fig. 7.9 Cross showing the repulsion experiment

On the basis of his experiments, Bateson gave his coupling and repulsion hypothesis.

According to this, coupling and repulsion was due to the tendency of genes to inherit together.

Conclusion

- So from above experiment, it is clear that if there is no crossover, all the alleles on a single chromosome would segregate together and would end up in same gamete. Hence, the coupling occurs.
- However during repulsion, the two dominant or recessive genes that come from different parents tend to remain separated.

Types of linkage

According to Morgan *et. al.*, the linkage can be

(i) **Complete or Perfect** It is found in all those cases, where genes remain together in the same chromosome for at least two generations, e.g. genes for bent wings (bt) and shaven bristles (srn) on 4th chromosome in mutant of *Drosophila.*

(ii) **Incomplete or Imperfect** It is found in all those cases, where genes remain together within the same chromosome for less than two generations. This linkage is very common and has been studied in almost all the organisms.

LINKAGE MAPS

- The graphic representation of the relative distances between the genes in a linkage group is called the **linkage map** or **chromosomal map** or **genetic map** or **crossover maps.**
- These are expressed in terms of percentage of crossing over and given for a single group of chromosomes.
- First chromosomal map was given by **Strutevant** and **Morgan**. It was the graphic representation of five genes on X-chromosome of *Drosophila.*

Construction of linkage map

The method of construction of linkage map includes following steps

Determination of linkage groups and total number of genes

- By carrying out hybridisation experiments between wild and mutant strains, we can determine total number of genes of any species.
- By the same technique, it can also be determined that how many phenotypic traits remain always together (linked) and consequently their determiners (genes) during the course of inheritance.
- Thus, different linkage groups of a species can be worked out.

Determination of map distance

- It is done with the help of test crosses. These test crosses can be
  - **Two point** test crosses which are helpful in detecting single crossover.
  - **Three point** crossovers which are helpful in detecting double crossovers.
- The map distances are calculated after knowing the total number of genes in each linkage group and percentage of crossing over between them.
- This percentage of crossing over is also known as **crossover frequency**. It is considered as the main parameter to calculate the map distance and show a linear relationship between genes.
- It is calculated with the help of following formula

$$\text{Crossover\%} = \frac{\text{Number of recombinants}}{\text{Total number of offsprings}} \times 100$$

Each crossover event unusually results in 50% recombinant gametes and 50% parental gametes.

- The figure given below is showing linkage between two genes, A and B.

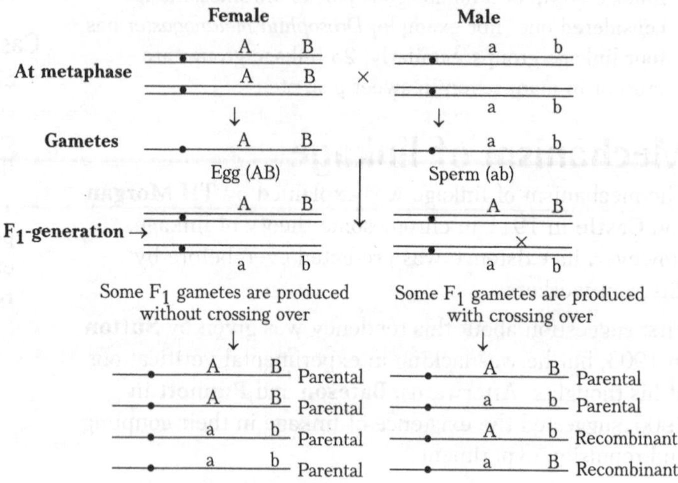

Fig. 7.10 Linkage between any genes A and B

Map unit

- An arbitrary unit of measurement called **map unit** is used to describe the distances between the linked genes.
- One map unit represents the linear distance within which one per cent crossing over takes place, i.e.

  1 map unit = 1% of crossing over
- One map unit is now referred to as **cM** (centiMorgan) in the honour of Morgan's contribution.

  1 cM = 100% crossing over

For better understanding, it is suggestive to go through following examples.

Example 7.1 A dihybrid having genotype AaCc is crossed with its double recessive parent, i.e. aacc. The results of F_2-generation are

(a) 37% dominant genes at both the loci (AAcc)
(b) 37% recessive genes at both the loci (aacc)
(c) 13% dominant genes at 1st locus and recessive at IInd (Ac/ac)
(d) 13% recessive genes at 1st locus and dominant at IInd (ac/ac)

Find out the approximate distance between genes A and C from the results given.

Among the members of F_2-generation, the last two groups are produced by single crossovers, i.e. crossover between genes A and C. It can be seen as

A— —a Cross over A— —a After separation A— —a
C— —c C— —c c— —C
crossover types

Here, the percentage of crossovers is 13% each. Thus, total number of crossover gametes are 13 + 13 = 26%. This means the distance between locus A and locus C is estimated to be 26 map units or cM.

Example 7.2 Three genes A, B and C are present within the same linkage group. A test cross is performed between trihybrid AaBbCc and its recessive parent aabbcc. Following results are obtained in F_2-generation.

(a) **Parental type,** i.e.

(i) ABC/abc = 36% (ii) abc/abc = 36%

Total parental types = 72%

(b) **Crossover type I** between locus A and B, i.e. single crossovers

(i) Abc/abc = 9% (ii) aBc/abc = 9%

Total single crossover types between A and B (Region 1) is 9 + 9 = 18%

(c) **Crossover type II** between locus B and C, i.e. single crossover

(i) ABc/abc = 4% (ii) abC/abc = 4%

Total single crossover types between locus B and C (region 2) is equal to 4 + 4 = 8%

(d) **Crossover type III** between (A–B) and (B–C), i.e. double crossover

(i) AbC/abc = 1% (ii) aBc/abc = 1%

Total double crossover type between locus (A–B) and (B – C) is equal to 1 + 1 = 2%

The given crossovers can be explained by following figures

(a) **Parental type**

(b) **Crossover type I**, i.e. between locus A and B

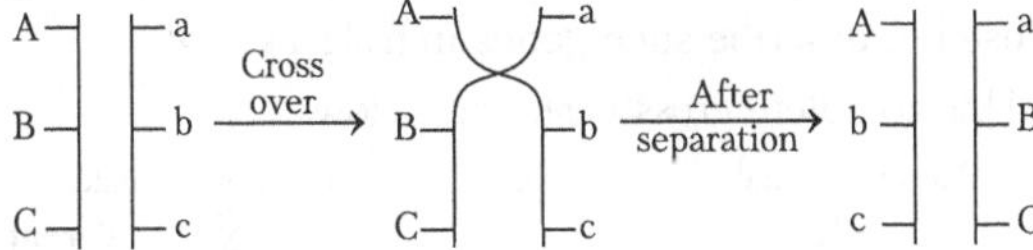

(c) **Crossover type II**, i.e. between locus B and C

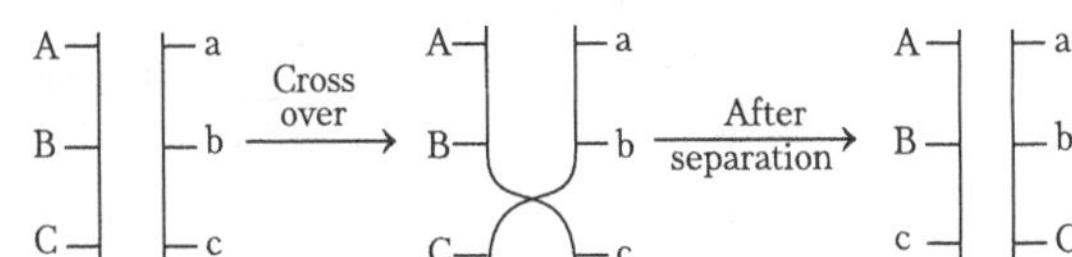

(d) **Crossover type III**, i.e. double crossover

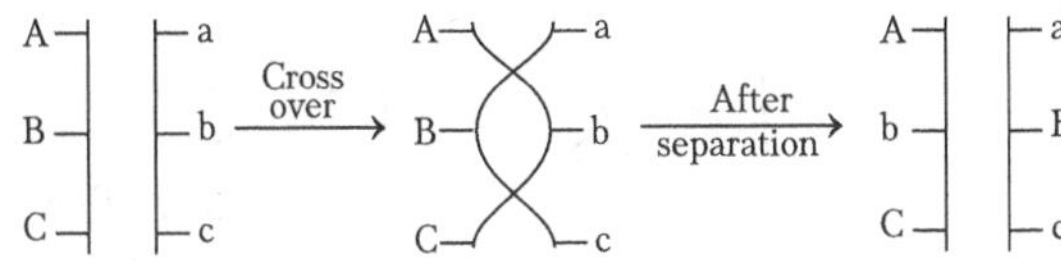

Now, the distance between gene locus A and gene locus B is % single crossovers in the region +% double crossovers in the region = 18+ 2 = 20 map units or cM.

Likewise, distance between gene locus B and C is = 8+ 2 = 10 map units or Morgan or cM.

From the above two distances, the distance between genes A and C can be calculated as

Distance between A and B + Distance between B and C = 20 + 10 = 30 map units.

Alternatively

Distance between A and C can also be calculated directly as follows

(Single crossover percentage between locus A and B) +
(Single crossover percentage between locus B and C)
2 × double crossover percentage between (A – B) and (B – C).

Example 7.3 The distance between genes A and B is 20 map units, B and C is 10 map units and A and C is 30 map units. Based on the given information, find out the possible order of genes A, B and C.

Let us assume that gene A is present in the middle, i.e.

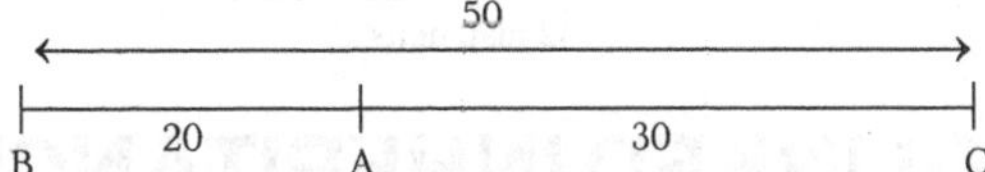

From this order, the distance between B and C comes out to be 50 map units, which is not in accordance with our findings (B – C = 10 cM).

Let us assume that C is present in middle, i.e.

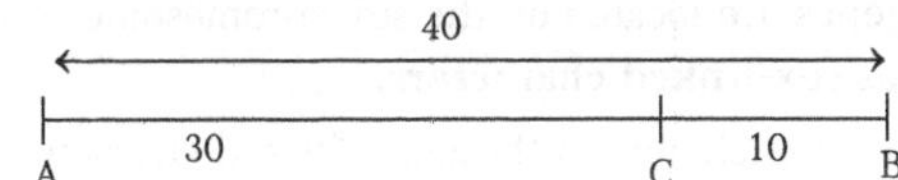

From this order, also the distance between A and B comes to be 40 map units, which is not in accordance with our findings (A – B = 20 cM).

Let us assume that B is present in the middle as shown below

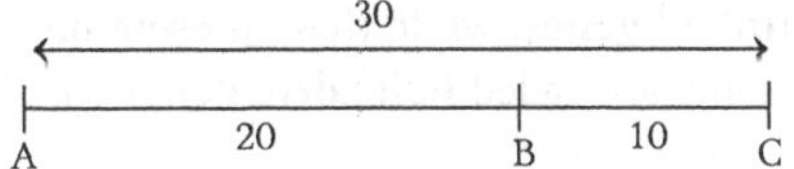

This arrangement satisfies all the conditions, i.e.

A – B = 20 Map units
B – C = 10 Map units
A – C = 30 Map units

Hence, the correct order of genes is A, B and C as seen above.

Example 7.4 Three map segments are given in the figure below. Based on these segments, construct a complete genetic map.

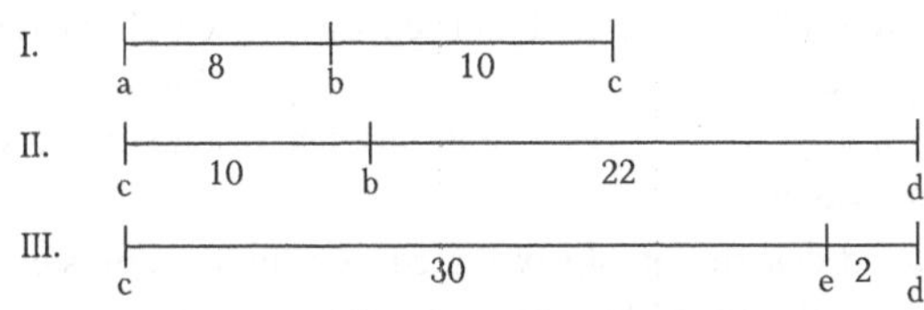

We can superimpose the give map segments by aligning the genes shared in common as

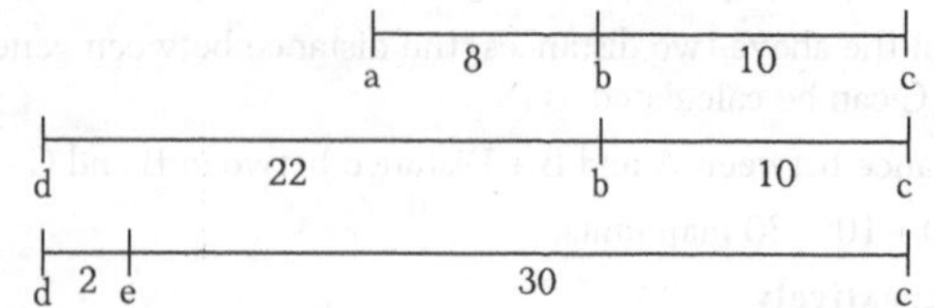

Now, we can combine them finally as

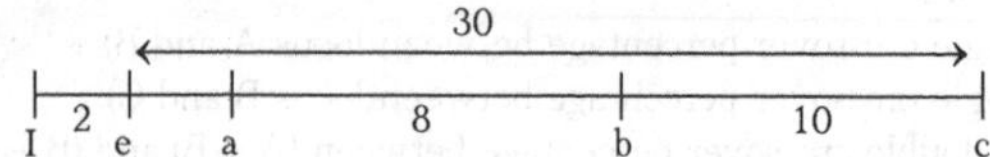

Distance between a and e = 30 − 8 − 10 = 12 map units.

Distance between c and d = 30 + 2 = 32 map units.

Thus, the combined map looks like

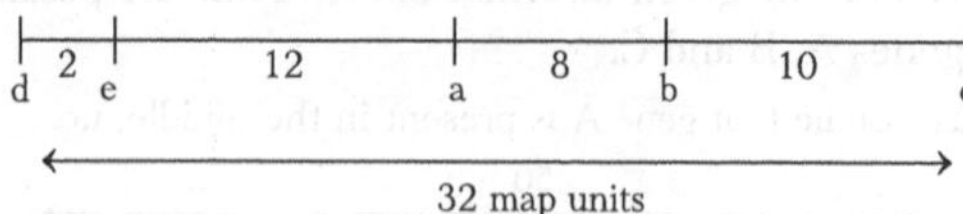

SEX-LINKED INHERITANCE

- Sex chromosomes are primarily concerned with the determination of sex. However, sex chromosomes also carry genes for other characters. The somatic characters whose genes are located on the sex chromosomes are known as **sex-linked characters**.
- The genes which govern these sex-linked characters are known as **sex-linked genes** and the phenomenon of their inheritance is known as **sex-linked inheritance**, e.g. haemophilia, colour blindness in human.
- The sex-linked genes located on X-chromosomes are called **X-linked genes**, while those present on Y-chromosome are called **holandric genes** (Greek, *holes* - whole; *andros* - makes).
- There are certain characters that are not linked to sex chromosomes, but are limited to one sex only. Such characters are known as **sex-limited** and **sex-influenced traits.**
- These differ from one another in the fact that sex-limited character is not seen totally in one sex, while sex-influenced character is seen more frequently in one sex than in the other.
- The genes for sex-limited and sex-influenced character are present in autosomes, but their expression is determined by the presence or absence of one of the sex chromosomes.
- Detailed description of sex-linked, sex-limited and sex influenced traits of humans is given in next chapter.

Concept of sex-linked inheritance by TH Morgan

The concept of sex-linked inheritance was introduced by **TH Morgan** in 1910 while working on *Drosophila melanogaster.*

Morgan experiment on *Drosophila*

- In *Drosophila*, sometimes a sudden appearance of one white-eyed in the culture of wild red-eyed *Drosophila* is noticed. Morgan crossed this white-eyed male with red-eyed female. This cross led to the formation of F_1 flies that were red-eyed.
- It indicates that the gene for white-eye colour is recessive to red-eye colour.
- When the F_1 flies were self-crossed, the red and white-eyed individuals appeared in the ratio of 3 : 1. Here, all white-eyed individuals were male, while red-eyed individuals were both male and female. No females with white-eyed were seen.
- Morgan concluded on the basis of this experiment that gene for eye colour is located on X-chromosome.
- The female flies will have white-eye colour only when both the X-chromosomes contain gene for white-eye, i.e. homozygous recessive condition. On the other hand, if a female fly contains either one X-chromosome with gene for white-eye colour or both the X-chromosomes with gene for red-eye colour, the fly will have red coloured eyes.
- In males, however one X-chromosome with gene for white eye colour gives white eyed males. The term hemizygous is used to describe such genes in male sex.
- This complete cross is shown below

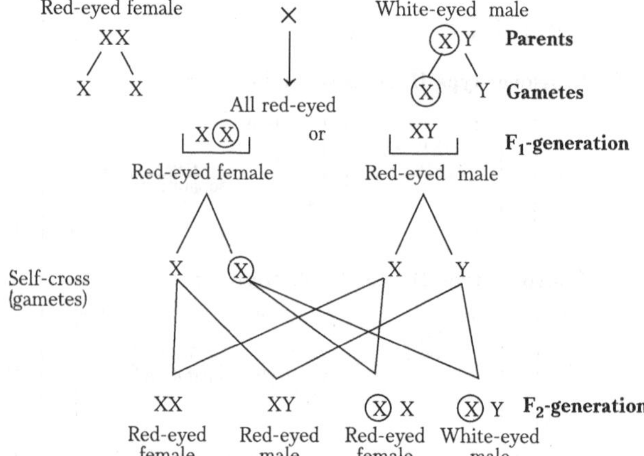

Fig. 7.11 Showing sex-linked inheritance in Drosophila

In a reciprocal cross, Morgan crossed a red-eyed male to a white-eyed female. Here, the F_1-generation individuals showed the presence of white-eyed members also. This reciprocal cross is shown below

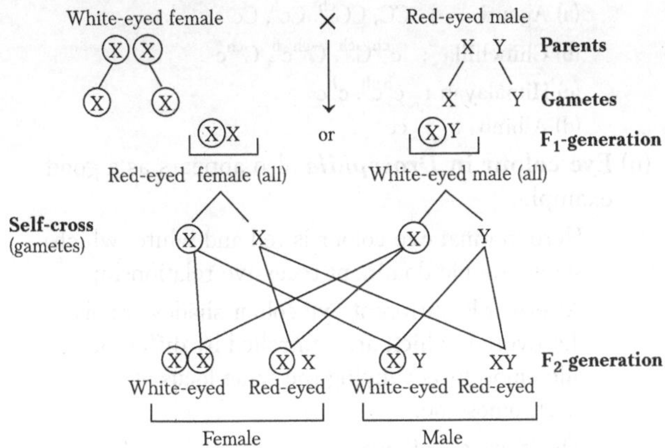

Fig. 7.12 Showing sex- linked cross in Drosophila

- Thus, here all the results of the cross are absolutely different from the previous cross.
- The difference lies in appearance of both the traits of eye colour in equal proportions in both the sexes of F_2-generation.

Conclusion

- Based on the results of both the crosses, Morgan concluded that eye colour gene is linked to sex and is located on the X-chromosome.
- Inheritance of this X-chromosome occurs in a *criss-cross* manner. It means that a male transmits his characteristics to his grandson through his daughter (carriers), while a female transmits the characteristic to her grand daughter through her son.

CHECK POINT 7.2

1. Linkage and crossing over are
   (a) inversely proportional to each other
   (b) directly proportional to each other
   (c) not related to each other
   (d) some phenomena
2. Which of the following is suitable for experiments on linkage?
   (a) AABB × aabb (b) AaBb × AaBb
   (c) AABB × aaBB (d) AAbb × AaBB
3. Assume that a crossover and resulting chiasma occurred between two gene loci 100% of the time. What would be the percentage of recombinant chromosomes among the progeny?
   (a) 100% (b) 50% (c) 25% (d) 75%
4. There are three genes a, b, c percentage of crossing over between a and b is 20%, b and c is 28% and a and c is 8%. What is the sequence of genes on chromosome?
   (a) b, a, c (b) a, b, c (c) a, c, b (d) None of these
5. In a linear chromosome, map distances between 4 loci is as follows
   a - b 10%, a - d 3%, b - c 4% and a - c 6%.
   The crossover frequency between c and d is
   (a) 4 to 12% (b) 3 or 9%
   (c) 9% (d) 3%
6. Which one of the following is a sex-linked character?
   (a) White-eye in *Drosophila*
   (b) Duffy blood group in human beings
   (c) AB blood group in human beings
   (d) All of the above

MULTIPLE ALLELISM

- Genes usually occur in two allelic forms or allelomorphs. For example, the genes for tall and dwarf characters of pea plant consists of two alleles. Here, one of them is called **normal** or **wild type**, while another is mutant type.
- Some genes however, may occur in more than two allelic forms, i.e. a gene can mutate several times to produce several alternative expressions. Such genes are called **multiple alleles**.
- The multiple alleles can be defined as a set of 3, 4 or more alleles, which arose as a result of mutation of the normal gene and occupy the same locus in the homologous chromosomes.

Characteristics

A mutant gene series is said to be multiple allele only if it possesses following characteristics

- Occupy same locus in homologous chromosome pair.
- Due to their presence on the same locus, they do not exhibit the phenomenon of crossing over in themselves.
- They always regulate same characteristic but with a variable degree of efficiency.
- Within a multiple series, a wild type is always dominant over normal genes and others may be dominant or intermediate.
- When any two of the mutant multiple alleles are crossed, the phenotype is mutant type and not the wild type.

Multiple alleles in plants

Several examples of multiple alleles are seen in maize.

(i) **Colour locus on chromosome 9**, that controls colour and have at least three alleles.
- C^I = Inhibitor of colour
- C^i = Responsible for full colour in the presence of two genes A and R
- c = Expresses colourless condition

(ii) **R locus on chromosome 10**, which is a complex locus, controlling anthocyanin colour of seed as well as the plant colour. Following four alleles are identified on this locus.
- R^r for coloured seed and coloured (red) plant
- R^g for coloured seed and green plant
- r^r for colourless seed and coloured (red) plant
- r^g for colourless seed and green plant

Later, these are designated in following ways as they control two independent functions

R^r = SP
R^g = SP
r^r = sP
r^g = sp

According to some authors and scientists, the genes in above written examples are closely linked rather than considered as multiple alleles. But as the possibility of crossing over is zero in between them, so these can be considered as multiple alleles.

Multiple alleles in animals

Following are some of the examples of multiple alleles in animals.

(i) Among animals, **coat colour in rabbit** is considered as the best example of multiple alleles. It is controlled by following genes
- Fully coloured or agouti (wild type) = C
- Chinchilla pattern (uniform light grey pattern) = C^{ch}
- Himalayan pattern (body white with extremities grey) = c^h
- Albino (pure white) = c
- The gene C is dominant over all other alleles.
- Chinchilla is recessive to full colour but dominant to others.
- Similarly, Himalayan pattern is dominant only over albino pattern and albino pattern is seen only in homozygous recessive state.
- Thus, different phenotypes and their possible genotypes are as follows
  (a) Agouti : CC, CC^{ch}, Cc^h, Cc
  (b) Chinchilla : $c^{ch}C^{ch}$, $C^{ch}c^h$, $C^{ch}c$
  (c) Himalayan : c^hc^h, c^hc
  (d) Albino : cc

(ii) **Eye colour in *Drosophila*** also appears as a good example.
- Here, normal eye colour is red and white, which shows simple dominant recessive relationship.
- Afterwards, different eye colour shades are also discovered, which are controlled by different allelomorphs occupying the same locus at X-chromosome.
- These are as follows
  - Apricot colour : w^a
  - Blood colour : w^{bl}
  - Cherry colour : w^{ch}
  - Ivory colour : w^i
  - Pearl colour : w^p
  - Tinged colour : w^t
- With wild type as red = W and recessive = w, these all patterns show intermediate inheritance when brought together.

(iii) ABO blood group in humans also serves as very good example of multiple alleles. This is described in detail in the next chapter.

Complementation
- It refers to the relationship between two different strains of an organism in which both have homozygous recessive mutations that produce the same phenotype.
- When a cross is made between two homozygous recessive mutants and if the result is wild type F_1 progeny, the mutant alleles are said to complement one another or to exhibit complementation.
- The complementation reveals whether two mutants belong to the same allelic pair or different allelic pair.

Various other allelic phenomenons

1. Isoalleles
- It is possible that several alleles either wild or mutant may exhibit within the same phenotypic range. Such alleles that have the ability to express themselves within the same phenotypic range are called **isoalleles**.
- For example, in *Drosophila*, several alleles exhibit red-eye colour, i.e. W^{+s}, W^{+c}, W^{+g}, etc.

2. Pseudoalleles
- Usually, alleles of a gene occupy same locus in the homologous pair and no crossing over takes place between them.

- However in some cases, there is a possibility that different genes may also occupy loci very close to each other. As a result of this, these genes are normally inherited together.
- Such genes that behave like multiple alleles and have minimum chances of crossing over are called **pseudoalleles.**
- For example, eye colour in *Drosophila*, bristle length, hairless bristles and ebony body.

CYTOPLASMIC INHERITANCE

- **Oscar Hertwig** in 1870s proposed that the units of inheritance are present in nucleus. Afterwards, the role of DNA and chromosomal inheritance of characteristics was properly understood.
- **Dr. Sanger** and **his colleagues** in 1950 suggested that there are some systems present outside the nucleus, i.e. in cytoplasm, which may also play important role in continuity and transmission of characteristics.
- These systems are capable of self-reproduction and alterations. This unique phenomena are named as **cytoplasmic inheritance** as in them, transmission of characters takes place through cytoplasm.
- Examples of such systems include plastids, mitochondria, Kappa particles in *Paramecium*, etc.
- These total self-replicating hereditary materials present in cytoplasm is called **plasmon,** while their cytoplasmic units of inheritance are described as **plasma genes.**

Dissimilarity between cytoplasmic and nuclear inheritance

The cytoplasmic inheritance is different from normal nuclear inheritance. The basis of this difference is the unequal contribution made by father and mother in fertilisation. The zygote receives most of its cytoplasm from the egg and very little or no cytoplasm from the sperm. Thus, we can say that extranuclear inheritance has following three distinct features

- It is more or less **maternal inheritance**, i.e. here only the female parent contributes towards inheritance. But in **nuclear inheritance**, both the parents contribute equally towards inheritance.
- Due to the participation of female only, the result of reciprocal crosses is not the same in case of cytoplasmic inheritance.
- The cytoplasmic hereditary units are denoted by α, β and γ, while nuclear hereditary units are denoted by a, b and c, etc.

Examples of cytoplasmic inheritance

Many examples of cytoplasmic inheritance are seen in both haploid and diploid organisms.

In yeast

Yeast have two varieties, i.e. the normal white variety and mutant red variety.

It was shown by **B Ephrussi** and others that the factor or gene for red colour is located in cytoplasm and its inheritance takes place through cytoplasmic inheritance.

In rusts

In some cases of rust, the size of rust spots is found to depend on agents which are transmitted through the egg only. Hence, agents responsible for the inheritance of such rust spots in rusts are considered as the example of cytoplasmic inheritance.

In plants

Some interesting examples of cytoplasmic inheritance in plants are discussed below

(i) ***Mirabilis jalapa***

- In these plants, the plastids are self-replicating bodies and their inheritance was first of all reported by **Correns** in 1908. These plants have complete, green, variegated (with various colours) and colourless leaves within the same plant.
- It is noted that if seeds were taken from an entirely green branch, they will germinate into complete green plants.
- Similarly, seeds from variegated leaves give rise to variegated plants only.

(ii) ***Oenothera***

- The evening primrose provides an interesting variant of plastid inheritance. In two species of *Oenothera,* i.e. *O. hookeri* and *O. muricata* normal green plants are seen.
- However, reciprocal crosses between them may result in deviations from expected phenotypes as shown below

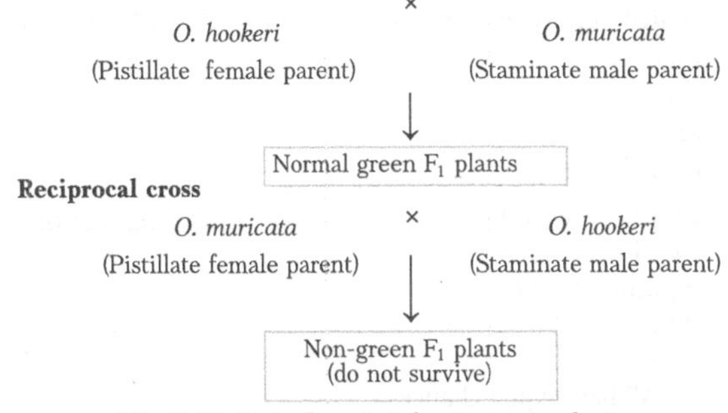

Fig. 7.13 Cytoplasmic inheritance in plants

The reason for such a difference in reciprocal crosses is seen due to the fact that *Oenothera muricata* plastids have the ability to develop normally in the presence of *hookeri* nucleus, whereas *hookeri* plastids do not have such capability.

In animals

Some interesting examples of cytoplasmic inheritance in animals are discussed below

(i) **In snails**

- The inheritance of shell coiling in *Limnaea* shows clearly visible maternal influence. Snails exhibit two types of coiling of their shells.
  - Coiling towards right hand side, i.e. **dextral.**
  - Coiling towards left hand side, i.e. **sinistral.**
- The inheritance of shell coiling is shown below

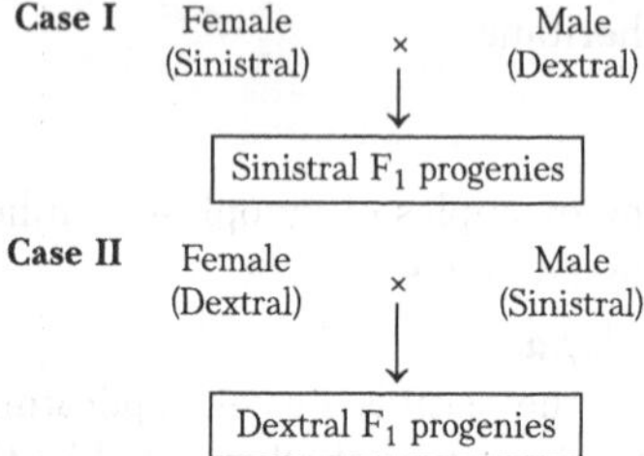

(ii) **In *Drosophila***

- It was discovered by **L Heritier** and **Teissier.**
- In these flies, one strain shows more sensitivity towards CO_2. This means that these are comparatively easily immobilised by exposing them to CO_2.
- This sensitive trait is regulated by a heat labile substance present in cytoplasm called **sigma.**

(iii) **In mice**

- Mammary cancer or breast tumour in these animals has been found to be maternally transmitted.
- Recent evidences indicate that this character is transmitted *via* mother's milk as a protein called **milk factor.**

(iv) **In *Paramecium***

- **TH Sonneborn** and his associates reported inheritance of certain self-duplicating, double membrane bound cytoplasmic particles called **kappa particles** in these protozoans.
- In *P. aurelia*, two strains are reported. One of these secretes toxic substance **paramecin** and called as **killer,** while the other one does not secrete paramecin and called as **sensitive.**
- The killer strain can secrete paramecin due to the presence of kappa particles in them.
- It was found out that the sensitive strain is killed if it comes in contact with paramecin.
- When these two strains of *Paramecium* undergo conjugation for longer duration (abnormal type), exchange of nuclear as well as cytoplasmic material took place.
- As a result of this, kappa particles also enter in sensitive species through cytoplasmic exchange. Thus, the sensitive strain is converted into killer strain.
- Another most interesting example of cytoplasmic inheritance in *Paramecium* is seen as the inheritance of **genetic determiner or sex factor or fertility factor** or **episome.**

CHECK POINT 7.3

1. Multiple alleles
(a) have the minimum chances of crossing over
(b) occupy same locus in homologous chromosome pair
(c) exhibit themselves within the same phenotype
(d) regulate different characteristic but with a variable degree of efficiency

2. Which genotype does not show chinchilla pattern in rabbit?
(a) $C^{ch}\,c^{ch}$
(b) CC
(c) C^{ch}
(d) $C^{ch}\,c$

3. Which of the following has the maximum chances of crossing over?
(a) Multiple alleles
(b) Isoalleles
(c) Pseudoalleles
(d) All have equal chances

4. When a certain character is inherited only through the female parent, it probably represents the case of
(a) incomplete dominance
(b) cytoplasmic inheritance
(c) Mendelian nuclear inheritance
(d) multiple plastid inheritance

5. The result of reciprocal crosses is not the same of cytoplasmic inheritance because
(a) plastids take part in crossing over
(b) only female parent contributes towards inheritance
(c) only male parent contributes towards inheritance
(d) recombination is not taking place

6. Which is not an example of cytoplasmic inheritance?
(a) Plastid inheritance
(b) Kappa particle inheritance
(c) Sigma particle inheritance
(d) Female sterility in maize

MUTATION

- The term mutation was introduced by **Hugo de Vries**. He defined mutations as large spontaneous inheritable changes, which occur suddenly in naturally reproducing populations.
- de Vries proposed mutation theory of evolution in his book the '*Mutation theory*' published in 1903. Another biologist named **Dobzhansky** stated that mutation is a mistake or misprint in cell division.
- It is defined as any heritable change in the genetic makeup of an individual. It is a sudden change of a gene or chromosome from one form to another. It may be visible as a discontinuous variation in the genotype and phenotype of an organism.
- Mutations produce an alteration in the character under the control of certain mutated gene. In addition to recombination, mutation is another phenomenon that leads to change in visible appearance of an organism.
- Changes due to mutation include changes in chromosomes either in number or in structure, i.e. **chromosomal mutations** and changes in the structure or composition of genes, i.e. **gene mutations.**
- In general, chromosomal mutations are also called **macromutation** and gene mutations are also called **micromutations** or **point mutations.**

Effects of mutation

- By going through the mechanism of gene expression, it can be understood that the sequences of amino acids in an enzyme depends upon the sequence of nucleotides in *m*RNA, which in turn depends upon the sequence of nucleotides in DNA. Thus, any change in the sequence of nucleotides in DNA affect the sequence of amino acids in an enzyme (or polypeptide chain).
- Such a change in polypeptide chain would also affect the traits controlled by that enzyme.

Silent mutation

Any gene mutation, which does not result a change in phenotypic expression is called **silent mutation**. These mutations may be silent due to following reasons.

- **Due to degeneracy of code**, i.e. more than one codon specify same amino acid. Hence, any change in codon may not result into alteration in amino acid. Thus, change in trait is not visible.
- **Due to inssufficient change in codon**, i.e. the change in codon may result into alteration in amino acid as well as in the polypeptide chain. But, this change is insufficient to modify the function of protein appreciably.
- **Due to mutation in non-functional gene**, i.e. the mutation occurs in a gene which is no longer functional or the protein which is not required by the organism for rest of the life.
- **Due to suppressor gene**, i.e. a simultaneous presence of suppressor mutations which may cause the mutation to be silent.

Chromosomal aberrations (Macromutation)

It is of following two types

I. Variations in chromosome number

The mutations arising due to variations in chromosome number from the normal diploid set are called **heteroploidy**.

These can be categorised into the following types

1. Euploidy

- The euploidy designates genome containing chromosomes that are multiple of some basic number (X).
- Here, the variation occurs in sets. Hence, the euploids contain balanced sets of chromosomes.
- The euploidy can be either **monoploidy**, i.e. variation of haploid set of chromosomes or **polyploidy**, i.e. variation to more than two sets of chromosomes.
- The polyploidy can be further divided into **triploidy** ($3n$), **tetraploidy** ($4n$), **pentaploidy** ($5n$), **hexaploidy** ($6n$), etc., types.

Monoploidy (Haploidy)

- These organisms contain only one set of chromosomes and thus, are hemizygous in nature.
- The monoploids are normally smaller in size and have less vigour than corresponding diploids.

Polyploidy

- They occur in nature due to failure of chromosomal separation during anaphase due to non-disjunction.
- The polyploids may be classified as primary and secondary.
- A **primary polyploid** is always even numbered because it arises by doubling of chromosomes of a particular organism.

  For example, $2n \xrightarrow[\text{To}]{\text{Doubled}} 4n$ or $3n \xrightarrow[\text{To}]{\text{Doubled}} 6n$, etc.
- A **secondary polyploid** arises by the crossing between organisms of different ploidy levels.
  For example,

  $4n$ (primary) crossed with $2n \xrightarrow{\text{To gives}} 3n$ (secondary)
- Depending upon the source of additional chromosome sets, the polyploids are of following three types
  (i) **Autopolyploids** These are the polyploids formed by the duplication of same genome. They are relatively rare in nature and can be produced artificially, e.g. doob grass (*Cyanodon dactylon*) is

an autotriploid and rye (*Secale cereale*) is an autotetraploid. Besides duplication, the autopolyploids can also be originated by any of the following ways

- By the union of diploid gametes produced in the absence of meiosis.
- By abnormal mitosis in diploid zygote ($2n \times 2$ = autotetraploid).
- By the union of a haploid gamete with the diploid gamete ($n + 2n$ = autotriploid).
- By a cross between a tetraploid and a diploid parent ($4n + n$ = autopentaploid).
- By fertilisation of an egg with two sperms ($n + 2 \times n$ = autotriploid).

The features of autopolyploids include

- These are larger than the diploids due to increased cell size (gigas effect).
- Flowering is delayed but flowers are comparatively larger.
- Seeds are few but larger in size.
- Their growth rate is slow due to slow rate of division.
- With the increase in cell size, water content is also increased causing reduced osmotic pressure and loss of resistance against frost.
- Autotetraploids show wrinkled leaves, dwarfing or weakling.
- Auto-octoploids or above have very low survival value.

(ii) **Allopolyploids** These are polyploids in which the chromosome sets are non-homologous and are initially derived from two different species.

These are derived from a heterozygous stock. Therefore, they contain different genomes that have come together during hybridisation.

The features of allopolyploids are as follows

- The alloploidy may result in immediate species formation. If the genomes of the two species are similar or almost similar, then a fertile hybrid may be formed. But if the genomes are dissimilar, then the hybrid will be sterile because synapsis will not take place in it.
- If the doubling of chromosomes takes place in the hybrid of second case (sterile) discussed above, then the resulting allotetraploid will be fertile and consists of chromosomes, which can undergo regular pairing.
- ***Raphanobrassica*** was the first known **allotetraploid** reported by Russian geneticist Karpechenko (1928). This plant is a hybrid of *Raphanus* (radish) and *Brassica oleracea* (cabbage).

(iii) **Autoalloploids** When autopolyploidy combines with allopolyploidy, it results into autoallopolyploidy.

- For example, if a tetraploidy ($4n$) arising by alloploidy undergoes chromosome doubling by autoploidy, an octoploid ($8n$) may result.
- Similarly, if two different autotetraploids undergo hybridisation followed by chromosome doubling, this will result into autoallopolyploid.

Induced polyploidy

It has been possible to induce polyploidy experimentally. The basic principle is to affect spindle formation during mitosis and thus, achieve doubling of chromosomes. The artificial polyploidy has been brought about by

- **High temperature**, e.g. in maize.
- **Decapitation**, e.g. in tomatoes.
- **Chemicals**, e.g. application of colchicine in plants. Colchicine interferes with spindle formation, but does not affect the division of chromosome. This chromosome division without cytoplasmic division results in the doubling of chromosome number. Other chemicals used for this purpose include acenaphthene, indole acetic acid, etc.

2. Aneuploidy

- Aneuploids were first discovered by **Bridges** in 1916. It is seen where the variations in individual chromosomes occur.
- Aneuploid plants and animals have incomplete genomes. These can be of two types namely,

(i) **Hyperploids**, i.e. those which have one or more chromosomes in addition to the normal diploid genome.

(ii) **Hypoploids**, i.e. those which have one or more chromosomes less than the normal diploid genome.

The following table shows most of the different types of aneuploids.

Table 7.1 Different types of aneuploidy

Types	Chromosome numbers
Diploid (normal)	$2n$
Hyperploids	
(i) Trisomics	$(2n+1)$
(ii) Double trisomic	$(2n+1+1)$
(iii) Tetrasomic	$(2n+2)$
(iv) Pentasomic	$(2n+3)$
Hypoploids	
(i) Monosomics	$(2n-1)$
(ii) Nullisomics	$(2n-2)$
(iii) Double monosomics	$(2n-1-1)$

- Important features related to aneuploids are
  (a) These may arise by any of the following two methods
    - By the union of gametes where one gamete contains an unbalanced number of chromosomes.
    - By perpetuation of a cell, in which more chromosomes are added or lost due to the failure of mitosis during anaphase-I.
  (b) These rarely survive and are much less viable than euploids.
  (c) The aneuploids can be true or false. In **true aneuploids**, there are complete genomes along with a fraction of other genome, while the **false aneuploids** contains supernumerary chromosomes.

II. Variations in chromosome structure

The variations in the chromosome structure may arise due to the following four processes

1. Deletion and deficiency 2. Duplication
3. Translocation 4. Inversion

An outline of all the four processes is given below

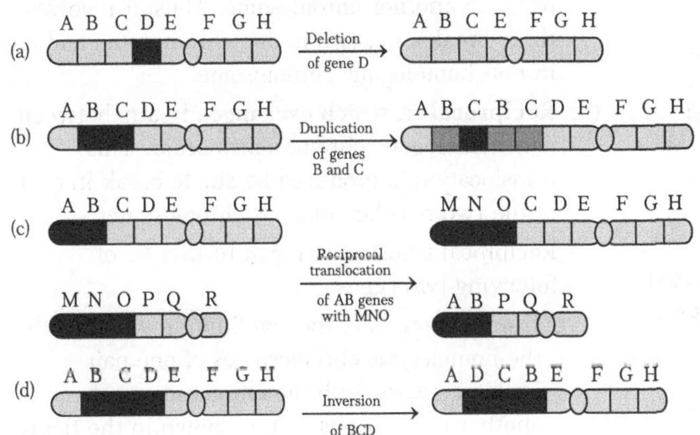

Fig. 7.14 Diagram showing the different forms of chromosomal mutations

1. Deletion and deficiency

- The deficiency is basically the absence of a chromosomal portion in terminal or interstitial regions, resulting into the loss of genes. Depending upon the length of lost the lost segment, the number of lost genes may vary from one to many. The process which results into deficiency is called **deletion**.
- Various features related to deletion are as follows
  - Deletion and deficiency are synonymous but a distinction is often made. The loss of terminal chromosomal segment is often described as deficiency, whereas the loss in intermediary position segment is designated as deletion.

Bridges (1917), first observed a deficiency in the bar locus of *Drosophila.*

  - In terminal deletions, a terminal section of a chromosome is lost and it is resulted by only one break.
  - The intercalary or interstitial deletion results from two breaks in chromosome followed by reunion of broken ends.
  - The part between the breaks is eliminated as shown below

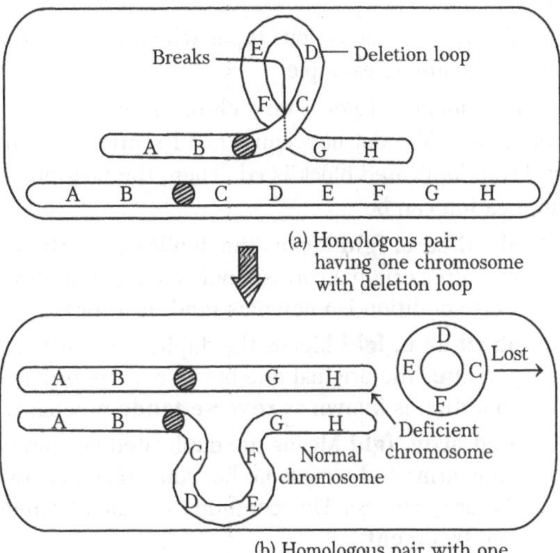

Fig. 7.15 Diagram showing deletion (Outline)

- The break in chromosomes may be caused by several agents like chemicals, drugs and radiations.
- Genenally in chromosomes, the union of broken ends may be **restitutional** (i.e. restoration of original structure) or **non-restitutional** (i.e. resulting to structural changes). In the cases of deletion, a non-restitutional union is seen.
- Deletions can be detected during pairing of homologous chromosomes.
- The genetic effect of deletion or deficiency is seen in the form of **pseudodominance** as it allows recessive genes to express itself phenotypically.
- In human, the **cat's Cry syndrome** occurs due to the deletion or deficiency in 5th chromosome.
- In plants, deletion is not easily transmitted to the offsprings. This is because the pollens with deletions in chromosomes are found to be sterile.
- The works of **Creighton** and **McClintock** has shown that in maize, small deficiencies are retained and inherited from one generation to the other.

2. Duplication

- The presence of one block of genes more than once in a haploid complement is known as **duplication**. This additional block is known as **repeat.**
- The duplication can arise by any of the following two possibilities
    - By the attachment of deleted piece from one chromosome to other.
    - By unequal crossing over in homologous chromosome.

Types

- Duplications are of various types which can be explained by following simple example.
- If the sequence of genes on a chromosome is abcde. fghi (the dot between e and f represents centromere) and the duplicated block is cd. Then, the possibilities of duplication can be
    - **ab cd cd e. fghi** Means the duplicated portion is situated just after original corresponding section of chromosome. This condition is known as **tandem repeat.**
    - **ab cd dc e. fghi** Means the duplicated portion is situated just after the original one but in reverse order. This condition is known as **reverse tandem repeat.**
    - **a cd bcde. fghi** Means the duplicated portion is on the same arm of chromosome but some distance away from the original site. This condition is called **homobrachial displacement.**
    - **a b cd e. f cd ghi** Means the duplicated portion is on the different arm of chromosome. This condition is known as **heterobrachial displacement.**
    - **k l m n o. pcd qr** Means the duplicated segment is repeated on a non-homologous chromosome. This condition is known as **transposition** or **displaced duplication.**

Features

Duplication have following features

- The duplicated block may have its own centromere in that case, it is considered as an **extrachromosomal duplication.**
- As duplication is possible at various positions within a chromosome or outside on any other chromosome, the possibility of **'position effects'** may also be there.
- The position effect is defined as the phenotypic changes in the expression of a gene which are due to the differences in the position of genes.

Note *The above two structural changes (i.e. deletion and duplication) in chromosome involve change in the number of genes on a chromosome, while rest two changes (i.e. translocation and inversion) involve only changes in the sequences of genes on a chromosome.*

3. Translocation

- The process of transfer of a part of chromosome or a block of genes from one chromosome to a non-homologous chromosome followed by its rearrangement is known as **translocation.**
- It occurs due to irregularities during crossing over. In the process, breaks in the chromosomes are followed by their union.
- The phenomenon of translocation is of common occurrence. It can be studied in *Drosophila, Oenothera,* maize and man.

Types

The translocation can be of following types

(i) **Simple** in which a small segment of a chromosome is added to the end of other non-homologous chromosomes. This type of translocation is very rare in nature and is caused by a single break in one chromosome only.

(ii) **Shift** in which an interstitial segment of one chromosome is broken off and inserted within the break in another chromosome. Thus, it involves three breaks, i.e. two in one chromosome and one in non-homologous chromosome.

(iii) **Reciprocal** in which exchange of parts between non-homologous chromosomes occur. This translocation is produced by single break in each of the two non-homologous chromosomes. Reciprocal translocation can further be of following two types

- **Homozygous**, i.e. the condition in which both the homologous chromosomes of one pair exchange parts with the chromosomes of another homologous pair as shown in the figure below

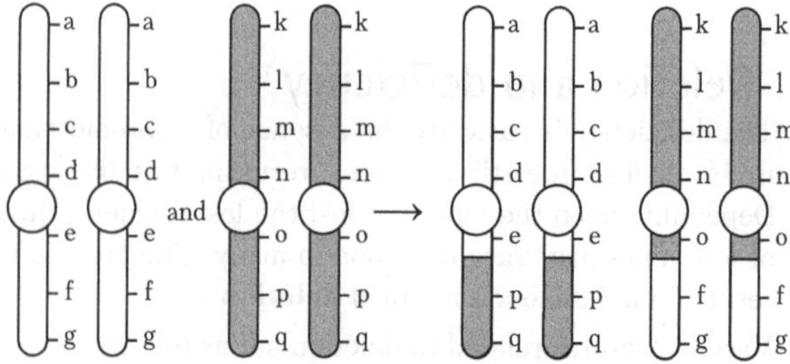

Fig. 7.16 *Translocation (homozygous)*
Please note that the segment exchange is visible in both the chromosomal branches simultaneously.

- **Heterozygous**, i.e. the condition in which only one member of different homologous pairs exchange their parts as shown in figure below

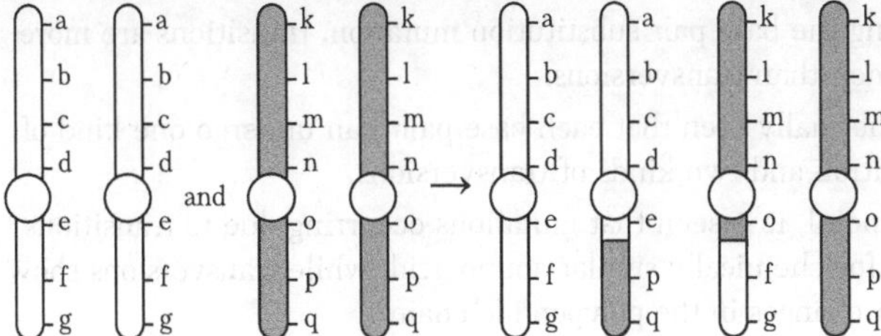

Fig. 7.17 Translocation (Heterozygous)
Please note that the segment exchange is visible in one chromosomal branch only.

(iv) **Multiple** in which more than two pairs of non-homologous chromosomes exchange their parts.

Identification of translocation during cell division

- In heterozygous reciprocal translocation, the two normal and two translocated chromosome pairs to form a cross-shaped configuration during the pachytene stage of meiosis instead of bivalent formation as shown below

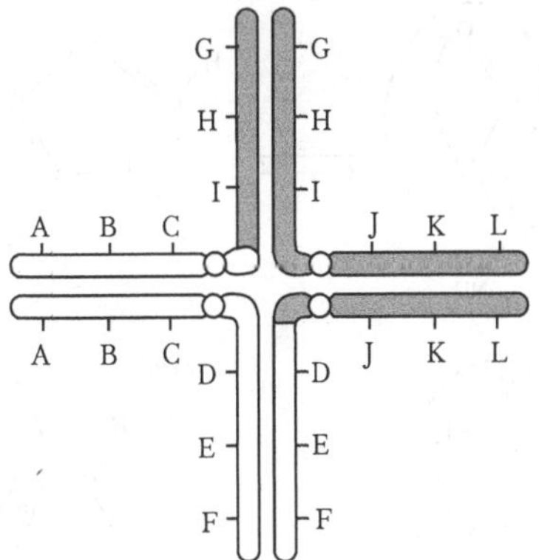

Fig. 7.18 Bivalent formation

- At the completion of terminalisation, the cross opens out to form a ring or a figure of 8 as shown below

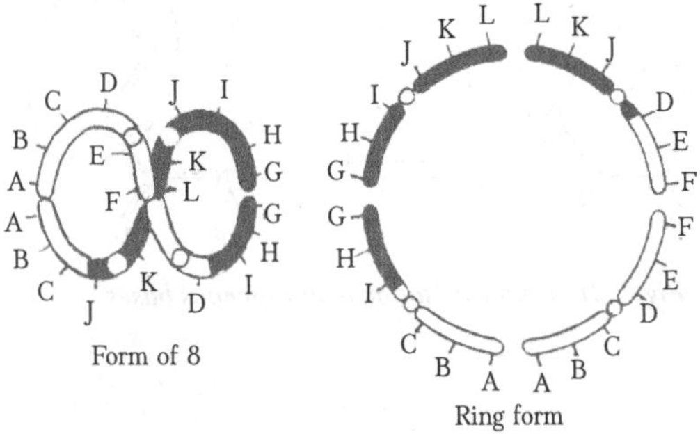

Fig. 7.19 Figure of 8 and ring in terminalisation

Robertsonian translocation

- Sometimes whole arm fusion occurs in the non-homologous chromosomes. It is called Robertsonian translocation. It is an eucentric reciprocal translocation where the break in one chromosome is near the front of the centromere and break in the other chromosome is immediately behind its centromere.
- The resultant smaller chromosome consists of largely inert heterochromatic material containing no essential genes. This chromosome tends to become lost thus, Robertsonian translocation results in a reduction of chromosome number.
- It is believed that Robertsonian translocation had contributed in the evolvement of human beings (46 chromosomes) from common ape ancestors (48 chromosomes).

4. Inversion

During inversion, a section of chromosome gets changed after the rotation through 180° on its own axis. Thus, the order of genes in the section become reversed.

The inversions are of following two types

(i) **Pericentric** in which inverted segment includes the centromere.

(ii) **Paracentric** in which the centromere is not included in inverted segment.

Mechanism

Inversions arise by the formation of loops on a chromosome. Breaks occur at the point of intersection of loops and then, reunion of broken ends takes place, resulting into inversion as shown below

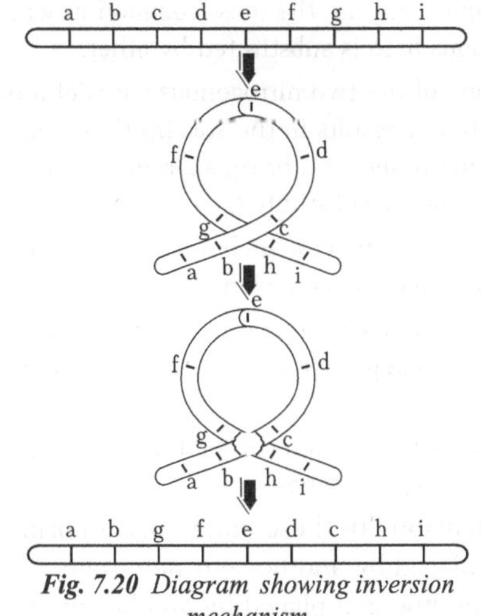

Fig. 7.20 Diagram showing inversion mechanism

Features

- Inversion occurring in a single chromosome is called **chromosomal inversion**, whereas that occurring in both the members of a homologous pair is called **allelosomal inversion**.

- Allelosomal inversion occurring in the same arms of homologous pair are called **allelobrachial**, while that occurring in different arms of homologous pair is called **heterobrachial.**
- Chromosomal inversion may also be called **heterozygous**, while allelosomal inversion may also be called **homozygous.**

Significance

- Inversions help in origin of new species.
- It provides the proof for crossing over and support the view that only two out of the four chromatids undergo crossing over.
- Inversions reduce the chances of crossing over. Thus, they are restricting the recombinations of gene loci.

Gene mutations
(Micromutation or Point mutation)

- Point mutations were first recorded by **Seth Wright** in 1791, when he noticed a lamb with exceptionally short legs (Ancon) in his flock of sheep.
- These mutations involve alterations in the structure of genes, i.e. modification in the structure of DNA. These mutations are also called **intragenic mutation.**
- Point mutations are mainly of following two types

1. Base pair mutation

- These mutations are the most common in which one nitrogenous base is substituted by other.
- When one of the two nitrogenous bases of a pair is substituted, it results in the substitution of other base also during replication or repair replication. Thus, a complete pair is substituted.
- The result of change of such a base pair is seen in the form of a changed codon.
- If the mutated codon specifies another amino acid, then the polypeptide chain is also affected by this change.
- This base pair mutation can be further categorised into following two types
  - (i) **Transitions** In these mutations, a purine base is replaced by another purine or one pyrimidine is replaced by another pyrimidine.
  - (ii) **Transversion** In these mutations, a purine is replaced by a pyrimidine and *vice-versa*.

Features

Important features related with base pair point mutation are as follows

- Among the base pair substitution mutation, transitions are more common than transversions.
- It is normally seen that each base pair can undergo one kind of transition and two kinds of transversions.
- In general, it is seen that mutations occurring due to transitions code for chemically similar amino acid, while transversions show larger changes in the polypeptide chain.
- If base pair insertion results into change in one amino acid of the polypeptide chain, the mutation is called **mis-sense mutation.**
- Transitions may arise due to tautomerisation of nitrogenous bases as shown below

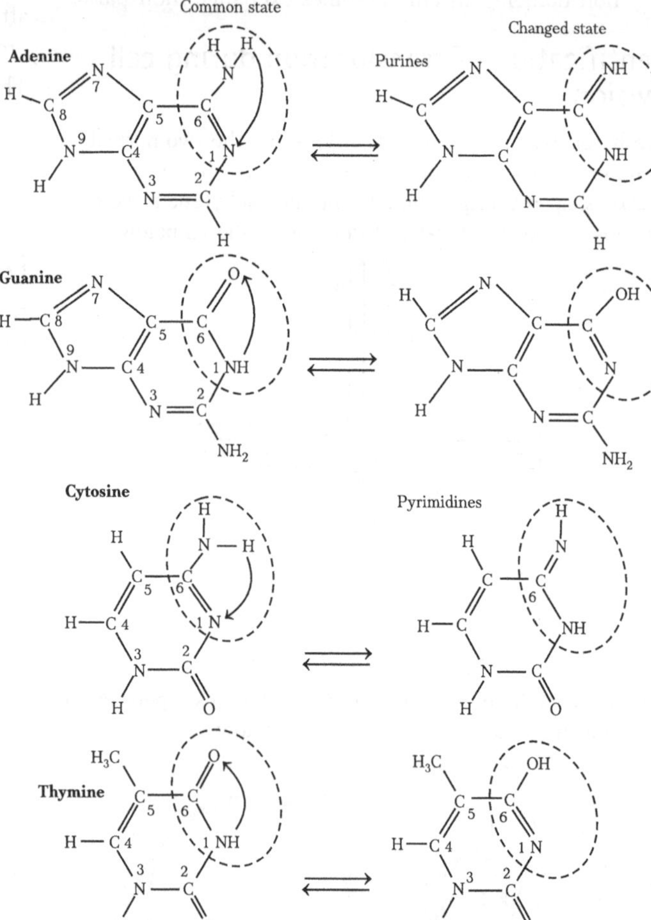

Fig. 7.21 Tautomerisation in nitrogenous bases

- On the other hand, if a single base substitution modifies a codon to termination (non-sense) codon, e.g. CAG→ UAG, the mutation is called **non-sense mutation.** Such polypeptide chain may terminate at the point of mutation.
- Although transition and transversion, both can cause non-sense mutations, but the chances of mis-sense mutation are usually greater.
- **A non-sense mutation near the 5′ end of DNA template** results into a very small polypeptide chain, which are biologically inactive.
- **A non-sense mutation near the 3′ end of DNA template** does not affect the polypeptide chain, except this chain will be smaller than the normal chain.
- **A mis-sense mutation at the termination codon** (i.e. in which a non-sense codon is converted into a sense codon, e.g. UAA is converted to AAA) results into an infinitely long polypeptide chain. Such chains are also biologically inactive most of the times.

2. Frameshift mutation

The name frameshift mutation is derived from the fact that there is a shift in reading frame either backward or forward. In these mutations, there occurs a deletion or insertion of one or more nitrogenous bases.

It occurs by following ways

(i) **Simple deletion** It is the removal of one or more nitrogenous bases from a nucleotide chain. As the code is commaless, the complete reading of frame after deletion gets shifted towards right as shown below

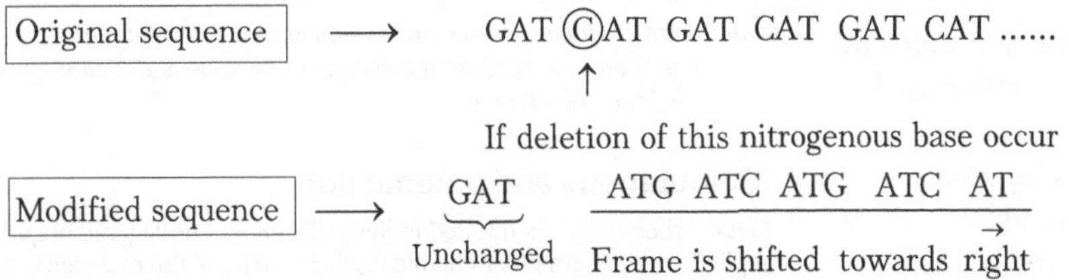

(ii) **Simple insertion** It is the addition of one or more nitrogenous bases to the nucleotide chain. Here, again as the code is commaless, the complete reading frameshifts towards left as shown below

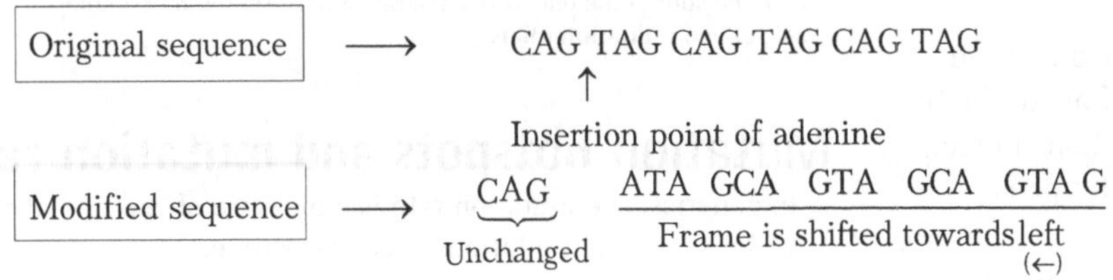

(iii) **Simultaneous deletion and insertion** If simultaneous deletion and insertion of nitrogenous bases is seen, then the shift in reading frame will be visible only between the deletion and insertion points as shown below

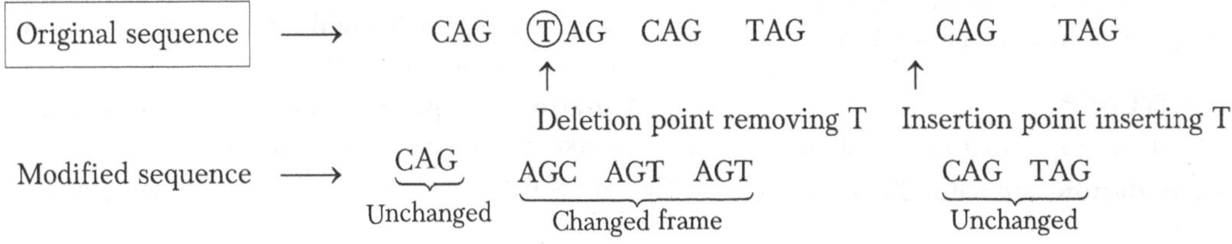

Some other types of mutations

Based upon various other parameters like cell types, effects on phenotypes, etc., mutations can be further classified as follows

Based on cell types

(i) **Germinal mutations** These are those mutations which occur in the germinal cells before differentiation of gametes or in a gamete or a zygote. These mutations affect the complete organism.

(ii) **Somatic mutations** These are those mutations which occur in the somatic cells of our body. These mutations affect some parts of an organism.

Based on the method of detection

A classification based upon the methods of detection of mutations are categorised as follows

(i) **Morphological mutations** involve alterations in external characteristics. Thus, can be detected by appearance only.

(ii) **Lethal mutations** are genotypic alterations which lead to the death of an individual.

(iii) **Biochemical mutations** are identified by a deficiency which can be overcome by supplying chemical compound for which the mutant is deficient.

(iv) **Resistant mutations** are identified by their ability to grow in the presence of an antibiotic like streptomycin, ampicillin, cycloheximide, etc., or a pathogen to which wild type is susceptible.

(v) **Conditional mutation** allows the mutant phenotype to be expressed under certain conditions called **restrictive conditions**. These conditions are contrary to normal conditions, which are called **permissive conditions**.

Based on occurrence

These are generally of two types that are as follows

(i) **Spontaneous mutations** are naturally occurring mutations.

(ii) **Induced mutations** are artificially generated mutations.

Based on their effects on phenotype

(i) **Lethal** that causes death of individual.

(ii) **Subvital** that reduces the chances of survival of an organism.

(iii) **Supervital** that results to the improvement of biological fitness under certain conditions.

All these changes are possible only because of the change in structure of enzymes controlling various biological activities of organisms.

Mutagens

Mutations can be artificially produced by certain agents called mutagens or **mutagenic agents**. Mutagens are usually of following two types

(i) **Physical mutagens**, e.g. X-rays, γ-rays, α-rays, β-rays, etc.

(ii) **Chemical mutagens**, e.g. nitrous acids, acridine, alkylating agents, base analogues, etc.

Note *Base analogues are structures similar to the normal nitrogenous bases, e.g. 5-bromo uracil is an analogue of thymine and 2 aminopurine is an analogue of adenine.*

Comutagens and potentiation

Certain chemicals when tested individually are not mutagenic but when applied with certain other chemicals, these increase the mutagenic activity. Such chemicals are called as comutagens.

These chemicals work on the phenomenon of potentiation, i.e. the enhancement of one agent by another so that the combine effect is greater than the sum of the effects of each one alone. Therefore, comutagens are also called **radio-potentials**.

Mutation hotspots and mutation rate

- In genetics, the mutation rate is a measure of the rate at which various types of mutations occur over time.
- The rate of spontaneous mutations is generally low, ranging from 10^{-7} to 10^{-12} per organism.
- The mutation rate can be calculated under two heads namely
  (i) **Mutation rate at individual loci**, i.e. chances of mutation for an individual locus.
  (ii) **Mutation rate per genome**, i.e. chances of mutation to be taken collectively for a complete genome.
- The rate of detectable mutations in an average gene is 1 in 10^6.
- Mutations occur much more frequently in certain regions of genome. These regions are called as **mutation hotspots**.

CHECK POINT 7.4

1. Failure of cytokinesis after telophase stage of cell division results in an increase in a whole set of chromosomes in an organism, this phenomenon is called
(a) aneuploidy (b) polyploidy (c) tetraploidy (d) All of these

2. Which of the following chromosomal mutation are most likely to take place, when homologous chromosomes are undergoing synapsis?
(a) Inversion and translocation
(b) Deletion and duplication
(c) Inversion and deletion
(d) Translocation and duplication

3. Which of the following chromosomal alterations does not alter genic balance but may affect phenotype because of differences in gene expression?
(a) Deletion (b) Inversion
(c) Duplication (d) Both (a) and (c)

4. If the DNA codons are ATG ATG ATG and a cytosine base is inserted at the beginning, which of the following will result?
(a) CA TGA TGA TG (b) C ATG ATG ATG
(c) CAT GAT GAT G (d) A non-sense mutation

5. If a mutation occurs in a gamete, it would influence
(a) only a single individual
(b) sterility in the progeny
(c) all successive generations of the parents
(d) only the particular sex of the progeny, whose gamete had undergone mutation

6. In the context of evolution, what is the most important source of new mutations?
(a) Exposure to X-ray
(b) Exposure to chemicals
(c) The mispairing of chromosomes during meiosis
(d) Errors during DNA replication

EXAM POINTS

- Chromosomal theory of inheritance was proposed by Sutton and Boveri. **[NEET 2020]**
- Experimental verification of the chromosomal theory of inheritance was done by Morgan. **[NEET 2020]**
- To make chromosomal studies easier, chromosomes are classified into certain groups like A to G. So, the chromosome number 21, 22 and Y are listed in 'G' group. **[JIPMER 2019]**
- In the construction of genetic maps, map unit or centiMorgan is a unit or distance between genes on chromosomes, representing 1% crossover. **[NEET 2019]**
- The frequency of recombination between gene pairs on the same chromosome as a measure of the distance between genes was explained by Alfred Sturtevant. **[NEET 2019]**
- Chromosome walking is used in genetic mapping. **[JIPMER 2019]**
- In human male, there is absence of one X-chromosome, presence of XY chromosome and absence of Barr body. **[JIPMER 2019]**
- XX-XO method of sex-determination is seen in grasshopper. **[NEET 2019, AIIMS 2018]**
- XX-XY method of sex-determination is seen in female homogamety. **[NEET 2019]**
- ZW-ZZ method of sex-determination is female heterogamety. **[NEET 2019]**
- In male grasshoppers, 50% of sperms have no sex chromosome. **[NEET 2019]**
- In domesticated fowls, sex of progeny depends on the type of egg rather than sperm. **[NEET 2019]**
- Human males have one of their sex chromosomes much shorter than the other. **[NEET 2019]**
- Male fruitfly is heterogametic. **[NEET 2019]**
- XYY composition is supermale. **[JIPMER 2018]**
- Tightly linked genes on the same chromosome show higher recombinations. **[AIIMS 2018]**
- Genes far apart on the same chromosome show very few recombinations. **[AIIMS 2018]**
- Genes loosely linked on the same chromosome show similar recombination. **[AIIMS 2018]**
- The non-allelic genes for red hair and prickles are usually inherited together. The genes for red hair and prickles located on the same chromosome in close association. **[AIIMS 2018]**
- The distance between the genes on the chromosomes is measured by using recombination frequency. **[EAMCET 2016]**
- In a test cross involving F_1 dihybrid flies, more parental type offspring were produced than the recombinant type offspring. This indicates the two genes are linked and present on the same chromosome. **[NEET 2016]**

Chapter Exercises

(A) Topical Exercise

Chromosomal Theory of Inheritance and Sex-Determination in Animal and Plants

1 The chromosomal theory of heredity means that
(a) chromosomes are composed of genes
(b) chromosomes are made up of DNA and protein
(c) genes are located on the chromosome
(d) All of the above

2 Consider the following statements.
I. Sutton and Boveri noted that the behaviour of chromosomes was parallel to the behaviour of genes.
II. Sutton gave chromosomal theory of inheritance and he united the knowledge of chromosomal segregation with Mendelian principle of segregation.

Choose the correct option.
(a) Statement I is true, but II is false
(b) Statement I is false, but II is true
(c) Both statements I and II are true
(d) Both statements I and II are false

3 Which of the following statements are correct?
(a) Sex chromosomes are also called as allosomes
(b) Autosomes are chromosomes having somatic characters
(c) Sex chromosomes X and Y were discovered by Stevens and Wilson
(d) All of the above

4 X-chromosome is designated as sex chromosome due to its involvement in
(a) determination of sex (b) producing female child
(c) Both (a) and (b) (d) None of these

5 In both XO and XY type of sex-determining mechanisms, males produce two different types of gametes
(a) Either with or without X-chromosome
(b) Some gametes with X-chromosome and some with Y-chromosome
(c) Both (a) and (b)
(d) None of the above

6 Haploids are used for researches because
(a) they contain only one chromosome
(b) they contain two sets of chromosomes
(c) they contain three sets of chromosomes
(d) they contain only one set of chromosomes

7 In a certain taxon of insects, some have 17 chromosomes and the others have 18 chromosomes. The 17 and 18 chromosomes bearing organisms are **[NCERT Exemplar]**
(a) males and females, respectively
(b) females and males, respectively
(c) all males
(d) all females

8 ZZ/ZW type of sex-determination is seen in **[NCERT Exemplar]**
(a) platypus (b) snails
(c) cockroach (d) peacock

9 Genic balance theory of sex-determination stated by CB Bridges is related to
(a) *Drosophila melanogaster* (b) Rumex
(c) Snapdragon (d) None of the above

10 In *Drosophila*, the sex is determined by
(a) the ratio of pairs of X-chromosomes to the pairs of autosomes
(b) whether the egg is fertilised or develops parthenogenetically
(c) the ratio of number of X-chromosomes to the set of autosomes
(d) X and Y-chromosomes

11 If the ratio between X-chromosomes and complete set of autosome is 0.5. Then, the individual will be
(a) female (b) superfemale
(c) male (d) supermale

12 *Drosophila* flies with XXY genotype are females, but human beings with such genotype are abnormal males. It shows that
(a) Y-chromosome is essential for sex-determination in *Drosophila*
(b) Y-chromosome is female determining in *Drosophila*
(c) Y-chromosome is male determining in human beings
(d) Y-chromosome has no role in sex-determination either in *Drosophila* or in human beings

13 Choose the incorrect statement.
(a) ZW-ZZ type of sex-determination is opposite of XX-XY type
(b) In *Drosophila,* $X/A > 1$ superfemale
(c) A fruitfly exhibiting superior male traits is gynandromorph
(d) In humans, females produce homomorphic X-chromosomes

14 Gynandromorphism in certain flies is the result of
(a) non-disjunction of X-chromosome
(b) repeated and sudden changes in both X and Y-chromosomes
(c) misdivision of chromosomes whereby one of the X-chromosome gets lost
(d) failure of X and Y-chromosomes to separate during gamete formation at the first zygotic division

15 Choose the incorrect matched pair.
(a) *Melandrium* - Environmental sex-determination
(b) *Neurospora* - Single gene effect
(c) *Lacerta sexicola* - Diploid females
(d) Ants - Haplo-diploidy mechanism

Crossing Over, Linkage and Sex-Linked Inheritance

16 Crossing over brings about
(a) recombination of genes
(b) no significant change
(c) study offspring
(d) cytoplasmic reorganisation

17 Crossing over occurs at
(a) 2 strand stage (b) 4 strand stage
(c) Both (a) and (b) (d) None of these

18 Crossing over that results in genetic recombination in higher organisms occurs between
(a) sister chromatids of bivalent
(b) non-sister chromatids of a bivalent
(c) two daughter nuclei
(d) two different bivalents

19 Crossing over occurs at four strands stage. This was proved by the observation that
(a) usually two gametes resulting from meiosis are recombinants
(b) all the four gametes resulting from meiosis are recombinants
(c) chiasmata are seen only at four strands stage
(d) chiasmata are seen only at two strands stage

20 What would be segregation pattern of ascospores in *Neurospora asci* in case of 'crossing over' of the type given below?
(a) ab, ab, ab, ab, AB, AB, AB, AB
(b) Ab, Ab, Ab, Ab, aB, aB, aB, aB
(c) Ab, Ab, aB, aB, aB, aB, aB, Ab, Ab
(d) aB, aB, ab, ab, AB, AB, Ab, Ab

21 Recombination describes
(a) generation of parental gene combinations
(b) generation of non-parental gene combinations
(c) generation of both parental and non-parental gene combinations
(d) None of the above

22 Lack of independent assortment of two genes A and B in fruitfly *Drosophila* is due to
(a) repulsion
(b) recombination
(c) linkage
(d) crossing over

23 *Drosophila* has four pairs of chromosomes. How many linkage groups does female *Drosophila* has (male *Drosophila* has 5 linkage groups)
(a) 4 (b) 8
(c) 3 (d) 5

24 Morgan coined the term linkage to describe
(a) generation of non-parental gene combinations
(b) association of genes on a chromosome
(c) physical status of gene combinations
(d) generation of parental gene combinations

25 Complete linkage in *Drosophila* males
(a) results in the absence of crossovers
(b) results in total absence of genetic recombination under normal control
(c) means that sperms produced are only of two types
(d) results in all the genes in a particular linkage group mapping at the same point

26 Two genes R and Y are located very close on the chromosomal linkage map of maize plant. When RRYY and rryy genotypes are hybridised then F_2-generation will show
(a) higher number of the recombinant types
(b) segregation is expected in 9:3:3:1 rate
(c) segregation in 3:1 ratio
(d) higher number of parental types

27 Morgan carried out several crosses in *Drosophila* to study genes that were sex-linked. Those crosses were
(a) monohybrid (b) dihybrid
(c) trihybrid (d) None of these

28 Which of the following will not result in variations among siblings? **[NCERT Exemplar]**
(a) Independent assortment of genes
(b) Crossing over
(c) Linkage
(d) Mutation

29 According to Morgan, when the two genes in a dihybrid cross were situated on the same chromosome
(a) the proportion of parent gene combinations were much higher than the non-parental type
(b) the proportion of parent gave combination were lower than the non-parental type
(c) the proportion of parent and non-parental combinations were equal
(d) Either (b) or (c)

30 Which of the following genetic events represent a case of incomplete linkage?
(a) Inheritance between gene, so that one gene prevents expression of other genes
(b) A condition, in which the phenotype effect of a gene's alleles are simultaneously expressed in the heterozygote
(c) Occasional separation of two genes on the same chromosome by a recombinant event
(d) Expression of heterozygous phenotype, which is distinct form and often intermediate to that of either parent

31 According to chromosome theory of linkage of Morgan and Castle,
(a) strength of linkage between two successive genes is inversely proportional to distance between two genes
(b) genes lie in a linear order in the chromosomes
(c) linked genes are arranged in *cis* or *trans* manner
(d) All of the above

32 *Drosophila* is used in genetic studies because
(a) its chromosome complement is simple
(b) a single mating produces over 100 offsprings
(c) life cycle time is small (10-20 days)
(d) All of the above

33 All genes located on the same chromosome
(a) form different groups depending upon their relative distance
(b) form one linkage groups
(c) will not form any linkage groups
(d) form interactive groups that affect the phenotype

34 A linkage group is explained as
(a) different groups of genes located on the same chromosomes
(b) all the linked genes of a chromosome
(c) all genes of a chromosome
(d) None of the above

35 Genetic map
(a) shows the stages during the cell division
(b) shows the distribution of various species in a region
(c) establishes sites of the genes on a chromosome
(d) establishes the various stages in gene evolution

36 Concept of gene mapping was first suggested by
(a) Morgan (b) Bridges
(c) Avery (d) Sturtevant

37 Unit of distance between genes in a chromosome is known as
(a) cDNA (b) nanometer (c) centiMorgan (d) spacer

38 If gene frequency between genes a and c is 2%, b and c is 13%, b and d is 6%, a and b is 15%, c and d is 19%. What will be the sequence of these genes in a chromosome?
(a) a, b, c, d (b) a, c, b, d
(c) d, b, a, c (d) a, d, b, c

39 In *Drosophila*, red-eyed colour is dominant to white and is sex-linked. What results would you expect from a cross between a red-eyed male and a white-eyed female?
(a) All females red-eyed and males white-eyed
(b) All males and females red-eyed
(c) All females white-eyed and males red-eyed
(d) All offsprings white-eyed

40 The loci of genes A and B are on different chromosomes. A dihybrid autotetraploid plant of genotype AA aa BB bb is self-pollinated. Assume that only diploid gametes are formed and that the loci A and B are very close to their respective centromere (chromosome segregation). Find the phenotypic expectations of the progeny.
(a) 1225 AB : 35Ab : 35aB : 1ab
(b) 1130 AB : 24Ab : 24aB : 1ab
(c) 936 AB : 14Ab : 14aB : 1ab
(d) 890 AB : 13Ab : 13aB : 1ab

41 In tomato, three pairs of genes are located on a chromosome of these each two are linked. There is 8% recombination between the genes for tallness (T) and smooth surface (S). There is 20% recombination between tallness and oval-shape (O) of the fruit and 12% between oval-shape fruit and smooth fruit surface. The correct sequence of the genes is
(a) S-O-T (b) S-T-O (c) T-S-O (d) O-T-S

42 In maize, coloured endosperm (C) is dominant over colourless (c) and full endosperm (S) is dominant over shrunken (s). When a dihybrid of F_1-generation was test crossed, it produced four phenotypes in the following percentage.
Coloured full 48%, coloured shrunken 5%, colourless full 7%, colourless shrunken 48%. From this data, what would be the distance between the two non-allelic genes?
(a) 48 units (b) 12 units (c) 7 units (d) 5 units

43 Geneticist plot the relative locations of genes on chromosomes by which of these methods?
(a) Exposing animals to radiations
(b) Calculating the number of genes
(c) Using powerful microscope
(d) Determining the frequency of crossovers (crossing over)

44 In a cross in *Drosophila*, the heterozygous animal with grey body (b+) and long wing (vg+) with black body and vestigial wings, the progeny has the animals in the following ratio – grey vestigial 24 : grey long 126 : black long 26 : black vestigial 124. What is the frequency of recombinants in the population?
(a) 14.5 (b) 17.5 (c) 16.7 (d) 15.8

45 Based on the relative proportion of parental and recombinant phenotypes in the test cross progeny involving two recessive genes r (round) and y (yellow) controlling the seed shape and seed colour respectively, the observed percent recombinant is 10. The distance between r and y is

(a) 10 map units (b) 20 map units
(c) 30 map units (d) 40 map units

46 Individuals homozygous for cd genes were crossed with wild type ++. The F_1 dihybrid, thus produced was test crossed. It produced progeny in the following ratio ++ 900, +d115, cd 880, c + 105. What is the distance between c and d genes?

(a) 47 units (b) 88 units
(c) 11 units (d) 5.75 units

47 In a cross between genotype Ab and ++, 1700 out of 2000 individuals were of parental type. The distance between A and B is

(a) 35 map units (b) 45 map units
(c) 30 map units (d) 15 map units

48 When two genetic loci produce identical phenotypes in *cis* as well as *trans* position, they are considered to be

(a) pseudoalleles (b) parts of the same gene
(c) multiple alleles (d) different genes

49 The test cross of a F_1 individual with genotype (++/ab) produced the following offsprings ++/ab 10, ab/ab 10, +a/ab 40, +b/ab 40. Based on this data, predict the configuration of F_1 heterozygous.

(a) *trans*-configuration (b) *cis*-configuration
(c) Both (a) and (b) (d) None of these

50 Alfred Sturtevant to measure the distance between genes and mapped their position on the chromosome used the frequency of

(a) recombination between gene pairs on the two different chromosomes
(b) recombination between gene pairs on the same chromosome
(c) gene pairing on two different chromosomes
(d) gene pairing on the same chromosome

51 Linkage map of X-chromosome of fruitfly has 66 map units with yellow body gene (y) at one end and bobbed hair (b) at the other end. The recombination frequency between y and b gene would be

(a) 66% (b) ≤ 50% (c) > 50% (d) 100%

52 The distance between the genes A, B, C and D in mapping units are $A-D=3.5$, $B-C=1$, $A-B=6$, $C-D=1.5$, $A-C=5$. Find out the sequence of arrangement of these genes.

(a) ACDB (b) ABCD (c) ACBD (d) ADCB

53 In Morgan's experiments on linkage, the percentage of white eyed, miniature-winged recombinants in F_2-generation is

(a) 1.3 (b) 37.2 (c) 62.8 (d) 73.2

54 Distance between the genes and percentage of recombination shows **[NCERT Exemplar]**

(a) a direct relationship
(b) an inverse relationship
(c) a parallel relationship
(d) no relationship

55 Linkage and cytological maps for the same chromosome

(a) are both based on mutant phenotypes and recombination data
(b) may have different sequences of genes
(c) have both the same sequences of genes and intergenic distances
(d) have the same sequences of genes, but different intergenic distances

56 In rabbit, two recessive genes produce a solid body colour and long hair in contrast to dominant spotted body colour and short hair. The result of a cross between heterozygous spotted short haired rabbit to solid long haired rabbit gives spotted, short haired 48, spotted long haired 5, solid short haired 7, solid long haired 40, total 100. In terms of crossover units, how far are there two genes on the chromosome?

(a) 40 map units (b) 7 units
(c) 12 map units (d) 48 map units

57 If two genes 'a' and 'b' are linked and show 20% recombination, the proportion of gametes produced in F_1 by a dihybrid ++/ab derived from a cross between ++/++ and ab/ab would be

(a) ++ 20 : ab 20 : + a 20 : +b 20
(b) ++ 80 : ab 20
(c) ++ 50 : ab 50
(d) ++ 40 : ab 40 : +a 10 : +b 10

58 *Criss-cross* inheritance in *Drosophila* led to the discovery of

(a) law of independent assortment
(b) extrachromosomal inheritance
(c) lethal gene
(d) sex-linked inheritance

59 When the dominant alleles or wild type say AB are present on one chromosome and its alternative recessive alleles a b are located on the other homologous chromosome AB/ab, then the linkage is said to be in

(a) repulsion phase (b) coupling phase
(c) neutral phase (d) dominant phase

60 'Bent', a dominant sex-linked allele B, in the mouse results in a short, crooked tail. Its recessive allele, b produces normal tails. If a normal tailed female is mated to a bent-tailed male, what phenotypic ratio should occur in the F_1?

(a) ♀ bent, ♂ normal (b) ♀ normal, ♂ bent
(c) ♀ bent, ♂ bent (d) ♀ normal, ♂ normal

61 Offsprings resemble their parents, but are not exactly like them. This is so, because of

(a) variation produced by crossing over at the time of gamete formation
(b) variation produced by chance and distribution of chromosomes to the two poles during meiosis-I
(c) Both (a) and (b)
(d) mingling of maternal and paternal characters

Multiple Allelism and Cytoplasmic Inheritance

62 The genes which seem to behave like alleles and have minimum chances of crossing over are called

(a) isoalleles (b) pseudoalleles
(c) Both (a) and (b) (d) multiple alleles

63 When alleles exhibit themselves within the same phenotype, it is

(a) pseudoalleles (b) multiple alleles
(c) isoalleles (d) None of these

64 Different mutations referrable to the same locus of a chromosome gives rise to

(a) multiple alleles (b) pseudoalleles
(c) polygenes (d) oncogenes

65 The maximum number of chromosomes in a flowering plant is $2n = 265$ in *Poa litorosa.* The minimum number (*Drosophila*) is

(a) $2n = 4$ (b) $2n = 14$
(c) $2n = 2$ (d) $2n = 16$

66 Inheritance of characters not located in the gene, but the young one resembling only the female part is due to

(a) cytoplasmic inheritance (b) chromosomal inheritance
(c) plastid inheritance (d) epigenesis

67 Genes present in the cytoplasm of eukaryotic cells, are found in

(a) mitochondria and inherited *via* egg cytoplasm
(b) lysosomes and peroxisomes
(c) Golgi bodies and smooth endoplasmic reticulum
(d) plastids and inherited *via* male gamete

68 What form of inheritance does a trait in human have, which is found in the siblings of parents, where the female has the trait, but is never found in siblings of parents, where only the male has the trait?

(a) X-linked inheritance
(b) Y-linked inheritance
(c) Autosomal inheritance
(d) Maternal (extranuclear) inheritance

69 When an albino plant of maize female is crossed with a normal green male plant, all plants in the progeny are albino because

(a) albinism is dominant over green characters
(b) plastids are inherited through maternal plants
(c) green plastids of male parent become maternal
(d) crossing results in structural change in green plants

70 Cytoplasmic male sterility in maize is the phenotypic manifestation of the interactions between

(a) cytoplasmic factors and male sterility genes
(b) cytoplasmic factors and male fertility nuclear genes
(c) chloroplast genes and nuclear genes
(d) mitochondrial and chloroplast genes

71 In multifactorial inheritance

(a) many characters are influenced by a simple gene
(b) many genes influence a simple character
(c) more than one allele of a gene is necessary to produce the effect
(d) one gene incompletely dominates the effect of its allele

72 Cytosterility in the pollen of maize is due to

(a) extrachromosomal inheritance
(b) complementary genes
(c) nuclear inheritance
(d) hypostasis

73 In *Mirabilis,* normal leaves (I) and variegated leaves (II) colour occur in different plants. If (II) male is crossed with (I) female, normal leaves occur in the hybrid. But (I) male is crossed with (II) female variegated leaves occur. It is an instance of

(a) cytoplasmic inheritance
(b) disjunction
(c) inversion
(d) epistasis

Mutation

74 Alteration in chromosomes results in

(a) abnormalities or aberrations
(b) recombination or abnormalities
(c) aberrations or replication
(d) replication or recombination

75 The phenomenon of mutation results in
(a) alteration of DNA sequences
(b) changes in the genotype of an organism
(c) changes in the phenotype of an organism
(d) All of the above

76 Mutations are mainly responsible for
(a) maintaining genetic continuity
(b) increasing population rate
(c) controlling variation in organisms
(d) controlling extinction of organisms

77 Which one of the following statements is correct as applied to the occurrence of mutations?
(a) Mutations are encountered in all forms of life including virus and bacteria
(b) Mutations occur in all forms of life except in such viruses, which have RNA as their genetic material
(c) Mutations take place only in such forms, which are under selection pressure
(d) Mutations occur only when the organisms are subjected to mutagenic agents

78 Choose the incorrect statement.
(a) Mutation in germ cells can be detected only in the next generation
(b) Mutations do not result in hybrid vigour
(c) The creation of mutation is called mutagenesis
(d) Mutation is more common when it is present in recessive condition

79 Mutation is a
(a) change, which affects the parents only but never inherited
(b) change, which affects the offspring of F_2-generation only
(c) factor responsible for plant growth
(d) change that is inherited

80 Consider the following statements.
I. The site in the gene, at which the mutations occur with usually high frequency are hotspots.
II. In nature, the rate of mutation is 1×10^{-7}.
Choose the correct option.
(a) Statement I is true, but II is false
(b) Statement I is false, but II is true
(c) Both statements I and II are true
(d) Both statements I and II are false

81 The point mutation occurs due to
(a) change in the base pairs of DNA
(b) change in a single base pair of DNA
(c) alteration in the base pairs of DNA
(d) aberrations in the base pairs of DNA

82 A micromutation is
(a) addition of chromosome (b) deletion of chromosomes
(c) change in gene (d) polyploidy

83 Inheritable mutations can be studied by
(a) generating a pedigree of a family
(b) pureline breeding
(c) Punnett square
(d) using chemical mutagens

84 The DNA sequence of *lac* gene shows a mutation where the middle base of a triplet code has been substituted. However, the gene does not show any mutation and expresses normal. This may be due to
(a) suppressor mutation (b) silent mutation
(c) wobbling of *t*RNA (d) degeneracy of codon

85 Choose the incorrect pair.
(a) Exchange of segments between non-homologous chromosome – Translocation
(b) When a mutation is limited to the substitution of one nucleotide pair of DNA – Point mutation
(c) The smallest element or subdivision of a gene, which can be affected by a mutation – Recon
(d) Conditions of a karyotype $2n \pm 1$ and $2n \pm 2$ – Aneuploidy

86 X-rays cause mutations by
(a) changing the chromosome morphology
(b) rupturing the nuclear envelope
(c) breaking the spindle fibres
(d) inducing the karyokinesis

87 Consider the following statements.
I. Chromosomal aberrations are commonly observed in cancer cells.
II. The alteration in chromosomes results due to loss of a segment of DNA and gain of a segment of DNA.
Choose the correct option.
(a) Statement I is true, but II is false
(b) Statement I is false, but II is true
(c) Both statements I and II are true
(d) Both statements I and II are false

88 Recessive mutations are expressed normally in
(a) homozygous condition
(b) heterozygous condition
(c) has to express always since it is a mutation
(d) neither in homozygous nor in a heterozygous condition

89 A mutational event, which changes the codon UGG to UAG is known as
(a) non-sense mutation (b) point mutation
(c) mis-sense mutation (d) frameshift mutation

90 Errors during DNA replication, repair or recombination can lead to base pair substitutions. Such changes are called
(a) mutagens
(b) saltatory changes
(c) spontaneous mutations
(d) conditional mutations

91 Haploids are more suitable for mutation studies than the diploids. This is because
(a) haploids are reproductively more stable than diploids
(b) mutagens penetrate in haploids more effectively than in diploids
(c) haploids are more abundant in nature than diploid
(d) all mutations, whether dominant or recessive are expressed in haploids

92 Which of the following mutational events is most difficult to detect?
(a) Auxotrophic mutations
(b) Lethal mutations
(c) Dominant mutations
(d) Recessive non-lethal mutations

93 The reason why some mutations, which are harmful do not get eliminated from gene pool is that
(a) they are dominant and show up more frequently
(b) they have future survival value
(c) they are recessive and carried by heterozygous individuals
(d) genetic drift occurs because of a small population

94 Dominant mutations are easier to detect than recessive mutations because they
(a) are always lethal and so their appearance is unmistakable
(b) are expressed in both homozygotes and heterozygotes
(c) occur at a higher frequency
(d) are always neutral in their effect

95 Microorganisms have been very useful in elucidating different effects of the mutations because
(a) they have short lifespan and many generations may be studied within a limited period
(b) they are haploid and therefore, express all the mutations induced in them
(c) they can be easily cultured under controlled condition on simple and defined media
(d) All of the above

96 Haploids are able to express both recessive and dominant alleles/mutations because there are
(a) many alleles for each gene
(b) two alleles for each gene
(c) only one allele for each gene in the individual
(d) only one allele in a gene

97 Certain chemicals when tested individually are not mutagenic, but when applied together, these increase the frequency of mutation. Such chemicals are called as
(a) comutagens (b) radio-potentials
(c) mutagen (d) Both (a) and (b)

98 Mutational events, which result in the deletion or addition of nucleotide bases in DNA, thereby causing gross changes in the amino acid sequences of proteins are termed as
(a) point mutations
(b) forward and backward mutations
(c) transversions
(d) frameshift mutations

99 Rearrangement of a group of genes within the chromosome in such a way that their order in the chromosome is same but position is different is referred to as
(a) inversion (b) translocation
(c) deletion (d) interchange

100 The exchange of chromosomal parts between non-homologous chromosomes is known as
(a) translocation (b) transcription
(c) transduction (d) translation

101 A *m*RNA with 6 codons (for chain initiation, termination and amino acid) is included in the rectangle shown in the given figure. The different types of mutations, indicated as *A*, *B*, *C* and *D* are respectively

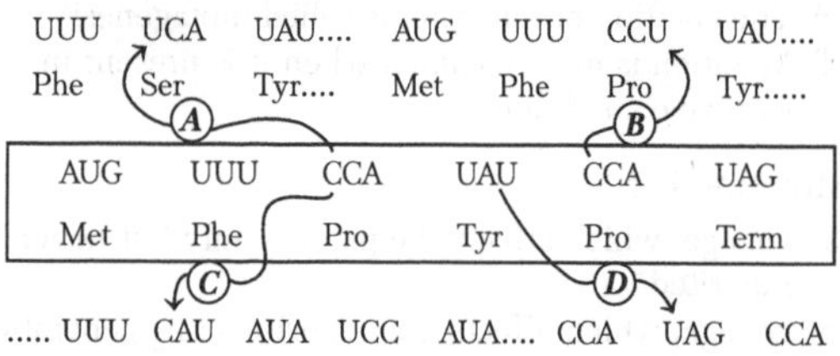

(a) silent, mis-sense, non-sense and frameshift
(b) silent, mis-sense, frameshift and non-sense
(c) mis-sense, silent, non-sense and frameshift
(d) mis-sense, silent, frameshift and non-sense

102 Type of gene mutation, which involves the replacement of purine with pyrimidine or *vice-versa* or the substitution of one type of base with another type of base is
(a) transition (b) transduction
(c) translation (d) transversion

103 Before a deletion occurred, the gene sequence was ABCDEF, now it is
(a) ABDBEF
(b) FEDCBA
(c) ABDEF
(d) ABEDCF

104 A segment of the DNA has a base sequence AAG GAG GAC CAA CCA. Which of the following sequences represents a frameshift mutation?

(a) AGG AGG ACC ACC CA
(b) AAG GCG GAC CCA AC
(c) ACG GAC GAC CAG CCA
(d) AAG GAG GAC CAA CCA

105 Which of the following shows silent mutations if *m*RNA strand has AUG UAU CCA UAU CCA UAC codons?

(a) AUG UAU GCC AUA UCC AUA
(b) AUG UAU UGA UAU CCA UAG
(c) AUG UAU CCU UAU CCA UAC
(d) AUG UAU UCA UAC CCA UAG

106 The trisomic condition ($2n+1$) found in mongoloid idiots would arise most easily from

(a) translocation (b) inversion
(c) triploidy (d) non-disjunction

107 After a mutation at a genetic locus, the character of an organism changes due to the change in

(a) protein structure
(b) DNA replication
(c) protein synthesis pattern
(d) RNA transcription pattern

108 If the haploid number of chromosome is 10. Then, what is a tetrasomic number?

(a) 20 (b) 10
(c) 22 (d) 40

109 Given below is a representation of a kind of chromosomal mutation. What is the kind of mutation represented?

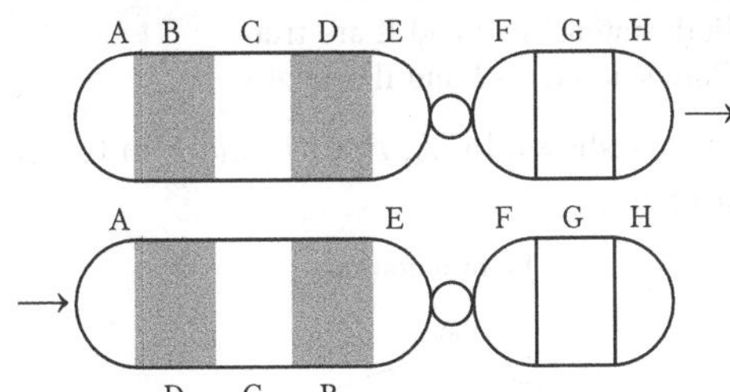

(a) Deletion (b) Duplication
(c) Inversion (d) Reciprocal translocation

110 Choose the incorrect statement regarding deletions.

(a) Can be detected during the pairing of homologous chromosomes
(b) Their genetic effect can be seen in the form of pseudodominance
(c) In plants, they can be easily transmitted to offsprings
(d) None of the above

111 Choose the incorrect match.

(a) Translocation – Change in gene sequence
(b) Inversion – Reversed gene sequence
(c) Reverse tandem – Translocation
(d) All of the above

112 A segment of DNA has the triplet base sequence AAC, GAC, AGC, CGC, ACA and AAA. Due to mutation, the first base only got deleted. Then the likely effect of this on the coding of DNA segment is that

(a) there will be complete change in the types and sequence of amino acids
(b) polypeptide will have one amino acid less
(c) there will be no change in polypeptide chain formed
(d) the first amino acid will be different

113 Which of the following mutations is likely to cause the greatest impact on the expression of a gene?

(a) Insertion of a base pair in the middle of the coding sequence
(b) Deletion of a base pair in the middle of the coding sequence
(c) Changing a base pair in the middle of the coding sequence
(d) Deletion of a base pair in the second codon of the coding sequence

114 Aneuploidy is a term used where

(a) zygotic chromosome number is multiple of 3 of gametic number
(b) zygote chromosome number is multiple of 2 of gametic number
(c) zygote chromosome number is multiple of 4 of gametic number
(d) zygote has abnormal number of chromosomes

115 Mutations used in agriculture are

(a) lethal and recessive
(b) artificially induced and recessive
(c) lethal and dominant
(d) None of the above

116 Euploidy is best explained by

(a) exact multiple of a haploid set of chromosomes
(b) one chromosome is less than the haploid set of chromosomes
(c) one chromosome is more than the haploid set of chromosome
(d) one chromosome is more than the diploid set of chromosomes

117 If the haploid number of chromosomes in a plant is 12, then the number of chromosomes in monosomic condition is

(a) 25 (b) 23
(c) 22 (d) 26

118 Polyploidy leads to rapid formation of new species because of
(a) isolation
(b) development of multiple sets of chromosomes
(c) mutation
(d) genetic recombination

119 When an additional copy of a chromosome is included in an individual, the condition is called
(a) monosomy (b) trisomy
(c) triploid (d) None of these

120 A ring of three chromosomes and six bivalents are observed in pea plant. What type of cytological abnormality is present in this plant?
(a) Triploid (b) Primary trisomic
(c) Secondary trisomic (d) Inversion homozygote

121 Which of the following represents an amphidiploid condition?
(a) A polyploid containing genetically different chromosome sets derived from two or more species
(b) A polyploid species, in which the genomes have been derived from the same original species
(c) A plant derived by doubling the chromosomes of F_1 hybrid of two species
(d) A plant having a chromosome number, which is not an exact multiple of the haploid number

122 Which of the following organisms is known as an allopolyploidy?
(a) A polyploid formed by the union of two distinct chromosome sets with subsequent doubling of chromosome number
(b) A polyploid containing genetically different chromosome sets derived from two or more species
(c) A polyploid, where the chromosome number is not an exact multiple of its haploid number
(d) A polyploid having identical sets of genome

123 One of the reasons why haploids are considered more suitable than diploids for the study of mutation is that the haploids
(a) have shorter generation time
(b) have small number of chromosomes
(c) allow expression of recessive mutations immediately (or in first generation)
(d) can be obtained in large number to give correct estimate of mutation theory

124 Different species of *Rhododendron* have somatic chromosome numbers of 26, 39, 52, 78, 104 and 156. By what means does evolution appear to be taking place in this genus?
(a) Aneuploidy (b) Hyperploids
(c) Euploidy (d) Autoalloploidy

125 Consider the following conditions.
I. Monoploidy
II. Hypoploidy
III. Polyploidy
IV. Hyperploidy
Which among these are euploidy?
(a) I and II (b) II and III
(c) Only IV (d) I and III

126 A species or type of a plant derived from doubling the chromosome of F_1 hybrid of two similar species is known as
(a) autopolyploid (b) amphidiploid
(c) autodiploid (d) hexaploid

127 Abyssinian oat is a tetraploid with 28 chromosomes. The common cultivated oat is a hexaploid in the same series. How many chromosomes do the common oat possess?
(a) 28 (b) 34 (c) 38 (d) 42

128 Application of colchicine to a vegetative bud of a homozygous tall diploid tomato plant (DD) caused development of a tetraploid branch. What is the genotype of the somatic cells of this branch?
(a) DDD (b) DDDD (c) DDdd (d) DdDd

129 Consider the following statements.
I. Polyploidy means occurrence of more than diploid sets of chromosome.
II. Polyploidy can be induced by the application of colchicine.
Choose the correct option.
(a) Statement I is true, but II is false
(b) Statement I is false, but II is true
(c) Both statements I and II are true
(d) Both statements I and II are false

130 What are shown by *A*, *B*, *C*, *D* and *E* in the given figure?

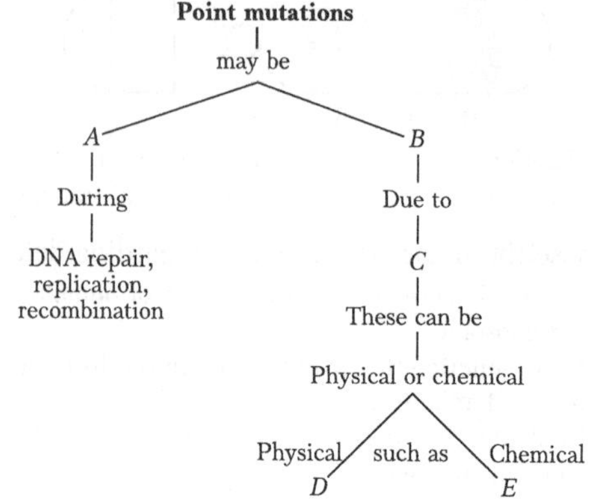

(a) *A*-Spontaneous, *B*-Artificial, *C*-Mutagens, *D*-Radiation like X-rays, *E*-Base analogues, HNO_2
(b) *A*-Induced, *B*-Artificial, *C*-Mutagens, *D*-HNO_2 *E*-X-rays
(c) *A*-Spontaneous, *B*-Artificial, *C*-Mutagens, *D*-X-rays, *E*-Base analogues, HNO_2
(d) *A*-Artificial, *B*-Spontaneous, *C*-Mutagens, *D*-Radiation like X-rays, *E*-Base analogues, HNO_2

131 First definite proof of mutagenic action (effect) of X-rays was discovered or given by or the person known to use X-rays to cause mutation is
(a) Leeuwenhoek
(b) Hooper
(c) Lister
(d) Muller

132 In man, which of the following genotypes and phenotypes may be the correct result of aneuploidy in sex chromosomes?
(a) 22 pairs + XXY males
(b) 22 pairs + XX females
(c) 22 pairs + XY females
(d) None of the above

(B) Cumulative Exercise

(Assorted Questions of the Chapter for Advanced Level Practice)

1 A scientist found that a particular gene was mutated, but the polypeptide coded by this gene had not changed. Which of the following mutation is probably involved?
(a) Deletion of one nucleotide
(b) Addition of a nucleotide
(c) Substitution of a nucleotide
(d) Addition of three nucleotides, which form a codon

2 Match the following columns.

	Column I		Column II
A.	XX-XO method of sex-determination	1.	Female heterogametic
B.	1.5 X/A ratio	2.	Turner's syndrome
C.	Karyotype 45	3.	Hemiptera
D.	ZW-ZZ method of sex-determination	4.	Metafemale

Codes

	A	B	C	D
(a)	2	4	1	3
(b)	3	4	2	1
(c)	4	1	2	3
(d)	1	4	2	3

3 Genes A and B are linked 12 map units apart. A heterozygous individual, whose parents were AAbb and aaBB, would be expected to produce gametes in the following frequencies

(a) 44% AB	6% Ab	6% aB	44% ab
(b) 6% AB	44% Ab	44% aB	6% ab
(c) 12% AB	38% Ab	38% aB	12% ab
(d) 6% AB	6% Ab	44% aB	44% ab

4 A cross of a wild type red-eyed female *Drosophila* with a violet-eyed male produces all red-eyed offsprings. If the gene is sex-linked, what should the reciprocal cross (violet-eyed female × red-eyed male) produce (Assume that the red allele is dominant to the violet allele)?
(a) All violet-eyed flies
(b) 3 red-eyed flies to 1 violet-eyed
(c) A 1:1 ratio of red and violet-eyes in both males and females
(d) Red-eyed females and violet-eyed males

5 What would happen if in a gene encoding, a polypeptide of 50 amino acids has UAC and its 25th position mutated to UAA?
(a) A polypeptide of 49 amino acids will be formed
(b) A polypeptide of 25 amino acids will be formed
(c) A polypeptide of 24 amino acids will be formed
(d) Two polypeptides of 24 and 25 amino acids will be formed

6 Match the following columns.

	Column I		Column II
A.	Monoploidy	1.	$2n-1$
B.	Monosomy	2.	$2n+1$
C.	Nullisomy	3.	$2n+2$
D.	Trisomy	4.	$2n-2$
E.	Tetrasomy	5.	n
		6.	$3n$

Codes

	A	B	C	D	E
(a)	5	1	4	2	3
(b)	5	2	4	1	3
(c)	6	5	3	4	2
(d)	2	1	3	6	5

7 Select the incorrect statement from the following.
(a) Linkage is an exception to the principle of independent assortment in heredity
(b) Galactosemia is an inborn error of metabolism
(c) Small population size results in random genetic drift in a populaiton
(d) Baldness is a sex-limited trait

8 In the given cross in *Drosophila*, if selfing of F_1-generation is made, the result observed by Morgan was

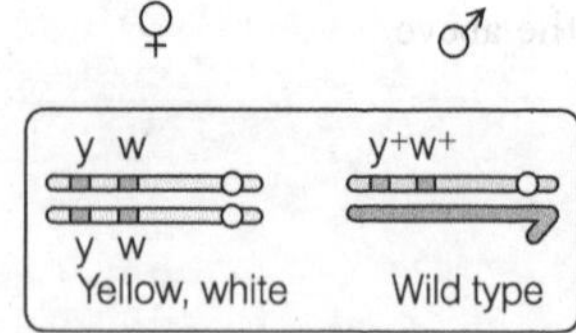

(a) Brown bodies and white eyed – 37.2%
(b) Brown bodies and yellow eyed – 1.3%
(c) Yellow bodies and red eyed – 0.65%
(d) White bodies and brown eyed – 1.3%

9 In *Drosophila*, the following crossing over percentages were found.

Gene	Gene	Crossing over %
bi	ec	1.4
bi	fa	3.9
wi	ec	4.0
wi	fa	1.5

What is the order of these genes?
(a) bi-ec-fa-wi (b) bi-ec-wi-fa
(c) ec-bi-fa-wi (d) ec-bi-wi-fa

10 Bateson used the terms coupling and repulsion, while discovering linkage in *Lathyrus.* If A, B are dominant alleles and a, b are recessive alleles of two genes, parental crosses in coupling and repulsion phases can be written as follows

	Coupling	**Repulsion**
(a)	AABB, aabb	AAbb, aaBB
(b)	AABB, aabb	AABB, AAbb
(c)	aaBB, aabb	AAbb, aabb
(d)	AAbb, aaBB	AbBa, aabb

11 You map four bacteriophage genes by recombination. The recombination frequencies between the four genes are shown in the table below. What is the order of the genes along the chromosome?

Genes	A	B	C	D
A	–	0.18	0.1	0.2
B		–	0.15	0.37
C			–	0.24
D				–

(a) ABCD (b) BADC (c) CABD (d) DACB

12 The experiment shown in the figure below has been carried out by Morgan to show the phenomenon of linkage and recombination.
If in cross I, genes are tightly linked and in cross II, genes are loosely linked, then what will be the percentage of recombinants product in cross I and cross II, respectively?

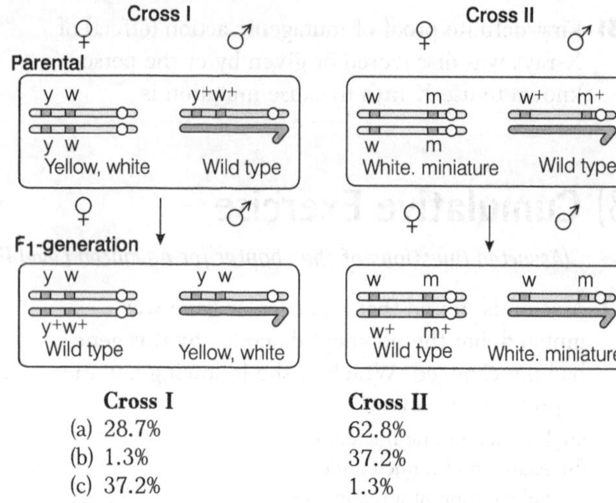

	Cross I	**Cross II**
(a)	28.7%	62.8%
(b)	1.3%	37.2%
(c)	37.2%	1.3%
(d)	62.8%	98.7%

13 In a test cross of Pp Qq plant, the following progeny is obtained
Pp Qq = 500
Pp qq = 50
pp Qq = 100
pp qq = 350
What is the distance between genes p and q?
(a) 15 cM (b) 10 cM
(c) 25 cM (d) 50 cM

14 The following cross was conducted by Morgan on *Drosophila.*

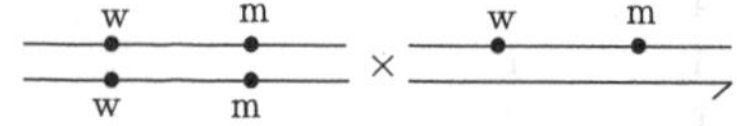

In F_2-generation, progeny had parental and recombinant traits in the ratio of 62.8 : 37. 2. What percentage of F_2 progeny would have the given condition?

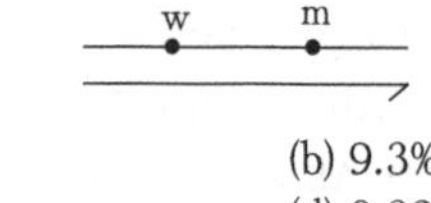

(a) 15.7% (b) 9.3%
(c) 24.68% (d) 0.32%

15 The number of linkage groups in a sperm and ovum of human is respectively
(a) 24, 23 (b) 23, 22
(c) 23, 23 (d) 23, 24

16 Consider among following statements regarding multiple alleles.

I. Influence the different characters.
II. Have arisen as a result of mutation of the normal gene.
III. Exhibit the phenomenon of crossing over in itself.
IV. Occupy the same locus in the homologous chromosomes.

Choose the correct option.

(a) I and II (b) II and III (c) II and IV (d) I and IV

17 Which of these statements represent reason for silent mutations?

I. More than one codon specify same amino acid.
II. Simultaneous presence of suppressor mutations.
III. The change in codon.
IV. Presence of activator genes.

Choose the correct option.

(a) I, II and III (b) II and IV (c) III and IV (d) I and III

18 Mendel conducted a number of crosses and studies but could never discover linkage. What could be the reason for this?

I. Some genes are linked but they are too far apart for crossing over to be distinguished from independent assortment.
II. Linked genes were never tested for the same time in same cross.
III. The seven genes were present on the 7 chromosomes.
IV. The genes underwent mutation during subsequent crossings.

Choose the correct option.

(a) I and II (b) II and III (c) III and IV (d) Only IV

19 Individual homozygous for cd genes were crossed with wild type (++). The F_1 hybrids thus produced was test crossed and progenies produced in following ratio ++- 450, cd - 440, +d - 58, +c -54.

Calculate the distance between c and d genes.

(a) 5.75 units (b) 11.2 units
(c) 45 units (d) 44 units

20 Match the following columns.

Column I (Chromosome aberrations)		Column II (Consequences)	
A.	Intercalary deficiency	1.	Transfer of part of chromosome to non-homologous segment
B.	Duplication	2.	Centromere is not involved
C.	Paracentric inversion	3.	Presence of same genes in chromosome in more than two doses
D.	Translocation	4.	Two breaks followed by reunion and deletion

Codes

	A	B	C	D
(a)	4	3	1	2
(b)	4	3	2	1
(c)	1	2	3	4
(d)	2	3	1	4

21 Which of the following statements are correct regarding crossing over?

I. It provides its results as variations, which are new material of evolutionary changes in nature.
II. It helps in the construction of linkage maps.
III. It affords a proof for linear arrangement of genes.
IV. It helps in the cytoplasmic inheritance.

Codes

(a) I, II and III (b) II and IV
(c) III and IV (d) Only IV

22 Which of the following mechanisms can explain the determination of sex?

I. Genic balance mechanism
II. Haplo-diploidy mechanism
III. Cytoplasmic inheritance
IV. Sex-linked inheritance

Codes

(a) I and II (b) III and IV
(c) Only IV (d) I, II and III

23 Match the following columns.

Column I	Column II
A. Traits close enough together on a chromosome.	1. Linkage
B. The exchange occurring between homologous areas of the chromosome during meiosis.	2. Carrier
C. A defective allele on the non-sex chromosomes that causes a disease.	3. Recombination

Codes

	A	B	C
(a)	1	3	2
(b)	3	2	1
(c)	1	2	3
(d)	2	1	3

24 Consider the following statements regarding linkage.

I. The linked genes are located on the same chromosome.
II. Crossing over between linked genes is rare.
III. Linked genes are always inherited together.
IV. Linked genes affect the percentage of homozygosity following hybridisation.

Choose the option containing correct statements.

(a) I and III (b) I, II and III
(c) II, III and IV (d) I, III and IV

25 If a plant were trisomic for one of its chromosomes and these chromosomes carried the alleles A, A^1 and A^2, respectively, how many types of gametes can be produced?

(a) 3 (b) 4 (c) 6 (d) 12

26 Match the following columns.

	Column I		Column II
A.	A chromosome fragment lost during meiotic recombination	1.	Inversion
B.	A 'picture' of a set of chromosome	2.	Karyotype
C.	A piece of the chromosome that gets flipped during recombination	3.	Deletion
D.	Movement of a piece of one chromosome to another	4.	Duplication
E.	Repeated DNA sequences produced by unequal crossing over	5.	Translocation

Codes

	A	B	C	D	E
(a)	3	2	1	5	4
(b)	1	2	3	4	5
(c)	4	3	2	1	5
(d)	5	4	3	2	1

27 Which of the following are correct?

I. An inversion is produced, when there are two breaks in a chromosome and the intercalary segment reunites in reverse order.

II. Reciprocal translocations involve mutual exchange of chromosome segments between two pairs of non-homologous chromosomes.

III. In paracentric inversion, inverted segment includes centromere.

IV Inversion occurring in both the members of homologous pair is called chromosomal inversion.

Codes

(a) I and II (b) III and IV
(c) II and III (d) Only IV

28 Which of the following statements are correct?

I. Point mutations involve deletion of a part of chromosome.

II. When a purine base is replaced by another purine and pyrimidine by another pyrimidine, it is transition.

III. In frameshift mutations, one nitrogenous base is substituted by other.

IV. When a purine is replaced by a pyrimidine and *vice-versa*, it is called transversion.

Codes

(a) I and II (b) II and IV
(c) III and IV (d) Only IV

29 Match the following columns.

Column I	Column II
A. Non-disjunction	1. A segment of the sequence is turned over and reinserted
B. Translocation	2. Exchange of material between non-homologous chromosomes
C. Inversion	3. A portion of the message is completely lost
D. Duplication	4. Certain sequences are copied more often than others
E. Deletion	5. Chromosomes fail to sort properly during meiosis

Codes

	A	B	C	D	E
(a)	5	2	1	4	3
(b)	4	1	5	2	3
(c)	3	2	1	4	5
(d)	2	3	4	1	5

Assertion and Reason

Direction (Q. Nos. 30-38) *In each of the following questions, a statement of Assertion (A) is given followed by corresponding statement of Reason (R). Of the statements, mark the correct answer as*

(a) Both A and R are true and R is the correct explanation of A
(b) Both A and R are true, but R is not the correct explanation of A
(c) A is true, but R is false
(d) A is false, but R is true
(e) Both A and R are false

30 **Assertion** (A) According to Bridges, the Y-chromosome is responsible only for the fertility of sex and not for sex-determination in *Drosophila.*

Reason (R) According to Bridges in *Drosophila,* autosomes are responsible for feminine characteristics.

31 **Assertion** (A) In *Habrobracon,* only haploid males are seen.

Reason (R) The unfertilised eggs only develop to males in this wasp. The fertilised eggs on the other hand always develop into females.

32 **Assertion** (A) In *Drosophila,* one strain shows more sensitivity towards CO_2.

Reason (R) The sensitivity is due to the presence of a heat labile substance within the cytoplasm called sigma.

33 Assertion (A) If both the chromosomes of a homologous pair contain dominant gene representation then the condition is known as *trans*.

Reason (R) The condition defined above is in response with crossing over.

34 Assertion (A) Somatic or mitotic crossover is never reported by any scientist.

Reason (R) The meiotic crossover produces patches of crossover tissue between the normal cells.

35 Assertion (A) XX-XY mechanism of sex determination occurs in human beings.

Reason (R) In humans, the X-chromosome is longer than Y-chromosome.

36 Assertion (A) During mutation, a gene may undergo a sudden change in expression due to the change in composition.

Reason (R) Some genes mutate more than one and have more than two alleles.

37 Assertion (A) Frameshift mutation is a gene mutation.

Reason (R) Gene mutation is also called point mutation.

38 Assertion (A) HJ Muller (1927) is first person who demonstrated the use of physical mutagens and got Nobel Prize in 1946.

Reason (R) X-rays, gamma rays are commonly used for producing mutations artificially.

(C) Medical Entrances' Gallery

(Collection of Questions Asked in NEET & in Various Medical Entrance Exams)

1 Chromosomal theory of inheritance was proposed by **[DUMET 2011, NEET 2020]**

(a) Sutton and Boveri (b) Bateson and Punnett
(c) TH Morgan (d) Watson and Crick

2 Experimental verification of the chromosomal theory of inheritance was done by **[NEET 2020, Kerala CEE 2011]**

(a) Sutton (b) Boveri (c) Morgan (d) Mendel

3 To make chromosomal studies easier, chromosomes are classified into certain groups. So, the chromosome number 21, 22 and Y are listed in **[JIPMER 2019]**

(a) A (b) D (c) E (d) G

4 What map unit (centiMorgan) is adopted in the construction of genetic maps? **[NEET 2019]**

(a) A unit of distance between two expressed genes representing 100% crossover
(b) A unit of distance between genes on chromosomes, representing 1% crossover
(c) A unit of distance between genes on chromosomes, representing 50% crossover
(d) A unit of distance between two expressed genes representing 10% crossover

5 The frequency of recombination between gene pairs on the same chromosome as a measure of the distance between genes was explained by **[NEET 2019]**

(a) Gregor J Mendel (b) Alfred Sturtevant
(c) Sutton-Boveri (d) TH Morgan

6 Which one of them is odd with respect to human male? **[JIPMER 2019]**

(a) Absence of one X-chromosome
(b) Addition of one X-chromosome
(c) Presence of XY-chromosome
(d) Absence of Barr body

7 Match the items of Column I with Column II.

	Column I	Column II
A.	XX-XO method of sex-determination	1. Turner's syndrome
B.	XX-XY method of sex-determination	2. Female heterogamety
C.	Karyotype-45	3. Grasshopper
D.	ZW-ZZ method of sex-determination	4. Female homogamety

Codes **[NEET 2019]**

	A	B	C	D
(a)	2	4	1	3
(b)	1	4	2	3
(c)	3	4	1	2
(d)	4	2	1	3

8 Chromosome walking is **[JIPMER 2019]**

(a) used in genetic mapping
(b) observed during mitosis
(c) to see position of ribosomes on nuclear membrane
(d) to check the expression of mutant genes

9 Select the incorrect statement. [NEET 2019]
(a) In male grasshoppers, 50% of sperms have no sex chromosome
(b) In domesticated fowls, sex of progeny depends on the type of sperm rather than egg
(c) Human males have one of their sex chromosome much shorter than the other
(d) Male fruitfly is heterogametic

10 Which one of the following conditions correctly describes the manner of determining the sex? [AIIMS 2018, CBSE AIPMT 2011]
(a) Homozygous sex chromosomes (ZZ) determine female sex in birds
(b) XO type of sex chromosomes determines male sex in grasshopper
(c) XO condition in humans as found in Turner's syndrome determines female sex
(d) Homozygous sex chromosomes (XX) produce males in *Drosophila*

11 XYY → composition [JIPMER 2018]
(a) superfemale (b) hermaphrodite
(c) male (d) supermale

12 Select the incorrect statements from the options given below.
I. Tightly linked genes on the same chromosome show higher recombinations.
II. Genes far apart on the same chromosome show very few recombinations.
III. Genes loosely linked on the same chromosome show similar recombinations.
Choose the correct option. [AIIMS 2018]
(a) I and II (b) II and III
(c) I and III (d) I, II and III

13 **Assertion** (A) The non-allelic genes for red hair and freckles are usually inherited together.
Reason (R) The genes for red hair and freckles located on the same chromosome in close association. [AIIMS 2018]
(a) Both A and R are true and R is the correct explanation of A
(b) Both A and R are true, but R is not the correct explanation of A
(c) A is true, but R is false
(d) Both A and R are false

14 In a test cross involving F_1 dihybrid files, more parental type offspring were produced than the recombinant type offspring. This indicates [NEET-I 2016]
(a) chromosomes failed to separate during meiosis
(b) the two genes are linked and present on the same chromosome
(c) Both of the characters are controlled by more than one gene
(d) the two genes are located on two different chromosomes

15 The distance between the genes on the chromosomes is measured by using [EAMCET 2016]
(a) pleiotropy (b) allele frequency
(c) codominance (d) recombination frequency

16 The mechanism that causes a gene to move from one linkage group to another is called [NEET-II 2016; CBSE AIPMT 2015]
(a) inversion (b) duplication
(c) translocation (d) crossing over

17 The term linkage was coined by [CBSE AIPMT 2015]
(a) TH Morgan (b) T Boveri
(c) GJ Mendel (d) W Sutton

18 Match the following columns.

Column I	Column II
A. ABO blood group	1. Landsteiner and Weiner
B. Rh-factor	2. Morgan and Castle
C. Sex linkage in *Drosophila*	3. Landsteiner
D. Chromosomal theory of linkage	4. TH Morgan

Codes [Chhattisgarh PMT 2015]

	A	B	C	D
(a)	3	1	4	2
(b)	4	1	3	2
(c)	2	1	4	3
(d)	3	2	4	1

19 A point mutation that changes a codon specifying an amino acid into a stop codon is called a [Chhattisgarh PMT 2015]
(a) non-sense mutation
(b) deletion mutation
(c) frameshift mutation
(d) mis-sense mutation

20 A species has $2n = 16$ chromosomes. How many chromosomes will be found per cell in each of the following mutant species?
I. Monosomic II. Autotriploid
III. Trisomic IV. Double monosomic
V. Nullisomic
The correct sequence of chromosomes for (I to V) are [Chhattisgarh PMT 2015]
(a) 15, 24, 17, 14, 14 (b) 24, 32, 18, 40, 12
(c) 16, 22, 14, 21, 16 (d) 26, 34, 20, 42, 14

21 If an inheritable mutation is observed in a population at high frequency, it is referred to as [KCET 2015]
(a) sequence annotation (b) DNA polymorphism
(c) linkage (d) expressed sequence tag

22 *Drosophila* with the genotype AAA+XX is **[EAMCET 2015]**
(a) normal male (b) normal female
(c) intersex (d) metamale

23 Which one of the following information is essential to determine the genetic map distance between two genes located on the same chromosome? **[WB JEE 2015]**
(a) Length of the particular chromosome
(b) Number of genes present in the particular chromosome
(c) Number of nucleotides in the particular chromosome
(d) Percentage of crossing over or recombinant frequency between the two genes

24 Conditions of a karyotype $2n + l - 2$ and $2n + l - 2$ are called **[J&K CET 2015]**
(a) aneuploidy (b) polyploidy
(c) autopolyploidy (d) monosomy

25 Genes for cytoplasmic male sterility in plants are generally located in **[J&K CET 2015]**
(a) nuclear genome (b) mitochondrial genome
(c) chloroplast genome (d) cytosol

26 Which is gynandromorph type of animal? **[Gujarat CET 2015]**
(a) *Drosophila* (b) Beetles
(c) Silkworms (d) All of these

27 Choose the incorrect statement. **[Kerala CEE 2014]**
(a) Failure of segregation of chromatids during cell division results in aneuploidy
(b) Additional copy of X-chromosome in males results in Klinefelter's syndrome
(c) Closely located genes in a chromosome always assort independently resulting in recombinants
(d) According to Mendel, recessive character never blend in heterozygous condition
(e) Failure of cytokinesis after DNA replication result in polyploidy

28 The frequency of crossing over occurring between two genes located on the same chromosome depends on **[WB JEE 2014]**
(a) length of the chromosome
(b) position of the centromere
(c) activities of two genes
(d) distance between two genes

29 Which of the following factor was used by Alfred Sturtevant to measure the distance between the genes and mapped their position on the chromosome? **[UK PMT 2014]**
(a) Total recombination
(b) Frequency of recombination
(c) Parental gene combination
(d) Non-parental combination

30 Choose the incorrect statement. **[Kerala CEE 2014]**
(a) In grasshoppers, besides autosomes males have only one X-chromosome, whereas females have a pair of X-chromosomes
(b) In XY type of sex-determination, both males and females have same number of chromosomes
(c) In *Drosophila*, males have one X and one Y-chromosome, whereas females have a pair of X-chromosome besides autosomes
(d) In birds, females have one Z and one W-chromosomes, whereas males have a pair of Z-chromosomes besides autosomes
(e) In insects with XO type of sex-determination, all sperms bear X-chromosome besides autosomes

31 Which of the following statement is not true of two genes that show 50% recombination frequency? **[NEET 2013]**
(a) The genes may be on different chromosomes
(b) The genes are tightly linked
(c) The genes show independent assortment
(d) If the genes are present on the same chromosome, they undergo more than one crossover in every meiosis

32 Who is known as Father of Radiation Genetics? **[AIIMS 2013]**
(a) Slatyer (b) Charles Elton
(c) Taylor (d) HJ Muller

33 Depending upon the distance between any two genes which is inversely proportional to the strength of linkage, cross over will vary **[Manipal 2013]**
(a) 50 – 100% (b) 0 – 50%
(c) 75 – 100% (d) 100 – 150%

34 Mutations can be induced with **[CBSE AIPMT 2011]**
(a) IAA (b) ethylene
(c) gamma radiations (d) infrared radiations

35 The chromosomal number in the meiocytes of housefly is **[Kerala CEE 2011]**
(a) 8 (b) 12 (c) 21 (d) 23
(e) 34

36 Allelic sequence variations where more than one variant (allele) at a locus in a human population with a frequency greater than 0.01 is referred to as **[Kerala CEE 2011]**
(a) incomplete dominance (b) multiple allelism
(c) SNP (d) EST
(e) DNA polymorphism

37 The loss of chromosomal segment is due to **[Kerala CEE 2011]**
(a) polyploidy (b) deletions
(c) duplications (d) inversions
(e) transversion

38 The chromosome constitution $2n-2$ of an organism represents **[DUMET 2011]**
(a) monosomic (b) nullisomic
(c) haploid (d) trisomic

39 Chimera is produced due to **[DUMET 2011]**
(a) somatic mutations (b) reverse mutations
(c) lethal mutations (d) pleiotropic mutations

40 During a process of chromosomal mutation, a student saw a chromosomal pair as a figure of 8. The most probable process expected for the above phenomenon is **[WB JEE 2011]**
(a) deletion (b) duplication
(c) inversion (d) translocation

41 Which of the following is not considered as mutagen? **[OJEE 2011]**
(a) Lower temperature (b) X-rays
(c) Higher temperature (d) UV rays

42 Change in single base pair **[OJEE 2011]**
(a) may not change the phenotype
(b) quickly change the phenotype
(c) change the natural process
(d) None of the above

43 Polyploid derived from two different species is called **[WB JEE 2011]**
(a) autopolyploid (b) triploid
(c) allopolyploid (d) monoploid

ANSWERS

Check Point 7.1

1. (a)	2. (a)	3. (c)	4. (c)	5. (c)	6. (c)

Check Point 7.2

1. (a)	2. (a)	3. (b)	4. (a)	5. (b)	6. (a)

Check Point 7.3

1. (b)	2. (b)	3. (c)	4. (b)	5. (b)	6. (d)

Check Point 7.4

1. (b)	2. (b)	3. (b)	4. (c)	5. (c)	6. (d)

(A) Topical Exercise

1. (d)	2. (c)	3. (d)	4. (a)	5. (c)	6. (d)	7. (a)	8. (d)	9. (a)	10. (a)
11. (c)	12. (c)	13. (c)	14. (a)	15. (a)	16. (a)	17. (b)	18. (b)	19. (a)	20. (b)
21. (b)	22. (c)	23. (a)	24. (b)	25. (a)	26. (d)	27. (b)	28. (c)	29. (a)	30. (c)
31. (d)	32. (d)	33. (b)	34. (b)	35. (c)	36. (d)	37. (c)	38. (b)	39. (a)	40. (a)
41. (c)	42. (b)	43. (d)	44. (c)	45. (a)	46. (c)	47. (d)	48. (a)	49. (a)	50. (b)
51. (b)	52. (d)	53. (b)	54. (a)	55. (d)	56. (c)	57. (d)	58. (d)	59. (b)	60. (a)
61. (c)	62. (d)	63. (d)	64. (a)	65. (a)	66. (a)	67. (a)	68. (d)	69. (b)	70. (b)
71. (b)	72. (a)	73. (a)	74. (a)	75. (d)	76. (c)	77. (a)	78. (d)	79. (d)	80. (c)
81. (b)	82. (c)	83. (b)	84. (b)	85. (c)	86. (a)	87. (c)	88. (a)	89. (a)	90. (c)
91. (d)	92. (d)	93. (c)	94. (b)	95. (d)	96. (c)	97. (d)	98. (d)	99. (a)	100. (a)
101. (d)	102. (d)	103. (c)	104. (a)	105. (c)	106. (d)	107. (a)	108. (c)	109. (c)	110. (c)
111. (c)	112. (b)	113. (d)	114. (d)	115. (b)	116. (a)	117. (b)	118. (b)	119. (b)	120. (b)
121. (c)	122. (a)	123. (c)	124. (c)	125. (d)	126. (a)	127. (d)	128. (b)	129. (c)	130. (a)
131. (d)	132. (a)								

(B) Cumulative Exercise

1. (c)	2. (b)	3. (b)	4. (d)	5. (c)	6. (a)	7. (d)	8. (b)	9. (a)	10. (a)
11. (d)	12. (b)	13. (a)	14. (a)	15. (c)	16. (c)	17. (a)	18. (a)	19. (b)	20. (b)
21. (a)	22. (a)	23. (a)	24. (b)	25. (c)	26. (a)	27. (a)	28. (b)	29. (a)	30. (c)
31. (d)	32. (b)	33. (c)	34. (d)	35. (b)	36. (b)	37. (b)	38. (b)		

(C) Medical Entrances' Gallery

1. (a)	2. (c)	3. (d)	4. (b)	5. (b)	6. (a)	7. (c)	8. (a)	9. (b)	10. (b)
11. (d)	12. (d)	13. (a)	14. (b)	15. (d)	16. (c)	17. (a)	18. (a)	19. (a)	20. (a)
21. (b)	22. (d)	23. (d)	24. (a)	25. (b)	26. (d)	27. (c)	28. (d)	29. (b)	30. (e)
31. (b)	32. (d)	33. (b)	34. (c)	35. (b)	36. (e)	37. (b)	38. (b)	39. (a)	40. (d)
41. (a)	42. (a)	43. (c)							

Explanations

(A) Topical Exercise

13 (*c*) Statement in option (c) is incorrect and can be corrected as A gynandromorph possesses half of male characters and half of female characters. These are known as sex mosaic.
Rest other statements are correct.

15 (*a*) Option (a) is incorrect matched pair and can be corrected as
In *Melandrium*, XX-XY type of sex-determination is seen.
Rest options are correct matched pairs.

38 (*b*)

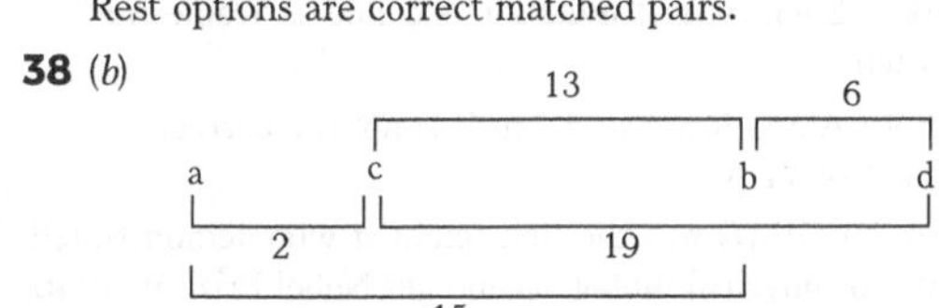

Thus, correct sequence is a, c, b, d.

41 (*c*) Frequency of recombination α distance between genes.

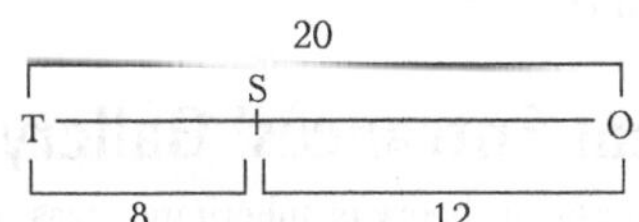

Thus, sequence of genes is TSO.

44 (*c*) Total number of recombinants $= 24 + 26 = 50$

Total number of progeny = 300.

RF $= \dfrac{50}{300} \times 100 = 16.7\%$

46 (*c*) Total number of progeny = 2000

Recombinant progeny = 220

$= \dfrac{220}{2000} \times 100 = 11$ map unit.

47 (*d*) If 1700 are of parental type, then remaining 300 are recombinant distance between genes is directly proportional to the percentage of recombinants or recombinant frequency.
Recombinant Frequency (RF)

$= \dfrac{\text{Total number recombinants}}{\text{Total offspring}} \times 100$

$= \dfrac{300}{2000} \times 100 = 15$ cM or 15 map unit.

52 (*d*)

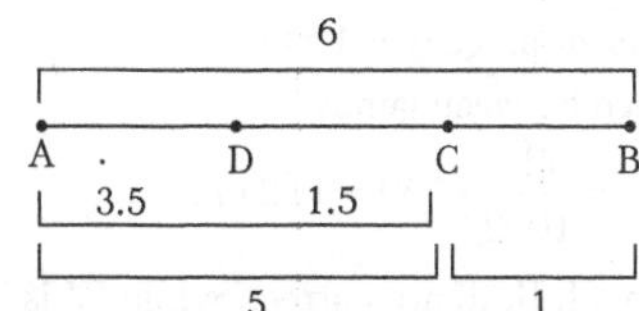

Thus, the correct sequence is ADCB.

78 (*d*) Statement in option (d) is incorrect and can be corrected as Mutation is more common when it is present in dominant gene. Thus, it can be expressed in both homozygous and heterozygous conditions.
Rest of the statements are correct.

85 (*c*) Option (c) is incorrect pair and can be corrected as The smallest element of a gene, which can be affected by a mutation is called muton.
Rest of the options are correct pairs.

108 (*c*) Tetrasomic condition $= 2n + 2$

$= (2 \times 10) + 2 = 22$

110 (*c*) Statement in option (c) is incorrect and can be corrected as Deletion mutations are not heritable in plants because pollens with deletions are mostly sterile.
Rest of the statements are correct about deletions.

111 (*c*) Option (c) is incorrect match and can be corrected as
Reverse tandem is a type of duplication in which the duplicated portion is situated at original site in reverse order.
Rest options are correct match pairs.

117 (*b*) Monosomy $= 2n - 1$

$= (2 \times 12) - 2 = 23$

(B) Cumulative Exercise

7 (*d*) Statement in option (d) is incorrect and can be corrected as
Baldness is sex-influenced trait.
Rest statements are correct.

9 (*a*)

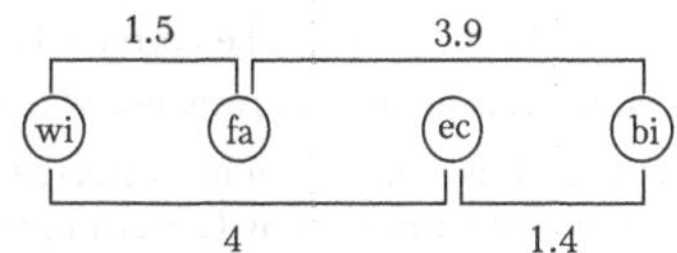

Thus, correct answer is bi-ec-fa-wi.

13 (*a*) Number of recombinants = 100 + 50 = 150
Total number of progeny = 1000
$$RF = \frac{150}{1000} \times 100 = 15 \text{ cM}$$
[RF = Distance between genes]

18 (*a*) Statement I and II are correct while III and IV are incorrect. Incorrect statements can be corrected as
Mendel could not find out linkage because all of his experimental characters of pea were not linked. They were present far apart from each other on four different chromosome.

19 (*b*) Number of recombinatns = 58 + 54 = 112
Total number of pregeny = 1002
RF = Distance between genes
$$= \frac{112}{1002} \times 100 = 11.2 \text{ units.}$$

21 (*a*) Statements I, II, III are correct, while IV is incorrect. Incorrect statement can be corrected as
Crossing over has no role in cytoplasmic inheritance.

24 (*b*) Statements I, II, III are correct, while IV is incorrect. Incorrect statement can be corrected as
Linked genes do not undergo hybridisation and thus, they do not affect homozygosity.

27 (*a*) Statements I and II are correct, while III and IV are incorrect. Incorrect statements can be corrected as
- In paracentric inversion, centromere is not involved.
- Inversion occurring in both the members of homologous pair is called allelosomal inversion.

28 (*b*) Statements II and IV are correct, while I and III are incorrect. Incorrect statements can be corrected as
- In point mutations, one nitrogenous base is substituted by other.
- In framestift mutations, entire reading frame gets shifted either backward or forward due to the insertion or deletion of one or more nitrogenous bases.

30 (*c*) A is true, but R is false. R can be corrected as
According to Bridges, autosomes are responsible for masculine characteristics. While X-chromosomes determine the feminine characteristics.

31 (*d*) A is false, but R is true. A can be corrected as
Habrobracon have both diploid and haploid males. The diploid males are produced by fertilised eggs.

32 (*b*) Both A and R are true, but R is not the correct explanation of A.
CO_2 sensitivity is regulated by the presence of heat labile factor sigma, i.e. which is responsible for the inheritance of CO_2 sensitivity only.

33 (*c*) A is true, but R is false. R can be corrected as
The *trans* condition is defined in response with linkage.

34 (*d*) A is false, but R is true. A can be corrected as
Somatic crossover was reported by C Stern in somatic cells of *Drosophila* and G Pontecarvo in fungus *Aspergillus* nodules and it is the somatic or mitotic crossover which produces such patches.

35 (*b*) Both A and R are true, but R is not the correct explanation of A.
XX-XY mechanism of sex-determination occurs in human beings as well as *Drosophila.* In this, XX zygotes become females, while XY becomes male. The size of X and Y-chromosomes is not similar, X is longer than Y-chromosome.

36 (*b*) Both A and R are true, but R is not the correct explanation of A.
Mutation is a heritable change in the nucleotide sequence (gene) of a chromosome. A gene has two alternative forms, i.e. alleles, one being dominant and the other is recessive. Here, one allele is wild and other is mutant. The mutant form is developed from wild form due to mutation.

37 (*b*) Both A and R are true, but R is not the correct explanation of A.
A gene mutation or point mutation is the result of a change in the nucleotide sequence of the DNA molecule in a particular region of the chromosome.
The addition or deletion of a base changes the way in which the code is read after the point of addition or deletion. Such type of mutation is called as 'frameshift' mutation.

38 (*b*) Both A and R are true, but R is not the correct explanation of A.
HJ Muller (1927) was the first scientist who demonstrated the use of physical mutagens and got Nobel Prize in 1946. A variety of agents increases the frequency of mutation, such agents are called mutagens.
They include chemical mutagens and radiations like X-rays, γ-rays and UV-rays.

(C) Medical Entrances' Gallery

1 (*a*) Chromosomal theory of inheritance was proposed by Sutton and Boveri independently in 1902.
The two workers found a close similarity between the transmission of hereditary traits and behaviour of chromosomes while passing from one generation to the next through gametes.

2 (*c*) Sutton and Boveri proposed chromosomal theory of inheritance, but it was experimentally verified by Thomas Hunt Morgan. According to this theory, genes are the units of heredity and are found in the chromosomes.

3 (*d*) To make chromosomal studies easier, chromosomes are classified into 7 groups, i.e. A to G. The chromosome number 21, 22 and Y are listed in G group.
Group A contains 1-3 chromosomes
B contains 4-5 chromosomes
C contains 6-12 chromosomes and X-chromosome
D contains 13-15 chromosomes
E contains 16-18 chromosomes
F contains 19-20 chromosomes
G contains 21-22 chromosomes and Y-chromosome

4 (*b*) In the construction of genetic maps, map unit or centiMorgan is a unit or distance between genes on Chromosomes, representing 1% crossover.

i.e. 1 map unit = 1% crossover

Hence, the genetic distance between genes is based on average number of crossover frequency between them.

5 (*b*) Alfred Sturtevant was the first to explain the concept of chromosomal mapping. It is drawn on the basis of recombination frequency between gene pairs on the same chromosome. This frequency is directly proportional to the distance between these two genes.

It can be used to determine the exact location of a gene on the chromosome.

6 (*a*) Option (a) is incorrect because

In human male karyotype, one 'X' and one 'Y' chromosome are present.

8 (*a*) Chromosome walking is used in genetic mapping. It is a method of positional cloning used to find, isolate and clone a particular allele in a gene library.

It is DNA based method of genetic mapping in which the chromosome is analysed by extending one tip to reach the other. This involves systematically moving along the chromosome from a known location to an unknown location.

9 (*b*) The statement in option (b) is incorrect and can be corrected as

In domesticated fowls, sex of progeny depends on the type of egg rather than type of sperm. In fowls, the females are heterogametic and produce two types of eggs containing either (A+Z) or (A+W) chromosomes. The males are homogametic and produce only one type of sperm containing (A + Z) chromosomes.

Rest of the statements are correct.

10 (*b*) The statement in option (b) is correct.

XO type of sex chromosomes determines the male sex in grasshoppers. This type of sex-determination comes under XX-XO type. It is common in cockroaches, grasshoppers and bugs. The female has two homomorphic sex chromosomes, XX and is homogametic. It produces similar eggs, each with one X-chromosome. The male has one chromosome only and is heterogametic. It produces two types of sperms, i.e. gynosperms with X and androsperms without X.

Rest of the statements are incorrect and can be corrected as

- In birds, the females are heterozygous and represented as ZW.
- Female sex in humans is represented as XX.
- In *Drosophila,* males are heterogametic, i.e. XY.

11 (*d*) The individuals having XYY chromosomes are known as supermales. They have an additional Y-chromosome. They suffer from poly Y-male syndrome. These individuals are characterised by abnormal height, mental retardation, antisocial behaviour and criminal bent of mind.

12 (*d*) All the statements are incorrect and can be corrected as

- Tightly linked genes on the same chromosome get inherited together and show less or no recombination.
- Genes far apart on the same chromosome show higher recombinations.
- Genes loosely linked on the same chromosome show high recombinations than tightly linked ones.

Thus, option (d) is correct.

13 (*a*) Both A and R are true and R is the correct explanation of A.

Genes situated in the same chromosomes are said to be linked. All genes in a single chromosome form a linkage group and usually pass it into the same gamete and are inherited together as a result of linkage.

These genes do not show independent assortment, e.g. genes for red hair and freckles are linked genes.

14 (*b*) When two genes in a dihybrid cross are situated on the same chromosome, the proportion of parental gene combinations are much higher than the non-parental or recombinant type as linked genes are inherited together in offspring.

15 (*d*) The distance between two genes on the chromosomes is measured by using recombination frequency. Morgan and Sturtevant stated that frequency of recombination between two linked gene is directly proportional to the distance between them.

16 (*c*) Translocation is the process causing a gene to move from one linkage group to another. It is the separation of a chromosome segment and its union to a non-homologous chromosome. It is of two types, i.e. simple and reciprocal. In simple translocation, one chromosome shows deletion or deficiency, while a non-homologous chromosome comes to have an additional segment.

In reciprocal translocation, two non-homologous chromosomes exchange segments between themselves to create new linkage groups in both the chromosomes.

Hence, option (*c*) is correct.

20 (*a*) Given, $2n = 16$

So, the number of haploid chromosomes → 8

I. Monosomic = $2n - 1 = 16 - 1 = 15$

II. Autotriploid = $3n = 3 \times 8 = 24$

III. Trisomic = $2n + 1 = 16 + 1 = 17$

IV. Double monosomic = $2n - 1 - 1 = 16 - 1 - 1 = 14$

V. Nullisomic = $2n - 2 = 16 - 2 = 14$

∴ The correct sequence of chromosomes for (I to V) are 15, 24, 17, 14, 14.

21 (*b*) Polymorphism can be defined as variation in individuals at genetic level. It can be inherited from parents to their children.

23 (*d*) Alfred H Sturtevant, one of Morgan's students, used the frequency of recombination or percentage of crossing over between gene pairs on the same chromosome as a measure of the distance between genes and mapped their position on the chromosome.

This technique is based on the assumption that the farther apart two genes are on a chromosome, the higher the probability that a crossover will occur between them.

26 (*d*) These are the animals, which have characteristics of both male and female individuals. These are mainly found in insects and the term gynandromorph is commonly used in entomology.

27 (*c*) Statement in option (c) is incorrect and can be corrected as
According to Mendel, during meiosis, chromosomes assort independently into gametes, such that the segregation of alleles of one gene is independent of alleles of another gene. This is stated as in Mendel's third law and is known as the law of independent assortment.
This law always holds true for genes that are located on different chromosomes, but for genes closely related on the same chromosome, it does not always hold true.

28 (*d*) The frequency of crossing over occurring between two genes located on the same chromosome is directly proportional to the distance between the two genes. Hence, closer the two genes are to one another on a chromosome, the greater will be their chance of being inherited together. In contrast, genes located away from each other on same chromosome are more likely to be separated during recombination. Other factors given in the options such as length of chromosome, position of centromere and activities of two genes does not have any relation with crossing over and recombination.

29 (*b*) Alfred Sturtevant used the frequency of recombination between gene pairs on the same chromosome as a measure of the distance between genes and mapped their position on the chromosome.

30 (*e*) Statement in option (e) is incorrect and can be corrected as
In XO type of sex-determination in insects, all sperms do not bear X-chromosomes. Males have only one X-chromosome and females have a pair of X-chromosomes. Eggs fertilised by sperms having X-chromosome become females and those fertilised by sperms that do not have X-chromosome become males.

31 (*b*) Statement in option (b) is not true and can be corrected as
The tightly linked genes on chromosomes show 100% parental types and 0% recombinants. Two genes that undergo independent assortment indicated by a recombinant frequency of 50% are present on non-homologous chromosomes located far apart in a single chromosome. As the distance between two genes increases, crossover frequency increases and more recombinant gametes, while fewer parental gametes are seen.

33 (*b*) The crossing over can never exceed above 50% . It ranges from 0-50%.

34 (*c*) Gamma radiations are ionising radiations and are physical mutagens. They are used as mutagens, when nucleus is deep seated, e.g. seeds, stem cuttings, etc. Sharbati Sonora variety of wheat has been developed by the effect of gamma radiations on 'Sonora 64' variety (Mexican dwarf wheat variety).

35 (*b*) The gamete mother cells ($2n$) are called meiocytes, which undergo meiosis to form gametes (n). The chromosome number in the meiocytes ($2n$) of housefly is 12.

37 (*b*) Deletion is a chromosomal aberration in which there is loss of a chromosomal segment.

38 (*b*) Nullisomic $= 2n-2$

Monosomic $= 2n-1$

Trisomic $= 2n+1$

Haploid $= n$

Thus, option (b) is correct.

40 (*d*) In the process of translocation, a figure of 8 is visible sometimes when the chromosomal pair undergo terminalisation process.

41 (*a*) Mutations can be induced by a number of agents called mutagens.
- **Physical mutagen** are UV rays, X-rays, cosmic rays, high temperature.
- **Chemical mutagens** are 5 bromouracil, proflavin.

42 (*a*) Change in single base pair may not change the phenotype. The codon is triplet and degenerate.

43 (*c*) A polyploid having two or more distinct genomes usually produced by chromosome doubling of interspecific hybrids is called allopolyploid or interspecific polyploid.

CHAPTER 08

Gene, Its Expression and Regulation

We already know that the hereditary units which are transmitted from one generation to next generation are called **genes**. It is a fundamental unit of genetic material.

Gene expression is the process by which the information present in an individual's gene is used as per their requirement of traits or characters. Cellular processes that control the rate and manner of gene expression are studied under gene regulation.

In this chapter, we will explore the details of genetic material, its type, basic molecular structure of gene, its condensed form, i.e. DNA, its synthesis, expression and regulation.

GENETIC MATERIAL

It is the material through which genetic information passes from a parent cell to its daughter cells. It also controls the formation and expression of traits in different organisms.

Properties of a genetic material

For any molecule to act as a genetic material, following criteria are required to be fulfilled

- It should be present in every cell and its amount should be same in all the somatic cells.
- It should be stable structurally as well as chemically.
- It should be able to generate its replica and must have the ability to pass its copies into its progeny.
- It should be able to provide scope for slow changes so as to allow adaptation and evolution to occur in organisms.
- It should be able to express information in the form of Mendelian characters.

Inside

DNA as the genetic material

Considering the above mentioned requirements for a molecule to act as a genetic material, two nucleic acids, i.e. RNA and DNA can be considered as a compatible genetic material.

It is so because

- Both of these are found in every cell of an organism.
- Both of these are able to direct their duplications because of base pairing and complementarity.

Experiments to prove DNA as the genetic material

Following experiments were conducted time to time to prove that DNA is the genetic material.

Griffith experiment

- **F Griffith** (1928) conducted an experiment using *Diplococcus pneumoniae*, a bacterium that causes pneumonia in mammals. This bacterium exists in two strains, i.e. S-strain and R-strain.
- **S-strain** is virulent, i.e. pathogenic. Bacterium of this strain have a mucopolysaccharide coat and produces smooth shiny colonies.
- **R-strain** is non-virulent, i.e. non-pathogenic. Bacterium of this strain does not possess coat and produces rough colonies when grown on a culture plate.

Procedure

Following four investigations were done to check the genetic material

1. S-strain → Injected in mice → Mice dies due to pneumonia
2. R-strain → Injected in mice → Mice survived and did not get diseased
3. Heat killed S-strains → Injected in mice → Mice survived
4. S-strain (heat killed) + R-strain (live) → Injected into mice → Mice died

Observation

- When a mixture of heat-killed S-strain and live R-strain bacteria were injected in the mice it died, while nothing was happened to mice when heat killed S-strain was injected alone.

Conclusion

- This was confirmed that the presence of heat-killed S-strain bacteria had caused a transformation of R-strain bacteria into virulent bacteria. But, the substance that had caused this transformation was not explained.

Experiment of Avery, MacLeod and McCarty

- Three scientists **Avery, MacLeod and McCarty** (1944) revealed after their experiment that the chemical nature of the transforming substance was DNA.
- They showed that DNA isolated from S-strain could itself confer the pathogenic properties to R-strain. This fact suggested that DNA possesses the genetic properties. The outline of their experiment is given below

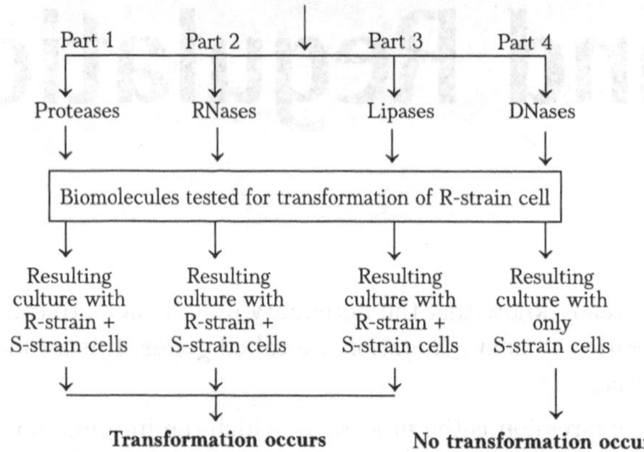

***Fig. 8.1** Summary of Avery, MacLeod an McCarty experiment, which demonstrate that DNA is the transforming material*

Observation

- In the extract contained DNA digesting enzyme, i.e. DNase, transformation did not occur. But on the other hand, transformation occurred in the extract containing other enzymes.
- It was suggested that DNA is the genetic material.

Experiment of Hershey and Chase

- **Alfred Hershey** and **Martha Chase** gave another definitive evidence for DNA as genetic material in 1952.

Procedure

- In this experiment, some T_2 bacteriophages were grown on the medium containing radioactive sulphur (^{35}S) and some on the medium containing radioactive phosphorus (^{32}P).
- Bacterium grown of radioactive sulphur (^{35}S), got ^{35}S incorporated in their protein coats, as DNA does not contain sulphur. Thus, these bacteria become labelled with ^{35}S in their protein coats.
- Bacterium grown on radioactive phosphorus (^{32}P), got ^{32}P incorporated in their DNA as phosphorus is the main constituent of DNA. Thus, these bacteria become labelled with ^{32}P in their DNA.

- After this, following three steps were carried out
  (i) **Infection** Both type of labelled phages were allowed normally to infect cultured bacteria separately.
  (ii) **Blending** These bacterial cells were agitated in a blender. As the result, the contact between bacteria and viruses was broken.
  (iii) **Centrifugation** The virus particles were separated from bacteria by centrifugation.

Observation

- After centrifugation, bacterial cells showed the presence of radioactive DNA labelled with ^{32}P.
- However, the radioactive protein labelled with ^{35}S was appeared in the medium outside bacterial cells.

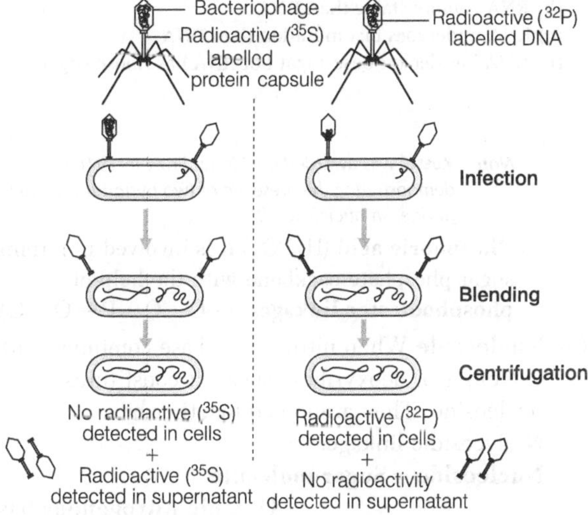

Fig. 8.2 Hershey and Chase experiment

Conclusion

- Presence of DNA labelled with ^{32}P in bacterial cell proved that phage DNA was entered into the bacterial cell.
- Presence of proteins labelled with ^{35}S in the medium outside the bacterial cell proved that phage protein coat was not entered into the bacterial cell. These were removed at the time of blending from the bacterial cell wall.
- Thus, DNA was proved to be the infective part of virus and also supposed to carry all genetic informations.

RNA as the genetic material

- RNA was the first genetic material to be originated.
- Due to high reactivity, RNA is very unstable. DNA is beleived to be evolved from RNA with chemical modifications that make it more stable. Being double stranded with complementary strand, DNA resist changes by evolving a process of repair.
- It was first demonstrated by A Gierer and G Schramm in 1956 by their experiments conducted on tobacco plant.
- Another approach was taken by H Fraenkel Conrat and B Singer. They showed that it is RNA not protein in TMV particles that cause infection.
- It was suggested that RNA molecules were the first biocatalysts to carryout the important biochemical reactions in the living world such as metabolism, translocation, splicing, etc.

DNA *vs* RNA

DNA is the genetic material in most organisms except in plant viruses and some animal viruses where RNA acts as genetic material.

This superiority of DNA as a genetic material in most organisms is due to the following facts that

- It is chemically less reactive than RNA, due to the absence of 2′–OH group which makes RNA highly reactive, labile and easily degradable.
- DNA is much more stable than RNA due to the presence of thymine instead of uracil.
- Being stable, DNA undergoes slow mutation for evolution and adaptation rather than faster mutation which takes place in RNA and results in lethality in higher lifeforms.
- Further more, due to its stability, DNA is not susceptible to undergo changes during different stages of life cycle, age or with change in metabolism of the organism.

Confirmatory facts regarding DNA as the genetic material

The existence of DNA as the genetic material is further confirmed by the following facts

- The total DNA content in all diploid cells of an organism of a species is same.
- The gametes contain half the amount of DNA present in their parent cells or in the somatic cells.
- Fertilisation (syngamy) doubles the amount of DNA. Thus, the zygote contains same amount of DNA as that was present in parent cell.
- During cell metabolism, it is only DNA which maintains its integrity while RNA, proteins, etc., loses it. DNA loses its integrity only during mutational processes.
- DNA composition is same in all the organisms of a species, but it differs also in organisms belonging to different species.
- Mutations are the result of either change in the structure of DNA or change in the amount of DNA in an organism.
- Cells with similar hereditary origin have DNA of similar composition.

CHECK POINT 8.1

1. In order to enable a chemical to serve as a genetic material, it is essential that the chemical should be
(a) able to duplicate itself
(b) able to form itself into long spiral molecules
(c) a compound of pyrimidines and purines
(d) easily changed

2. During Griffith's experiment following observations were done. Choose the correct one.
(a) S-strain injected into the mice $\rightarrow$ Mice live
(b) R-strain injected into the mice $\rightarrow$ Mice dies
(c) Heat killed S-strains injected into the mice $\rightarrow$ Mice live
(d) Both (a) and (b)

3. Transformation efficiency of bacteria (as in the experiment of Avery *et. al*) would not be there, if the transforming material is treated with
(a) lipase (b) ribonuclease
(c) protease (d) DNase

4. If a virus is grown with radioactive ^{35}S, it will show radioactivity in
(a) DNA (b) RNA
(c) protein (d) All of these

5. A bacteriophage with radioactive DNA and radioactive protein when infect a bacterium, the radioactivity inside the bacterium will be seen in
(a) bacterial DNA
(b) bacterial protein
(c) Both (a) and (b)
(d) All parts of bacterial cell

6. Which of the following is not a difference between DNA and RNA?
(a) DNA is less reactive than RNA
(b) RNA is more stable than DNA
(c) RNA undergoes fast mutation than DNA
(d) DNA has deoxyribose sugar but RNA has ribose sugar

DEOXYRIBONUCLEIC ACID (DNA)

- DNA was discovered by **Friedrich Meischer** in 1869 from the nucleus of the pus cells found in discarded bandages in the Franko-Prussian war and from Salmons sperm. He called it **'nuclein'**.
- Nuclein was named nucleic acid by **Altmann** in 1889 due to its slightly acidic nature. Besides chromosome, it is also found in cell organelles like mitochondria, chloroplast, etc.
- The DNA of all plants, animals, polyomavirus, bacteriophage T_2, T_4 and T_6 is **double-stranded**, while that of bacteriophage $\phi \times 174$ is **single-stranded.**

The detailed study of DNA has been discussed earlier in chapter biomolecules and enzymes, exploring biology, volume I, still an outline of its structure is given here also.

Structure of DNA

An outline of the DNA structure is as follows

(i) DNA is a long heteropolymer of deoxyribonucleotides.

(ii) Each deoxyribonucleotide is composed of deoxyribose sugar, nitrogenous base and phosphoric acid.

(a) **Deoxyribose sugar** It is a pentose sugar in which oxygen is absent at position 2C-atom.

(b) **Nitrogenous bases** They are of two types

- **Purines** Adenine (A) and guanine (G) constitute the purines, which are dicyclic in nature.
- **Pyrimidines** The most commonly found pyrimidines in DNA are thymine (T) and cytosine (C). In RNA, uracil (U) is present instead of thymine (T). These are monocyclic.

Note *Kossel was awarded the Nobel Prize in 1910 for demonstrating the presence of two pyrimidines and two purines in nucleic acids.*

(c) **Phosphoric acid** (H_3PO_4) It is involved in forming sugar phosphate backbone with the help of **phosphodiester linkages** (—C—O—P—O—C).

(iii) **Nucleoside** When nitrogenous base combines with C-atom-1 of deoxyribose sugar, it constitutes a nucleoside. They are joined together by N-glycosidic linkage.

Nucleoside = Sugar molecule + Organic nitrogenous base

(iv) **Nucleotides** A nucleotide is formed by the union of a phosphate group with nucleoside by phosphodiester bond.

Nucleotide = Nucleoside + Phosphate group

Watson and Crick model of DNA

The outline of Watson and Crick model of DNA is as follows

- DNA molecule consists of two helically twisted strands connected together by base pairs. The alignment of these strands is antiparallel or opposite.
- Each strand consists of a backbone made up of alternating deoxyribose sugar and phosphate. The phosphate joins the two sugars through a phosphodiester bond.
- The arrangement of sugars gives polarity to DNA. As both the strands are antiparallel, so sugar placement is opposite to each other.

This sugar placement gives following 2 ends to each strand.

(a) 3′ end, i.e. the end having 3rd C-atom of sugar at the top.

(b) 5′ end, i.e. the end having 5th C-atom of the sugar at the top.

- The nitrogenous bases are stacked inside the helix. Each nitrogenous base pair with that of the opposite strand through hydrogen bonds (H-bonds).
- Their is a specificity in base pairing. **Adenine** (A) always pairs up with **thymine** (T) by **two H-bonds** and **guanine** (G) always pairs up with **cytosine** (C) by **three H-bonds**. This pairing of purines with pyrimidines leads to a uniform width of DNA throughout its length (20 Å).
- The two strands are interwined in a clockwise direction, i.e. in the form of a right-handed helix and have antiparallel arrangement as shown in figure below

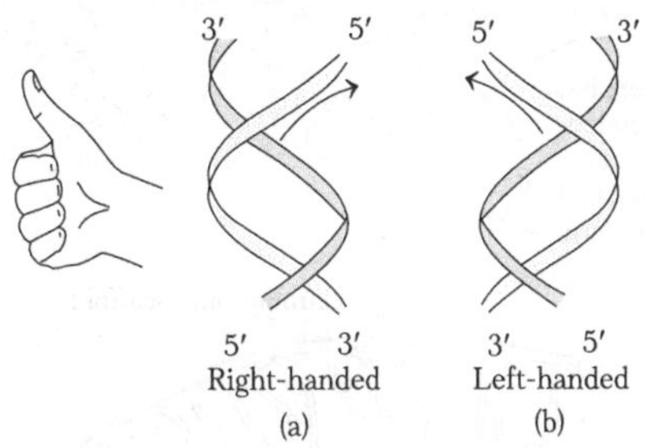

***Fig. 8.3** Structure of DNA showing antiparallel arrangement of the two strands : (a) showing right handed helix and (b) showing left handed helix*

- Notice that one polynucleotide chain runs in $5' \rightarrow 3'$ direction and the other in $3' \rightarrow 5'$ direction so that, the 3′-end of one chain lies besides the 5′-end of other chain.
- The twisting of strand results into **major** (deep) and **minor** (shallow) **groove**. A complete turn measures 34 Å with a distance of 3.4 Å or 0.34 nm between two successive base pairs.
- There are present 10 base pairs per turn. Each successive nucleotide turns 36° in horizontal plane from the previous one. The tilt of base pair to the normal axis of the helix is 6.3°. The above description is given with respect to a typical A-DNA.

Chargaff's rule

Erwin Chargaff (1950) made quantitative analysis of DNA and showed that the composition of DNA molecules varied in complex ways depending upon the source of DNA. He proposed base equivalence rule or Chargaff's rule, which states that

- For a double-stranded DNA, the proportion of adenine is always equal to that of thymine and the proportion of guanine is always equal to that of cytosine, i.e. A = T and G = C.

  It follows that an equal proportion of purines and pyrimidines is always seen in a double-stranded DNA, i.e. $A + G = T + C$ *or* $\frac{A + G}{T + C} = 1$
- The $\frac{(A + T)}{(G + C)}$ ratio is low in primitive organism, but higher in advanced organism.

  Chargaff's equivalence rule has been found to apply almost universally in different organisms, which can be seen in the table 8.1.

Table 8.1 Haploid DNA contents and base composition of DNA of some organisms

Organisms	Haploid DNA content (pg = 10^{-12} g)	Purines		Pyrimidines		(A+G) / (C+T) ratio
		Adenine (%)	Guanine (%)	Cytosine (%)	Thymine (%)	
Animals						
Man	3.2	31.0	19.1	18.4	31.5	1.00
Cattle	2.8	28.7	22.2	22.0	27.2	1.03
Drosophila melanogaster	0.18	27.3	22.5	22.5	27.6	0.99
Plants						
Maize	7.5	25.6	24.5	24.6	25.3	1.00
Tobacco	1.2	29.7	19.8	20.0	30.4	0.98
Neurospora crassa (fungi)	0.046	23.0	27.1	26.6	23.3	1.00
Bacteria						
Diplococcus pneumoniae	0.002	30.3	21.6	18.7	29.5	1.08
Escherichia coli	0.0047	24.6	25.5	25.6	24.3	1.00
Viruses						
Bacteriophage T_2	0.0002	32.6	18.2	16.6	32.6	1.03
Bacteriophage λ	0.000055	26.0	23.8	24.3	25.8	0.99

Packaging of DNA helix in chromosomes

- The length of DNA in a human diploid cell is 6.6×10^9 bp $\times 0.34 \times 10^{-9}$ m = **2.2 m.** This length is far greater than the dimension of typical nucleus which is approximately 10^{-6} m. Similarly, the length of prokaryotic DNA is about 1.36 mm which is placed in a cell having size 1 μm.
- The long sized DNA is accommodated in the smaller area through packaging or compaction. It occurs by the folding and attachment of DNA with basic protein, i.e. non-histone proteins in prokaryotes and histone proteins in the case of eukaryotes.

1. DNA packaging in prokaryotes

- In prokaryotes, DNA is not scattered throughout the cell. It is found in the cytoplasm in supercoiled stage.
- The coils are maintained by RNA and non-histone proteins called **polyamines**. These proteins are positively charged, which can hold the negatively charged DNA firmly. This packaged structure of DNA is called **nucleoid** or **genophore** or **prochromosome.**

2. DNA packaging in eukaryotes

- To explain the packaging of DNA in eukaryotes, many models were proposed including **'Folded-fibre model'** by **EJ Dupraw** (1965) and **'Nucleosome model'** by **RD Kornberg** (1974), etc.
- The most accepted model is of **Kornberg.** It explains that DNA (negatively charged) is tightly bound to an equal mass of histones (positively charged) which forms a repeating array of DNA particles, called **nucleosomes.**
- According to this model, the mitotic chromosomes are made up by the coiling of a large cylindrical fibre called **unit fibre.**
- This fibre is presumed to be formed by following three levels of coiling as follows
  (i) **First level** At this level, DNA coils as the string of nucleosomes, i.e. a beaded string-like structure.
  (ii) **Second level** The string of nucleosomes is then coiled into 30 nm diameter solenoid having about six nucleosomes per turn.
  (iii) **Third level** The solenoid is further coiled into a super solenoid with a diamter of 400 nm and a wall of 30 nm. This super solenoid structure is the unit fibre. The super solenoid undergoes further coiling to produce a chromatin fibre of 30-80 nm and then a chromatid of 700 nm.
  Chromatin is held over a scaffold of Non-Histone Chromosomal (NHC) proteins. The chromatid further coils to form chromosomes of about 1400 nm diameter.
- All the above mentioned levels are shown in the figure below

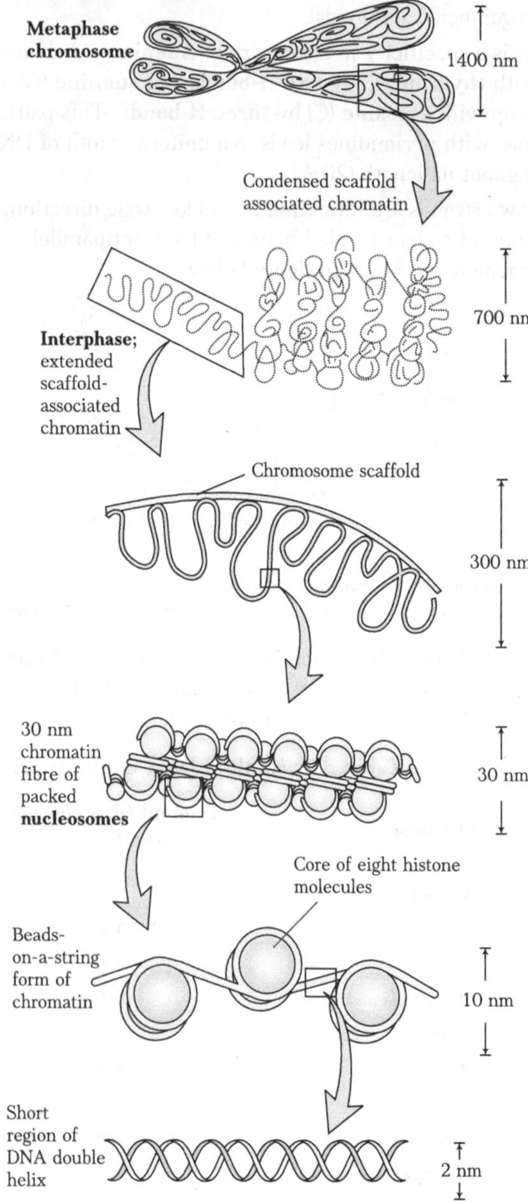

Fig 8.4 Model of the packaging of chromatin and the chromosome at metaphase

Replication of DNA

- The process by which a DNA molecule makes its identical copies is known as **DNA replication.** It takes place in S-phase of interphase.
- The three possible ways of DNA replication are conservative, semiconservative and dispersive modes as shown below

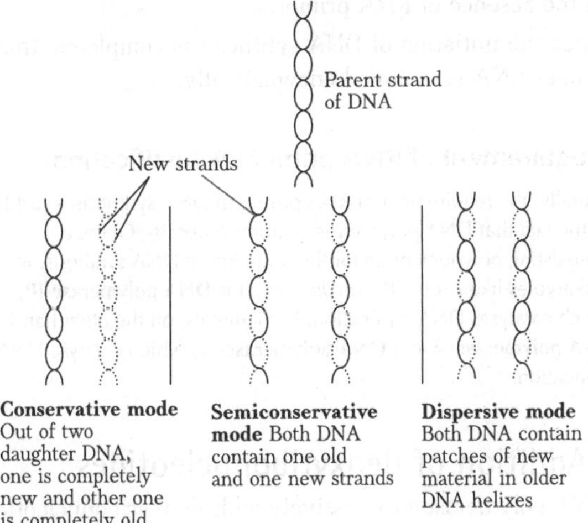

Fig. 8.5 The three theoretically possible modes of DNA replication

- Out of these, the semiconservative mode of DNA replication is universally accepted because there are several evidences in support of this model.
- The idea of semiconservation DNA replication was also given by **Watson** and **Crick** after they explained the DNA structure.

The experimental proof of semiconservative replication

The following experiments suggest that DNA replication is semiconservative.

(i) **Matthew Meselson and Franklin Stahl experiment** (1988) They varified semiconservative nature of DNA replication in a series of experiments. They used isotopically labelled DNA and a form of (specialised isopycnic) density gradient centrifugation.

The stepwise procedure used in the experiment is given below

- They cultured *E. coli* in the medium containing a heavy isotope of nitrogen (N^{15}) instead of commonly occurring and lighter (N^{14}).
- *E. coli* cells that were grown on N^{15} medium were washed and transferred to N^{14} containing medium and were allowed to grow for specific length of time.
- Heavy DNA (N^{15}) was separated from the lighter DNA (N^{14}) by centrifugation in CsCl (cesium chloride) density gradient.
- The DNA that was extracted from the culture after 1st generation had a hybrid or intermediate density. DNA extracted from the culture after another generation, i.e. 2nd generation was composed of equal amount of hybrid DNA ($N^{14}N^{15}$) and light DNA ($N^{14}N^{14}$).
- Subsequent generations produced greater number of light DNA molecules, however the quantity of hybrid DNA remained constant.

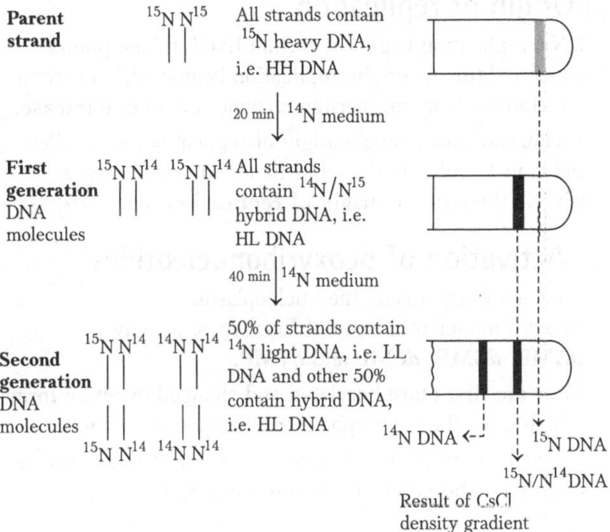

Fig. 8.6 Meselson and Stahl experiment

- **Conclusion** Results of the experiment provided the possibility that DNA replication is a semiconservative process as there is a subsequent increase in the amount of lighter DNA and constancy in hybrid DNA as the experiment progresses.

(ii) **Cairn's autoradiography experiment** (1963) In this experiment, heavy isotope of hydrogen [H^3] was used to replace thymine with tritiated thymidine in DNA molecule. Cairn also proposed a model for replication in circular DNA.

(iii) **Taylor experiment** (1969) He proved semiconservative mode of chromosome replication in eukaryotes using tritiated thymidine in the roots of *Vicia faba* (faba beans).

The machinery of DNA replication

- The process of replication in living cells requires a set of enzymes and among these **DNA dependent DNA polymerase** is the major one.

- It is highly efficient in polymerising about 2000 bp per second.
- The whole machinery of DNA replication with all the enzymes is collectively called **replisome.**
- DNA replication in eukaryotes is semiconservative, semi-discontinuous and bidirectional as compared to the semiconservative, bidirectional and continuous one in prokaryotes.

Mechanism

The process of DNA replication involves the following steps

(i) Origin of replication

- DNA replication begins at certain fixed unique points called **origin.** At origin, replication begins with a nick or incision made by an incision enzyme, i.e. **endonuclease.**
- Prokaryotes have single origin of replication. It is called ***ori* C** in *E. coli.* On the other hand, eukaryotes have several thousand of **origin of replication** called ***ori.***

(ii) Activation of deoxyribonucleotides

- It occurs freely inside the nucleoplasm. Deoxyribonucleotides are of four types, namely ***d*AMP**, ***d*GMP**, ***d*CMP** and ***d*TMP**.
- They are first phosphorylated and changed to active forms which have three phosphate residues instead of one.
- Formed triphosphates then act as a substrate and provides energy for the polymerisation of nucleotides.

(iii) Unwinding of DNA helix

- DNA double helix is unwinded by enzyme **helicase.**It is ATP dependent enzyme and acts on hydrogen bonds of DNA strand. The separated strands are stabilised by **Single-Stranded Binding Proteins** (SSBPs).
- The unwinding of DNA imposes tension or strain on the distal end of DNA molecule. This tension is released by the enzyme **topoisomerase.** This enzyme causes nicking and resealing of DNA strand.
- Alongwith topoisomerase, bacteria possess another enzyme called **DNA gyrase**, which can introduce negative super coils.
- Unwinding of DNA helix into two strands results in the formation of Y-shaped structure, called **replication fork.**

(iv) Formation of primer strand

- Initiation of DNA synthesis always requires a smaller segment of RNA called **RNA primer.** It is synthesised at 5′ end of new DNA strand with the help of DNA specific RNA polymerase enzyme called **primase.**
- Formation of RNA primer constitutes the initiation phase of DNA synthesis. DNA polymerase cannot add nucleotides in the absence of RNA primer.
- Once the initiation of DNA synthesis is completed, this primer RNA is removed enzymatically.

Requirement of RNA primer : A Justification

Actually, the requirement of RNA primer in DNA synthesis is justified by the fact that DNA polymerase requires a free 3′—OH of a pre-existing polynucleotide for the initiation of DNA synthesis. In prokaryotes like *E. coli, B. subtilis,* etc., it is **DNA polymerase-III,** which catalyses DNA replication. In mammals, on the other hand, it is **DNA polymerase-** δ and **DNA polymerase-** α, which catalyse DNA replication.

(v) Addition of deoxyribonucleotides

- DNA polymerase progressively adds deoxyribonucleotides to the 3′—OH end of the newly synthesised polypeptide chain.
- Prokaryotes have three major types of DNA polymerase namely III, II and I. All of them possesse 3′ $\rightarrow$ 5′ exonuclease activity. In eukaryotes, five types of DNA polymerases are found, i.e. α, β, γ, δ and ε .

(vi) Activity of DNA polymerase

- Two strands of a double helix are antiparallel to each other, i.e. one runs in the 5′ $\rightarrow$ 3′ direction, while the other has opposite 3′ $\rightarrow$ 5′ polarity.
- DNA polymerase-III synthesises DNA in 5′ $\rightarrow$ 3′ direction only. This means that the strand with 3′ $\rightarrow$ 5′ polarity serves as a template for continuous DNA synthesis and called **leading strand.**
- Other strand with 5′ $\rightarrow$ 3′ polarity forms the loop structure. This loop inverts the orientation of the template. DNA strand that is synthesised on this loop is fragmented or discontinuous and it is known as **lagging strand.**
- On this strand, discontinuous DNA synthesis takes place and formed fragments are called **okazaki fragments.**

Leading and lagging strands, and Okazaki fragments are shown in the figure below

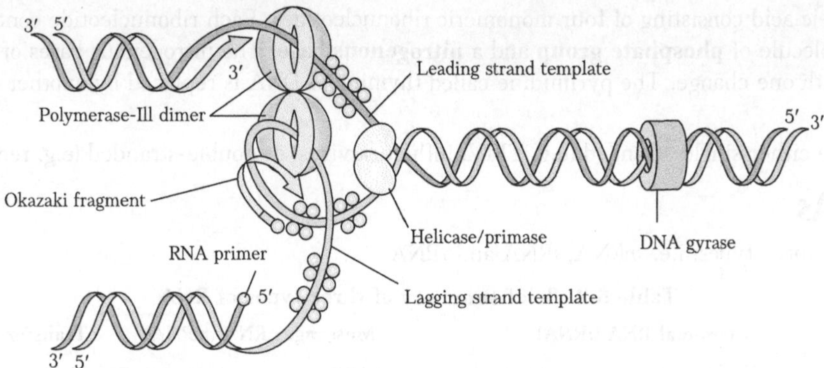

Fig 8.7 Summary of DNA synthesis at a single replication fork showing various enzymes and proteins essential for the process

(vii) Elongation of new strand

- The enzyme DNA polymerase-I degrades the RNA primer and simultaneously catalyses the synthesis of short DNA segments to replace the primer.
- This segment is then joined to main DNA strand by **DNA ligase enzyme.**

Summary of enzymes involved in DNA replication process and their role is given below

Protein	Role
Helicase	Unwinds the double helix
Primase	Synthesises RNA primers
Single-strand binding protein	Stabilises single-stranded regions
DNA gyrase (topoisomerase)	Relieves torque or strain
DNA polymerase-III	Synthesises DNA ($5' \rightarrow 3'$)
DNA polymerase-I	Erases primer and fill gaps
DNA ligase	Joins the ends of DNA segments

Proofreading and DNA repair

- Sometimes during replication, a wrong base is introduced erroneously. To compensate such inaccuracies, DNA polymerase possesses $3' \rightarrow 5'$ exonuclease activity. Thus, it detects and excises a mismatched nucleotide. This process is known as proofreading.

CHECK POINT 8.2

1. Choose the incorrect bonding for DNA.
   (a) Hydrogen bonding
   (b) Phosphodiester bonding
   (c) Disulphide bonding
   (d) All of the above

2. The difference between nucleoside and nucleotide is the lack of ...*A*... . The difference between DNA and RNA is the presence of ....*B*... in RNA.
   (a) *A*-phosphate group, *B*-uracil
   (b) *A*-sugar, *B*-adenine
   (c) *A*-hydroxyl group, *B*-guanine
   (d) *A*-base, *B*-cytosine

3. Who amongst the following scientists had no contribution in the development of the double helix model for the structure of DNA?
   (a) Rosalind Franklin (b) Maurice Wilkins
   (c) Erwin Chargaff (d) Meselson and Stahl

4. If the percentage of A and G is 30%, the percentage of T and C is
   (a) 40% (b) 70%
   (c) 30% (d) 50%

5. A bacterium *E. coli* with completely radioactive DNA was allowed to replicate in a non-radioactive medium for two generations. What % of the bacteria should contain radioactive DNA?
   (a) 100% (b) 50%
   (c) 25% (d) 12.5%

6. The replication of DNA in eukaryotes commences from
   (a) one end of chromatid extending to the other end
   (b) the centromeres to either of the ends of chromatids
   (c) several sites along the DNA of the chromatid simultaneously
   (d) both ends of the chromatid simultaneously

RIBONUCLEIC ACID (RNA)

It is a polymeric nucleic acid consisting of four monomeric ribonucleotides. Each ribonucleotide contains a **pentose sugar** (D-ribose), a molecule of **phosphate group** and a **nitrogenous base**. The nitrogenous bases of RNA are same as that found in DNA with one change. The pyrimidine called thymine of DNA is replaced by another pyrimidine called uracil in RNA.

RNA molecule may be either single-stranded (e.g. TMV, influenza virus) or double-stranded (e.g. reoviruses).

Types of RNAs

The RNA is mainly of three types, i.e. *m*RNA, *t*RNA and *r*RNA.

Table 8.2 Brief summary of three types of RNA

Characters	Ribosomal RNA (*r*RNA)	Messenger RNA (*m*RNA)	Transfer RNA (*t*RNA)
Weight	Heaviest	Heavy	Light
Percentage of total RNA of cell	~ 80%	3-5%	10-20%
Sedimentation coefficient	28S, 18S, 5.8S, 23S, 16S, 5S	8S	3.8S
Number of nucleotides	5S RNA: 120 nucleotides. 16-18S RNA : 1,600 to 2,500 nucleotides. 23-28S RNA : 3,200 to 5,500 nucleotides.	*E. coli* : 900 to 1,500 nucleotides.	73-93 nucleotides.
Molecular weight	23S RNA : 1.1×10^6 30S RNA : 0.55×10^6	500000	25000-30000
Unusual bases	Small amount of methylated bases. (*E. coli* 1 per 100-150 nucleotides)	Small amount of unusual bases.	High content of unusual bases. (*E. coli* 1 per 30-40 nucleotides)
Site of synthesis	Derived from nucleolar DNA.	Synthesised in nucleus on DNA template.	Synthesised in nucleus on DNA template.
Beginning of synthesis	Synthesis begins at gastrulation and increases as development proceeds.	Some *m*RNA is found in the ovum. New *m*RNA is synthesised during early cleavage.	*t*RNA synthesis occurs at the end of cleavage stages.
Base of relationship DNA	No obvious base relationship to DNA. *r*RNA is formed from small sections of DNA.	*m*RNA shows base relationship to DNA. It is formed from all sections of DNA.	Same as in *r*RNA.
Function	Unpaired base may bind *m*RNA and *t*RNA to ribosomes.	Convey genetic information from DNA of chromosomes to the ribosomes, where it takes part in protein synthesis.	Adapter for attaching amino acids to *m*RNA template.

Messenger or Template RNA (*m*RNA)

- The name messenger RNA was proposed by **Jacob** and **Monod** (1961). It is always single-stranded, without any base pairing. Infact, base pairing in *m*RNA strand destroys its biological activity.
- It brings instructions from the DNA for the formation of particular type of polypeptide. Therefore, it is also called as **informational** or **genetic RNA**.

Structure

- The structural components of *m*RNA are given below
  - CAP (at 5′ end)
  - Non-coding region 1
  - Initiation codon (AUG)
  - Coding region
  - Termination codon
  - Non-coding region 2
  - Poly-A sequence (at 3′ end)
- The **cap** is present at the 5′ end and controls the rate of protein synthesis. Without the cap, *m*RNA molecules bind very poorly to ribosomes. The cap is rich in methyl residues which protects *m*RNA from enzymatic degradation.

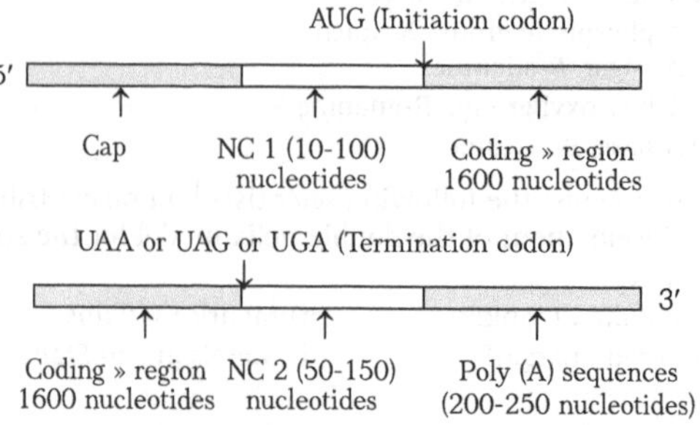

Fig. 8.8 Structure of mRNA

- The cap is followed by **non-coding region 1** or **Untranslated Regions (UTRs) 1**, it consists of 10 to 100 nucleotides. This region is rich in A and U residues. It does not have the ability to translate protein.
- The non-coding region terminates at the **initiation codon** AUG (sometimes GUG or UUG also) in both prokaryotes and eukaryotes.
- After the initiation codon, the **coding region** begins which contains an average of about 2500 nucleotides. Actually, the length of coding region depends upon the length of polypeptide chain.
- The coding region terminates at **termination codon**, i.e. either of UAA, UAG, UGA.
- The termination codon is followed by **non-coding region 2** (NC 2), containing 50-150 nitrogenous bases.
- The 3′ terminus of *m*RNA contains a **poly** (A) **sequence** or **tail region** present after NC 2 which contains 200-250 residues. Tail region protects the *m*RNA from cellular enzymes and helps in the detachment from ribosome.
- The length of *m*RNA decreases with age. This sequence may have some role in the stabilisation of *m*RNA.
- The *m*RNA of prokaryotes is considered as metabolically unstable as it does not stay longer in their body. On the other hand, the *m*RNA of eukaryotes is considered as metabolically stable.

Types

- **Monocistronic** These *m*RNA molecules contain the coding sequence for one polypeptide. These contain only one initiation site and are found in eukaryotes.
- **Polycistronic** These *m*RNA molecules transcript or encode several genes of a metabolic pathway. They can initiate protein synthesis at any internal position and these are found in prokaryotes.

> **RNA**
>
> The transcribed *m*RNA in eukaryotes is found to be about 20% greater than its original length. This greater RNA is called *hn*RNA (heterogeneous nuclear RNA). According to **Weinberg** (1973), all those RNA which have sedimentation coefficient more than 8S are called *hn*RNA.

Ribosomal RNA (*r*RNA)

- It is the basic constituent of ribosomes and develops from the nucleolar organiser region of chromosomes in eukaryotes. It is most abundant (70-80% of total), stable and insoluble RNA.

Structure

- The structure of *r*RNA depends upon various factors like ionic strength, pH, temperature, etc.
- At low ionic strength, *r*RNA is seen as a compact rod or coil and with increasing ionic strength, it occurs in the form of extended regions and shows helical regions.

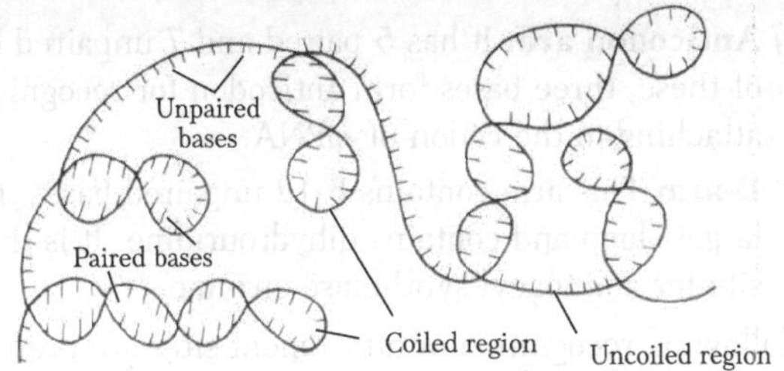

Fig. 8.9 Secondary structures of ribosomal RNA

Types

- *r*RNA of eukaryotes are of four types, i.e. 28S, 18S, 5.8S and 5S. Prokaryotic ribosomes have three types of *r*RNA, i.e. 23S, 16S and 5S. The 23 S *r*RNA and 5 S *r*RNA occur in 50 S ribosomal subunit, while 16S *r*RNA occurs in 30S ribosomal subunit of 70S ribosomes of prokaryotes.
- 3′ end of 18S *r*RNA has nucleotides complementary to cap region of *m*RNA. 5S *r*RNA and surrounding protein complex provide binding sites for *t*RNA.

Table 8.3 Types of *r*RNA

Types of RNA	Molecular weights	Numbers of nucleotides	Types
High MW *r*RNA	Over one million	3,000-5,500	21-29S
High MW *r*RNA	Below one million	1,200-2,500	12-18S
Low MW *r*RNA	Near about 40,000	Approximately 120	5S

Transfer RNA or Soluble RNA (*t*RNA or *s*RNA)

The first person to determine the base sequence of a *t*RNA molecule of yeast was **Robert Holley**.

Structure

To explain the structure of *t*RNA, a clover leaf model was proposed by **Holley** (1965). This model is considered as the primary structure.

This structure contains five arms each with a loop and a stem.

(i) **Acceptor stem** The first arm contains stem only, i.e. this arm is without loop and contains 7 paired bases and 4 unpaired bases. It contains amino acid binding site over it. This site lies at the 3′-end (opposite to the anticodon) and possesses a CCA—OH group. The 5′-end of this stem bears Guanine (G).

(ii) **TψC arm** It has 7 unpaired bases, out of which ψ (pseudouridine) and *r*T (ribothymidine) are unusual bases. This loop is the site for ribosome attachment.

(iii) **Variable arm** It is not present in all *t*RNAs. It consists of about 3-21 nucleotides. Its length is variable due to variability in nucleotide composition.

(iv) **Anticodon arm** It has 5 paired and 7 unpaired bases. Out of these, three bases form anticodon for recognising and attaching to the codon of *m*RNA.

(v) **D-arm** This arm contains 8-12 unpaired bases. It has the largest loop and contains dihydrouridine. It is the binding site for aminoacyl synthetase enzyme.

So, following recognition or attachment sites are present on *t*RNA.

(a) Amino acid binding site - at acceptor atom
(b) Ribosme recognition site - at TψC arm
(c) Aminoacyl synthetase binding site - at D arm
(d) Anticodon - for the attachment with *m*RNA

Complete molecular primary structure of *t*RNA is given below

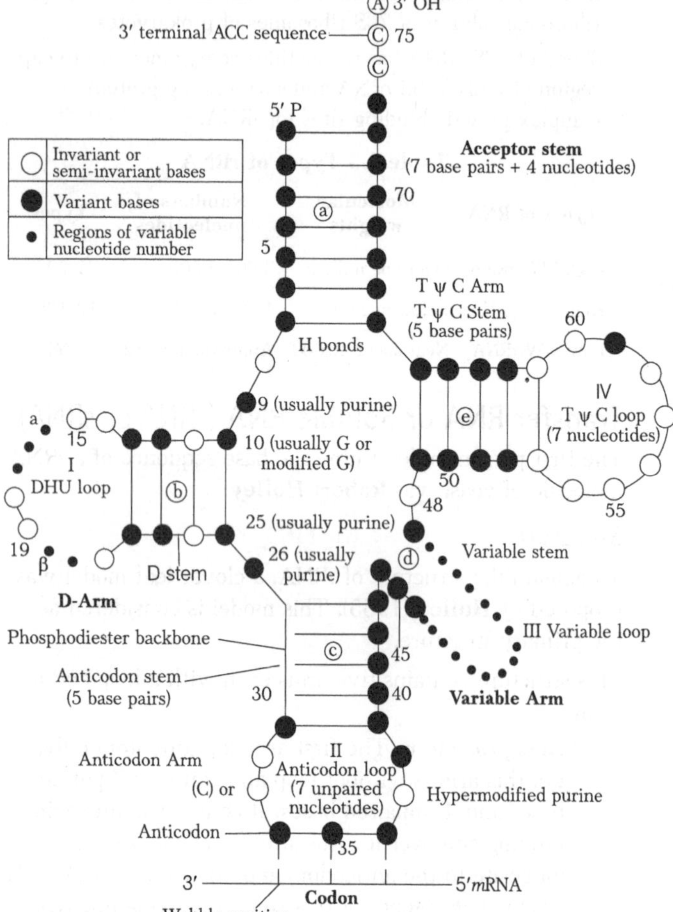

Fig. 8.10 tRNA : Clover leaf structure fully worked out by Holley et. al. (1965) from yeast alanine tRNA

The electron density maps has revealed the presence of tertiary structure in *t*RNA. This tertiary structure is formed due to hydrogen bonds present between

(a) Nitrogenous bases
(b) Bases and ribose phosphate backbone
(c) Ribose phosphate backbone residues itself

Tertiary structure of *t*RNA is given below

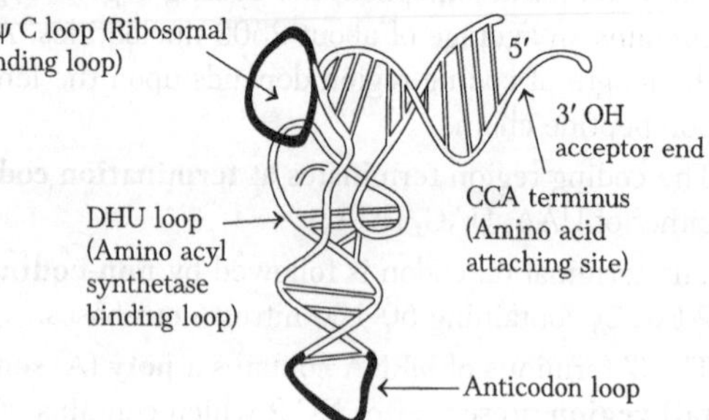

Fig. 8.11 The tertiary structure of tRNA

- Only 0.025% part of total DNA content codes for *t*RNA. The *t*RNAs carry amino acids for initiation codon and called **initiator *t*RNA** or **adapter RNA.** This adapter role was assigned to *t*RNA by **Francis Crick.**

Table 8.4 Differences between DNA and RNA

DNA	RNA
It is the main genetic material in almost all living organisms.	RNA is the genetic material of some viruses only.
It is usually double-stranded. However in certain viruses, DNA is also found to be single-stranded (e.g. $\phi \times 174$).	Most cellular RNA is single-stranded. However, some viruses, e.g. reovirus, have double-stranded RNA.
The pentose sugar is deoxyribose.	The pentose sugar is ribose.
The common organic bases are adenine, guanine, cytosine and thymine.	The common organic bases are adenine, guanine, cytosine and uracil.
Adenine pairs with thymine and guanine with cytosine.	Adenine pairs with uracil and guanine with cytosine.
Pairing of bases is present throughout the length of the helix.	Pairing of bases is present only in the helical region, or completely absent, e.g. in *m*RNA.
There are fewer uncommon bases.	There are more uncommon bases.
It is present in different form, i.e. A, B, C and D forms.	There are three types of RNA, i.e. messenger, ribosomal and transfer RNA.

DNA	RNA
Most of the DNA is found in the chromosomes. Some DNA is also found in the cytoplasm, e.g. in mitochondria and chloroplasts.	Ribosomal RNA is formed from the chromosomes and is found in the nucleolus and cytoplasm, *m*RNA and *t*RNA are also formed from the chromosomes and are found in cytoplasm.
Denaturation (melting) is partially reversible.	Complete and practically instantaneous reversibility of the process of melting.
DNA on replication forms DNA and on transcription forms RNA.	Usually, RNA does not replicate or transcribe exept in certain viruses where RNA can synthesise RNA chain.
Genetic messages are usually encoded in DNA.	The usual function of RNA is to help in translating messages encoded in DNA into proteins.
DNA consists of a large number of nucleotides, which may range up to 4.3 million.	RNA consists of fewer nucleotides, which may range up to 12000.

GENE AND ITS SUBUNITS

Johanssen (1909) defined gene as an elementary unit of inheritance, which can be assigned to a particular trait. Based on his studies on T_4-phage, the terms 'cistron', 'recon' and 'muton' were proposed by American geneticist **S Benzer** in 1957 to describe the three acceptable definitions of a gene.

(i) **Cistron** is the functional gene. It is defined as the segment of DNA consisting of base sequence that codes for a polypeptide chain, *t*RNA, *m*RNA or *r*RNA molecule. It contains upto 30,000 pairs of nucleotide.

(ii) **Muton** is defined as the gene segment which is capable of undergoing mutation. Number of base pair or lengthwise, it is considered as the smallest gene segment.

(iii) **Recon** is defined as the gene segment capable of undergoing recombination.

C Yanofsky (1967) have shown that Benzer's muton is equivalent to a single nucleotide and his recon to the distance separating two adjacent nucleotides. The cistron, recon and muton are the gene segments in descending order of their size.

Interpretation of genes

Various interpretation of genes are as follows

(i) **Housekeeping genes** or **Constitutive genes** These are the genes, which constantly express themselves in a cell because their products are required for the normal cellular activities, e.g. genes for glycolysis, ATPase, etc.

(ii) **Non-constitutive genes** or **Luxury genes** These genes do not always express themselves in a cell. They are switched on or off according to the requirements of cellular activities, e.g. gene for nitrate reductase in plants, lactose system in *Escherichia coli*, etc.

Non-constitutive genes are further of following two types

(a) **Inducible genes** These genes get switched on in response to the presence of a chemical substance or inducer, which is required for the functioning of the product of gene activity, e.g. nitrate for nitrate reductase.

(b) **Repressible genes** These genes continue to express themselves till a chemical (often an end product) inhibits or represses their activity. Inhibition by an end product is known as **feedback repression.**

(iii) **Multigenes** (Multiple gene family) It is a group of similar or nearly similar genes for meeting the requirements of time and tissue specific products, e.g. globin gene family.

(iv) **Repeated genes** The genes which occur in multiple copies, e.g. histone genes, *t*RNA genes, *r*RNA genes, actin genes, etc.

(v) **Single copy genes** These genes are present in single copies and occasionally seen 2-3 times. They form 60-70% of the functional genes.

(vi) **Pseudogenes** These genes have homology to functional genes, but are unable to produce functional product due to intervening non-sense codons, insertions, deletions and inactivation of promoter regions, e.g. of *sn*RNA genes.

(vii) **Processed genes** These are the eukaryotic genes, which lack introns. These genes are probably formed due to reverse transcription or retroviruses.

(viii) **Split genes** These genes were discovered by **Sharp** and **Roberts**. Split genes possess extra or non-essential regions interspersed with essential or coding regions. The non-coding parts are called **introns** or **spacer DNA** or **Intervening Sequence** (IVS). Essential or **coding** parts are called **exons.** Transcribed intronic regions are removed before RNA pass into cytoplasm. Split genes are the characteristic of eukaryotes.

(ix) **Overlapping gene** The nucleotide sequence of these genes overlaps with the expressible nucleotide sequence of another gene. In this way, a nucleotide sequence may make a contribution to the function of one or more gene products. These genes are usually seen in smaller organisms like bacteria.

(x) **Transposons** These are also known as **jumping genes.** Transposons were first discovered by McClintock (1965) through an analysis of genetic instability in maize.

These are the segments of DNA which can move from one place in the genome to another. In human beings, the most common type of transposons belong to Alu family. The transposon causes mutations like insertions, deletions and translocations.

(xi) **Structural genes** These genes have encoded information for the synthesis of chemical substances which is required for cellular machinery. The chemical substances may be

- Structural proteins, e.g. collagen, elastin, actin and tubulin proteins, etc.
- Enzymes
- Proteinaceous hormones, e.g. insulin, growth hormone, parathyroid hormone.
- Antibodies, antigens, certain toxins, blood coagulation factors, etc.

(xii) **Regulatory genes** These genes are meant for controlling the functions of structural genes. The important regulatory genes are promoters, terminators, operators and repressor.

Functions of genes

Following two functions are attributed to genes

- Inheritance of characters from one generation to another.
- Expression of inherited characters in any one generation.

Connectivity between the genes, enzymes and characteristics

- In early 1902, **Archibald Garrod** suggested that there is a relationship between inheritance and metabolic diseases on the basis of his studies on alkaptonuria disease. He introduced the phrase, i.e. 'inborn error of metabolism' to explain this relationship.
- He observed that the family members often had the same disorder due to the lack of certain enzymes.
- Since, enzymes were considered as proteins only at that time thus, he was the first person to establish a link between genes and proteins.
- The following experiments were carried out to understand this connectivity

1. One gene-one enzyme hypothesis

- This hypothesis was put forward by **Beadle** and **Tatum** in 1948.
- They conducted experiments on the nutritional strains of pink mould, *Neurospora crassa.*
- The wild type *Neurospora crassa* is called **prototroph.**
- These grow on simple nutrient medium and has the ability to synthesise all its cellular components.
- An organism that is unable to synthesise a particular cellular metabolite (like an amino acid) is called **auxotroph.**
- Beadle and Tatum produced arginine auxotrophs (unable to synthesise arginine), through steps that are shown in the following pathway

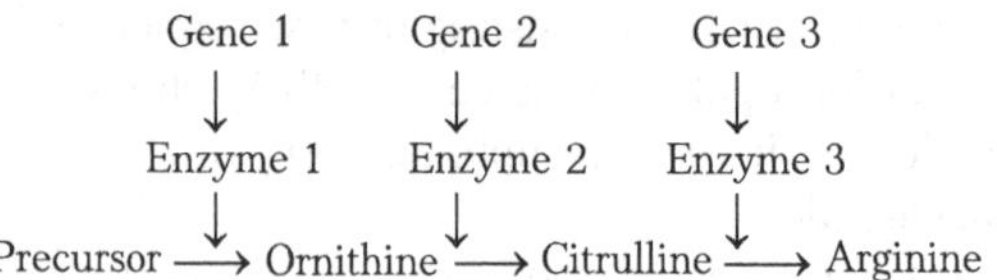

- Beadle and Tatum concluded that each gene is responsible for producing a single enzyme that in turn, affects a single step in the above metabolic pathway.
- A defective enzyme resulted due to a defective or mutant gene.
- Hence, a gene expresses its effect by controlling the synthesis of an enzyme.

2. One gene-one polypeptide hypothesis

- According to this hypothesis, the information enclosed in one gene is sufficient to form one polypeptide only.
- To check the idea of Beadle and Tatum, **Pauling** and **Itano** decided to see the sequential difference in the proteinaceous part of haemoglobin of a person suffering from sickle-cell anaemia and the haemoglobin of normal person.
- They carried out their investigation in the following steps
  (i) They subjected haemoglobin collected from normal as well as sickle-cell anaemic individual to electrophoresis. It is the procedure that separates molecules according to their sizes, density and charge.
  (ii) The difference in the migration rate of both the haemoglobin towards the positive pole was observed.
  (iii) It was noticed that the haemoglobin showed separation into two bands, out of which one corresponds to the normal haemoglobin and the other corresponds to the sickle-cell trait. On this basis, Pauling and Itano concluded that a mutation leads to the change in the structure of haemoglobin protein.

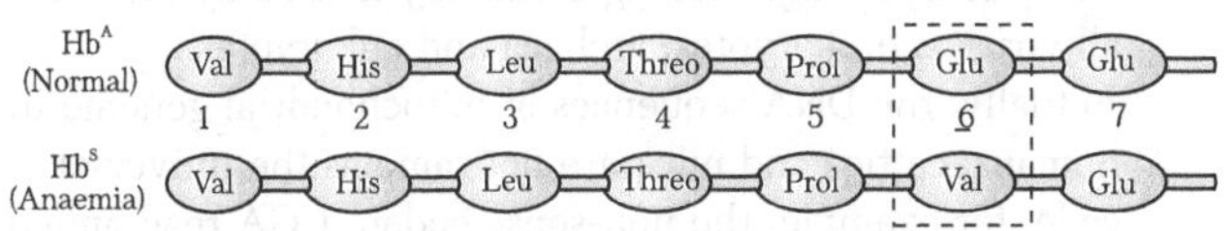

Fig. 8.12 Portion of polypeptide chains of Hb^A and Hb^S

Interpretation

Haemoglobin contains two types of polypeptide chains designated as α and β. As shown above, the difference in haemoglobin lies in β-chain at the position 6. This suggests that there must be one gene for each such type of chain. Hence, the one gene-one enzyme theory was revised and modified as one gene-one polypeptide hypothesis.

Central dogma

- This central dogma of molecular biology was proposed by **Crick** (1958). It is the centralised diagrammatic representation of connectivity between DNA and polypeptide.
- It states that there is one way or unidirectional flow of information from master copy DNA to working copy RNA (transcription) and from working copy RNA to building plan of polypeptide chain (translation).

$$\text{DNA} \xrightarrow{\text{Transcription}} m\text{RNA} \xrightarrow{\text{Translation}} \text{Polypeptide chain (protein)}$$

It is also written as follows

$$\text{DNA} \xrightarrow{\text{Replication}} \text{DNA} \xrightarrow{\text{Transcription}} m\text{RNA} \xrightarrow{\text{Translation}} \text{Polypeptide}$$

- During this, transcription or RNA synthesis occurs over DNA and translation or protein synthesis occurs over ribosomes.
- In eukaryotes, these two processes are separated in time and space. This protects DNA from respiratory enzymes and RNAs degradation from nucleases.
- During the formation of RNA from DNA, information is passed on in the language of nucleotide sequence.
- However, from RNA to protein, the information is passed on in the language of amino acid sequence.
- This can be seen in the given figure below

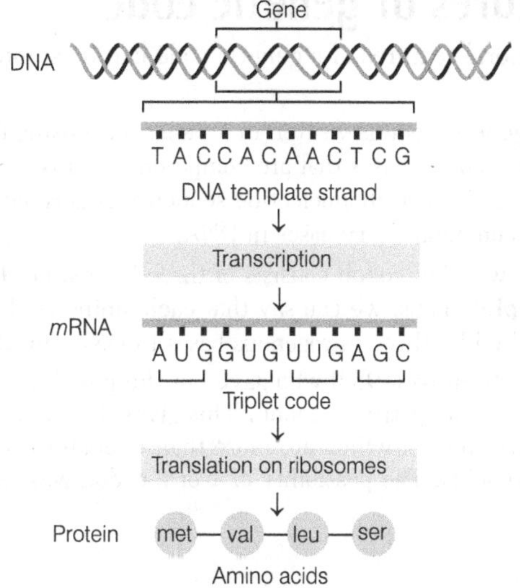

Fig. 8.13 Transfer of information from DNA to protein (An outline view)

Central dogma reverse

- **Temin** and **Baltimore** (1970s) reported the existence of 'RNA dependent DNA polymerase' which could synthesise DNA from a single-stranded RNA template. This gave rise to the concept of **central dogma reverse** or **teminism** suggesting that information flow can also take place from RNA-DNA.

$$\circlearrowleft \text{DNA} \underset{\text{Reverse transcription}}{\overset{\text{Transcription}}{\rightleftharpoons}} \text{RNA} \circlearrowleft \xrightarrow{\text{Translation}} \text{Polypeptide}$$

- **D Baltimore** (1970) also described the presence of reverse transcriptase enzyme in RNA tumour viruses.

GENETIC CODE

- More than 200 amino acids are found in nature, but only 20 are used in protein synthesis. To specify these 20 amino acids, four nitrogenous bases are present in a DNA molecule.
- Several doubts arose on how it is possible that the 20 amino acids are encoded by only four nitrogenous bases? The most accepted theory to solve this doubt was given by **FH Crick**.
- According to this theory, there exists a genetic code, which is made up of these four nitrogenous bases. This code is considered as the smallest unit to code one amino acid.
- Genetic code is defined as the nucleotide sequence of nitrogenous bases, which specifies the amino acid sequence in a polypeptide molecule.

Features of genetic code

The general features of a genetic code can be summarised as follows

- The genetic code is written in a linear form using the ribonucleotide bases that are composed by *m*RNA molecule as 'letters'. This ribonucleotide sequence is derived from their complementary bases in DNA.
- Each 'word' of codon consists of three letters, i.e. **the codon is triplet**. Thus, we can say that each amino acid is specified by three nitrogenous bases in DNA and RNA.
  It was **Gamow** (1954) who gave out the possibility of three letter codon or triplet codon. This gives $4 \times 4 \times 4 = 64$ codons, in total which are more than enough to code for 20 amino acids. The possibility of 1 or 2 codon was rejected as possible combinations from 1 or 2 nitrogenous bases are much lesser than required 20 codons.
- The genetic code is **non-ambiguous** and **specific**, because a particular codon always codes for the same amino acid.
  But in certain rare cases, the genetic code is found to be ambiguous, i.e. some codons code for different amino acids under different conditions, for example the codon UUU, normally codes for phenylalanine, but it may also code for isoleucine, leucine or serine, when ribosomes are treated with streptomycin.
- The genetic code is said to be **commaless**, i.e. no internal punctuations (commas) is used in the code.
- The code is **non-overlapping**, i.e. any single ribonucleotide at a specific location within *m*RNA is the part of only one triplet.
- The code has **polarity**, i.e. a code has fixed starting and termination ends. These ends are 3′ and 5′ end depending upon the placement of *m*RNA.
- The code is almost **universal**, i.e. with only minor exceptions, a single coding dictionary is used by almost all viruses, prokaryotes, archaea and eukaryotes. Actually, the DNA sequences of mitochondrial genome in humans, cattles and mice are not same as the universal code, for example, the non-sense codon, UGA read amino acid tryptophan, AUA codes for methionine rather than isoleucine, etc.
- The code is **degenerate,** i.e. a given amino acid can be specified by more than one codon. This is the case for 18 out of 20 amino acids as seen in the table given below

Second base

First base	U		C		A		G		Third base
U	UUU, UUC	Phenyl-alanine (Phe) F	UCU, UCC, UCA, UCG	Serine (Ser) S	UAU, UAC	Tyrosine (Tyr) Y	UGU, UGC	Cysteine (Cys) C	U, C
	UUA, UUG	Leucine (Leu) L			UAA	Stop codon	UGA	Stop codon	A
					UAG	Stop codon	UGG	Tryptophan (Trp) W	G
C	CUU, CUC, CUA, CUG	Leucine (Leu) L	CCU, CCC, CCA, CCG	Proline (Pro) P	CAU, CAC	Histidine (His) H	CGU, CGC, CGA, CGG	Arginine (Arg) R	U, C
					CAA, CAG	Glutamine (Gln) Q			A, G
A	AUU, AUC, AUA	Isoleucine (Ile) I	ACU, ACC, ACA, ACG	Threonine (Thr) T	AAU, AAC	Asparagine (Asn) N	AGU, AGC	Serine (Ser) S	U, C
	AUG	Methionine (Met) start codon M			AAA, AAG	Lysine (Lys) K	AGA, AGG	Arginine (Arg) R	A, G
G	GUU, GUC, GUA, GUG	Valine (Val) V	GCU, GCC, GCA, GCG	Alanine (Ala) A	GAU, GAC	Aspartic acid (Asp) D	GGU, GGC, GGA, GGG	Glycine (Gly) G	U, C
					GAA, GAG	Glutamic acid (Glu) E			A, G

Wobble hypothesis

- The occurrence of more than one codon per amino acid is called **degeneracy**. **Crick** (1966) proposed a hypothesis to explain the degeneracy of code known as wobble hypothesis.
- Usually, the multiple codons specifying an amino acid differ by only one base, i.e. the third or **3′ base of the codon**. This third base is called **wobble base**.
- The wobble base of a codon lacks specificity. To tackle this change in codon-anticodon pairing, the base in the first position of anticodon is usually unusual, e.g. inosine, etc.
- These unusual bases are able to pair up with more than one nitrogen base at the same position, e.g. inosine can pair with A, C and U.
- This specialised pairing between the unusual base of *t*RNA and wobble base of *m*RNA is called **wobble pairing.**

Initiation and termination codons

- Among the codons, certain codons contain start and stop signals, i.e. certain triplets are necessary to initiate and to terminate translation.
- **Initiation codon is AUG** in most of the cases and it codes for methionine (met) in eukaryotes and for N-formyl methionine (f-met) in prokaryotes.
- GUG also serves as initiation codon in bacterial protein synthesis. It codes for valine. This codon also found to initiate protein synthesis when the normal AUG codon is lost by deletion or parallel processes.
- There are three termination codons, i.e. UAG, UGA and UAA these codons are also called as **Amber, Opal** and **Ochre**, respectively. The termination codons do not code for any amino acid, hence, they cause termination of polypeptide chain and release the chain. These are also called **non-sense codons**.

Amber, Ochre and Opal

UAG was first set of non-sense mutation. It was discovered by **Richard Epstein** and **Charles Steinberg**. They named it Amber mutation on their friend's name **Harris Bernstein** (whose last name means Amber in German).

UAA was the second stop codon mutation to be discovered. It was named ochre (colour name) to match with amber mutant. Similarly, opal (UGA) name was given to match with above name.

Contributions of Nirenberg, Methaei and HG Khorana regarding genetic code

- **Nirenberg** and **Methaei** in 1961 proved the triplet code existence by experiments. They synthesise artificial *m*RNA, which contained only one nitrogenous base, i.e. uracil.
- This synthetic poly-U sequence was then placed in a cell free system containing protein synthesising enzymes and 20 amino acids.
- **Dr. HG Khorana** also derived a technique for artificially synthesising *m*RNA with repeated sequences of known nucleotides.
- During the procedure, a small polypeptide molecule was produced, which was formed by the linking of phenylalanine. This suggested that UUU is the codon for phenylalanine.
- Similarly, it was also found that the synthetic poly-A *m*RNA gave polylysine peptide chain and poly-C sequence gave polyproline.
- Such a polynucleotide chain of *m*RNA formed of single type of nucleotides is known as **homopolymer chain.**
- Nirenberg and his associates discovered co-polymers, i.e. formed by two or more bases, e.g. ACA, CAA, CCA, etc.
- Nirenberg, Holley and Khorana shared the Nobel Prize of 1968 for their contributions.

CHECK POINT 8.3

1. In a double-stranded DNA, the sequence of base pairs in one strand are AGCTAAGC. What is the complementary sequence on the *m*RNA strand?
(a) TCGATTCG (b) UCGAUUCG
(c) AGCTAAGC (d) CAUTAUCG

2. Gene and cistron show which of the following relationship?
(a) A gene is a cistron with particular function
(b) One cistron comprises many genes
(c) Gene is physical moiety, while cistron is physiological one
(d) One gene can have many cistrons

3. During transfer of genetic information in the form of protein, codon and anticodon belong to
(a) DNA, *m*RNA and *t*RNA respectively
(b) *m*RNA, DNA and *t*RNA respectively
(c) DNA, *t*RNA and *m*RNA respectively
(d) *t*RNA, *m*RNA and DNA respectively

4. Which is related to teminism?
(a) DNA $\rightarrow$ RNA $\rightarrow$ Protein
(b) RNA $\rightarrow$ DNA $\rightarrow$ Protein $\rightarrow$ *m*RNA
(c) DNA $\rightarrow$ RNA $\rightarrow$ Protein $\rightarrow$ DNA
(d) None of the above

5. A genetic code is a
(a) sequence of nitrogenous bases on *m*RNA
(b) sequence of nitrogenous bases on *t*RNA
(c) sequence of nitrogenous bases on *r*RNA
(d) sequence of nitrogenous bases on DNA

6. In a genetic code, the process of degeneracy is that
(a) one codon has many meanings
(b) many codons have same meaning
(c) two codons only share many amino acids
(d) third base is not stable

GENE EXPRESSION

- It is the process by which information contained in genes is decoded to produce other molecules that determine the phenotypic traits of organisms.
- The process is initiated when the information contained in the base sequence of DNA is copied into a molecule of RNA and is used to determine the linear order of amino acids in a polypeptide chain.
- The principal steps in expression of gene are as follows
  - *m*RNA molecules are synthesised from DNA. This process of *m*RNA formation is called **Transcription.** It is carried out with the help of enzyme, RNA polymerase. DNA strand on which this process takes place is called **template strand**. Resultant *m*RNA has base sequence complimentary to that of DNA template.
  - In the nucleus of eukaryotic cells, the *m*RNA usually undergoes chemical modifications called **RNA processing.**
  - The processed *m*RNA molecule is used to specify the sequence in which amino acids are joined together to form a polypeptide chain.
  - This production of an amino acid sequence from an RNA base sequence is called **translation** and the resultant protein is called the **gene product**.

Transcription

- It is the process of copying genetic information from one strand (antisense or template strand) of DNA into *m*RNA.
- It is worth noticing that the principle of complementarity also governs the trascription with the exception of adenosine which pairs with uracil instead of thymine.
- But unlike the replication, in transcription, only a segment and a strand of DNA is copied into RNA due to following reasons
  (i) If both the strands of DNA act as template, then the genetic information transfer machinery gets more complicated. These would code for RNA molecule with different sequences and the protein produced would be different.
  (ii) If both strand act as template, then both of them will generate RNA that would be complementary to each other. Thus, a double-stranded RNA will be produced, which cannot be translated into protein.

Structure of transcription unit

A segment of DNA that takes part in transcription is called **transcription unit.**

It has following three components.

(i) Structural gene

- The DNA strand that has the 3′ → 5′ polarity acts as template and referred to as **template strand** or **antisense (–) strand**, as it has sequence complimentary to RNA transcript.
- The other strand which has the 5′→ 3′ polarity and the sequence similar to RNA is referred to as **coding strand.** This strand does not code for anything. It is also known as **sense (+) strand** due to its sequence similarity with RNA transcript.

(ii) Promoter

- This region is present upstream of structural gene at 5′ of the coding strand. This sequence provides the site for binding RNA polymerase. The template and coding strands of DNA are defined by the promoter site.
- This site is AT rich region **(TATA box)**. In bacteria, this region is called **Pribnow box** and in eukaryotes, this region is called the **Hogness box.**
- This region contains the sequence of two folds symmetry in which sections of DNA on either side of a particular point are symmetrical, i.e. the sequences in these sections are **palindromic.**

(iii) Terminator

- This region is present downstream of structural gene at 3′ end of the coding strand. It usually defines the end of transcription process.
- The schematic presentation of complete transcription unit is given below

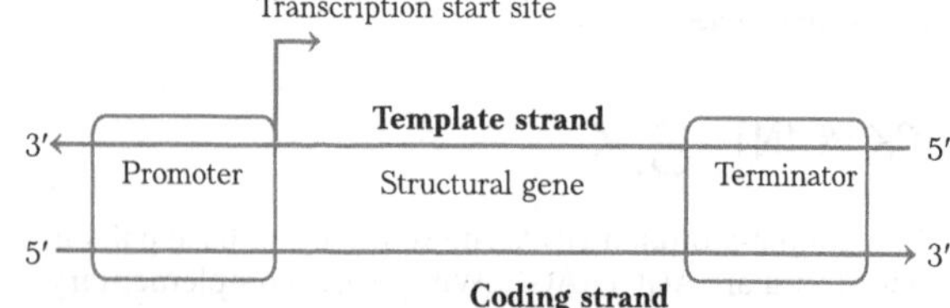

Fig. 8.14 Schematic structure of a transcription unit

- The inheritance of a character is also affected by promoter and regulatory sequence of a structural gene. Thus, **regulatory sequences** are sometimes defined as regulatory genes, even though these sequences do not code for any RNA or protein.

Process of transcription

The mechanism of RNA synthesis was worked out in the late 1950s by the American investigations **Jerard Hurwitz, Samuel B Weiss** and **Audrey Stevens** by independent *in vitro* experiments.

In prokaryotic cell

- In prokaryotes, this process occurs in cytoplasm and a single RNA polymerase controls the synthesis of all types of cellular RNA, e.g. in *E. coli*, same RNA polymerase catalyses the synthesis of *m*RNA, *t*RNA and *r*RNA.
- This **RNA polymerase** (holoenzyme) is very large and consists of following five units
  - Two α subunits-bind to regulatory proteins
  - One β-subunit-bind to RNA nucleoside subunits
  - One β′-subunit-bind to DNA template σ (sigma) factor-recognise start signal on DNA.
  - The first four subunits, i.e. the two α, β and β′ forms the core enzyme., The σ factor is not firmly attached to the core enzyme which means it can be easily isolated. The core enzyme is only capable of catalysing the process of **elongation.**
- The process of prokaryotic transcription occurs in following steps
  - The sigma factor directs RNA polymerase in selecting the initiation sites (promoter). RNA polymerase (σ factor + core enzyme) binds to promoter region of the DNA and begins the process of transcription.
  - Once RNA molecule becomes 8-9 bases long, σ factor is released from the RNA polymerase.
  - The β and β′ subunits help RNA polymerase in unwinding of DNA molecule. The core enzyme moves along the DNA, binds a nucleoside triphosphate that pairs with next DNA base and opens DNA helix as it moves.
  - Once the polymerase reaches the terminator region, a chain terminating protein called **rho (ρ) factor stop RNA synthesis**. The nascent RNA and RNA polymerase fall off and it results in the **termination of trascription**. All these steps are shown in the figure below

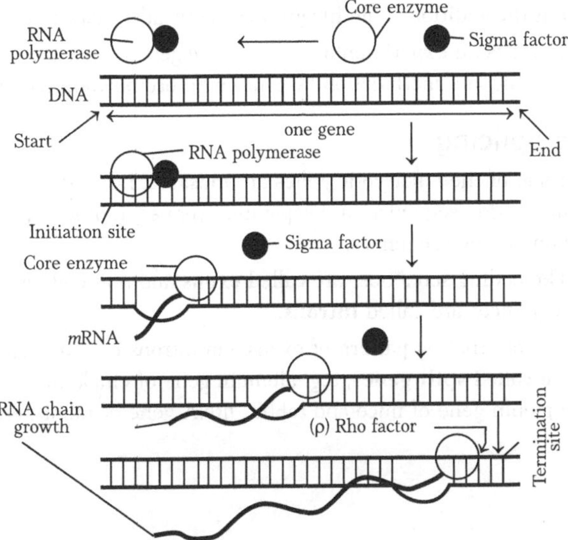

Fig. 8.15 Transcription process in prokaryotes

Note • *One more factor, i.e. psi (ψ) factor is also isolated from E. coli and causes preferential transcription of DNA coding for rRNA. The ψ factor requires entire enzyme for its functioning.*

- *The core enzyme in bacterium, Bacillus subtilis have seven polypeptide chains, i.e. β, β′, α, α′, δ, ω_1 and ω_2.*
- *Sometimes the translation can begin much before the mRNA is fully transcribed due to lesser space in smaller oganisms. Thus, the transcription and translation can be coupled in bacteria.*

In eukaryotic cell

- It occurs within the nucleus under the direction of three separate forms of RNA polymerase. **Eukaryotic RNA polymerase** exists in three unique forms, each of which trancribes different types of genes as shown below

Table 8.5 RNA polymerase in eukaryotes

Polymerase forms	Products	Locations
I	*r*RNA	Nucleolus
II	*m*RNA, *sn*RNA	Nucleoplasm
III	5S *r*RNA, *t*RNA	Nucleoplasm

- The mechanism of transcription can be broadly divided into following steps

(i) Promoter recognition

- The RNA polymerase binds to a DNA sequence of 20-200 nucleotides in length. This sequence is called **promoter.**
- Adenine or Guanine is often the first nucleotide in this transcript.
- The promoters of genes of RNA polymerase-II contain three distinct regions which are centered at sites lying between-25 bp and-100 bp. These regions are as follows
  - (a) **TATA or Goldberg-Hogness box** It is 7 bp long and least effective of three regions. It is located 20 bp upstream to starting point.
  - (b) **CAAT box** It contains about 70-80 bp and includes ACAATCT base composition.
  - (c) **GC box** It contains about 60-100 bp and includes GGGCGG base composition.
- The strength of the binding of RNA polymerase to different promoters varies greatly.
- In eukaryotes, in addition to the promoter sequences, there are also other DNA sequences called **enhancers.**
- These interact with promoter to determine the extent of transcription and result in the differences in the extent of gene expression from one gene to another.
- The promoters typically require accessory proteins for active transcription by RNA polymerase.

(ii) Chain initiation

- After the initial binding step, the RNA polymerase unwinds the DNA double helix. This inturn causes the separation of strand that is to be transcribe from its complementary strand. The separated strand is now available for *m*RNA formation *via* RNA polymerase. This strand is called **template strand.**

- *m*RNA synthesis is initiated and proceeds in the 5′ →3′ direction. The other strand of DNA (5′ – 3′) is known as **antisense strand.** It does not take part in transcription.

(iii) Chain elongation

- RNA polymerase moves progressively along the transcribed DNA strand.
- The nucleotides are added continuously to the growing RNA chain.

(iv) Chain termination

- When RNA polymerase reaches a chain termination sequence, the transcription stops.
- The newly synthesised RNA molecule and the polymerase are released.
- In eukaryotes, two kinds of termination events are known,
  (a) **Self terminating events**, which depend only on the nucleotide sequence in the DNA template.
  (b) **Protein regulated termination** that requires some specific proteins for the termination.

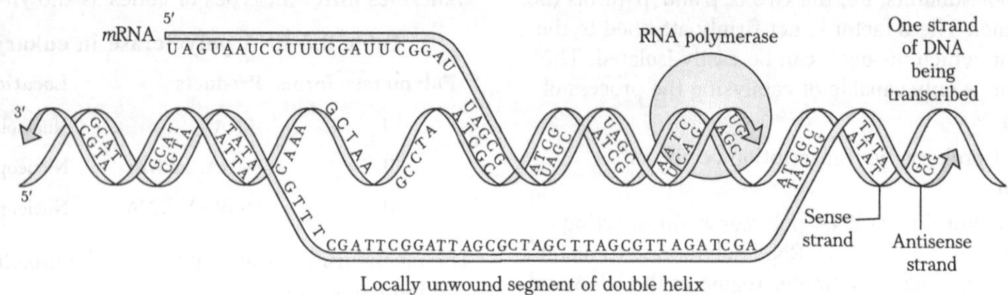

Fig 8.16 Transcription or messenger RNA synthesis

RNA processing

- The initially formed RNAs are often larger than the functional RNAs. These are called **pre *m*RNAs** or **primary transcript.**
- It is found only in the nucleus and known as **heterogeneous nuclear RNA** (*hn*RNA) as defined by **Weinberg** (1973).
- These RNA molecules are of variable size and are complexed with proteins, forming heterogeneous nuclear Ribonucleoprotein Particles (*hn*RNPs).
- RNA processing or maturation is required to convert primary transcript of all types of RNAs into functional RNAs. The process of maturation of eukaryotic *m*RNA from primary *m*RNA transcripts is known as **'RNA processing'**.

The steps of RNA processing are as follows

(i) Capping

- This involves the formation of a cap at the 5′ end by the condensation of guanylate residues. Technically, this cap is formed by the modification of GTP into 7-methyl guanosine.

(ii) Tailing

- Addition of tail at 3′ end occurs in the form of adding poly (A) or polyadenylate sequence. This sequence consists of 180-200 nucleotides and its addition takes place with the help of enzyme poly (A) synthetase.
- This poly (A) sequence supposes to play role in stabilising *m*RNA.

(iii) Methylation

- It is the addition of methyl group to a few adenylate residues.
- There is an experimental evidence suggesting that the capping and methylation take place before polyadenylation.

(iv) Splicing

- Some of the eukaryotic genes are **mosaics**, i.e. coding nucleotide sequences are separated from each other by non-coding sequences.
- The coding sequences are called **exons** and non-coding sequences are called **introns.**
- The alternating pattern of exons and introns bearing genes are called **split genes**, e.g. albumin gene of chicken, β-globin gene of mice and rabbit, *t*RNA gene of rabbit, etc.

- The primary transcript of a typical eukaryotic genes contains introns as well as exons. The introns are removed from this primary transcript or pre *m*RNA by a process called **RNA splicing.**

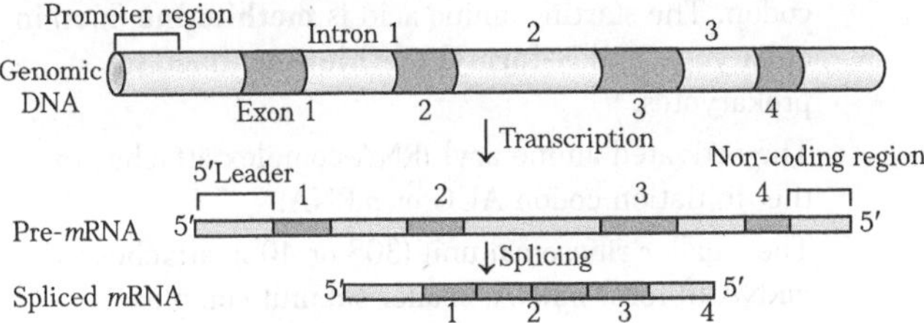

Fig. 8.17 Split gene with transcription and splicing

- The process of splicing involves two successive transesterification reactions in which phosphodiester linkages within the pre *m*RNA are broken and then new linkage is formed.
- The complete process is carried out with the help of a large complex called **spliceosome.** The complex comprises about 150 proteins and five RNAs and is similar in size to a ribosome.
- The five RNAs present here are called **small nuclear RNAs** (*sn*RNAs), each of these are 100-300 nucleotides long and complexed with many proteins. These RNA protein complexes are called **small nuclear ribonuclear proteins** or ***sn*RNPs** or **pronounced as 'snurps'**.
- The process of splicing can have following self-explanatory five possibilities
  - (i) Normal
  - (ii) Exon skipped
  - (iii) Exon extended
  - (iv) Intron retained
  - (v) Alternative exons

Self-splicing in *Tetrahymena* : Ribozymes

- In the splicing of a ribosomal RNA precursor in a ciliate *Tetrahymena*, **the intron is found to work as an enzyme in** catalysing the splicing reaction.
- This self-splicing in *Tetrahymena* RNA molecule was the first example of a RNA molecule that could function as an enzyme in catalysing a chemical reaction.
- Such enzymatic RNA molecules are usually called as **ribozymes.** These are first and foremost non-proteinaceous enzymes.
- For the discovery of ribozymes, **Thomas Cech** got the Nobel Prize in 1986.

Exonic Splicing Enhancer (ESE) and Intronic Splicing Enhancer (ISE)

These are specialised proteins having the tendency to enhance splicing at nearby splice sites when bind to specific sites.

Alternative splicing and isoforms

When two or more functional *m*RNAs are developed from a single primary transcript due to the differences in splicing pattern, their splicing is called **alternative splicing.**

Thus, through alternative splicing, multiple protein products can be produced from a single gene. These different proteins are called **isoforms.**

Translation

- It is the simply known as the process of protein synthesis from *m*RNA. In this process, the genetic information present in *m*RNA directs the sequence of specific amino acid to form a polypeptide chain. The cellular factory responsible for synthesising the protein is ribosome.
- When the smaller subunit of ribosome encounters an *m*RNA, the process of translation begins.
- The complete process have following steps
  1. Activation of amino acids
  2. Transfer of activated amino acids to *t*RNA
  3. Initiation of polypeptide chain synthesis
  4. Elongation of polypeptide chain
  5. Termination of polypeptide chain formation

1. Activation of amino acids

- The activation of amino acids takes place through their carboxyl groups. In the presence of ATP, each amino acid combines with its specific aminoacyl-*t*RNA synthetase. It produces aminoacyl adenylate enzyme complex.
- The complete reaction is as follows

$$\text{Amino acid} + \text{ATP} + \underset{\text{Aminoacyl synthetase}}{\text{Enzyme}} \xrightarrow{Mg^{2+}} \underset{\text{Aminoacyl adenylate enzyme complex}}{\text{Enzyme}} \text{—Amino acid—AMP} + \text{PPi}$$

This step is also known as **aminoacylation of *t*RNA.**

- Any cell has atleast 20 aminoacyl synthetase enzymes for 20 amino acids. Each enzyme is specific and attaches with the specific amino acid without any error.

- Activating enzymes used in this process are substrate specific, but some activator enzymes can activate more than one amino acid, e.g. **isoleucine tRNA synthetase** can also activate **valine.**
- The series of events are displayed in the following diagram

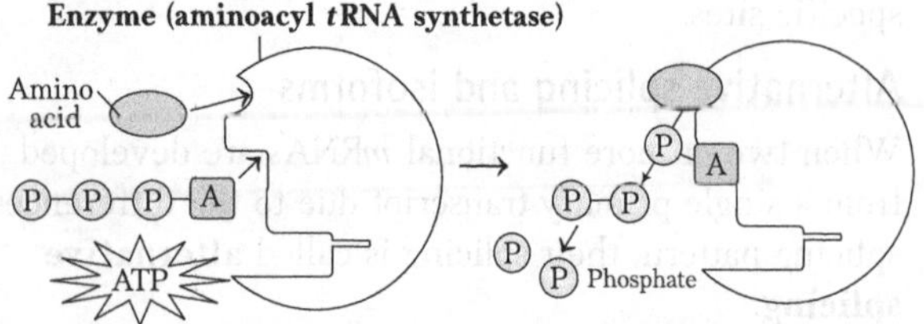

Fig. 8.18 Amino acid activation

2. Transfer of activated amino acid to tRNA

- In this step, the amino acids are attached to the tRNA by high energy bonds. These bonds are formed between the carboxyl group of amino acid and 3′-hydroxy terminal of ribose of terminal adenosine of CCA and of tRNA.
- The complete reaction is carried out by the enzyme **synthetase**, which has two active sites, i.e. one for tRNA and another for specific amino acid molecule.
- The complete reaction is given below

Enzyme—Amino acid—AMP + tRNA ⟶
Aminoacyl adenylate and enzyme

Amino acid tRNA + AMP + Enzyme
Aminoacyl tRNA

- The series of events are displayed in following diagram

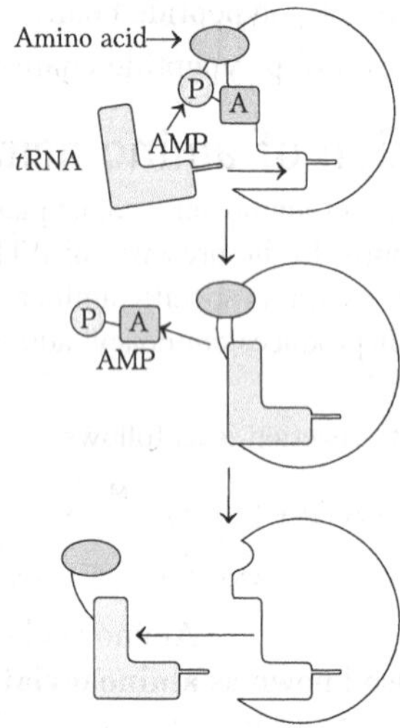

Fig. 8.19 Transfer of active amino acid to tRNA

- The aminoacyl tRNA moves towards the ribosomes, i.e. the site of protein synthesis with mRNA.

3. Initiation of polypeptide chain synthesis

The steps of chain initiation are as follows

- Aminoacyl-tRNA complex is specific for the initiation codon. The starting amino acid is **methionine** (met) in eukaryotes and **N-formyl methionine** (fmet) in prokaryotes.
- The activated amino acyl tRNA complex attaches to the initiation codon AUG or mRNA.
- The smaller ribosomal unit (30S or 40S) attaches to mRNA to form mRNA smaller subunit complex.
- This complex is shown in the diagram below

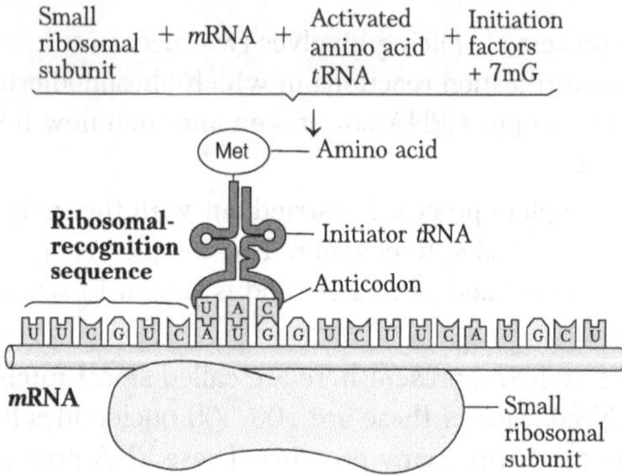

Fig. 8.20 Joining of smaller ribosomal unit with mRNA and initiator tRNA

- The larger subunit then joins the smaller subunit to form complete translation initiation complex. Initiation factors are necessary to bring all the components of translation initiation complex together.
- These factors join the small subunit of ribosome at the start of the process and leave when large subunit of ribosome joins the small subunit.
- First amino acid tRNA complex occupies the P-site of ribosome. Mg^{2+} also takes part in this process.
- The translation initiation complex is shown below

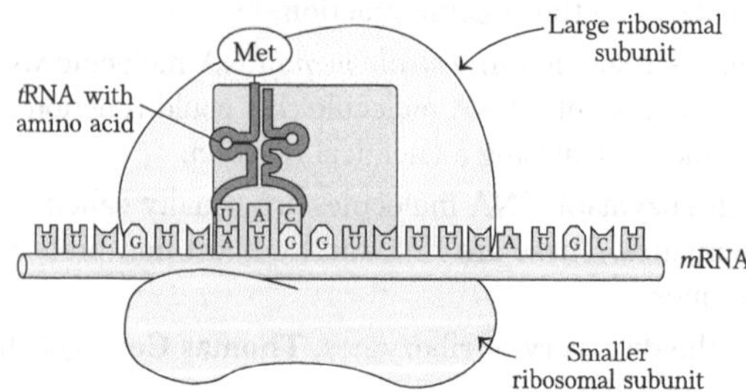

Fig. 8.21 Joining of larger subunit of ribosome to smaller subunit to form initiation complex

Initiation Factors

In **prokaryotes**, three initiation factors IF-1, IF-2 and IF-3 are required for initiation of protein synthesis, while in **eukaryotes**, the initiation factors are eIF-2, eIF-2′, eIF-2a$_1$, eIF-2a$_2$, eIF-2a$_3$ (Ochoa; 1976). **Anderson** (1975) named these **eukaryotic initiation factors** as IF-MP, IF-M1, IF-M2A, IF-M 2B α, IF-M2B β and IF-M3.

4. Elongation of polypeptide chain

The elongation of polypeptide chain involves the following steps

(i) Codon recognition

- After the formation of complete ribosome (*m*RNA-*t*RNA) complex, an aminoacyl acceptor site (A-site) is established next to the P-site.
- It exposes *m*RNA codon next to the intiation codon.
- The second amino acid *t*RNA-complex now occupies the A-site of larger ribosomal subunit.

(ii) Peptide bond formation

- First step is followed by the **peptide bond formation** between both the amino acids present at P-site as well as A-site.
- The enzyme, which helps in the process of peptide bond formation is **peptidyl transferase.**
- Ribosome acts as catalyst for peptide bond formation. The bond formation is simultaneous with the transfer of amino acid from P-site to A-site.

(iii) Translocation

- After peptide bond formation, translocation occurs, involving the movement of second amino acid *t*RNA-complex from A-site to P-site.
- In actual sense, this involves the movement of ribosome relative to *m*RNA in 5′ → 3′ direction.
- The initiator *t*RNA molecule is unloaded from the ribosome. As a result of translocation, the P-site becomes vacant and second amino acid *t*RNA-complex along with 'met' or 'fmet' occupies the P-site.

(iv) Growing polypeptide chain

- Subsequently, the third amino acid *t*RNA-complex occupies the A-site. This is followed by peptide bond formation, transfer of chain and translocation in the similar manner, resulting to a chain of three amino acids.

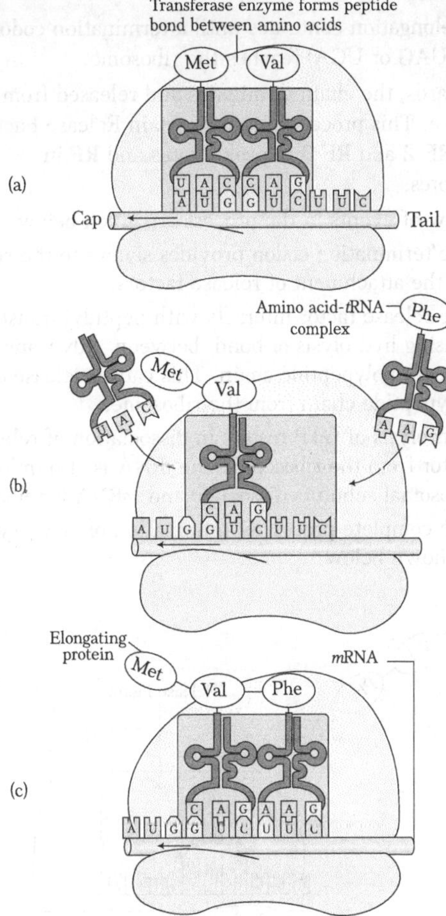

Fig. 8.22 Chain elongation

Elongation factors

The process of elongation requires soluble proteins called **Elongation Factors** (EFs). These were named as **EF-T** and **EF-G** in **prokaryotes**. It was found EF-T contains two proteins, which were named separately as EF-Tu and EF-Ts . Among the **eukaryotes**, elongation factors are named as **EF-1** and **EF-2**, corresponding to EF-T and EF-G.

EF-Tu and EF-Ts are required for binding aminoacyl *t*RNA to ribosome, while EF-G is involved in the translocation of *m*RNA. This is the reason only that EF-G is also called **translocase**.

5. Termination of polypeptide chain formation

- Chain elongation continues until a termination codon (UAA, UAG or UGA) reaches the ribosome.
- Afterwards, the chain terminates and released from the ribosome. This process requires certain Release Factors, i.e. **RF-1, RF-2** and **RF-3** in prokaryotes and **RF** in eukaryotes.
- The flow of events in the process are given below
  - The termination codon provides signals to the ribosome for the attachment of release factors.
  - The release factor interacts with peptidyl transferase, causing hydrolysis of bond between *t*RNA and nascent polypeptide chain. This causes release of polypeptide chain from the ribosome.
  - Hydrolysis of GTP results in dissociation of release factor from the ribosome. The *t*RNA is also unloaded, ribosomal subunits dissociate and *m*RNA is released.
  - The complete process of termination of chain synthesis is shown below

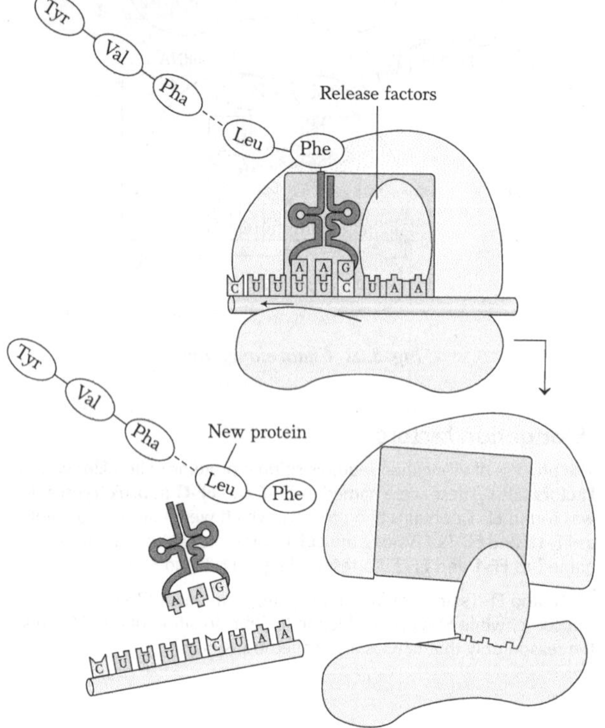

Fig. 8.23 Termination of chain synthesis

Ribosome recycling

- Termination is the last step of protein biosynthesis which requires the combined action of the **ribosome recycling process.**
- After the release of polypeptide chain and the release factors, the ribosome is still bound to the *m*RNA and is left with two deacylated *t*RNAs (at A and P-sites).
- To participate in a new round of polypeptide synthesis, the *t*RNAs and *m*RNA must be removed from the ribosome and ribosome must dissociate into large and smaller subunits. These all events collectively referred to as ribosome recycling.

REGULATION OF GENE EXPRESSION

- It is the mechanism of switching off and switching on the genes, depending upon the requirement of the cells and the stage of development. Because of this regulation, only certain proteins are synthesised as few as 5-10 molecules, while others are formed as more than 1,00,000 molecules per cell.
- There are many possible control points for the regulation of gene expression.
- Some important control points of expression of gene are discussed below
  - **DNA rearrangement** It is the change in the gene expression. It depends upon the position of DNA sequence in the genome.
  - **Transcriptional regulation** It is done by controlling the initiation or termination of RNA chain synthesis. The transcription is regulated in 'On' and 'Off' manner so that the gene products are produced only when needed.
  - **RNA processing** or **Regulation** It is done through RNA splicing or its alternative patterns.
  - **Stability of *m*RNA** It occurs because the *m*RNAs that persist in the cell have long-lasting effects than those that are degraded rapidly.
  - **Translational control** of polypeptide chain synthesis.

Control of gene expression in prokaryotes

- A hypothesis for protein synthesis regulation in prokaryotes was given by **F Jacob** and **J Monod** of Pasteur Institute in Paris.

- For this, they were awarded with Nobel Prize in 1965 (Medicine). This hypothesis is known as **Operon Model**. It was given on the basis of their studies related to the enzyme β-galactosidase in *E. coli*.
- An operon is the part of DNA, which acts as single regulated unit and consists of following components

(i) Structural gene (Cistrons)

- These are the segments of DNA, which carry codes for the synthesis of proteins. These genes determine the primary structure of a polypeptide chain by having the coding sequence of amino acids in them.
- For example, the *lac* operon of *E. coli* contains three structural genes, i.e. *Z*, *Y* and *A*.
  (a) **Gene-*Z*** contains 3063 base pairs and codes for the **enzyme β-galactosidase**, which hydrolyses lactose into glucose and galactose.
  (b) **Gene-*Y*** contains 800 base pairs and codes for **β-galactose permease,** a membrane bound carrier protein which helps in the transfer of metabolites.
  (c) **Gene-*A*** contains 800 base pairs and codes for **enzyme β-galactose transacetylase**, an enzyme that transfers an acetyl group from acetyl Co-A to β-galactosidase.

(ii) Operator gene

- It controls the function of structural genes and lies next to it. Operator gene is the segment of DNA which exercises the control over transcription.
- The repressor substance of regulator gene has an affinity for operator gene.
- Binding of repressor with regulator prevents RNA polymerase to form the initiation complex.
- In other words, we can say that the operator gene works like 'on' and 'off' switches in protein synthesis.

(iii) Promoter gene

- It is located adjacent to the operator gene. It is the DNA segment at which RNA-polymerase binds.
- It initiates the transcription of the structural genes and controls the rate of *m*RNA synthesis.
- The main site in promoter region of *lac* operon is CRP site, i.e. cyclic AMP receptor protein, which is essential for binding RNA polymerase to the promoter site.
- **Pribnow** (1975) suggested three essential elements in promoter region, i.e. a recognition sequence, a binding sequence and an *m*RNA initiation site.

(iv) Regulator gene

- This gene is involved in controlling the expression of one or more other genes *via* syntheis of a negative or repressor and a positive or inducer substances.

(a) Repressor

- It is a protein synthesised by regulator gene.
- It is meant for blocking the operator gene so that the structural gene is unable to form *m*RNA.
- The repressor may be active or inactive (aporepressor).
- The active repressor is normally seen in an inducible systems, while aporepressor is seen in repressible system.

(b) Inducer

- It is a substance or hormone or some other metabolite which after coming in contact with the repressor, changes its conformation.
- Thus, repressor is inactivated and repressor-inducer complex is formed.
- Due to the formation of this complex, inducer is unable to bind with operator.
- In *lac* operon, lactose (actually allolactose or metabolite of lactose) acts as inducer.
- The regulator, promoter and operator genes together are called the **control genes.**

Types of operon system

Following two types of operon systems are seen in prokaryotes.

(i) **Inducible system** In these systems, the operon remains switched off normally, but becomes functional in the presence of an inducer, e.g. *lac* operon in *E. coli.*

Here, inducer induces enzyme synthesis.

The regulation of protein synthesis in inducible systems is given below

- **Case I When inducer is absent**, so regulator gene produces active repressor, which binds to operator gene and blocks transcription thus, blocking the protein synthesis.
- **Case II When inducer is present**, regulator gene produces active repressor which forms inducer-repressor complex. Thus, it does not bind and block the operator gene. If operator gene is free, *m*RNA synthesis goes on, which afterwards results into protein synthesis.

(ii) **Repressible system** In these systems, regulator normally produces aporepressor or inactive repressor. This aporepressor normally functions in the presence of another substance called corepressor. The corepressor is normally a metabolite, which has the affinity for repressor. Its concentration controls transcription in the cell. The regulation of protein synthesis in repressible systems is given below

- **Case I When corepressor is absent,** regulator gene produces aporepressor, which does not have affinity for the operator gene. Hence, it does not bind and block operator. When operator gene is free, transcription goes on, thus, protein synthesis also goes on.
- **Case II When corepressor is present,** the aporepressor produced by regulator gene combines with corepressor to form active repressor. This active repressor then binds to operator gene and blocks it. Due to the blockage of operator, no transcription takes place, thus, protein synthesis does not occur.

Note *The inducible operons generally function in* ***catabolic pathways*** *and the repressible operons in* ***anabolic pathways.***

Mechanism of inducible operon (*lac* operon)

It can be studied under following two headings

Switch off mechanism

- When the inducer is absent or it level falls off, the active repressor protein associates ifself with the operator gene and blocks it. Thus, no transcription of *m*RNA by structural gene can take place and thus, there is no enzyme synthesis. This complete procedure, is shown below as points (1) to (5).

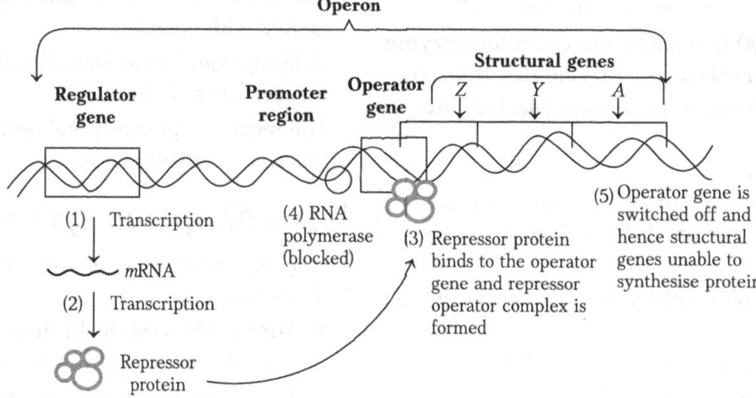

Fig. 8.24 Mechanism of lac operon when gene is switched off, i.e. in the absence of inducer

Switch on mechanism

- In the presence of an inducer (i.e. lactose), the repressor has a higher affinity for the inducer than that of operator gene.
- Now let us understand this mechanism by taking *E. coli* in consideration.
- When lactose is added to *E.coli* culture, a few lactose molecules are carried into the cells by enzyme lactose permease, as small amounts of this enzyme are always present in the cell even when the operon is not working. These few lactose molecules are converted into **allolactose** (an isomer of lactose) molecules, which act as an **inducer** and binds to the **repressor.** As the repressor inducer complex is formed, it fails to join with operator gene of the operon. Thus, operator gene

becomes free and the RNA polymerase can move from the promoter to the structural genes. Thus, the enzyme synthesis takes place. The complete procedure is shown below as points (1) to (7).

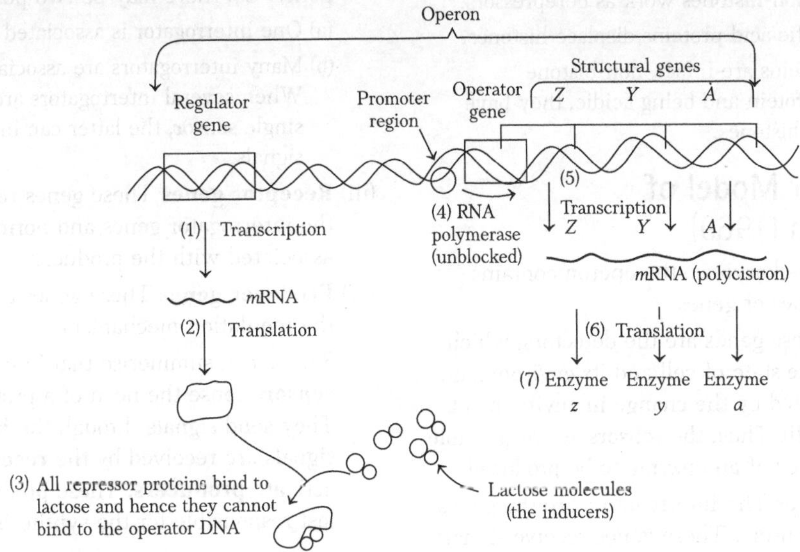

Fig. 8.25 Mechanism of lac operon when gene is switched on, i.e. in the presence of inducer

Note **CAP** *It is an activator called Catabolite Activator Protein (CAP). It exerts a positive control in lac operon because in its absence, RNA polymerase is unable to recognise promoter gene. CAP activates lac genes only when glucose is absent.*

Mechanism of repressible operon
(Tryptophan operon)

- In this operon, three enzymes are necessary for the synthesis of amino acid, tryptophan. These enzymes are synthesised by the activity of five different genes, i.e. trpA, trpB, trpC, trpD and trpE in coordinated manner.
- The addition of tryptophan, however stops the production of these enzymes.
- Tryptophan when added binds to the aporepressor as corepressor. This **aporepressor-corepressor complex** binds to operator gene and blocks the function of RNA polymerase. So, transcription would not occur.
- Thus, the system is known as **repressible system**.

Control of gene expression in eukaryotes

- The control of gene expression is complex in eukaryotic cell as operons are controlled by more than one promoter region and also the gene regulation takes place by different mechanisms.
- Here, histones play major role in gene regulation in the following manner
  (i) Histones are gene repressors. They mask the gene activity in non-specific manner. As histones are responsible for the supercoiling of DNA in eukaryotes, so, the RNA polymerase molecule would not be able to move along the super coiled DNA. Hence, no transcription is possible.
  (ii) The removal of histones from the genic site is necessary to produce a protein. For the removal of histones, two possibilities are suggested.
  (a) **Frenester's model** (1965)
  - According to this model, histones are removed from a particular genic site with the help of nuclear polyions.
  - These form complexes with histones. Thus, they permit the separation of DNA strand in a random manner.
  - Gene specific derepressor RNA hybridises with the non-transcribing DNA strand, thus, stabilising it in open position.
  - This supports the other DNA strand and permits it to transcribe *m*RNA.

(b) **Paul** (1971) ***et. al.* and Stein *et. al.* model**

- In this model, non-histones work as derepressors.
- The gene specific acid proteins displace histones.
- These acid proteins are infact, non-histone chromosomal protein and being acidic, they have affinity for the histones.

Operon-Operator Model of Britton-Davidson (1969)

According to them, in eukaryotes, the operon contains following four basic types of genes

(i) **Sensor genes** These genes are the detectors, which are sensitive to the state of cell and its environment. These are stimulated by the change in environment (or state of the cell). Thus, the sensors are responsible for sensing the need of an enzyme to be produced.

(ii) **Interrogator genes** The interrogators are the genes associated with sensors. These genes receive signals from the sensor genes and transmit it to the other genes. So, there may be two possibilities,

(a) One interrogator is associated with one sensor.

(b) Many interrogators are associated with one sensor. When several interrogators are associated with a single sensor, the latter can initiate a variety of signals.

(iii) **Receptor genes** These genes receive signals from the interrogator genes and normally remains associated with the producer.

(iv) **Producer genes** These genes are output control of the regulation mechanism.

So, we can summerise that in eukaryotes, when the **sensors** sense the need of a protein to be produced. They send signals through the **interrogator**. These signals are received by the **receptors,** which in turn, activate **producers.** These producers are at last responsible for the synthesis of protein.

CHECK POINT 8.4

1. The linkages involved in the process of splicing are
   (a) hydrogen linkages
   (b) disulphide linkages
   (c) phosphodiester linkages
   (d) ionic linkages
2. During transcription, the RNA polymerase holoenzyme binds to a gene promoter and assumes a saddle-like structure. What is its DNA-binding sequence?
   (a) TTAA (b) AATT
   (c) CACC (d) TATA
3. With regard to mature *m*RNA in eukaryotes,
   (a) exons and introns do not appear in the mature RNA
   (b) exons appear but introns do not appear in the mature RNA
   (c) introns appear, but exons do not appear in the mature RNA
   (d) both exons and introns appear in the mature RNA
4. A prokaryotic gene of 600 nucleotides long can code for a polypeptide chain of about, how many amino acids?
   (a) 100 (b) 200 (c) 300 (d) 600
5. In the absence of β-galactosidase, transcription of
   (a) *lac-A* is not possible
   (b) *lac-Y* is not possible
   (c) *lac-Z* is not possible
   (d) All of the above
6. RNA polymerase, which is on the promoter, moves to the structural genes to transcribe them. However, it happens with
   (a) RNA polymerase shifts first to regulator gene
   (b) inducer binds to structural genes
   (c) there is repressor on the operator
   (d) there is no repressor on the operator

EXAM POINTS

- A molecule that can act as a genetic material must fulfil the traits like; it should be able to express itself in the form of 'Mendelian characters'. It should be able to generate its replica and it should provide the scope for slow changes that are required for evolution. **[NEET 2016]**
- Hershey and Chase experimentally proved that DNA is the genetic material in bacteriophage. **[NEET 2019, 17]**
- The term nuclein for the genetic material was used by Meischer. **[NEET 2020]**
- If the distance between two consecutive base pairs is 0.34 nm and the total number of base pairs of a DNA double helix in a typical mammalian cell is 6.6×10^9 bp then the length of the DNA is approximately 2.2 meter. **[NEET 2020]**
- In the polynucleotide chain of DNA, a nitrogenous base is linked to the — OH of 1°C pentose sugar. **[NEET 2020]**
- Purines found in both DNA and RNA are Adenine and Guanine. **[NEET 2019]**
- Adenylic acid, cytidylic acid and guanylic acid, are all nucleotides. **[AIIMS 2019]**
- In DNA, if 20% bases are adenine then pyrimidines are 50%. **[JIPMER 2019]**
- Ribose + Uracil + Phosphate = Ribonucleotide. **[JIPMER 2018]**
- Linker DNA is attached to H_1. **[JIPMER 2018]**
- DNA fragments are negatively charged. **[NEET 2017]**
- The association of histone H1 with a nucleosome indicates the DNA is condensed into chromatin fibre. **[NEET 2017]**
- Chargaff's rule is not applicable to RNA. **[CBSE AIPMT 2015]**
- During DNA replication, supercoiling is relaxed by DNA topoisomerase. **[JIPMER 2019]**
- The experimental proof for semiconservative replication of DNA was first shown in a bacterium. **[NEET 2018]**
- DNA replication in bacteria occurs prior to fission. **[NEET 2020]**
- Taylor conducted the experiments to prove semiconservative mode of chromosome replication on *Vicia faba*. **[NEET 2016]**
- Cistron is equivalent to structural gene. **[Manipal 2012, NEET 2016]**
- DNA dependent RNA polymerase catalyses transcription on one strand of DNA which is called the template strand. **[NEET-II 2016, Kerala CEE 2014]**
- RNA polymerase is the enzyme that facilitates the opening of DNA helix during transcription. **[NEET 2020]**
- RNA polymerase-I transcribes *r*RNA, RNA polymerase-II transcribes *hn*RNA and RNA polymerase-III transcribes *t*RNA. **[NEET 2019]**
- In the process of transcription in eukaryotes, the RNA polymerase-I transcribes *r*RNAs-28S, 18S and 5.8S. **[NEET 2019]**
- The three steps of transcription are initiation, termination and elongation. **[AIIMS 2019]**
- In eukaryotes, transcription occurs in nucleus. In bacteria, transcription and translation occur in cytoplasm. **[AIIMS 2019]**
- 7mG is present at 5'end of eukaryotic *m*RNA. **[JIPMER 2018]**
- Spliceosomes are not found in the cells of bacteria. **[NEET 2017]**
- *hn*RNA undergoes two additional processes. Out of them, capping is the process in which an unusual nucleotide (methyl GTP) is added to the 5' end of molecule. **[JIPMER 2017]**
- Genetic variation cannot be effectively brought about by amplification. **[JIPMER 2019]**
- *r*RNA is the most abundant in animal cell. **[NEET 2017]**
- 23S *r*RNA acts as structural RNA as well as ribozyme in bacteria. **[NEET 2016]**
- A complex of ribosome attached to a single strand of RNA is known as polysome. **[NEET 2016]**
- The first phase of translation is aminoacylation of *t*RNA. **[NEET 2020]**
- *t*RNA binds to *m*RNA through anticodon loop. **[JIPMER 2019]**
- The premature termination of polypeptide synthesis due to stop codon can be overcome *via* compensatory mutation in *t*RNA. This genetic phenomenon is called extragenic suppression. **[AIIMS 2017]**
- Selenocystein is the 21st amino acid. **[JIPMER 2018]**
- Codons of glycine are GGU, GGC, GGA and GGG. **[AIIMS 2018]**
- The genetic code of arginine are CGU, CGC, CGA. **[AIIMS 2019]**
- A genetic code is degenerate, non-overlapping and non-ambiguous. **[NEET 2019]**
- The feature of genetic code that allows bacteria to produce human insulin by recombinant DNA technology is that the genetic code is nearly universal. **[NEET 2019]**
- UAA, UAG, and UGA are stop codon. **[JIPMER 2019]**
- AUG is a start codon. **[NEET 2016]**
- Structural genes, an operator and a promoter are all parts of an operon. **[NEET 2018]**
- A repressor protein is attached to the operator. **[JIPMER 2018]**
- Multigenes are globin gene, inducible genes produce nitrate reductase, overlapping genes are B, E and K in $\phi \times 174$, structural gene produces insulin. **[AIIMS 2018]**
- In the *lac* operon model, lactose molecule function as inducers, which bind with the repressor protein. **[JIPMER 2017]**
- Gene regulation governing lactose operon of *E. coli* that involves the *lac i* gene products is negative and inducible because repressor protein prevents transcription. **[CBSE AIPMT 2015]**
- *i* gene produces repressor, *z* gene produces β -galactosidase, *a* gene produces transacetylase and *y* gene produces permease. **[NEET 2019]**
- The human genome contains 3164.7 million nucleotide bases. Their repeated sequences makeup very large portion of the human genome. The chromosome I has most genes (2968) and Y has the fewest (231). **[AIIMS 2019]**

Chapter Exercises

(A) Topical Exercise

Genetic Material in Organisms

1 Genetic material is
(a) any nucleic acid
(b) a nucleic acid made from a nucleic acid template that has been or is capable of being used as a template in replication
(c) a nucleic acid that is capable of being used as a template in transcription
(d) a nucleic acid that is capable of being used as a template in replication and transcription

2 The properties of genetic material is
(a) it should express in parents but not in offspring
(b) it should replicate itself
(c) it should not change at all
(d) All of the above

3 The genetic material should be stable enough to not to change with
I. age
II. different stages of life cycle
III. change in physiology of the organism
Choose the correct option.
(a) I and II (b) Only II (c) Only III (d) I, II and III

4 Consider the following statements.
I. The transformation experiment on *Diplococcus pneumoniae* was performed by Frederick Griffith.
II. The transformation experiment on *Diplococcus pneumoniae* gave first undoubted evidence that DNA is the genetic material.
Choose the correct option.
(a) Statement I is true, but II is false
(b) Statement I is false, but II is true
(c) Both statements I and II are true
(d) Both statements I and II are false

5 The scientists Avery, MacLeod and McCarty are famous for
(a) identifying RNA as genetic material
(b) giving chemical nature of RNA
(c) revealing chemical nature of transforming principle
(d) giving double helical structure of DNA

6 The isotopes used by Hershey and Chase were
(a) ^{59}Iron and ^{15}Nitrogen
(b) ^{131}Iodine and ^{45}Calcium
(c) ^{15}Nitrogen and ^{14}Carbon
(d) ^{35}Sulphur and ^{32}Phosphorus

7 Viruses grown in the presence of radioactive phosphorus contained radioactive DNA, but not radioactive protein because
(a) DNA contains phosphorus, but protein does not
(b) DNA contains deoxyribose sugar, but protein does not
(c) protein contains radioactive sulphur, but DNA does not
(d) protein contains radioactive carbon, but DNA does not

8 Protein cannot be a genetic material because it is not
(a) a large molecule
(b) ubiquitous
(c) having diversity and specificity
(d) able to replicate

9 Consider the following statements.
I. The first genetic material to be originated was RNA.
II. The difference between RNA and DNA lives both in their base and sugar.
Choose the correct option.
(a) Statement I is true, but II is false
(b) Statement I is false, but II is true
(c) Both statements I and II are true
(d) Both statements I and II are false

DNA Structure

10 Choose the correct option.
I. Nucleotides present in one spiral of DNA are ....*A*.... .
II. Nucleotides present in a DNA of 20,000 base pairs are ....*B*.... .
III. Number spirals (twins or helices) present in a DNA of 2000 base pairs is ....*C*... .
(a) *A*-5, *B*-400, *C*-2000
(b) *A*-20, *B*-4000, *C*-200
(c) *A*-10, *B*-40, *C*-4000
(d) *A*-25, *B*-100, *C*-45.5

11 Choose the incorrect pair.
(a) Sugar and phosphate – Joined by phosphodiester bonds
(b) Nitrogenous base and sugar – Joined by glycosidic bond
(c) Single ring nitrogen base – Thymine
(d) Deoxyribose and ribose – Hexoses

12 The pyrimidines found in RNA are
(a) Adenine, guanine
(b) Thymine, cytosine
(c) Uracil, cytosine
(d) Adenine, uracil

13 The fact that a purine base always paired through hydrogen bonds with a pyrimidine base leads to, in the DNA double helix **[NCERT Exemplar]**
(a) the antiparallel nature
(b) the semiconservative nature
(c) uniform width throughout DNA
(d) uniform length in all DNA

14 Consider the following statements.
I. Glycosidic bonds form between 1′C of sugar and position 1-N in pyrimidine.
II. In a DNA strand, the nucleotides are linked together by phosphodiester bonds.
Choose the correct option.
(a) Statement I is true, but II is false
(b) Statement I is false, but II is true
(c) Both statements I and II are true
(d) Both statements I and II are false

15 Chargaff's rule is applicable to
(a) single-stranded RNA
(b) single-stranded DNA and RNA
(c) single-stranded DNA
(d) double-stranded DNA

16 DNA is a polymer of nucleotides which are linked to each other by 3′-5′ phosphodiester bond. To prevent polymerisation of nucleotides, which of the following modifications would you choose? **[NCERT Exemplar]**
(a) Replace purine with pyrimidines
(b) Remove/Replace 3′ OH group in deoxyribose
(c) Remove/Replace 2′ OH group with some other group in deoxyribose
(d) Both (b) and (c)

17 While analysing the DNA of an organism, a total number of 5386 nucleotides were found out of which the proportion of different bases were Adenine = 29%, Guanine = 17%, Cytosine = 32%, Thymine = 17%. Considering the Chargaffs rule it can be concluded that
(a) it is a double-stranded circular DNA
(b) it is single-stranded DNA
(c) it is a double-stranded linear DNA
(d) No conclusion can be drawn

18 What are proteosomes?
(a) Complexes of *sn*RNA and proteins that excise introns
(b) Small, positively charged proteins that form the core of nucleosomes
(c) Enormous protein complexes that degrade unneeded proteins in the cell
(d) Complexes of transcription factors whose protein-protein interactions are required for enhancing gene transcription

19 Choose the incorrect statement.
(a) Examples of right handed helix are A and B DNAs
(b) The DNA coiled in prokaryotes are maintained by non-histone protein and polyamines
(c) Phosphorus is present in nitrogenous bases
(d) The most accepted model for the DNA packaging in eukaryotes is nucleosome model

Replication of DNA

20 Experiments using N^{15} (heavy nitrogen) to confirm the semiconservative replication of DNA were carried out by
(a) Meselson and Stahl (b) Hershey and Chase
(c) Beadle and Tatum (d) Watson and Crick

21 A DNA molecule of *Escherichia coli* is heavy (full labelled with N^{15}) and is allowed to duplicate in a medium containing N^{14}. After one generation, the two daughter strand molecules have
(a) same density, but do not resemble their parent DNA
(b) different densities, but resemble their parent DNA
(c) different densities and also do not resemble the parent DNA
(d) both the strands are same in density, but do not resemble to their parent DNA

22 If Meselson and Stahl's experiment is continued for four generations in bacteria, the ratio of $N^{15}/N^{15}: N^{15}/N^{14}: N^{14}/N^{14}$ containing DNA in the fourth generation would be **[NCERT Exemplar]**
(a) 1:1:0 (b) 1:4:0 (c) 0:1:3 (d) 0:1:7

23 A bacterium containing 100% N^{15} nitrogen bases is allowed to replicate in a medium containing N^{14} bases. After one round of duplication, the result would be
(a) all individuals would be identical to parents
(b) all individuals would be radioactive, but the percentage of radioactivity in DNA would be 50%
(c) only 50% individuals would be radioactive
(d) all individuals would be similar to parents, but different among themselves

24 Discontinuous synthesis of DNA occurs in one strand, because
(a) DNA molecule being synthesised is very long
(b) DNA dependent DNA polymerase catalyses polymerisation only in one direction (5′ → 3′)
(c) It is a more efficient process
(d) DNA ligase has to have a role

25 A fragment formed at the lagging strand during DNA synthesis is
(a) polymerase fragment (b) RNA fragment
(c) Okazaki fragment (d) epimerase activity

26 The Okazaki fragments in DNA chain growth
I. polymerise in the 3′ to 5′ direction and forms replication fork.
II. prove semiconservative nature of DNA replication.
III. polymerisation in the 3′ to 5′ direction and forms replication.
Choose the correct option.
(a) Only I (b) I and II
(c) I, II and III (d) Only III

27 The DNA strand that has the polarity 3′ → 5′ and acts as a template, is also referred to as
(a) coding strand (b) leading strand
(c) Both (a) and (b) (d) All of these

28 Choose the incorrect pair.
(a) Unwinding of DNA double helix – Helicase
(b) DNA formation – RNA polymerase
(c) Joining of Okazaki fragments – DNA ligase
(d) Polymerase which primers and fills gap – DNA Polymerase-I

RNA and Its Types

29 Which of the following are the functions of RNA?
(a) It is carrier of genetic information from DNA to ribosomes synthesising polypeptides
(b) It carries amino acids to ribosomes
(c) It is a constituent component of ribosomes
(d) All of the above

30 The RNA which carries hereditary information in riboviruses and viroids is known as
(a) genomic RNA (b) genetic RNA
(c) antisense RNA (d) All of these

31 Consider the following statements.
I. *t*RNA is the smallest RNA.
II. *t*RNA has the function of adopter for attaching amino acids over *m*RNA template.
Choose the correct option.
(a) Statement I is true, but II is false
(b) Statement I is false, but II is true
(c) Both statements I and II are true
(d) Both statements I and II are false

32 A ribozyme is an
(a) exception to the one gene-one RNA molecule axiom
(b) enzyme that adds the 5′ cap and poly (A) tail to *m*RNA
(c) example of rearrangement of protein domains caused by RNA splicing
(d) RNA molecule that functions as an enzyme

33 Choose the correct statement(s).
(a) The genomic RNA is double-stranded in wound tumour virus
(b) RNA which constitutes 5% of the total RNA is *m*RNA
(c) *t*RNA is the soluble RNA
(d) All of the above

34 Choose the correct gene function.
(a) DNA formation (b) Protein synthesis
(c) RNA formation (d) None of these

35 Functional unit of DNA that is responsible for coding specific gene product
(a) regulatory gene (b) *Z*-gene
(c) cistron (d) *A*-gene

36 Consider the following statements.
I. The smallest unit of genetic material which when mutated produces a phenotypic effect is muton.
II. Length of *m*RNA that carries information for complete polypeptide synthesis is cistron.
Choose the correct option.
(a) Statement I is true, but II is false
(b) Statement I is false, but II is true
(c) Both statements I and II are true
(d) Both statements I and II are false

37 Regulatory genes are genes that
(a) code for repressor proteins
(b) are transcribed continuously
(c) are not contained in the operon they control
(d) All of the above

38 Genes that are involved in turning off or on the transcription of a set of structural genes are called
(a) polymorphic genes (b) operator genes
(c) reductant genes (d) regulatory genes

39 One gene-one polypeptide hypothesis was proposed by
(a) Linus Pauling (b) v Ingram
(c) Beadle and Tatum (d) Brenner

40 Central dogma of genetic information was modified by the discovery of
(a) reverse transcriptase
(b) DNA polymerase
(c) RNA polymerase
(d) ligase

41 The sequence of events mentioned below are symbolised by alphabets. Choose the correct answer, where the alphabets are matched with the processes

$$\text{RNA} \xrightarrow{A} \text{DNA} \xrightarrow{B} \text{DNA} \xrightarrow{C} m\text{RNA} \xrightarrow{D} \text{Polypeptide}$$

(a) *A* – Replication, *B* – Transformation, *C* – Transcription, *D* – Translation
(b) *A* – Reverse transcription, *B* – Replication, *C* – Transcription, *D* – Translation
(c) *A* – Replication, *B* – Transcription, *C* – Translation, *D* – Transduction
(d) *A* – Reverse transcription, *B* – Translation, *C* – Transcription, *D* – Replication

42 Teminism is
(a) a reverse central dogma
(b) a central dogma of molecular biology
(c) a circular flow of hereditary material
(d) an effect of cytoplasm on functioning of DNA

43 Nobel Prize to A Kornberg and S Ochoa was given for
(a) artificial synthesis of DNA and RNA
(b) theory of natural selection
(c) one gene-one enzyme theory
(d) mutation theory

Genetic Code

44 The salient feature of genetic code is
(a) one codon codes for only one amino acid
(b) some amino acids are coded by more than one codon
(c) a codon is made up of three nucleotides
(d) All of the above

45 Genetic code translates the language of
(a) RNA into that of proteins
(b) proteins into that of RNA
(c) amino acids into that of RNA
(d) RNA into that of DNA

46 There are 64 codons in genetic code dictionary because
(a) there are 64 types of *t*RNAs found in the cell
(b) there are 44 meaningless and 20 codons for amino acids
(c) there are 64 amino acids to be coded
(d) genetic code is triplet

47 Consider the following statements.
I. Each codon present on *m*RNA and anticodon present on *t*RNA is composed of a set of three out of U, C, A, G.
II. The codon in *m*RNA is readed in a contiguous fashion because there are no punctuations.
Choose the correct option.
(a) Statement I is true, but II is false
(b) Statement I is false, but II is true
(c) Both statements I and II are true
(d) Both statements I and II are false

48 The genetic code is
I. universal　　II. commaless
III. degenerate　　IV. ambiguous
Codes
(a) I and II　　(b) III and IV
(c) I, II and III　　(d) II, III and IV

49 Because most of the amino acids are represented by more than one codon, the genetic code is said to be
(a) deaminated　　(b) commaless
(c) degenerate　　(d) overlapping

50 Out of 64 codons, only 61 codes for the 20 different amino acids. This character of genetic code is called
(a) degeneracy
(b) non-ambiguous nature
(c) redundancy nature
(d) overlapping

51 Consider the following statements.
I. UAA, UAG and UGA are known as non-sense codon.
II. Non-sense codon terminates the message of gene controlled protein synthesis.
Choose the correct option.
(a) Statement I is true, but II is false
(b) Statement I is false, but II is true
(c) Both statements I and II are true
(d) Both statements I and II are false

52 When TMV-RNA is used for infection, the amino acid sequence of the coat protein of the progeny is the same whether the host is *Zinnia* or tobacco. This proves that the genetic code is
(a) degenerate　　(b) universal
(c) unidirectional　　(d) non-overlapping

53 Which one of the following pairs of codons is correctly matched with their function or the signal for the particular amino acid?
(a) GUU, GCU – Alanine
(b) UAG, UGA – Stop
(c) AUG, ACG – Start/ Methionine
(d) UUA, UCA – Leucine

54 Which of the following groups of codons, code for amino acid serine?
(a) CUU, CUC, CUA and CUG
(b) UAU, UAC, UGU and UGC
(c) UCU, UCC, UCA and UCG
(d) UGU, UGC, UGA and UAG

55 Which one of the following pairs is correctly matched with regard to the codon and the amino acid coded by it?
(a) UUA-valine　　(b) AAA-lysine
(c) AUG-cysteine　　(d) CCC-alanine

56 Which among the following codon does not code for valine (val)?
(a) GUC　　(b) GUA
(c) GCA　　(d) GUG

57 A phenomenon, where the third base of *t*RNA at its 5′ end can pair with a non-complementary base of *m*RNA is called
(a) universality　　(b) collinearity
(c) degeneracy　　(d) wobbling

58 What becomes established from the wobble hypothesis?
(a) Process of peptide chain elongation
(b) Economy of the number of *t*RNA molecules
(c) Process of peptide chain initiation
(d) Process of peptide chain termination

59 Whose experiments cracked the DNA and discoverd unequivocally that a genetic code is a triplet?
(a) Nirenberg and Mathaei (b) Hershey and Chase
(c) Morgan and Strutevant (d) Beadle and Tatum

60 Khorana and his colleagues synthesised RNA molecule with repeating sequence of UG nitrogenous bases (UGUGUGUGUGUG). It produced a tetrapeptide with alternating sequence of cysteine and valine. It proves that the codon for cysteine and valine is
(a) UGG and GUU (b) UUG and GGU
(c) UGU and GUG (d) GUG and UGU

Transcription

61 The process of copying genetic information from one strand of the DNA into RNA is termed as
(a) translation (b) transamination
(c) replication (d) transcription
(e) deamination

62 The sequences of nucleotides in yeast, a little away from the starting point, which are responsible for transcription are
(a) TGTG AAA (b) TAT GGG
(c) TATAAAA (d) GAGAAAA

63 The strand of DNA acting as template for *m*RNA transcription is
I. coding strand
II. non-coding strand
III. sense strand
IV. anti-sense strand
Choose the correct option.
(a) I and III (b) I and IV
(c) II and IV (d) II and III

64 In a transcription unit, the activity of RNA polymerase at a given promoter is in turn regulated by interaction with accessory proteins, which affect its ability to
(a) recognise start sites
(b) bind to initiator
(c) terminate the polypeptide chain
(d) release the polypeptide chain

65 The gene, which produces *m*RNA has specific start and stop signals, which have the same structure whether they are read from left to right or right to left. This is because
(a) the base sequence is the same either way
(b) they have the same base repeated many times
(c) they have only one base
(d) they have only one codon

66 During transcription, the nucleotide sequence of the DNA strand that is being coded is ATACG, then the nucleotide sequence in the *m*RNA would be
(a) TATGC (b) TCTGG
(c) UAUGC (d) UATGG

67 RNA polymerase
(a) is the protein responsible for the production of ribonucleotides
(b) is the enzyme that creates hydrogen bonds between nucleotides on the DNA template strand and their complementary RNA nucleotides
(c) is the enzyme that transcribes exons, but does not transcribe introns
(d) begins transcription at a promoter sequence and moves along the template strand of DNA, elongating the RNA molecule in a $5' \rightarrow 3'$ direction

68 When *m*RNA is synthesised on DNA, the unwanted DNA regions are removed and regions coding for amino acids are joined together, this process is called as
(a) capping (b) tailing
(c) termination (d) splicing

69 Select the correct statement about the structural gene in a transcription unit in bacteria.
(a) The structural gene in a transcription unit in bacteria could be said as polycistronic
(b) In bacteria, the structural gene has *m*RNA that can encode more than one polypeptide separately within the same RNA molecule
(c) The structural gene in a transcription unit in bacteria could be said as monocistronic
(d) All of the above

70 Unlike the process of replication, which one set in the total DNA of an organism get duplicated, in transcription
(a) only a segment of DNA and only one of the strands is copied into RNA
(b) only a segment of DNA, but both the strands are copied into RNA
(c) the complete DNA with both the strands is copied into RNA
(d) None of the above

71 The promoter site and the terminator site for transcription are located at **[NCERT Exemplar]**
(a) 3′ (downstream) end and 5′ (upstream) end, respectively of the transcription unit
(b) 5′ (upstream) end and 3′ (downstream) end, respectively of the transcription unit
(c) the 5′ (upstream) end
(d) the 3′ (downstream) end

72 If the sequence of nitrogen bases of the coding strand of DNA in a transcription unit is
5'-A T G A A T G-3',
the sequence of bases in its RNA transcript would be
(a) 5′-A U G A A U G - 3′
(b) 5′-U A C U U A C-3′
(c) 5′-C A U U C A U - 3′
(d) 5′-G U A A G U A-3′

73 Regulatory protiens are the accessory proteins that interact with RNA polymerase and affect its role in transcription. Which of the following statements is correct about regulatory protein? **[NCERT Exemplar]**
(a) They only increase expression
(b) They only decrease expression
(c) They interact with RNA polymerase, but do not affect the expression
(d) They can act both as activators and as repressors

74 During transcription, holoenzyme RNA polymerase binds to a DNA sequence the DNA assumes a saddle-like structure at that point. What is that sequence called?
(a) CAAT box (b) GGTT box
(c) AAAT box (d) TATA box

75 Consider the following statements.
I. Reverse transcriptase is RNA dependent RNA polymerase.
II. The process of reverse transcription was discovered by Temin and Baltimore.
Choose the correct option.
(a) Statement I is true, but II is false
(b) Statement I is false, but II is true
(c) Both statements I and II are true
(d) Both statements I and II are false

76 In eukaryotes during transcription,
(a) RNA polymerase-I transcribes *r*RNAs
(b) RNA polymerase-II transcribes precursor of *m*RNA
(c) RNA polymerase-III is responsible for transcription of *t*RNA, 5 *sr*RNA and *sn*RNA
(d) All of the above

77 Which of the following is not involved in the formation of a eukaryotic transcription initiation complex?
(a) Transcription factors (b) *sn*RNA
(c) RNA polymerase-II (d) Promoter

78 All of the following would be found in a eukaryotic cell except
(a) *m*RNA
(b) *r*RNA
(c) simultaneous transcription and translation
(d) *sn*RNA

79 Which of the following is transcribed and then translated to form a protein product?
(a) Gene for *t*RNA
(b) Intron
(c) Gene for a transcription factor
(d) Leader and trailer

80 Eukaryotic RNA polymerase-III catalyses the synthesis of
(a) *m*RNA (b) *t*RNA and 5 S *r*RNA
(c) 188 *r*RNA (d) 5S *r*RNA

81 During elongation of polypeptide chain, sigma factor is
(a) functionless
(b) retained for specific function
(c) released for reuse
(d) required during closing of chain

82 In some viruses, DNA is synthesised by using RNA as template. Such a DNA is called **[NCERT Exemplar]**
(a) A-DNA (b) B-DNA
(c) *c*DNA (d) *r*DNA

83 Consider the following statements.
I. Segments of *m*RNA removed during splicing are introns.
II. Exon segments rejoined after splicing by RNA ligase.
Choose the correct option.
(a) Statement I is true, but II is false
(b) Statement I is false, but II is true
(c) Both statements I and II are true
(d) Both statements I and II are false

84 Which of the following steps in transcription is catalysed by RNA polymerase? **[NCERT Exemplar]**
(a) Initiation
(b) Elongation
(c) Termination
(d) All of the above

85 Which of the following statements are incorrect?
(a) During transcription, the RNA that forms from DNA is *m*RNA
(b) The RNA type which helps in the processing of *r*RNA and *m*RNA in the nucleus is *sn*RNA
(c) The transcription of cluster of genes coding for protein is controlled by regulator, promoter and operator
(d) Sigma factor is a component of DNA polymerase

86 Which of the following is true for RNA processing?
(a) Exons are excised before the *m*RNA is translated
(b) Assemblies of protein and *sn*RNPs, called spliceosomes, may catalyse splicing
(c) The RNA transcript that leaves the nucleus may be much longer than the original transcript
(d) Large quantities of *r*RNA are assembled into ribosomes

Translation

87 The process of translation requires
(a) transfer of genetic information from a polymer of nucleotides to a polymer of amino acids
(b) splicing, where the exons are removed and introns are joined in a defined order
(c) a nucleic acid is copied to form amino acids
(d) DNA that undergoes capping and tailing

88 Transfer RNA
(a) forms hydrogen bonds between its codon and the anticodon of *m*RNA in the A-site of a ribosome
(b) binds to its specific amino acid in the active site of an aminoacyl *t*RNA synthetase
(c) uses GTP as the energy source to bind its amino acid
(d) is translated from *m*RNA

89 When the amino acids are activated in the presence of ATP and linked to their cognate *t*RNA, the process is called
(a) activation of *t*RNA
(b) aminoacylation of *t*RNA
(c) initiation of *t*RNA
(d) None of the above

90 Which enzyme is responsible for the synthesis of *t*RNA?
(a) RNA replicase
(b) RNA polymerase
(c) Aminoacyl *t*RNA synthetase
(d) Ribosomal enzymes

91 During protein synthesis, the correct amino acid is brought to the ribosome and inserted in correct sequence in the growing polypeptide chain by
(a) base pairing between DNA and *m*RNA
(b) base pairing between *m*RNA codons and anticodon in *t*RNA
(c) interaction between two anticodons
(d) interaction between two triplet codons

92 Translocation involves
(a) the movement of the *t*RNA from the A-site to the P-site
(b) the movement of the *m*RNA strand one triplet length in the A-site
(c) the release of the unattached *t*RNA from the E-site
(d) All of the above

93 Several proteins may be produced at the same time from a single *m*RNA by
(a) the action of several ribosomes in a string called a polyribosome
(b) several RNA polymerase molecules working sequentially
(c) single peptides that associate ribosomes with rough ER
(d) the involvement of multiple spliceosomes

94 During translation initiation in prokaryotes, a GTP molecule is needed in
(a) association of 30 S, *m*RNA with formyl-met-*t*RNA
(b) association of 50 S subunit of ribosome with initiation complex
(c) formation of formyl-met-*t*RNA
(d) binding of 30 S subunit of ribosome with *m*RNA

95 During chain elongation, peptide bond is formed between carboxyl group of first and amino group of second amino acid by
(a) peptidyl transferase
(b) DNA ligase
(c) *Taq* polymerase
(d) helicase

96 In bacteria, the formation of peptide bond during translation is effected by
(a) lysozyme
(b) ribozyme
(c) nucleosome
(d) microsome

97 In protein synthesis, a polypeptide of five amino acids is synthesised. Which one of the following can be the correct polypeptide?
(a) Glycine – Valine – Methionine – Histidine – Lysine
(b) Methionine – Lysine – Glycine – Valine – Histidine
(c) Lysine – Methionine – Valine – Glycine – Histidine
(d) Valine – Methionine – Glycine – Histidine – Lysine

98 In *m*RNA, AUG is the initiating codon and UAA, UAG and UGA are terminating codons. Therefore, the polypeptide cannot be synthesised beyond any of these triplets to the end of *m*RNA, then which one of the following *m*RNA can be translated completely?
(a) AUG UUG UCC UGA UGG UAU
(b) AUG UUC UCC UGG UAA UAU
(c) AUG UAU UUC UGC CUG GUU
(d) AUG AGG UAU UUC UGA CUC

99 To initiate translation, the *m*RNA first binds to
(a) the smaller ribosomal subunit
(b) the larger ribosomal subunit
(c) the whole ribosome
(d) No such specificity exists

100 Which of the following will be translated into a protein?
(a) UAA AUG CCC TCC ATT ATG
(b) AUG CCC UCU AUA GUA GTC
(c) UAA CCC UCU AUA GUA GUC
(d) AUG CCC UCU AUG GUC UAG

101 Ribosome contains two sites in the large subunit for
(a) amino acid to bind
(b) polypeptide chain to terminate
(c) *m*RNA to initiate gene regulation
(d) amino acid to stop the gene expression

102 Which of the following is not true for an anticodon?
(a) It consists of three nucleotides
(b) It is the basic unit of the genetic code
(c) It extends from one end of a *t*RNA molecule
(d) It may pair with more than one codon, especially if it has the base inosine in its third position

103 Changes in a polypeptide after translation may involve the
(a) addition of sugars or lipids to certain amino acids
(b) action of enzymes to add amino acids at the beginning of the chain
(c) removal of poly (A) from the end of the chain
(d) addition of a 5′ cap of a modified guanosine residue

104 Which of the following is true about the terminator?
(a) The terminator is located towards 3′ end (downstream) of the coding strand
(b) The terminator usually defines the end of the process of transcription
(c) Both (a) and (b)
(d) None of the above

Regulation of Gene Expression

105 The expression of genes is regulated by
(a) metabolic conditions
(b) physiological conditions
(c) environmental conditions
(d) All of the above

106 Jacob and Monod studied lactose metabolism in *E. coli* and proposed operon concept, it is applicable for
(a) all prokaryotes
(b) all prokaryotes and some eukaryotes
(c) all prokaryotes and all eukaryotes
(d) all prokaryotes and some protozoans

107 Control of gene expression takes place at the level of **[NCERT Exemplar]**
(a) DNA replication (b) transcription
(c) translation (d) None of these

108 According to operon concept, the regulatory gene regulates biochemical reaction in a cell by
(a) inhibiting transcription
(b) inactivating enzymes
(c) inactivating replication
(d) inhibiting migration of *m*RNA

109 Inducible enzymes are
(a) usually involved in anabolic pathways
(b) produced when a small molecule inactivates the repressor protein
(c) produced when an activator molecule enhances the attachment of RNA polymerase with the operator
(d) regulated by inherently inactive repressor molecules

110 In *E. coli*, the *lac* operon gets switched on when
(a) lactose is present and it binds to the repressor
(b) repressor binds to operator
(c) RNA polymerase binds to the operator
(d) lactose is present and it binds to RNA polymerase

111 According to the *lac* operon concept which functional unit of the bacterial genetic material is responsible for suppressing the activity of the operator gene in the absence of lactose?
(a) Regulator gene
(b) Structural gene
(c) Promoter gene
(d) Repressor protein

112 Which of the following statements is correct?
(a) Glucose acts as inducer for *lac* operon
(b) Galactose acts as inducer for *lac* operon
(c) Glucose or galactose act as inducers for *lac* operon
(d) Glucose or galactose cannot act as inducers for *lac* operon

113 The RNA polymerase holoenzyme transcribes
(a) the promoter, structural gene and the terminator region
(b) the promoter and the terminator region
(c) the structural gene and the terminator regions
(d) the structural gene only

114 Wild type *E. coli* cells are growing in normal medium with glucose. They are transferred to a medium containing lactose only as the sugar. Which one of the following changes take place?
(a) The *lac* operon is repressed
(b) All operons are induced
(c) *E. coli* cells stop dividing
(d) The *lac* operon is induced

115 The complex CAP-*c*-AMP, which increases the affinity of RNA polymerase for *lac* operon promoter so that the *lac*-genes are transcribed, is formed in
(a) cytoplasm
(b) low glucose concentration
(c) high lactose concentration
(d) high glucose concentration

116 In an *E. coli* cell, according to the operon theory, an operator gene combines with
(a) inducer gene to 'switch on' structural gene transcription
(b) regulator gene to 'switch off' structural gene transcription
(c) regulator protein to 'switch off' structural gene transcription
(d) regulator protein to 'switch on' structural gene transcription

117 In *E. coli*, tryptophan switches off the *trp* operon by
(a) inactivating the repressor protein
(b) inactivating the gene for the first enzyme in the pathway by feedback inhibition
(c) binding to the repressor and increasing the latters affinity for the operator
(d) binding to the operator

118 In tryptophan synthesis pathway, tryptophan acts as a corepressor. What is its role as a corepressor?
(a) It prevents transcription of the genes of the operon
(b) It binds to the promoter that blocks the attachment of RNA polymerase
(c) It binds to the *trp* repressor to change it into its active form
(d) It binds to the operator gene at an allosteric site to switch off the operon

119 Addition of lactose in a culture of *E. coli* induces enzymes .... to breakdown the lactose into glucose and galactose.
(a) β-galactosidase and transacetylase
(b) transacetylase and permease
(c) β-galactosidase, permease, transacetylase
(d) None of the above

120 Which of the following is true about the promoter gene?
(a) The promoter is located towards 5′ end (upstream) of the structural gene
(b) Promoter is a DNA sequence that provides binding site for RNA polymerase
(c) The presence of promoter in a transcription unit defines the template and coding strands
(d) All of the above

121 The *lac* operon requires a 'helper' protein which, by binding to the promoter and by facilitating the attachment of RNA polymerase, accelerates the rate of transcription. The protein is
(a) amino acid activating enzyme
(b) essential metabolite
(c) inactive repression protein
(d) catabolite activator protein

122 *E. coli* cells with a mutated Z gene of the *lac* operon cannot grow in medium containing only lactose as the source of energy because
(a) in the presence of glucose, *E. coli* cells do not utilise lactose
(b) they cannot transport lactose from the medium into the cell
(c) the *lac* operon is constitutively active in these cells
(d) they cannot synthesise functional β-galactosidase

123 In eukaryotes, the structural gene in a transcription unit could be said as
(a) monocistronic
(b) polycistronic
(c) encoding only one polypeptide per RNA molecule
(d) Both (a) and (c)

124 Aporepressor is inactive repressor in tryptophan repressible operon system. It is generally a
(a) protein
(b) a substrate
(c) a metabolite
(d) may be protein

125 In eukaryotes, the regulation could be exerted at
(a) transcriptional and processing level
(b) processing and translational level
(c) transport of *m*RNA from nucleus to the cytoplasm
(d) All of the above

126 The control of gene expression is more complex in eukaryotic cells because the
(a) gene expression differentiates specialised cells
(b) the chromosomes are linear and more numerous
(c) operons are controlled by more than one promoter region
(d) inhibitory or activating molecules may not help to regulate transcription

127 Which process occurs in the regulation of gene expression in prokaryotes, but does not occur in the regulation of gene expression in eukaryotes?
(a) RNA is formed from the transcription of base triplets on DNA
(b) Translation of the *m*RNA starts as the 5′ end of the *m*RNA strand separates from the DNA template that transcribed it
(c) RNA polymerase synthesises RNA nucleotides in a 5′ to 3′ direction
(d) Polyribosomes help to produce many copies of polypeptides during translation

(B) Cumulative Exercise

(Assorted Questions of the Chapter for Advanced Level Practice)

1 In regulation of gene expression in prokaryotes,
I. lactose acts as the suppressor for gene expression.
II. tryptophan acts as the inducer for gene expression.
III. regulator gene is the one that produces the repressor molecule.
(a) Only I is correct
(b) Only II is correct
(c) Only III is correct
(d) Both I and II are correct

2 Match the following columns.

Column I	Column II
A. *t*RNA	1. Linking of amino acids
B. *m*RNA	2. Transfer of genetic information
C. *r*RNA	3. Nucleolar organising region
D. Peptidyl transferase	4. Transfer of amino acid from cytoplasm of ribosome

Codes

	A	B	C	D
(a)	4	2	3	1
(b)	1	4	3	2
(c)	1	2	3	4
(d)	1	3	2	4

3 During translation initiation is prokaryotes a GTP molecule is needed is
(a) formation of formyl-met-*t*RNA
(b) binding of 30S subunit of ribosome with *m*RNA.
(c) association of 30S *m*RNA with formyl met *t*RNA
(d) association of 50S subunit of ribosome with initiation complex

4 The main steps involved in the process of translation are
I. activation of amino acid.
II. initiation of polypeptide chain synthesis.
III. termination of polypeptide chain formation.
IV. transfer of polypeptide chain to *t*RNA.

Codes
(a) I and II (b) III and IV
(c) I, II and III (d) II, III and IV

5 Which of the following statements are correct?
I. The structural gene is the segment of DNA, which exercises a central over transcription.
II. The regulator gene is responsible for the synthesis of repressor.
III. The operator gene is the segment of DNA, which carries code for the synthesis of protein.
IV. The promoter gene is the DNA segment at which RNA polymerase binds.

Codes
(a) I and II (b) II and III
(c) III and IV (d) II and IV

6 Which of the following statements are correct?
I. Peptidyl transferase helps in the process of peptide bond formation.
II. The regulator, promoter and operator together called the control genes.
III. Polypeptide chain elongation continues until a termination codon reaches the ribosomes.
IV. Gene regulation in eukaryotes can be explained by *lac* operon model.

Codes
(a) I, II and III (b) II and IV
(c) III and IV (d) I and III

7 Consider the following statements.
The genetic codes are said to be degenerate and universal, which means that
I. Amino acids may have more than one codon.
II. All amino acids have more than one codon.
III. Codons are common for higher and lower organisms.
IV. Codons are not found in bacteria.

Codes
(a) I and III (b) I and II
(c) I, II and IV (d) I, II and III

8 Match the following columns.

Column I	Column II
A. Chargaff	1. Wilkins and Franklin
B. Replicon	2. Uptake of lactose
C. Permease	3. *hn*RNA
D. Split gene	4. Length of DNA
E. X-ray diffraction studies	5. (A+ G) = (C+T)

Codes

	A	B	C	D	E
(a)	5	4	2	3	1
(b)	5	4	1	3	2
(c)	5	4	2	1	3
(d)	5	1	2	3	4

9 If following is the sequence of nucleotides in *m*RNA, predict the sequence of amino acids coded by it

AUG UUU UUC UUC UUU UUU UUC

(a) Met-Phe-Phe-Phe-Phe-Phe-Phe
(b) Met-Phe-Leu-Leu-Phe-Phe-Leu
(c) Ser-Leu-Phe-Leu-Phe-Leu-Phe
(d) Arg-Leu-Leu-Leu-Leu-Leu

10 Which of the following pairs is correctly matched?

(a) Ribosomal RNA – Carries amino acids to the site of protein synthesis
(b) Transcription – Process by which protein is synthesised
(c) Translation – Process by which *m*RNA carries the information from the nucleus to ribosomes
(d) Anticodon – Site of a *t*RNA molecule that binds to the *m*RNA molecule

11 Practice using the dictionary of the genetic code and determine the amino acid sequence for a polypeptide coded by the following *m*RNA transcript (written 5′ → 3′)

AUGCCUGACUUUAAGUAG

(a) Met Pro Lys Asp Phe Stop
(b) Met Pro Asp Phe Lys Stop
(c) Pro Lys Met Phe Asp Stop
(d) Pro Met Lys Asp Phe Stop

12 Find the sequence of binding of the following aminoacyl *t*RNA complexes during translation to a *m*RNA transcribed by a DNA segment having the base sequence 3′-TACATGGGTCCG-5′. Choose the answer showing the correct order of alphabets.

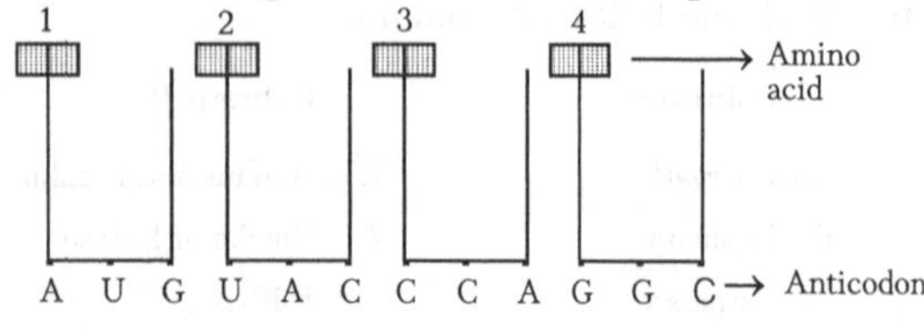

(a) 1, 2, 3, 4
(b) 2, 1, 3, 4
(c) 1, 2, 4, 3
(d) 2, 1, 4, 3

13 Which one of the following pairs is correctly matched?

(a) Frederick Griffith – Discovered the phenomenon of transformation
(b) Linus Pauling – Isolated DNA for the first time
(c) Francis Crick – Proposed one gene-one polypeptide hypothesis
(d) George Beadle – Proposed the concept of inborn errors

14 In the following diagrams of protein synthesis, name the stages (*A-D*).

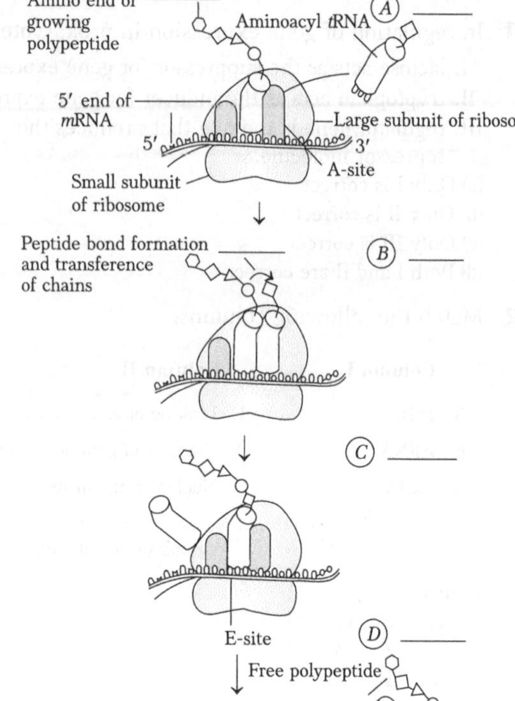

(a) *A*-Codon recognition, *B*-Peptide bond formation, *C*-Translocation, *D*-Termination
(b) *A*-Peptide bond formation, *B*-Translocation, *C*-Peptide chain elongation, *D*-Termination
(c) *A*-Codon recognition, *B*-Translocation, *C*-Peptide bond formation, *D*-Termination
(d) *A*-Peptide bond formation, *B*-Peptide chain elongation, *C*-Translocation, *D*-Termination

15 Match the following columns.

Column I	Column II
A. Structural gene	1. Joins the DNA segments
B. Operator gene	2. Unwinds the DNA double helix
C. Promoter gene	3. Synthesise RNA primers
D. DNA polymerase	4. Erase prime and fill gaps

Codes

	A	B	C	D
(a)	1	2	3	4
(b)	4	3	2	1
(c)	3	4	2	1
(d)	2	1	4	3

16 Match the following columns.

Column I	Column II
A. Chain elongation	1. Second stage of translation
B. Exons	2. Part of mature *m*RNA transcript
C. Genetic code	3. Set of 64 codons in *m*RNA
D. Introns	4. The parts removed from pre *m*RNA transcript before translation
E. Codon	5. Base triplet for amino acid

Codes

	A	B	C	D	E
(a)	1	2	3	5	4
(b)	5	4	1	2	3
(c)	5	4	3	2	1
(d)	1	2	3	4	5

17 Which of the following statement(s) is/are incorrect?

I. Six codons do not code for any amino acid.
II. Codon is read in *m*RNA in a contiguous fashion.
III. Three codons function as stop codons.
IV. The initiator codon AUG codes for methionine.

Choose the correct option.

(a) I, II and IV (b) I, II and III
(c) II, III and IV (d) Only I

18 Which one of the following statements is/are incorrect about the properties of DNA?

I. DNA is denatured when heated upto 70°C.
II. DNA shows high absorption of UV radiation at 260mμ.
III. DNA directly participates in protein synthesis.
IV. Pyrimidines of DNA are cytosine and thymine.

Codes

(a) I and II (b) II and III
(c) III and IV (d) Only III

19 Which of the following statements are related to the structure of double helical DNA?

I. The helix makes one complete spiral turn every 34 Å.
II. The diameter of the helix is 20 Å.
III. The distance between adjacent nucleotide is 3.4 Å.
IV. Each strand of helix has a backbone made up of alternating ribose sugar and phosphate.
V. The two adjacent sugar molecules are joined with phosphate by phosphodiester bond.

Codes

(a) I and II (b) I, II, III and V
(c) II and IV (d) III, IV and V

20 Select the two correct statements out of the four (I-IV) given below about *lac* operon.

I. Glucose or galactose may bind with the repressor and inactivate it.
II. In the absence of lactose, the repressor binds with the operator region.
III. The *z*-gene codes for permease.
IV. This was elucidated by Francois Jacob and Jacque Monod.

Codes

(a) I and II (b) II and IV
(c) III and IV (d) I and IV

21 Match the following columns.

Column I	Column II
A. Substance that induces	1. *r*RNA
B. Non-coding segment of DNA	2. Lactose
C. Forms part of the ribosome	3. Anticodon
D. *m*RNA as it leaves the DNA	4. Transcript
E. Part of *t*RNA	5. Intron

Codes

	A	B	C	D	E
(a)	2	5	1	4	3
(b)	5	4	3	2	1
(c)	1	2	3	4	5
(d)	3	1	4	5	2

22 Match the following columns.

Column I (Components of *lac* operon)	Column II (Functions)
A. Structural gene	1. Binding site for repressor protein
B. Operator gene	2. Codes for repressor protein
C. Promoter gene	3. Induces lactose transport from the medium
D. Regulator gene	4. Codes for enzyme proteins
	5. Binding site for RNA polymerase

Codes

	A	B	C	D
(a)	3	4	5	1
(b)	2	3	1	4
(c)	5	4	2	1
(d)	4	1	5	2

23 During translation, the activation of amino acids

I. takes place through their carboxyl groups.
II. continues until a termination codon reaches the ribosome.
III. is catalysed by its own activating enzyme called aminoacyl *t*RNA synthetase.
IV. involves movement of second amino acid *t*RNA complex from A-site to P-site.

Codes

(a) I and II
(b) II and III
(c) I and III
(d) II and IV

24 Match the following columns.

Column I	Column II
A. β-galactosidase	1. Hydrolysis of lactose
B. Permease	2. Increases permeability to β-galactosidase
C. Ligase	3. Joining of DNA fragments
D. Ribozyme	4. Peptide bond formation

Codes

	A	B	C	D		A	B	C	D
(a)	2	1	4	3	(b)	3	4	1	2
(c)	2	4	1	3	(d)	1	2	3	4

25 Match the following columns.

Column I	Column II
A. Chloramphenicol	1. Inhibits binding of aminoacyl *t*RNA to ribosome
B. Erythromycin	2. Inhibits interaction between *t*RNA and *m*RNA
C. Neomycin	3. Inhibits initation of translation
D. Streptomycin	4. Inhibits peptidyl transferase activity
E. Tetracycline	5. Inhibits translocation of *m*RNA along ribosomes

Codes

	A	B	C	D	E
(a)	1	2	3	5	4
(b)	3	1	5	4	2
(c)	2	3	4	1	5
(d)	4	5	2	3	1

26 Transcription

I. is the copying of a complementary *m*RNA on a DNA strand.
II. requires a template, activated precursors, a divalent metal ion and RNA polymerase.
III. is the first step in activation of amino acid.
IV. directs the order of specific amino acids to form a polypeptide or protein.

Codes

(a) I and II (b) III and IV
(c) I and III (d) II and IV

27 Match the following columns.

Column I	Column II
A. DNA structure	1. Muller and Stadler
B. Semiconservative replication of DNA	2. Beadle and Tatum
C. One gene-one enzyme theory	3. Watson and Crick
D. Induction of mutation	4. Meselson and Stahl

Codes

	A	B	C	D
(a)	1	2	3	4
(b)	3	4	1	2
(c)	3	4	2	1
(d)	4	3	2	1

28 Which of the following statement(s) is/are correct?

I. Introns are present in *m*RNA and exons are present in *t*RNA.
II. Codons are present in *m*RNA and anticodons in *t*RNA.
III. Every intron is a set of three terminator codons.
IV. Exons are present in eukaryotes, while introns are present in prokaryotes.

Codes

(a) I, II and III (b) Only II
(c) III and IV (d) II and IV

29 Match the following columns in codons with their respective amino acids and choose the correct answer from the codes given below.

Column I	Column II
A. UUU	1. Serine
B. GGG	2. Methionine
C. UCU	3. Phenylalanine
D. CCC	4. Glycine
E. AUG	5. Proline

Codes

	A	B	C	D	E
(a)	3	4	1	5	2
(b)	3	1	4	5	2
(c)	3	4	5	1	2
(d)	2	4	1	5	3
(e)	2	4	1	3	5

30 Consider the following statements.

I. *r*RNA provides the template for synthesis of proteins.
II. *t*RNA brings amino acids and reads the genetic code.
III. RNA polymerase binds to promoter and initiates transcription.
IV. A segment of DNA coding for polypeptide is called intron.

Choose the option containing correct statements.

(a) I and III
(b) I and II
(c) I, II and III
(d) II and III

Assertion and Reason

Direction (Q. Nos. 31-40) *In each of the following questions, a statement of Assertion (A) is given followed by the corresponding statement of Reason (R). Of the statements, mark the correct answer as*

(a) Both A and R are true and R is the correct explanation of A
(b) Both A and R are true, but R is not the correct explanation of A
(c) A is true, but R is false
(d) A is false, but R is true
(e) Both A and R are false

31 Assertion (A) The *t*RNA molecules possess anticodons.
Reason (R) It needs the message in the form of codon.

32 Assertion (A) *m*RNA attaches to ribosome through its 3′ end.
Reason (R) The *m*RNA has F-capsular nucleotide and bases of lagging sequence.

33 Assertion (A) DNA code is copied during the synthesis of *m*RNA.
Reason (R) *t*RNA moves out of nucleus and after attaching on ribosomes forms the template.

34 Assertion (A) A non-overlapping code means that a base in *m*RNA is not used for different codons.
Reason (R) In translating *m*RNA molecules, the codons do not overlap but are read sequentially.

35 Assertion (A) Proteins are polymers of amino acids.
Reason (R) Nucleic acids are polymers of nucleotides.

36 Assertion A single-strand of *m*RNA is capable of forming different polypeptide chains.
Reason Termination codons occur in *m*RNA.

37 Assertion (A) Reading codons and consequent translation into protein are functions of *t*RNA.
Reason (R) Anticodon can recognise the codon.

38 Assertion (A) Non-sense codons are responsible for terminating peptide chain.
Reason (R) They are not recognised by *t*RNA.

39 Assertion (A) Replication and transcription occur in the nucleus, but translation occurs in the cytoplasm.
Reason (R) *m*RNA is transferred from the nucleus into the cytoplasm where ribosomes and amino acids are available for protein synthesis.

40 Assertion (A) Amber codon is a termination codon.
Reason (R) If in a *m*RNA, a termination codon is present, the protein synthesis stops abruptly whether the protein synthesis is complete or not.

(C) Medical Entrances' Gallery

(Collection of questions asked in NEET & Various Medical Entrance Exams)

1 The first phase of translation is [NEET 2020]
(a) recognition of DNA molecule
(b) aminoacylation of *t*RNA
(c) recognition of an anticodon
(d) binding of *m*RNA to ribosome

2 If the distance between two consecutive base pairs is 0.34 nm and the total number of base pairs of a DNA double helix in a typical mammalian cell is 6.6×10^9 bp then the length of the DNA is approximately. [NEET 2020]
(a) 2.5 m (b) 2.2 m
(c) 2.7 m (d) 2.0 m

3 Name the enzyme that facilitates opening of DNA helix during transcription. [NEET 2020]
(a) DNA helicase (b) DNA polymerase
(c) RNA polymerase (d) DNA ligase

4 The term 'Nuclein' for the genetic material was used by [NEET 2020]
(a) Franklin (b) Meischer
(c) Chargaff (d) Mendel

5 In the polynucleotide chain of DNA, a nitrogenous base is linked to the – OH of [NEET 2020]
(a) 2′ C pentose sugar (b) 3′ C pentose sugar
(c) 5′ C pentose sugar (d) 1′ C pentose sugar

6 *E. coli* has only 4.6×10^6 base pairs and completes the process of replication within 18 minutes, then the average rate of polymerisation is approximately [NEET 2020]
(a) 2000 bp/s (b) 3000 bp/s (c) 4000 bp/s (d) 1000 bp/s

7 Purines found both in DNA and RNA are [NEET 2014, 2019]
(a) adenine and guanine (b) guanine and cytosine
(c) cytosine and thymine (d) adenine and thymine

8 What will be the sequence of *m*RNA produced by the following stretch of DNA? [NEET 2019]

3′ATGCATGCATGCATG5′ Template strand
5′TACGTACGTACGTAC3′ Coding strand

(a) 3′-AUGCAUGCAUGCAUG 5′
(b) 5′-UACGUACGUACGUAC 3′
(c) 3′-UACGUACGUACGUAC 5′
(d) 5′-AUGCAUGCAUGCAUG 3′

9 Which scientist experimentally proved that DNA is the sole genetic material in bacteriophage? **[NEET 2019]**
(a) Beadle and Tatum (b) Meselson and Stahl
(c) Hershey and Chase (d) Jacob and Monod

10 Which of the following are all nucleotides? **[AIIMS 2019]**
(a) Adenosine, cytidylic acid, cytosine
(b) Adenylic acid, cytidylic acid, guanylic acid
(c) Cytidine, adenine, adenylic acid
(d) Uracil, thymidine, thymidylic acid

11 In DNA, 20% bases are adenine. What percentage of bases are pyrimidines? **[JIPMER 2019]**
(a) 30% (b) 60% (c) 50% (d) 20%

12 During DNA replication, supercoiling is relaxed by **[JIPMER 2019]**
(a) primase (b) polymerase
(c) DNA topoisomerase (d) SSBPs

13 Which of the following is not true? **[JIPMER 2019]**
(a) β-galactosidase - *lac* operon
(b) Photorespiration - C_3-plants
(c) Krebs' cycle - mitochondrial matrix
(d) Southern hybridisation - related to identification of RNA sequence

14 Under which of the following conditions will there be no change in the reading frame of following *m*RNA? **[NEET 2019]**

5′AACAGCGGUGCUAUU3′

(a) Deletion of G from 5th position
(b) Insertion of A and G at 4th and 5th positions, respectively
(c) Deletion of GGU from 7th, 8th and 9th positions
(d) Insertion of G at 5th position

15 Which of the following features of genetic code does allow bacteria to produce human insulin by recombinant DNA technology ? **[NEET 2019]**
(a) Genetic code is redundant
(b) Genetic code is nearly universal
(c) Genetic code is specific
(d) Genetic code is not ambiguous

16 Match the following Column I (RNA polymerases) with Column II (their transcribed products).

Column I	Column II
A. RNA polymerase -I	1. *t*RNA
B. RNA polymerase -II	2. *r*RNA
C. RNA polymerase -III	3. *hn*RNA

Select the correct option from the following codes given below. **[NEET 2019]**

	A	B	C		A	B	C
(a)	1	3	2	(b)	1	2	3
(c)	2	3	1	(d)	3	2	1

17 From the following, identify the correct combination of salient features of genetic code. **[NEET 2019]**
(a) Universal, Non-ambiguous, Overlapping
(b) Degenerate, Overlapping, Commaless
(c) Universal, Ambiguous, Degenerate
(d) Degenerate, Non-overlapping, Non-ambiguous

18 In the process of transcription in eukaryotes, the RNA polymerase-I transcribes **[NEET 2019]**
(a) *m*RNA with additional processing, capping and tailing
(b) *t*RNA, 5S *r*RNA and *sn*RNAs
(c) *r*RNAs-28S, 18S and 5.8S
(d) precursor of *m*RNA, *hn*RNA

19 What initiation and termination factors are involved in transcription in eukaryotes? **[NEET 2019]**
(a) σ and ρ, respectively (b) α and β, respectively
(c) β and γ, respectively (d) α and σ, respectively

20 The genetic codes of arginine are **[AIIMS 2019]**
(a) CGU, CGC, CGA (b) CAU, CAC, CAA
(c) AGU, AGC, AAC (d) GAU, GAC, GAA

21

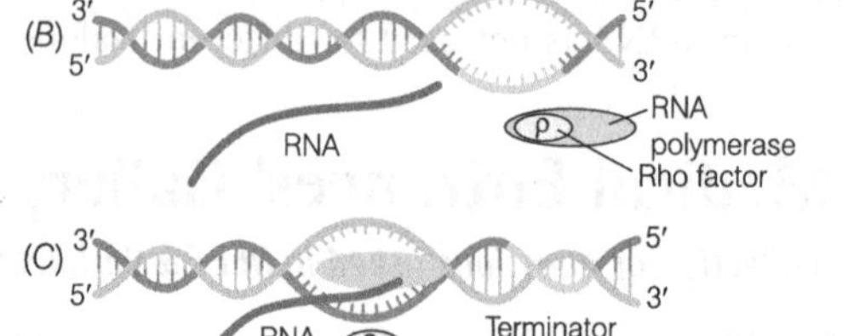

[AIIMS 2019]

Identify *A*, *B* and *C*.
(a) *A*- Elongation, *B*- Termination, *C*- Initiation
(b) *A*- Initiation, *B*- Termination, C- Elongation
(c) *A*- Initiation, *B*- Elongation, *C*- Termination
(d) *A*- Termination, *B*- Elongation, *C*- Initiation

22 **Assertion** (A) In eukaryotes, transcription occurs in nucleus.

Reason (R) In bacteria, transcription and translation occur in cytoplasm. **[AIIMS 2019]**
(a) Both A and R are true and R is the correct explanation of A
(b) Both A and R are true, but R is not the correct explanation of A
(c) A is true, but R is false
(d) Both A and R are false

23 Which of the following is not a stop codon? **[JIPMER 2019]**
(a) UAA (b) UAC (c) UAG (d) UGA

24 *t*RNA binds to *m*RNA through **[JIPMER 2019]**
(a) anticodon loop (b) TψC loop
(c) amino acid binding loop (d) D loop

25 Match the following columns in genes of the *lac* operon with their respective products.

Column I	Column II
A. *i* gene	1. β-galactosidase
B. *z* gene	2. Permease
C. *a* gene	3. Repressor
D. *y* gene	4. Transacetylase

Select the correct option from the codes given below. [NEET 2019]

	A	B	C	D
(a)	3	1	2	4
(b)	3	1	4	2
(c)	3	4	1	2
(d)	1	3	2	4

26 Select the wrong statement from the following. [AIIMS 2019]

(a) The human genome contains 3164.7 million nucleotide bases
(b) Less than 10% of the genome codes for protein
(c) Repeated sequences makeup very large portion of the human genome
(d) Chromosome 1 has most genes (2968) and Y has the fewest (231)

27 Genetic variation cannot be effectively brought about by [JIPMER 2019]

(a) transduction (b) mutation
(c) transformation (d) amplification

28 Select the correct match. [NEET 2018]

(a) TH Morgan - Transduction
(b) F_2 × Recessive parent - Dihybrid cross
(c) Ribozyme - Nucleic acid
(d) G Mendel - Transformation

29 The experimental proof for semiconservative replication of DNA was first shown in a [NEET 2018]

(a) plant (b) bacterium
(c) fungus (d) virus

30 Select the correct match. [NEET 2018]

(a) Matthew Meselson and F Stahl - *Pisum sativum*
(b) Alfred Hershey and Martha Chase - TMV
(c) Alec Jeffreys - *Streptococcus pneumoniae*
(d) Francois Jacob and Jacques Monod - *Lac* operon

31 What is ribonucleotide? [JIPMER 2018]

(a) Ribose + Uracil + Phosphate
(b) Deoxyribose + Uracil + Phosphate
(c) Deoxyribose + Thymine + Phosphate
(d) Ribose + Thymine + Phosphate

32 Linker DNA is attached to [JIPMER 2018]

(a) H1 (b) H2A
(c) H2B (d) H3

33 AGGTATCGCAT is a sequence from the coding strand of a gene. What will be the corresponding sequence of the transcribed *m*RNA? [NEET 2018]

(a) ACCUAUGCGAU (b) UGGTUTCGCAT
(c) AGGUAUCGCAU (d) UCCAUAGCGUA

34 Codons of glycine are [AIIMS 2018]

(a) CCU, CCC, CCA, CCG (b) CGU, CGC, CGA, CGG
(c) GGU, GGC, GGA, GGG (d) ACU, ACC, ACA, ACG

35 Which of the following *m*RNA can be translated? [JIPMER 2018]

(a) AUG, UGA, UUU (b) UAA, UAV, UGG
(c) UAG, UGA, UUV (d) UGA, UUV, UGG

36 Which is present at 5′ end of eukaryotic *m*RNA? [JIPMER 2018]

(a) Poly-A tail (b) Modified C at 5′
(c) 7 mG (d) Poly-C

37 Which is the 21st amino acid? [JIPMER 2018]

(a) Pyrrolysine (b) Selenocysteine
(c) Cysteine (d) Histidine

38 All of the following are parts of an operon except [NEET 2018]

(a) an enhancer (b) structural genes
(c) an operator (d) a promoter

39 To which of the following, repressor protein is attached? [JIPMER 2018]

(a) Operator (b) Inducer
(c) Promoter (d) Structural gene

40 Match the following columns.

Column I	Column II
A. Multigenes	1. Transposons
B. Inducible genes	2. Insulin
C. Overlapping genes	3. B, E and K in $\phi \times 174$
D. Structural genes	4. *Sn* RNA
	5. Globin gene
	6. Nitrate reductase

Codes [AIIMS 2018]

	A	B	C	D		A	B	C	D
(a)	1	3	5	2	(b)	5	6	3	2
(c)	4	5	6	1	(d)	1	2	5	4

41 In the *lac* operon model, lactose molecules function as [JIPMER 2017]

(a) inducers, which bind with the operator gene
(b) repressors, which bind with the operator gene
(c) inducers, which bind with the repressor protein
(d) corepressors, which bind with repressor protein

42 DNA replication in bacteria occurs [NEET 2017]
(a) during S-phase (b) within nucleolus
(c) prior to fission (d) just before transcription

43 Which one of the following RNAs should be most abundant in animal cell? [NEET 2017]
(a) *r*RNA (b) *t*RNA
(c) *m*RNA (d) *mi*RNA

44 DNA fragments are [NEET 2017]
(a) positively charged
(b) negatively charged
(c) neutral
(d) either positively or negatively charged depending on their size

45 The final proof for DNA as the genetic material came from the experiments of [NEET 2017)
(a) Griffith
(b) Hershey and Chase
(c) Avery, MacLeod and McCarty
(d) Har Gobind Khorana

46 The association of histone H1 with a nucleosome indicates [NEET 2017]
(a) transcription is occurring
(b) DNA replication is occurring
(c) the DNA is condensed into chromatin fibre
(d) the DNA double helix is exposed

47 Spliceosomes are not found in the cells of [NEET 2017]
(a) plants (b) fungi
(c) animals (d) bacteria

48 The premature termination of polypeptide synthesis due to stop codon can be overcome *via* compensatory mutation in *t*RNA. This genetic phenomenon is called [AIIMS 2017]
(a) extragenic suppression (b) intragenic suppression
(c) codon bias (d) true reversion

49 *hn*RNA undergoes two additional processes. Out of them in one process, an unusual nucleotide (methyl GTP) is added to the 5′ end of molecule. What would you called this? [JIPMER 2017]
(a) Tailing (b) Splicing
(c) Termination (d) Capping

50 Which of the following *r*RNAs act as structural RNA as well as ribozyme in bacteria? [NEET-II 2016]
(a) 5S *r*RNA (b) 18S *r*RNA
(c) 23S *r*RNA (d) 5·8S *r*RNA

51 Taylor conducted the experiments to prove semiconservative mode of chromosome replication on [NEET-II 2016]
(a) *Vinca rosea* (b) *Vicia faba*
(c) *Drosophila melanogaster* (d) *E. coli*

52 The equivalent of a structural gene is [NEET-II 2016; Manipal 2012]
(a) muton (b) cistron (c) operon (d) recon

53 DNA-dependent RNA polymerase catalyses transcription on one strand of the DNA which is called the [NEET-II 2016]
(a) template strand (b) coding strand
(c) alpha strand (d) antistrand

54 A molecule that can act as a genetic material must fulfil the traits given below, except [NEET-II 2016, Kerala CEE 2014]
(a) it should be able to express itself in the form of 'Mendelian characters'
(b) it should be able to generate its replica
(c) it should be unstable structurally and chemically
(d) it should provide the scope for slow changes that are required for evolution
(e) None of the above

55 A complex of ribosomes attached to a single strand of RNA is known as [NEET-I 2016]
(a) polymer (b) polypeptide
(c) Okazaki fragment (d) polysome

56 Which of the following statements is incorrect? [NEET-I 2016]
(a) Cellulose is a polysaccharide
(b) Uracil is a pyrimidine
(c) Glycine is a sulphur containing amino acid
(d) Sucrose is a disaccharide

57 Which one of the following is the start codon? [NEET-I 2016, Chhattisgarh PMT 2015]
(a) UGA (b) UAA (c) UAG (d) AUG

58 Match the following columns.

Column I	Column II
A. RNA Polymerase-I	1. *t*RNA, 5 S *r*RNA, *sn*RNA
B. RNA Polymerase-II	2. Transcribes all types of RNAs
C. RNA Polymerase-III	3. 28S, 18S and 5.8S RNAs
D. Bacterial RNA Polymerase	4. Precursor of *m*RNA
	5. Synthesis of DNA

Codes [EAMCET 2016, Karnataka CET 2015]

	A	B	C	D		A	B	C	D
(a)	3	1	5	4	(b)	2	5	3	1
(c)	3	4	1	2	(d)	1	3	5	2

59 *Escherichia coli*, in which both the strands of DNA are labelled with ^{15}N, is transferred to ^{14}N medium and allowed to replicate for two generations. Find out the number of hybrid DNA molecules in the second generation. [EAMCET 2016]
(a) One (b) Two
(c) Four (d) Eight

60 What is the amino acid sequence in the polypeptide segment translated from *m*RNA strand with base sequence of UCU-UGG-UGC-UGU-GGU? **[EAMCET 2016]**

(a) Arg-Phe-Tyr-Gly-Gly (b) Trp-Ser-Tyr-Cys-Gly
(c) Tyr-Cys-Ser-Gly-Cys (d) Ser-Trp-Cys-Cys-Gly

61 Which one of the following is not applicable to RNA? **[CBSE AIPMT 2015]**

(a) Complementary base pairing
(b) 5′ phosphorly acid 3′ hydroxyl ends
(c) Heterocyclic nitrogenous bases
(d) Chargaff's rule

62 Identify the correct order of organisation of genetic material from largest to smallest. **[CBSE AIPMT 2015]**

(a) Chromosome, gene, genome, nucleotide
(b) Genome, chromosome, nucleotide, gene
(c) Genome, chromosome, gene, nucleotide
(d) Chromosome, genome, nucleotide, gene

63 Gene regulation governing lactose operon of *E. coli* that involves the *lac* I gene products is **[CBSE AIPMT 2015]**

(a) positive and inducible because it can be induced by lactose
(b) negative and inducible because repressor protein prevents transcription
(c) negative and repressible because repressor protein prevents transcription
(d) feedback inhibition because excess of β-galactosidase can swich off transcription

64 In sea urchin DNA, which is double-stranded 17% of the bases were shown to be cytosine. The percentages of the other three bases expected to be present in this DNA are **[CBSE AIPMT, WB JEE 2015]**

(a) G/34%, A/24.5%, T/24.5%
(b) G/17%, A/16.5%, 5/32%
(c) G/17%, A/33%, T/33%
(d) G/8.5%, A/50%, T/24.5%

65 Semiconservative replication of DNA was first demonstrated in **[AMU 2015]**

(a) *Escherichia coli*
(b) *Streptococcus pneumoniae*
(c) *Drosophila melanogaster*
(d) *Salmonella typhimurium*

66 The enzyme used to join the fragments of DNA during the process of replication is **[AMU 2015]**

(a) DNA polymerase (b) DNA ligase
(c) endonuclease (d) helicase

67 6 (4-hydroxy-3 methyl- trans-2-butenylamine) purine is also called as **[AMU 2015]**

(a) methyl jasmonate (b) zeatin
(c) brassinolide (d) triacontanol

68 Which of the following is correct regarding RNA processing ? **[AMU 2015]**

(a) In capping, methylguanosine triphosphate is added to 3′ end of *hn*RNA
(b) RNA polymerase-I transcribes *t*RNA in eukaryotes
(c) In tailing, adenylate residues are added at 3′ end of *hn*RNA
(d) Three types of RNA polymerase catalyse the transcription of these different types of RNAs in most bacteria

69 Splicing is the process where **[AMU 2015]**

(a) exons are removed from growing *t*RNA strand
(b) introns are removed from growing polypeptide chain
(c) introns are removed from heterogeneous nuclear RNA
(d) exons are removed from *m*RNA

70 Identify this structure.

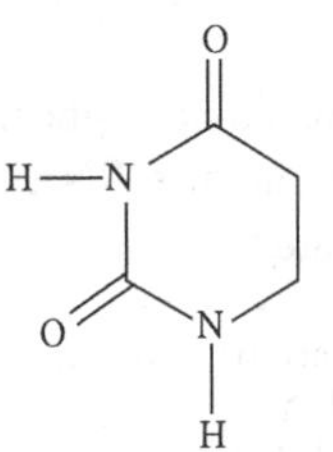

[Karnataka CET 2015]

(a) adynylic acid (b) uracil
(c) cholesterol (d) adenosine

71 Match the following columns.

Column I	Column II
A. VNTR	1. Largest gene
B. Introns and exons	2. DNA fingerprinting
C. Dystrophin	3. Bulk DNA
D. Satellite DNA	4. Splicing

Codes **[Karnataka CET 2015]**

	A	B	C	D
(a)	3	4	1	2
(b)	2	4	1	3
(c)	2	1	4	3
(d)	4	1	2	3

72 In 125 amino acid sequence, if the codon of 25th amino acid is mutated to UAA, then **[Karnataka CET 2015, Bihar CECE 2012]**

(a) a polypeptide of 24 amino acids is formed
(b) a polypeptide of 124 amino acids is formed
(c) no polypeptides are formed
(d) a polypeptide of 25 amino acids is formed

73 The codon AUG has dual function. It is initiation codon and also codes for **[Karnataka CET 2015]**

(a) phenylalanine (b) formaldehyde
(c) serine (d) methionine

74 The nitrogen base found only in DNA is also called **[Karnataka CET 2015]**

(a) uracil (b) 5-methyl uracil
(c) guanine (d) NH_4Cl

75 In a 3.2 kbp long piece of DNA, 820 adenine bases were found. What would be the number of cytosine bases? **[Karnataka CET 2015]**

(a) 780 (b) 1560
(c) 740 (d) 1480

76 A beads on a string-like chromatin with 200 beads or nucleosomes contains ...... bp of DNA. **[EAMCET 2015]**

(a) 80,000 (b) 40,000
(c) 20,000 (d) 10,000

77 **Assertion** (A) Transcription unit is often monocistronic in eukaryotes and polycistronic in prokaryotes.

Reason (R) Exons do not appear in mature RNA, introns appear in mature RNA. **[EAMCET 2015]**

(a) Both A and R are true and R is the correct explanation of A
(b) Both A and R are true, but R is not the correct explanation of A
(c) A is true, but R is false
(d) A is false, but R is true

78 Which is *A* and *B* in given diagram?

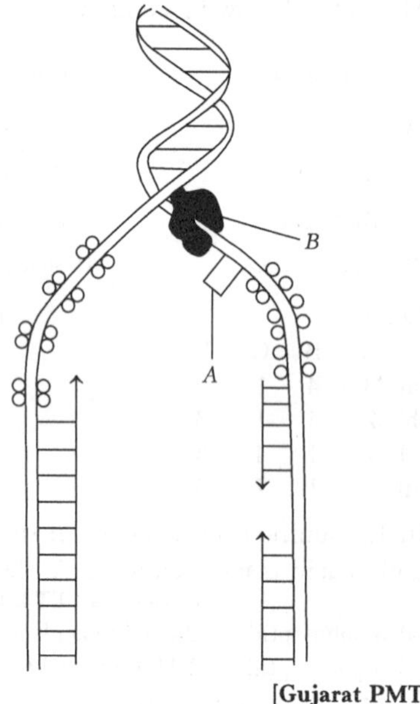

[Gujarat PMT 2015]

	A	*B*
(a)	Lagging strand	Movement of hellicase
(b)	RNA primer	DNA helicase
(c)	Single strand binding protein	DNA helicase
(d)	RNA primer	RNA helicase

79 Match the following columns.

Column I	Column II
A. A-DNA	1. 10 base pair per turn
B. B-DNA	2. 9.33 base pair per turn
C. C-DNA	3. 12 base pair per turn
D. Z-DNA	4. 11 base pair per turn

[Chhattisgarh PMT 2015]

Codes

	A	B	C	D
(a)	2	1	3	4
(b)	3	4	1	2
(c)	4	1	2	3
(d)	4	3	2	1

80 In translation, aminoacyl *t*RNA synthetase recognises the correct amino acid on the basis of **[Chhattisgarh PMT 2015]**

(a) COO group (b) NH_3 group
(c) H-atom (d) *R*-group

81 The *t*RNA anticodon 3′-UAC-5′ will pair with the *m*RNA codon **[WB JEE 2015]**

(a) 5′-AUU-3′ (b) 5′-UAC-3′
(c) 5′-AUG-3′ (d) 3′-GUA-5′

82 Select the correct option. **[CBSE AIPMT 2014]**

	Column I (Direction of RNA synthesis)	Column II (Direction of reading of the template DNA strand)
(a)	5′– 3′	3′ - 5′
(b)	3′ - 5′	5′ - 3′
(c)	5′ - 3′	5′ - 3′
(d)	3′ - 5′	3′ - 5′

83 Which one of the following is wrongly matched? **[CBSE AIPMT 2014]**

(a) Transcription — Writing information from DNA to *t*RNA
(b) Translation — Using information in *m*RNA to make protein
(c) Repressor — Binds to operator to stop enzyme protein synthesis
(d) Operon — Structural genes, operator and promoter

84 Transformation was discovered by **[CBSE AIPMT 2014]**

(a) Meselson and Stahl (b) Hershey and Chase
(c) F Griffith (d) Watson and Crick

85 What will be the number of histone molecules in a chromatin fibre having 50 nucleosomes? **[MHT CET 2014]**

(a) 400 (b) 449 (c) 500 (d) 1000

86 The sequence of nucleotides AUG CUU CUC indicates that it is a segment of **[MHT CET 2014]**
(a) sense strand of DNA
(b) anti-sense strand of DNA
(c) RNA
(d) polypeptide chain

87 Match the following columns.

	Column I (Chemical compounds)		Column II (Examples)
A.	Nitrogen base	1.	RNA
B.	Nucleoside	2.	Thymidylic acid
C.	Nucleotide	3.	Cytidine
D.	Nucleic acid	4.	Uracil

Codes **[Kerala CEE 2014]**

	A	B	C	D
(a)	1	2	3	4
(b)	1	3	2	4
(c)	4	3	2	1
(d)	4	2	3	1
(e)	1	3	4	2

88 In eukaryotic genes, coding sequences are called **[Kerala CEE 2014]**
(a) introns (b) exons
(c) regulatory sequence (d) repetitive DNA
(e) histones

89 Which site of the *t*RNA pairs through hydrogen bonding with the triplet codes on *m*RNA? **[Kerala CEE 2014**
(a) Codon (b) 5′ end of *t*RNA
(c) 3′ end of *t*RNA (d) Anticodon
(e) Amino acid acceptor end

90 Find the wrongly matched pair. **[Kerala CEE 2014]**
(a) Har Govind Khorana — Synthesised RNA molecules chemically
(b) George Gamow — Codon is triplet
(c) Meselson and Stahl — Regulation of gene expression
(d) Alec Jeffreys — DNA fingerprinting
(e) Frederick Sanger — Amino acid sequencing

91 If an inheritable mutation is observed in a population at high frequency, it is referred as **[Kerala CEE 2014]**
(a) DNA polymorphism
(b) expressed sequence tag
(c) sequence annotation
(d) linkage
(e) triplet codon

92 In eukaryotes, RNA polymerase-II transcribes **[Kerala CEE 2014]**
(a) *hn*RNA (b) 18S *r*RNA
(c) 28S *r*RNA (d) *t*RNA
(e) *sn*RNAs

93 Identify the wrong statement about DNA. **[Kerala CEE 2014]**
(a) The length of DNA is defined as the number of base pairs present in it
(b) Cytosine is common to both DNA and RNA
(c) In a nucleotide, the nitrogenous base is linked to a phosphate group
(d) Thymine is chemically 5-methyl uracil
(e) Deoxythymidine is a nucleoside

94 Which triplet codon does not have a *t*RNA associated with it? **[Kerala CEE 2014]**
(a) UAA (b) UUA (c) UUU (d) AUU
(e) GUU

95 Read the following statements and choose the correct statement(s).
I. RNA polymerase associates transiently with 'Rho' factor to initiate transcription.
II. In bacteria, transcription and translation take place in the same compartment.
III. RNA polymerase-I is responsible for transcription of *t*RNA.
IV. When *hn*RNA undergoes capping process, adenylate residues are added at 3′-end in a template independent manner.
V. *hn*RNA is the precursor of *m*RNA. **[Kerala CEE 2014]**

Codes
(a) Only II (b) II, III and IV (c) III and IV (d) I and IV
(e) I and V

96 Choose the correct statement. **[Kerala CEE 2014]**
(a) Haploid content of human DNA is 4.6×10^6 bp
(b) A nitrogenous base is linked to pentose sugar through phosphodiester linkage
(c) X-ray diffraction data of Maurice Wilkins and Rosalind Franklin was the basis of Watson and Crick's DNA model
(d) DNA is an acidic substance was first identified by Watson and Crick
(e) Ratios between adenine, thymine and guanine, cytosine are not constant.

97 Aminoacylation of *t*RNA is essential for **[Kerala CEE 2014]**
(a) replication of RNA (b) formation of peptide bond
(c) splicing (d) initiation of transcription
(e) termination

98 Which codon is not an indicator of completion of protein synthesis? **[WB JEE 2014]**
(a) UAG (b) AUG (c) UAA (d) UGA

99 If the sequence of bases in the coding strand of a double-stranded DNA is 5′-GTTCGAGTC-3′ the sequence of bases in its transcript will be **[WB JEE 2014**
(a) 5′-GACUCGAAC-3′ (b) 5′-CAAGCUCAG-3′
(c) 5′-GUUCGAGUC-3′ (d) 5′-CUGAGCUUG-3′

100 Which of the following processes was discovered by Lederberg and Tatum (1946)? **[WB JEE 2014]**
(a) Transduction (b) Transformation
(c) Asexual reproduction (d) Conjugation

101 Formation of polysome does not require **[WB JEE 2014]**
(a) *r*RNA (b) *m*RNA
(c) *t*RNA (d) *sn*RNA

102 The region of DNA sequence that provides binding site for RNA polymerase is **[J&K CET 2014]**
(a) terminator (b) structural gene
(c) origin sequence (d) promoter

103 In *lac* operon, if mutation occurs in the middle gene of the 'structural gene' then **[Gujarat CET 2014]**
(a) β-galactosidase will not be synthesised
(b) permease will not be synthesised
(c) transacetylase will not be synthesised
(d) lactose digestion will be rapid

104 Which option is correct for the amino acid and the total number of their genetic code? **[Gujarat CET 2014]**
(a) Val = 6, Pro = 6 (b) Arg = 6, His = 6
(c) Pro = 4, Thr = 4 (d) Thr = 4, Arg = 4

105 Which option shows correctly labelled region in the given diagram of DNA replication?

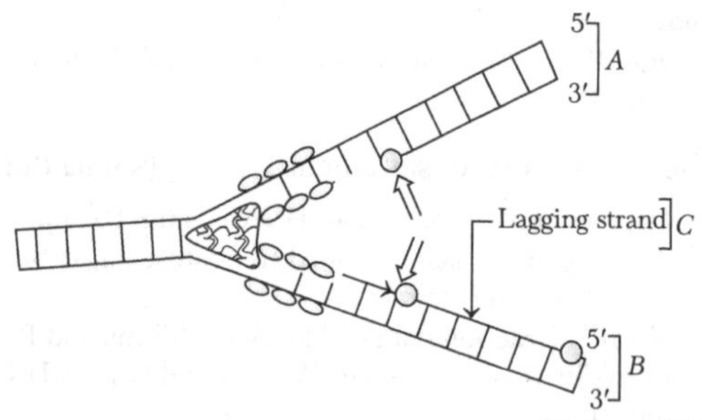

[Gujarat CET 2014]
(a) *A* and *C* (b) Only *C*
(c) *A* and *B* (d) *B* and *C*

106 If the codon GGU is reversed, the resulting codon will code for this amino acid **[EAMCET 2014]**
(a) Tyr (b) Trp (c) Leu (d) Thr

107 Match the following columns.

Column I		Column II
A.	Exon	1. Site for binding of RNA polymerase
B.	Capping	2. Coding sequence
C.	Tailing	3. Lagging stand
D.	Promoter	4. Methyl guanosine triphosphate
		5. Adenylate residues

Codes **[EAMCET 2014]**

	A	B	C	D		A	B	C	D
(a)	2	4	5	1	(b)	2	4	1	5
(c)	3	1	2	4	(d)	4	2	3	1

108 Identify the correct pair of combinations.
I. ^{14}C - Distinction between PS-I and PS-II.
II. ^{15}N - Semiconservation replication of DNA.
III. ^{35}S - Polypeptide synthesis.
IV. ^{32}C - Identification of chemical natrue of genetic material. **[EAMCET 2014]**
Codes
(a) II and III (b) II and IV (c) I and II (d) I and III

109 Assume that the occurrence of nitrogen bases in adjacent positions in a DNA strand is random. Identify the minimum number of nucleotides in a DNA strand where GAAT can occur once on the basis of probability. **[EAMCET 2014]**
(a) 512 (b) 256 (c) 4096 (d) 1024

110 The result of the following reaction/experiment carried out by Avery *et al.* on *Streptococcus pneumoniae* has proved conclusively that DNA is the genetic material **[Karnataka CET 2014]**
(a) live 'R' strain + DNA from 'S' strain + DNase
(b) heat killed 'R' stain + DNA from 'S' strain + DNase
(c) live 'R' strain + DNA from 'S' strain + RNase
(d) live 'R' strain + Denatured DNA of 'S' strain + Protease

111 Which of the following events would occur in *lac* operon of *E. coli* when the growth medium has high concentration of lactose? **[Karnataka CET 2014]**
(a) The structural genes fail to produce polycistronic *m*RNA
(b) The repressor protein binds to RNA polymerase and prevents translation
(c) The repressor protein attaches to the promoter sequence and derepresses the operator
(d) The inducer molecule binds to repressor protein and RNA polymerase binds to promoter sequence

112 Consider the following statements.
Statement I The primary transcript produced in eukaryotes is translated without undergoing any modification or processing.
Statement II The *hn*RNA in humans has exons and introns.
(a) Statement I is true, but II is false **[Karnataka CET 2014]**
(b) Statement I is false, but II is true
(c) Both statements I and II are true
(d) Both statements I and II are false

113 The diagram shows an important concept in the genetic implication of DNA. Fill in the blanks *A* to *C*. **[NEET 2013, AFMC 2012]**

$$\text{DNA} \xrightarrow{A} m\text{RNA} \xrightarrow{B} \text{Protein} \xrightarrow[C]{\text{Proposed by}}$$

(a) *A*-Translation, *B*-Transcription, *C*-Erwin Chargaff
(b) *A*- Transcription, *B*- Translation, *C*- Francis Crick
(c) *A*- Translation, *B*- Extension, *C*- Rosalind Franklin
(d) *A*- Translation, *B*- Replication, *C*- James Watson

114 Which enzyme/s will be produced in a cell in which there is a non-sense mutation in the *lac y*-gene? **[NEET 2013]**
(a) Lactose permease
(b) Transacetylase
(c) Lactose permease and transacetylase
(d) β-galactosidase

115 What would happen if in a gene encoding a polypeptide of 50 amino acid, 25th (UAC) is mutated to UAA? **[Bihar CECE 2012]**
(a) A polypetide of 49 amino acids will be formed
(b) A polypeptide of 25 amino acids will be formed
(c) A polypeptide of 24 amino acids will be formed
(d) Two polypeptides of 24 and 25 amino acids will be formed

116 The number of codons that code different amino acids is **[AMU 2012]**
(a) 16 (b) 31 (c) 61 (d) 64

117 Some amino acids are coded by more than one codon **[AMU 2012]**
(a) unambiguous (b) degenerate
(c) universal (d) initiator

118 What is not true for genetic code? **[Manipal 2012]**
(a) A codon in *m*RNA is read in a non-contiguous fashion
(b) It is nearly universal
(c) It is degenerate
(d) It is non-ambiguous

119 Okazaki is known for his contribution to the understanding of **[AIIMS 2012]**
(a) transcription (b) translation
(c) DNA replication (c) mutation

120 During replication of DNA, Okazaki fragments are formed in the direction **[BHU 2012]**
(a) $5' \rightarrow 3'$ (b) $3' \rightarrow 5'$ (c) $3' \rightarrow 3'$ (d) $5' \rightarrow 5'$

121 Which of the following amino acid codon was used by Khorana? **[BHU 2012]**
(a) Serine (b) Tryptophan
(c) Alanine (d) Valine

122 Which one of the following statement regarding *lac* operon is correct? **[BHU 2012]**
(a) *Lac* operon is inducible system
(b) *Lac* operon is repressible system
(c) *Lac* operon of *E.coli* contains four structural genes
(d) None of the above

123 Select the true statement. **[BHU 2012]**
(a) *m*RNA acts as template of *t*RNA synthesis
(b) DNA acts as template for protein synthesis
(c) *m*RNA acts as template for *c*DNA synthesis
(d) *m*RNA is inactive

124 Which antibiotic inhibits interaction between *t*RNA and *m*RNA during bacterial protein synthesis? **[Manipal 2012]**
(a) Neomycin
(b) Streptomycin
(c) Tetracycline
(d) Erythromycin

125 Out of 64 codons, the number of codons with GGG, is **[AMU 2012]**
(a) 1 (b) 2 (c) 4 (d) 6

126 Given below is a sample of portion of DNA strand giving the base sequence on the opposite strands. What is so special shown in it? **[CBSE AIPMT 2011]**
5′ – GAATTC – 3′
3′ – CTTAAG – 5′
(a) Deletion mutation
(b) Start codon at the 5′ end
(c) Palindromic sequence of base pairs
(d) Replication completed

127 Peptide synthesis inside a cell takes place in **[CBSE AIPMT 2011]**
(a) mitochondria (b) chromoplast
(c) ribosomes (d) chloroplast

128 Who was awarded Nobel Prize in 1959 for *in vitro* synthesis of polyribonucleocide? **[UP CPMT 2011]**
(a) Tatum (b) Darwin
(c) Kornberg (d) Khorana

129 Gene of bacteria and virus code for more than one polypeptide are called **[Odisha JEE 2011]**
(a) overlapping gene
(b) monocistronic gene
(c) polycistronic gene
(d) non-ambiguous gene

130 Methyl guanosine triphosphate is associated with **[Kerala CEE 2011]**
(a) point mutation (b) tautomerism
(c) capping (d) Okazaki fragments
(e) tailing

ANSWERS

Check Point 8.1

1. (a)	2. (c)	3. (d)	4. (c)	5. (a)	6. (b)

Check Point 8.2

1. (c)	2. (a)	3. (d)	4. (c)	5. (b)	6. (c)

Check Point 8.3

1. (b)	2. (d)	3. (a)	4. (d)	5. (d)	6. (d)

Check Point 8.4

1. (c)	2. (d)	3. (b)	4. (b)	5. (c)	6. (d)

(A) Topical Exercise

1. (d)	2. (b)	3. (d)	4. (c)	5. (c)	6. (d)	7. (a)	8. (d)	9. (c)	10. (b)
11. (d)	12. (c)	13. (b)	14. (c)	15. (d)	16. (b)	17. (b)	18. (b)	19. (c)	20. (a)
21. (b)	22. (d)	23. (b)	24. (b)	25. (c)	26. (d)	27. (b)	28. (b)	29. (d)	30. (d)
31. (c)	32. (d)	33. (d)	34. (b)	35. (c)	36. (c)	37. (d)	38. (d)	39. (c)	40. (a)
41. (b)	42. (a)	43. (a)	44. (d)	45. (a)	46. (d)	47. (c)	48. (c)	49. (c)	50. (a)
51. (c)	52. (b)	53. (b)	54. (c)	55. (b)	56. (c)	57. (d)	58. (b)	59. (a)	60. (c)
61. (d)	62. (c)	63. (c)	64. (a)	65. (a)	66. (a)	67. (d)	68. (d)	69. (c)	70. (a)
71. (b)	72. (a)	73. (d)	74. (d)	75. (c)	76. (d)	77. (b)	78. (d)	79. (c)	80. (b)
81. (a)	82. (c)	83. (c)	84. (b)	85. (d)	86. (b)	87. (a)	88. (b)	89. (b)	90. (b)
91. (b)	92. (a)	93. (a)	94. (a)	95. (a)	96. (b)	97. (b)	98. (c)	99. (a)	100. (d)
101. (a)	102. (b)	103. (c)	104. (b)	105. (d)	106. (a)	107. (b)	108. (a)	109. (b)	110. (a)
111. (a)	112. (d)	113. (d)	114. (d)	115. (b)	116. (c)	117. (c)	118. (c)	119. (c)	120. (d)
121. (d)	122. (d)	123. (d)	124. (a)	125. (d)	126. (a)	127. (b)			

(B) Cumulative Exercise

1. (c)	2. (a)	3. (c)	4. (c)	5. (d)	6. (a)	7. (a)	8. (a)	9. (a)	10. (d)
11. (b)	12. (b)	13. (a)	14. (a)	15. (a)	16. (d)	17. (d)	18. (d)	19. (b)	20. (b)
21. (a)	22. (d)	23. (c)	24. (d)	25. (c)	26. (a)	27. (c)	28. (b)	29. (a)	30. (d)
31. (b)	32. (e)	33. (c)	34. (b)	35. (b)	36. (b)	37. (a)	38. (a)	39. (a)	40. (a)

(C) Medical Entrances' Gallery

1. (b)	2. (b)	3. (c)	4. (b)	5. (d)	6. (c)	7. (a)	8. (b)	9. (c)	10. (b)
11. (c)	12. (c)	13. (d)	14. (c)	15. (b)	16. (c)	17. (d)	18. (c)	19. (*)	20. (a)
21. (b)	22. (b)	23. (b)	24. (a)	25. (b)	26. (b)	27. (d)	28. (c)	29. (b)	30. (d)
31. (a)	32. (a)	33. (c)	34. (c)	35. (a)	36. (c)	37. (b)	38. (a)	39. (a)	40. (b)
41. (c)	42. (c)	43. (a)	44. (b)	45. (b)	46. (c)	47. (d)	48. (a)	49. (d)	50. (c)
51. (b)	52. (b)	53. (a)	54. (c)	55. (d)	56. (c)	57. (d)	58. (c)	59. (b)	60. (d)
61. (d)	62. (c)	63. (b)	64. (c)	65. (a)	66. (b)	67. (b)	68. (c)	69. (c)	70. (b)
71. (b)	72. (a)	73. (d)	74. (b)	75. (a)	76. (b)	77. (c)	78. (b)	79. (c)	80. (d)
81. (c)	82. (a)	83. (a)	84. (c)	85. (b)	86. (c)	87. (c)	88. (b)	89. (d)	90. (c)
91. (a)	92. (a)	93. (c)	94. (a)	95. (e)	96. (c)	97. (b)	98. (b)	99. (c)	100. (d)
101. (d)	102. (d)	103. (b)	104. (c)	105. (b)	106. (b)	107. (a)	108. (a)	109. (b)	110. (a)
111. (d)	112. (b)	113. (b)	114. (d)	115. (c)	116. (c)	117. (b)	118. (a)	119. (c)	120. (a)
121. (a)	122. (a)	123. (c)	124. (c)	125. (a)	126. (c)	127. (c)	128. (c)	129. (b)	130. (c)

Explanations

(A) Topical Exercise

11 (*d*) Option (d) is incorrect and can be corrected as
Deoxyribose and ribose both are pentoses or pentose sugar.

16 (*b*) Polymerisation is defined as the process by which small molecules will join or bind together to generate a large molecule chemically. Thus, to avoid nucleotide polymerisation 3′OH group present in deoxyribose should be either replaced or removed.

17 (*b*) According to Chargaff rule, the adenine proportion is always equal to thymine and proportion of guanine is equal to cytosine. This law is applicable for double-stranded DNA. As in the question, proportion of adenine is not equal to thymine and proportion of guanine is not equal to cytosine, the DNA of the organism is single-stranded.

19 (*c*) Statement in option (c) is incorrect and can be corrected as
Phosphorus is not present in nitrogenous bases.

22 (*d*) Experiment performed by Meselson and Stahl was based on DNA semiconservative nature.
Now, keeping DNA semiconservative nature into consideration and beginning with the DNA strand that have N^{15} and then N^{14}, after the fourth generation there are 14 strands having N^{14} N^{14}, O strands having N^{15} N^{15} and 2 strands with N^{15} N^{14}.
Thus, the ratio will be 0 : 2 : 14 or 0 : 1 : 7.

28 (*b*) Option (b) is incorrect pair and can be corrected as
RNA formation- RNA polymerase

53 (*b*) Only the pairs of codon present in option (b) is correctly matched with their function or the signal for the particular amino acid.
Rest other options are not correctly matched with their function or the signal for the particular amino acid and can be corrected as

- GCC, GCU -Alanine
- AUG-Start/methionine
  ACG - Threonine
- UUA-Leucine
  UCA-Tyrosine

85 (*d*) Statement in option (d) is incorrect and can be corrected as
Sigma factor is a component of RNA polymerase.

86 (*b*) Statement in option (b) is true for RNA processing. Other statements are not true and can be corrected as

- Introns are excised before the *m*RNA is translated.
- The RNA transcript that leaves the nucleus may be much smaller than original transcript.
- Large quantities of *t*RNA are assembled into ribosomes.

(B) Cumulative Exercise

6 (*a*) Statements I, II and III are correct except statement IV. Incorrect statement can be corrected as
The gene regulation in prokaryotes can be explained by *lac* operon model.

7 (*a*) Statement I and III are correct. The genetic codes said to be degenerate because amino acids may have more than one codon. They are universal becaue codons for higher and lower organisms are common.
Thus, option (a) is correct.

9 (*a*) AUG codes Methionine (Met)
UUU codes Phenyl-alanine (Phe)
UUC codes Phenyl-alanine (Phe)
Thus, sequence of amino acid coded will be
Met-Phe-Phe-Phe-Phe-Phe-Phe

11 (*b*) The given sequence is

AUG CCU GAC UUU AAG UAG

AUG – Methionine (Met)
CCU – Proline (Pro)
GAC – Aspartic acid (Asp)
UUU – Phenyl alanine (Phe)
AAG – Lysine (Lys)
UAG – Stop
Thus, the amino acid sequence will be
Met-Pro-Asp-Phe-Lys-Stop

13 (*a*) The correctly matched pair can be seen in option (a). Other pairs are incorrectly matched and can be corrected as
Linus Pauling-Discovered proteins spiral structure.
Francis Crick -Gave model of DNA along with Watson.
George Beadle-Gave one gene-one enzyme hypothesis.

20 (*b*) Statements II and IV are correct while I and III are incorrect. Incorrect statements can be corrected as

- Galactose binds with the repressor and inactivate the operon.
- The *z*-gene codes for the enzymes, β-galactosidase which breaks lactose into glucose and galactose.

23 (*c*) Statement I and III are correct because
During translation, the activation of amino acids takes place through their carboxyl group. In the presence of ATP, each amino acid combines with its specific aminoacyl *t*RNA synthetase and get catalysed.
Thus, option (c) is correct.

30 (*d*) Statements II and III are correct while I and IV are incorrect. Incorrect statements can be corrected as

- *m*RNA provides the template for synthesis of protein.
- A segment of DNA coding for polypeptide is called exon.

31 (*b*) Both A and R are true, but R is not the correct explanation of A.
*t*RNA has anticodons, which read the message expressed in the form of codons in *m*RNA and occupy a specific place on *m*RNA. *t*RNA also recognises the amino acids.

32 (*e*) Both A and R are false and can be corrected as *m*RNA attaches itself to 30 S unit of ribosome through its 5′ end. This process is helped by G-cap nucleotide and bases of leader sequence present on *m*RNA where G-cap is present as in eukaryotes.

33 (c) A is true, but R is false.
Transcription involves transfer of genetic information from DNA to *m*RNA. It occurs in nucleus from where *m*RNA moves towards ribosome in cytoplasm for translation. The translation of protein synthesis involves the translation of language of nucleic acids (i.e. *m*RNA) into language of proteins.

34 (*b*) Both A and R are true, but R is not the correct explanation of A.
The genetic code is triplet, degenerate, commaless, non-ambiguous, universal and non-overlapping. The non-overlapping code means that a base in *m*RNA is not used for two different codons. For example, AUG AGC GCA are not read as AUG GAG (an overlap of two bases) or CGA GCA CA (overlapping of one base).

35 (*b*) Both A and R are true, but R is not the correct explanation of A.
Proteins are the polymers of amino acids. Two amino acids are linked with each other through peptide bonds. Nucleic acids (i.e. DNA and RNA) are the polymers of nucleotides. Two nucleotides are linked to each other through phosphodiester bonds.

36 (*b*) Both A and R are true, but R is not the correct explanation of A.
In prokaryotes, a single *m*RNA molecule may code for one or several polypeptide chains. If it carries the code for only polypeptide, the *m*RNA is 'monocistronic' and if it codes for two or more different polypeptides, the *m*RNA is 'polycistronic'. In eukaryotes, most *m*RNAs are monocistronic. Termination codons like UAA, UGA, UAG, etc., are present on *m*RNA and are capable to release the polypeptide chain.

37 (*a*) Both A and R are true and R is the correct explanation of A.
*t*RNA is present in cytoplasm. Its main function is to take desired amino acids to ribosomes during protein synthesis. Actually, *t*RNA contains an anticodon (i.e. a triplet of three nitrogenous bases), this reads codon present on *m*RNA, which comes from nucleus and on this bases, it takes up amino acids from cytoplasm.

38 (*a*) Both A and R are true and R is the correct explanation of A.
There are three codons, i.e. UAA, UAG, UGA, which are responsible for the termination of a polypeptide chain also known as stop codon because these triplets are not recognises by *t*RNA during the process of translation.

39 (*a*) Both A and R are true and R is the correct explanation of A.
Replication and transcription occur in the nucleus as all the raw material for DNA and RNA synthesis is present in the nucleus. From the nucleus, the transcribed *m*RNA moves to the cytoplasm where ribosomes and amino acids are available for protein synthesis.

40 (*a*) Both A and R are true and R is the correct explanation of A.
Amber codon is called termination codon because where this codon is present in the *m*RNA, the translation stops at that place.

(C) Medical Entrances' Gallery

1 (*b*) The first phase of translation is aminoacylation of *t*RNA, i.e. activation of amino acids and the formation of AA-*t*RNA complex. In the presence of an enzyme *t*RNA synthetase, the amino acid (AA) molecule is activated and then each amino acid is attached to the specific *t*RNA molecule at 3′/CCA end to form aminoacyl-*t*RNA complex. The reaction needs ATP. This process is thus called charging of *t*RNA or amino acylation of *t*RNA.

2 (*b*) The distance between two consecutive base pairs is 0.34 nm (0.34×10^{-9} m). The length of DNA double helix in a typical mammalian cell can be calculated by multiplying the total number of bp with distance between the two consecutive bp, i.e. 6.6×10^{9} bp $\times 0.34 \times 10^{-9}$m/bp = 2.2 m (the length of DNA).
Thus, option (b) is correct.

3 (*c*) RNA polymerase facilitates opening of DNA helix during transcription. RNA polymerase is the main transcription enzyme. Transcription begins when RNA polymerase binds to a promoter sequence near the beginning of a gene.
Other options are explained as
DNA helicases function in other cellular processes where double-stranded DNA must be separated, including DNA repair and transcription. DNA ligases help in joining breaks in the phosphodiester backbone of DNA that occur during replication. DNA polymerase does not function during transcription.

4 (*b*) The nucleic acid was first reported by Friedrich Meischer in 1869 from the nuclei of pus cells and was named nuclein.

5 (*d*) In a DNA polynucleotide chain, a nitrogenous base is linked to the hydroxy (—OH) of 1′ C pentose sugar.
It is represented in the structure given below

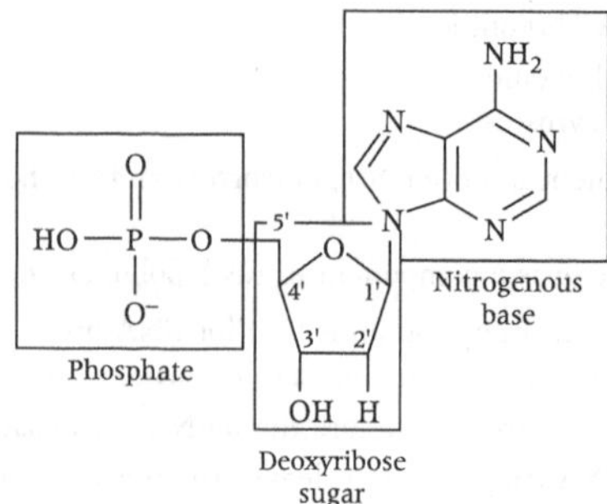

6 (*c*) *E. coli* has 4.6×10^{6} base pairs.
It completes replication process in 18 minutes, i.e. 18×60 seconds.

$$\text{Rate of polymerisation} = \frac{4.6 \times 10^6 \text{ bp}}{18 \times 60}$$
$$= \frac{4.6 \times 10^5}{18 \times 6} = \frac{46 \times 10^4}{108}$$
$$= \frac{460000}{108}$$
$$= 4259.25 \text{ bp/s}$$

or approximately 4000 bp/sec

Thus, the correct option is (c).

7 (*a*) Adenine and guanine are the purines which are found both in DNA and RNA. Purines are heterocyclic aromatic organic compounds consisting of a pyrimidine ring fused to an imidazole ring. Cytosine and thymine are the pyrimidines which are found in DNA. In case of RNA, thymine is replaced by uracil.

8 (*b*) The *m*RNA will be complementary to the DNA strand, but in RNA, uracil will be present in place of thymine. If the template strand is 3′-A T G C A T G C A T G C A T G -5′ then the base sequence of *m*RNA for the given DNA strand will be 5′ - U A C G U A C G U A C G U A C - 3′.

9 (*c*) Alfred Hershey and Martha Chase (1952) experimentally proved that DNA is the sole genetic material in bacteriophage. On the other hand, Beadle and Tatum (1940) experimentally showed one gene-one enzyme hypothesis using *Neurospora.* Meselson and Stahl first showed that DNA replicates semiconservatively through experiments on *E.coli.*

Jacob and Monod were first to explain *lac* operon.

10 (*b*) Adenylic acid, cytidylic acid and guanylic acid are nucleotides.

A nucleotide is composed of three components, nitrogen base (adenine cytosine, guanine), ribose sugar and a phosphate group. On the other hand, adenosine, cytidine, thymidine are nucleosides.

Uracil, cytosine and adenine are nitrogenous bases.

11 (*c*) According to Chargaff's rule, the amount of adenine is always equal to that of thymine and the amount of guanine is always equal to that of cytosine,

i.e. A = T and G = C. Also, the purines and pyrimidines are always in equal amounts, i.e., A + G = T + C. Given *ds*DNA has 20% adenine that means thymine will also be 20%. Since, as adenine pairs with thymine, together they form 40% of bases DNA and

cytosine and guanine together form 60% of bases of DNA. Hence, cytosine would be 60/2 = 30%.

Total percentage of pyrimidine bases (T +C) are 20 + 30 = 50%.

12 (*c*) During DNA replication, supercoiling is relaxed by DNA topoisomerase. These enzymes participate in the over winding or underwinding of DNA. Other options are explained as

SSBPs are Single Strand Binding Proteins which stabilise the unwound parental DNA.

Primase enzyme synthesises RNA primer on DNA template to initiate DNA synthesis.

Polymerase enzyme helps in synthesis of new DNA or RNA strand during replication.

13 (*d*) Option (d) is not correctly matched and can be corrected as Southern hybridisation technique is related to identification of DNA sequences. RNA sequences are identified by Northern hybridisation.

Other options are correctly matched.

14 (*c*) The reading frame of given *m*RNA will not change even after the deletion of GGU from 7th, 8th and 9th positions because removal of three of its multiple bases will not change the reading frame but will remove one or more amino acids.

However, the amino acid, glycine will not be formed at third position in this case which is being coded by GGU. In rest of the cases, insertion or deletion of one or two nucleotide bases would result in the complete alteration in the reading frame of *m*RNA.

15 (*b*) Bacteria are able to produce human insulin because genetic code is nearly universal in all organisms.

For example, the codon AGG specifies amino acid arginine in bacteria, animals and plants.

But there are also some exceptions to it, e.g. in human mitochondria, stop codon UGA specifies amino acid tryptophan.

17 (*d*) The correct combination of salient features of genetic code is Degenerate, Non-overlapping, Non-ambiguous. These are explained as one codon codes for only one amino acid, hence genetic code is unambiguous and specific.

Some amino acids are coded by more than one codon, hence the code is degenerate. The codon is read in *m*RNA in a contiguous fashion. There are no punctuations and overlapping.

18 (*c*) In the process of transcription (i.e. copying of genetic information from one strand of the DNA into RNA) in eukaryotes, the RNA polymerase-I transcribes *r*RNA - 28S, 18S and 5.8S.

On the other hand, *t*RNA, 5S*r*RNA are transcribed by RNA polymerase-III. RNA polymerase-II transcribes precursor of *m*RNA, *hn*RNA *sn*RNA.

19 (*) This question is not correct because out of the given initiation and termination factors, none is involved in transcription in eukaryotes. Only option (a) gives initiation and termination factors which are involved in transcription.

These factors (σ and ρ) initiate and terminate transcription in prokaryotes (not in eukaryotes). Initiation and termination factors involved in transcription in eukaryotes are General Transcription Factors (GTF IIA-TF II H) and Transcription Termination Factor-1 (TTF-1), respectively.

20 (*a*) Genetic code is a sequence of nucleotides in nucleic acid (DNA or RNA) that determines the amino acid sequence during protein synthesis.

Genetic codes for arginine are CGU, CGC, CGA and CGG. On the other hand CAU and CAC code for histidine. CAA and CAG code for glutamine. AGU and AGC code for serine. AAC codes for asparagine. GAU, GAC codes for aspartic acid. GAA codes for glutamic acid.

21 (*b*) Option (b) is correct, i.e. A-Initiation, B-Termination, C- Elongation.

In prokaryotes, transcription of all types of bacterial RNA is catalysed by a single DNA dependent RNA polymerase in three steps

Initiation It involves binding of RNA polymerase with the promoter site by associating with a initiation or sigma (σ) factor.

Termination In this step, RNA polymerase on reaching termination region separates and RNA falls off from transcription unit. This step is characterised by binding of termination or rho (ρ) factor with RNA polymerase, which marks termination of transcription.

Elongation This step involves elongation of RNA chain as the RNA polymerase travel in $5' \rightarrow 3'$ direction. This step is characterised by dissociation of 'σ' initiation factor from RNA polymerase.

22 (*b*) Both A and R are true, but R is not the correct explanation of A.

In eukaryotes, transcription, i.e. synthesis of RNA from DNA, occurs inside nucleus because the genetic material, DNA is enclosed inside the nuclear membrane in eukaryotes. Whereas, in prokaryotes like bacteria, the genetic material, DNA remains suspended within the cytoplasm, thus in prokaryotes, the process of transcription and translation occur in cytoplasm.

23 (*b*) UAC is not a stop codon. It codes for tyrosine amino acid. The last codon of a functional gene which helps in termination of the polypeptide chain, is termed as stop or termination codons. These are UAA, UAG and UGA.

24 (*a*) *t*RNA binds to *m*RNA through anticodon loop, as it bears the base complementary to those on *m*RNA being translated.

On the other hand, the amino acid loop of *t*RNA is involved in binding the respective amino acid. The TψC loop helps in binding the ribosomes, while the D loop of *t*RNA is the binding site for aminoacyl synthetase enzyme.

26 (*b*) Statement in option (b) is wrong. The correct form of statement is 'less than 2% of the genome codes for protein'. The content of the human genome is commonly divided into coding and non-coding DNA sequences. Coding DNA are those sequences that can be transcribed into *m*RNA and translated into protein, they occupy only a small fraction (< 2%) of genome. Non-coding DNA (introns) sequences do not encode proteins.

In most of organisms, more than 98% of human genome is composed of non-coding DNA (junk DNA).

Rest other statements are true.

27 (*d*) Genetic variation cannot be effectively brought about by amplification, it is a technique used in molecular biology, by which multiple copies of gene or DNA sequence is produced by *in vitro* methods.

It has no role in introducing genetic variation in organism. It just leads to increase in the frequency of a gene.

28 (*c*) Option (c) is correctly matched.

Ribozymes are RNA molecules having enzymatic activity, i.e. they are capable of catalysing specific biochemical reactions. Hence, they are nucleic acids with enzymatic function.

Other options are not correct matches and can be corrected as

- TH Morgan is known as the 'Father of Experimental Genetics'. He worked on linkage, crossing over, linkage maps, etc.
- F_2 is crossed with recessive parent in a test cross.
- Mendel is considered as the 'Father of Genetics'. He proposed the laws of inheritance.

29 (*b*) The experimental proof for semiconservative replication of DNA was first shown in a bacterium, *Escherichia coli*. It was shown by Meselson and Stahl (1958).

In this mode of replication, one strand of parent DNA is conserved in the progeny while the second is freshly synthesised. Meselson and Stahl proved this by using heavy isotope of nitrogen (N^{15}).

30 (*d*) Option (d) is correct match.

Jacob and Monod (1916) discovered the *lac* operon. An operon is a part of genetic material of DNA which acts as a single regulated unit. It possesses one or more structural genes, an operator gene, a promoter gene, a regulator gene and a repressor gene and inducer of corepressor.

Other options are not correct matches and can be corrected as

- Matthew Meselson and F Stahl discovered the semiconservative mode of DNA replication in *E. coli*.
- Alfred Hershey and Martha Chase used T_2-bacteriophage in their experiments to infect *E. coli* and proved that DNA is the genetic material.
- Alec Jeffreys (1984) invented the DNA fingerprinting technique which determines nucleotide sequences of certain areas of DNA, unique to each individual.

31 (*a*) Ribonucleotide is a nucleotide containing ribose as its pentose component, uracil as nitrogenous base and a phosphate.

It is considered as a molecular precursor of nucleic acids. In living organisms, the most common bases for ribonucleotides are adenine, guanine, cytosine and uracil.

Therefore, option (a), i.e. ribose + uracil + phosphate is correct.

32 (*a*) Linker DNA is attached to H1 histone protein (called plugging protein and acts as marker protein). It connects two adjacent nucleosomes and together they constitute a chromatosome. The latter gives rise to chromatin fibre after condensation.

33 (*c*) Coding strand is the one that codes for *m*RNA. It has same nucleotide sequence as that of *m*RNA except thymine (T) is replaced by uracil (U) in *m*RNA. So, the corresponding sequence of the transcribed *m*RNA is AGGUAUCGCAU.

34 (*c*) The codons of glycine are GGU, GGC, GGA, GGG. A genetic code is the smallest unit to code one amino acid. This genetic code is defined as nucleotide sequence of nitrogenous bases, which specifies the amino acid sequence in a polypeptide molecule. On the other hand, CCU, CCC, CCA, CCG are the codons of proline, CGU, CGC, CGA, CGG are of arginine and ACU, ACC, ACA, ACG are of threonine.

35 (*a*) Among the given options, only first one, i.e. AUG, UGA, UUU can be translated because it possesses an initiation codon, AUG which codes for methionine. Rest of the *m*RNA sequences start with termination codons, i.e. UAA (ochre), UAG (amber) and UGA (opal). Therefore, these cannot be translated.

36 (*c*) At the 5' end of eukaryotic *m*RNA, 7 mG (7-methyl Guanosine) is present. In eukaryotes, primary transcript is often larger than the functional RNAs. Therefore, post-transcription processing is required to convert primary transcript into functional RNAs.

It is of four types, cleavage, splicing, terminal additions and nucleotide modification. The terminal additions include capping and tailing. In capping, 7 mG is added to 5′ end of *m*RNA. In tailing, polyadenylation occurs which is the addition of poly-A tail to 3′ end of *m*RNA.

37 (*b*) Selenocysteine (Sec) is the 21st amino acid in the genetic code. This amino acid contains selenium. Pyrrolysine is the 22nd amino acid. Cysteine is a sulphur containing amino acid. Histidine is an α-amino acid.

38 (*a*) Except an enhancer, all the given components are parts of an operon. Enhancer sequences are present in eukaryotes that, when bound by specific proteins or transcription factors, enhance the transcription of an associated gene.

39 (*a*) Repressor protein is attached to operator gene. It is a regulatory protein synthesised by regulator gene. Repressor is meant for blocking the operator gene, so that the structural genes are unable to form *m*RNAs.

41 (*c*) Lactose or *lac* operon of *E. coli* is an example of inducible operon. Lactose is known to be an inducer and substrate for the enzyme β-galactosidase. It binds with the repressor protein forming inducer-repressor complex and changes it into a non-DNA binding state, thus activating the operon.

Thus, Option (c) is correct

42 (*c*) DNA replication in bacteria occurs prior to fission. It is a rapid process and requires DNA polymerase-III enzyme. In eukaryotes, DNA replication occurs during S-phase.

43 (*a*) *r*RNA is the most abundant RNA (70-80%) and it has 3-4 types, e.g. 23S, 28S, etc. In eukaryotic animal cells, four types of *r*RNA are found 28S, 18S, 5.8S and 5S. On the other hand, *t*RNA constitutes about 15% and *m*RNA about 2 - 5% of the total RNA content of the cell.

44 (*b*) DNA fragments are negatively charged molecules due to the presence of negatively charged phosphate (PO_4^-) group that constitutes every nucleotide.

45 (*b*) The final proof that DNA is the genetic material came from the experiments of Alfred Hershey and Martha Chase (1952). Griffith's experiment proved the existence of genetic material while Avery, MacLeod and McCarty worked to determine the biochemical nature of transforming principle.

46 (*c*) The association of H1histone with nucleosome indicates that DNA is condensed into chromatin fibre.

Refer to Ans. 32.

47 (*d*) Spliceosome is a large molecular complex found in nucleus of eukaryotic cells of plants, animals and fungi, etc. It is assembled from *sn*RNAs and protein complexes that play an important role in splicing of introns. Spliceosome is absent in prokaryotic cells like bacteria.

48 (*a*) Extragenic or intergenic suppression relieves the effect of a mutation in a gene at a different place within the genome.

It can be explained as a mutation disrupting the complementary interaction between protein molecules which can be compensated by a second mutation occurring at some place in the genome. It helps to restore a suitable alternative interaction between those molecules.

49 (*d*) The process of addition of methyl GTP at the 5′ end of *hn*RNA is known as capping. Enzyme guanyl transferase catalyses this process.

Cap is essential for the formation of *m*RNA-ribosome complex. Translation is not possible if cap is lacking, because cap is identified by 18S *r*RNA of ribosome unit.

50 (*c*) Bacterial cells use their 23S *r*RNA as an enzyme during protein synthesis. This is the only non-proteinaceous enzyme known so far.

51 (*b*) The use of radioactive thymidine to detect the semiconservative mode of replication of newly synthesised DNA in the chromosomes was performed on *Vicia faba* by Taylor and colleagues in 1969. This experiment proved that the DNA in chromosomes replicates semiconservatively.

52 (*b*) Gene that codes for either RNA or protein during protein synthesis process is known as structural gene. Therefore, cistron is considered equivalent of structural gene because it also encodes for polypeptids or proteins.

54 (*c*) A molecule that can act as a genetic material must be stable structurally and chemically.

Thus, option (c) is correct.

56 (*c*) Statement in option (c) is incorrect and can be corrected as Glycine is the simplest amino acid in which functional group *R* is replaced by hydrogen atom (H).

Rest options are correct.

60 (*d*) UCU-Serine, UGG-Tryptophan, UGC-Cysteine, UGU-Cysteine, GGU-Glycine

So, correct sequence for UCG-UGG-UGC-UGU-GGU will be Ser-Trp-Cys-Cys-Gly.

61 (*d*) Chargaff's rule is not applicable to RNA. It is the generalised formula about double-stranded DNA structure. The rule states that DNA from any cell of all organisms should have a 1:1 ratio (base pair rule) of pyrimidine and purine bases, i.e. the amount of guanine is equal to cytosine and the amount of adenine is equal to thymine. Further, complementary base pairing is sometimes, visible in RNA as well (in doubled-stranded RNAs of viruses) hence, option (a) is not taken into consideration.

63 (*b*) *Lac* I gene produces an inhibitor or repressor that induces negative regulation of *lac* operon. The repressor binds to the operator gene and represses promoter from binding to RNA polymerase. Repressor is meant to block the operator gene so that structural genes are unable to form *m*RNA thus, stopping the transcription of genes.

64 (*c*) Chargaff's rule states that purine and pyrimidine base pairs are present in equal amount in *ds*DNA, i.e. A = T, G = C

$$\therefore \quad \frac{A+T}{G+C} = 1$$

If cytosine = 17%

If A + G + C + T = 100 and G = C, A = T

then A + 17 + 17 + T = 100

$$A + T + 34 = 100$$
$$A + T = 100 - 34$$
$$A + T = 66$$
$$A = T = \frac{66}{2} = 33\%$$

Hence, if cytosine is 17% then G = 17% and A and T will be 33% each.

67 (*b*) Zeatin is found in corn and other plants as the free base, 6 (4-hydroxy-3 methyl-trans-2-butenylamine) purine, as well as in the form of ribonucleoside and ribonucleoside 5-phosphate.

68 (*c*) Option (c) is correct regarding RNA processing. Capping of the pre *m*RNA involves the addition of 7-methylguanosine to the 5′ end. Whereas in tailing, adenylate residues are added at 3′ end of *hn*RNA.

69 (*c*) In splicing, introns (non-coding regions) are removed from heterogeneous nuclear RNA and exons (coding regions) are joined to form a mature *m*RNA.

73 (*d*) The codon AUG has dual functions. It is an initiation codon and also codes for methionine while protein synthesis.

75 (*a*) According to Chargaff's equivalency rule.

$$\frac{A+G}{T+C} = 1$$
$$A = T$$
$$G = C$$

If A = 820 then T = 820

$$A + T = 820 + 820 = 1640$$
$$3.2\,\text{kbp} = 3200\text{ bp} \quad \therefore (1\text{kbp} = 1000\text{ bp})$$
$$G + C = 3200 - 1640$$
$$G + C = 1560$$

So, $\text{Cytosine} = \frac{1560}{2} = 780$

77 (*c*) A is true, but R is false, R can be corrected as

During the RNA splicing, introns are removed and exons are joined to form a contiguous coding. This makes mature *m*RNA ready for translation.

Eukaryotic *m*RNA molecules are monocistonic, containing the coding sequence only for one polypeptide. In prokaryotes, an individual bacterial *m*RNA molecules are polycistronic having transcripts of several genes.

78 (*b*) The figure depicts the process of DNA replication *A* is RNA primer. It is the starting point of DNA synthesis in the lagging strand *B* is DNA helicase that unwind the two strands during replication process.

80 (*d*) The enzyme aminoacyl *t*RNA synthetase read the genetic code present on the *m*RNA and accordingly identify the amino acids and attach with them on their functional group (*R*).

85 (*b*) Number of histone proteins in one nucleosome = 8 and between each nucleosome 1 linker histone (H_1) is present hence,

Total number of linker histone protein in so nucleosome = 49

So, in 50 nucleosome number of histone protein

$$= 50 \times 8 + 49$$
$$= 400 + 49 = 449$$

90 (*c*) Out of the pairs given in the option, all pairs the scientists with their discoveries correctly except, i.e. Meselson and Stahl because they supported the hypothesis that DNA replicates semiconservatively through experiments. Thus, option (c) is correct.

91 (*a*) In a population, if an inheritable mutation is observed at high frequency it is known as DNA polymorphism. Polymorphism is the variation in individuals at the genetic level. In an individual, DNA from every tissue, i.e. blood, skin, saliva, hair follicle, etc., show the same degree of polymorphism. It arises due to mutation and is inherited from parents to children.

92 (*a*) In nucleus, there are three RNA polymerases out of which RNA polymerase-II is responsible for the transcription of the *m*RNA precursor which is known as heterogeneous nuclear RNA (*hn*RNA). The process of transcription in eukaryotes is similar to that in the prokaryotes except some additional complexities.

93 (*c*) Statement in option (c) is wrong and can be corrected as

In a nucleotide, the 5′-OH of a nucleoside (rather than a nitrogen base) is linked to a phosphate group.

Rest statements are correct.

94 (*a*) Out of the triplet codon given in the options, UAA is the only codon that does not have a *t*RNA associated with it. This is because UAA is a stop codon and does not code for any amino acid. Other stop codons are UGA and UAG.

95 (*e*) Out of the statements given I and V are the correct options, remaining three are incorrect. These can be corrected as

- In bacteria, transcription and translation does not take place in same compartments they are instead coupled in the cytosol itself as there is no separation of nucleus and cytosol in bacteria therefore, translation starts much before the *m*RNA is fully transcribed.
- RNA polymerase I is responsible for the transcription of *hn*RNA (not *t*RNA).
- When *hn*RNA undergoes capping process, methyl guanosine triphosphate are added at 5′ end in a template independent manner.

96 (*c*) Among all the statements given about DNA. Only statement in option (c) is correct, while rest all others are incorrect. Incorrect statements can be corrected as

- Haploid content of DNA is 3.3×10^9 bp.
- A nitrogenous base is linked to a pentose sugar through N-glycosidic linkage.
- DNA is an acidic substance and was first identified by Frederick Meischer.
- Ratios between adenine, thymine, guanine, cytosine are constant.

99 (*c*) In the case of bases in the transcript, i.e. when *m*RNA is formed, the sequence will be 5′-GUUCGAGUC-3′, i.e. exactly similar to the coding strand except at the place of thymine (T) there will be uracil (U).

101 (*d*) In the options provided except *sn*RNA, which is used for splicing, all types of RNA, i.e. *m*RNA, *t*RNA and RNA are required for the formation of polysome during translation. Polysome or polyribosomes are a cluster of ribosomes that bound to *m*RNA during protein synthesis.

105 (*b*) According to the diagram given in the question only part that is correctly labelled is *C*, i.e. lagging strand because replication in lagging strand is opposite to leading strand with short Okazaki fragments being formed which later gets linked together.

106 (*b*) If the codon GGU is reversed, the resulting codon will be UGG, that codes for Trp (Tryptophan), GGU codes for Gly (Glycine).

108 (*a*) II and III are the correct pairs of combinations.

^{15}N isotope was used by Meselson and Stahl to experimentally determine the semiconservation method of DNA replication. S^{35} isotopes take part in protein synthesis, that is why it is also called as protoplasmic element.

109 (*b*) On this basis balance, the probability of minimum number of nucleotides in.

Singlet code = $(4) \times 1 = 4$

Doublet code = $4 \times 4 = 16$

Triplet code = $4 \times 4 \times 4 = 64$

Here, the code given in quadruplet (GAAT)

So, it will be $4 \times 4 \times 4 \times 4 = 256$ number of nucleotides.

112 (*b*) Statement I is false, but II is true.

Incorrect statement can be corrected as

The primary transcript contains both introns and exons and are non-functional. Therefore, they undergo a process of splicing for removing introns and joining exons in the proper order. It will further undergo post-transcriptional modifications, i.e. capping and tailing. After which a fully processed *hn*RNA is now called *m*RNA, is transported out of the nucleus for translation.

114 (*d*) If non-sense mutation occurs in *lac y*-gene on that time it forms only Z cistron and when Z cistron is translated it form β-galactosidase.

115 (*c*) UGA, UAG and UAA are three non-sense codons which do not code for any amino acid. If in a gene encoding a polypeptide of 50 amino acids, 25th is mutated for UAA then the chain will terminate at that place because it will become difficult to bring amino acid from amino acid pool. Hence, a polypeptide of 24 amino acids will be formed.

121 (*a*) By using synthetic DNA, Khorana *et. al.* prepared chains of polyribonuclotides with known repeated sequence of two or three nucleotides as poly CUC UCU CUC UCU.

Here, two codons repeated alternately. This dictates the formation of polypeptide chain having two amino acids alternatively, i.e. serine and leucine.

122 (*a*) Statement in option (a) is correct.

Lac operon is an inducible operon in which the presence of key metabolic substance, i.e. lactose induces transcription of structural genes.

Rest statements are incorrect and can be corrected as

- *Lac* operon consists of three structural genes.
- Tryptophan operon is a repressible operon, where repressor is inactive and it becomes active as DNA binding proteins complexed with corepressor.

123 (*c*) Option in statement (c) is true.

The enzyme reverse transcriptase is involved in the synthesis of *c*DNA (complementary DNA) from RNA by a process called reverse transcription. It was discovered by Temin and Baltimore. The presence of this enzyme changed the central dogma of protein synthesis into reverse DNA directly. It does not act as template for protein synthesis, but first synthesises *m*RNA which acts as template for protein synthesis.

130 (*c*) During post-transcriptional process, capping involves the addition of an unusual nucleotide, called methyl Guanosine Triphosphate (*m*GTP) to the 5′ end of *hn*RNA.

CHAPTER 09

Human Genetics

The basic principles of inheritance are equally applicable to man. However, human genetics cannot be studied like plants and animals. This is mainly because of the absence of controlled selective breeding, limited number of offsprings, long reproductive span, multiple traits, high percentage of heterozygosity in traits and modifying effects of diet and environment.

Sir Archibald Garrod (1909) was the first person to study human genetics, as he was the first person to link the black urine disease, alkaptonuria to a recessive Mendelian factor. Therefore, Garrod is also known as the **Father of Biochemical Genetics** and **Father of Human Genetics**.

In this chapter, we will deal with various aspects of human genetics including sex-determination, various human genetic disorders, pedigree analysis, etc.

HUMAN KARYOTYPE

The term 'karyotype' refers to the total chromosome complement of a cell. It represents the full set of chromosomes of a cell arranged with respect to size, shape and number. The diagrammatic representation of a karyotype in decreasing order of chromosomes is called **idiogram**.

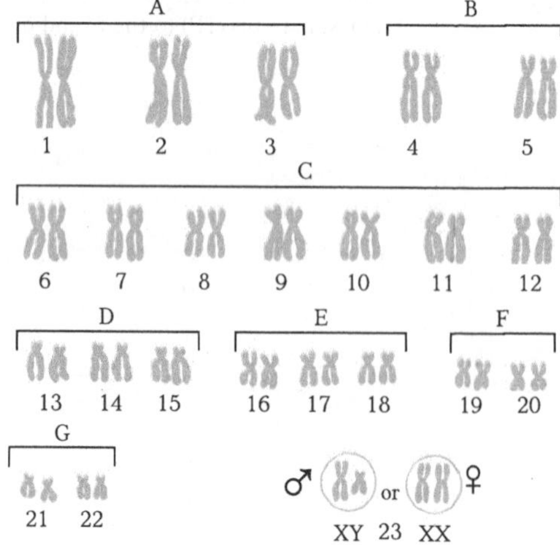

Fig. 9.1 Human karyotype (Male and female)

Human karyotypes are prepared from the nuclei of cultured white blood cells that are frozen at the metaphase stage of mitosis.

Inside

In this process, photographs of the chromosomes are arranged on a grid so that the homologous pairs are placed together. The homologous pairs are identified by their general shape, length and the banding pattern produced by a special staining technique. Idiograms of human male and female karyotypes are shown in figure 9.1.

Table 9.1 Characteristics of the chromosomes in human karyotype

Groups	Sizes	Shapes	Numbers in set
A.	Large	Metacentric, submetacentric	1-3
B.	Large	Submetacentric	4-5
C.	Medium	Submetacentric	6-12 and X
D.	Medium	Acrocentric	13-15
E.	Small	Submetacentric	16-18
F.	Small	Metacentric	19-20
G.	Smallest	Acrocentric	21-22 and Y

The **male karyotype** has 44 autosomes, a single X-chromosome and a Y-chromosome (44+XY), whereas the **female karyotype** shows two X chromosomes (44 + XX).

SEX-DETERMINATION IN HUMANS

As we know, the human females are homogametic and males are heterogametic.

Thus, females produce only one type of eggs, each with 22 autosomes and one X-chromosome. In contrast, males produce two types of spermatozoa, 50% with X-chromosome and 50% with Y-chromosome, in addition to 22 autosomes.

Inheritance

- Sex is determined at the time of fertilisation by the sperm that fertilises the egg.
- Y-chromosome bearing sperms produce male zygotes and X-chromosome bearing sperms produce female zygotes.
- So, X-chromosome bearing sperms are also called **gynosperms** and Y-chromosome bearing sperms are also called **androsperms**.
- Since, X-carrying and Y-carrying sperms are produced in 1:1 ratio, the average ratio of women and men in human population is 1:1.

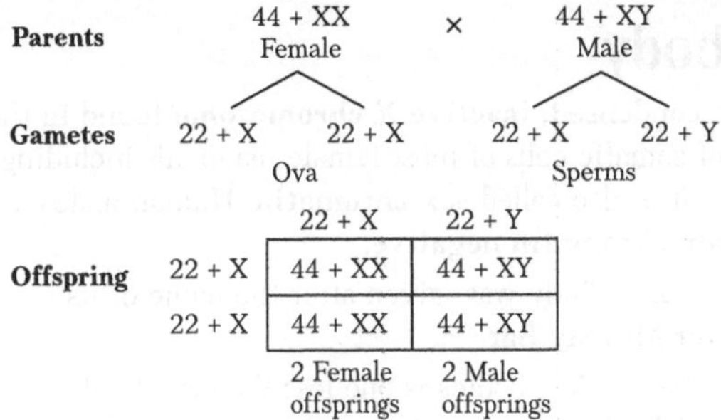

Fig. 9.2 Determination of sex in human beings

Process

- The key to sex-determination in humans is the **Sex-determining Region Y** (SRY) gene located on the short arm of the Y-chromosome.
- In the male, the Testis Determining Factor (TDF) is produced by SRY on the Y-chromosome.
- TDF induces the medulla of the embryonic gonads to develop into testes.
- In the absence of SRY on Y-chromosome, no TDF is produced.
- Lack of TDF allows the cortex of the embryonic gonads to develop into ovaries.
- If testes do not differentiate till the 6th week of embryonic life, the gonads differentiate into ovaries. Thus, female is a default sex. Diagrammatic representation of complete process is given below

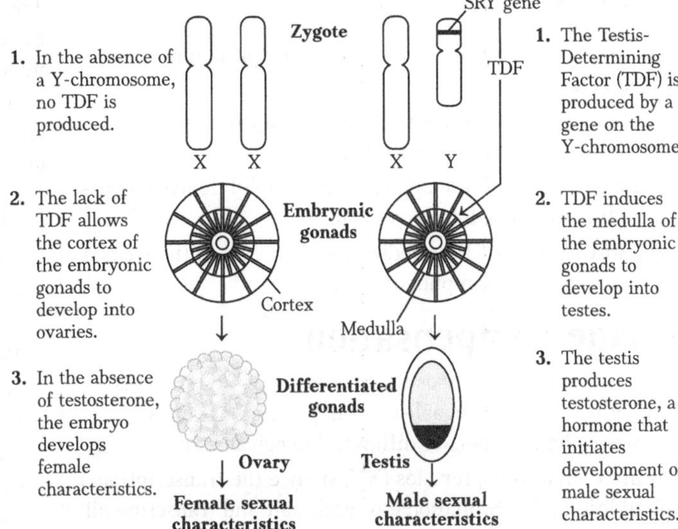

Fig. 9.3 Process of sex-determination in human beings

The functioning of male and female sexes in humans is closely associated with Barr bodies and dosage compensation phenomena.

Barr body

- It is the condensed, **inactive X-chromosome** found in the nuclei of somatic cells of most female mammals including humans. It is also called **sex-chromatin**. Human males are called **sex-chromatin negative**.
- The name Barr body was given after the name of its discoverer **Murray Barr**.
- The number of Barr bodies is one less than the total number of X-chromosomes present in an organism.
- A relation of X-chromosome number and Barr body number is given in the table below

Table 9.2 Chromosome number and number of Barr body

Chromosome numbers	Numbers of X chromosome (N)	Numbers of Barr body (N–1)
45, XY	1	0
45, X	1	0
46, XX	2	1
45, XXY	2	1
47, XXX	3	2
48, XXXY	3	2
48, XXXX	4	3
49, XXXXY	4	3

- These can be observed in the skin, oral epithelium and blood cells.
- Barr bodies appear as a circular, disc-shaped chromatin attached to the cell nuclear membrane.
- In a blood smear, these appear in neutrophil (leucocytes) as a small **drumstick** like projection.
- The justification of Barr bodies can be given on the basis of dosage compensation phenomenon.

Dosage compensation

- It is a term that describes the process by which humans and other mammals equalise the expression of genes between the members of different biological sexes.
- In these organisms, females (XX) silence the transcription of additional X-chromosome of each pair and transcribe all informations from the other expressed X-chromosome.
- This is done naturally to compensate the dose of X-chromosome products in all individuals irrespective to the number of X-chromosomes present in them.

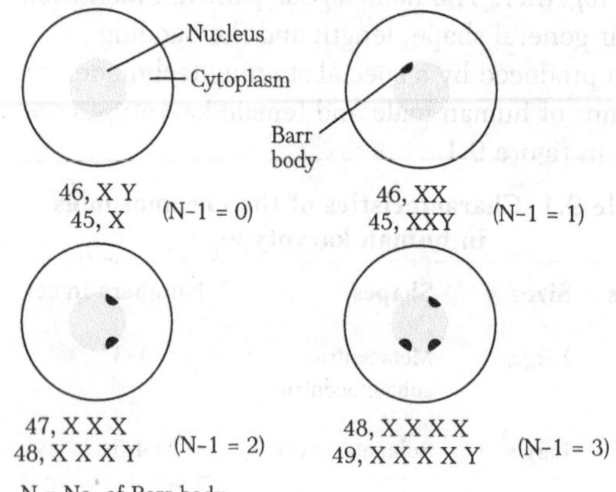

Fig. 9.4 Chromosome variations and Barr body

SEX-LINKED INHERITANCE

- In previous chapter, we have already studied about sex-linked, sex-limited and sex-influenced traits.
- In humans, inheritance of sex-linked traits can be studied by taking examples of sex-linked genetic disorders or diseases.
- The genes of sex-linked inheritance may be present on X-chromosome, Y-chromosome or on a homologous pair of both XY-chromosomes.

1. X-linked inheritance

The sex-linked disorders which are caused by recessive gene are located on the X-chromosome. These affect the males more than the females because there is no homologue of this gene present on the Y-chromosome to check its expression. Among these, the major ones are given below

(i) Inheritance of colour blindness

- **Dalton** first reported this disease in 1798. The sex-linked transmission of this disease was described by **Horner** in 1876.
- **Wilson** described the connectivity of this disease with X-chromosome in 1911.
- In this disease, the eyes of patients fail to distinguish red and green colours.
- Colour blindness is an X-linked recessive trait because the gene for the formation of colour sensitive cone cells are present on X-chromosome.

- The X-chromosome related inheritance of colour blindness is given below

Case I When a normal woman marries a colourblind man, all her sons and daughters would have normal colour vision, but when her daughters marry men with normal colour vision, some colourblind sons are born.

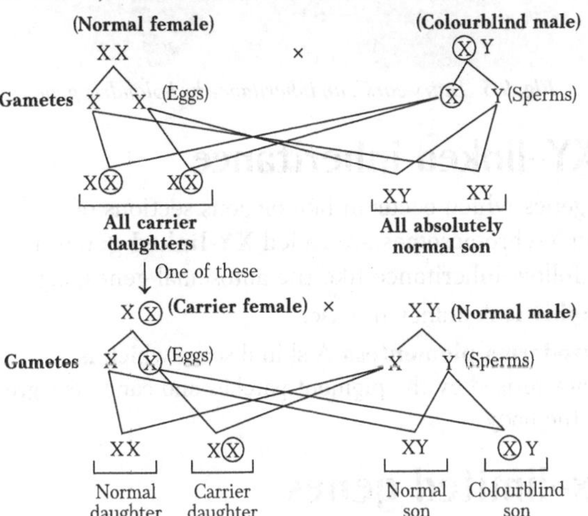

Conclusion The cross clearly indicates that if a woman with normal vision, whose father was colourblind, marries a normal man, then 50% of her sons will be colourblind and 50% of her daughters will be carriers.

> ### *Criss-cross* inheritance
> The recessive X-linked genes have characteristic of *criss-cross* inheritance. For example, male transmits his X-linked genes to his grandson through his daughter (**diagynic**) while a female transmits the traits to her grand daughter through her son (**diandric**).

Case II When a colourblind woman marries a normal man, all her sons show colour blindness and all her daughters have normal vision. But when these daughters marry a colourblind man, 50% of their sons as well as daughters are colourblind.

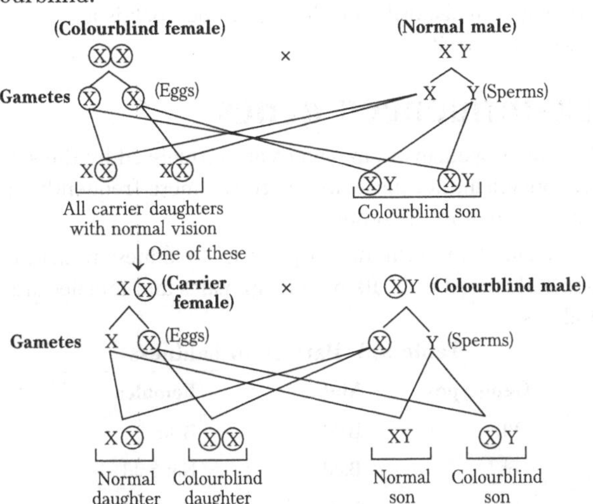

Conclusion The cross clearly indicates that if a woman with normal vision, whose mother was colourblind marries a colourblind man, 50% of her sons as well as daughters will be colourblind. Among the rest, 50% of their daughters will be carriers and sons will be absolutely normal.

Note
- *The inability to visualise red colouration is called **protanopia**, inability to visualise green colour is called **deuteranopia** and inability to visualise blue colouration is called **tritanopia**.*
- *Congenital colour blindness is called **dichromatism** or **daltonism**.*
- *Kalmus (1965) and Keats (1983) demonstrated two genes **protan** and **deutan** of X-chromosome responsible for red-green colour blindness.*

(ii) Inheritance of haemophilia

- It is also called **Bleeder's disease** and it is also a X-linked recessive disease.
- This disease was first studied by **John Otto** in 1803. It follows exactly same pattern of inheritance as colour blindness. The only difference here is that, the **haemophilic females do not survive**, i.e. the condition is lethal for females. It may be because of heavy blood loss even during menstruation.
- Likewise, the chances of homozygous girl being born in random mating are very low because the frequency of haemophilic male is about 1 in 10000.
- The most famous pedigree of haemophilia was discovered by **Haldane** in several interrelated **Royal families** of Europe. This had apparently arisen from a mutation in one parent of Queen Victoria of England (1819-1901).
- Haemophilia is of following types
  (a) **Haemophilia-A** It is characterised by the lack of **antihaemophilic globulin** (factor VIII) required for normal blood clotting. About 4/5th of the cases of haemophilia are of this type.
  (b) **Haemophilia-B** or **'Christmas disease'** It results from a defect in Plasma Thromboplastin Component (PTC or Factor IX).
  (c) **Haemophilia-C** or **Rosenthatl syndrome** It occurs due to the deficiency of clotting factor XI, i.e. Plasma Thromboplastin Antecedent (PTA). It is comparatively milder and rarer than haemophilia-A and B. In a patient of haemophilia, blood is deficient of thromboplastin, which is an important blood clotting factor.

(iii) Inheritance of night blindness

- It is also a recessive X-linked disorder and more common in males.
- Females become nightblind only when they receive defective two genes. Males suffer by the disease even by having a single gene for the defect.

- It is of following two types
  (a) **Congenital night blindness** It is caused due to visual purple deficiency that interferes with the functioning of the retinal rods.
  (b) **Acquired night blindness** It is not caused due to vitamin-A deficiency. It is not inherited like red-green colour blindness.

(iv) Inheritance of Duchenne muscular dystrophy

- In this disease, the mutated gene on X-chromosome is unable to produce a protein called **dystrophin.**
- This protein is believed to relay the nerve signals to the calcium storage organelle in the muscle cell.
- Due to its absence, calcium is not released from the muscle cells thus, leading to inhibition of muscle contraction.
- Hence, this disorder causes deterioration of muscles at an early age. Most patients are confined to wheel chairs by the age of 10 and they generally die by the age of 20.

(v) Inheritance of G-6-PD deficiency syndrome

- This disease is caused by the deficiency of **Glucose-6-Phosphate Dehydrogenase** (G-6-PD), which is essential for carrying out hexose monophosphate shunt.
- In the absence of G-6-PD, haemoglobin crystallises and erythrocyte membrane ruptures. Favism (allergy to fava beans) and certain drugs induce haemolysis in G-6-PD deficient persons.

2. Holandric or Y-linked inheritance

- In humans, the Y-chromosome is less than half of the length of X-chromosome and slightly longer than the smallest autosome. In most species, it possesses very few genes.
- Since, Y-chromosome is very small and does not contain many genes so, the Y-linked diseases are very rare. However, Y-chromosome deletions are frequent cause of male infertility.
- The tip of short arm of Y-chromosome is homologous to the tiny region at the tip of short arm of X-chromosome. This region contains at least two simply inherited traits. The rest of the part of Y-chromosome is called **non-homologous** part and the genes present on it are called **holandric genes**. These genes are inherited straight from father to son.
- About 17 genes are present on the Y-chromosome of humans, out of which gene for **hypertrichosis**, i.e. long hair growth on ear is the most common one.
- Other examples include porcupine skin, Testis Determining Factor (TDF), etc.

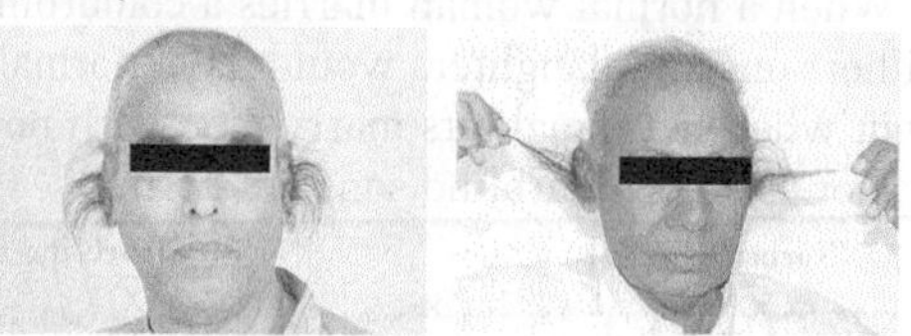

Fig. 9.5 'Hairy ears', an inheritance by holandric gene

3. XY-linked inheritance

The genes which occur in homologous sections of X and Y-chromosomes are called **XY-linked genes** and they follow inheritance like the autosomal genes, e.g.

- **Nephritis** A kidney disease.
- **Xeroderma pigmentosa** A skin disease which is characterised by the pigment patches and cancerous growth on the body.

Sex-limited genes

These genes are present on autosomes, but their expression is determined by the presence or absence of one or more sex hormones. Hence, their expression is limited to one sex only. For example,

- Beard development, deep voice and stout musculature are the characters which limit themselves in males.
- Similary, feminine voice, breast development and feminine musculature are the female limited characters.
- In man, some more traits have been considered as sex-limited, e.g. **premature baldness**, i.e. baldness in twenties and thirties. It is suggested that the premature baldness is controlled by certain genes that are expressed only in the presence of certain levels of androgenic hormones. This level is never attained in females, but can be reached easily in males.
- Among animals, brilliant plumage in peacock is a sex-limited trait.

Sex-influenced genes

- In some organisms, some genes are influenced by the sex of the organism, i.e. these are expressed more frequently in one sex than in the other.
- For example, inheritance of pattern of baldness in man is a sex-influenced trait. Its pattern in males and females are as follows

Table 9.3 Pattern of baldness

Genotypes	Males	Females
BB	Bald	Bald
Bb	Bald	Not bald
bb	Not bald	Not bald

- In comparison to sex-limited traits, here the frequency of expression is different. However, both (sex-limited as well as sex-influenced) are concerned with autosomes.
- It simply seems that the baldness pattern is dominant in male while it is recessive in female.
 Other examples of sex-influenced traits are as follows
  - **Forelock** areas of skin which completely lack pigment.
  - Absence of upper lateral incisor teeth.
  - **Hare lip**, a fissure in upper lip.
  - **Cleft palate**, a fissure in roof of mouth.
  - Stuttering involuntary repeats of letter or words.
  - Short index finger are more common and more severely influenced in human males.

Among other animals, horns in sheeps and spotting in cattle are considered as sex-influenced traits.

BLOOD GROUP INHERITANCE

- On the basis of antigens located on the surface of RBCs, several dozen blood groups have been defined.
- Each blood group system is determined by a set of different genes. These are as follows

ABO blood groups

Karl Landsteiner in 1900 identified three types of blood groups in humans, i.e. blood groups A, B and O.

Bernstein in 1925, discovered the inheritance of blood types A, B, AB and O. A set of three multiple alleles on the chromosome 9 is responsible for these four blood types. These four phenotypes are the result of the various combinations of three ABO alleles, i.e. I^A, I^B and i.

These combinations may give rise to following six genotypes.

Genotypes	Blood types	Antibodies present
I^AI^A	A	Anti-B
I^Ai	A	Anti-B
I^BI^B	B	Anti-A
I^Bi	B	Anti-A
I^AI^B	AB	None
ii	O	Anti-A and Anti-B

Inheritance

- Both I^A and I^B are dominant to i.
- Thus, blood group A will be expressed if the genotype is either $I^{A/A}$ or $I^{A/i}$.
- Similarly, blood group-B will be expressed if the genotype is either I^B/I^B or $I^{B/i}$.
- Heterozygous I^A/I^B individuals express blood group AB.
- People homozygous for the recessive i allele possesses blood group O.

***Note** AB blood group was discovered by **de Castello and Steini**.*

Codominance in ABO blood group

- The ABO blood group is a good example of codominance. Heterozygous I^A/I^B individuals have blood group AB.
- The antigen A (product of the I^A alleles) and the antigen B (product of the I^B alleles) are codominant.
- An individual who expresses blood group O, must possess i/i genotype. Each parent would have to be either homozygous for allele i or heterozygous, with i as one of the two alleles. Thus, blood group O could be obtained in following situation.
  (i) Both the parents are O (i /i× i /i)
  (ii) A ($I^{A/i} \times I^{A/i}$) or B ($I^{B/i} \times I^{B/i}$) to produce one fourth (i/i progeny)
  (iii) one could be A and one could be B ($I^{A/i}$ / $I^{B/i}$)

MN blood group system

- It is a blood group system found in humans, where antibodies are absent, but antigens are present.
- This blood group system was discovered by **Landsteiner** and **Levine** in 1927.
- They found that antigen M, N or both MN are present on the surface of RBC of human beings.
- No antibodies are however, formed in the blood plasma for these antigens.

Rh blood groups

- Rh-factor was first reported in RBCs of *Macaca* rhesus (rhesus monkey) by **Landsteiner** and **Wiener** in 1940.
- Individuals having Rh-factor are called **Rh positive**, while those lacking Rh-factor are called **Rh negative**.
- Apart from rhesus monkey, the Rh-factor is also found in humans. The percentage of Rh positive people in India is 97% of the population.

Inheritance

- The inheritance of Rh groups consists of at least three genes (C, D and E) located on the chromosome 1.
- Each of these have two alleles (C, c; D, d and E, e) thus, making a large number of genotypic combinations possible.
- The antigens formed by genes C and E are weak, i.e. they make only minimal immune response.
- Individuals of genotypes DD or Dd are said to be Rh positive (Rh^+) and those of genotype dd are said to be Rh negative (Rh^-).

CHECK POINT 9.1

1. A human showing two Barr bodies in the somatic cells would be
   (a) Only a male with one X-chromosome
   (b) Only a female with two X-chromosomes
   (c) Only a male having two Y-chromosomes
   (d) Either a male or a female having three X-chromosomes
2. A marriage between normal visioned man and colourblind woman will produce, which of the following types of offsprings?
   (a) Normal sons and carrier daughters
   (b) Colourblind sons and carrier daughters
   (c) Colourblind sons and 50% carrier daughters
   (d) 50% colourblind sons and 50% carrier daughters
3. A woman has a haemophilic son and three normal children. Her genotype and that of her husband with respect to this gene would be
   (a) XX and X^hY (b) X^hX^h and X^hY
   (c) X^hX^h and XY (d) X^hX and XY
4. How can a female be nightblind?
   (a) Both parents normal
   (b) Father normal, mother carrier
   (c) Father colourblind, mother carrier
   (d) Father colourblind, mother normal
5. The trait which is not influenced by sex is
   (a) hare lip (b) forelock
   (c) premature baldness (d) cleft palate
6. Parents with blood group O will have children with blood groups
   (a) A and O in ratio 1 : 4
   (b) Only O
   (c) B and O in the ratio of 1 : 4
   (d) A and B in equal ratio

METHODS USED TO STUDY HUMAN GENETICS

The study of human genetics is done by using the following methods

Pedigree analysis

Pedigree is a chart showing the record of inheritance of certain genetic traits for two or more ancestral generations of an individual.

Pedigree analysis helps in knowing the possibility of the presence of a trait in homozygous or heterozygous state in a particular offspring. During pedigree analysis, following points are to be kept in mind

- Inheritance of genes follows Mendelian principles.
- There are linkages and crossing overs.
- The principle of probability and chance of difference should always be taken into consideration.
- Various alternatives are thought and eliminated.

Some common symbols used in pedigree analysis are given below

Symbols	Used for	Symbols	Used for
□	Male	[siblings symbol]	Siblings
○	Female	[dizygotic twins symbol]	Dizygotic twins
◇	Sex designated or unspecified	[monozygotic twins symbol]	Monozygotic twins/Identical twins
[□][○]	Adopted	[no offspring symbol]	No offspring
◇ with p	Pregnancy	[arrow symbols]	Patient initiating genetic workup (proband, index case, consultand)
[deceased symbols]	Deceased	□+○—□	Two matings
■ ●	Affected with trait	[recessive allele symbols]	Recessive allele
[half-shaded symbols]	Carrier for trait	[half-shaded] or [half-shaded]	Heterozygous condition is sometimes shown by solid or darkening in half of the symbol
⊙	Carrier for X-linked trait	[still death symbol]	Still death
□—○	Mating	[divorced symbol]	Divorced or Separated
□═○	Consanguineous mating	□+○	Miscarriage or SAB

Note
- Roman numerals–Generation
- English numerals–Different members of one generation,
- Horizontal line between symbols–Parents
- Horizontal line above the symbols–Offspring
- Vertical line–Progeny
- SAB-Spontaneous Abortion.

Importance of pedigree analysis

- Pedigree analysis is important to know the possibility of a recessive allele which may create disorders like haemophilia, colour blindness, thalassemia, etc., in the progeny.
- It is used for studying inheritance of human traits like polydactyly (extra digits), syndactyly (fused digits) and brachydactyly (short digits), etc.
- It may indicate the usefulness or harmfulness of marriage between close relatives.
- It is used for genetic counselling.
- It is extensively used in medical research.

Population genetics

- The study of distribution and changes of allele frequency in a population is called **population genetics.**
- It uses various principles of probability and statistical tools.
- For autosomal dominant-recessive relationship, Hardy-Weinberg equation is applied directly, which is $(p+q)^2 = 1$

Twins

- These are two offsprings produced within the same pregnancy.
- These are born as a case during multiple births.
- The number of births may be three (triplets), four (quadruplets), five (quintuplets) or even more.

Types of twins

Following types of twins are of usual occurrence

(i) **Monozygotic twins**

- These twins are also known as **identical twins.**
- These twins arise when two blastomeres resulting from first cleavage of zygote completely separate from each other and develop into independent embryos.
- These twins possess similar sex and genotype.
- The identical twins possess 100% of the genes in common except for an occasional mutation.
- They provide an excellent opportunity to distinguish the effects of environment and heredity on the expression of trait.
- Similar traits in identical twins are considered as **hereditary** and the features in which they differ are regarded as **environmental traits.**

(ii) **Dizygotic twins**

- These twins are also known as **fraternal** or **non-identical twins.**
- These are produced by simultaneous fertilisation of two different eggs by two different sperms.
- These twins may either have same sex or different sexes and vary genetically. These twins are common in cattle like cow, sheep, goat, etc.
- The fraternal twins have an average 50% of their genes in common, like other siblings.

(iii) **Siamese twins**

- These twins are also known as **conjoint twins.**
- These twins can be monozygotic (more often) or dizygotic.
- The separation of these twins is incomplete and these are born attached and remain so even after.
- About one out of each 500 pairs of twins born may be joined together completely or in part.

Free Martins

- In cows and buffaloes, twins develop frequently.
- But sometimes in them, the placenta of the two dizygotic twins with opposite sexes develop blood vascular connections.
- Through this connection, the male hormones produced by male one are passed to the other female twin.
- They suppresses the differentiation of female twin internal organs, thereby making the female sterile.
- This sterile female mammal with masculinised behaviour and non-functioning ovaries is known as a free-martin. Its karyotype shows cells with XX/XY chromosomes.

HUMAN GENETIC DISORDERS

- Genetic disorders are defects that are caused by any genetic mechanism like Mendelian genes, multifactor genes, chromosomal aberrations and anomalies.
- In 1902, **Sir Archibald Garrod** and **William Bateson** scanned human population and found that several human disorders seem to be inherited like Mendelian genetics.

Some of the better known hereditary diseases along with the number of chromosome on which their genes are located are shown below

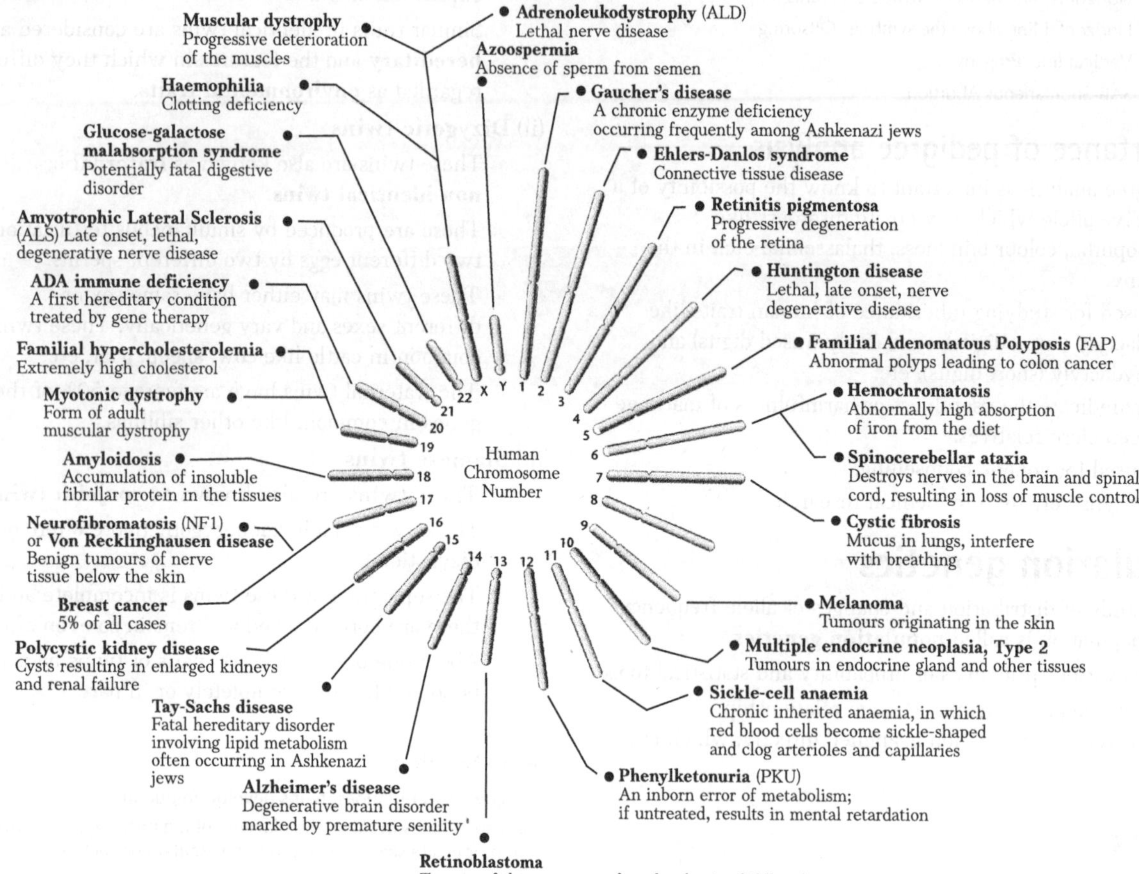

Fig. 9.6 The chromosomes of human being, showing the location of genes whose abnormal forms cause some of the better known hereditary diseases. Those inherited conditions that can be diagnosed using DNA analysis are indicated by (•)

Human genetic disorders can have following categorise

(i) **Human genetic disorders due to chromosomal abnormality**
  - (i) Autosomal disorders/abnormalities
  - (ii) Sex chromosomal disorders/abnormalities

(ii) **Human genetic disorders due to genic abnormality**
  - (i) Due to gene mutation in autosomes.
  - (ii) Due to gene mutation in sex chromosomesm, as discussed previously in the topic sex-linked inheritance.

Disorders due to chromosomal abnormality

- These genetic disorders are caused due to the absence or excess or abnormal arrangement of one or more chromosomes.
- These disorders are not inherited like Mendelian traits.
- Types of human genetic disorders due to chromosomal abnormality are as follows

I. Autosomal disorders/ Abnormalities

These genetic disorders arise due to abnormalities in autosomal chromosome number. Major ones among them are as follows

1. Down's syndrome (Mongolism, Mongolian idiocy, 21-trisomy)

- **Langdon Down** first reported Down's syndrome in 1866, but its cause was found by **Lejeune** in 1959.
- It is caused due to the presence of an extra chromosome number 21. The condition is seen because both the chromosomes of 21 position pass into a single egg due to non-disjunction.

- Thus, the egg instead of possessing 23 chromosomes, have 24 chromosomes and offspring has 47 chromosomes, i.e. 45+XY in male and 45+XX in female instead of 46. That is why, this syndrome is also known as **21-trisomy**.
- The women around 45 yrs of age are more likely to produce children having Down's syndrome as the incidence of non-disjunction is more common in aged women.
- The children born with Down's syndrome display following symptoms.
  - small round head
  - protruding furrowed tongue
  - permanently open mouth
  - broad hands with stubby fingers, protruding lower lip
  - flattened nasal bridge, broad forehead and Mongolian eyes
  - Gonads and genitalia are generally undeveloped low intelligence, short stature, defective heart and other organs and short life.

2. Patau's syndrome (13-trisomy)

- **Klaus Patau** reported this disorder in 1960.
- This syndrome is caused due to an extra chromosome number 13.
- It occurs in about 1 in 5000 live births.
- The affected person shows abnormalities such as polydactyly, mental retardation, anomalies in dermal pattern, small head and abnormalities of face, eye, low set deformed ears, small chin, cleft lip, cleft palate, etc.
- Death usually occurs within hours or days.

3. Edward's syndrome (18-trisomy)

- **John Hilton Edward** described Edward's syndrome in 1960. This disorder is caused due to an extra chromosome number 18.

  Thus, total number of chromosomes is 47.
- Females are mostly affected as compared to males.
- The frequency of this abnormality is about 1 per 500 live births.
- The affected person keeps the fingers tightly clenched against the palm of the hand.
- The patient is mentally retarded.
- The person is seen with long, but narrow skull, small face, short digits webbed neck, corneal opacity, deafness, small jaws, small sternum and pelvis.

4. Cri-Du-Chat (Cat cry) syndrome (5-monosomy or partial monosomy)

- This disorder was first described by **Lejeune** in 1963 in France.
- It is a very rare syndrome.
- The affected newborn cries-like mewing of a cat. This condition is caused due to a deletion in the short arm of the chromosome number 5.
- The patients have microcephaly, increased distance between eyes, moon face, severe mental deficiency, cat-like cry of neonate, small head and receding chin.

II. Allosomal (Sex-chromosomes) disorders/Abnormalities

- These are the genetic disorders which arise due to non-disjunction of sex chromosome during gametogenesis.
- This leads to abnormal number of sex chromosomes in the gametes.

These are as follows

1. Turner's syndrome

- **Henry H-Turner** first described this condition in 1938.
- The affected individual possesses 45 chromosomes (44 + OX) instead of 46. One in every 3000 children is a victim of Turner's syndrome.
- Such persons are sterile females who have
  - rudimentary ovaries
  - undeveloped breasts
  - short stature
  - small uterus
  - abnormal intelligence
  - do not ovulate or menstruate.

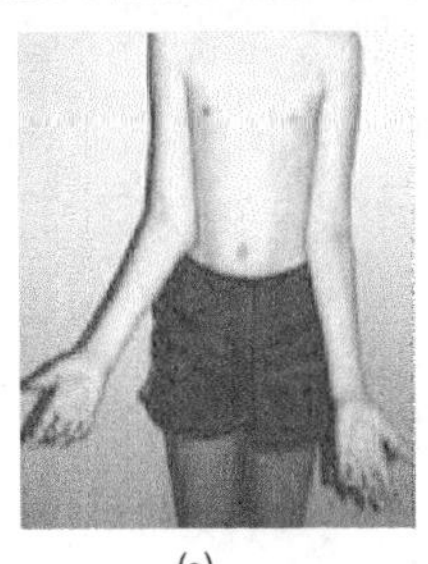

(a)

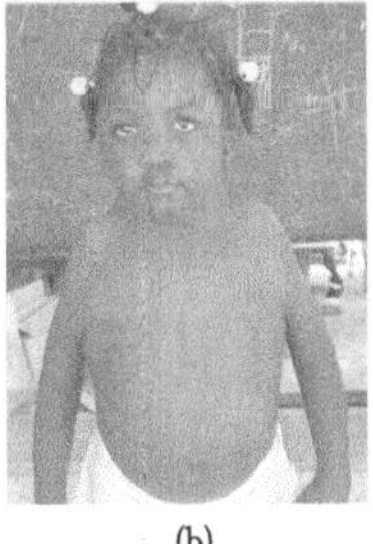

(b)

Fig. 9.7 Turner's syndrome, (a) Note the marked cubitus valgus, (b) Note the webbing of the skin in neck region

2. Noonan Syndrome (NS)

- This syndrome is used to be referred to as the male version of Turner's syndrome and is still sometimes described in this way.
- The genetic causes of Noonan syndrome and Turner syndrome are distinct.
- The syndrome is named after **Dr. Jacqueline Noonan**.
- The chromosomal complement of Noonan syndrome is 44+YO (45).

- The principal features include
  - congenital heart defect (typically pulmonary valve stenosis)
  - hypertrophic cardiomyopathy
  - short stature
  - learning problems
  - pectus excavatum, i.e. sinking of breast bone into chest
  - impaired blood clotting
  - a characteristic configuration of facial features including a webbed neck and a flat nose bridge.

3. Klinefelter's syndrome

- **HF Klinefelter** first described this condition in 1942.
- This genetic disorder occurs by the union of an XX egg and a normal Y sperm or normal X egg and abnormal XY sperm.
- The individual has 47 chromosomes (44 + XXY).
- Phenotypically these individuals are males, but they may show female secondary sexual characters and are usually sterile.
- Their important characteristics are
  - small testes
  - azoospermia
  - increased urinary elimination of gonadotropin
  - sparse body hair
  - long limbs
  - enlarged breasts (gynaecomastia)
  - feminine pitched voice

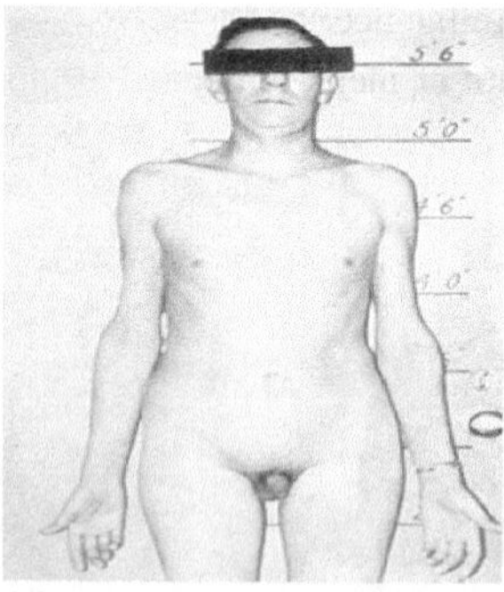

Fig. 9.8 Klinefelter's syndrome

Note *The superficially normal male genitalia, gynaecomastia and feminine distribution of the pubic.*

4. Poly X-females or Superfemales

- Superfemales have 47 (44+XXX), 48 (44+XXXX) or 49 (44+XXXXX) chromosomes.
- These females have abnormal sexual development and mental retardation.
- The symptoms become more severe with the increase in the number of X-chromosomes.

5. Jacobs syndrome or Supermales

- **PA Jacobs** gave details of this condition in 1965.
- These individuals have 47 (44+XYY) chromosomes.
- Males have characteristic abnormal tall height, criminal bent of mind and mental retardation.
- They have an over production of male sex hormone.
- These males are more aggressive than normal males.

Disorders due to genic abnormality

- These disorders are determined by mutations in a single gene.
- They are transmitted to the offspring as per Mendelian inheritance so, these diseases are also called **Mendelian human disorders.**

Diseases due to gene mutations in autosomes

These are of two types, i.e. **recessively inherited traits** and **dominantly inherited traits**. Some of these genetic disorders are given below

1. Phenylketonuria (PKU)

- In 1934, **A Folling** discovered this autosomal recessive mutation of gene on chromosome 12.
- This abnormal recessive gene causes the deficiency of liver enzyme, phenylalanine hydroxylase that converts phenylalanine into tyrosine.
- It causes the accumulation of phenylalanine to potentially toxic level in the body.
- The affected babies are normal at birth, but within a few weeks, there is rise in plasma phenylalanine level which inhibits the development of brain.
- Usually, by six months of life, severe mental retardation is evident.
- The affected person's muscles and cartilages of the legs become defective thus, the person experience inability to walk.

2. Alkaptonuria

- It was described by **Garrod** in 1908.
- Alkaptonuria is a recessive gene disorder. It is caused due to the deficiency of an **oxidase enzyme** required for the breakdown of **homogentisic acid.**
- This enzyme is also called **alkapton**, hence the disease is called alkaptonuria.
- In patients of alkaptonuria, homogentisic acid accumulates in the tissues and is also excreted in the urine.

- The most commonly affected tissues are cartilages, capsules of joints, ligaments and tendons.
- The urine of these patients, if allowed to stand for some hours in air, turns black due to the oxidation of homogentisic acid.

3. Neurofibromatosis (NF)

- This disease is also known as **Von Recklinghansen disease**.
- It is caused by a dominant gene on chromosome 17.
- The affected person may have ten spots on the skin which may later on increase in number and size.
- Neurofibromas (small benign tumours) grow in the nervous system.

4. Albinism

- It is an autosomal recessive mutation, caused due to deficiency of **tyrosinase enzyme**. It is a copper containing enzyme involved in the production of melanin.
- This enzyme normally converts the amino acid tyrosine to melanin through an intermediate product DHPA (**Dihydroxyphenylalanine**).
- The albino person cannot synthesise melanin which provides white or blonde colour to the skin and hair.
- In humans, there are two principal types of albinisms
  (a) **Occulocutaneous** affecting the eyes alongwith skin.
  (b) **Hair and ocular** affecting the eyes only.

5. Galactosemia

- This disease was first described by **Friedrich Goppert** in 1917.
- It is inherited as an autosomal recessive trait. The affected person is unable to convert galactose to glucose.
- This disease is caused due to the deficiency of the enzyme **Galactose-1- Phosphate Uridyltransferase** (GPUT).
- Milk is toxic to galactosemic infants and child usually dies at or near the age of 3 years.

6. Marfan's syndrome

- This disorder is caused due to dominant mutation resulting in the production of abnormal form of connective tissues and characteristics extreme looseness of joints.
- The long bones of the body grow longer and fingers become very long called **spider fingers** or **arachnodactyly**.
- The lenses in the eyes become displaced.

7. Gaucher's disease

- In this disease, the metabolism of fatty acid is impaired.
- This results in accumulation of lipid materials in the body tissues and blood.
- It is caused by a recessive gene which inhibits the activity of an enzyme, **glucocerebrosidase**.
- Consequently, there is accumulation of cerebroside (a sphingolipid).
- Enlargement of the spleen and some limb bones also occurs in this disease.

8. Tay-Sachs disease (TSD)

- This disease is named after scientists **Warren Tay** who first reported it in 1881 and **Bernard Sach** who later on described the first pathological description of the disease in 1887. Tay-Sachs disease is also called **infantile amaurotic idiocy.**
- It is a rare autosomal recessive gene disorder.
- In this disease, there is absence of a gene on the chromosome 15 that encodes for **hexosaminidase-A enzyme.**
- Due to the absence of this enzyme, a fatty substance or lipid called **ganglioside** accumulates abnormally in cells, especially in the nerve cells and causes progressive damage to the cells.
- Children with Tay-Sachs disease are born normal, but develop severe brain and spinal cord damage later due to the disorder in fat metabolism.
- Individual with this disease die at the age of 2-4 yrs.
- These is no cure for this disease and hence, there is no surviver.

9. Sickle-cell anaemia

- It is a genetic disorder caused by a defective allele (Hb^A) on chromosome 11 which produces β-chain of adult haemoglobin. In defective haemoglobin, **glutamine at 6th place of β-chain is replaced by valine.**
- In homozygous condition, the disorder kills the individual. However, in heterozygous condition, it leads to haemolytic anaemia under conditions of oxygen deficiency.
- The red blood cells of such individuals become elongated and curved to become sickle-shaped and do not transport oxygen efficiently. They are further removed by spleen, thus causing severe anaemia.
- Genetically, the heterozygous condition is represented by Hb^A and Hb^S.

  Hb^A represents normal haemoglobin, while Hb^S represents modified haemoglobin. The inheritance of these genes follow normal Mendelian approach.

10. Huntington's disease/Huntington's chorea

- It is a dominant autosomal disorder caused due to an allele on short arm of chromosome 4.
- It produces an inhibitor of brain cell metabolism.
- The symptoms of this disease may start at the age of 15-40 yrs, but can also occur in older persons.

- The symptoms include atrophy in the parts of brain resulting in respiratory irregularity, faulty articulation of speech, irregular arrhythmic movement of limbs, etc.

11. Thalassemia

- This disorder is caused due to the reduced synthesis of either α or β-chains of haemoglobin, likewise the disease is designated as α or β-thalassemia.
- β- thalassemia was first described by **Cooley**. Hence, it is also called **Cooley's anaemia** or **thalassemia major**.
- The reduced synthesis of β-chains leads to the accumulation of α-chains which cause damage to the precursors of red blood corpuscles in the bone marrow.
- Person homozygous for the β-thalassemia gene on chromosome 11 suffer from severe haemolytic anaemia.
- Heterozygous persons are also not normal, but exhibit the defect in a less severe form called **thalassemia minor**.
- α-thalassemia is controlled by two genes, i.e. HBA2 and HBA1 on chromosome 16.

12. Alzheimer's disease

- It is a chronic neurodegenerative disorder.
- It is caused by the accumulation of amyloid protein plaques in the brain resulting in the degeneration of neurons.
- It is common in Down's syndrome (21 trisomy) patients.
- The gene for the **Amyloid Precursor Protein** (APP) is present on chromosome 21.
- Various other genes are also linked to Alzheimer's disease, but these genes only predict the susceptibility to disease.
- This disease is characterised by dementia, i.e. mental deterioration, leading to loss of memory.
- It is common in the age group of 65 years and above.

13. Cystic Fibrosis (CF)

- The disorder was formarly called **mucoviscidosis.**
- It is a recessive autosomal disorder which arises due to the alleles present on chromosome 7.
- People with cystic fibrosis have elevated levels of sodium and chloride ions in the sweat. It is due to the failure of chloride ion mechanism in the body.
- This further causes the accumulation of thick mucus in lungs and airways, leading to blockage and secondary infection.
- In most cases of cystic fibrosis, there is impairment of pancreatic and liver functions. This disorder is common in Caucasian population.

14. Taste blindness of PTC

- This is a genetic trait not a disease, discovered by **Fox** in 1932.
- PTC (Phenyl Thiocarbamide) is a compound of nitrogen, carbon and sulphur with sour taste.
- About 30% of the people lack the ability to taste PTC which is transmitted by a dominant gene T.
- The genotypes TT and Tt are tasters of PTC, while tt are non-tasters or tasteblind persons.

GENOMICS

- The term was coined by **Thomas Roderick** in 1986.
- It is the study of genomes through analysis, sequencing and mapping of genes and non-cistronic areas with the study of their functions.
- It is comparatively a new branch of biology. The study of genomics is classified into following 3 classes
  - (i) **Structural genomics** which involves mapping and sequencing of genomics.
  - (ii) **Functional genomics** which involves identification of the function of a particular gene.
  - (iii) **Application genomics** which involves the use of genomics information for crop improvement.

Human Genome Project (HGP)

- Human body is made up of about 100 trillion cells grouped into over 260 types.
- Every cell contains the same number of chromosomes and the same kind of genome.
- With the establishment of genetic engineering techniques, a very ambitious project of sequencing human genome was launched in the year 1990.
- The project was completed with the help of automated DNA sequencing machines in 2003.
- The project was coordinated by US Department of Energy and National Institute of Health. Additional contributions came from UK, Japan, France, Germany, China and others.

Goals of HGP

The objectives of HGP are as follows

- Mapping the whole human genome at the level of nucleotide sequences.
- To store the information gathered from the project in databases and develop tools for data analysis.
- To solve any Ethical, Legal or Social Issue (ELSI) which may arise from the project.

Methodologies

Two major approaches were taken in the project as follows

(i) First approach was focussed on identifying all the genes that were expressed as RNA. These genes were referred as **Expressed Sequence Tags** (ESTs).

(ii) Other approach took a blind approach of simply sequencing the whole set of genome that contained the coding and non-coding sequence. The functions to different regions in this sequence were assinged afterwards. This was referred as **sequence annotation**.

- For sequencing, total DNA of the cell was isolated through techniques like electrophoresis and converted into random fragments (RFLP) of relatively smaller sizes. Then, these were cloned in suitable host using specialised vectors and suitable techniques like **PCR**.
- The cloning resulted into amplification of each piece. The commonly used hosts were bacteria and yeast. The vectors used were **BAC**, i.e. Bacterial Artificial Chromosome and **YAC**, i.e. Yeast Artificial Chromosome.
- Resulting fragments were sequenced by using automated DNA sequencers. These sequencers work on the principle of the methodology developed by **F Sanger**.
- The resulting sequences were then arranged based on some overlapping regions present in them. For this overlapping, sequences were generated. For alignment of these sequences, specialised computer based programmes were developed. An outline of this procedure is given below

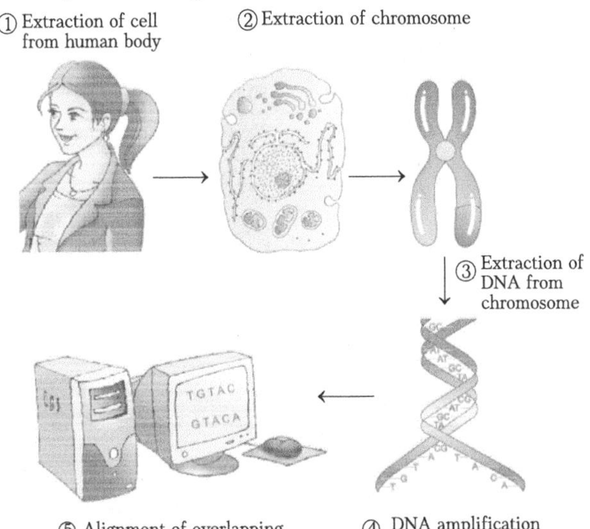

Fig. 9.9 A representative diagram of human genome project

- The sequence of human chromosome 1 was completed in May, 2006. This was last to be completed of the 24 chromosome. In this project, 22 autosomes, one X and one Y-chromosome were sequenced.
- For assigning genetic and physical maps of the genome information, polymorphism of restriction endonuclease recognition sites and some repetitive DNA sequences or microsatelites were used.

Salient features of HGP

These are as follows

- The human genome contains about 3.2 billion base pairs. Fruitfly (*Drosophila melanogaster*) has 132 million base pairs. This is 1/24 of the total length of the human genome.
- HGP has found out that the human genome carries about 30000-40000 genes. The number is the same as present in mouse and double the number of genes in fruitfly.
- The size of genome or number of genes is unrelated with the complexity of body organisation. Lily plant has 18 times more DNA than human genome. Inspite of this fact, lily produces fewer proteins than human beings.
- Chomosome 1 has most genes (2968 genes) and the Y has fewest (231 genes).
- Eukaryotes contain mostly split genes having long non-coding areas or introns. Further, not more than 10% of the genome contains coding areas or exons. The remaining DNA is non-coding having either pseudogenes or repeated sequences.
- The part of DNA which contains repeated sequences is called **satellite DNA**. This satellite DNA is of several types. One of them is moderately repetitive sequences of 150-300 base pairs. They include transposons and *Alu* elements. **Minisatellite sequences** are 11-60 base pairs long hypervariable repeat sequences. They are VNTRs used in DNA fingerprinting. Over a million copies of Simple Sequence Repeates (SSR) or microsatellites occur in the genome. They have 5-8 base pairs. These repeated sequences are called **junk DNA**.
- About 99.9% of DNA of human population is identical, so that genomically, all human beings are exactly the same.
- The length of different human genes varies widely. Generally, it is over a few thousand base pairs in length. β-globin and insulin genes are less than 10 kilo base pair long. The **longest gene of human body is that of Duchenne Muscular Dystrophy on X-chromosome**. It is 24000 kilo base pair long. The **smallest gene is that of Testis Determining Factor** (TDF), a holandric gene (present on Y-chromosome). It is only 14 base pairs long.

Prospects and implications of HGP

Prospects and implications of HGP are as follows

- Studying the genes that will cause reversion of cancerous cells to normal cells.
- It will be possible to study interactions between various genes.
- It holds promise of healthier and longer living, designer drugs and genetically modified diets according to the needs of individual human beings.
- There are more than 1200 genes that cause common cardiovascular ailments, endocrine diseases like diabetes, Alzheimer's disease and other neurological disorders, cancers, etc. After taking their snapshots, it will be possible to know the method to alter them and remove the possibility of the disorders.
- Single gene defects produce a number of hereditary diseases. Their exact location, reason for defect and method of correcting the same can be found out.

SOME USEFUL BRANCHES OF GENETICS

These include eugenics, euthenics, euphenics and genethics.

Eugenics

- A British scientist **Sir Francis Galton** in 1883 coined the term eugenics.
- Galton is known as the **'Father of Eugenics'**. This branch of science deals with the improvement of human race genetically.
- Eugenics can be divided into two types
  (i) **Positive eugenics** in which future generations are improved by encouraging the inheritance of better or desired traits.
  (ii) **Negative eugenics** in which reproduction of people having defective or undesirable traits is restricted.

Euthenics

It is the science associated with improvement of human race by improving the environmental conditions such as better nutrition, unpolluted ecological conditions, education and sufficient amount of medical facilities. So, in other words, we can say that it is the science of learning to live well.

Euphenics

It is the science of making phenotypic improvements to humans after birth. The term euphenics was given by **AC Pai** in 1974 for symptomatic treatment of human genetic disease especially, inborn errors of metabolism.

Genethics

It is the study of ethical issues that arise out of the science of genetics and the uses of genetic technologies.

Intelligence Quotient (IQ)

The ratio between actual (chronological) age and mental age multiplied with 100 is known as **Intelligence Quotient** or IQ.

So, it is the mental competence in relation to the chronological age in humans.

$$IQ = \frac{\text{Mental age}}{\text{Actual age}} \times 100$$

Different levels of Intelligence Quotient (IQ)

Categories	IQ
Genius	140 or more
Superior	110-139
Average	90-110
Ordinary	80-90
Dull	70-80
Moron	50-70
Imbecile	25-50
Idiot	0-25

CHECK POINT 9.2

1. Identify the correct choice for given symbols (*A* and *B*)

(a) *A*–Consanguineous mating, *B*–Mating
(b) *A*–Mating, *B*–Mating between relatives
(c) *A*–Mating, *B*–Consanguineous mating
(d) Both (b) and (c)

2. Monozygotic twins are born because
(a) two sperms fertilise four ova
(b) two sperms fertilise two ova
(c) two blastomeres separate after first cleavage
(d) None of the above

3. Free Martin condition is observed in
(a) dizygotic twins
(b) monozygotic twins
(c) Both (a) and (c)
(d) None of the above

4. Down's syndrome is related to
(a) increase in chromosome number of 21st pair
(b) decrease in chromosome number of 21st pair
(c) increase in chromosome number of 18th pair
(d) decrease in chromosome number of 18th pair

5. Cri-du-chat syndrome in humans is caused by the
(a) fertilisation of an XX egg by normal Y-bearing sperm
(b) loss of half of the short arm of chromosome 5
(c) loss of half of the long arm of chromosome 5
(d) trisomy of 21st chromosome

6. Albinism is known to be due to an autosomal recessive mutation. The first child of a couple with normal skin pigmentation was an albino. What is the probability that their second child will also be albino?
(a) 50% (b) 75%
(c) 100% (d) 25%

7. The technique/process not used in HGP was
(a) PCR (b) cloning
(c) DNA fingerprinting (d) electrophoresis

EXAM POINTS

- The heterochromatinised X-chromosome is called Barr body, it is attached with the nuclear membrane. The inactivation of X-chromosome is called lyonisation. **[EAMCET 2016]**
- X-linked recessive gene disorder describes haemophilia. **[NEET 2016]**
- A hereditary disease, which is never passed on from father to son is X-chromosomal linked disease because male has only one X-chromosome that is inherited from his mother further and passed to his daughter. **[J&K CET 2012]**
- More men suffer from colour blindness then women because men are hemizygous and one defective gene is enough to make them colourblind. **[Karnataka CET 2011]**
- Colour blindness and haemophilia are caused by two genes located on X-chromosome, both are X-linked recessive traits. **[WB JEE 2012, Odisha JEE 2012]**
- Double line in pedigree analysis shows consanguineous marriage. **[Karnataka CET 2015]**
- Down's syndrome is characterised by 21 trisomy. **[Chhattisgarh PMT 2015, AMU 2015]**
- Karyotype of Down's syndrome has 47 chromosomes. **[JIPMER 2019]**
- Non-disjunction in meiosis results in trisomy. **[JIPMER 2018]**
- A disease caused by an autosomal primary non-disjunction is Down's syndrome. **[NEET 2017]**
- An abnormal human baby with 'XXX' sex chromosomes is born due to the formation of abnormal ova in the mother. **[AMU 2015]**
- Down's syndrome is an example of aneuploidy of autosome. **[Karnataka CET 2014]**
- The human female with Turner's syndrome has 45 chromosomes with XO. **[CBSE AIPMT 2014]**
- Klinefelter's syndrome is the genetic disorder in which an individual has an overall masculine development, gynaecomastia and is sterile. **[NEET 2019]**
- Gynaecomastia is seen in Klinefelter's syndrome. **[JIPMER 2019]**
- Person suffering from Klinefelter's syndrome have 44A + XXY chromosome setup. **[EAMCET 2015, RPMT 2014]**
- In Klinefelter's syndrome, each cell in the affected person has three sex chromosomes XXY. **[NEET 2019]**
- The best example of pleiotropy is phenylketonuria. **[NEET 2020]**
- Phenylketonuria is a recessive hereditary disease caused due to deficiency of liver enzyme, phenylalanine hydoxylase which convert phenylalanine into tyrosine. **[Kerala CEE 2014, AIIMS 2018]**
- In sickle-cell anaemia, substitution of glutamic acid molecule by valine molecule takes place at position 6 of the β-chain of haemoglobin. **[Chhattisgarh PMT 2015, Karnataka CET 2014, Kerala CEE 2014]**
- The gene of sickle-cell anaemia is inherited by autosomes. **[WB JEE 2013]**
- Cri-du-chat syndrome in human is caused by the loss of half of the short arm of chromosome 5. **[UP CPMT 2015]**
- In α-thalassemia, the gene HBA1 is located on the chromosome 16. **[EAMCET 2014]**

Chapter Exercises

(A) Topical Exercise

Human Karyotype, Sex-Determination and Sex-linked Inheritance

1 Consider the following statements.
I. Garrod is known as Father of Human Genetics.
II. Karyotype represents full set of chromosome.
Choose the correct option.
(a) Statement I is true, but II is false
(b) Statement I is false, but II is true
(c) Both statements I and II are true
(d) Both statements I and II are false

2 Consider the following statements.
I. Barr bodies in human is one less than the total number of X-chromosomes.
II. Human males are sex-chromatin negative.
Choose the correct option.
(a) Statement I is true, but II is false
(b) Statement I is false, but II is true
(c) Both statements I and II are true
(d) Both statements I and II are false

3 Dysgenics is the study of
(a) evolution in man
(b) improving human race
(c) chromosomal mutations
(d) undesirable traits of the human race and the gene causing them

4 What all are the chances of colourblind daughters and sons being born in a marriage of normal man marrying a normal woman whose father was colourblind?
(a) All sons are normal and daughters are colourblind
(b) Both the sons and daughters are phenotypically normal
(c) Both the sons and daughters are colourblind
(d) 50% of sons are colourblind and all daughters are phenotypically normal

5 Gene for colour blindness is located on
(a) Y-chromosome (b) 13th chromosome
(c) X-chromosome (d) 21st chromosome

6 A colourblind girl is rare and can be born when
(a) her father is colourblind and mother has normal vision but her mother's father (maternal grandfather) is colourblind
(b) her mother is colourblind, even if father has normal vision
(c) even when both her parents have normal vision provided the grand parents were colourblind
(d) her mother is colourblind and her father had normal vision, but her paternal grandfather (father's father was colourblind)

7 Parents are colourblind. What is the phenotype of grandsons in F_2-generation?
(a) 50% colourblind and 50% normal
(b) All normal
(c) All colourblind
(d) All are carriers

8 If both parents of a male child are normal, what are the chances of the child being colourblind?
(a) It is impossible
(b) It is possible only if mother's father was colourblind
(c) It is possible only if father's mother was colourblind
(d) It is possible even when all the four grandparents have normal vision

9 Which is incorrect about colour blindness?
(a) This is due to defect in either red or green cone of eye resulting in failure to discriminate between red and green colour
(b) A daughter will not normally be colourblind, unless her mother is a carrier and her father is colourblind
(c) If female has X^CX then it is called carrier, but when male has X^CY then it will be colourblind
(d) The son of a woman who carries the gene has 25% chance of being colourblind

10 Mr. Phillips is colourblind. What is the probability of his male child inheriting this disease from him?
(a) 100% (b) 25% (c) 50% (d) 0%

11 Men are usually colourblind than women because
(a) man suffers from vitamin-A deficiency
(b) Y-chromosome in man has the genes for this character
(c) genes are located on sex-chromosomes
(d) character is dominant in men and recessive in women

12 Haemophilia, an X-linked recessive disease is caused due to the deficiency of
(a) blood plasma and vitamin-K
(b) blood platelets and haemoglobin
(c) lack of clotting material and vitamin-K
(d) All of the above

13 The daughter born to haemophilic father and normal mother could be
(a) normal (b) carrier
(c) haemophilic (d) None of these

14 If a boy's father has haemophilia and his mother has one gene for haemophilia, what is the chance that the boy will inherit the disease?
(a) 100% (b) 50% (c) 0% (d) 75%

15 Mary's father has haemophilia and her husband is also haemophilic. What is the chance of her daughter having this disease?
(a) 0% (b) 50% (c) 100% (d) 25%

16 It is normally impossible for a
(a) haemophilic father to pass the gene to his son
(b) carrier mother to pass the gene to her son
(c) haemophilic father to pass the gene to his daughter
(d) carrier mother to pass the gene to her daughter

17 Of a normal couple, half of sons are haemophilic and half of daughters are heterozygous. The genes for this disease in couple are located on
(a) Both X-chromosomes of mother
(b) Y-chromosomes of father
(c) One X-chromosome of mother and X-chromosome of father
(d) Both sex chromosomes of the father

18 One child is haemophilic (sex-linked trait), while its fraternal twins brother is normal. Which one of the following informations is most appropriate?
(a) Haemophilic child is male
(b) The other child is female and the father is haemophilic
(c) Child is monozygotic twin
(d) The mother must have been heterozygous

19 A woman with two genes, one for haemophilia and one for colour blindness on one of its X-chromosome, marries a normal man. The progeny will be
(a) All sons haemophilic and colourblind
(b) 50% haemophilic and colourblind sons and 50% normal sons
(c) All daughter haemophilic and colourblind
(d) 50% haemophilic daughters and 50% colourblind daughters

20 A person whose father is colourblind marries a lady, whose mother is daughter of a colourblind man. Their children will be
(a) All sons are colourblind
(b) Some sons normal and some daughters are colourblind
(c) All sons and daughters are colourblind
(d) All daughters are normal

21 A man known to be the victim of haemophilia marries a normal woman whose father was known to be bleeder, then it may be expected that
(a) all their children will be bleeders
(b) half of their sons will be bleeders
(c) one fourth of their children will be bleeders
(d) all will be normal

22 Consider the following statements.
I. Both colour blindness and haemophilia are sex-linked recessive traits.
II. In sex-linked recessive traits, heterozygous or carrier female transmit disease to sons.
Choose the correct option.
(a) Statement I is true, but II is false
(b) Statement I is false, but II is true
(c) Both statements I and II are true
(d) Both statements I and II are false

Blood Group Inheritance

23 Consider the following statements.
I. Karl Landsteiner identified blood groups A, B and O.
II. Blood contains two types of proteinaceous substances.
Choose the correct option.
(a) Statement I is true, but II is false
(b) Statement I is false, but II is true
(c) Both statements I and II are true
(d) Both statements I and II are false

24 When both parents are of blood type AB, they can have children with
(a) A, B, AB and O blood types
(b) A, B and AB blood types
(c) A and B blood types
(d) A, B and O blood types

25 A man with type A blood married a woman, who has type AB blood. We do not know either the man is homozygous or heterozygous for the I allele. Which one of the following types in the progeny of this couple would indicate that the man is heterozygous?
(a) O (b) A (c) B (d) AB

26 Father has blood group A and mother's blood group is B. Both are heterozygous. If they have identical twins, the percentage probability of both twins having blood group A is
(a) 100% (b) 50%
(c) 25% (d) 6.25%

27 A person with type A blood group may safely receive a transfusion of
(a) type AB
(b) type AB and type O
(c) type AB and type AB
(d) type A and type O

28 In man, four phenotypes of blood groups are due to the presence of antigen 'A' and antigen 'B' on the surface of RBCs. The chromosome that has the gene to control these antigens is
(a) X-chromosome (b) 9th chromosome
(c) 7th chromosome (d) 21st chromosome

29 Consider the following statements.

I. Agglutinogens A and B are found in plasma membrane of RBC.

II. Agglutination may lead to organ failure.

Choose the correct option.

(a) Statement I is true, but II is false
(b) Statement I is false, but II is true
(c) Both statements I and II are true
(d) Both statements I and II are false

30 Which one of the following conditions is caused due to Rh-factor incompatibility?

(a) AIDS (b) Turner's syndrome
(c) Erythroblastosis foetalis (d) Sickle-cell anaemia

31 Erythroblastosis foetalis occurs

(a) when the mother is Rh negative and the child is Rh positive
(b) when the father and child both are negative, but the mother is positive
(c) when the mother and child both are Rh positive, but the father is Rh negative
(d) when the mother and father are Rh positive, but the child is Rh negative

32 A Rh^- mother carrying a Rh^+ child then

(a) antibody formed in mother's blood is transmitted against the erythrocytes of subsequent foetus
(b) the RBC of foetus destroys the antibodies present in mother's blood
(c) antigens produced in mother's blood are transmitted against the antibodies in the foetus blood
(d) antigens produced in foetus blood are transmitted against the antigens present in mother's blood

Pedigree Analysis

33 Which option is incorrect with respect to pedigree analysis?

(a) It helps to trace the inheritance of specific trait
(b) It confirms that DNA is carrier of genetic information
(c) It helps to understand the trait is dominant or recessive
(d) It confirms that the trait is linked to one of the autosome

34 Given below is a pedigree chart showing the inheritance of a certain sex-linked trait in human.

Generation - I

Generation - II

Generation - III

Unaffected male　Unaffected female

Affected male　Affected female

The trait traced in the above pedigree chart is

(a) dominant X-linked (b) recessive X-linked
(c) dominant Y-linked (d) recessive Y-linked

35 Match the following columns and choose the correct option from the codes given below.

	Column I		Column II
A.	□—○	1.	Consanguineous mating
B.	□═○	2.	Affected female
C.	◇	3.	Mating
D.	□┬○ with □ below	4.	Unaffected female
E.	○	5.	Parents with male child unaffected
		6.	Sex unspecified

Codes

	A	B	C	D	E
(a)	3	1	2	5	4
(b)	2	1	6	3	4
(c)	3	4	1	5	2
(d)	3	1	6	5	4

36 Identify the type of inheritence in the given diagram.

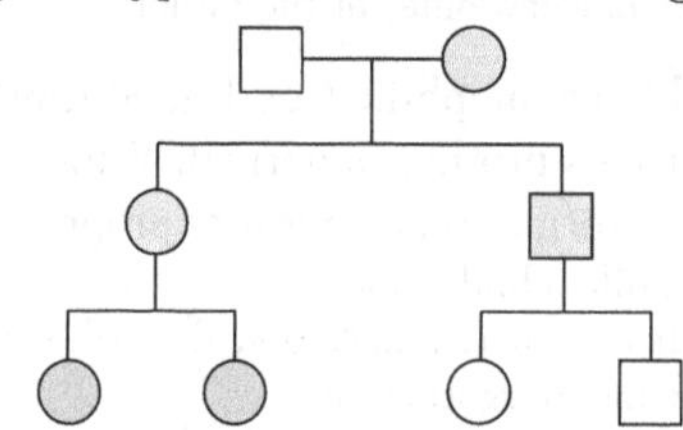

(a) dominant X-linked
(b) recessive X-linked
(c) dominant Y-linked
(d) cytoplasmic or mitochondrial inheritance

37 In this pedigree, which of the progeny is younger?

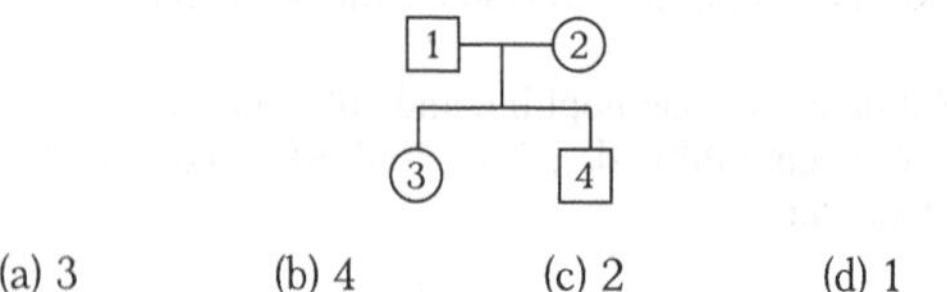

(a) 3 (b) 4 (c) 2 (d) 1

38 Given below is a pedigree chart showing the inheritance of a certain sex-linked trait in human.

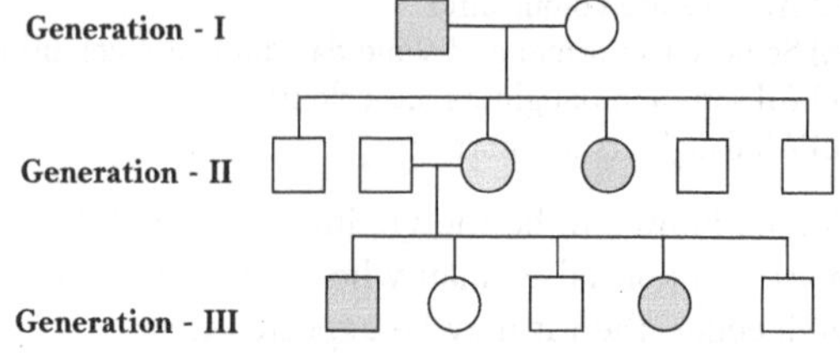

The trait traced in above pedigree is

(a) dominant X-linked (b) recessive X-linked
(c) dominant Y-linked (d) recessive Y-linked

39 Match the following column and choose the correct option from the codes given below.

	Column I		Column II
A.	Vertical line	1.	Spontaneous abortion
B.	SAB	2.	Different members of one generation
C.	Roman numerals syndrome	3.	Progeny
D.	English numerals	4.	Generation

Codes

	A	B	C	D
(a)	3	1	4	2
(b)	4	1	2	3
(c)	3	1	2	4
(d)	1	2	3	4

40 This pedigree is of a rare trait, in which children have extra fingers and toes. Which one of the following patterns of inheritance is consistent with this pedigree?

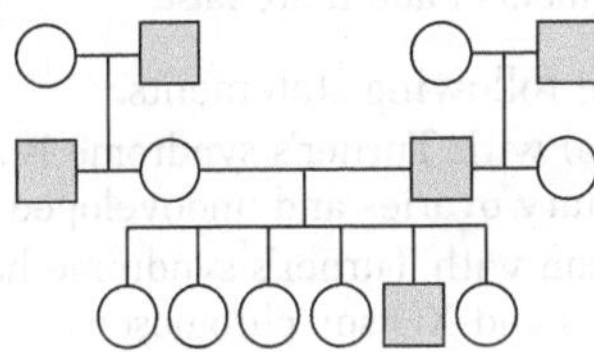

(a) Autosomal recessive (b) Autosomal dominant
(c) Y-linkage (d) Sex-linked recessive

41 Which one of the following patterns of inheritance is consistent with the pedigree? Assume that trait is rare.

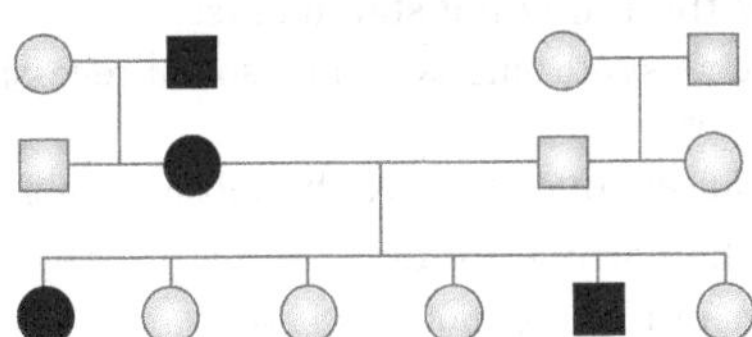

(a) Autosomal recessive (b) Autosomal dominant
(c) Y-linkage (d) sex-linked recessive

42 Given below is a pedigree chart of a family with five children. It shows the inheritance of attached ear lobes as opposed to the free ones. The squares represent the male individuals and circles the female individuals.

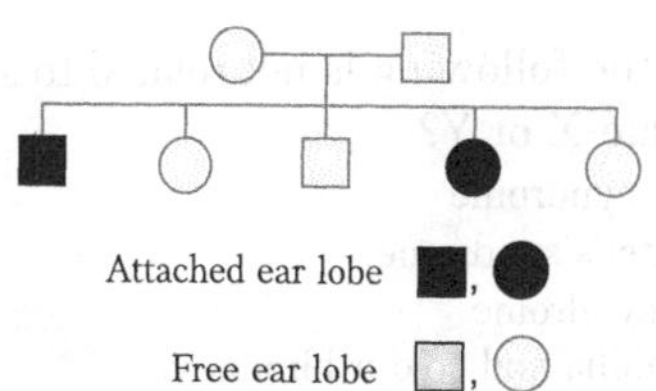

Which one of following conclusions drawn is correct?
(a) The parents are homozygous recessive
(b) The trait is Y-linked
(c) The parents are homozygous dominant
(d) The parents are heterozygous

43 From the pedigree of a family given below, it is clear that trait is inherited as dominant autosomal trait. What will be the genotype of mother and father?

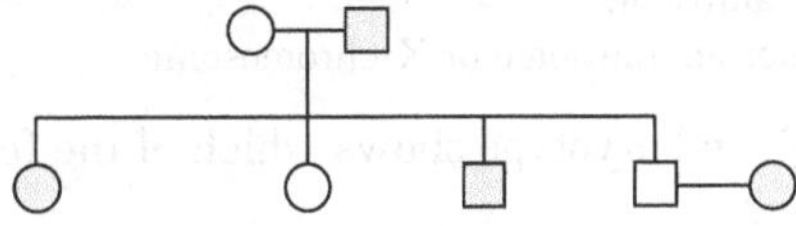

(a) Mother is aa and father is Aa
(b) Father is AA and mother is aa
(c) Father is Aa and mother is Aa
(d) None of the above

44 The diagram given below show the inheritance of haemophilia in a family. What will be the genotype of the individual marked M?

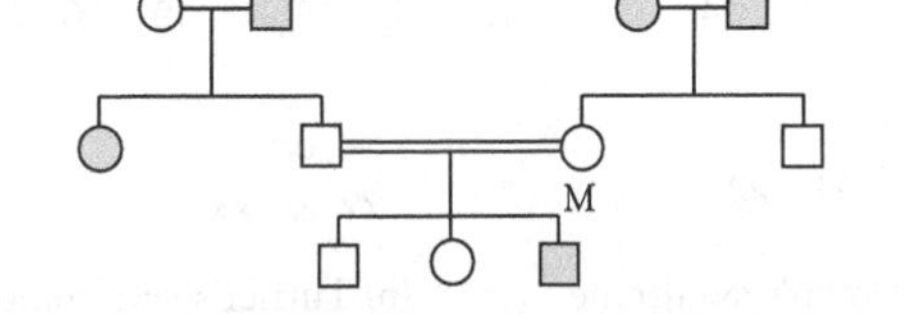

(a) M – XY (b) M – XX (c) M – X^hX^h (d) M – X^hX

45 Study the pedigree chart given below.

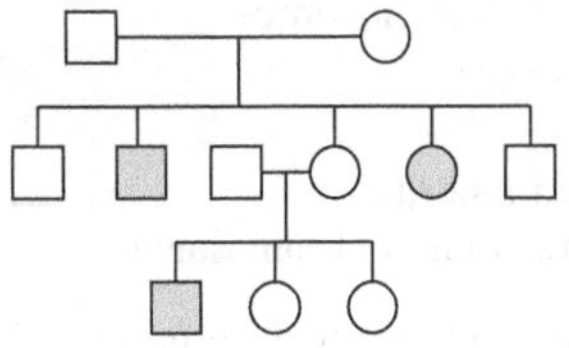

What does it show?
(a) Inheritance of a sex-linked inborn error of metabolism like phenylketonuria
(b) Inheritance of a condition like phenylketonuria as an autosomal recessive trait
(c) The pedigree chart is wrong as this is not possible
(d) Inheritance of a recessive sex-linked disease like haemophilia

46 If husband is PTC taster and wife is PTC non-taster. Their daughters are non-tasters, but their son is taster. This is not related with a sex-linked trait. Out of four a, b, c, d which pedigree is correct?

(a)
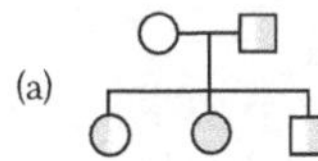

(b)
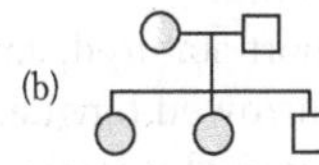

(c)
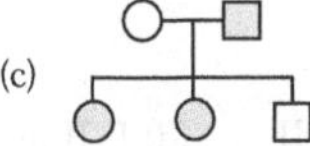

(d)
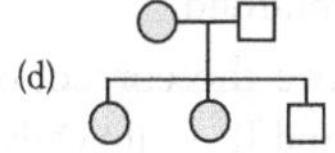

Chromosomal Disorders

47 Usually, the recessive character is expressed only when present in a double recessive condition. However, single recessive gene can express itself in human beings when the gene is present on
(a) the X-chromosome of the female
(b) the X-chromosome of the male
(c) any autosome
(d) either an autosome or X-chromosome

48 The given karyotype shows which of the following disease?

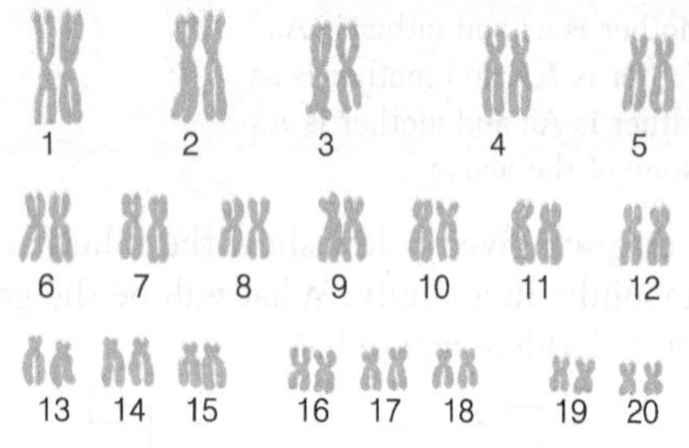

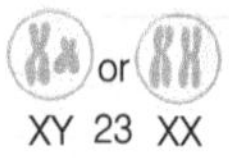

(a) Down's syndrome (b) Turner's syndrome
(c) Klinefelter's syndrome (d) Edward's syndrome

49 Which of the following mechanism is involved in causing Down's syndrome?
(a) Crossing over
(b) Linkage
(c) Sex-linked inheritance
(d) Non-disjunction of chromosomes

50 Consider the following statements.
I. Mongolism, Patau's syndrome and Edwards's syndrome are caused due to autosomal abnormalities.
II. In Down's syndrome or Mongolism, the affected person possesses an extra chromosomes.
Choose the correct option.
(a) Statement I is true, but II is false
(b) Statement I is false, but II is true
(c) Both statements I and II are true
(d) Both statements I and II are false

51 What is true for an individual from Down's syndrome?
I. Short statured, small round head.
II. Furrowed tongue, palm crease.
III. Physical psychomotor and mental development is retarded.
Choose the correct option.
(a) I and II (b) Only III (c) Only II (d) I, II and III

52 Match the following columns.

	Column I	Column II
A.	Mongolism	1. XYY
B.	Jacob's syndrome	2. 21-trisomy
C.	Patau's syndrome	3. 18-trisomy
D.	Edward's syndrome	4. 13-trisomy

Codes

	A	B	C	D		A	B	C	D
(a)	1	2	3	4	(b)	4	3	2	1
(c)	2	1	3	4	(d)	2	1	4	3

53 Consider the following statements.
I. Chromosome number in Down's syndrome is 47.
II. Epicanthus is the symptom of Down's syndrome.
Choose the correct option.
(a) Statement I is true, but II is false
(b) Statement I is false, but II is true
(c) Both statements I and II are true
(d) Both statements I and II are false

54 Consider the following statements.
I. Individual with Turner's syndrome is a female with rudimentary ovaries and undeveloped breasts.
II. The person with Turner's syndrome has 44 autosomes and XO sex chromosome.
Choose the correct option.
(a) Statement I is true, but II is false
(b) Statement I is false, but II is true
(c) Both statements I and II are true
(d) Both statements I and II are false

55 Consider the following statements.
I. Turner's syndrome is an autosomal recessive disorder.
II. I is causeal due to XXX chromosomal abnormality.
Choose the correct option.
(a) Statement I is true, but II is false
(b) Statement I is false, but II is true
(c) Both statements I and II are true
(d) Both statements I and II are false

56 Mental retardation is not related with
(a) trisomy 21
(b) phenylalanine hydrolase
(c) myelinisation of neuron
(d) additional Y-chromosome

57 Which of the following is not related to sex chromosome-X or Y?
(a) Turner's syndrome
(b) Klinefelter's syndrome
(c) Down's syndrome
(d) Haemophilia and colour blindness

58 Down's syndrome and Turner's syndrome occur in human beings due to
(a) monosomic and nullisomic conditions, respectively
(b) monosomic and trisomic conditions, respectively
(c) trisomic and monosomic conditions, respectively
(d) trisomic and tetrasomic conditions, respectively

59 Go through the given genetic disorders.
I. Down's syndrome II. Edward's syndrome
III. Patau's syndrome IV. Turner's syndrome
Which ones are due to trisomy of chromosome?
(a) I and II (b) II and III (c) I, II and III (d) Only IV

60 An abnormality in men who are always sterile due to improper development of testis because of an additional X-chromosome (47-XXY) is known as
(a) Huntington's disease (b) Marfan syndrome
(c) Klinefelter's syndrome (d) Turner's syndrome

61 Excessive growth of hair on the pinna is a feature found only in males because
(a) the female sex hormone oestrogen supresses the character in females
(b) the gene responsible for the character is present on the Y-chromosomes only
(c) the gene responsible for the character is recessive in females and dominant only in males
(d) the character is induced in males as males produce testosterone

62 The 'Cri-du-chat' syndrome is caused by change in chromosome structure involving
(a) deletion (b) duplication
(c) inversion (d) translocation

63 Which of the following abnormalities, results from an unnatural presence of a Barr body?
(a) Turner's syndrome (b) Down's syndrome
(c) Klinefelter's syndrome (d) All of the above

64 Edward's syndrome is an abnormality leading to mental deficiency caused by trisomy of chromosome number
(a) 18 (b) 9 (c) 15 (d) 5

65 Match the following columns.

Column I	Column II
A. Down's syndrome	1. An additional sex chromosome
B. Cri-du-chat syndrome	2. Loss of a part of chromosome 5
C. Klinefelter's syndrome	3. Absence of sex chromosome
D. Turner's syndrome	4. Presence of an extra chromosome
	5. Presence of two extra chromosomes

Codes

	A	B	C	D		A	B	C	D
(a)	4	2	1	3	(b)	5	4	2	1
(c)	4	2	5	3	(d)	4	2	3	1

66 Which of the following conditions in human is correctly matched with its chromosomal abnormality linkage?
(a) Down syndrome – 44 autosomes + XO
(b) Colour blindness – Y-linked
(c) Klinefelter's syndrome – 44 autosomes + XXY
(d) Erythroblastosis fetalis – X-linked

67 Spermatogenesis is absent in person suffering from
(a) Klinefelter's syndrome (b) Down's syndrome
(c) Turner's syndrome (d) Thalassemia

68 Consider the following abnormalities due to changes in sex chromosome number.
I. Turner's syndrome II. Klinefelter's syndrome
III. Cri-du-chat syndrome IV. Down's syndrome
Codes
(a) I and III (b) II and IV (c) III and IV (d) I and II

69 The chromosomal pattern of individual is shown here. This individual is suffering from

	Column I		Column II
A.	Mental retardation	1.	Down's syndrome
B.	Gynaecomastia	2.	Klinefelter's syndrome
C.	Rudimentary ovaries	3.	Phenylketonuria
D.	Partially open mouth	4.	Turner's syndrome

Codes

	A	B	C	D		A	B	C	D
(a)	1	2	3	4	(b)	4	1	2	3
(c)	3	2	4	1	(d)	3	4	1	2

70 Recognise the figure and find out the correct matching.

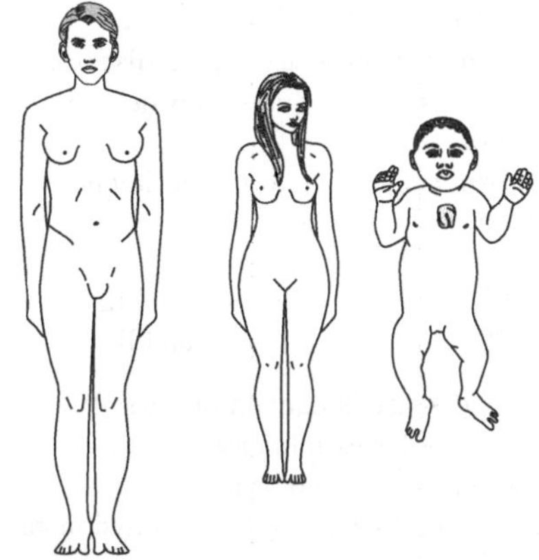

(a) A–Down's syndrome, B–Turner's syndrome, C–Klinefelter's syndrome
(b) A–Klinefelter's syndrome, B–Turner's syndrome, C–Down's syndrome
(c) A–Turner's syndrome, B–Down's syndrome, C–Klinefelter's syndrome,
(d) A–Turner's syndrome, B–Klinefelter's syndrome, C–Down's syndrome

Mendelian Disorders

71 A person is suffering from disease phenylketonuria, which is an autosomal recessive disease. Which of these is lacking in the person?
(a) Homogentisic acid (b) Phenylalanine hydroxylase
(c) Ceruloplasmin (d) Cystine

72 Consider the following statements.
I. In infants, there is rise in plasma phenylalanine level which inhibits brain development.
II. The muscles and cartilages of the affected person become defective.

Choose the correct option.
(a) Statement I is true, but II is false
(b) Statement I is false, but II is true
(c) Both statements I and II are true
(d) Both statements I and II are false

73 Which of the following is/are correct with respect to alkaptonuria?
I. This is due to accumulation of homogenetisic acid.
II. It is a recessive gene disorder.

Choose the correct option.
(a) Statement I is true, but II is false
(b) Statement I is false, but II is true
(c) Both statements I and II are true
(d) Both statements I and II are false

74 Which of the following is not a symptom of alkaptonuria?
(a) Darkening of cartilage of ear
(b) Darkening of urine
(c) Deposition of alkapton causing arthritis
(d) Convolusions and tremors

75 Which of the following is/are incorrect?
I. Albinism in man is sex-linked disease.
II. Albinism is caused due to physical mutation by radiation.
III. Albinism occurs due to the deficiency of tyrosinase enzyme.

Codes
(a) I and III (b) II and III
(c) Only III (d) I and II

76 Tay-Sachs disease is caused due to
(a) deficiency of hexosaminidase-A
(b) absence of tyrosinase enzyme
(c) absence of enzyme phenylalanine hydroxylase
(d) None of the above

77 Which of the following is true?
I. The mutant haemoglobin of sickle-cell anaemic individual undergo polymerisation under low oxygen tension causing sickling of RBC.
II. Individuals heterozygous for sickle-cell anaemia ($Hb^S Hb^A$) are resistant towards malaria.

Codes
(a) Only I
(b) Only II
(c) Both I and II
(d) None of the above

78 Sickle-cell anaemia has not been eliminated from the African population because it
(a) is controlled by recessive genes
(b) is not a fatal disease
(c) provides immunity against malaria
(d) is controlled by dominant genes

79 Which of these statements about Huntington's disease is correct?
(a) Genetic tests to detect the presence of the allele responsible for Huntington's disease do not exist at this time
(b) The onset of Huntington's disease is typically between birth and 3 yrs of age
(c) There is currently no effective treatment of Huntington's disease
(d) Huntington's disease is caused by the expression of a recessive allele

80 Phenylketonuria, Huntington's disease and sickle-cell anaemia are caused respectively due to disorders associated with
(a) chromosome 7, chromosome 11 and chromosome 12
(b) chromosome 12, chromosome 4 and chromosome 11
(c) chromosome 7, chromosome 12 and chromosome 11
(d) chromosome 4, chromosome 7 and chromosome 11

81 A woman with cystic fibrosis (an autosomal condition), marries her first cousin. What is the risk that their first child will have cystic fibrosis?
(a) 1/4 (b) 1/2 (c) 3/4 (d) 1/8

82 Read the following statements and find out the incorrect statement.
(a) Alpha thalassemia is controlled by two closely linked genes HBA1 and HBA2 on chromosome 11 of each parent and it is observed due to mutation or deletion of one or more of the four genes
(b) Beta thalassemia is controlled by a single gene HBB on chromosome 11 of each parent
(c) Beta thalassemia is also called Cooley's anaemia or thalassemia major
(d) None of the above

83 Consider the following statements.
I. Thalassemia is caused due to excess synthesis of either of α-β-chain of haemoglobin.
II. Person homozygous for β-thalassemia suffer severe haemolytic anaemia.

Choose the correct option.
(a) Statement I is true, but II is false
(b) Statement I is false, but II is true
(c) Both statements I and II are true
(d) Both statements I and II are false

Genomics

84 Who coined the term 'genomics'?
(a) Thomas Roderick
(b) Jeffreys *et. al.*
(c) Griffith
(d) All of the above

85 Consider the following statements.
I. The term genome refers to the total genetic constitution of an organism.
II. Genome is a complete copy of genetic information (DNA) or one complete set of chromosomes (haploid) of an organism.
Choose the correct option.
(a) Statement I is true, but II is false
(b) Statement I is false, but II is true
(c) Both statements I and II are true
(d) Both statements I and II are false

86 Consider the following statements.
I. Functional genomics involves, mapping, sequencing and analysis of genome.
II. Structural genomics deals with the study of functions of all gene sequences and their expression in organisms.
Choose the correct option.
(a) Statement I is true, but II is false
(b) Statement I is false, but II is true
(c) Both statements I and II are true
(d) Both statements I and II are false

87 Which of the following is the application of genomics?
(a) Genomics is used in agriculture to develop transgenic crops having more desirable characters
(b) Genetic markers developed in genomics have applications in forensic analysis
(c) Genomics can lead to introduce new gene in microbes to produce enzymes, therapeutic proteins and even biofuels
(d) All of the above

88 The full form of HGP is
(a) Human Genome Project (b) Human Gene Profile
(c) Horse Genome Project (d) None of these

89 Consider the following statements.
I. Human genome project was completed in the year 2000.
II. 4.0 million base pairs are present in human genome.
Choose the correct option.
(a) Statement I is true, but II is false
(b) Statement I is false, but II is true
(c) Both statements I and II are true
(d) Both statements I and II are false

90 Consider the following statements.
I. A field of biology explored by hGP is Eugenics.
II. The human Genome Project (hGP) was initiated in 1990.
Choose the correct option.
(a) Statement I is true, but II is false
(b) Statement I is false, but II is true
(c) Both statements I and II are true
(d) Both statements I and II are false

(B) Cumulative Exercise

(Assorted Questions of the Chapter for Advanced Level Practice)

1 A couple has 6 children, 5 are girls and 1 is boy. The percentage of having a girl on next time is
(a) 10% (b) 20% (c) 50% (d) 100%

2 Match the following columns.

	Column I		Column II
A.	Tetrasomy	1.	45 chromosomes
B.	Patau's syndrome	2.	$2n+2$
C.	Turner's syndrome	3.	Down's syndrome
D.	Mongolian idiocy	4.	Trisomy of 18 chromosome
E	Edward's syndrome	5.	Trisomy of 13 chromosome

Codes

	A	B	C	D	E
(a)	2	5	1	3	4
(b)	1	2	4	5	3
(c)	3	1	2	4	5
(d)	4	5	3	2	1

3 Observe the pedigree chart given below.

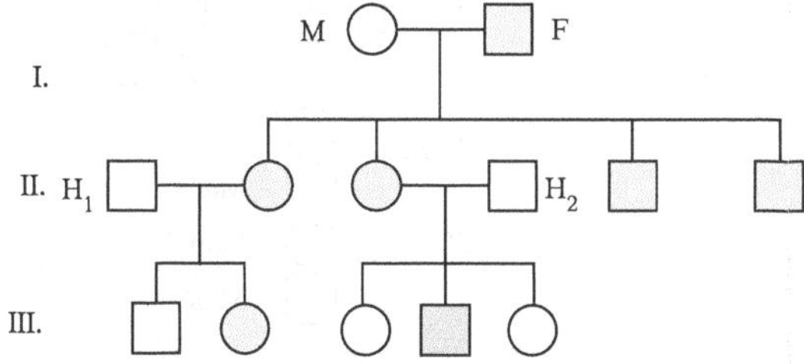

In the above pedigree, the genotypes of father (F), mother (M) in the 1st generation and husbands (H_1 and H_2) of daughters in the IInd generation are
(a) F—AA, M—AA, H_1 —Aa, H_2 —aa
(b) F—AA, M—aa, H_1—AA, H_2 —AA
(c) F—aa, M—Aa, H_1 —Aa, H_2 —Aa
(d) F—AA, M—aa, H_1 —aa, H_2 —aa

4 Choose the correct set of statements from the following.

I. Phenylketonuria is an inborn error of metabolism.
II. Haemophilia is not a congenital disease.
III. Bleeder's disease is known as Royal family disease.
IV. Dizygotic twins are common in human beings.

Codes

(a) I and II (b) II and III
(c) I and III (d) III and IV

5 Select the correct bases of DNA, RNA and amino acid of beta chain resulting in sickle-cell anaemia.

	DNA	RNA	Amino acids
(a)	CTC/GAG	GUG	Glutamic acid
(b)	CAC/GAG	GUG	Valine
(c)	CAC/GTC	GAG	Valine
(d)	CTC/GAG	GUG	Valine

6 Pick out the correct statements.

I. Haemophilia is a sex-linked recessive disease.
II. Down's syndrome is due to aneuploidy.
III. Phenylketonuria is an autosomal dominant gene disorder.
IV. Phenylketonuria is an autosomal recessive gene disorder.
V. Sickle-cell anaemia is an X-linked recessive gene disorder.

Codes

(a) I, III and V (b) I and III
(c) II and V (d) I, II and IV

7

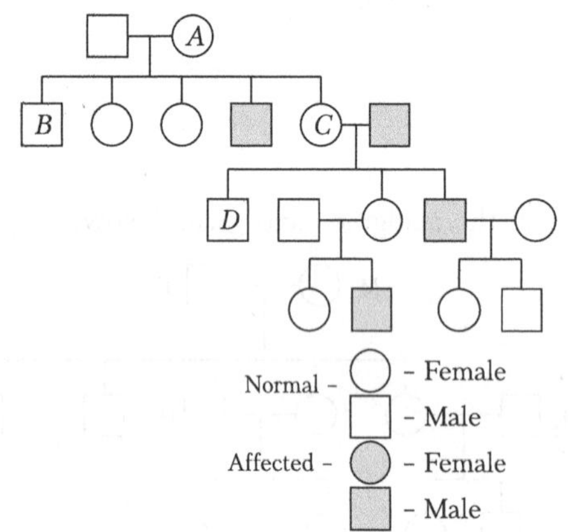

In the above pedigree, assume that no outsider marrying in, carry a disease. Write the genotypes of *C* and *D*.

(a) X^CY and X^CX^C
(b) X^CX and XY
(c) XY and X^CX^C
(d) X^CX^C and X^CX

8 Study the two cases carefully. The correct interpretation of the two cases is

Cases	Mother	Father	Children
Case I	With disease	Normal	Sons always with disease
Case II	With disease	Normal	Sons and daughters could show disease

(a) Case I - X-linked recessive disease
Case II - autosomal recessive disease
(b) Case I - Y-linked recessive disease
Case II - X-linked recessive disease
(c) Case I and II - X-linked recessive disease
(d) Case I - X-linked dominant disease
Case II - autosomal dominant disease

9 Consider the following statements.

I. Failure of segregation of chromatids during cell division results in aneuploidy.
II. Chromosomal disorders are mainly determined by alteration or mutation in a single gene.
III. Thalassemia and cystic fibrosis are Mendelian disorders.
IV. Sickle-cell anaemia is a X-linked trait.

Choose the correct option.

(a) I and III alone are correct
(b) I, III and IV alone are correct
(c) III and IV alone are correct
(d) II and IV alone are correct

10 Recognise the figure and find out the correct matching.

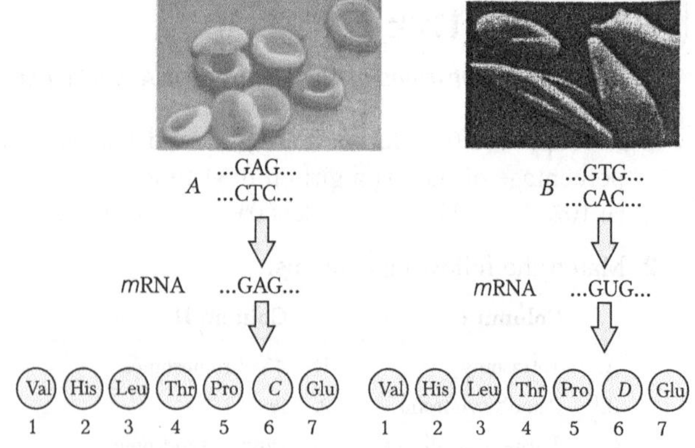

(a) *A*-Normal Hb (A) gene, *B*-Sickle-cell Hb (S) gene, *C*-Glu, *D*-Val
(b) *A*-Sickle-cell Hb (S) gene, *B*-Normal Hb (A) gene, *C*-Glu, *D*-Val
(c) *A*-Normal Hb (A) gene, *B*-Sickle-cell Hb (S) gene, *C*-Val, *D*-Glu
(d) *A*-Sickle-cell Hb (S) gene, *B*-Normal Hb (A) gene, *C*-Glu, *D*-Val,

11 Which is incorrect about thalassemia?
(a) This blood disease is transmitted from parents to the offspring when both the partners are unaffected carrier for the gene (heterozygous)
(b) The defect is due to either mutation or deletion which ultimately results in reduced rate of synthesis of one of the globin chains that makeup haemoglobin
(c) This causes the formation of abnormal haemoglobin molecule resulting into anaemia which is characteristic of the disease
(d) Thalassemia differs from sickle-cell anaemia in that the former is a qualitative problem of synthesising an incorrectly functioning globin while the latter is a quantitative problem of synthesising too few globin molecules

12 The gene for brown eyes is dominant over the gene for blue eyes. Following are given some statements.
I. For the child to be blue-eyed, at least one parent should be blue-eyed.
II. Both parents with blue eyes will have a blue-eyed child.
III. Blue-eyed person will always show both the alleles different from brown-eyed person.
IV. Identical twins of blue-eyed parents will both have either blue or brown eyes.
V. For the child to be brown-eyed, one parent should be brown eyed.

The correct statements are
(a) I, IV and V
(b) II and V
(c) II and III
(d) I and III

13 A couple got their first daughter quite normal, but the mother was unable to deliver the second child because after conception and before parturition, the embryo gets destroyed in womb. The reason may be that
(a) male and female have Rh + ve
(b) male has Rh + ve and female Rh − ve
(c) male has Rh − ve and female Rh + ve
(d) Both have Rh − ve

14 A mother with B blood group has two children, one with A blood group and other with O blood group. Her husband has O blood group. The correct sentence regarding the above data is the
(a) husband is not the father of both the children
(b) husband is the father of both the children
(c) husband must be the father of child with O blood group and may be father of child with A blood group
(d) husband could be the father of child with O blood group, but not the father of child with A blood group

15 Read the following statements and choose the correct option.
I. In phenylketonuria, the affected person does not secrete the enzyme to convert phenylalanine to tyrosine.
II. Possibility of male becoming haemophilic is extremely rare.
III. Myotonic dystrophy is an autosomal dominant.
(a) I and III alone are wrong
(b) II alone is wrong
(c) II and III alone are wrong
(d) III alone is wrong

16 In human, red-green colour blindness is recessive and sex-linked, while albinism is recessive and autosomal. A marriage between two homozygous parents, a normal visioned albino woman and a colourblind and normally pigmented man will produce children
(a) who are all phenotypically normal visioned and have normal pigmentation
(b) half of whom are colourblind and other half having normal vision and all of them having normal pigmentation
(c) all of whom have normal vision, but half of whom are albino and the other half with normal pigmentation
(d) of four categories normal visioned pigmented; normal visioned albino; colourblind, pigmented; colourblind, albino; all in equal proportions

17 A man with certain disease marries a normal woman. They have eight children (three daughters and five sons). All the daughters suffer from their father's disease, but none of the sons is affected. Which of the following mode of inheritance do you suggest for this disease?
(a) Sex-limited recessive (b) Autosomal dominant
(c) Sex-linked dominant (d) Sex-linked recessive

18 Read the following statements.
I. Mendelian disorders are mainly determined by alteration or mutation in the single gene.
II. Chromosomal disorders are caused due to the absence or excess or abnormal arrangement of one or more chromosomes.
III. Aneuploidy arises due to chromosomal non-disjunction.
IV. Sickle-cell anaemia is X-linked disorder.
V. Haemophilia is an autosomal recessive disorder.

How many of the above statements are correct?
(a) Two (b) Three (c) Four (d) Five

19 Match the human genetic disorders in Column I with the causative abnormal chromosomes in Column II.

Column I	Column II
A. Sickle-cell anaemia	1. Sex-linked (X-chromosome)
B. Colour blindness	2. Autosomal chromosome 7
C. Phenylketonuria	3. Autosomal chromosome 11
D. Cystic fibrosis	4. Autosomal chromosome 4
E. Huntington's disease	5. Autosomal chromosome 12

Codes

	A	B	C	D	E
(a)	3	5	1	2	4
(b)	5	1	2	3	4
(c)	4	1	5	2	3
(d)	3	1	5	2	4

20 Sickle-cell anaemia is an autosomal linked recessive trait that can be transmitted from parents to the offspring when both the partners are carriers for all the genes or heterozygous.

The disease is controlled by a single pair of allele, Hb^A and Hb^S. Identify *X*, *Y* and *Z*.

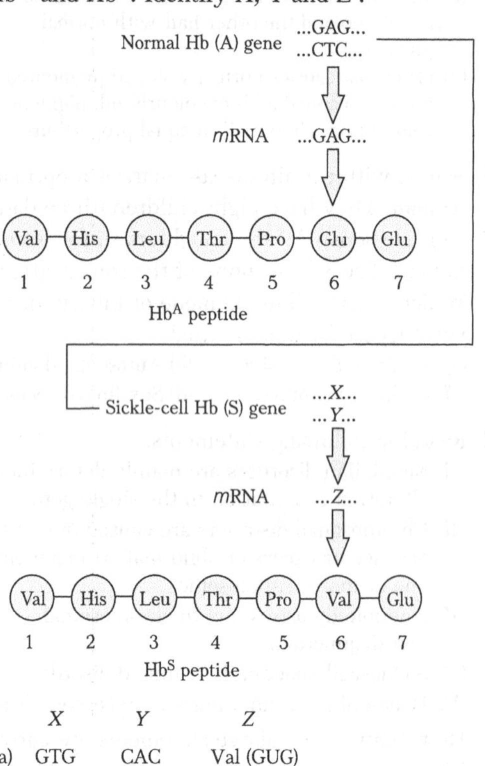

	X	*Y*	*Z*
(a)	GTG	CAC	Val (GUG)
(b)	CAC	CTC	Val (GUG)
(c)	GTA	GAG	Val (GUG)
(d)	GTC	GAC	Val (GUG)

21 One of the following is a mismatch.
(a) Down's syndrome – Autosomal aneuploidy
(b) Klinefelter's syndrome – XO complement
(c) Haemophilia – Sex-linked
(d) Turner's syndrome – Females with retarted sexual development

22 In a family, father had a trait, but mother did not. All their sons and daughter had this trait. The same trait was found in some grand-daughters, through daughter were married to the normal persons. Choose the correct pedigree chart for this condition.

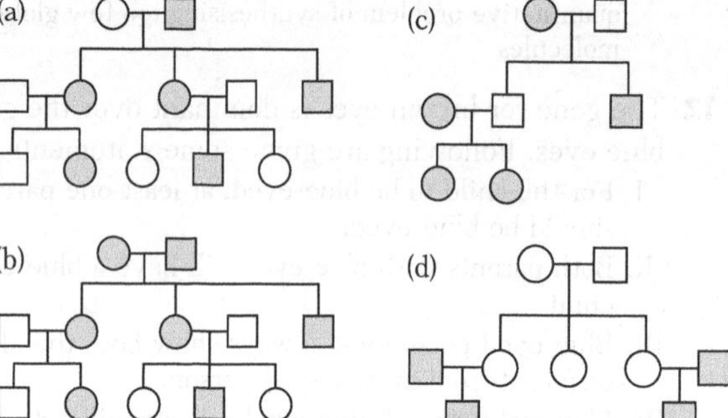

23 In man with the following genotypes and phenotypes may be the correct result of aneuploidy in sex chromosomes?
(a) 22 pairs + XXY – Males
(b) 22 pairs + XX – Females
(c) 22 pairs + XXXY – Females
(d) 22 pairs + Y – Females

24 Match Column I with Column II and select the correct answer using codes given below.

Column I (Syndromes)	Column II (Chromosomal abnormalities)
A. Patau's syndrome	1. 44 + XXY = 47
B. Klinefelter's syndrome	2. 44 + X = 45
C. Down's syndrome	3. 46 + 1 = 47, chromosome 13th
D. Turner's syndrome	4. 46 + 1 = 47, chromosome 21st

Codes

	A	B	C	D		A	B	C	D
(a)	1	2	3	4	(b)	4	3	2	1
(c)	3	2	4	1	(d)	3	1	4	2

25 Read the following statements.
I. 44 + XXY results in Klinefelter's syndrome.
II. Individuals with Klinefelter's syndrome has overall masculine development, are sterile and also show gynaecomastia.
III. 44 + XO results in Turner's syndrome.
IV. Individuals with Turner's syndrome possess most of the secondary sexual characters.

V. Individuals, with Turner's syndrome are sterile with rudimentary ovaries.

Which of the above statements are correct?

(a) I, II, III and V (b) Only III
(c) IV and V (d) III, IV and V

26 Which of the following were the main aims of project?

I. Mapping the entire human genome at the level of nucleotide sequence.
II. To store the information collected from the project in databases.
III. To develop tools and techniques for the analysis of the data.
IV. Transfer of the related technologies to the private sectors such as industries.
V. Taking care of the legal, ethical and social issues which may rise from project.

(a) I, II and IV (b) II, III and V
(c) I and V (d) I, II, III, IV and V

27 Match the following columns.

	Column I (Pedigree symbols)		Column II (Refers to)
A.	□	1.	Death
B.	○	2.	Five unaffected offspring
C.	◇	3.	Sex unspecified
D.	◇ (S)	4.	Female
E.	⧄ ⦸	5.	Male

Codes

	A	B	C	D	E
(a)	1	2	5	4	3
(b)	1	2	4	3	5
(c)	1	2	3	4	5
(d)	5	4	3	2	1

28 Sita and Ram have their first child. Sita knows her blood type is A, but Ram does not know his blood type. However, Ram knows that both his mother and father have type B blood. The first child is a boy named Kush. Kush has type O blood. Sita and Ram do not understand how this happened. Which of the following is the best explanation?

(a) Sita's genotype is AA and Ram's genotype is OO, thus skip expresses the O phenotype
(b) Sita's genotype is AO and Ram's genotype is OO, thus skip expresses the O phenotype
(c) Because Ram's parents are both type B, Ram is not Kush's father
(d) Kush's blood type will need to be checked after his first month of life, if Sita and Ram want to know his blood type, as it takes about a month for the blood type to develop in a newborn child

29 In a family, father had a particular trait, but mother did not show it. Their two sons are normal, but their daughter had that trait. The daughter was married to a normal person and her daughter has the trait.

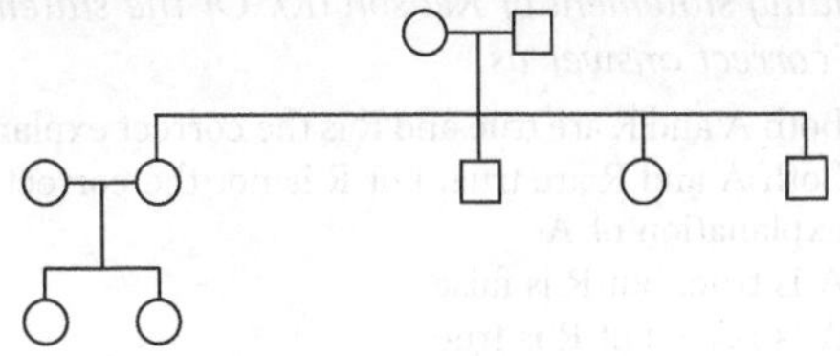

Pick out the correct representation.

(a) ○Aa × aa□

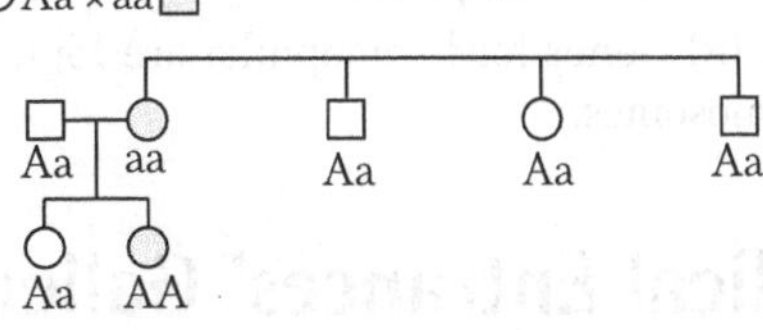

(b) ○AA×aa□

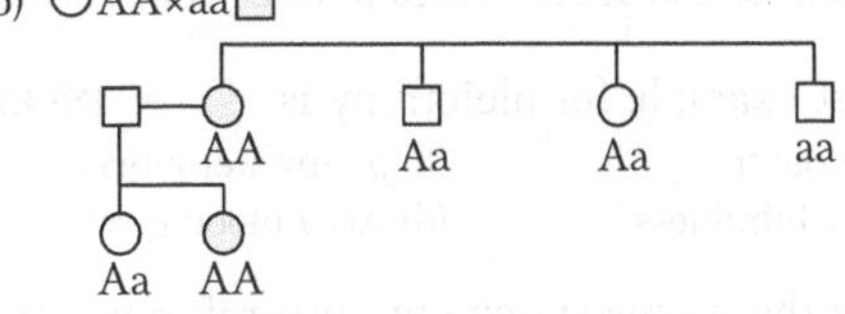

(c) ○aa × □AA

Aa aa AA Aa AA

AA aa

(d) ○aa × □Aa

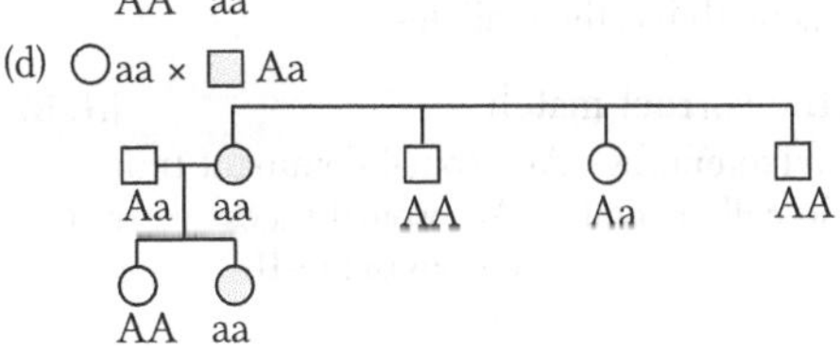

30 What will be the phenotypic sex of the following organisms on the basis of the sex chromosomal constitution indicated against each organism?

Organism constitutions	Sex chromosomes
I Human being	XO
II *Drosophila*	XO
III Human being	XXY
IV *Drosophila*	XXY

Select the correct answer using the codes given below.

	Male	Female
(a)	I and III	II and IV
(b)	III and IV	I and II
(c)	II and IV	I and III
(d)	II and III	I and IV

Assertion and Reason

Direction (Q. Nos. 31-34) *In each of the following questions, a statement of Assertion (A) is given followed by corresponding statement of Reason (R). Of the statements, mark the correct answer as*

(a) Both A and R are true and R is the correct explanation of A
(b) Both A and R are true, but R is not the correct explanation of A
(c) A is true, but R is false
(d) A is false, but R is true
(e) Both A and R are false

31 **Assertion** (A) Haemophilia rarely affects the woman.
Reason (R) Genes for haemophilia are found in X-chromosomes.

32 **Assertion** (A) Mother may be a carrier for haemophilia.
Reason (R) The father is always a carrier for haemophilia.

33 **Assertion** (A) Inheritance of holandric genes is always from father to son.
Reason (R) Holandric genes are found on Y-chromosome.

34 **Assertion** (A) In humans, female sex is determined by XX-chromosome.
Reason (R) Male sex is determined by XY-chromosome.

(C) Medical Entrances' Gallery

(Collection of Questions Asked in NEET & in Various Medical Entrance Exams)

1 The best example for pleiotropy is **[NEET 2020]**
(a) skin colour (b) phenylketonuria
(c) colour blindness (d) ABO blood group

2 Identify the wrong statement with reference to the gene 'I' that controls ABO blood groups. **[NEET 2020]**
(a) A person will have only two of the three alleles
(b) When I^A and I^B are present together, they express same type of sugar
(c) Allele 'i' does not produce any sugar
(d) The gene (I) has three alleles

3 Select the correct match. **[NEET 2020]**
(a) Phenylketonuria - Autosomal dominant trait
(b) Sickle-cell anaemia - Autosomal recessive trait, chromosome-II
(c) Thalassemia - X-linked
(d) Haemophilia - Y-linked

4 In which genetic condition, each cell in the affected person, has three sex chromosomes XXY? **[NEET 2019]**
(a) Thalassemia (b) Klinefelter's syndrome
(c) Phenylketonuria (d) Turner's syndrome

5 Karyotype of Down's syndrome has how many chromosomes? **[JIPMER 2019, UP CPMT 2013]**
(a) 43 (b) 46
(c) 47 (d) 45

6 Gynaecomastia is present in which syndrome? **[JIPMER 2019, NEET 2019]**
(a) Turner's (b) Klinefelter's
(c) Down's (d) None of these

7 **Assertion** (A) Down's syndrome, Klinefelter's syndrome and Turner's syndrome are chromosomal disorders.
Reason (R) In Klinefelter's syndrome, females are sterile. **[AIIMS 2019]**
(a) Both A and R are true and R is the correct explanation of A
(b) Both A and R are true, but R is not the correct explanation of A
(c) A is true, but R is false
(d) Both A and R are false

8 What is the genetic disorder in which an individual has an overall masculine development gynaecomastia and is sterile ? **[NEET 2019]**
(a) Klinefelter's syndrome
(b) Edward's syndrome
(c) Down's syndrome
(d) Turner's syndrome

9 A normal woman whose father was colourblind, marries a normal man. What kinds of children can be expected and in what proportion? **[AIIMS 2018]**
(a) All daughters normal, 50% of sons colourblind
(b) All daughters normal, all sons colourblind
(c) 50% daughters colourblind, all sons normal
(d) All daughters colourblind, all sons normal

10 **Assertion** (A) Phenylketonuria is recessive hereditary disease caused by body's failure to oxidise an amino acid phenylalanine to tyrosine, because of defective enzyme.

Reason (R) It is characterised by in the presence of phenylalanine acid in urine.
[AIIMS 2018, Kerala CEE 2014]

(a) Both A and R are true and R is the correct explanation of A
(b) Both A and R are true, but R is not the correct explanation of A
(c) A is true, but R is false
(d) Both A and R are false

11 Non-disjunction in meiosis results in **[JIPMER 2018]**
(a) trisomy
(b) normal diploid
(c) gene mutation
(d) None of these

12 Thalassemia and sickle-cell anaemia are caused due to a problem in globin molecule synthesis. Select the correct statement. **[NEET 2018]**
(a) Both are due to a qualitative defect in global chain synthesis
(b) Both are due to a quantitative defect in globin chain synthesis
(c) Thalassemia is due to less synthesis of globin molecules
(d) Sickle-cell anaemia is due to a quantitative problem of globin molecules

13 A disease caused by an autosomal primary non-disjunction is **[NEET 2017]**
(a) Down's syndrome
(b) Klinefelter's syndrome
(c) Turner's syndrome
(d) Sickle-cell anaemia

14 A man whose father was colourblind marries a woman, who had a colourblind mother and normal father. What percentage of male children of this couple will be colourblind? **[AIIMS 2017]**
(a) 25% (b) 0%
(c) 50% (d) 75%

15 Pick out the correct statements.
I. Haemophilia is a sex-linked recessive disease.
II. Down's syndrome is due to aneuploidy.
III. Phenylketonuria is an autosomal recessive gene disorder.
IV. Sickle-cell anaemia is an X-linked recessive gene disorder. **[NEET-II 2016]**
(a) II and IV (b) I, III and IV
(c) I, II and III (d) I and IV

16 If a colourblind man marries a woman who is homozygous for normal colour vision, the probability of their son being colourblind is
[NEET-II 2016, WB JEE 2014]
(a) 0 (b) 0.5
(c) 0.75 (d) 1

17 Which one of the following statements is wrong with reference to Barr bodies? **[EAMCET 2016]**
(a) The heterochromatinised X-chromosome is called Barr body
(b) The inactivation of X-chromosome is called lyonisation
(c) The extra X-chromosome undergoes heterochromatinisation and becomes active during early embryonic development
(d) The heterochromatinised X-chromosome remains attached with the nuclear membrane

18 In the following human pedigree, the filled symbols represent the affected individuals. Identify the type of given pedigree.

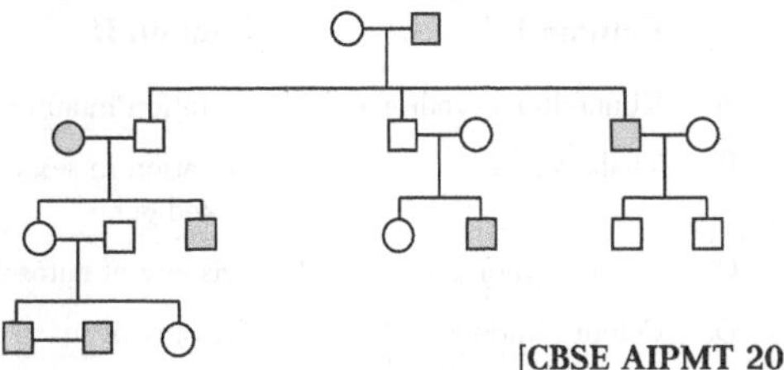

[CBSE AIPMT 2015]
(a) autosomal dominant (b) X-linked recessive
(c) autosomal recessive (d) X-linked dominant

19 A colourblind man marries a woman with normal sight, who has no history of colour blindness in her family. What is the probability of their grandson being colourblind? **[CBSE AIPMT 2015]**
(a) 0.5 (b) 1 (c) Nil (d) 0.25

20 With respect to phenylketonuria identify which statement is not correct? **[Karnataka CET 2015]**
(a) It is a case of aneuploidy
(b) It is an example of pleiotropy
(c) Caused due to the autosomal recessive trait
(d) It is an error in metabolism

21 Double lines in pedigree analysis show
[Karnataka CET 2015]
(a) unaffected offspring (b) sex unspecified
(c) normal mating (d) consanguineous marriage

22 Three copies of chromosome 21 in a child with Down's syndrome have been analysed using molecular biology technology to detect any possible DNA polymorphism with reference to different alleles located on chromosome 21. Results showed that out of 3 copies 2 of the chromosomes of the child contain the same alleles as one of the mother's alleles. Based on this when did the non-disjunction event most likely occur? **[Karnataka CET 2015]**
(a) Paternal meiosis-I
(b) Maternal meiosis-I
(c) Paternal meiosis-II
(d) Maternal meiosis-II

23 A person with 44A + XXY chromosome setup has gynaecomastia and are Barr body positive. They have symptoms of **[EAMCET 2015, Rajasthan PMT 2014]**
(a) Turner's syndrome (b) Klinefelter's syndrome
(c) Down's syndrome (d) Edward's syndrome

24 Find out the mismatched pair. **[EAMCET 2015]**
(a) Lyonisation — Liane Russell and Mary Lyon
(b) Y-chromosome — Stevens and Wilson
(c) X-body — Henking
(d) Shotgun sequencing — Jeffreys

25 Match the items in Column I with those in Column II and choose the correct answer.

	Column I		Column II
A.	Klinefelter's syndrome	1.	Mutation in autosomal gene
B.	Thalassemia	2.	Mutation in sex chromosome linked gene
C.	Down's syndrome	3.	Trisomy of autosome
D.	Colour blindness	4.	Trisomy of sex chromosome

Codes **[WB JEE 2015, Rajasthan PMT 2014]**

	A	B	C	D		A	B	C	D
(a)	1	2	3	4	(b)	2	3	4	1
(c)	3	4	1	2	(d)	4	1	3	2

26 Which one of the following statements is relevant to sex-linked characters? **[WB JEE 2015]**
(a) They always follow *criss-cross* inheritance
(b) They do not follow *criss-cross* inheritance
(c) They are mostly present on Y-chromosome
(d) They are only present on X-chromosome

27 Match the following columns I, II with III.

Column I	Column II	Column III
A. Sickle-cell anaemia	1. Due to recessive PP genes	(i) Arrangement of valine in place of glutamic acid
B. Phenylketonuria	2. Due to the absence of homogentisic oxidase enzyme	(ii) Inborn error of metabolism
C. Alkaptonuria	3. Follows Mendelian principles	(iii) Urine turns black when exposed to air
D. Thalassemia	4. Characters caused by homozygous recessive genes	(iv) The required haemoglobin is not generated in the blood.

Codes **[Gujarat CET 2015]**

	A	B	C	D
(a)	3-(iii)	1-(ii)	4-(i)	2-(iv)
(b)	4-(i)	1-(ii)	2-(iii)	3-(iv)
(c)	4-(i)	3-(iii)	1-(iv)	2-(ii)
(d)	2-(iv)	3-(iii)	1-(ii)	4-(i)

28 Down's syndrome is characterised by **[AMU 2015, Chhattisgarh PMT 2015]**
(a) 19 trisomy
(b) 21 trisomy
(c) one X-chromosome
(d) two X and one Y-chromosome

29 An abnormal human baby with 'XXX' sex chromosomes was born due to **[AMU 2015]**
(a) formation of abnormal sperms in the father
(b) formation of abnormal ova in the mother
(c) fusion of two ova and one sperm
(d) fusion of two sperms and one ovum

30 In sickle-cell anaemia, substitution of glutamic acid molecule by valine molecule takes place at **[Chhattisgarh PMT 2015, Kerala CEE 2015]**
(a) position 6 of the α-chain of haemoglobin
(b) position 6 of the β-chain of haemoglobin
(c) position 5 of the β-chain of haemoglobin
(d) position 5 of the α-chain of haemoglobin

31 If a boy's father has haemophilia and mother is heterozygous, what is the chance that the boy will inherit haemophilia disease? **[Chhattisgarh PMT 2015]**
(a) 50% (b) 25%
(c) 75% (d) 100%

32 A human female with Turner's syndrome **[CBSE AIPMT 2014]**
(a) has 45 chromosomes with XO
(b) has one additional X-chromosome
(c) exhibits male characters
(d) is able to produce children with normal husband

33 A couple, both carriers for the gene sickle-cell anaemia planning to get married, wants to know the chances of having anaemic progeny. **[MHT CET 2014]**
(a) 100% (b) 75%
(c) 50% (d) 25%

34 Which of the following is correctly matched? **[MHT CET 2014]**

	Column I	Column II		Column III
(a)	Thalassemia	A. XO	(i)	Flat nose, simian crease
(b)	Down's syndrome	B. 42 AA + XY	(ii)	Webbing of neck
(c)	Turner's syndrome	C. 44 AA + XXX	(iii)	Anaemia, jaundice
(d)	Klinefelter's syndrome	D. 44 AA + XXY	(iv)	Tall thin eunuchoid

35 Match the following columns.

	Columns I		Columns II
A.	Down's syndrome	1.	45 X
B.	Edward's syndrome	2.	47, XX + 13
C.	Klinefelter's syndrome	3.	47, XX+ 18
D.	Patau's syndrome	4.	47, XX, + 21
E.	Turner's syndrome	5.	17, XXY

Codes [EAMCET 2014]

	A	B	C	D	E
(a)	3	4	2	1	5
(b)	2	3	4	5	1
(c)	4	3	5	2	1
(d)	4	2	5	3	1

36 In alpha thalassemia, the gene HBAl is located on the chromosome [EAMCET 2014]
(a) 8 (b) 22 (c) 9 (d) 16

37 Down's syndrome is an example for [Karnataka CET 2014]
(a) aneuploidy of sex chromosome
(b) aneuploidy of autosome
(c) syndrome caused due to gene mutation
(d) loss of one sex chromosome from the diploid set

38 In the given pedigree, the shaded individuals are homozygous recessive for colour blindness. What is the genotype of individual *B* ?

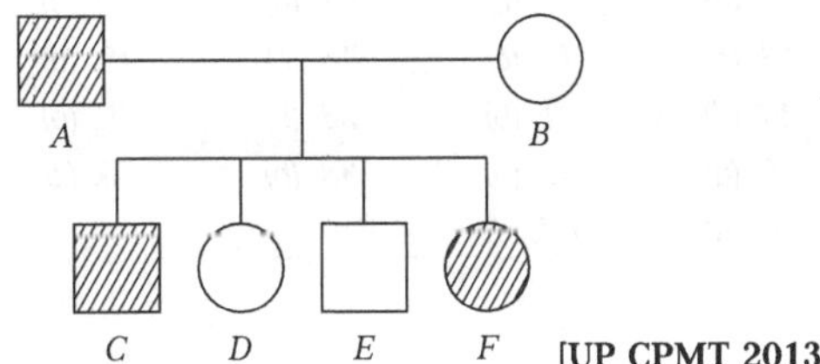

[UP CPMT 2013]

(a) Heterozygous
(b) Homozygous recessive
(c) Homozygous dominant
(d) None of these

39 Haemophilia is related to [OJEE 2013]
(a) albinism
(b) sickle-cell anaemia
(c) colour blindness
(d) thalassemia

40 The gene of sickle-cell anaemia is inherited by [WB JEE 2013]
(a) blood cells (b) bone cells
(c) sex chromosomes (d) autosomes

41 Represented below is the inheritance pattern of a certain type of traits in humans. Which one of the following conditions could be an example of this pattern?

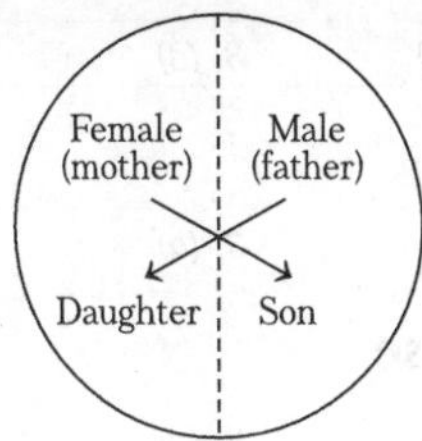

[CBSE AIPMT 2012]

(a) Phenylketonuria (b) Sickle-cell anaemia
(c) Haemophilia (d) Thalassemia

42 A normal-visioned man whose father was colourblind, marries a woman whose father was also colourblind. They have their first child as a daughter. What are the chances that this child would be colourblind? [CBSE AIPMT 2012]
(a) 100% (b) 0% (c) 25% (d) 50%

43 A woman with albinic father marries an albinic man. A proportion of her progeny is [AIIMS 2012]
(a) 2 normal:1 albinic (b) all normal
(c) all albinic (d) 1 normal:1 albinic

44 Which pairs of the following diseases are caused by two genes located on human X-chromosomes? [WB JEE 2012]
(a) Colour blindness and phenylketonuria
(b) Colour blindness and haemophilia
(c) Colour blindness and albinism
(d) Colour blindness and hypertrichosis

45 Cri-du-chat' syndrome in humans is caused by the [UP CPMT 2012]
(a) fertilisation of an XX egg by a normal Y-bearing sperm
(b) loss of half of the short arm of chromosome 5
(c) loss of half of the long arm of chromosome 5
(d) trisomy of 21st chromosome

46 A hereditary disease, which is never passed on from father to son is [J&K CET 2012]
(a) X-chromosomal linked disease
(b) autosomal linked disease
(c) Y-chromosomal linked disease
(d) None of the above

47 More men suffer from colour blindness than women because [KCET 2011]
(a) women are more resistant to disease than men
(b) the male sex hormone testosterone causes the disease
(c) the colourblind gene is carried on the Y-chromosome
(d) men are hemizygous and one defective gene is enough to make them colourblind

ANSWERS

Check Point 9.1

1. (d) 2. (c) 3. (d) 4. (c) 5. (c) 6. (b)

Check Point 9.2

1. (d) 2. (c) 3. (a) 4. (a) 5. (b) 6. (d) 7. (c)

(A) Topical Exercise

1. (c) 2. (c) 3. (d) 4. (d) 5. (c) 6. (a) 7. (c) 8. (b) 9. (d) 10. (d)
11. (d) 12. (c) 13. (b) 14. (b) 15. (b) 16. (a) 17. (c) 18. (d) 19. (b) 20. (b)
21. (b) 22. (c) 23. (c) 24. (b) 25. (c) 26. (c) 27. (d) 28. (b) 29. (c) 30. (c)
31. (a) 32. (a) 33. (b) 34. (a) 35. (d) 36. (d) 37. (b) 38. (a) 39. (a) 40. (c)
41. (b) 42. (d) 43. (c) 44. (d) 45. (d) 46. (d) 47. (b) 48. (a) 49. (d) 50. (c)
51. (d) 52. (d) 53. (c) 54. (c) 55. (d) 56. (c) 57. (c) 58. (c) 59. (c) 60. (c)
61. (b) 62. (a) 63. (c) 64. (a) 65. (a) 66. (c) 67. (a) 68. (d) 69. (c) 70. (b)
71. (b) 72. (c) 73. (c) 74. (d) 75. (d) 76. (a) 77. (c) 78. (c) 79. (c) 80. (b)
81. (d) 82. (a) 83. (b) 84. (a) 85. (c) 86. (d) 87. (d) 88. (a) 89. (d) 90. (b)

(B) Cumulative Exercise

1. (c) 2. (a) 3. (d) 4. (c) 5. (b) 6. (d) 7. (b) 8. (a) 9. (a) 10. (a)
11. (d) 12. (b) 13. (b) 14. (d) 15. (b) 16. (a) 17. (c) 18. (b) 19. (d) 20. (a)
21. (b) 22. (a) 23. (a) 24. (d) 25. (a) 26. (d) 27. (d) 28. (b) 29. (d) 30. (d)
31. (b) 32. (c) 33. (a) 34. (b)

(C) Medical Entrances' Gallery

1. (b) 2. (b) 3. (b) 4. (b) 5. (c) 6. (b) 7. (c) 8. (a) 9. (a) 10. (b)
11. (a) 12. (c) 13. (a) 14. (c) 15. (c) 16. (a) 17. (c) 18. (c) 19. (d) 20. (c)
21. (d) 22. (b) 23. (b) 24. (d) 25. (d) 26. (d) 27. (b) 28. (b) 29. (b) 30. (b)
31. (a) 32. (a) 33. (d) 34. (d) 35. (c) 36. (d) 37. (b) 38. (b) 39. (c) 40. (d)
41. (c) 42. (b) 43. (d) 44. (b) 45. (b) 46. (a) 47. (d)

Explanations

(A) Topical Exercise

10 (*d*) If Mr. Phillips is colourblind then the chances of his male child inheriting this disease is 0% because it is X-linked recessive disease, Y-chromosome does not carry gene for colour vision.

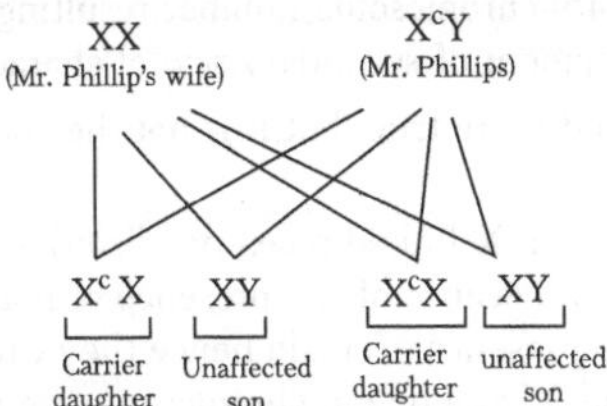

Though, his daughters will be carrier, but his sons can never inherit this disease.

14 (*b*) If a boy's father has haemophilia and his mother has one gene of haemophilia then, following offsprings would produce.

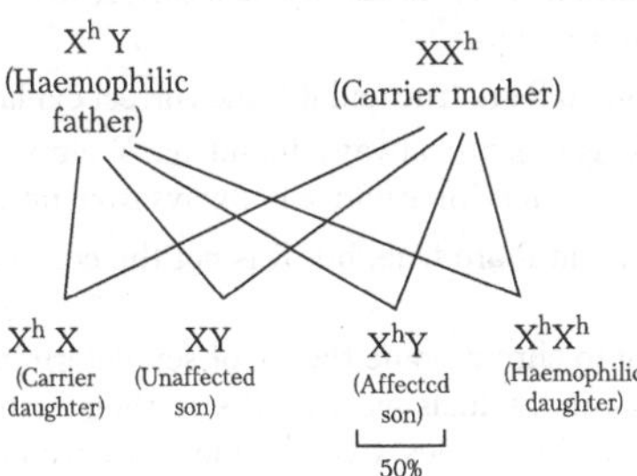

Hence, there are 50% chances that the boy will inherit the disease.

15 (*b*) If Mary's father is haemophilic then she can be a carrier, it can be expained as

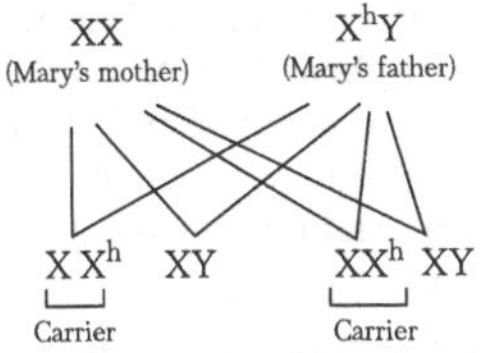

If she is carrier and her husband is a haemophilic, then

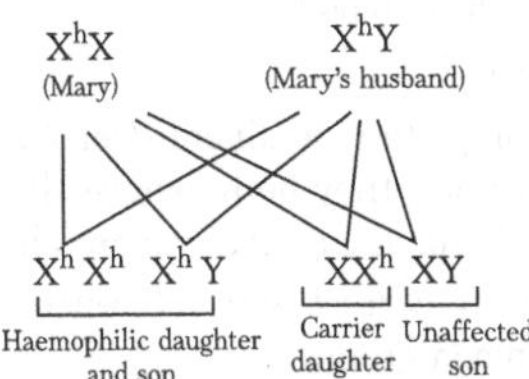

Hence, there are 50% chances that her daughter can be a carrier and 50% chance of her daughter having disease.

26 (*c*)

$I^A i$ (Father) × $I^B i$ (Mother)

Gametes: I^A, i and I^B, i

F_1-generation

♀ \ ♂	I^A	i
I^B	I^AI^B	I^Bi
i	I^Ai	ii

Thus, there is 25% chance of blood group A in offspring.

34 (*a*) Since, all the daughters are affected and inherited the disease from affected father, the given trait is dominant X-linked.

36 (*d*) Cytoplasmic mitochondrial inheritance is the inheritance in which the trait pass only form mother to all o their offsprings.

40 (*c*) From the pedigree chart, it is visible that the males are the only ones who are affected and it is the clear evidence of Y-linked disease.

41 (*b*) Autosomal dominant traits do not skip any generation and affect both males and females equally.

42 (*d*) As it is visible in the pedigree chart that trait skips generation, the unaffected parents hare diseased progeny which means that trait is present in recessive condition in parents. Thus, parents are heterozygous for the recessive trait and serve as carrier for it.

44 (*d*) The genotype of the individual 'M' has to be X^hX, i.e. she has to be the carrier, so as to produce an individual who is affected in the last generation.

46 (*d*) People having the ability to taste the bitter compound Phenyl Thiocarbamide or PTC, are PTC tasters whereas, for some people, PTC seems tastes and such are called PTC non-taster. The inability to taste PTC is an autosomal recessive genetic disorder, i.e. it occurs when the allele for this trait is present in homozygous recessive condition.

Pedigree D shows correct representation for this in which wife is affected and husband is unaffected. The daughters may be affected because they will inherit (one autosome) from the mother and the other one from father which may also hare the allele for PTC trait.

55 (*d*) Both statements I and II are false and can be corrected as Turner's syndrome is sex chromosome disorder in which female lacks one X-chromosome and thus, possesses XO condition.

67 (*a*) Option (a) is mismatch and can be corrected as

The person affected with Klinefelter's syndrome has long limbs. Rest options are correct match pairs.

75 (*d*) Statement I and II are incorrect and can be corrected as Albinism is autosomal recessive mutation, caused due to deficiency of tyrosinase enzyme. It is copper containing enzyme involved in the production of melanin.

79 (*c*) Statement in option (c) is correct.

Huntington's disease is an autosomal disorder occur due to an allele on short arm of chromosome 4. The symptoms of this disease include atropy in the parts of brain, resulting in irregular breathing, irregular rhythmic movement of limbs, etc.

This disease may start at the age of 15-40 yrs, but can also occur in older person.

Currently there is no effective treatment to cure this disease.

86 (*d*) Both the statement I and II are false and can be corrected as

Structural genomics involves mapping, sequencing and analysis of genome. Functional genomics involve identification of the function of a particular gene.

89 (*d*) Both the statement I and II are false and can be corrected as

Human genome project was completed in the year 2003.

3.2 billion base pairs are present in human genome.

90 (*b*) Statement I is false, but II is true. Incorrect statement can be corrected as

A field of biology explored by hGP is bioinformatics.

81 (*d*) The genotype of affected woman is cc. Her parents are obligate carriers (cc) and one of her grand parent must also be a carrier. Her first cousin then has a 1/4 chance being a carrier. He has 1/2 % chance of transmitting his (c) allele if it is present.

So, the chances of child being a patent of cystic fibrosis is

$$\frac{1}{4} \times \frac{1}{2} = \frac{1}{8}$$

(B) Cumulative Exercise

4 (*c*) Statements I and III are correct while II and IV are incorrect. Incorrect statements can be corrected as

- Haemophilia is a congenital disorder.
- Dizygotic twins are common in animals like cow, buffaloes, etc.

6 (*d*) Statements I, II and IV are correct, while III and V are incorrect. Incorrect statements can be corrected as

- Phenylketonuria is an autosomal recessive gene disorder.
- Sickle-cell is a chromosomal disorder which occurs due to defective haemoglobin where glutamine at 6th place is replaced by valine.

9 (*a*) Statements I and III are correct, while II and IV are incorrect. Incorrect statements can be corrected as

- Genetic disorders are determined by the alteration or mutation in a single gene.
- Sickle-cell anaemia is chromosomal disorder, which occurs due to replacement of valine instead of glutamine in 6th place.

11 (*d*) Statement in option (d) is incorrect about thalassemia and can be corrected as

Sickle-cell anaemia differ from thalassemia in that the former is a qualitative problem of synthesising an incorrectly functioning globin while the latter is a quantitative problem of syntheising few globin molecules.

Rest statements are correct about thalassemia.

15 (*b*) Statement II alone is false and can be corrected as Possibility of female becoming haemophils is extremely rare.

18 (*b*) Statements IV and V are incorrect and can be corrected as sickle-cell anaemia is chromosomal disorder, which occurs to replacement of valine instead of glutamine in 6th place. Haemophil is X-linked recessive disease.

25 (*a*) All statements are correct except statement IV. Incorrect statement can be corrected as

Turner's syndrome is a chromosomal disorder which occurs due to deamination of one X-chromosome in female, i.e. 44A + XO (45) chromosome number resulting in underdevelopment of secondary sexual characters.

31 (*b*) Both A and R are true, but R is not the correct explanation of A.

Haemophilia is a X-linked recessive disorder but it rarely affects women because of the presence of homozygous chromosome present in female hence they can be carrier but in males, one 'X' and one Y-chromosome are present hence, they are more prone to this disorder.

32 (*c*) A is true, but R is false because

Females have two X-chromosomes (XX). They may be carrier for haemophilic gene, while males have only single X-chromosome (XY), so cannot be a carrier for haemophilic gene.

33 (*a*) Both A and R are true and R is the correct explanation of A.

Holandric genes are always found on Y-chromosome of the male. Hence, their inheritance is always from father to the son.

34 (*b*) Both A and R are true, but R is not the correct explanation of A.

According to chromosome theory of sex-determination, male and female individuals would differ in their chromosome constitution. In females, two chromosomes are homomorphic (XX) and in males, these are heteromorphic (XY).

(C) Medical Entrances' Gallery

1 (*b*) The best example for pleiotropy is phenylketonuria, which occurs in humans. In pleiotropy, a single gene can exhibit multiple phenotypic expressions. This gene is called pleiotropic gene. In phenylketonuria, a single gene mutation that codes for enzyme phenylalanine hydroxylase is seen. This manifests itself through phenotypic expression characterised by mental retardation, a reduction in hair and skin pigmentation.

2 (*b*) When I^A and I^B are present together, they express same type of sugar is wrong statement with reference to the gene (I) that controls ABO blood group.

It can be corrected as

I^A and I^B are completely dominant over I^O, but when I^A and I^B are present together, they both express their own types of sugar and thus behaving as codominant alleles.

Rest statement are correct with reference to the gene 'I' that controls ABO blood group.

3 (*b*) Option (b) is correct match whereas options (a), (c) and (d) are incorrect. Incorrect matches can be corrected as

Phenylketonuria is an autosomal recessive disorder. Due to this disorder, enzyme phenylalanine hydroxylase is not synthesised. This enzyme is required for conversion of

phenylalanine (PA) into tyrosine. If enzyme production stops, the concentration of PA in body tissue increases, this accumulated PA gets converted into phenyl pyruvic acid which is responsible for damaging the brain.
Thalassemia is an autosomal recessive disorder. It is of two types depending upon which protein chain of haemoglobin gets synthesised or not synthesised in a defective manner.
Haemophilia is an X-linked disorder in which the clotting time is delayed.

4 (*b*) Klinefelter's syndrome is a genetic condition in which each cell in the affected person contains three sex chromosomes XXY. It is caused due to the presence of an additional copy of X-chromosome resulting into a karyotype of 47, XXY. Such individuals are sterile.

5 (*c*) Karyotype of people suffering from Down's syndrome is 47 chromosomes (45 + XY in males, 45 + XX in females) instead of 46. It is caused due to the presence of an extra chromosome number 21, thus it is also known as 21st trisomy.

6 (*b*) Gynaecomastia is present in Klinefelter's syndrome. It is swelling of the breast tissue in boys or men, caused by an imbalance of the hormones oestrogen and testosterone. It is commonly found in males affected with Klinefelter's syndrome. Klinefelter's syndrome is the most common sex chromosomal disorder in males. It also characterised by low testosterone and reduced muscle mass, facial and body hair.

7 (*c*) A is true, but R is false because
Down's syndrome, Klinefelter's syndrome and Turner's syndrome are chromosomal disorders.
But in Klinefelter's syndrome, males are sterile as individual possess 47 chromosomes (44 + XXY).

Down's syndrome It is also called 21st trisomy. It occurs due to the non-disjunction of 21st chromosome during meiosis. It is an autosomal aneuploidy caused by the presence of extra chromosomes number 21 (45 + XY in male, 45 + XX in female).

Turner's syndrome It is due to monosomy. The individual has (44 + XO) instead of 46 chromosomes. The females become sterile.

8 (*a*) In Klinefelter's syndrome, individual has overall masculine development, gynaecomastia and is sterile. This condition is represented as 44 + X (47) due to the presence of an extra X-chromosome in males.
Other options are explained as

- Edward's syndrome is 18 trisomy and it causes severe developmental delay.
- Down's syndrome is 21 trisomy and it is identified as Mongolism due to the short stature of affected individual.
- Turner's syndrome is characterised by a missing X-chromosome in females. It causes sterility in females.

9 (*a*) A normal woman whose father was colourblind, marries a normal man.

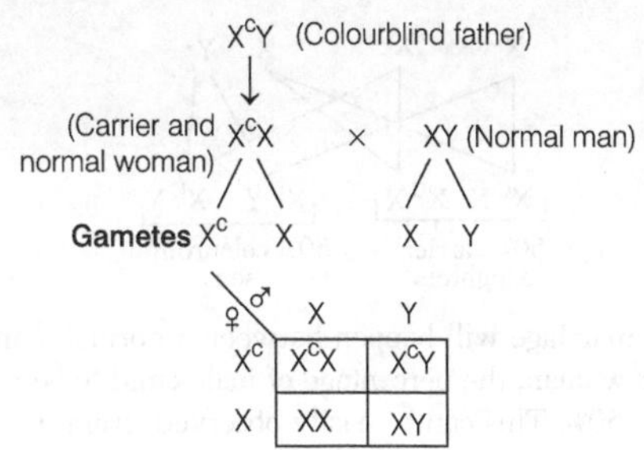

X^CX = (50% carrier daughters)
XX = (50% normal daughters)
X^CY = (50% colourblind sons)
XY = (50% normal sons)

Therefore, we can expect all daughters normal, 50% of sons colourblind.

10 (*b*) Both A and R are ture, but R is not the correct explanation of A.
Phenylketonuria is due to deficiency of liver enzyme phenylalanine hydroxylase, which converts phenylalanine into tyrosine. It occurs in people, who are homozygous recessive. It results with a high level of phenylalanine in blood, tissue fluids and urine.

11 (*a*) Non-disjunction in meiosis results in trisomy, i.e. the presence of three copies of a chromosome rather than the normal two. Such individuals have 47 chromosomes instead of 46. Some examples of such abnormalities include Down's syndrome (21 trisomy), Patau's syndrome (13 trisomy) and Edward's syndrome (18 trisomy).

12 (*c*) Statement in option (c) is correct.
Thalassemia is caused due to less synthesis of the globin chains of haemoglobin. Anaemia is the main feature of this disease. Rest of the statements are incorrect and can be corrected as
Thalassemia differs from sickle-cell anaemia in that the former is a quantitative problem of synthesising few globin molecules, while the latter is a qualitative problem of synthesising an incorrectly functioning globin.

13 (*a*) Down's syndrome occurs due to an autosomal primary non-disjunction. In this, there is the presence of an additional copy of chromosome number, 21 (trisomy of 21st chromosome) in humans.

14 (*c*) Colourblindness is an autosomal recessive genetic disorder, as gene for it is present on X-chromosome. According to the situation given in the question, a man whose father was colourblind will be XY normal likewise a woman whose mother was colourblind and father was normal will be a carrier as shown in the figure

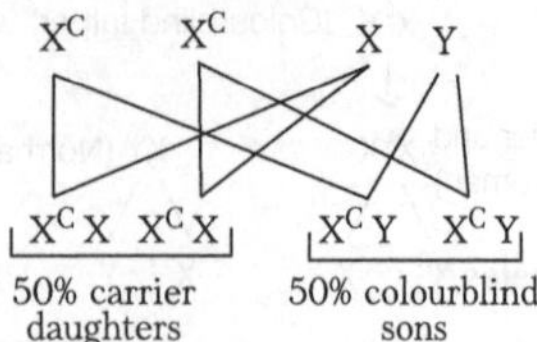

When marriage will happen between a normal man and a carrier woman, the percentage of male child to be colourblind will be 50%. This can be easily observed from the cross given below

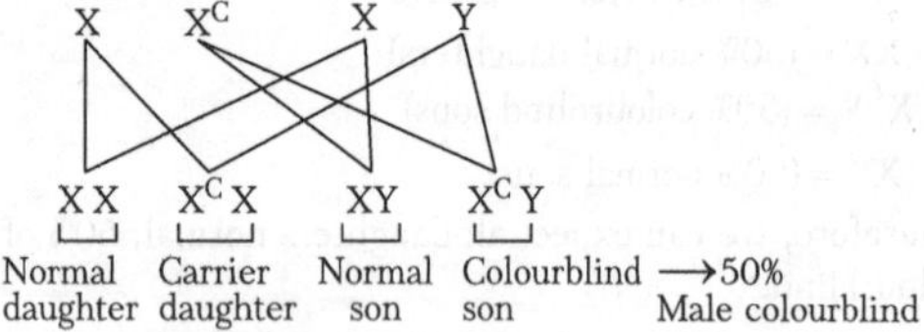

15 (*c*) All statements are correct except statement IV. Incorrect statement can be corrected as

Sickle-cell anaemia is an autosomal recessive gene disorder in which sickle-celled RBCs are formed instead of normal ones. They carry very less content of O_2 as their haemoglobin is malformed. The person suffering from this disease shows symptoms of anaemia.

16 (*a*) If a colourblind man marries a woman who is homozygous for normal colour vision, the probability of their son being colourblind is zero. Colour blindness is a recessive sex-linked trait in which the eye fails to distinguish between red and green colour. In females, colour blindness appears only when both sex chromosomes carry recessive gene (X^CX^C). However, in human males, the defect appears due to single recessive gene (X^CY) because Y-chromosome does not carry gene for colour vision. This disease shows *criss-cross* inheritance.

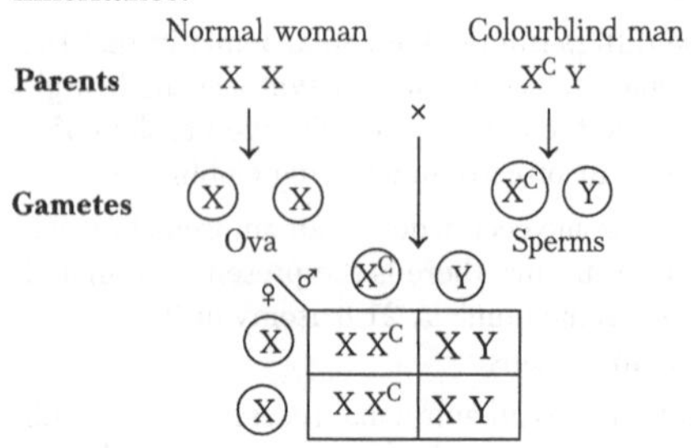

Thus, there is zero probability of son being colourblind. Hence, option (a) is correct.

17 (*c*) Statement in option (c) is wrong with reference to Barr bodies and can be corrected as

The extra X-chromosome although change into Barr body in somatic cells, but it becomes active in later stages of life. Genetic balance between male and female is maintained by inactivation of X-chromosome. This one chromosome undergoes heterochromatisation in all somatic cells. But, it becomes active in germ cells, producing female gemetes. Rest statements are correct with reference to Barr bodies.

18 (*c*) The given pedigree shows the autosomal recessive disorder. In this disorder, the individual inherits two mutated genes, one from each parent. This disorder is usually passed on by two carriers. Health is rarely affected, but individual have one mutated gene (recessive gene) and one normal gene (dominant gene) for the condition. The carriers have a 25% chance of having an unaffected child with normal genes, 50% chance of having an unaffected child who is also a carrier and a 25% chance of having an affected child with recessive genes.

19 (*d*) When a colourblind man (X^CY) marries a woman with normal sight (XX), who has no family history of colour blindness, all of their sons will be normal pure and all of their daughters will be carriers as shown below.

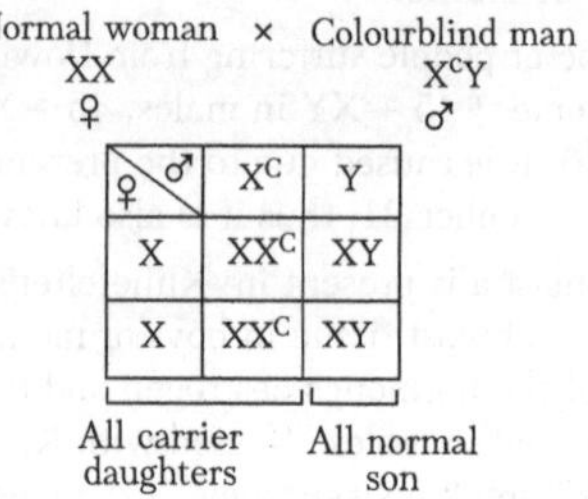

So, in the next generation, the children of all of their sons will be normal in all conditions (except the case in which the wife involved is not carrier neither colourblind) for carrier daughters.

(i) If they marry to a normal man, 50% of their grandsons will become colourblind as

Carrier woman XX^C ♀ × Normal man XY ♂

♀ \ ♂	X	Y
X	XX	XY
X^C	X^CX	X^CY ⟵ Colourblind son

(ii) If carrier daughter marries to a colourblind man, 50% of their grandson will be colourblind along with 50% of the grand daughter while rest 50% of the grand daughters will be carriers as

Carrier woman XX^C ♀ × Colourblind man X^CY ♂

♀ \ ♂	X^C	Y
X	XX^C Carrier	XY Normal
X^C	X^CX^C Colourblind	X^CY Colourblind
	Daughters	Son

So, in both the above cases, the result shows that 50% of grandsons will be colourblind which in terms of over all progenies (son + daughters) comes as 25% thus, confirming the probablity as 0.25.

22 (*b*) Non-disjunction of chromosome is the failure of homologous chromosome to separate during meiosis-I. As same alleles come from mother side, so non-disjunction may be during maternal meiosis-I.

24 (*d*) Option (d) is mismatched pair and can be corrected as Shotgun sequencing or Shot cloning or Sanger sequencing is developed by Frederick Sanger. It is a method used for sequencing long DNA strands.

Rest options are matched pairs.

26 (*d*) Statement in option (d) is relevant to sex-linked character. Sex-linked characters are the X-linked characters (the term sex-linked is presently referred to as X-linked). Their inheritance is due to the X-linked gene.

Only X-linked recessive characters follow *criss-cross* pattern of inheritance or skip-generation inheritance. In *criss-cross* inheritance, character is inherited to the second generation through the carrier of first generation.

30 (*b*) Sickle-cell anaemia is an example of point mutation in the β-haemoglobin gene that converts GAG codon to GUG at the position 6 of β-chain. This codes amino acid valine in place of glutamic acid.

31 (*a*)

Carrier mother × Haemophilic father

XX^h X^hY

XX^h	XY	X^hX^h	X^hY
Carrier daughter	Normal son	Haemophilic daughter and son	

So, the chances are 50% that children will have haemophilia.

33 (*d*) It is clear from the condition given that the parents are carrier of the disease. Sickle-cell anaemia is an autosomal linked recessive trait which gets transmitted from parents to offsprings, when both the partners are carrier for the gene. According to the situation given in the question, the cross is given below

Carrier mother Carrier father

X^SX X^SY

↓ ↓

X^S X X^S Y **Gametes**

♀ \ ♂	X^S	Y
X^S	X^SX^S (Affected daughter) (anaemic)	X^SY (Carrier son)
X	X^SX (Carrier daughter)	XY (Normal son)

Thus, the chances of getting anaemic progeny is only 25%, i.e. daughter will only be affected.

34 (*d*) The only correctly matched pair is of Klinefelter's syndrome.

Other options are incorrectly matched pairs and can be corrected as

- Thalassemia – Blood disorder-Anaemia, jaundice
- Down's syndrome – 45 + XX Female, 45 + XY Male — Flat nose, simian crease
- Turner's syndrome – 45 + XO – Webbing of neck

36 (*d*) In α-thalassemia, the gene HBA1 is located on chromosome 16. In this, the synthesis of alpha globin chain is reduced or absent.

37 (*b*) Down's syndrome is an example for aneuploidy of autosome was described by J Langdon Down (1866). It occurs due to the additional copy of chromosome number 21 or trisomy of chromosome 21.

38 (*b*) In the given pedigree, *B* represents the female carrier for colour blindness. Colour blindness is due to recessive gene carried on X-chromosome. A pedigree is a family tree or chart made of symbols and lines that represents a patient's genetic family history. Females are represented by circles and males by squares.

39 (*c*) Haemophilia is related to colour blindness, both are X-linked recessive diseases. The gene for both is found on X-chromosome only. Albinism, sickle-cell anaemia and thalassemia are autosomal diseases.

41 (*c*) Haemophilia could be an example of this pattern. It is a sex-linked or X-linked disease. The gene of haemophilia goes to son from mother and to daughter from father. In this disease, the blood fails to clot when exposed to air resulting in continuous bleeding that leads to death.

42 (*b*) Colour blindness is an X-linked disease. So, woman whose father was colourblind will be carrier for the disease.

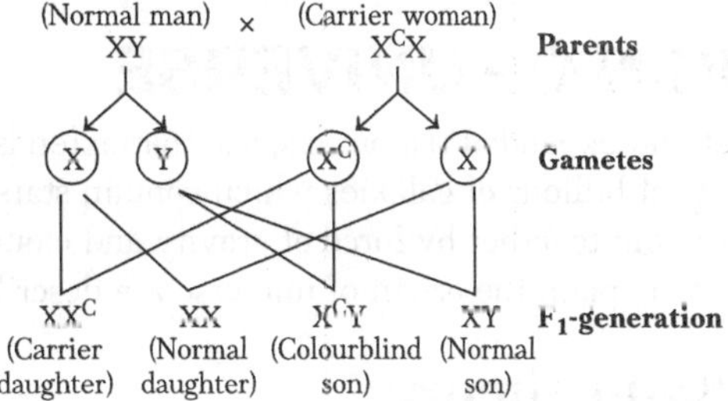

So, possibility of a colourblind daughter, i.e. X^CX^C in F_1-generation is 0%.

43 (*d*) Albinism is a recessive trait, so woman will be carrier. If she marries an albinic man, 50% progeny will be albinic, 50% will be carrier.

Thus, option (d) is correct.

44 (*b*) Colour blindness and haemophilia are caused by two genes located on X-chromosome, both are X-linked recessive traits.

45 (*b*) Cri-du-chat syndrome in humans is caused by a conspicuous deletion in the short arm of 5th chromosome. These individuals are severely impaired and their crying (cat-like) gives the syndrome its name.

46 (*a*) Man has only one X-chromosome that is inherited to his daughter. Therefore, a hereditary disease, which is X-chromosomal linked is never passed on from father to son.

CHAPTER 10

Origin of Life

The two important aspects of life are its origin and evolution. The branch of life science, which deals with both of these aspects is called **evolutionary biology**.

It is difficult to go back in time and observe the origin and evolution of life. However, it is quite clear that life was originated in following 3 broad steps

I. Origin of universe and earth

II. Origin of life

III. Evolution of life

The universe and earth was supposed to have originated about 4.5 billion years back. **Big Bang theory** and **Solar Nebular hypothesis** are the two most accepted theories regarding it.

ORIGIN OF UNIVERSE

The vast and expanded region in space that extends to infinity is called **universe**. It consists of billions of galaxies which contain stars, planets and rocks. All of these are held together by force of gravity and clouds of gas and dust. Some theories to explain the origin of universe are described below

Big Bang theory

This theory was proposed by **Abbe Lemaitre** in 1931. Major facts related to this theory are given below

- The universe is very old and formed almost **20 billion years ago** as a result of a huge thermonuclear explosion, i.e. Big Bang.
- As a result of this explosion, cataclysmic eruption of hot, energy-rich subatomic particle took place.
- In a very short span of time, the simplest gases, i.e. hydrogen and helium were formed.
- As the universe expanded and its temperature cooled down further, the materials condensed under the influence of gravity to form stars and planets that resulted in the formation of numerous galaxies.
- Among these, our galaxy is a bright wheeling disc containing about 100 billion stars and is called as **milky way**.

Inside

Solar Nebular hypothesis

This theory was given by **Immanuel Kant** in 1753. It is the most widely accepted theory regarding the origin of universe. Major facts related to this theory are given below

- According to this theory, about **4.5 billion years ago**, our solar system was created from the gaseous clouds called **solar nebula**. It started to collapse under the force of its own gravity and became a flattened spinning disc of atoms and particles.
- Its central region heated up and become a star, known as the 'sun'.
- Later on, the atoms and dust grains orbiting the centre of gaseous disc got aggregated into clumps and grew into planets such as Mercury, Venus, Earth, Mars, Jupiter, Saturn, Uranus and Neptune.
- The origin of earth is also understood by this theory.

ORIGIN OF EARTH

The earth is one of the eight planets (previously nine) revolving around the sun. It is approximately 8000 miles in diameter and 6.6×10^{21} tonnes in weight.

It is estimated that earth have been formed 4.5 billion years ago from the left over dust and gases of the sun. Initially, it was in the form of a solidified red-hot cloud containing free atoms and having approximate temperature of 5000°-6000° C.

Primitive reducing atmosphere on the earth

- Early earth had **no atmosphere** or gaseous envelope around it.
- Surface of earth was in molten state, which after cooling resulted in huge emission of gases like carbon dioxide, water vapours, methane and ammonia.
- UV rays coming from the sun reacted with water vapours to form hydrogen and oxygen.
- Hydrogen being lighter got escaped. Oxygen combined with ammonia and methane to form water, carbon dioxide and nitrogen gas. Therefore, free oxygen was not present on early earth. This kind of atmosphere is referred as **reducing atmosphere**.
- In a reducing atmosphere, a lesser amount of energy is required to form carbon rich molecules and therefore, it helped in the origin of life.
- It is also believed that there was no degradation of any organic compounds arising in primitive earth due to unavailabilty of oxygen.

Distinction between primitive atmospheric and recent (modern) atmospheric conditions of earth is given below

Contents	Primitive atmosphere	Recent atmosphere
Nature	Reducing	Oxidising
Gases (dominant)	Methane (CH_4), ammonia (NH_3), hydrogen (H_2), water (H_2O), etc.	Nitrogen, oxygen (O_2), carbon dioxide (CO_2), etc.
Free oxygen	Absent	Present
Free hydrogen	Present	Almost absent
Origin of life	Favourable to origin of life	Not favourable to origin of life
Ultraviolet (UV) rays and cosmic rays	Reaching directly to earth's surface	Absorbed by ozone layer
Temperature	High	Normal
Rainfall and electric storms	High	Normal

ORIGIN OF LIFE

There were many thoughts put forward by scientists to explain the origin of life on earth. These thoughts or theories are categorised into following two types, i.e. ancient theories and modern theories.

Ancient theories of origin of life

Some of the most important ancient theories are discussed below

Theory of special creation

This theory was given by **Father Saurez** and supported by **Milton.** It states that life was created by some supernatural power (God). The first man was Adam, while the first woman was Eve. The two most popular views regarding this theory are as follows

(i) **Hindu Mythology** Hindus believed that the world was created by Brahma and Manu was the first man, whereas the first woman was Shradha.

(ii) **Genesis of 'Bible'** According to 'Bible' published in 16th century, God created the world in six days. The earth and heaven were created on first day, while humans were created on the day six.

This theory is a belief as there is no experimental support either to approve or disprove it.

Modern theory of origin of life

- This theory is also known as **modern theory** or **abiogenic origin** or **naturalistic theory** or **physico-chemical** evolution.
- It was given as a hypothesis by **AI Oparin** and supported by **JBS Haldane.**
- According to this theory, life originated on the earth after a long period of 'abiogenic molecular evolution' extended over some 3 billion years.
- Origin of life on the earth took place as a result of physico-chemical changes that brought about a gradual evolution of inorganic and organic compounds. This is called **chemical evolution** or **chemogeny**. It was followed by **biological evolution** or **biogeny.**

Deep sea vents hypothesis (1993 and 2003)

- According to this most recent hypothesis, life was originated in deep sea hydrothermal vents.
- These hydrothermal vents are submarine hot springs in which sea water seeps through the cracks in bottom until the water comes close to hot magma.
- This super heated water is expelled forcibly and carries a variety of molecules.
- These molecules include mainly hydrogen sulphide (H_2S), methane (CH_4), iron and sulphide ions. The positive charge of the sulphide ions would have acted as a magnet for the negatively charged organic molecules.
- This hypothesis of origin of life became popular due to the new science of genomics especially, ribosomal RNA (*r*RNA) sequencing. It suggests that the ancestors of today's prokaryotes are most closely related to the bacteria that live on the deep sea vents, i.e. the Archaebacteria.
- The primitive sea was alkaline. The presence of salts like NaCl in the body fluids of animals confirms that life originated in primitive oceans.

Process of origin of life according to modern theory

- In the process of origin of life, it is believed that some organic molecules were formed from the water and some other components of primordial earth's atmosphere.
- These molecules included nucleic acids, amino acids, short proteins and lipids. Some molecules of RNA possess enzymatic properties.
- Thus, in the primitive atmosphere, these may have catalysed the assembly of copies of themselves from the nucleotides in earth's water.
- These RNAs are considered to be the forerunners of life.
- Later on, some protein-lipid microspheres enclosing these RNA molecules may have formed.
- These first cell like organisms were called **protocells**. These protocells later gave rise to various forms of life *via* diversification.

- All these events are summerised in the below given figure

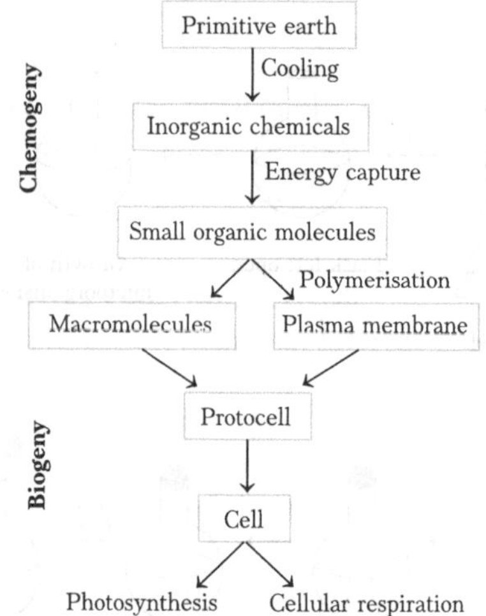

Fig. 10.4 Chemical and biological evolution

- Thus, chemogeny, followed by biogeny were responsible for origin of life.

Chemogeny or Chemical evolution

In this phase of origin of life, several organic and inorganic molecules were formed.

This chemical evolution or chemogeny had occurred in following steps

1. Atomic phase

- Due to very high temperature (5000°-6000°C), early earth had all the elements in the form of free atoms like hydrogen, oxygen, carbon, nitrogen, sulphur and phosphorus (lightest atoms).
- As the earth began to cool and condense, the atoms were segregated in three concentric masses, according to their weight as shown below

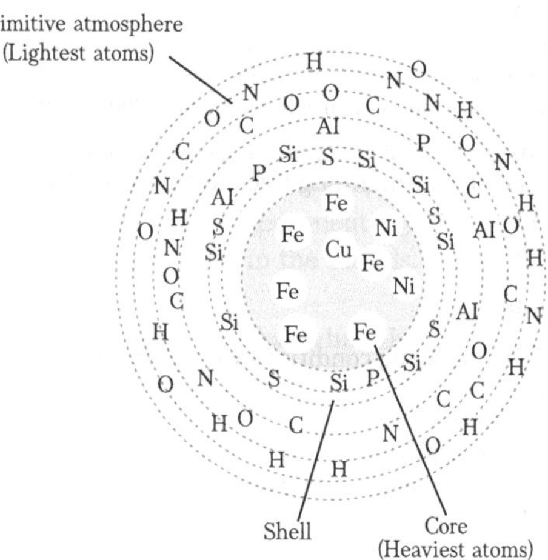

Fig. 10.5 The atomic phase

- These atoms are indispensable for the formation of protoplasm.
- The heavier elements like copper (Cu), nickel (Ni), iron (Fe), etc., passed to the core of the earth.
- Intermediate elements like silicon, aluminium passed to the middle.
- The lighter elements remained on the surface and in the atmosphere of earth.

2. Formation of early molecules

- Hydrogen atoms were the most reactive free atoms among all the elements present in the earliest atmosphere.
- The gradual fall in the surface temperature allowed hydrogen and other lighter earth's elements to interact with each other.
- As a result of this, lighter elements such as **water** (H_2O), **methane** (CH_4), **ammonia** (NH_3), **hydrogen cyanide** (HCN) and **oxides of carbon** were formed.
- During the formation of water, all free oxygen disappeared and the environment became reducing.
- Initially, water existed in the form of super heated steam that on cooling became hot rainwater and evaporated again.
- This rainwater ultimately accumulated in the depressions of earth and formed oceans, lakes and rivers, etc.

3. Formation of simple organic molecules

- Later, the oceans and lakes became rich in salts by dissolving large amounts of early compounds like ammonia (NH_3), methane (CH_4), hydrogen cyanide (HCN), nitrides, carbides, various gases and elements into water.
- Methane (CH_4) was probably the first organic compound and hydrogen cyanide was formed later.
- The formation of HCN was the most important event for the origin of life on earth.
- The high concentration of these simple organic compounds in the sea water induced them to react with each other and produced some unsaturated hydrocarbons such as ethylene, acetylene, aldehydes, ketones, alcohols and organic acids.
- As a result of further interaction of these hydrocarbons, some simple organic compounds such as simple sugars (e.g. glucose, ribose, deoxyribose, etc.), nitrogenous bases, (e.g. purines and pyrimidines), amino acids, fatty acids and glycerols were formed.
- The energy required for these reactions came from the following sources
  (i) **Solar radiations** like ultraviolet (UV) light rays, cosmic rays and X-rays, etc.
  (ii) **Electrical discharge** from lightning.
  (iii) **High energy radiations** from radioactive unstable isotopes on primitive earth.

4. Formation of larger organic molecules

- Later, by the polymerisation of simple organic compounds, larger organic molecules were formed in the primitive atmosphere.
- Amino acids polymerised into peptides and polypeptides, sugar molecules into polysaccharides and glycerol and fatty acids into fat.
- Nucleotides were formed by the combination of nitrogenous bases, sugars and phosphates.
- All of these reactions took place without enzymes, ribosomes and other cell components.

5. Formation of complex organic compounds

- A number of hydrocarbons, purines and pyrimidine bases, amino acids, fatty acids, sugars and other organic compounds accumulated in the primitive seas.
- This was followed by the polymerisation of larger organic molecules into complex organic molecules.
- Nucleic acids (DNA or RNA) were formed by the spontaneous polymerisation of nucleotides, accompanied by the loss of water molecules.
- ATP, the energy rich molecule was formed by the addition of triphosphate to adenine.
- **JBS Haldane** used the term **prebiotic soup** for oceanic water containing mixture of simple organic compounds, while **Darwin** used the term **warm little pond** for the same.

Which came first RNA or protein?

It is a matter of great controversy among biologists that which came first RNA or protein. There are three views regarding this problem and all scientists can be divided into three camps on this basis

1. **RNA world** The group of scientists, who focus on RNA as the first molecule. RNA world group feels that without a hereditary molecule, other molecules could not have formed consistently. This view is supported by the discovery of **ribozyme**, a **catalytic RNA molecule**, which have the ability to act like enzymes.
2. **Protein world** scientists, of this group argues that without enzymes (which are proteins), nothing could replicate at all. They are in view that the nucleotide is very complex molecule therefore, it cannot be formed spontaneously.
3. **Peptide-Nucleic Acid** (PNA) **world** This group of scientists focus on the combination of RNA and protein. The PNA world believed that there must have been a pre-RNA world, where the peptide, nucleic acid were the basis for life. PNA is simple and able to self-replicate.

Miller and Urey's experiment in the support of chemogeny

- The first experimental support to **Oparin-Haldane's theory of origin of life** came from **Urey** and **Miller's experiment** in 1953.
- They conducted an experiment on evolution to prove the biochemical origin of life. In 1953, Miller built an apparatus of glass tubes and flasks in the laboratory.

- He created an atmosphere containing hydrogen (H_2), ammonia (NH_3), methane (CH_4) and water vapour (H_2O) in one big flask and allowed condensed liquid to accumulate in another small flask.
- The ratio of **methane, ammonia** and **hydrogen** taken in the large flask was 2 : 1 : 2. This complete arrangement is shown below

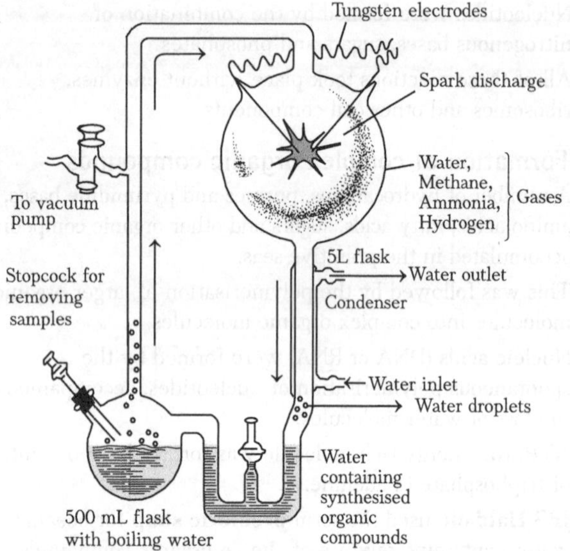

Fig. 10.6 Miller's experimental apparatus

- Energy was supplied to the apparatus by heating the liquid as well as by electric sparks from tungsten's electrodes in the large flask. These conditions of apparatus resembled the atmosphere present on the early earth.
- The experiment was conducted continuously for about one week and then the chemical composition of the liquid inside the apparatus was analysed.

Analysis and observations of Miller's experiment

After continuous heating, cooling, circulation and electrical discharge, Miller obtained an acid turbid red liquid. This liquid was a mixture of a variety of compounds shown table below

Table 10.1 Products formed under prebiotic conditions

Carboxylic acids	Nucleic acid bases	Amino acids	Sugars
Formic acid	Adenine	Glycine	Straight and branched
Acetic acid	Guanine	Alanine	Pentoses and hexoses
Propionic acid	Xanthine	α-amino butyric acid	
Straight and branched fatty acids (C_4-C_{10})	Hypoxanthine	Valine	
Glycolic acid	Cytosine	Leucine	
Lactic acid	Uracil	Isoleucine, proline	
Succinic acid		Aspartic acid, serine, threonine	

Miller concluded that the way abiotic synthesis occurred in the simulated experimental conditions, it may also have occurred in the primitive atmospheric conditions.

Several other scientists also conducted similar experiments by slightly changing the starting materials and sources of energy like UV rays and became successful in generating more or less similar products.

CHECK POINT 10.2

1. Major facts in favour of vent hypothesis are
   (a) Archaebacteria, KOH
   (b) Mycoplasma, NaCl
   (c) Mycoplasma, KOH
   (d) Archaebacteria, NaCl
2. Group of elements present in the core of primitive earth were
   (a) H, O, C
   (b) Si, Al, P
   (c) Cu, Ni, Fe
   (d) N, Si, Al
3. Which of the following appeared later when the earth cooled down to a temperature below 100°C?
   (a) Lithosphere (b) Atmosphere
   (c) Stratosphere (d) Hydrosphere
4. During the origin and evolution of life, key biological compounds were progressively synthesised in ocean with the help of energy obtained from
   (a) combustion of certain compounds
   (b) UV light only
   (c) lightning and ultraviolet light
   (d) lightning only
5. Which of the following has replaced methane of the primitive atmosphere as the major carbon containing compounds of the present day earth's atmosphere?
   (a) Carbon dioxide
   (b) Coal
   (c) Carbon monoxide
   (d) Hydrocarbon
6. Miller synthesised simple amino acids from which one of the following mixture in his experiment?
   (a) H_2, O_2, N_2 (2 : 1 : 2) and H_2O
   (b) CH_4, NH_3, H_2 (2 : 1 : 2) and H_2O
   (c) H_2, O_2, N_2 (1 : 2 : 1) and H_2O
   (d) CH_4, NH_3, H_2 (1 : 2 : 1) and H_2O

Biogeny or Biological evolution

It includes the formation of coacervates, protocells origin of prokaryotes and eukaryotes *via* diversification, etc.

Biological evolution took place in following steps

1. Formation of coacervates and microspheres

The large organic molecules synthesised abiotically on the primitive earth were considered to be the precursors of certain colloidal prebiotic aggregates.

These colloidal aggregates were called **coacervates** by **Oparin** and **microspheres** by **Sydney Fox**.

A comparison of both of these is given below

Coacervates	Microspheres
They consist of proteins, nucleoproteins and organic molecules in various combinations.	They consist of protein like structure with branched amino acids called **proteinoids.**
They exhibit a double membrane layer made up of fatty acids.	They also exhibit double layer which is devoid of fatty acids.
They were formed by mixing oppositely charged colloids (e.g. gum arabic and gelatin)	These were formed when artificially produced organic compounds were mixed with cold water.
They show growth by accumulation of various substances and action of enzymes.	They developed the ability of binary fission and budding for further growth.
These are unstable and disintegrate with time.	These are stable and exhibit uniformity.

Coacervates could even divide by budding like bacteria. Thus, more complex microspheres and coacervates functioned as pre cells or pre-bionts.

2. Formation of protocells or Eobionts or Protobionts

- With the formation of nucleoproteins, coacervates and likewise molecules changed into first living cells or protocells. These protocells in the ancient ocean represented the beginning of life.
- Protocells or Protobionts are nucleoproteinoid molecules having free-living genetic material.
- They were similar to the present day mycoplasma and virus. These were heterotrophs obtaining energy and nutrients from the organic molecules.
- Some protobionts also had chromophores in their membrane. Chromophores are the molecules that absorb visible light. The oldest fossil cells were similar to heterotrophic bacteria (prokaryote).

3. Origin of prokaryotes

- The protobionts later gave rise to monerans, which in turn gave rise to prokaryotes like bacteria and cyanobacteria, etc.
- The fossils of these primitive protobiont (*Eubacterium isolatum*) have been obtained from the rocks, in Africa about 3 billion years back.
- The first prokaryotic unicells had naked DNA and protein manufacturing machinery as protoribosomes.
- They were **anaerobes** and **chemoheterotrophs**, which obtained organic molecules from the outside, for body structuring and energy requirements.

4. Evolution of various modes of nutrition in prokaryotes

This can be studied chronologically under following steps

Step 1 Origin and evolution of chemoheterotrophs

- The first living organisms were chemoheterotrophs, which obtained energy by the fermentation of complex organic substances present in sea broth.
- These organisms multiply rapidly and increase in number. Due to which, the nutrients from sea water began to the disappear. This led to the evolution of
  (a) **Parasitic** mode of nutrition in which organisms obtain energy from other similar organisms.
  (b) **Saprophytic** mode of nutrition in which organisms depend on dead bodies and decaying cells for nourishment.

Step 2 Origin and evolution of chemoautotrophs

- These organisms obtained their energy by the process of fermentation.
- They resemble our present day anaerobic bacteria, e.g. nitrifying bacteria, sulphur bacteria and yeast.
- These were the forerunners of photosynthetic cells which released large amount of carbon dioxide in the atmosphere that paved way for the utilisation of carbon dioxide in photosynthesis.

Step 3 Origin and evolution of anaerobic photoautotrophs

- The first photoautotrophs were anaerobic. These had the ability to trap sunlight for energy and obtained carbon from carbon dioxide.
- In the mean time, evolution of chlorophyll molecule enabled some protocells to utilise light energy and synthesise carbohydrates.
- Although, they did not had the ability to use water and did not release oxygen in the atmosphere.

- They were similar to present day sulphur bacteria, in which hydrogen was used in food manufacturing and sulphur was released as a waste product.
- Perhaps, this was the initiation of autotrophism.
- Thus, the first photoautotrophs performed anoxygenic photosynthesis, e.g. *Chlorobium* and *Rhodopseudomonas.*

Step 4 Origin and evolution of aerobic photoautotrophs

- These photoautotrophs were developed about 3300-3500 million years ago due to the accumulation of carbon dioxide in the atmosphere and formation of chlorophyll molecule.
- Initially, they were comparable with present day cyanobacteria or blue-green algae.
- These had the ability to use water as hydrogen donor and carbon dioxide as a source of carbon in oxygenic photosynthesis.
- So, we can say that these were oxygen producing photosynthesisers, which released free oxygen in the atmosphere.

Stromatolites

- These are fossilised microbial mats consisting of layers of filamentous prokaryotes and trapped sediments. Microbial mats are layered microbial community, which contains **cyanobacteria** in the **uppermost layer**, **anoxygenic phototrophic bacteria** in **subsequent layers** and **chemoorganotrophic, especially sulphate-reducing bacteria in the lower layers**. It develops in a variety of environment especially, in hot springs.
- Stromatolites provide evidence for microbial life on the early earth. It can be concluded that the ancient stromatolites were formed by filamentous phototrophic bacteria, perhaps relatives of the green non-sulphur bacterium, *Chloroflexus*.
- The oldest known stromatolites were found in a rock about 3.5 billion years old from the Warrawoona group in Western Australia.

5. Oxygen revolution

- As number of photoautotrophs had increased, oxygen was liberated in the sea and atmosphere.
- Dominated methane and ammonia of primitive atmosphere reacted with free oxygen and get transformed into carbon dioxide and free nitrogen.
- Aerobic respiration was the prokaryotic adaptation which occurred during oxygen revolution.

Ozone layer formation

- As oxygen accumulated in the atmosphere, the UV light changed some of oxygen into ozone as

$$2O_2 + O_2 \rightarrow 2O_3$$

- This ozone formed a layer in the atmosphere to block the ultraviolet light. Thus, the visible light left as the only main source of energy.

6. Origin of eukaryotes

- The rising level of atmospheric oxygen due to oxygen revolution led to the appearance of first one-celled eukaryotic organisms.
- These eukaryotic cells had evolved from the prokaryotes and Archaebacteria like protocells in ancient ocean about 1500 million years ago (oldest known eukaryotic fossil is about 1.5 billion years old).
- There are following two views regarding the mode of origin of eukaryotes

I. Symbiotic or Endosymbiotic origin

- According to this view, **Lynn Margulis** explained that the oxygen respiring bacteria was developed from mutual association between a predator and primitive aerobic bacteria.
- This predator cell became the first eukaryotic animal cell. The complete outline of development is shown in the figure given below

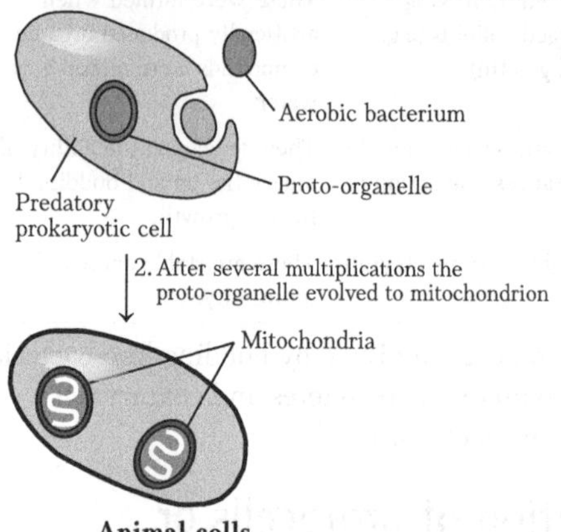

Fig. 10.7 Probable origin of mitochondria and animal cell

Similarly, the predator cells, which captured both aerobic bacteria and photosynthetic blue-green algae became the first eukaryotic plant cell as shown below

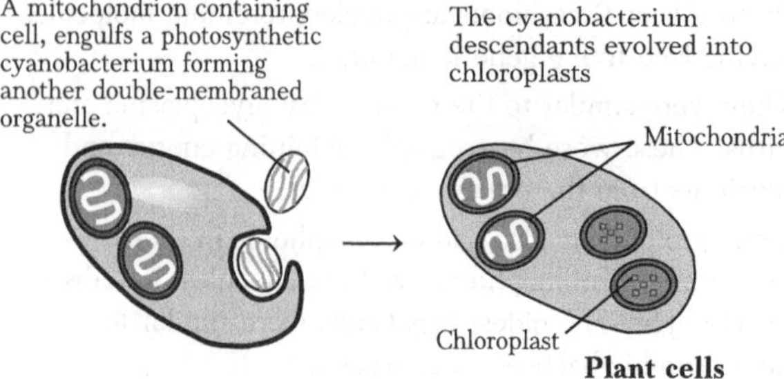

Fig. 10.8 Probable origin of chloroplast and plant cell

Evidences of endosymbiotic evolution are given below

- Mitochondria and chloroplasts are double membrane bound cell organelles. The inner membrane probably evolved from the plasma membrane of engulfed bacterium and outer membrane from the plasma membrane or endoplasmic reticulum of the host cell.
- The ribosome of mitochondria, chloroplast and bacteria are similar in size.
- Cristae of mitochondria resemble the folded membranes in various groups of bacteria.
- Mitochondria and chloroplast both possess circular DNA that is similar to bacterial DNA.

II. Origin by invagination

According to this theory, organelles of eukaryotic cells might have evolved by the invagination of surface membrane of primitive prokaryotic cells.

Role of ribozymes in origin of life

- Ribozyme is a catalytic RNA (*r*RNA), which has the ability to act as an enzyme.
- It was first found in *Tetrahymena* (a ciliated protozoan) as a self-splicing 413 nucleotide long intron.
- In 1983, another catalytic RNA (ribozyme) containing 377 nucleotides was obtained from *E. coli*.
- Ribozymes are considered as those very first living molecules, which catalysed their own replication without the involvement of protein. So, these can also be called as **RNA replicases**.

EVOLUTION OF LIFEFORMS

Evolution is defined as the act of unrolling or gradual changes from one generation to another.

Evolution is classified into following four types

- **Microevolution** Small changes in a gene pool for a reatively shorter period, i.e. one or two generations.
- **Macroevolution** These are continuous changes occurring over a long period of time, e.g. fossil records exhibit macroevolution.
- **Megaevolution** Origin of a whole new biological group.
- **Quantum evolution** Evolution which occurs with systematic mutation.

We will discuss evolution in detail in our next chapter.

Life on other planets

The Oparin-Haldane theory of origin of life raises the possibility of life on other planets of solar system where atmospheric conditions are similar to that, present on the earth at the time of origin of life. For example,

- **Moon** lacks both water and an atmosphere. This does not show any sign of life due to the absence of water vapours.
- **Mercury** is extremely hot due to its nearness to the sun and also lacks atmosphere.
- Conditions of **Venus** are not well-known. Therefore, there is no possibility of existence of life on these planets.
- **Jupiter**, **Saturn**, **Uranus** and **Neptune** have dense atmosphere made up of thick clouds of helium, hydrogen, ammonia and methane. These are similar to primitive atmosphere of the early earth. These atmospheric conditions suggest the possibility of life on these planets.
- However, very low temperature (-200°-400°F) is an adverse condition for life. **Pluto** is also very cold.
- **Mars** is the only planet, where life could be supported. Its atmosphere consists of nitrogen, carbon dioxide and water vapours, temperature is 30°-60°C at daytime.
- Scientists from different countries including India are trying to find out the sign of life on Mars and other planets. The photos sent by **Mariner-9 of America** have shown the possibility of the existence of life on Mars, but photos sent by **Viking** in 1976 had made this possibility doubtful.

Study of meteorites and origin of life

During the study of space, biologists regarding meteorites revealed that the space contains some chemical compounds which can form life. Some of these observations with respect to origin of life are as follows

- Meteorites contain amino acids and polynucleotides similar to DNA.
- DNA found in meteorites were of chemical origin and had identical strands instead of complementary strands found in the DNA of organisms.
- The polynucleotides were found in meteorites, which fell in Ukraine in 1889.

CHECK POINT 10.3

1. A coacervate is
   (a) a nucleoprotein in nature
   (b) a mixture of ammonia and water
   (c) a colloidal suspension in water
   (d) a mixture of contemporary bioproteins
2. Which of the following is not found in a lipid coacervate droplet or a proteinoid microsphere?
   (a) The ability to grow
   (b) A nucleus
   (c) A two-layer boundary
   (d) Division by pinching in two layers
3. It is believed that the first organisms, which inhabited earth's surface were
   (a) mixotrophs
   (b) chemotrophs
   (c) heterotrophs
   (d) autotrophs
4. Which of the following is a nucleoproteinoid molecule having free-living gene?
   (a) Protobionts (b) Microspheres
   (c) Coacervates (d) Cephalin
5. Which of the following is the chief reason showing that the protocell was probably a fermenter?
   (a) It did not have any enzymes
   (b) The atmosphere did not have any oxygen
   (c) Atmosphere was oxidising
   (d) None of the above
6. Bacteria that obtain energy by oxidising inorganic hydrogen sulphide. They use this energy to build organic molecules from carbon obtained from the carbon dioxide in the seawater. These bacteria are
   (a) photoheterotrophs (b) chemoautotrophs
   (c) photoautotrophs (d) chemoheterotrophs

EXAM POINTS

- After 500 million years of formation of earth, life appeared on this planet. **[NEET 2020]**
- Abiogenesis means spontaneous generation. **[BHU 2012]**
- According to the theory of spontaneous generation, life originated from decaying and rotting matter like straw, mud, etc. **[COMEDK 2015]**
- Oparin and Haldane proposed that the first form of life could have come from pre-existing non-living organic molecules. **[UP CPMT 2011]**
- At the time of origin of life, O_2 was absent in the atmosphere. **[Rajasthan PMT 2011]**
- Miller and Urey conducted the experiment on evolution to prove biochemical origin of life. **[BCECE 2012, UP CPMT 2008]**
- SL Miller produced amino acids by mixing CH_4, H_2, NH_3 and water vapour at 800°C. **[BCECE 2015, NEET 2020]**
- The earliest organisms that appeared on the earth were anaerobic chemoautotrophs. They were first autotrophic organisms. **[NEET-I 2016]**
- The first catalytic molecule during evolution of life was *r*RNA. **[BCECE 2015]**
- The correct sequence of events in the origin of life is

  Synthesis of organic monomers
  ↓
  Synthesis of organic polymers
  ↓
  Formation of protobionts
  ↓
  Formation of DNA based genetic systems **[NEET 2016]**

Chapter Exercises

(A) Topical Exercise

Origin of Universe, Origin of Earth

1 The branch of science which deals with the study of universe is called
(a) universology
(b) evolutionary biology
(c) cosmology
(d) astrology

2 Find the incorrect match.
(a) Origin of universe - 15-20 million years ago
(b) Origin of galaxy - 100 billion years ago
(c) Origin of solar system - 4.5 million years ago
(d) Origin of earth - 4.5 billion years ago

3 Consider the following statements.
I. Big Bang hypothesis was proposed by Lemaitre.
II. The age of Big Bang is likely to be in the order of 10^5 year.
Choose the correct option.
(a) Statement I is true, but II is false
(b) Statement I is false, but II is true
(c) Both statements I and II are true
(d) Both statements I and II are false

4 According to the Big Bang theory, the gaseous clouds which created solar system were
(a) hydrogen and helium (b) solar nebula
(c) milky way (d) methane and ammonia

5 Universe originated about 15 billion years ago by
(a) a thermonuclear explosion
(b) fusion
(c) gravity
(d) destruction of atmosphere

6 Who discovered solar nebula?
(a) Abbe Lemaitre (b) Kant
(c) Louis Pasteur (d) None of these

7 The solar system was created by the collapse of solar nebula. Solar nebula was the
(a) gaseous cloud
(b) solid ball of soil
(c) liquid of water and minerals
(d) solid iron

8 Consider the following statements.
I. The stellar distances are measured in light years.
II. There was reducing environment on primitive atmosphere.
Choose the correct option.
(a) Statement I is true, but II is false
(b) Statement I is false, but II is true
(c) Both statements I and II are true
(d) Both statements I and II are false

9 Temperature in the interior of the sun is 20000000°C. The reason for this high temperature is
(a) various exothermic reactions are taking place
(b) fusion reactions converting hydrogen of sun to helium
(c) collision of particles releasing energy
(d) None of the above

10 There was no degradation of any organic compounds arising in primitive earth because
(a) atmosphere was absent
(b) atmosphere was highly reducing
(c) atmosphere was highly oxidising
(d) None of the above

11 In primordial atmosphere, when the living organism evolved the respiration process was
(a) aerobic as it released more energy
(b) anaerobic because early atmosphere contained little or no oxygen
(c) aerobic as it was more complex
(d) anaerobic as it released more energy

12 The atmosphere of the earth at the time of origin of life was
I. reducing
II. did not contain free oxygen
III. oxidising
IV. similar to recent atmosphere
Codes
(a) I and II (b) III and IV
(c) II and III (d) II and IV

Ancient Theories of Origin of Life

13 Theory of special creation states that
(a) God is the creator of life
(b) origin of life is supernatural or vitalistic event at a particular time in the past
(c) life is immutable and has not changed ever since its origin
(d) All of the above

14 Who proposed the Theory of Cosmozoic Origin?
(a) Richter and Arrhenius
(b) Urey and Miller
(c) Haeckel
(d) Lamarck

15 The formation of living and non-living world simultaneously is the main feature of
(a) theory of panspermia
(b) theory of cosmozoic origin
(c) theory of catastrophism
(d) theory of abiogenesis

16 Which of the following is true about cosmozoan theory?
(a) Life is coeternal with matter without any beginning
(b) Origin of life is extraterrestrial
(c) Life originated once or several times in various parts of galaxy
(d) All of the above

17 Which of the following is a factor against the theory of panspermia?
(a) Non-conductive conditions of extremely low temperature and lack of atmosphere in interplanetary space to life
(b) Very high flux of cosmic and ultraviolet radiation from the sun
(c) Ultra dryness in interplanetary space
(d) All of the above

18 The idea of spontaneous generation was supported by
(a) Anaximus (b) Anaximander
(c) Empedocles (d) Pasteur

19 Which one of the following theories is also called theory of abiogenesis?
(a) Theory of special creation
(b) Theory of spontaneous generation
(c) Theory of cosmozoic origin
(d) Theory of catastrophism

20 Which of the following is an example of theory of spontaneous generation?
(a) Frog could arise from moist soil
(b) Frog could arise from parent frog
(c) Frog could arise from fishes
(d) None of the above

Theory of Biogenesis

21 The most widely accepted view for origin of life is
(a) biogenesis (b) abiogenesis
(c) biochemical origin (d) biopoiesis

22 The theory of spontaneous generation of life was refuted by
I. Francesco Redi
II. Louis Pasteur
III. Lazzaro Spallanzani
IV. van Helmont

Codes
(a) Only III (b) II and III
(c) III and IV (d) I, II and III

23 Which of the following theory accepted that microorganisms come only from other microorganisms?
(a) Theory of abiogenic origin
(b) Theory of abiogenesis
(c) Theory of biogenesis
(d) Theory of cosmozoic origin

24 In Francesco Redi's experiment
I. maggots developed in uncovered jar.
II. maggots developed in jar covered by muslin cloth.
III. maggots developed in tightly sealed jar.
Choose the correct option.
(a) Only II (b) Only I
(c) I and II (d) Only III

25 Pasteur's experiments and similar ones that followed convinced most people that spontaneous generation of life did not happen because
(a) Pasteur did not boil his flask for a long time
(b) Pasteur's swan-necked flasks ruled out the objection that spoiled air could have contaminated his experiments
(c) Pasteur was extremely meticulous
(d) Pasteur used very fine mesh screens to cover his flasks

26 Who said that the organisms develop from pre-existing organisms?
(a) Louis Pasteur (b) Aristotle
(c) AI Oparin (d) Haldane

27 Pasteur succeeded in disproving the spontaneous generation theory because
(a) he was lucky
(b) he was ingenious in drawing out the neck of the glass flasks so as to provide access to air but not to microorganisms
(c) of the fact that sample of yeast taken by him was dead
(d) of the clean surroundings of his laboratory

28 Mark the correct statement.
(a) L Spallanzani stated that air carried microorganisms
(b) Father Saurez discarded the view of special creation
(c) L Pasteur did his experiments on flesh
(d) F Redi put forward the theory of special creation

29 Match the following columns.

Column I	Column II
A. Catastrophism	1. Cuvier
B. Origin of species	2. Suarez
C. Special creation	3. Darwin

Codes

	A	B	C
(a)	2	1	3
(b)	3	2	1
(c)	1	2	3
(d)	1	3	2

Modern Theory of Origin of Life and Chemical Evolution

30 Modern theory of origin of life is also known as
(a) naturalistic theory
(b) abiogenesis
(c) physico-chemical evolution
(d) All of the above

31 Naturalistic theory was given by
(a) Darwin and Haldane (b) Abbe Lemaitre
(c) Oparin and Haldane (d) Saurez and Kant

32 Terrestrial or abiogenic origin of life interprets that the life arose
(a) by a series of sequential chemical reactions
(b) from pre-existing life
(c) spontaneously from lifeless matter
(d) coexternally with matter

33 During primitive times, oceans contained
I. fishes
II. algae
III. water
IV. ammonia, methane and minerals
Choose the correct option.
(a) II and III (b) I and IV (c) I and II (d) III and IV

34 The concept of chemical evolution is based on
(a) crystallisation of chemicals
(b) interaction of water, air and clay under intense heat
(c) the effect of solar radiation on chemicals
(d) possible origin of life by the combination of chemicals under suitable environmental conditions

35 As the earth started condensing, which of the following passed to core of the earth?
(a) Silicon (b) Aluminium
(c) Nickel (d) All of the above

36 The presence of salts (NaCl and other) in the animal body fluids gives an inference that life originated in the
(a) rainwater (b) primitive ocean
(c) salt solutions (d) None of these

37 Most probably now, no origin of life is taking place in the way as occurred on primordial earth because
(a) free oxygen may react with most intermediate compounds
(b) free hydrogen is absent
(c) water vapour is absent
(d) free oxygen is poisonous

38 In the early earth, organic acids were produced by the combination of H_2 with
(a) ammonia and methane (b) hydrogen
(c) organic matter (d) sulphates and nitrates

39 In the ancient atmosphere, free nitrogen, oxygen and carbon dioxide were not present because
(a) of the large amount of hydrogen and high temperature
(b) carbon would have combined with hydrogen to form methane
(c) any free oxygen would have combined with iron, silicon, aluminium, etc., to form minerals of the earth's crust
(d) All of the above

40 The energy source for the creation of the first organic compounds came from
(a) electronic discharge
(b) UV light
(c) high temperature from volcanoes
(d) All of the above

41 The complex organic compounds that may have first evolved in the direction of origin of life on earth may have been
(a) proteins and amino acids
(b) proteins and nucleic acids
(c) urea and nucleic acids
(d) urea and amino acids

42 The most important event for the origin of life on earth was the formation of
(a) hydrogen cyanide (b) calcium carbonate
(c) nitric acid (d) None of these

43 Evolution of the DNA → RNA → Protein, system was a milestone because the protocell
(a) could now reproduce
(b) was a heterotrophic fermenter
(c) pass on genetic information
(d) needed ATP for requirement of energy

44 The first genetic material was most likely to be
(a) DNA polymer
(b) protein enzyme
(c) DNA oligonucleotide
(d) RNA polymer

45 As per theory of chemosynthetic generation, what was the sequence of origin of life?
(a) Amino acids – Nucleoproteins – Chlorophyll
(b) Nucleoproteins – Amino acids – Chlorophyll
(c) Nucleoproteins – Chlorophyll – Amino acids
(d) Amino acids – Chlorophyll – Nucleoproteins

46 Which of the following explanations accounts for the statements. 'It has yet not been possible to create life'?
(a) Most molecules are known except a few
(b) Nature and molecular organisation is complex and not completely understood
(c) All molecules of life have not been identified as yet
(d) Some molecules are organic and others are inorganic in nature

47 Why do scientists think that the RNA and not DNA, was the first gene?
(a) RNA can store information and acts as an enzyme
(b) DNA copies itself but cannot store information
(c) DNA did not exist in early cells
(d) RNA sometimes forms a double helix

48 Consider the following statements.
I. The term prebiotic soup and warm little pond given by Darwin and Haldane have same meaning.
II. According to deep sea vents hypothesis, primitive sea was alkaline.
Choose the correct option.
(a) Statement I is true, but II is false
(b) Statement I is false, but II is true
(c) Both statements I and II are true
(d) Both statements I and II are false

Miller Experiment

49 Chemical theory of origin of life was given by
(a) Stanley Miller
(b) Spallanzani
(c) Oparin and Haldane
(d) Louis Pasteur

50 The Oparin-Haldane hypothesis on the origin of life was experimentally proved by
(a) Louis Pasteur (b) Urey and Miller
(c) Malthus (d) Plato

51 According to Oparin and Haldane, transformation of lifeless chemicals into living matter extended over some
(a) 1 billion years (b) 2 billion years
(c) 3 billion years (d) 4 billion years

52 According to Oparin, which one of the following was present in the primitive atmosphere?
I. Methane II. Hydrogen
III. Water vapour IV. Oxygen
Codes
(a) Only I (b) Only IV
(c) II and IV (d) I, II and III

53 Which hypothesis on the origin of life states that the proteins, lipids and other complex organic molecules are formed when energy from the sun and other sources causes chemical reactions among gases in earth's prehistoric atmosphere?
(a) Self-replicating molecules
(b) Biogenesis
(c) Miller and Urey's experiment
(d) Spontaneous generation

54 Miller conducted his experiment in an apparatus containing methane, ammonia and hydrogen in the ratio of
(a) 2 : 5 : 4 (b) 2 : 1 : 2 (c) 5 : 4 : 1 (d) None of these

55 Which of the following is correct with respect to Miller's experiment?
I. The category of molecules produced were organic monomers.
II. Amino acids were formed at the end of experiment.
Choose the correct option.
(a) Statement I is true, but II is false
(b) Statement I is false, but II is true
(c) Both statements I and II are true
(d) Both statements I and II are false

56 In the Miller-Urey experiment, the control setup was different from the actual experimental setup in
(a) presence of oxygen in control setup
(b) ratio of gases used in chamber
(c) presence or absence of energy source
(d) types of gases used in reaction mixture

57 Which of these did Stanley Miller place in his experimental system to show that the organic molecules could have arose from the inorganic molecules on the primitive earth?
(a) The primitive gases
(b) Purines and pyrimidines
(c) Microspheres
(d) Protocells

58 Which of the following type of sugar was present in turbid red liquid?
(a) Straight chain sugars (b) Pentoses
(c) Hexoses (d) All of these

59 Apart from Miller and Urey, who produced complex compounds from simpler compounds to prove theory of physico-chemical evolution?
(a) Fox (b) Dobzhansky
(c) Calvin (d) Both (a) and (c)

Biological Evolution and Evolution of Lifeforms

60 The term coacervates was given by
(a) Sydney Fox (b) Oparin
(c) Stanley (d) Haldane

61 Under certain conditions, scientists have obtained cell-like structures. These are known as
(a) microbes (b) protists
(c) coacervates (d) prebiotic soup

62 Coacervates containing nucleoprotein and surrounded by several nutritive substances and covered by a surface membrane represents

(a) protocells (b) liposome
(c) pre-cells (d) microsphere

63 Coacervates can divide like bacteria by the process of

(a) fragmentation (b) fission
(c) budding (d) Both (b) and (c)

64 Consider the following statements.

I. Protocells were similar to the present day virus and eukaryotes.
II. The proteinoid colloidal aggregate obtained by Sydney Fox are microspheres.

Choose the correct option.

(a) Statement I is true, but II is false
(b) Statement I is false, but I is true
(c) Both statements I and II are true
(d) Both statements I and II are false

65 Which of these gives a possible sequence of organic chemicals prior to the protocell?

(a) Inorganic gases, amino acids, polypeptide, microsphere
(b) Inorganic gases, nucleotides, nucleic acids, genes
(c) Water, salts, protein, oxygen
(d) Both (a) and (b)

66 An evolving coacervate like system would have needed a controlled and constant source of energy for

(a) maintaining their organisation
(b) making large complex molecules
(c) organising these molecules into structural patterns
(d) All of the above

67 How is biological evolution distinct from the chemical evolution?

(a) Biological evolution preceded chemical evolution during origin of life
(b) Not all organisms on earth undergo biological evolution
(c) Biological evolution is not affected by mutation
(d) Biological evolution happens when organisms could replicate

68 Consider the following statements.

I. The age of oldest sedimentary rock is about 2.7-3.2 billion year.
II. The oldest eukaryotic fossil is about 1.5 billion year old.

Choose the correct option.

(a) Statement I is true, but II is false
(b) Statement I is false, but II is true
(c) Both statements I and II are true
(d) Both statements I and II are false

69 The first organisms to appear on earth were more like plants because

(a) plants are simpler (b) plants are more
(c) plants do photosynthesis (d) None of these

70 The main difference between prokaryotic and eukaryotic cell is that in the prokaryotic cell there is no

I. nucleus with a nuclear membrane.
II. mitochondria and chloroplasts.
III. cell wall.
IV. genetic material.

Codes

(a) Only I (b) Only II
(c) I and II (d) I and III

71 The first autotrophic organisms were

(a) chemoautotrophic that never release oxygen
(b) photoautotrophic that were aerobic
(c) chemoautotrophic that were aerobic
(d) photoautotrophic that were anaerobic

72 The heterotrophic hypothesis helps us to understand

(a) definition of the term life
(b) difference between living and non-living
(c) increasing complexity moving from the atom to the simple molecule to complex proteins to living organisms, populations, societies and communities
(d) All of the above

73 What prokaryotic adaptation occurred during the oxygen revolution and opened up the possibility for energy demanding multicellular lifeforms?

(a) Electron transport systems
(b) Anaerobic fermentation
(c) Aerobic respiration
(d) Photosynthesis

74 The reason of presence of free oxygen in the earth's atmosphere, whereas absence of free oxygen at the time of origin of life is

(a) catalytic activity of animals
(b) photosynthetic activity of plants
(c) heating of the earth
(d) None of the above

75 Which of the following modes of nutrition is most primitive?

(a) Chemoautotroph
(b) Chemoheterotroph
(c) Anaerobic photoautotroph
(d) Aerobic photoautotroph

76 The discovery of virus has placed the problem of the origin of life in new light and it is believed that the higher forms of life have descended from

(a) free-living viruses (b) free-living bacteria
(c) free-living Protozoa (d) free-living Metazoa

77 The fossilised microbial mats which consist of filamentous prokaryotes and trapped sediments are

(a) stromatolites (b) sulphur bacteria
(c) saprophytes (d) None of these

78 Consider the following statements.

I. Archaebacteria are the oldest living fossil.
II. Stromatolites, the first found fossils were cyanobacteria.

Choose the correct option.

(a) Statement I is true, but II is false
(b) Statement I is false, but II is true
(c) Both statements I and II are true
(d) Both statements I and II are false

79 Choose the correct option regarding fossils.

I. Fossil records usually exhibit macroevolution.
II. Ribozymes are considered as molecular fossil.
III. The oldest fossil cells are about same size of modern prokaryotes.

Codes

(a) Only I (b) Only III
(c) II and III (d) I, II and III

80 The polynucleotides were found in which of the following meteorites which fell in Ukraine?

(a) Muchison meteorite (b) Mighi meteorite
(c) Meteorite (d) Both (a) and (b)

81 Which of these is a true statement?

(a) Eukaryotes evolved before prokaryotes
(b) Prokaryotes evolved before eukaryotes
(c) The true cell evolved before the protocell
(d) Prokaryotes did not evolve until 1.5 billion years ago

82 Which of the following is the strongest evidence that prokaryotes evolved before eukaryotes?

(a) Meteorites that have struck the earth
(b) Abiotic experiments that constructed liposomes in the laboratory
(c) Liposomes look like prokaryotic cells
(d) The oldest fossilised cells resemble prokaryotes

83 Which of the following statements does not explain the usefulness of study of the origin and evolution of life?

(a) The human species is most evolved, so no harm can be done to us
(b) We know that life can exist anywhere else as well
(c) We learn that human beings have the responsibility to conserve nature
(d) We learn about the unity and diversity of living organisms

(B) Cumulative Exercise

(Assorted Questions of the Chapter for Advanced Level Practice)

1 In what respect, the heterotroph hypothesis differs from the early ideas of spontaneous generation?

(a) It assumed that spontaneous generation was a continuous process that could happen even today
(b) The idea of spontaneous generation maintained that complex organisms could arise suddenly from non-living matter
(c) The heterotroph hypothesis assumes that a very simple organism evolved slowly from non-living matter and this occurred in the primitive environmental conditions
(d) In all of the above conditions

2 In Spallanzani's experiment, one set of flasks had access to air through holes in the cork and the other set did not. In the set having access to air, the contents showed abundant growth of microorganisms. What inference would you draw from this experiment?

(a) Spontaneous generation does not need air
(b) Spontaneous generation requires contact with air
(c) The contents of the flask had not been boiled thoroughly
(d) Spontaneous generation is impossible, if there is no spore source like air

3 What is the difference between spontaneous generation and biogenesis?

(a) Biogenesis supposes that the non-living materials can produce life, while spontaneous generation follows the idea that living things come only from the other living things
(b) Spontaneous generation and biogenesis both support the theory that non-living materials are the source of living organisms
(c) Spontaneous generation proposes that the non-living materials can produce life, biogenesis follows the idea that living things come only from other living things
(d) Spontaneous generation applies only to plants and how they produce life, while biogenesis applies to animals and how they produce life

4 The endosymbiotic theory states that ......; one piece of evidence supporting this theory is the fact that ....

(a) the first hereditary material was RNA; mitochondria and chloroplasts have heredity based on RNA
(b) the genomes of complex animals came in part from the genomes of invading pathogens; the human genome contains the complete genomes of 120 viruses and 10 bacteria
(c) mitochondria and chloroplasts originated as ingested organelles; prokaryotes, mitochondria and chloroplasts have their own DNA
(d) over the time, parasites evolve to resemble their hosts; the DNA of human parasites contains segments of human DNA

5 Which of the following statements are correct about the characteristics of protobionts, like microspheres as envisaged in the abiogenic origin of life?

I. They exhibit simple reproduction.
II. They could separate the combinations of molecules from the surroundings.
III. They were partially isolated from the surroundings.
IV. They could maintain an internal environment.

Codes

(a) I and II (b) II and III
(c) III and IV (d) I, II, III and IV

6 In 1953, SL Miller created primitive earth conditions in the laboratory and gave experimental evidence for origin of first form of life from pre-existing non-living organic molecules. The primitive earth conditions created include **[NCERT Exemplar]**

(a) low temperature, volcanic storms, atmosphere rich in oxygen
(b) low temperature, volcanic storms, reducing atmosphere
(c) high temperature, volcanic storms, non-reducing atmosphere
(d) high temperature, volcanic storms, reducing atmosphere containing CH_4, NH_3, etc

7 Which of the following is correct about microspheres?

I. Protobionts made of polypeptides are called microspheres.
II. They show division by binary fission.
III. Viruses are exactly similar to the microspheres.
IV. Bacteria are exactly similar to the microspheres.

Codes

(a) I and III (b) I and II
(c) III and IV (d) I, II and III

8 Which of the following gives a possible sequence of organic chemicals prior to protocell?

I. Inorganic gases, amino acids, polypeptides, microsphere.
II. Inorganic gases, nucleotides, nucleic acids, genes.
III. Water, salts, proteins, oxygen.
IV. Protein, salts, oxygen, water.

Codes

(a) I and II (b) Only III
(c) I and III (d) III and IV

9 The sequence of origin of life may be

(a) Inorganic materials → Organic materials → Colloidal aggregate → Eobiont → Cell
(b) Organic materials → Inorganic materials → Colloidal aggregate → Eobiont → Cell
(c) Inorganic materials → Organic materials → Eobiont → Cell → Colloidal aggregate
(d) Organic materials → Inorganic materials → Eobiont → Cell → Colloidal aggregate

10 The given diagram represents Miller's experiment. Choose the correct combination of labelling for *A*, *B*, *C* and *D*.

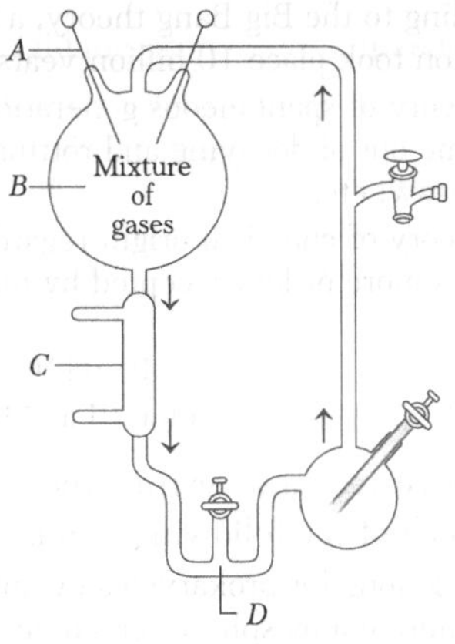

(a) *A*-Electrodes, *B*-$NH_3 + H_2 + H_2O + CH_4$, *C*-Condensor, *D*-U-trap
(b) *A*-Electrodes, *B*-$NH_3 + H_2 + CO_2 + CH_3$, *C*-Vacuum pump, *D*-U-trap
(c) *A*-Electrodes, *B*-$NH_3 + H_2O$, *C*-Condensor, *D*-Vacuum pump
(d) *A*-Electrodes, *B*-$NH_3 + H_2 + H_2O + CH_4$, *C*-Boiling water, *D*-Vaccum pump

11 Match the following columns.

	Column I		Column II
A.	Cyanobacteria	1.	The first organisms to evolve oxygen
B.	Chemoheterotrophs	2.	Organisms that can grow with or without oxygen
C.	Facultative anaerobes	3.	Obtained energy from fermentation of organic molecules
D.	Obligate anaerobes	4.	Organisms that are poisoned by oxygen

Codes

	A	B	C	D		A	B	C	D
(a)	1	3	2	4	(b)	1	2	3	4
(c)	2	3	1	4	(d)	2	1	3	4

12 Which of the following discoveries would force scientists to revise their present theories regarding the origin of life on earth?

I. The earth is found to be billion years old, rather than 4.6 billion.
II. Polypeptides can catalyse replication of small RNA molecules.
III. There was a lot of oxygen gas in the atmosphere 4 billion years ago.
IV. Minerals in lava catalyse formation of polypeptides from amino acids.

Codes

(a) I and III (b) I and IV (c) II and III (d) Only III

ANSWERS

Check Point 10.1

1. (a)	2. (c)	3. (a)	4. (d)	5. (c)	6. (a)

Check Point 10.2

1. (d)	2. (c)	3. (c)	4. (c)	5. (a)	6. (b)

Check Point 10.3

1. (d)	2. (b)	3. (b)	4. (a)	5. (b)	6. (b)

(A) Topical Exercise

1. (c)	2. (b)	3. (a)	4. (a)	5. (a)	6. (b)	7. (a)	8. (c)	9. (b)	10. (a)
11. (b)	12. (a)	13. (d)	14. (a)	15. (b)	16. (d)	17. (d)	18. (b)	19. (b)	20. (a)
21. (c)	22. (d)	23. (c)	24. (c)	25. (b)	26. (a)	27. (b)	28. (a)	29. (d)	30. (d)
31. (c)	32. (a)	33. (d)	34. (d)	35. (c)	36. (b)	37. (a)	38. (a)	39. (d)	40. (d)
41. (b)	42. (a)	43. (a)	44. (d)	45. (a)	46. (b)	47. (a)	48. (c)	49. (c)	50. (b)
51. (c)	52. (d)	53. (c)	54. (b)	55. (c)	56. (c)	57. (a)	58. (d)	59. (d)	60. (b)
61. (c)	62. (a)	63. (c)	64. (c)	65. (d)	66. (d)	67. (d)	68. (c)	69. (c)	70. (c)
71. (d)	72. (d)	73. (c)	74. (b)	75. (b)	76. (a)	77. (a)	78. (c)	79. (d)	80. (d)
81. (b)	82. (d)	83. (a)							

(B) Cumulative Exercise

1. (d)	2. (d)	3. (c)	4. (c)	5. (d)	6. (d)	7. (b)	8. (c)	9. (a)	10. (a)
11. (a)	12. (d)	13. (d)	14. (c)	15. (c)	16. (d)	17. (a)	18. (c)	19. (b)	20. (b)
21. (c)	22. (d)	23. (d)	24. (b)						

(C) Medical Entrances' Gallery

1. (d)	2. (c)	3. (c)	4. (c)	5. (b)	6. (d)	7. (b)	8. (a)	9. (c)	10. (c)
11. (d)	12. (c)								

Explanations

(A) Topical Exercise

3 (*a*) Statement I is true, but II is false. Incorrect statement can be corrected as

The age of Big Bang is likely to be in the order of 10^{10} year.

18 (*b*) The idea of spontaneous generation was supported by Anaximander, Aristotle, Plato, etc.

According to this theory, life originated from the non-living (lifeless) materials automatically.

25 (*b*) Pasteur by his swan-necked flask experiment, ruled out the objection that spoiled air could have contaminated his experiment.

In his experiment, no growth of microorganisms in the broth was observed even through when it was in direct contact with the air, due to the seal formed by the condensed water.

After the swan-neck was broken, colonies of microorganisms could be seen growing.

Hence, it was concluded that growth of microorganisms was not spontaneous and was possible due to contamination.

35 (*c*) Due to very high temperature, early earth had all elements in the form of free atoms like hydrogen, oxygen, carbon, etc., which segregated as per their weight when the earth condensed. Heavier elements like Ni, Cu, Fe, etc. passed to the core, intermediate ones like Si, Al, etc., passed to the middle and lighter ones remained at the surface and in the atmosphere of the earth.

39 (*d*) The primitive atmosphere of the earth was reducing and rich in water vapour, CO_2, CO and H_2. The greenhouse gases absorbed infrared radiations and contributed to an increased temperature.

The high temperature, along with UV light and lightening gave way to reactions occurring between the above components.

O_2 did not occur in free state as it readily combined with elements like Si and Fe, forming respective oxides.

Hydrogen combined with free O, N and C, forming H_2O, CH_4, NH_3 and HCN.

Thus, option (d) is correct.

58 (*d*) In the millers experiment after comtinuous heating, cooling circulation and electrical discharge, miller obtained an acid turbid red liquid which was a mixture of compounds including carboxylic acids like formic acid, succinic acid, Acetic acid etc, Nucleic acid bases like Adenine Guanine, Cytosine, Uracil etc. Amino acids like Glycine, Valine, Alanine etc and sugars like pentoses and Hexoses.

71 (*d*) The first autotrophs were photoautotrophs that were anaerobic and they used to perform anoxygenic photosynthesis.

(B) Cumulative Exercise

13 (*d*) Statements I, III and IV are correct, while II is incorrect. Incorrect statement can be corrected as

According to Big Bang theory, a thermonuclear explosion took place 20 billion years ago.

16 (*d*) Statements I, II and IV are true, while III is false. Incorrect statement can be corrected as

Francesco Redi and Lazzaro Spallanzani supported the theory of biogenesis.

17 (*a*) Both A and R are true and R is the correct explanation of A.

Theory of chemical evolution states that life originated from pre-existing non-living organic molecules and the formation of life was preceded by chemical evolution. The conditions on primitive earth which favoured chemical evolution were high temperature (4800°C), volcanic storms and a reducing atmosphere that contained CH_4, NH_3, water vapours, etc.

18 (*c*) A is true, but R is false because

Each coacervate was a cluster of macromolecules surrounded by a membrane. According to Oparin, coacervates were the sole living molecules which gave rise to cells.

19 (*b*) Both A and R are true, but R is not the correct explanation of A.

First living cell is named protocell or eobiont or protobiont, which evolved into prokaryotic cell.

20 (*b*) Both A and R are true, but R is not the correct explanation of A.

With the addition of oxygen into the atmosphere, methane and ammonia began to disappear as they got oxidised forming carbon dioxide and nitrogen, respectively.
These events ultimately transformed the ancient reducing, oxygen free atmosphere into the modern oxidising atmosphere with plenty of free oxygen. As more oxygen accumulated in the atmosphere. Ozone began to appear in the top layers. It developed in the presence of high energy radiations.

21 (*c*) A is true, but R is false because

Coacervates and microspheres are believed to be the presursors of life. The coacervates contain mainly proteins, polysaccharides and some water. As these coacervates do not have lipid outer membrane hence, they cannot reproduce.

22 (*d*) A is false, but R is true. A can be corrected as
Earth is about 4.5 billion years old. Primitive earth had no atmosphere and contained water vapours, CH_4, CO_2, NH_3. Life appeared 500 million years back after the formation of earth.

23 (*d*) A is false, but R is true. A can be corrected as

Coacervates were aggregates of organic biomolecules surrounded by film of water molecules. These lacked definite membrane, but did exhibit some life like characters.
Microspheres were non-living collections of organic macromolecules, double-layered and formed from proteinoids, by heating a mixture of amino acids at 180°C.

24 (*b*) Both A and R are true, but R is not the correct explanation of A.

The theory of special creation states that God created life by his divine act of creation. This theory lacked scientific evidences and thus was not accepted.

Theory of spontaneous generation states that life originated from decaying and rotting matter like straw, mud, etc. Louis pasteur rejected the theory of spontaneous generation and demonstrated that life came from pre-existing life forms.

(C) Medical Entrances' Gallery

1 (*d*) The correct option is (d) because
In 1953, SL Miller created electric discharge in a closed flask containing CH_4, H_2, NH_3 and water vapours at 800°C.

2 (*c*) During the course of evolution, earth probably formed about 4.5 billion years ago. After its formation life appeared about 500 million years ago in oceans. The first living forms were believed to be heterotrophs and used to derive nutrition from external sources.

4 (*c*) Both statements I and II are true.
The earliest organisms that appeared on the earth were anaerobic chemoautotrophs. Chemoautotrophs were the first autotrophic organisms. They were unable to perform photolysis of water and never released oxygen, e.g. sulphur bacteria.

10 (*c*) Modern theory of origin of life was proposed by AI Oparin and JBS Haldane. As per this theory, origin of life is the result of long series of physico-chemical changes. They brought about chemical evolutions and biological evolution.

11 (*d*) It is suggested that the large organic molecules that were formed abiotically in the primitive earth, came together spontaneously and due to intermolecular attractions among them, large colloidal aggregates called coacervates were formed. An envelope of water molecules formed around each such aggregate due to hydrophilic nature of these compounds.

12 (*c*) Primitive atmosphere of earth was reducing. It contained methane, ammonia, hydrogen and water vapour. There was no free oxygen (O_2) in it.

CHAPTER 11

Evidences of Evolution

The evidences for evolution indicate that how present day forms have arisen by gradual changes from pre-existing forms and how the complexed forms have been evolved from the simpler forms. The evidences of biological evolution are derived from many lines of study. Out of these, some significant convincing evidences for the occurrence of descent with modification come from the following lineage

1. Morphology and comparative anatomy
2. Embryology
3. Connecting links
4. Palaeontology
5. Geographical distribution or Biogeography
6. Taxonomy
7. Biochemistry and physiology
8. Cytology
9. Genetics

Inside

EVIDENCES FROM MORPHOLOGY AND COMPARATIVE ANATOMY

This lineage includes following evidences

1. From homologous organs and homology

Organs having similar embryonic origin and basic structure, but which may or may not perform the similar function, are known as **homologous organs**. This relationship between the structures of different groups of organisms is called **homology** or **divergent evolution**. It indicates common ancestry.

Types of homology

(i) **Phylogenetic homology** existing between different species e.g. pentadactyl limbs of air breathing vertebrates.

(ii) **Sexual homology** existing between the sexes of same species, e.g. between testes of man and ovaries of a woman, likewise between penis of man and clitoris of woman.

(iii) **Serial homology** existing between the organs of same individuals occupying different levels of the body, e.g. arm and leg of man.

Homology in animals

The examples of homology observed in animals are as follows

(i) **Forelimbs of vertebrates** For example, whale's or seal's front flipper, bat's wing, cat's paw, horse's front leg, human hand and bird's wings share similar bone structure, but functionally these are dissimilar and adapted for different functions, as shown below

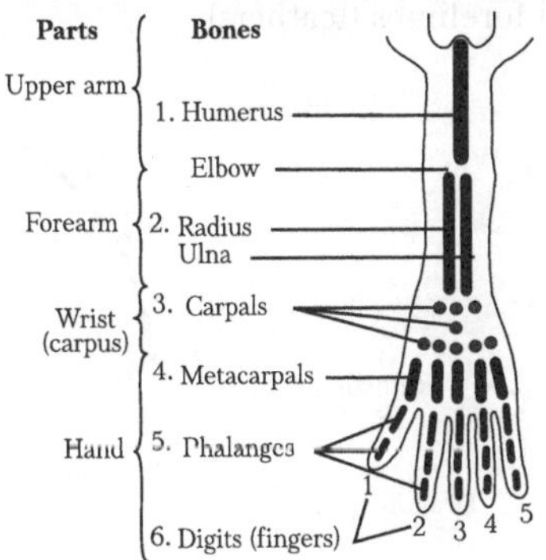

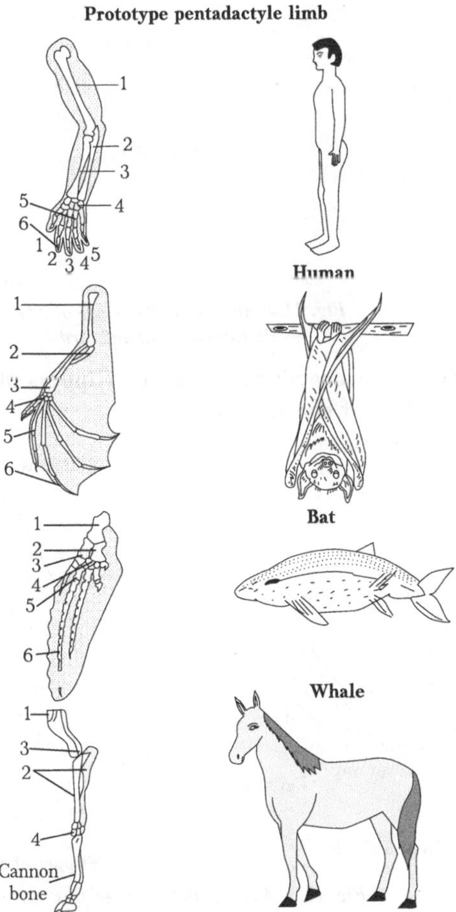

Fig 11.1 Homology of forelimbs in vertebrates

Similar homology is seen in their hindlimbs.

(ii) **Brain in vertebrates** From fishes to mammals, brain constitutes the similar parts, i.e. olfactory lobes, cerebral hemispheres, optic lobes, cerebellum, medulla and so on. Thus, it shows homology.

(iii) **All insect legs** consist of five parts, i.e. coxa, trochanter, femur, tibia and tarsus, Even their sequencing in all the insect is same. However, legs of insects may vary functionally.

Homology in plants

The examples of homology in plants are as follows

(i) In general, all the plant leaves are homologous.

(ii) Parts of flowers, i.e. sepals, petals, stamens and carpels are all homologous structures.

(iii) Leaves modified as thorns (*Bougainvillea*) and tendrils (*Cucurbita*) both arise in axillary positions and are modified branches.

(iv) Phyllode of *Opuntia* and cladode of *Asparagus* are also homologous as both are modified stems to perform the function of photosynthesis.

(v) Tendrils of wild pea are homologous to entire leaves, while that of *Smilax* sp. and *Clematis* are homologous to stipules and petioles, respectively.

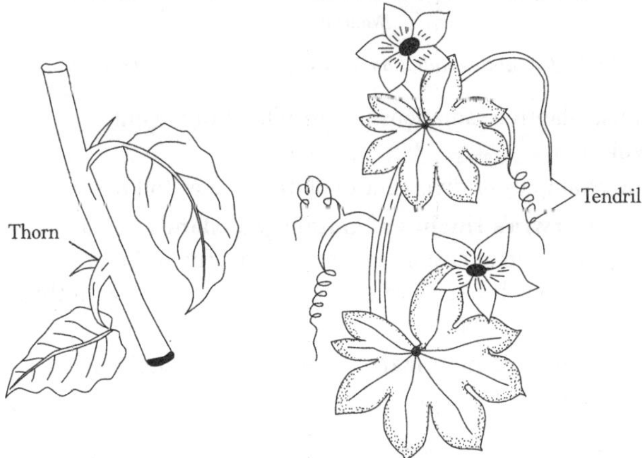

Fig. 11.2 Homologous structure: Thorn of Bougainvillea and tendril of Cucurbita

Adaptive radiation (Divergent evolution)

HF Osborn (1898) developed this concept. It refers to 'the development of different functional structures from a common ancestral form'.

So in divergent evolution, a same basic organ becomes specialised to perform different functions. It helps the organism to adapt different environmental conditions, prevailing in the habitat, e.g. forelimbs of marsupial vertebrates as shown below

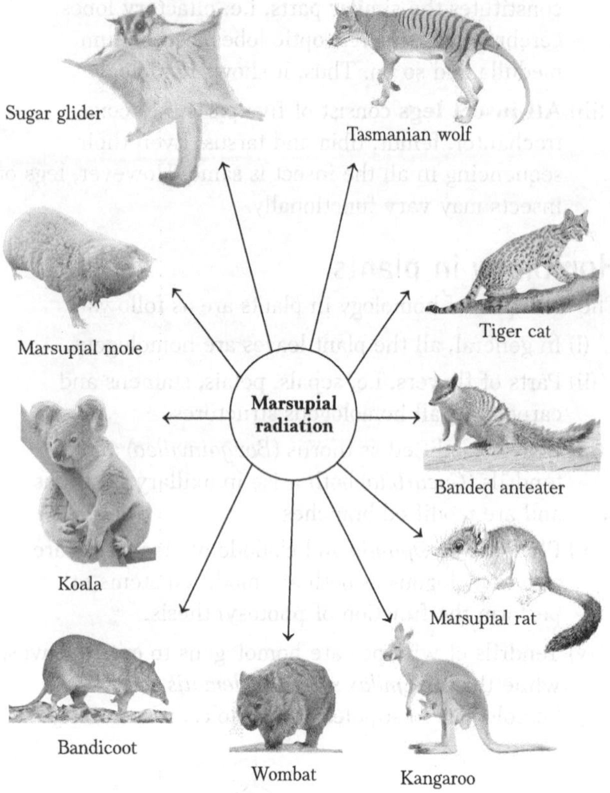

Fig 11.3 Adaptive radiation in forelimbs of marsupial vertebrate

Thus, adaptive radiations is a results of divergent evolution.

The examples of divergent evolution are as follows

(i) **Darwin's finches of Galapagos islands** had a common ancestors as a seed eater finch. Later on, various beaks were evolved in accordance with their feeding habits.

(ii) **Limbs of mammals** are also good examples of divergent evolution.

2. From analogous organs and analogy

In contrast to homologous organs, the analogous organs are different in their basic structure and developmental origin, but perform similar functions.

This relationship between the structures of different groups of animals due to their similar functions is called **analogy**.

Analogy in animals

Examples of analogy in animals are as follows

(i) **Wings of insects Patagium of *Pteranodon*, bats** and **birds** show analogy as both are flat structures, well-adapted for flight. However, their basic structure is different as insects wings are formed from their integument (chitin), while the wings of birds and patagium of *Pteranodon* and bats are their modified forelimbs (feathers).

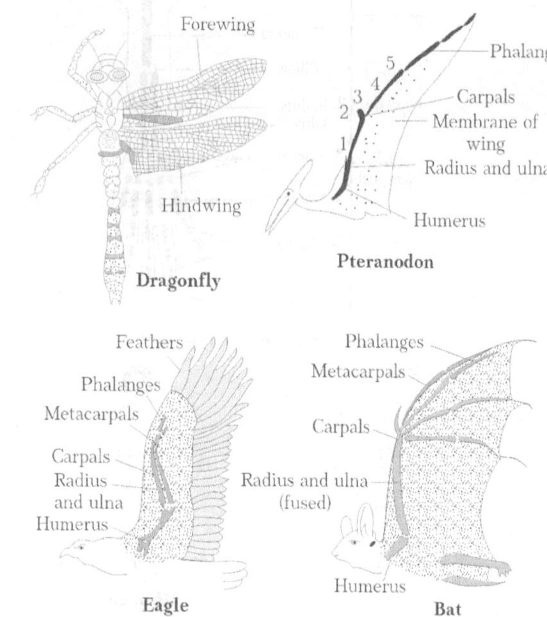

***Fig. 11.4** Analogy in the wings of insects Pteranodon, bat and bird*

(ii) Similar analogy is seen between **flippers of dolphin** and **fins of shark.**

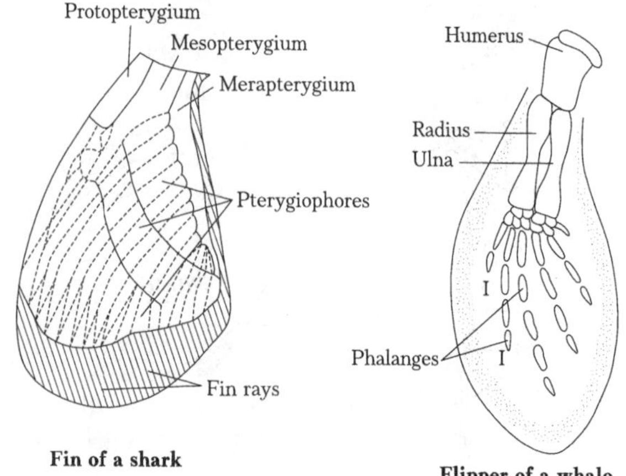

***Fig. 11.5** Analogy in the paired fins*

(iii) **Tracheae of an insect** and **lungs of the vertebrates** both are adapted for gaseous exchange and both are analogous as tracheae are ectodermal in origin, whereas the lungs are endodermal in origin.

Analogy in plants

Examples of analogy in plants are as follows

(i) Leaf of a plant and cladode of *Ruscus* are analogous organs. Both look alike and perform the function of photosynthesis, but are different in origin as cladode is a modified stem.

(ii) Sweet potato *(Ipomoea batatas)* is an underground tuberous root and potato *(Solanum tuberosum)* is an underground stem. Both are the modifications and meant for the storage of food. These are, therefore, analogous.

Adaptive convergence (Convergent evolution)

- In adaptive convergence, separate lineages show similar morphology under the influence of similar environmental factors.
- This leads to the formation of **homeomorphs**, i.e. species of distinct lineages showing close resemblance in overall morphology. Thus, such kind of adaptive convergence leads to **convergent evolution.**
- Marsupial mammals in Australia are a good example to study adaptive convergence and convergent evolution.
- They exhibit adaptive convergence with placental mammal.
- A comparison of Australian marsupials with placental mammals is given below

Placental mammals	Australian marsupial
Mole	Marsupial mole
Mouse	Marsupial mouse
Flying squirrel	Flying phalanger
Wolf	Tasmanian wolf
Lemur	Spotted cuscus
Bobcat	Tasmanian tiger cat

Table 11.1 Differences between homologous and analogous organs

Homologous organs	Analogous organs
These have similar basic plan and origin.	These have different basic plan and origin.
These are adapted to perform different functions.	These are adapted to perform similar functions.
These confirm divergent evolution.	These confirm convergent evolution.

3. From vestigial organs

- The degenerated, rudimentary organs which are non-functional in the possessor, but were functional in their ancestors and related animals are called **vestigial organs**. There are more than 90 vestigial organs in the human body.
- Some examples in humans are coccyx (tailbone), nictitating membrane (3rd eyelid), caecum, vermiform appendix, wisdom teeth, body hair, auricular muscles, mammary glands in males, etc.
- Vestigial organs are present in some other animals also, e.g. splint bones in horse, hindlimbs and pelvic girdle in python, wings and feathers in flightless birds, etc.

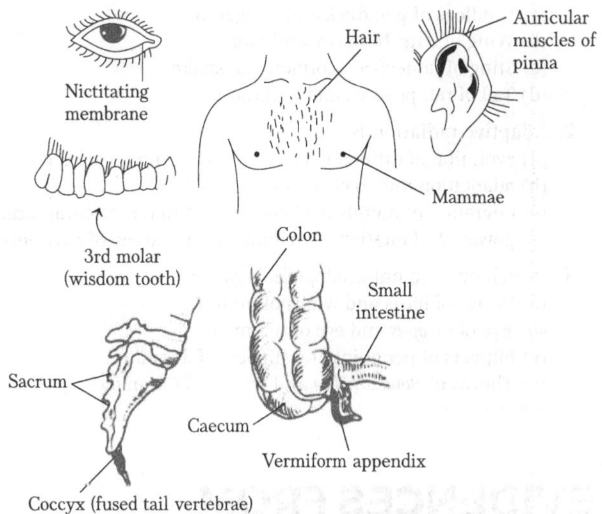

Fig 11.6 Some vestigial organs in human body

4. From atavism or Reversion

It is the sudden reappearance or refunctioning of some ancestral organs, which have either completely disappeared or are present as vestigial organs. It supports the idea that living organisms have the ability to retract or even loose non-functional structures. For example

- Long and dense body hair.
- Development of power of moving pinna in some individuals.
- Birth of a human baby with a small tail
- Presence of additional mammae in some individuals.

Atavism may also be observed in plants like in *Citrus* leaf, the lamina is separated from wing petiole by means of a joint or constriction.

Sometimes the winged part of the petiole is enlarged to produce two lateral leaflets thus, making the leaf trifoliolate.

It shows that *Citrus* leaf was once trifoliolate compound, but during evolution, two leaflets have degenerated.

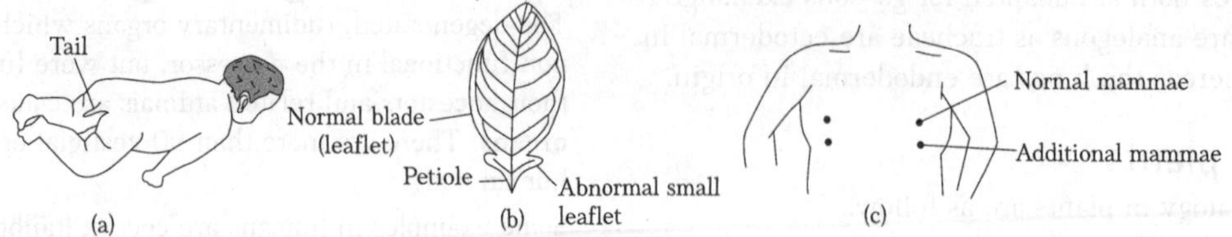

Fig 11.7 Atavism : (a) A baby with tail, (b) A citrus leaf two extra leaflets, (c) Additional mammae

CHECK POINT 11.1

1. Which one of the following sets include all homologous organs?
   (a) Hindlegs of pig, duck and kangaroo
   (b) Wing of bats, butterfly and bird
   (c) Sting of honeybee, scorpion and snake
   (d) Tail of rat, peacock and cockroach
2. Adaptive radiation is
   (a) evolution of different species from a common ancestor
   (b) adaptation due to geographical isolation
   (c) migration of members of species to different geographical area
   (d) power of adaptation of an individual to variety of environment
3. Which one are not analogous organs?
   (a) Wings of birds and wings of butterfly
   (b) Eye of *Octopus* and eye of mammals
   (c) Flippers of penguins and flippers of dolphin
   (d) Thorns of *Bougainvillea* and tendril of *Cucurbita*
4. In adaptive convergence,
   (a) separate lineages show similar morphology
   (b) separate morphology have similar lineages
   (c) environmental factors do not play any role
   (d) Both (a) and (c)
5. Which of the following is not a vestigial organ in human?
   (a) Ear pinna muscle
   (b) Nictitating membrane
   (c) Mammary glands in males
   (d) Knee bone
6. An example, which best explain the atavism is
   (a) leaves and stem of plants
   (b) wisdom tooth
   (c) vermiform appendix
   (d) long, thick and dense body hair

EVIDENCES FROM EMBRYOLOGY

Embryology It may also provide evidences for organic evolution. These evidences which are based on the comparative study of the embryos of various animals are given below

1. From homology in early embryonic development

A common pattern of development is found in all the multicellular organisms. It is observed at various stages as described below

- The development of embryo starts from unicellular zygote or fertilised egg.
- The zygote undergoes repeated cleavage or cell division to form a solid structure called **morula**.
- The morula divides to form **blastula**, which is a single-layered hollow structure.
- This blastula finally develops into **gastrula**, which is two to three-layered structure.
- The animals with two-layered gastrula are termed as **diploblastic**, e.g. in coelenterates. The animals in which three-layered gastrula is found, are known as **triploblastic**, e.g. frog, lizard, etc.
- These two or three layers of gastrula are termed as **primary germ layers**, which give rise to the entire animal. Thus, the similar early embryonic development shows close relationship among all the multicellular organisms.

2. From resemblance among vertebrate embryos

If a comparative study of embryos of vertebrates at same age is done, it is observed that they resemble one another.

Some similarities in early embryonic stages are as follows

- Presence of gill clefts, notochord, tail, rudimentary eyes and ears, etc., in all vertebrates from fishes to mammals.
- Notochord is replaced by vertebral column in all adult vertebrates.

- Gills are replaced by lungs in adult amphibians, reptiles and mammals.

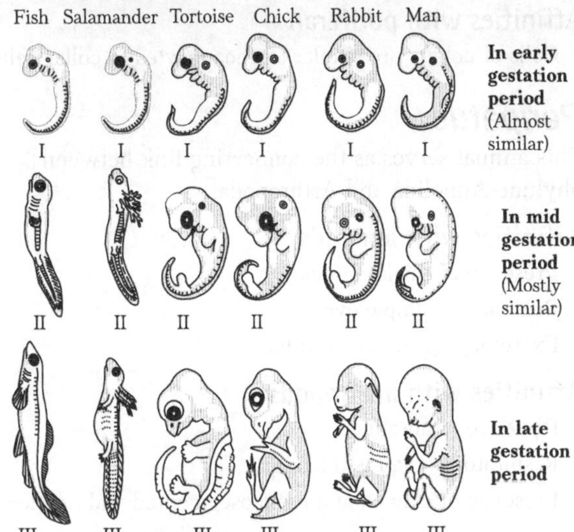

Fig. 11.8 Depicting the remarkable similarity in the early embryos of some vertebrates

3. From resemblance among invertebrate larvae

Annelids and molluscs possess a similar type of larva called **trochophore**. Similarly, echinoderms and hemichordates also have similar larvae that indicate common ancestry.

4. From progressive metamorphosis

The Ammocoete larva of *Lamprey* resembles the adult form of Amphioxus or *Branchiostoma* in most of the details. These are possible only if we presume that *Lamprey* has evolved from *Branchiostoma* like animals.

5. From retrogressive metamorphosis

The adult ascidians (e.g. *Herdmania*) are derived through the process of retrogressive metamorphosis of tadpole larvae. Due to this, most of their chordate characters are lost yet, they may show some chordate affinities.

In these organisms, the larvae have helped in establishing phylogenetic relationship. The ascidian tadpole larva is free-swimming and possesses all the three chordate characters, i.e. notochord, nerve cord and myotomes. Thus, free-swimming nature of larva and presence of all chordate characters justify the inclusion of these animals in Chordata.

Some other examples of developmental evidences of evolution are listed below

- Presence of fish-like characters, e.g. gills, gill slits, tail, tail fin, lateral line and sense organs in tadpole larva of frog.
- Adult frogs excrete urea, whereas tadpoles excrete ammonia as in fishes.
- Birds generally excrete uric acid, but embryos excrete ammonia first and urea later on.
- Presence of filamentous green algae like structure, i.e. protonema during development of *Funaria* (moss).
- Pteridophytes, primitive gymnosperms and animals have flagellated sperms and they depend on water for fertilisation.

6. From neoteny

The condition in which larvae fail to undergo metamorphosis, instead develop gonads and attain sexual maturity is called neoteny.

Reproduction in such larval forms is called **paedogenesis**, e.g. axolotl larvae of *Ambystoma.* Both these processes development of new morphological forms.

7. From temporary embryonic structures

Some structures are temporary in embryos, which remain absent in adults, e.g.

- Bird embryo has tooth buds and gill clefts, which remain absent in adults. This shows that the birds may have evolved from toothed ancestors, which were lost during evolution.
- The embryo of whale possesses hairs, which remain absent in adults. These hairs are shed before birth.

8. From recapitulation theory or biogenetic law

Karl Ernst von Baer (Father of Modern Embryology) in 1828 published the **Baer's law** or **von Baer's law** of embryology to explain the details of embryological development. He discredited the conceptions of recapitulation theory published in 1811 by **Friedrich Meckel.**

The important statements proposed in this law were as follows

- During development, general characters appear before specialised characters in following manner
  More general → Less general → Specialised
- During development, an animal progressively departs from the specific forms of other animals.
- Organisms of different groups share resemblance among their embryonic forms.

In 1866, **Ernst Haeckel** postulated biogenetic law or recapitulation theory by combining the ideas of Darwin's evolution and Baer's law.

Biogenetic law states that 'the ontogeny recapitulates phylogeny', i.e. development of the embryo is the recapitulation (repeatition) of phylogeny (the ancestral sequence).

EVIDENCES FROM CONNECTING LINKS

A connecting link demonstrates characteristics of more than one group of organisms. These connecting links are helpful in establishing continuity in the series by proving that one group has evolved from the other.

Some Important connecting links

Some examples of connecting links are given below

Viruses

These are the connecting links between living and non-living.

Affinities with non-living organisms

- These can be crystallised like inorganic and organic compounds.
- Completly unable to respond to external stimuli.
- Complete lack of metabolism.

Affinities with living organisms

- Undergo mutation and show recombination and heritability.
- Have the ability to reproduce in living cells.

Euglena

This protist serves as the connecting link between the animals and plants.

Affinities with animals

- Locomotion through flagella.
- Holozoic mode of nutrition is also present.

Affinities with plants

- Has chloroplasts and synthesise food through photosynthesis.
- Common nutrition is holotypic or autotrophic.

Proterospongia

This organism shares the characteristic of phylum-Protozoa and Porifera.

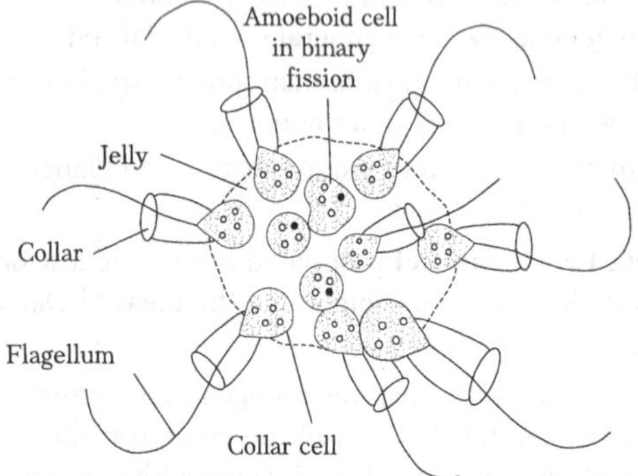

Fig. 11.9 Proterospongia haeckelii

Affinities with protozoan

- Unicellular colonial body structure.

Affinities with poriferan

- Cells of colony are similar to choanocytes or collar cells.

Peripatus

This animal serves as the connecting link between phylum-Annelida and Arthropoda.

Affinities with annelids

- Presence of thick cuticle.
- Presence of simple eyes.
- Excretory organ is nephridia.

Affinities with arthropods

- Presence of antennae.
- Respiratory organ is trachea.
- Presence of clawed and pseudosegmented walking legs.

Neopilina

This animal is the connecting link between Annelida and Mollusca.

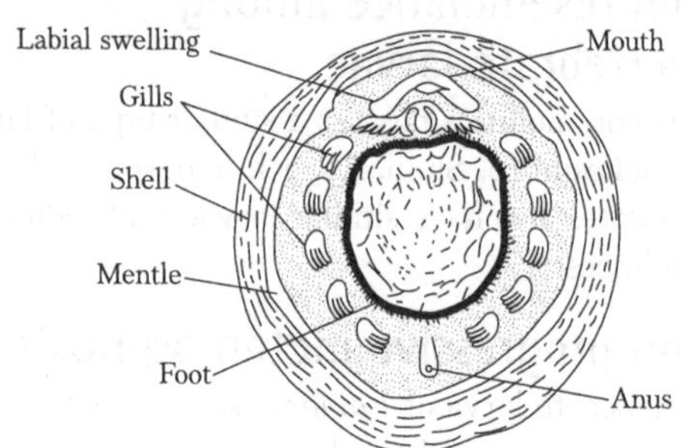

Fig. 11.10 Neopilina

Affinities with annelids

- Presence of trochophore larva.
- Egg divides by spiral cleavage.
- Presence of ctenidia, nephridia.

Affinities with molluscs

- Soft and dorsoventrally flattened body.
- Presence of shell or mantle.
- Presence of a flat muscular foot.

Balanoglossus

This animal is the connecting link between non-chordates and chordates.

Affinities with chordates

- Presence of notochord.
- Presence of a dorsal hollow nerve cord.
- Presence of pharyngeal gill slits.

Affinities with non-chordates

- Dorsal positioning of heart.
- Nervous system is poorly developed and forms epidermal nerve plexus.

Chimaera

- This fish serves as a connecting link between bony and cartilaginous fishes.

Affinities with bony fishes

- Presence of four pairs of gills.
- Presence of small mouth with fleshy lips.
- Cloaca remains absent.
- Anus and urinogenital apertures are separate.
- Presence of an operculum.

Affinities with cartilaginous fishes

- Presence of ventral mouth.
- Presence of cartilaginous endoskeleton.
- Pelvic claspers present in males.
- Presence of two dorsal fins.
- Placoid scales present in young ones.

Lung fishes (*Protopterus*)

These fishes are the connecting links between the fishes and amphibians.

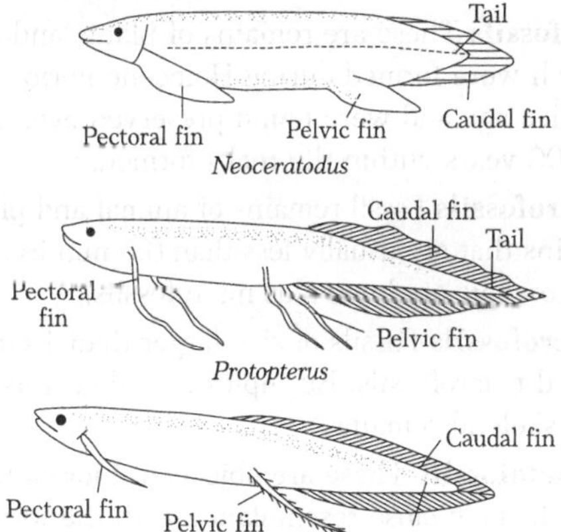

Fig. 11.11 Lung fishes

Affinities with fishes

- Fish like appearance.
- Presence of paired fins.
- Presence of dermal scales.
- Presence of gills.
- Presence of lateral line sensing system.
- Ear is represented by internal ear only.

Affinities with amphibians

- Presence of internal nostrils.
- Presence of lungs, i.e. modified air bladders.
- Heart with imperfectly divided auricle.

Prototheria

Echidna (spiny anteater) and *Ornithorhynchus* (platypus) are connecting link between reptiles and mammals.

Affinities with reptiles

- Presence of cloaca.
- Eggs with reptilian structure and development.
- Embryonic development is also similar to reptiles.

Affinities with mammals

- Presence of hairs.
- Presence of mammary glands.
- Milk production to nourish their children.

Missing link

These are the transitional fossil forms which show characters of two different groups of animals.

Archaeopteryx

It is a connecting link between reptiles and birds.

Fossils of this animal were found in the rocks of Cretaceous period by **Andreas Wagner** (1861) in Germany.

Affinities with reptiles

- Jaws with homodont (similar) teeth.
- Long lizard like tail with 20 free caudal vertebrae.
- Bones were not pneumatic.
- Cervical vertebrae were, 9 19. i.e. not 7.
- Vertebral centrum was amphicoelus.
- Cervical were abdominal ribs were present.
- Sternum was weak or absent.
- Scales are present.
- Carpals and metacarpal were free.
- Pelvic girdle had an elongated ilium and backwardly directed pubis.

Affinities with birds

- Presence of feathers.
- Forelimbs were modified as wings.
- Rounded braincase.
- Beak was present.
- Bones in the skull were intimately fused.
- Bones of limb and girdle were bird like.
- Tibia and fibula were separate.
- V-shaped furcula was present.

Note *Some other missing links are*

- *Lycaenops and Cynognathus — Between reptiles and mammals*
- *Seymouria — Between amphibians and reptiles*
- *Ichthyostega — Between fishes and amphibians*

CHECK POINT 11.2

1. Choose the option with supportive evidence for evolution from comparative embryology?
   (a) All plants seed look alike
   (b) All embryos arise from the union of egg and sperm
   (c) Different species have different embryos
   (d) Different species develop along the pattern set by their common ancestor
2. Which of the following is the correct sequence during character development of animal according to von Baer's law?
   (a) More number → Less number → Fused
   (b) More number → Fused → Less number
   (c) Fused → Less number → More number
   (d) Less number → Fused → More number
3. Viruses are considered as non-living because they do not show
   (a) reproduction (b) heredity
   (c) metabolism (d) mutation
4. A living connecting link that provides evidence of organic evolution is
   (a) *Sphenodon* between reptiles and birds
   (b) *Archaeopteryx* between reptiles and birds
   (c) lung fishes between pisces and reptiles
   (d) duck billed platypus between reptiles and mammals
5. Which of the following option is incorrect?
   (a) *Peripatus* is a connecting link between annelids and molluscs
   (b) *Neopilina* is a connecting link between molluscs and annelids
   (c) *Protopterus* is a connecting link between pisces and amphibians
   (d) *Prototherians* is connecting link between reptile and mammals
6. *Archaeopteryx* is considered missing link because
   (a) it has pneumatic bones (b) it has feathers
   (c) it is a fossil organism (d) it has a long tail

EVIDENCES FROM PALAEONTOLOGY

- Study of fossils of plants and animals that lived in prehistoric times provide solid evidences of evolution.
- **Fossils** are the material remains (bones, teeth, shells) or traces (physical or chemical) of ancient organisms. According to **Charles Lyell**, fossil is 'complete body or traces of body of animal or plant buried and preserved by the natural causes'. This study of fossils is called **Palaentology**.
- **Leonardo da Vinci** (1452-1519), an Italian painter is known as the **'Father of Palaeontology'** and **Baron Georges Cuvier** (1769-1832) is known as **'The Founder of Modern Palaeontology'**.
- Cuvier was a Palaeontologist and an Anatomist, who in 1812 proposed the **'Theory of Catastrophism'** to explain the concepts such as origin of life, appearance and disappearance of dinosaurs and other species on the basis of fossil records.

Fossil records in India

India has a number of fossil plant and animal deposits surviving about 35000 million years ago. Institute of Palaeobotany' (Lucknow), was established by the initiative of Prof. Birbal Sahni (Father of Indian Palaeobotany). It has records of about 20 million years old fossil forests (fossil parks).
Some famous **fossil parks** in India are

- Indroda Dinosaur and Fossil Park, Gujarat
- Ghughua Fossil Park, Madhya Pradesh
- National Fossil Wood Park, Santhanur Tamil Nadu
- Shivalik Fossil Park, Himachal Pradesh

Types of fossils

(i) **Body fossils** These are hard parts of an organism, which provide details of shape and function of actual organisms such as bone, teeth, shell, etc.

(ii) **Subfossils** These are remains of plants and animals, which were formed during Holocene period after the last ice age and were found preserved even after 10000 years within the rocks formed.

(iii) **Microfossils** Fossil remains of animal and plant origins that are usually less than 0.5 mm in size, i.e. microscopic are known as microfossils.

(iv) **Macrofossils** Fossils of size larger than 1 cm are called macrofossils. Examples include corals, claws and skeletal remains.

(v) **Pseudofossils** These are objects of inorganic origins, which show close resemblance with the forms of organic origin and are found in sedimentary rocks.

(vi) **Unusual fossils** Fossils formed as a result of combination of events and conditions. These fossils result in all or most of the organisms getting preserved in the rock such as, *Archaeopteryx* and woolly mammoth.

(vii) **Trace fossils** These are the fossils of footprints and trails, left in mud by the organisms living in the past such as dinosaur's footprint. Trace fossils are also known as **ichnofossils**.

(viii) **Coprolites** These are the fossils of droppings of animal faecal matter. Sizewise, these are as small as faecal pellets of sea snail or as large as coprolites of dinosaurs, crocodiles and mammals.

Formation of fossils

- Generally fossils are preserved in sedimentary rocks. These are formed when parts of dead organisms decay with the passage of time and get replaced by inorganic materials like pyrites, silica and calcium carbonate, etc. This mineral replacement is called **petrification.**
- The hard parts of the body (i.e. bone, teeth, shell, etc.) are preserved more readily than soft parts, into these rocks. For example, there are instances of entire tree trunks being preserved in the **'Petrified forests' of Arizona.**
- Fossils are also formed by processes other than petrification. Like an organism may get buried intact in preservatives like resins, snow, oil, tar, volcanic, ash, etc. Sometimes, the organism particularly when buried in rapidly hardening mud, decays completely and the space it occupies, becomes filled with another kind of material. This process of fossilisation is called **mould formation.**
- A common type of plant fossil where the internal structure is lost, leaving a thin carbon film which gives the outline of the original plant. This kind of fossil formation is called **impression.**

Living fossils

These are living organisms that are similar in appearance to their fossilised distant ancestors and usually have no extinct close relatives, e.g. coelacanth or *Ginkgo*, crocodile, *Neopilina, Tuatara, Nautilus*, Australian and African lung fish, etc.

Determination of age of fossils

Age or dating of fossils can be determined by following methods

1. Radioactive decay methods

The age of fossils or rocks can be determined by decay or conversions of various radioactive isotopes into other elements with passage of time. This conversion takes place at different durations in different radioactive elements.

Table 11.2 List of radioactive elements to determine age of fossils

Isotopes	**Transformed isotopes**	**Half-life** (in yrs)	**Used for range** (in yrs)
Carbon (C^{14})	Nitrogen (N^{14})	5730	Hundred-30 thousand
Potassium (K^{40})	Argon (Ar^{40})	1.3 billion	1 lakh–4.5 billion
Rubidium (Rb^{87})	Strontium (Sr^{87})	47 billion	10 million–4.5 billion
Uranium (U^{238})	Lead (Pb^{207})	4.5 billion	10 million–4.6 billion
Thorium (Th^{232})	Lead (Pb^{206})	710 million	10 million–4.6 billion

Radioactive decay method has an error factor of less than 10%. Radioactive decay methods may be of following types

(i) **Radioactive carbon (C^{14}) dating method**

This method was discovered by **WF Libby.**

- In this method, dating of fossil sample is done after checking C^{14} sample quantity in it.
- C^{14} has the half-life of 5730 years.
- This method is useful only to determine the age of actual remains and is ineffective for the evaluation of moulds, casts or impressions.

(ii) **Radioactive clock method** This method was discovered by **Boltwood** (1907) and is based on the disintegrating property of other radioactive elements.

- This method is used for finding the age of those fossils, which cannot be calculated using carbon dating method.
- These elements disintegrate at a steady rate into a stable substance.

(iii) **Uranium-argon method** In this method, the age of rock is calculated by estimating the uranium and lead quantity. This method is particularly useful for igneous rocks containing minerals and is useless for determining the age of sedimentary rocks and fossils directly.

(iv) **Potassium-argon method** This is the most recent method to estimate the age of fossils.

- The age of earliest known fossil of hominids in East Africa have been estimated by this method only.
- The transformation of radioactive Potassium (K^{40}) to Argon (Ar^{40}) and Rubidium (Rb^{87}) to Strontium (Sr^{87}) has been used for dating fossil bearing rocks of any age and any type. It is because, a greater concentration of potassium is found in most rocks.
- Thus, it is a more accurate method of dating fossils than Uranium, which is a relatively rare element. It is also possible to date very old rocks, e.g. over 3 billion years by this method.

2. Electron Spin Resonance (ESR) method

- It is a relatively new, more precise and most accurate method of dating. ESR is used mostly to date calcium carbonate in limestone, corals, fossil teeth, molluscs and egg shells. It can also be used to date quartz and flint.
- Palaeoanthropologists have used ESR mostly to date samples from the last 300,000 years. However, it potentially could be used for much older samples also.
- Since within the process, the magnetic field progressively changes with the time in a predictable way so, it provides another atomic clock or calendar that can be used for dating purposes.

Geological time scale

- Careful observation or study of geological time scale also provides evidences of evolution. It represents complete lifespan of earth, i.e. 4600 million years.
- The geological time scale has been divided into **eras.** These eras are divided into **periods** and periods are further divided into **epochs.**
- Thus, the arrangement of these eras, periods and epochs according to their approximate dates in million of years forms the geological time scale.
- **Giovanni Arduino**, an Italian scientist was the first to develop geological time scale in 1760.

Table 11.3 Geological time scale with notes on events in the evolution of life and environment

Era	Period	Epoch	Time from beginning of period to present in millions of years	Geological and climatic conditions	Flora (Plant life)	Fauna (Animal life)
Cenozoic (Age of mammals)	Quaternary (Age of man)	Recent (Holocene)	0.01	End of last ice age, climate warmer, climatic zones distinct.	Dominance of herbs.	Modern man, development of human cultures.
		Pleistocene	2	Periodic continental glaciers in North.	Increase of herbs, great decrease of woody plants.	Primitive man, extinction of many large mammals.
	Tertiary	Pliocene	2-5	Cool and temperature climate away from equator, continuous rise of mountains of Western-North America.	Decline of forests, spread of herbs and grassland.	Abundance of mammals, elephant, horses and camels, etc. Humans evolving.
		Miocene	5-24	Cooling of climate	Development of grasses, reduction of forests.	Mammals at height of evolution, first man-like apes.
		Oligocene	24-33	Lands lower, climate warmer.	Worldwide tropical forests, rise of monocots and flowering plants.	Archaic mammals extinct, appearance of modern mammals.
		Eocene	33-55	Zoned climatic belts well-established.	Extension of angiosperms.	Placental mammals diversified and specialised, hoofed mammals and carnivores established.
		Palaeocene	55-65	Development of climatic belts.	Modernisation of angiosperms.	Evolutionary explosion of mammals.
Rocky mountain revolution (Little destruction of fossils)						
Mesozoic (Age of reptiles)	Cretaceous		65-144	Birth of modern reptiles, development of climatic diversity.	Rise of flowering plants especially monocotyledons, decrease of gymnosperms.	**Dinosaurs** became extinct, toothed birds became extinct, beginning of teleost fishes and **first modern birds appeared,** archaic mammals common.
	Jurassic		144-206	Culmination of worldwide warm climates.	Cycades and conifers common, appearance of first known flowering plants.	Dominance of dinosaurs, **appearance of first toothed birds**, spread of reptiles, rise of insectivorous marsupials.
	Triassic		206-248	Continents exposed, world subtropical climates.	Gymnosperms dominant, declining towards the end, extinction of seed fern.	Transition of reptiles to mammals, rise of progressive reptiles and egg laying mammals, extinction of primitive amphibians.

Appalachian revolution (Some loss of fossils)					
	Permian –	248-290	Rise of continents, climate became arid and varied, glaciation in Southern hemisphere.	Dwindling of ancient plants, decline of lycopods and horsetails.	Extinction of ammonites and trilobites, abundance of primitive reptiles, **appearance of mammals like reptiles,** decline of amphibians.
	Carboniferous –	290-323	Uniform climate throughout world.	Great forests of seed-ferns and gymnosperms (great tropical coal forests).	Amphibians dominanted on land, insects common, **appearance of first reptiles.**
	–	323-354	Climate uniform, humid at first, cooler later, spread of tropical seas.	Mosses and seed ferns dominant, gymnosperms increasingly widespread (early coal forest).	Rise of insects, sea lilies at peak, spread of ancient sharks. **Golden age of amphibians.**
Palaeozoic (Age of ancient life)	Devonian –	354-417	Broad distribution of uniform climates, increased temperature.	First forests, first **gymnosperms** and first known liverworts, horsetails and ferns.	Diversification in fishes, sharks and lung fishes abundant, evolution of amphibians. **Golden age of fishes.**
	Silurian –	417-443	Slight climate cooling, extensive continental seas.	First known land plants club mosses appeared, algae dominant.	Wide expansion of invertebrates **first insects,** rise of fishes.
	Ordovician –	443-490	Warm climate, great submergence of land.	Land plants probably first appeared, marine algae abundant.	First indication of fishes; corals and **trilobites** abundant, diversified molluscs.
	Cambrian –	490-544	Climate became progressively warmer.	Blue-green algae fungi and bacteria, **first fossils of plant life.**	Invertebrates numerous and varied, most modern phyla established.
Second great revolution (Considerable loss of fossils)					
Proterozoic (Era of early life)	–	544-2500	Cool climate, volcanic eruptions, repeated glaciations.	Primitive aquatic plants algae, fungi and bacteria.	Shelled protozoans, coelenterates, flatworms, primitive annelids.
First great revolution (Considerable loss of fossils)					
Archaeozoic (Era of dawn of life)	–	2500-4600	Great volcanic activities, no recognisable fossils, indirect evidence of living things form some sedimentary deposits of organic material in rocks, e.g. *Eubacterium isolatum, Archaeospheroides barbertons.*		

Geological history of earth

The geological history of earth, i.e. the time since the birth of earth to the present can be interpreted by means of a geological clock. It is a graphic aid to help us visualise time. It is a 24 hours clock that represents the initial events that brought about the formation of earth upto now.

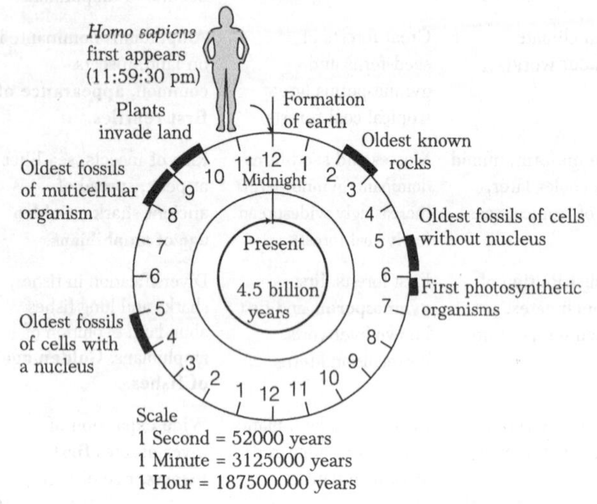

EVIDENCES FROM BIOGEOGRAPHY

- Based on biogeographical patterns, phylogenetic relationships can be established between different species.
- Scientists believe that millions of years ago, all continents were in the form a single land mass. Later, due to continental drift various continents were formed.
- On the basis of variable environmental conditions prevailing on the different continents, these became independently developed into different biogeographical regions.
- For instance, although similar climatic conditions occur in Brazil, India and Africa, yet elephants and rhinoceros occur only in India and Africa and not in Brazil.

Plate Tectonics Theory or Continental Drift

This theory was given by **Alfred L Wegener** (1929).

It can be summarised in following points to explain the changes during the course of earth's history and development of various biogeographical regions.

- During Carboniferous period (about 375 million years ago), all the present day continents existed in the form of a single, giant landmass called **pangea**.
- Pangea existed till about 200 million years ago, i.e. fill the beginning of Mesozoic era, This was surrounded by ancestral Panthalassa ocean (Pacific ocean) and ancestral Tethys sea (Mediterranean sea).
- During the end of Triassic period (about 180 million years ago), Pangaea splitted into two parts
  - **Laurasia** Northern half landmass consisting of North America, Europe and Asia.
  - **Gondwana** Southern half landmass consisting of South America, Australia, Africa, India and Antarctica.
- During Jurassic period (about 135 million years ago), South America separated from Africa and drifted towards West.
- About 40 million years ago, India separated, moved from North and rammed into Asia. At the same time, Tibetan Plateau and Himalayan mountains uplifted as a result of collision.
- North Atlantic and Indian ocean increased in size due to the rotation of land masses.
- During the end of Mesozoic era, North America drifted from Europe and Madagascar isolated from Eastern Africa.

EVIDENCES FROM TAXONOMY

- One can conclude similarities and common ancestry by studying phylogenetic taxonomy and fill gaps in evolutionary sequence.
- During classification, organisms are grouped according to their resemblance and placed into taxonomic groups with simple organisation leading towards the complex organisms.
- There was no difference among animals and plants during origin of unicellular stage of organisms.
- Thus *Euglena,* a unicellular organism is a common ancestor of both animals and plants.
- After appearance of unicellular plants and animals, complexity increased gradually.
- Consequently, diploblastic animals evolved, followed by triploblastic, acoelomate and coelomate animals.

EVIDENCES FROM BIOCHEMISTRY AND PHYSIOLOGY

The biochemical composition reactions and physiological reactions provide the following most convincing evidence indicating common ancestry.

(i) **Metabolism** Anabolic reactions like photosynthesis, protein synthesis, carbohydrate, fat and biosynthesis of various organic molecules and catabolic reactions like respiration and breakdown of macromolecules occur in all living beings ranging from bacteria to man and in all plants and animals. Beside these, energy in all living beings is released by the biological oxidation and is stored in the form of ATP.

(ii) **Enzymes** Most of the enzyme catalysed biochemical reactions are same in bacteria to man and plants, e.g. enzymes of glycolysis and Krebs' cycle are almost similar in both plants and animals. Similarly, trypsin and amylase enzymes are also same in all the animals.

(iii) **Hormones** Some hormones of vertebrates are similar chemically as well as functionally. However, thyroxine and insulin like hormones can be used interchangeably, e.g. cattle/porine insulin can be used for human treatment and human thyroxine can be used for metamorphosis in a frog tadpole.

(iv) **Cytochrome-*c*** It is a respiratory pigment found in all eukaryotic cells, which is a part of electron transport system. Cytochrome-*c* accepts H^+ in all eukaryotic cells.
The amino acid sequence of cytochrome-*c* molecule in humans and chimpanzee is nearly identical, whereas that of *Neurospora* differs from human's cytochrome-*c* at few amino acids.

(v) **Blood group** Four types of blood groups, A, B, AB and O are found in human, whereas apes have only A and B type. Monkeys lack such type of blood groups. This indicates that the humans are closer to apes than monkeys

(vi) **Blood and lymph** The composition and physiological role of blood, lymph and tissue fluid are similar in all vertebrates, thus indicating evolutionary relationship between vertebrates.

(vii) **Haemoglobin** It is a conjugated protein having two alpha chains, each with 141 amino acids in man and two beta chains, each with 146 amino acids in man. There is single amino acid difference between the human and gorilla haemoglobin chain and 26 amino acids between the human and horse, whereas a difference of 10 amino acids is seen between human and pig's haemoglobin. These all comparisons help in comparing the distance between two different species.

(viii) **Serological tests** These are tests done to study serum and other bodily fluids in animals. In serological tests, close similarity is found in species of a single genus, while genera of the same family show moderate reaction. Families of the same order show slight reaction but detectable similarity. This indicates that closely related organisms show more similarity in protein structure and function.

EVIDENCES FROM CYTOLOGY

Some evidences from cytology are given below

- The cells of all organisms (except minor differences) have almost same basic pattern of organisation with cell organelles like ER, mitochondria, cell membrane, Golgi body, nucleus, etc.
These similarities provide evidence for common ancestry.
- Protoplasm of all the organisms (physical basis of life) have carbon, hydrogen, oxygen and nitrogen.
- Cells are the building blocks, forming tissues of both the plants and animals.
- DNA and rarely RNA is the genetic material in all the organisms. The packaging of DNA is also common with all organisms. This shows common ancestry and origin of all organisms.
- The same genetic code having triplet codons is found from the viruses to man and all living beings have same amino acids for same codons.

EVIDENCES FROM GENETICS

- Genetics draws the final evidence for evolution because genes are inherited generation after generation by means of chromosomes which are the carriers of genetic information.
- Mutation and variations produce changes in genes and these changed genes determine the character in different direction than the original.
- The forces of natural selection and isolation operate on these changed genes and the useful mutations get accumulated permanently for the development of new species and varieties. For phylogeny, some specific *r*RNA sequences are also used.

CHECK POINT 11.3

1. The study of fossil show/confirms
   (a) that life form varied over time and restricted to certain time span
   (b) that new terms of life arose at the same time in history of earth
   (c) the theory of 'theory of Panspermia'
   (d) the theory of spontaneous generation
2. The age of fossils or dating of fossils can be best estimated by
   (a) radioactive carbon (C^{14}) dating method
   (b) radioactive nitrogen method
   (c) electron spin resonance method
   (d) Both (a) and (c)
3. If 60,000 years old fossil was recovered from igneous rock, then which of the following method would have been used to find its age?
   (a) Uranium-argon method (b) Carbon -14 method
   (c) Potassium-argon method (d) Both (a) and (b)
4. The correct order of the geological eras, from most ancient to most recent is
   (a) Palaeozoic, Cenozoic, Mesozoic
   (b) Precambrian, Mesozoic, Cenozoic, Palaeozoic
   (c) Palaeozoic, Mesozoic, Cenozoic
   (d) Cenozoic, Mesozoic, Palaeozoic
5. Archaeozoic era is considered as the age of
   (a) appalachian revolution
   (b) first great revolution
   (c) rocky mountain revolution
   (d) second great revolution
6. All organisms share the same genetic code. This commonality is the evidence that
   (a) the evolution is occurring now
   (b) the convergent evolution has occurred
   (c) the evolution occurs gradually
   (d) all the organisms have descended from a common ancestor

EXAM POINTS

- Organs with similar structure and origin are called homologous organs. **[AIIMS 2018, EAMCET 2014]**
- Flipper of whale is homologous to the wing of bird. **[NEET 2016, 2014]**
- The formation of two species from one ancestral species is known as divergent evolution. **[Karnataka CET 2015]**
- Eyes of *Octopus*, bat and man are example of divergent evolution. **[NEET 2018]**
- The similarity of bone structure in the forelimbs of many vertebrates is an example of homology. **[NEET 2018]**
- Forelimbs of cat, lizard used in walking, forelimbs of whale used in swimming and forelimbs of bats used in flying are the examples of homologous organs. **[CBSE AIPMT 2014]**
- Thorns of *Bougainvillea* and tendrils of *Cucurbita* are example of divergent evolution. **[KCET 2014]**
- Organs with dissimilar structure are called analogous organs. **[AIIMS 2018, EAMCET 2014]**
- Wings of bat and wings of pigeon are analogous structures. **[CBSE AIPMT 2014]**
- The wings of a bird and the wings of an insect are analogous structure and represent convergent evolution. **[CBSE AIPMT 20105]**
- Similarities in organisms with different polymer indicates convergent evolution. **[UP CPMT 2012]**
- The eye of *Octopus* and eye of cat show different patterns of structure, yet they perform similar function. This is an example of analogous organs that have evolved due to convergent evolution. **[NEET 2013]**
- Analogous structures are a result of convergent evolution. **[NEET 2016, 2017]**
- Flippers of penguin and dolphins are example of convergent evolution. **[NEET 2020]**
- The process by which organisms with different evolutionary history evolve similar phenotypic adaptations in response to a common environmental challenge is called convergent evolution. **[NEET 2013]**
- Evolution of different species in a given area starting from a point and spreading to other geographical areas is called adaptive radiation. **[CBSE AIPMT 2012]**
- Area with many type of vacant habitat will lead to adaptive radiation when a population of species invades a new area. **[NEET 2019]**
- In Australia, marsupials and placental mammals have evolved to share many similar characteristics. This type of evolution may be referred to as convergent evolution. **[NEET 2019]**
- Vermiform appendix arises from caecum. **[AMU 2015]**
- Embryological support for evolution was disapproved by Karl Ernst von Baer. **[NEET 2020]**
- Evolutionary history of an organism is known as phylogeny. **[UP CPMT 2012]**
- Recapitulation theory was given by Haeckel. **[OJEE 2013]**
- Evolutionary convergence is characterised by the development of a common set of characteristics in groups of different ancestry. **[BCECE 2012]**
- Biogenetic law is given by Haeckel states that 'ontogeny recapitulates phylogeny'. **[AMU 2012]**
- Connecting link between fish and amphibia is lungfish, *Protopterus*. **[Chhattisgarh PMT 2015]**
- Cretaceous period witnessed the maximum diversity of reptiles. **[Chhattisgarh PMT 2015]**
- 3125000 years are considered in one minute in geological clock. **[Gujarat CET 2015]**

Chapter Exercises

(A) Topical Exercise

Evidences From Homology and Analogy

1 Homologous organs have
(a) same origin, but different functions
(b) different origin, but same functions
(c) neither same origin nor same functions
(d) different origin and different functions

2 Serial homology is exhibited by
(a) the organs of same individual occupying different levels of the body
(b) the organs of different organisms with same function
(c) the organs of different organisms at same level
(d) All of the above

3 Which one of the following sets includes all homologous organs?
(a) Hindleg of pig, duck and kangaroo
(b) Wings of bat, butterfly and birds
(c) Sting of honeybee, scorpion and snake
(d) Tail of rat, peacock and cockroach

4 In the following figures, the given structures are

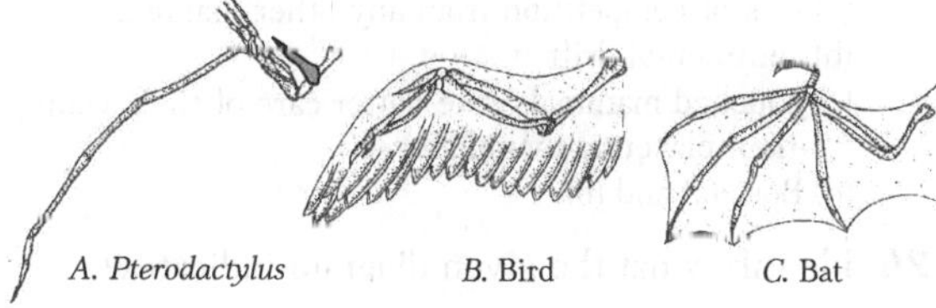

(a) analogous
(b) homologous
(c) Both *A* and *B* are analogous
(d) Both *B* and *C* are homologous

5 Homologous organs are
(a) tails of birds, monkey and scorpion
(b) stings of honeybee, scorpion and fangs of snake
(c) wings of butterfly, flying fish and bird
(d) paddle of whale, front legs of horse and arms of human/legs of duck, hindlimbs of pig, hindlimbs of kangaroo

6 Being mammals, whale, dolphin, bat, monkey and horse have some important common characters, but they also show conspicuous differences. This is due to the phenomenon of
(a) normalisation
(b) genetic drift
(c) convergence
(d) divergence

7 An important evidence in favour of organic evolution is the occurrence of
(a) homologous and vestigial organs
(b) analogous and vestigial organs
(c) homologous organs only
(d) homologous and analogous organs

8 Which of the following sets contain only homologous organs?
(a) Whale's flipper, horse's forelimb, human hand
(b) Wings of butterfly, crow and insect
(c) Horse's forelimb, insect wing, human hand
(d) Vermiform appendix, body hair and patella

9 Identify the incorrect statement about homology.
(a) Heart and brain of vertebrates are homologous organs
(b) Homologous structures are a result of divergent evolution
(c) Stipules of *Lathyrus aphaca* and petiole of *Acacia* are homologous structures
(d) Richard Owen introduced the term homologous organs

10 Diagram given below indicates

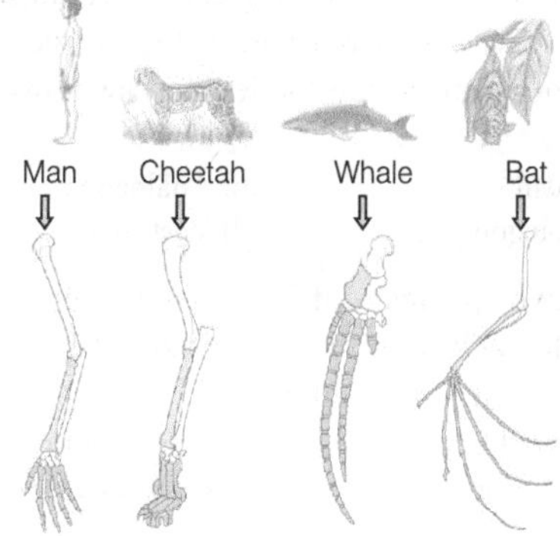

(a) analogous organs
(b) homologous organs
(c) convergent evolution
(d) All of the above

11 The bones of forelimbs of whale, bat, cheetah and man are similar in structure, because **[NCERT Exemplar]**
(a) one organism has given rise to another
(b) they share a common ancestor
(c) they perform the same function
(d) they have biochemical similarities

12 The different wings of the different animals in the given figures are

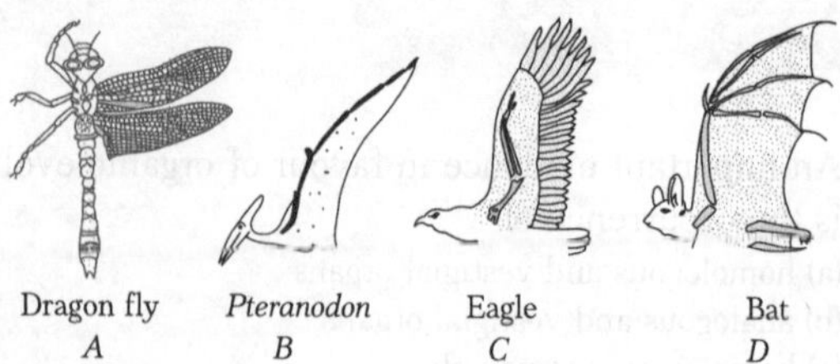

(a) all homologous
(b) all analogous
(c) *B*, *C* and *D* are homologous and *A* is analogous to all
(d) *B*, *C*, *D* are analogous

13 Which of the following is incorrect about analogous organs?
(a) They show superficial resemblance, though their internal structures are quite different
(b) They have similar function
(c) They are a result of convergent evolution
(d) They always develop in related organism

14 In some organisms, the existence of analogous structures (wings of insects and bat, jointed legs of insects and vertebrates) is due to the phenomenon of
(a) convergent evolution (b) divergent evolution
(c) organic evolution (d) genetic drift

15 Which one of the following terms would most correctly describe the relationship between the flight organs of animals like locust, bat, swallow and flying fish?
(a) Atavism (b) Analogous
(c) Homologous (d) Vestigial

16 When two species of different genealogy come to resemble each other as a result of adaptation, the phenomenon is termed as
(a) divergent evolution (b) microevolution
(c) coevolution (d) convergent evolution

17 Convergent evolution is illustrated by ...*A*... and ...*B*... .

	A	*B*
(a)	rat	dog
(b)	bacterium	protozoan
(c)	starfish	cuttle fish
(d)	dogfish	whale

18 In Africa, there is a species of bird called the yellow-throated longclaw. It looks almost exactly like the meadowlark found in North America, but they are not closely related. This is an example of
(a) uniformitarianism (b) artificial selection
(c) gradualism (d) convergent evolution

19 What is the supportive evidences for evolution from comparative anatomy?
(a) All antelopes have four legs
(b) Most animals have a head
(c) Similar gene sequences code for similar proteins
(d) Diverse species have homologous structures

20 Which one of the following sets of structures includes only analogous organs?
(a) Hindlegs of horse, grasshopper and bat
(b) Hands of man, monkey and kangaroo
(c) Mandibles of cockroach, mosquito and honeybee
(d) Wings of butterfly, housefly and bat

21 An example of analogous organ is
(a) tubers of potato and sweet potato
(b) tubers of *Dahlia* and sweet potato
(c) tubers of potato and Jerusalem artichoke
(d) All of the above

22 Flippers of penguin and dolphin are considered analogous though they are modified forelimbs because of the
(a) absence of certain bones
(b) development from different lineages
(c) structural differences
(d) functional differences

23 The pouched mammals of Australia survived because of
(a) lack of competition from any other mammal
(b) continental drift
(c) pouched mammals take better care of their young ones than placental mammals
(d) Both (a) and (b)

24 Identify what the given diagram indicates?

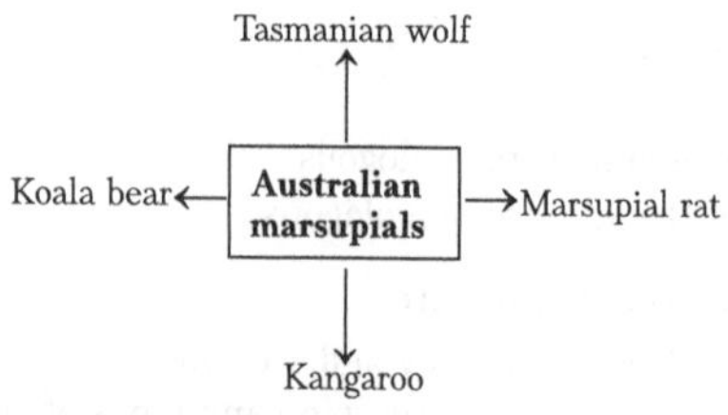

(a) Convegent evolution
(b) Divergent evolution
(c) Recapitulation
(d) Parallel evolution

25 Adaptive radiations refer to
(a) adaptation due to geographical isolation
(b) evolution of different species from a common ancestor
(c) migration of members of a species to different geographical areas
(d) power of adaptation in an individual to a variety of environments

Vestigial Organs and Atavism

26 Which of the following is a correct set of vestigial organs?
(a) Wisdom teeth and ear pinna
(b) Scalp muscles and premolars
(c) Pineal gland and vermiform appendix
(d) Auricular muscles and wisdom teeth

27 Which of the following are not vestigial organs in human beings?
(a) Scalp muscles and third molars
(b) Rudimentary ear muscles and coccygeal vertebrae
(c) Ear pinna, patella and olecranon process
(d) Vermiform appendix and nictitating membrane

28 Which one of the following is the vestigial organ in human beings?
(a) Nictitating membrane (b) Spleen
(c) Femur (d) Tibia

29 Identify the vestigial organ in the given figure.

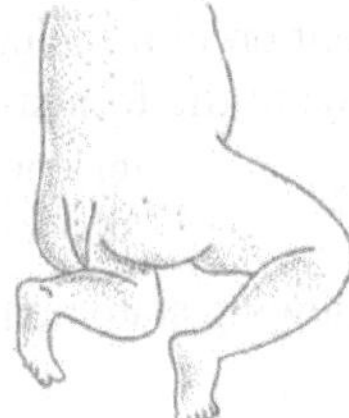

(a) Vermiform appendix (b) Auricular
(c) Coccyx (d) Plica semilunaris

30 Consider the following statements.
I. Vestigial organ present in greenland whale is pelvic girdle and hindlimb.
II. Tail vertebrae, auricular muscles, scalp muscles are example of vestigial organs.

Choose the correct option.
(a) Statement I is true, but II is false
(b) Statement I is false, but II is true
(c) Both statements I and II are true
(d) Both statements I and II are false

31 A baby has been born with a small tail. It is the case of exhibiting
(a) retrogressive evolution (b) mutation
(c) atavism (d) metamorphosis

Evidences from Embryology

32 Identify the incorrect statement about the embryological evidences of evolution.
(a) Ammocoete larva of *Lamprey* resembles the adult form of Amphioxus
(b) Bird embryo has tooth buds and gill cleft, which are not found in adult animal
(c) Several bryophytes pass through a filamentous protonema stage
(d) Tadpole larva of *Herdmania* lacks the notochord, which is present in the adult stage

33 Embryological support for evolution given by Ernst Haeckel includes the
(a) presence of hair all over the body in adult human
(b) absence of tail bone and presence of wisdom tooth
(c) absence of vestigial gill slits in human's embryo
(d) presence of row of vestigial gill slits in embryo of all vertebrates

34 In the developmental history of mammalian heart, it is observed that it passes through a two-chambered fish like heart, three-chambered frog like heart and finally four-chambered stage. To which hypothesis can the above cited statement be approximated?
(a) Biogenetic law (b) Hardy-Weinberg law
(c) Lamarck's principles (d) Mendelian principles

35 '*Ontogeny Recapitulates Phylogeny*' is narrated in which of the evidences for organic evolution?
(a) Palaeontological evidence
(b) Physiological evidence
(c) Embryological evidence
(d) Anatomical evidence

36 The ammocoete larva of *Lamprey* resembling the adult Amphioxus indicates
(a) progressive metamorphosis
(b) neoteny
(c) retrogressive metamorphosis
(d) Both (b) and (c)

37 Appearance of teeth in the embryo of a bird proves that the
(a) ontogeny repeats phylogeny
(b) evolution has taken place
(c) birds have evolved from reptiles
(d) All of the above

Evidences from Connecting Links and Missing Links

38 Identify the animal in the given figure. It is a connecting link between

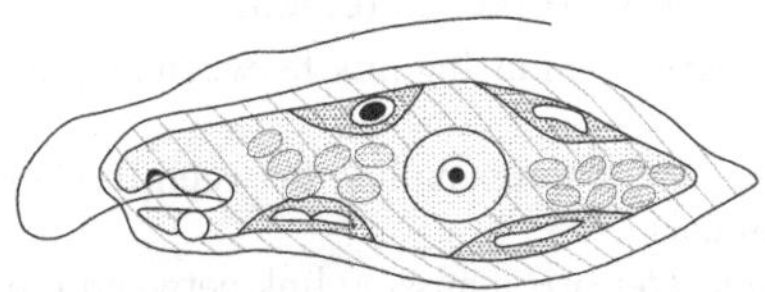

(a) *Euglena*; animals and plants
(b) Virus; non-living and living
(c) *Euglena*; non-living and living
(d) Virus; animals and plants

39 *Peripatus* is a connecting link between
(a) Ctenophora and Platyhelminthes
(b) Mollusca and Echinodermata
(c) Annelida and Arthropoda
(d) Coelenterata and Porifera

40 *Chimaera* is a connecting link between
(a) bony and cartilaginous fish
(b) reptiles and amphibians
(c) fishes and amphibians
(d) None of the above

41 Echidna and *Ornithorhynchus* are the connecting links between
(a) amphibians and Aves (b) mammals and amphibians
(c) reptiles and mammals (d) reptiles and amphibians

42 *Archaeopteryx* is a missing link. Its fossil was discovered by Andreas Wagner from the rocks of
(a) Jurassic period
(b) Pliocene period
(c) Cretaceous period
(d) Holocene period

43 Consider the following statements with respect to *Archaeopteryx*.
I. Forelimbs are modified into wings.
II. Connecting link between birds and reptiles.
Choose the correct option.
(a) Statement I is true, but II is false
(b) Statement I is false, but II is true
(c) Both statements I and II are true
(d) Both statements I and II are false

44 Which of the following characteristic of *Archaeopteryx* show affinities with birds?
I. Round braincase
II. Free carpals and metacarpals
III. Presence of scales
IV. Separate tibia and fibula
V. Fused skull bone
Choose the correct option.
(a) I, II and III
(b) I, IV and V
(c) II, III and V
(d) III, IV and V

45 Identify the incorrect statement.
(a) *Seymouria* is a missing link between amphibians and reptiles
(b) *Lycaenops* is a missing link between reptiles and mammals
(c) *Archaeopteryx* is a missing link between reptiles and Aves
(d) *Ichthyostega* is a connecting link between non-chordates and chordates

Evidences from Palaeontology

46 Palaeontology is the study of fossils and is in support of evolution. Such an evidence is
(a) a complete evidence of evolution
(b) an incomplete evidence of evolution
(c) incomplete evidence in India and complete in Europe
(d) the statement is wrong

47 Palaeontology does not help in
(a) reconstruction of phylogeny
(b) studying various forms and structures of endangered species
(c) providing missing links between two groups of organisms
(d) studying habits of extinct organisms

48 Sometimes, the remains of a dead animal escape destruction and become buried in sediment of ash or survives under heating, crushing or folding.
The sediments or rock becomes elevated as a part of the landscape destructive erosion by water or wind and the object becomes exposed or dug out and comes to the attention of a zoologist. Such a phenomenon leads to the formation of
(a) a new species (b) a new animal
(c) a fossil (d) no, this is not possible

49 Which of the following statement/s about fossils is/are correct?
(a) Fossils are useful in constructing the evolutionary history of an organism
(b) Fossils help in understanding the habit of extinct organisms
(c) Fossils provide the connecting links between two groups of organisms
(d) All of the above

50 Fossils in which the internal structure is absent but a thin carbon film indicates the outline of the external features is
(a) actual remains (b) moulds
(c) imperssions (d) casts

51 To justify that fossil '*A*' is older to '*B*', one of the following can be selected.
(a) Fossil '*B*' is in more deeper layers
(b) Fossil '*B*' shows homology and analogy with '*A*'
(c) Fossil '*A*' was found in more deeper sedimentation
(d) None of the above

52 Fossilisation occurs, where
(a) organisms are buried and preserved by natural processes
(b) animals are destroyed by environment
(c) animals are destroyed by scavengers
(d) animals are buried by natural processes

53 The fossils are dated by their presence in different layers of earth, the method being considered is
(a) stratigraphic position
(b) amount of calcium residue
(c) association with other animals
(d) radioactive carbon contents

54 Which of the following are fossils?
(a) Pollen grains buried in the bottom of peat bogs
(b) The petrified cast of clam's burrow
(c) The impression, a clam shell made in mud, preserved in mudstone
(d) All of the above

55 Consider the following statements.
I. Fossils present in the lower strata of earth are older than those present in upper strata.
II. The study of fossils in different sedimentary layers indicates the geographical period in which they existed.

Choose the correct option.
(a) Statement I is true, but II is false
(b) Statement I is false, but II is true
(c) Both statements I and II are true
(d) Both statements I and II are false

56 Consider the following statements with respect to fossil.
I. They are remains of decayed and decomposed body parts.
II. They are remains of hard part of lifeforms that existed in that part of earth.

Choose the correct option.
(a) Statement I is true, but II is false
(b) Statement I is false, but II is true
(c) Both statements I and II are true
(d) Both statements I and II are false

57 Footprints, trails, tracks and tunnels of various organisms made in mud are rapidly filled in with sand and covered by sediments. This is an example of which of the following types of fossil?
(a) Coprolites (b) Imprints
(c) Gastroliths (d) Petrified fossils

58 Ichnofossil is an alternative term used for
(a) trace fossil
(b) macrofossil
(c) body fossil
(d) coprolites

59 A living fossil among given options is
(a) *Tuatara*
(b) *Neopilina*
(c) *Nautilus*
(d) All of the above

60 Casts are fossils in which
(a) dead bodies of plants and animals are found deep in the sea
(b) body parts of dead plants and animals get incorporated into the ice
(c) the cavities of the mould get filled with minerals and harden
(d) body parts get deposited on the soft mud of an oceanic floor

61 Which of the following is an incorrect statement?
(a) Fossilised faecal material of animals is known as coprolites
(b) Petrified fossils are formed by the replacement of organic parts by mineral deposits
(c) Fossils of pollens are called palynofossils
(d) Frozen fossils of woolly mammoths found buried in the ice of Siberia are an example of moulds

62 The most accurate method for dating of fossils is
(a) radioactive carbon dating
(b) uranium lead method
(c) electron spin resonance method
(d) potassium argon method

63 The oldest evidence of life on earth, although controversial, is
(a) the fossilised remains of simple plants that are over 5 billion years old
(b) 3.8 billion years old rocks with isotopes of carbon that seem to represent the metabolic activity of the organisms
(c) the mineralised remains of tiny animals
(d) the fossilised remains of cellular colonies dating from about 3 million years ago

64 A radioactive isotope has a half-life of 1.2 billion years. As measured by the presence of the isotope and its stable decay product, a rock originally contained 10 g of the radioactive isotope and now contains 1.25 g. How many years old is the rock?
(a) 10,000 years
(b) 12 billion years
(c) 3.6 billion years
(d) 0.3 billion years

Geological Time Scale

65 What is the strongest evidence that protobionts may have formed spontaneously?
(a) The fossil record found in the stromatolites
(b) The discovery of ribosomes, showing that prebiotic RNA molecules may have been autocatalytic
(c) The production of organic compounds within a laboratory apparatus simulating conditions of early earth
(d) The relative case with which liposomes can be synthesised in laboratories

66 In Miocene,
(a) mammals reached a peak of evolution
(b) reptiles reached a peak of evolution
(c) gymnosperms were dominant
(d) birds were dominant

67 Jurassic period of the Mesozoic era is characterised by
(a) gymnosperms are dominant plants and first birds appear
(b) radiation of reptiles and origin of mammals like reptiles
(c) dinosaurs become extinct and angiosperms appear
(d) flowering plants and first dinosaurs appear

68 In the Mesozoic era, the correct sequence of the periods, beginning with the earliest, is
(a) Triassic, Jurassic, Cretaceous
(b) Jurassic, Cretaceous, Triassic
(c) Cretaceous, Triassic, Jurassic
(d) Triassic, Cretaceous, Jurassic

69 Which of the following is an incorrect statement?
(a) Angiosperms appeared on earth during the Triassic period of the Mesozoic era
(b) Dinosaurs became extinct in the Cretaceous period
(c) Mammals and dinosaurs originated almost at the same time in the Triassic period
(d) Trilobites were the extinct ancestors of the present day arthropods

70 Cenozoic era is known as an age of
(a) amphibians and lycopods
(b) marine invertebrates
(c) reptiles and gymnosperms
(d) mammals and modern flora

71 Match the options given in Column I with Column II.

Column I		Column II
A. 350 million years ago	1.	*Ichthyosaurs* were formed
B. 200 million years ago	2.	Sea weeds and few plants existed
C. 320 million years ago	3.	Invertebrates were formed and active
D. 500 million years ago	4.	Jawless fish evolved

Codes

	A	B	C	D		A	B	C	D
(a)	4	1	3	2	(b)	4	1	2	3
(c)	1	4	2	3	(d)	2	1	3	4

72 The study of fossils is useful evidence of evolution as it suggests
(a) life originated spontaneously from non-living matter
(b) life came on earth as spores or panspermia from other planets
(c) new forms of life arose at the same time in the history of earth
(d) lifeforms varied over time and certain lifeforms are restricted to certain geological time spans

73 Match the following columns.

	Column I		Column II
A.	Carboniferous	1.	Dinosaurs dominated over earth
B.	Cretaceous	2.	Dinosaurs became extinct, origin of angiosperms
C.	Ordovician	3.	Age of amphibians, origin of reptiles
D.	Jurassic	4.	Molluscs diversification

Codes

	A	B	C	D		A	B	C	D
(a)	3	2	4	1	(b)	1	2	3	4
(c)	4	1	2	3	(d)	2	3	4	1

74 Identify the incorrect match.
(a) Age of pisces – Devonian period
(b) Age of amphibians – Carboniferous period
(c) Age of reptiles – Permian period
(d) Age of dinosaurs – Jurassic period

75 Which of the following is a mismatch?
(a) Ordovician period – Age of giant molluscs
(b) Cambrian period – Origin of trilobites
(c) Devonian period – Origin of Pisces
(d) Permian period – Origin of mammals like reptiles

76 Choose the correct order in which the evolution of plant forms occurred through geological periods.
(a) Chlorophyte ancestor → *Rhynia* type plant → Psilophyton → Tracheophyte ancestor
(b) Psilophyton → *Rhynia* type plants → Tracheophyte ancestors → Chlorophyte ancestors
(c) *Rhynia* type plants → Chlorophyte ancestors → Tracheophyte ancestors → Psilophyton
(d) Chlorophyte ancestors → Tracheophyte ancestors → *Rhynia* type plants → Psilophyton

Evidences from Biogeography, Taxonomy, Biochemistry, Physiology, Cytology and Genetics

77 Alfred Wallace divided earth into six major biogeographical realms. Two such realms separated by high mountain ranges are
(a) Oriental and Ethiopian (b) Palaearctic and Oriental
(c) Palaearctic and Nearctic (d) Nearctic and Neotropical

78 Consider the following statements.
I. Effectiveness of hormones such as thyroxine and insulin of one vertebrate on another supports biochemical evidence for the evolution of living organisms.
II. Short tail in some humans represents atavism.
Choose the correct option.
(a) Statement I is true, but II is false
(b) Statement I is false, but II is true
(c) Both statements I and II are true
(d) Both statements I and II are false

79 Molecular homology deals with
(a) The different types of nucleic acids and proteins in closely related animals
(b) The similarities in anatomical structures of different organisms
(c) The similarities in anatomical structures of closely related animals
(d) The similarities of base sequence in nucleic acid and proteins of different organisms

80 Evolutionary convergence is the development of
(a) common set of characters in closely related groups
(b) common set of characters in the group of different ancestry
(c) random mating
(d) dissimilar characters in the closely related groups

81 Biochemical similarities are based on study of
(a) similarities in carbohydrates of organisms
(b) similarities in fat (fatty acid) of organisms
(c) similarities in protein and genes of organisms
(d) All of the above

82 We would predict that two very distantly related species like blue birds and alligators probably share
(a) most of the same DNA sequences
(b) more DNA sequences than a blue bird and a duck
(c) relatively few DNA sequences
(d) all the same DNA sequences

83 Current theories of prebiotic evolution are based on evidence for all of the following except the abiotic
(a) production of small organic molecules
(b) production of liposomes
(c) formation of oligopeptides
(d) origin of DNA-protein interactions

84 Consider the following statements.
I Comparative anatomy and morphology show similarities and differences among organisms of today and those that existed years ago.
II Different aged rock sediments contain fossils of different lifeforms who probably died during the formation of the particular sediment.

Choose the correct option.
(a) Statement I is true, but II is false
(b) Statement I is false, but II is true
(c) Both statements I and II are true
(d) Both statements I and II are false

(B) Cumulative Exercise

(Assorted Questions of the Chapter for Advanced Level Practice)

1 Match the following columns.

Column I	Column II
A. Atavism	1. Thorns of *Bougainvillea* and tendrils of *Cucurbita*
B. Vestigial organs	2. Leaf of a plant and cladode of *Ruscus*
C. Analogous organs	3. Pelvic girdle in python
D. Homologous organs	4. Development of power of moving pinna in some persons

Codes

	A	B	C	D		A	B	C	D
(a)	4	3	2	1	(b)	1	2	3	4
(c)	3	1	2	4	(d)	2	4	3	1

2 Which of the following statements about geological time scale are correct?
I. Origin of first seed plant occurred in Carboniferous period.
II. Angiosperms appeared in Cretaceous period.
III. There was complete absence of living organisms in Azoic era.
IV. Precambrian period comprises about 87% of the geological time scale.

Codes
(a) I and III (b) II and IV
(c) Only III (d) I, II, III and IV

3 Identify what is indicated in the given diagram?

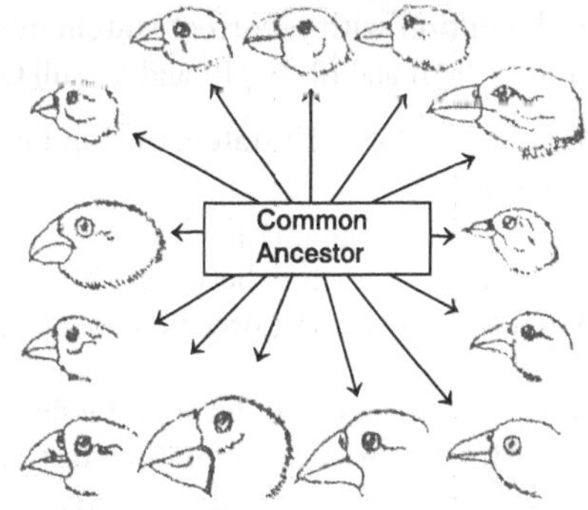

I. Recombination
II. Adaptive radiation
III. Ecological succession
IV. Different species of penguins by mutation

Choose the correct option.
(a) Only I (b) Only III
(c) Only IV (d) Only II

4 Identify the geological time periods marked as *A*, *B*, *C* and *D*.

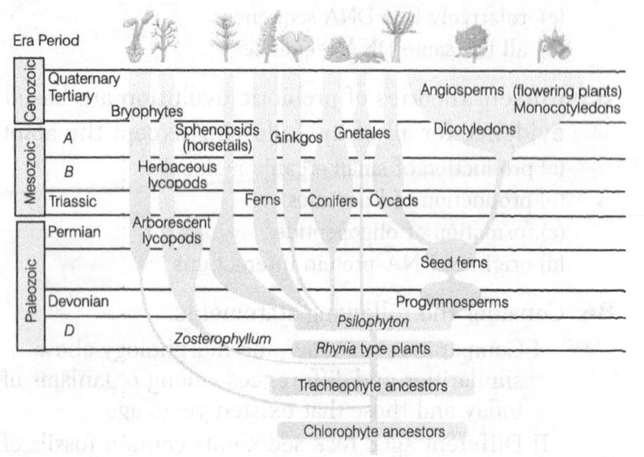

	A	*B*	*C*	*D*
(a)	Cretaceous	Carboniferous	Jurassic	Silurian
(b)	Silurian	Jurassic	Cretaceous	Carboniferous
(c)	Cretaceous	Jurassic	Carboniferous	Silurian
(d)	Jurassic	Silurian	Carboniferous	Cretaceous

5 Consider the following statements.

I. Neoteny is the reproduction of axolotl larva.
II. Biogenetic law states that, 'Ontogeny is recapitulation of phylogeny'.
III. Virus is a connecting link between plants and animals.
IV. Most of the enzymes catalysed biochemical reactions are same from bacteria to man and plants.
V. The composition and physiological role of blood, lymph and tissue fluid are different in all vertebrates.

Choose the option with incorrect statements.

(a) I and II (b) II and III (c) III and V (d) Only IV

6 Find the true (T)/false (F) statements and choose the correct option.

I. *Archaeopteryx* is the missing link because it is a fossil and has characters between birds and reptiles.
II. Origin of first mammals occurred about 220 million years ago.
III. Dinosaurs first appeared during Jurassic period.
IV. Most of the fossils occur in sedimentary rocks.

	I	II	III	IV
(a)	T	T	T	T
(b)	F	T	F	T
(c)	T	T	F	T
(d)	T	F	T	F

7 Which of the following is an incorrect statement?

(a) *Triceratops* and *Pteranodon* are extinct reptiles
(b) Australian marsupials are examples of adaptive radiation
(c) The half-life of C^{14} is 70,000 years
(d) von Baer is called the Father of Modern Embryology

8 Mark the incorrect statement.

(a) Giant ferns fell to form coal deposits
(b) In 1938, a fish caught in South Africa happened to be a coelacanth, which was thought to be extinct
(c) Amphibians lay thick-shelled eggs, which do not dry up in sun unlike those of reptiles
(d) By 500 million years ago, invertebrates were formed and active

9 Fossils are studied for

I. tracing evolutionary history of organisms.
II. studying extinct organisms.
III. establishing genetic relationships.
IV. DNA fingerprinting of new species only.

Codes

(a) I and II (b) II and III (c) III and IV (d) I and III

10 Read the following statements and choose the incorrect statements.

I. Around 350 million years ago, fish with stout and strong fins could move on land and go back to water and were called lobefins.
II. About 65 million years ago, the dinosaurs suddenly disappeared from the earth.
III. Invertebrates were formed 350 million years ago.
IV. Giant ferns were present, but they fell to form coal deposits slowly.

Codes

(a) I and II (b) II and III (c) III and IV (d) Only III

11 Identify the periods *A-D* in the diagram given below.

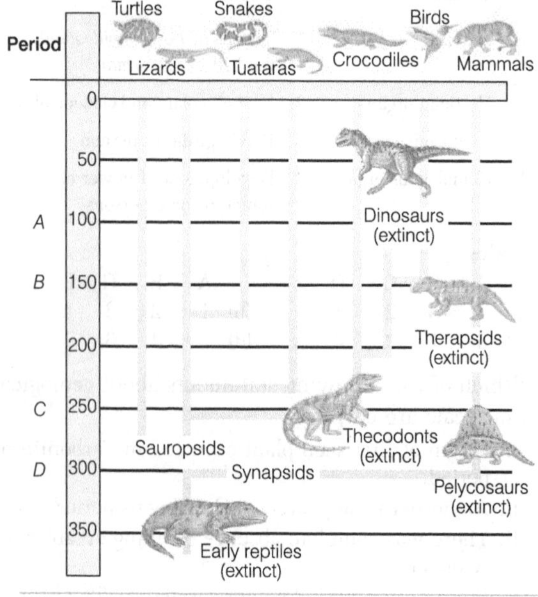

	A	*B*	*C*	*D*
(a)	Cretaceous	Jurassic	Permian	Carboniferous
(b)	Cretaceous	Permian	Jurassic	Carboniferous
(c)	Cretaceous	Permian	Jurassic	Cretaceous
(d)	Cretaceous	Triassic	Tertiary	Carboniferous

12 Match the following columns.

	Column I	Column II
A.	*Euglena*	1. Connecting link between bony fishes and cartilaginous fishes
B.	*Peripatus*	2. Connecting link between non-chordates and chordates
C.	*Chimaera*	3. Connecting link between animals and plants
D.	*Balanoglossus*	4. Connecting link between reptiles and mammals
E.	*Platypus*	5. Connecting link between annelids and arthropods

Codes

	A	B	C	D	E
(a)	1	2	3	4	5
(b)	3	5	1	2	4
(c)	2	5	1	4	3
(d)	4	3	2	1	5

13 Identify the correct statements.

I. The eye of *Octopus* and the eye of cat are analogous organs that have evolved due to convergent evolution.
II. Trilobites appeared and disappeared, respectively, during the Silurian and Carboniferous periods.
III. Dinosaurs were present during the Mesozoic Era.
IV. The origin of first toothed birds took place in the Jurassic period.

Codes

(a) I and II (b) III and IV
(c) II and IV (d) I, III, and IV

14 Mark the incorrect among the following.

I. Evolution of unicellular organisms occurred in the Proterozoic era.
II. Mammals and birds were originated in the Cenozoic era.
III. Mesozoic era is called the 'Age of Reptiles'.
IV. Dinosaurs originated during the Triassic period along with primitive mammals.

Codes

(a) I, II and III (b) I, III and IV
(c) II, III and IV (d) I, II, and IV

15 Read the following statements.

I. Birbal Sahni is the Father of Indian Palaeobotany.
II. Sweet potato (root modification) and potato (stem modification) are examples of analogous organs.
III. Convergent evolution is seen between lemur and spotted cuscus.
IV. The first organisms that invaded land were insects.
V. Jawless fish evolved around 500 million years ago.

Which of the above statements are incorrect?

(a) I and II (b) II and III
(c) IV and V (d) II and IV

16 Mark the incorrect statement from the following.

(a) The process of evolution of different species in a given geographical area starting from a point and literally radiating to other areas of geography is called adaptive radiation
(b) French biologist Lamarck had said that evolution of life forms had occurred but it is driven by use and disuse of organs
(c) A study of fossils in different sedimentary layers of rocks indicates the geographical period in which they existed
(d) Tendrils in different plants are examples of convergent evolution leading to homologous organ development

17 Read the following statements.

I. The presence of gill slits in the embryos of all vertebrates support the theory of recapitulation.
II. Around 65 million years ago, some of the land reptiles went back to water and evolved into fish like reptiles, called *Ichthyosaurs.*
III. Dinosaurs became extinct 200 million years ago.
IV. The first mammals were like shrews.

Which of the above statements are incorrect?

(a) I and II (b) II and III (c) III and IV (d) I and IV

18 Which of the following is a correct statement?

(a) Homologous organs explain convergent evolution
(b) The modern day amphibians that live on land and in water are supposed to have evolved from lobefins
(c) Echidna is connecting link between reptiles and birds
(d) Vermiform appendix is an example of atavistic character

19 Match the options given in Column I with those given in Column II.

	Column I		Column I
A.	Homologous organs	1.	Presence of long canines
B.	Analogous organs	2.	Nipples in males
C.	Vestigial organs	3.	Leaves of plants and cladode of *Ruscus*
D.	Atavism	4.	Mouth parts of cockroach and butterfly

Codes

	A	B	C	D		A	B	C	D
(a)	1	2	3	4	(b)	4	3	2	1
(c)	2	4	1	3	(d)	4	3	1	2

20 Match the following columns.

Column I		Column II
A. The collection of preserved remains of ancient organisms.	1.	Embryology
B. A method for determining the age of natural material based upon the decay of radioactive elements.	2.	Molecular biology
C. The study of the physical form of organisms.	3.	Fossils record

Column I		Column II
D. The study of how organisms develop from fertilised eggs.	4.	Radiometric dating
E. The study of the biomolecules responsible for the development and patterns seen in organisms.	5.	Morphology

Codes

	A	B	C	D	E
(a)	1	2	3	5	4
(b)	4	1	3	5	2
(c)	3	4	5	1	2
(d)	2	3	1	4	5

21 Consider the following statements and select the correct option stating which one is true (T) and which one is false (F).

I. *Tyrannosaurus* was the biggest dinosaur about 20 feet in height and had huge fearsome dagger-like teeth.
II. Some land reptiles went back into water to evolve into fish like reptiles probably 200 million years ago.
III. According to the theory of spontaneous generation, 'panspermia' was transferred from different planets from outer space, to earth.
IV. According to Darwin, there has been gradual evolution of lifeforms.
V. Homology is based on convergent evolution, while analogy refers to a situation exactly opposite.

	I	II	III	IV	V
(a)	T	T	T	F	F
(b)	T	F	T	F	F
(c)	T	T	F	T	F
(d)	T	T	T	T	F

Assertion and Reason

Direction (Q. Nos. 22-31) *In each of the following questions, a statement of Assertion (A) is given followed by corresponding statement of Reason (R). Of the statements, mark the correct answer as*

(a) Both A and R are true and R is the correct explanation of A
(b) Both A and R true, but R is not the correct explanation of A
(c) A is true, but R is false
(d) A is false, but R is true
(e) Both A and R are false

22 **Assertion** (A) *Ginkgo biloba* is a living fossil.
Reason (R) It has persisted and remains unchanged for the past several million years, while its relatives disappeared.

23 **Assertion** (A) Homologous organs have common ancestry and similar function.
Reason (R) Analogous organs have unlike origin and dissimilar function.

24 **Assertion** (A) Third molars and hairs on body in humans are examples of atavism.
Reason (R) Atavism is the reappearance of disappeared ancestral characters.

25 **Assertion** (A) Archaeozoic era contains abundant fossils.
Reason (R) Life originated in Palaeozoic era.

26 **Assertion** (A) Petrified fossils contain hard parts of organisms.
Reason (R) Moulds and casts lack the remains of organisms.

27 **Assertion** (A) Comparative biochemistry provides a strong evidence in favour of common ancestry of living beings.
Reason (R) Genetic codes are applicable universally.

28 **Assertion** (A) From evolutionary point of view, human gestation period is believed to be shortening.
Reason (R) One major evolutionary trend in human has been the larger head undergoing relatively faster growth rate in the foetal stage.

29 **Assertion** (A) Amphibians have evolved from fishes.
Reason (R) *Archaeopteryx* is a fossil linking fishes and amphibians.

30 **Assertion** (A) During development, general characters appear before specialised characters.
Reason (R) Embryos of different groups resemble with each other in early developmental stages.

31 **Assertion** (A) Claspers of cartilaginous fishes are analogous to human penis.
Reason (R) Both act as a copulatory organ and transfer the sperms into female.

(C) Medical Entrances' Gallery

(Collection of questions Asked in NEET & Various Medical Entrance Exams)

1 Flippers of penguins and dolphins are example of **[NEET 2020]**
(a) convergent evolution (b) industrial melanism
(c) natural selection (d) adaptive radiation

2 Embryological support for evolution was disapproved by **[NEET 2020]**
(a) Alfred Wallace (b) Charles Darwin
(c) Oparin (d) Karl Ernst von Baer

3 In Australia, marsupials and placental mammals have evolved to share many similar characteristics. This type of evolution may be referred to as **[NEET 2019]**
(a) adaptive radiation (b) divergent evolution
(c) cyclical evolution (d) convergent evolution

4 A population of a species invades a new area. Which of the following conditions will lead to adaptive radiation? **[NEET 2019]**
(a) Area with large number of habitats having very low food supply
(b) Area with a single type of vacant habitat
(c) Area with many types of vacant habitats
(d) Area with many habitats occupied by a large number of species

5 Among the following sets of examples for divergent evolution, select the incorrect option. **[NEET 2018]**
(a) Brain of bat, man and cheetah
(b) Heart of bat, man and cheetah
(c) Forelimbs of man, bat and cheetah
(d) Eye of *Octopus,* bat and man

6 The similarity of bone structure in the forelimbs of many vertebrates is an example of **[NEET 2018]**
(a) convergent evolution (b) analogy
(c) homology (d) adaptive radiation

7 Choose the correct statements with reference to organic evolution.
I. Flippers of whale and wings of bat exhibit analogy.
II. Wings of butterfly and wings of bird exhibit homology.
III. Organs with dissimilar structure are called analogous organs.
IV. Organs with similar structure and origin are called homologous organs. **[EAMCET 2014, AIIMS 2018]**

Codes
(a) I and IV (b) I and III (c) III and IV (d) II and IV

8 Which of the following represents order of horse?
(a) *Equidae* (b) Perissodactyla **[NEET 2017]**
(c) *Caballus* (d) *Ferus*

9 Analogous structures are a result of **[NEET-I 2016]**
(a) convergent evolution (b) shared ancestry
(c) stabilising selection (d) divergent evolution

10 Which of the following structures is homologous to the wing of a bird? **[NEET-I 2016]**
(a) Wing of a moth (b) Hindlimb of rabbit
(c) Flipper of whale (d) Dorsal fin of a shark

11 The wings of a bird and the wings of an insect are **[CBSE AIPMT 2015]**
(a) homologus structures and represent divergent evolution
(b) analogous structures and represent convergent evolution
(c) phylogenetic strutures and represent divergent evolution
(d) homologus structures and represent convergent evolution

12 The formation of two species from one ancestral species is known as **[Karnataka CET 2015]**
(a) convergent evolution (b) phyletic evolution
(c) allopatry (d) divergent evolution

13 Connecting link between fish and Amphibia is **[Chhattisgarh PMT 2015]**
(a) Lungfish, *Protopterus* (b) *Latimeria*
(c) *Seymouria* and *Sphenodon* (d) All of these

14 One of the following period witnessed the maximum diversity of reptiles **[Chhattisgarh PMT 2015]**
(a) Cretaceous (b) Jurassic (c) Pleistocene (d) Triassic

15 Vermiform appendix arises from **[AMU 2015]**
(a) caecum (b) colon (c) rectum (d) ileum

16 How many years are considered in one minute in Geological clock? **[Gujarat CET 2015]**
(a) 190000 years (b) 187500000 years
(c) 3125000 years (d) 52000 years

17 Forelimbs of cat, lizard used in walking, forelimbs of whale used in swimming and forelimbs of bats used in flying are an example of **[CBSE AIPMT 2014]**
(a) analogous organs (b) adaptive radiation
(c) homologous organs (d) convergent evolution

18 Which one of the following are analogous structures?
(a) Wings of bat and wings of pigeon **[CBSE AIPMT 2014]**
(b) Gills of prawn and lungs of man
(c) Thorns of *Bougainvillea* and tendrils of *Cucurbita*
(d) Flippers of dolphin and legs of horse

19 Choose the wrong statement. **[Kerala CEE 2014]**
(a) Louis Pasteur demonstrated that life comes only from pre-existing life
(b) SL Miller observed that electric discharge in a flask containing CH_4, H_2, NH_3 and water vapour at 800°C formed amino acids
(c) Flippers of penguins and dolphins are examples for homology
(d) Homology indicates common ancestry
(e) Analogous structures are the result of convergent evolution

20 Thorns of *Bougainvillea* and tendrils of *Cucurbita* are example for **[Karnataka CET 2014]**
(a) convergent evolution (b) divergent evolution
(c) adaptive evolution (d) coevolution

21 The process by which organisms with different evolutionary history evolve similar phenotypic adaptations in response to a common environmental challenge, is called **[NEET 2013]**
(a) natural selection (b) convergent evolution
(c) non-random evolution (d) adaptive radiation

22 The eye of *Octopus* and eye of cat show different patterns of structure, yet they perform similar function. This is an example of **[NEET 2013]**
(a) homologous organs that have evolved due to divergent evolution
(b) analogous organs that have evolved due to convergent evolution
(c) analogous organs that have evolved due to divergent evolution
(d) homologous organs that have evolved due to convergent evolution

23 Recapitulation theory was given by **[Odisha JEE 2013]**
(a) Haeckel (b) Misra
(c) Weismann (d) Lamarck

24 Which one of the following options gives one correct example each of convergent evolution and divergent evolution? **[CBSE AIPMT 2012]**

	Convergent evolution	Divergent evolution
(a)	Eyes of *Octopus* and mammals	Bones of forelimbs of vertebrates
(b)	Thorns of *Bougainvillea* and tendrils of *Cucurbita*	Wings of butterfly and birds
(c)	Bones of forelimbs of vertebrates	Wings of butterfly and birds
(d)	Thorns of *Bougainvillea* and tendrils of *Cucurbita*	Eyes of *Octopus* and mammals

25 Evolution of different species in a given area starting from a point and spreading to other geographical areas **[CBSE AIPMT 2012]**
(a) adaptive radiation (b) natural selection
(c) migration (d) divergent evolution

26 Sequence of which of the following is used to know phylogeny? **[AFMC 2012]**
(a) *m*RNA (b) *r*RNA
(c) *t*RNA (d) DNA

27 Similarities in organisms with different polymer indicates **[UP CPMT 2012]**
(a) microevolution (b) macroevolution
(c) convergent evolution (d) divergent evolution

28 Evolutionary history of an organism is known as **[UP CPMT 2012]**
(a) ancestry (b) palaeontology
(c) ontogeny (d) phylogeny

29 Biogenetic law is given by Haeckel states that **[AMU 2012]**
(a) ontogeny recapitulates phylogeny
(b) phylogeny recapitulates ontogeny
(c) ontogeny and phylogeny go together
(d) there is no relationship between phylogeny and ontogeny

30 An evolutionary pattern characterised by a rapid increase in the number and kinds of closely related species is called **[AMU 2012]**
(a) convergent evolution (b) divergent evolution
(c) adaptive radiation (d) parallel evolution

31 Evolutionary convergence is characterised by **[BCECE 2012]**
(a) development of dissimilar characteristics in closely related groups
(b) replacement of common characteristics in differentiation groups
(c) development of a common set of characteristics in groups of different ancestry
(d) development of characteristics by random mating

32 Study of fossils is called **[MHT CET 2011]**
(a) Organic evolution (b) Herpetology
(c) Cytology (d) Palaeontology

33 Which one among the following is an example for homology? **[Kerala CEE 2011]**
(a) Eye of *Octopus* and mammals
(b) Tuber of sweet potato and potato
(c) Wings of butterfly and birds
(d) Flippers of penguins and dolphins
(e) Thorn and tendrils of *Bougainvillea* and *Cucurbita*

34 Homologous organs indicate the **[Rajasthan PMT 2011]**
(a) convergent evolution (b) parallel evolution
(c) common descendent (d) natural selection

35 Fossilised faecal materials of animals are known as **[J&K CET 2011]**
(a) coprolites (b) compressions
(c) moulds (d) casts

36 Wings of birds and wings of flies perform similar functions, so they are examples of **[J&K CET 2011]**
(a) homologous organ (b) analogous organ
(c) evolutionary organ (d) paralogous organ

37 Analogous structures are **[DUMET 2011]**
(a) anatomically different, but performing similar functions
(b) anatomically similar, but performing different functions
(c) anatomically similar and functioning similarly
(d) anatomically different and functioning differently

ANSWERS

Check Point 11.1

1. (a)	2. (a)	3. (d)	4. (a)	5. (d)	6. (d)

Check Point 11.2

1. (d)	2. (a)	3. (c)	4. (d)	5. (a)	6. (c)

Check Point 11.3

1. (a)	2. (d)	3. (b)	4. (c)	5. (b)	6. (d)

(A) Topical Exercise

1. (a)	2. (a)	3. (a)	4. (b)	5. (d)	6. (d)	7. (a)	8. (a)	9. (c)	10. (b)
11. (b)	12. (c)	13. (d)	14. (a)	15. (b)	16. (d)	17. (d)	18. (d)	19. (d)	20. (d)
21. (a)	22. (b)	23. (d)	24. (b)	25. (b)	26. (d)	27. (c)	28. (a)	29. (c)	30. (c)
31. (c)	32. (d)	33. (d)	34. (a)	35. (c)	36. (a)	37. (d)	38. (a)	39. (c)	40. (a)
41. (c)	42. (c)	43. (c)	44. (b)	45. (d)	46. (a)	47. (b)	48. (c)	49. (d)	50. (c)
51. (c)	52. (a)	53. (a)	54. (d)	55. (c)	56. (c)	57. (b)	58. (a)	59. (d)	60. (c)
61. (d)	62. (c)	63. (b)	64. (c)	65. (c)	66. (a)	67. (a)	68. (a)	69. (a)	70. (d)
71. (b)	72. (d)	73. (a)	74. (c)	75. (c)	76. (d)	77. (b)	78. (c)	79. (d)	80. (b)
81. (c)	82. (c)	83. (d)	84. (c)						

(B) Cumulative Exercise

1. (a)	2. (d)	3. (d)	4. (c)	5. (c)	6. (c)	7. (c)	8. (c)	9. (a)	10. (d)
11. (a)	12. (b)	13. (d)	14. (b)	15. (c)	16. (d)	17. (b)	18. (b)	19. (b)	20. (c)
21. (d)	22. (a)	23. (e)	24. (d)	25. (e)	26. (b)	27. (b)	28. (e)	29. (c)	30. (a)
31. (a)									

(C) Medical Entrances' Gallery

1. (a)	2. (d)	3. (d)	4. (c)	5. (d)	6. (c)	7. (c)	8. (b)	9. (a)	10. (c)
11. (b)	12. (d)	13. (a)	14. (a)	15. (a)	16. (c)	17. (c)	18. (a)	19. (c)	20. (b)
21. (b)	22. (b)	23. (a)	24. (a)	25. (a)	26. (b)	27. (c)	28. (d)	29. (a)	30. (c)
31. (c)	32. (d)	33. (e)	34. (c)	35. (a)	36. (b)	37. (a)			

Explanations

(A) Topical Exercise

9 (*c*) Statement in option (c) is incorrect and can be corrected as

Stipules of *Lathyrus aphaca* and petiole of *Acacia* are analogous structures.

Rest statements are correct about homology.

13 (*d*) Statement in option (d) is incorrect and can be corrected as

Analogous organs always develop in unrelated organisms. Rest statements are correct about analogous organs.

32 (*d*) Statement in option (d) is incorrect and can be corrected as

Tadpole larva of *Herdmania* possesses notochord.

Rest statements are correct about the embryological evidences of evolution.

45 (*d*) Statement in option (d) is incorrect and can be corrected as

The missing link between non-chordates and chordates is *Balanoglossus*.

61 (*d*) Statement in option (d) is incorrect and can be corrected as Frozen fossils of woolly mammoths found buried in the ice of Siberia are an example of unusual fossils.

Rest statements are correct.

69 (*a*) Statement in option (a) is incorrect and can be corrected as During the triassic period, gymnosperms were dominant. Angiosperms appeared during the Paleocene period.

74 (*c*) Option (c) represents incorrectly matched pair and can be corrected as

Mesozoic period is considered as the age of reptiles.

75 (*c*) Option (c) is mismatched and can be corrected as Origin of Pisces was observed in Ordovician period.

(B) Cumulative Exercise

5 (*c*) Statements III and V are incorrect and can be corrected as

- Viruses are the connecting link between living and non-living.
- The composition and physiological role of blood, lymph and tissue fluid are same in all vertebrates.

Rest statements are correct.

6 (*c*) Only statement III is false and can be corrected as Dinosaurs first appeared during Triassic period.
Rest statements are true. Thus, option (c) is correct.

7 (*c*) Statement in option (c) is incorrect and can be corrected as
- The half-life of C^{14} is 5730 years.

Rest statements are correct.

8 (*c*) Statement in option (c) is incorrect and can be corrected as
- Amphibians do not produce amniotic eggs, i.e. eggs with shell. Reptiles produce thick shelled eggs.

Rest statements are correct.

10 (*d*) Only statements III is incorrect and can be corrected as Invertebrates were formed 500 million years ago.
Rest statements are correct.

13 (*d*) Statements I, III, IV are correct whereas II is incorrect. Incorrect statement can be corrected as
Trilobites appeared in Ordovician period and disappeared in Permian period.

15 (*c*) Statements IV and V are incorrect and can be corrected as
- The first organisms that invaded land were amphibians.
- Jawless fish evolved 350 million years ago.

Rest statements are correct.

16 (*d*) Statement in option (d) is incorrect and can be corrected as
- Tendrils in different plants are examples of divergent evolution.

Rest statements are correct.

17 (*b*) Statements II and III are incorrect and can be corrected as
- Fish like reptiles called *Ichthyosaurs* evolved 200 million years ago.
- Dinosaurs became extinct around 65 million years ago.

Rest statements are correct.

18 (*b*) Statement in option (b) is correct. Rest statements are incorrect and can be corrected as
- Homologous organs explain divergent evolution.
- Echidna is a connecting link between reptiles and mammals.
- Vermiform appendix is an example of vestigial organ.

21 (*d*) Only statement V is false and can be corrected as
- Homology is based on divergent evolution, while analogy is based on convergent evolution.

Rest statements are true.

22 (*a*) Both A and R are true, and R is the correct explanation of A.
Ginkgo biloba is a living fossil because it is unchanged for many hundred years, while its relatives disappeared.
Rest statements are true.

23 (*e*) Both A and R are false and can be corrected as
Homologous organs are those, which have the same essential structure that they inherit from common ancestors though they may be very differently modified for performing different functions.
For example, in case of whales, hindlimbs are only represented internally and are not apparent externally, the forelimbs are modifed into paddles and retain the bones of the shoulder, forearm, wrist and fingers all of which are enclosed in a fin-shaped sac; the head is fish like, but possesses all the mammalian bones. Analogous organs are structurally different organs, which get modified to perform similar functions.

24 (*d*) A is false, but R is true because
Atavism is the reappearance of certain ancestral characters, which have either disappeared or are reduced. There are present some examples of atavism in human being *viz* the power of moving pinna in some persons, greatly developed canine teeth, exceptionally long dense hair, short tail in some babies, etc. Third molars and hair on the body are the examples of vestigial organs.

25 (*e*) Both A and R are false and can be corrected as
The rocks of the Archaeozoic era (4600 million years) do not contain fossils, as there was no life at that time.
Life originated in the precambrian era.

26 (*b*) Both A and R are true, but R is not the correct explanation of A.
Replacement of organic parts by mineral deposits is called petrification of fossils. These fossils are termed as petrified fossils. These consist of only the hard parts of extinct organisms. Moulds are hardened and fossilised mud that surround an extinct individual.
Sometimes, a mould is found with petrified fossil of the individual also. Such fossils are termed as casts.

27 (*b*) Both A and R are true, but R is not the correct explanation of A.
Genetic codes are applicable universally because a codon specifies the same amino acid from a virus to a tree or human beings. Convincing evidences of common ancestry also comes from the similarities in the biochemical composition, reactions and physiological activities of living beings like metabolic process, enzymes, cytochrome-*c*, hormones, haemoglobin, lymph, etc.

28 (*e*) Both A and R are false and can be corrected as
The human would require more gestation period (should have been 21 months as compared to 9 months and will increase). Similarly, the head size is increasing (especially the frontal brain), hence growth rate needs to increase, but surprisingly most of the brain growth occurs after birth till 2 years (when the anterior fontanellae close at 18 months) and some more till 30 years when finally the cranial sutures close.
Thus, an increase in brain/skull size would require increase in gestation period.

29 (*c*) A is true, but R is false.
Amphibians have evolved from fishes. Lung fishes are the connecting link between fishes and amphibians.
Archaeopteryx is a connecting link or transitional stage between the reptiles and birds, as it possesses both reptilian as well as avian characters.

30 (*a*) Both A and R are true and R is the correct explanation of A.
von Baer is known as Father of Modern Embryology. He put forward Baer's law in 1828, which states that during development, general characters appear before specialised characters.
Development characters develop through
More general → Less general → Specialised.

During development, an animal departs progressively from the form of other animals.

Organisms of different groups resemble each other at embryonic stage.

31 (*a*) Both A and R are true and R is the correct explanation of A.

Claspers are posterior extensions of each of the pelvic fin in male cartilaginous fishes and penis is the external copulatory organ in humans. These serve as copulatory organ to channel semen in female's cloaca during mating.

(C) Medical Entrances' Gallery

3 (*d*) In Australia, marsupials and placental mammals have evolved to share many similar characteristics. This type of evolution is referred to as convergent evolution.

Convergent evolution is represented by the presence of similar adaptive functional structures in unrelated groups of organisms. For example, a number of marsupials, each different from the other evolved from an ancestral stock, but all within the Australian island continent. Also, marsupials in Australia resemble placental mammals in the rest of the world, they evolved in isolation after Australia separated from other continents.

4 (*c*) Adaptive radiation occurs when a population of a species invades a new area because it provides organisms of a population a new habitat with plenty of niche spaces. Darwin's finches represent one of the best examples of this phenomenon.

Thus, option (c) is correct.

5 (*d*) Option (d) is incorrect and can be corrected as

Eyes of *Octopus*, bat and man are examples of analogous organs which show convergent evolution. Divergent evolution results in homologous structures. These organs have the same fundamental structure but are different in functions. Structural homology is seen in brain, heart and forelimbs of man, bat and cheetah.

6 (*c*) The similarity of bone structure in the forelimbs of many vertebrates is an example of homology. The homologous organs have the same fundamental structure but are adapted to perform different functions, e.g. forelimbs of man, cheetah, whale and bat.

Other options are explained as follows

Analogous organs show convergent evolution. These organs have similar functions but are different in their structural details and origin. Development of different functional structures from a common ancestral form is called adaptive radiation.

7 (*c*) Statements III and IV are correct with reference to organic evolution. Statements I and II are incorrect and can be corrected as

- Flippers of whale and wings of bat are homologous structures. Since, they have the same embryonic origin and basic structure but they do not perform same function.
- The wings of butterfly and birds are analogous organs as they have different structural plan and developmental origin. However, they perform similar functions in different organisms.

8 (*b*) The order of horse is Perissodactyla. Order being the higher taxon of classification exhibits the few similar characters of families. The order-Perissodactyla includes odd toed mammals, e.g. *Equus asinus* (donkey), *Rhinoceros indicus* (the great one-horned rhinoceros).

13 (*a*) Lungfish, *Protopterus* is a connecting link between fish and amphibians.

Other options are explained as

Latimeria also is a connecting link between fish and amphibians, but is a non-living fossil.

Seymouria and *Sphenodon* is a connecting link between amphibians and reptiles.

19 (*c*) All the given statements are correct except (c).

Incorrect statement can be corrected as

Flippers of penguins and dolphins are analogous organs because these are functionally similar, but are anatomically different. This results in the convergent evolution.

23 (*a*) Ernst Haeckel – Recapitulation theory
Weismann – Continuity of germplasm.
Lamarck – Inheritance of acquired characters

Thus, option (a) is correct.

24 (*a*) Convergent evolution involves the independent development of similar structures in organisms that are not directly related. It is represented by analogous organs, e.g. eyes of *Octopus* and mammals, wings of insects and birds.

In divergent evolution, same basic organ becomes adapted by specialisation to perform different functions. It is represented by homologous organs, e.g. forelimbs of vertebrates (like seal's flipper, bat's wing, cat's paw, horse's front leg and human hand), thorns of *Bougainvillea* and tendrils of *Cucurbita*.

25 (*a*) The diversification of an ancestral group into two or more species in different habitats is called divergent evolution. When this involves large number of species to occupy different niches, this is called adaptive radiation.

Adaptive radiation is the process of evolution of different species in a given geographical area starting from a species of animals or plants and literally radiating to other areas of geography (habitats). Darwin's finches represent one of the best examples of this phenomenon. Australian marsupials are another example of adaptive radiation.

26 (*b*) The genes for *r*RNAs tend to be highly conserved and are often employed for phylogenetic studies, e.g. 16 S *r*RNA is used in reconstructing phylogenies, due to the slow rates of evolution of genes of this region.

28 (*d*) Phylogeny (Gr. *Phylon*-tribe or race; *geneia*-origin) is the origin and diversification of any taxon or the evolutionary history of its origin and diversification. It is usually represented as a diagrammatic phylogenetic tree (that traces putative evolutionary relationships), i.e. dendrogram.

32 (*d*) Palaeontology – Study of fossils
Cytology – Study of cell structure and function
Herpetology – Study of reptiles and amphibians

Organic evolution – The sequence of events involved in the evolutionary development of a species or taxonomic group of organisms.

Thus, option (d) is correct.

34 (*c*) Homologous organs are those organs, which have the same basic structure, but different functions. These show common descendent and divergent evolution, while analogous organs show convergent evolution.

CHAPTER 12

Theories of Evolution

It is believed that in due course of time, the ancestral species living in different regions of earth adapted to their environment and gradually evolved. This led to the formation of separate species that we see today. Based on the evidences of evolution, many scientists have proposed their theories or hypotheses to explain the mechanism of evolution.

In this chapter, we will try to explore a few, most revolutionary theories that have been put forward by some of the great scientists of their times. To begin with, the chronology of some important contributions on evolution is given below

Table 12.1 History of evolutionary thoughts

Greek and medieval period	
Democritus	Living things arose by spontaneous generation from the slime of the earth.
Thales (640-556 BC)	All life originated in water.
Aristotle (384-322 BC)	Proposed theory of continuous and gradual evolution from the lifeless matter. Based on his observations of animals, recognised a 'scala naturae' for animals.
Age of speculation (1400-1790)	
John Ray (1627-1705)	Developed concept of species.
Carolus Linnaeus (1707-1778)	Formalised binomial classification system. Suggested genera were created separately and species were the variants of them.
Buffon (1707-1788)	Suggested that different types of animals had different origins at different times. Recognised influence of external environment. Believed in acquired inheritance.
James Hutton (1726-1797)	Theory of uniformatarianism. Calculated the age of earth in millions of years.

Inside

1 Lamarck and Lamarckism : Theory of inheritance of acquired characters
2 Darwinism or Darwin's theory of evolution
3 Mutation theory of Hugo de Vries
4 Modern synthetic theory of evolution

Age of Formulation (1790-1900)	
Erasmus Darwin (1731-1802)	Life arose from one single 'filament' made by God. The filaments are evolved by the acquired characteristics. Refused the preformation of human.
Jean Baptiste Lamarck (1744-1829)	The concept of use and disuse of organs. Inheritance of acquired characteristics, environment acts on organisms, phenotypic changes are passed on to offsprings.
George Cuvier (1769-1832)	Established palaeontological evidence. Fossils are the results of 'catastrophes' by which new species arose.
William Smith (1769-1838)	Opposed Cuvier's theory of catastrophism on the basis of continuity of similar species in related strata.
Charles Lyell (1797-1875)	Demonstrated the progressive history of fossil evidence.
Charles Darwin (1809-1882)	Influenced by Lyell and Malthus, established the theory of evolution by means of natural selection.
Alfred Russel Wallace (1823-1913)	Similar theory to Darwin, but his theory did not include human.
August Weismann (1834-1914)	Showed that the reproductive cells of animals are distinct and therefore, unaffected by the influences acting on somatic tissues. Gave the theory of germplasm.
Hugo de Vries (1848-1935)	Recognised existence of mutations, which were heritable, as a basis for discontinuous variation and regarded species as arising by mutation.
Developments of 20th Century	
HJ Muller (1927)	Genotype can be altered by X-rays, induced mutation.
RA Fischer (1930)	No difference between change investigated by geneticists and change shown in the fossil record.

The most important theories of evolution include Lamarckism, Darwinism, mutation theory and modern synthetic theory, etc.

LAMARCK AND LAMARCKISM : THEORY OF INHERITANCE OF ACQUIRED CHARACTERS

- The first attempt to explain origin of species and their adaptation to the environment was done by French naturalist, **Jean Baptiste de Lamarck** (1744-1829). He gave the first theory of evolution known as **Lamarckism** or the theory of inheritance of acquired characters.
- The theory states that all changes, which organisms acquire during their lifetime, are transmitted to their offsprings by the process of inheritance.
  Lamarck believed that a nervous fluid within each species helps to progress up. The more strongly exercised organs attract more of the 'nervous fluid' which in turn, enlarges these organs and such alterations are inherited.
- Lamarck published this theory in his famous book ***'Philosophie Zoologique'*** in 1809, the same year of Darwin birth. He also introduced certain terms such as invertebrates, vertebrates and Annelida.

Postulates of Lamarckism

The theory of inheritance of acquired characters was explained by Lamarck using following four main postulates.

1. Internal vital force

Organisms and their organs have a natural tendency to continuously increase in size, generation after generation. For example, the ancestors of present day giraffes had small neck and forelimbs. However, the internal vital force helped them to increase their size and becomes relatively larger in due course of time.

2. Effect of environment and new needs

Continuous changes in the environmental conditions directly influence the nature, habits, ways of living of an organism and their structural organisation.

For example,

- Early giraffes used to feed on the grasses and other surface plants of an area. With time, the climate of this area became arid. As a result, the grasses and other surface vegetation dried up, leaving only a few taller trees.

- Thus, the leaves of these tall trees were the only food available to ancestors. It is called **doctrine of appetency** or **desires.**

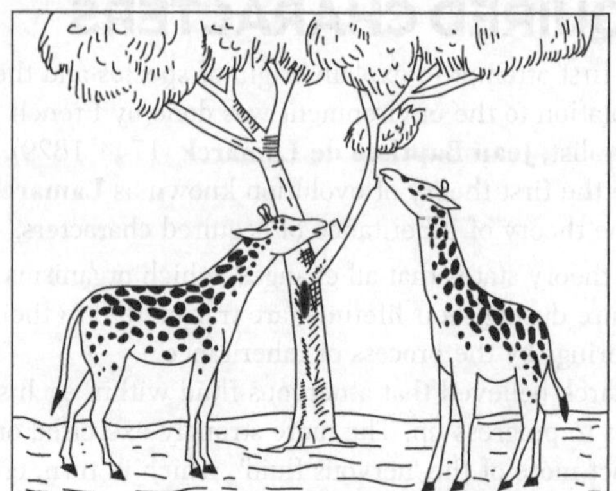

Early giraffes probably had short necks which they stretched to reach to tall trees, when the grasses dried up due to climate change.

3. Use and disuse of organs

The growth of less used parts decline, while that of better used parts progresses.

For example,

- To fulfil their new needs, the giraffes continuously stretched their necks to reach to the taller trees. As the neck was comprehensively used to reach to the trees, its permanent elongation took place and the character was acquired.

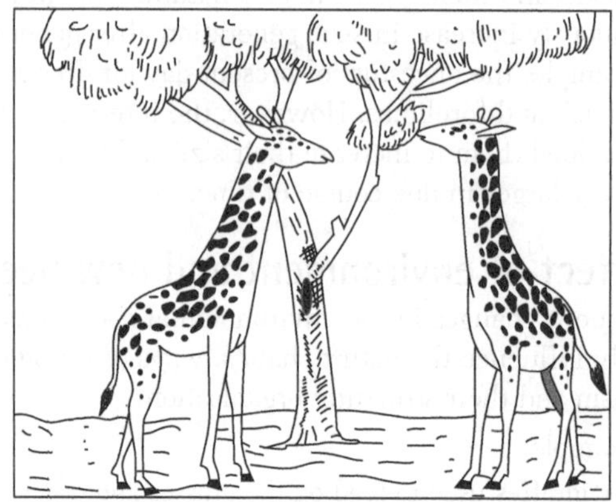

Their offsprings also had longer necks that they stretched to reach food.

4. Inheritance of acquired characters

The growth of organs (either better or poorer) acquired during lifetime of an organism is heritable.

As in case of giraffes, where the acquired character, i.e. long neck was transmitted in next generations.

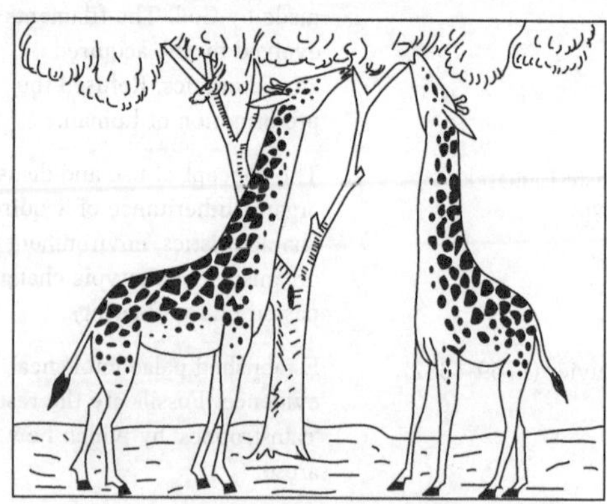

Eventually, the continued stretching of the neck resulted in today's long-necked giraffe.

Other examples in favour of Lamarckism

(i) **Snakes** The present day limbless snakes with long slender body were developed from the limbed ancestors. It is due to continued disuse of limbs and stretching of their body to suit their creeping mode of locomotion and fossorial mode of living.

(ii) **Aquatic birds** Ducks, geese like aquatic birds were developed from their terrestrial ancestors by the inheritance of acquired characters like reduction of wings due to their continued disuse, development of webs between their toes for wading purposes, etc. These changes were mainly induced due to the deficiency of food on land and severe competition.

(iii) **Flightless birds** The flightless birds like ostrich developed from their flying ancestors due to continued disuse of wings as they were found in well protected areas with plenty of food.

(iv) **Flat fishes** These are deep sea fishes present at the bottom of sea where there is no sunlight. They led an inactive life, lying on one side of the body.

(v) **Whales** They lost their hindlimbs as the consequence of their disuse.

(vi) **Wading birds** They developed long legs through the generations of sustained stretching to keep the body above the water level, e.g. Jacana bird.

(vii) **Cave dwellers** Eyes are reduced in cave dwellers (moles) since, they live underground.

(viii) **Emergent hydrophytes** In emergent hydrophytes like *Ranunculus aquatilis*, all the submerged leaves are dissected while the emerged ones are simply lobed. When the plant is grown out of water, all the leaves are undissected.

There are other effects also that exemplify the Lamarckian theory such as

- vestigial organs in some living animals.
- strong claws and canines in carnivores.
- sensitive skin and tactile points on the ventral side of the body.
- callosities of palm in hard workers.

Evidences in favour of Lamarckism

Evidences in favour of Lamarckism or theory of inheritance of acquired characters are given below

- **Sumner** (1990) performed an experiment on mice. According to him, the mice kept in warmer environments develop longer tails and larger ear pinna as compared to those kept in cooler environments. This trait was also inherited in next generations.
- **McDougall** (1938) trained mice to come and go using a similar path for 40-45 generation. He observed that the later generations needed less training.
- **Pavlov** (1897) also trained some dogs to come to food on hearing bell. He observed that the successive generations needed less training.
- **Paul Kammerer** (1924) kept *Salamandra maculosa* having yellow and black spots on body in two different environments, i.e. yellow and black background. The animals grown in yellow background had larger yellow spots while those in black background had larger black spots. This characteristic was also acquired in next generations.
- In normal course of life, usually somatic cells produce somatic cells while germ cells produce germ cells. However, during vegetative propagation of plants and regeneration in animals, germ cell can be produced from somatic cells.
- Radish is a biennial crop in cold countries, but it completes its growth in a year in tropical areas.
- European peach, which is deciduous becomes evergreen in India.

Criticism of Lamarckism

Lamarckism or theory of inheritance of acquired characters was criticised due to the following reasons

- Blind, deaf and lame parents do not produce abnormal, i.e. blind, deaf or lame offsprings.
- Wounds evenscans of parents do not appear in their offsprings.
- Despite the use of iron shoes to keep their feet short by Chinese women, their young ones at birth have normal feet size.
- One of the famous objection to Lamark's theory came from a German biologist, **August Weismann** (1890). He cut the tail of newborn mice for 22 generation but could neither get a tailless mice nor the mice developed shorter tail.

Theory of germplasm

Theory of continuity of germplasm (1892) was proposed by August Weismann (1834-1914).
Based on his observations, he suggested that the changes which occur only in the germplasm are inherited by the offsprings, whereas those in the somatoplasm are not transmitted to next generation.

Neo-Lamarckism

A group of scientists further studied Lamarckian theory and some of them like **Alfred Giard, WL Tower, ED Cope, Richard Goldschmidt, George Henslow, H Spencer, Ernst Haeckel**, etc., supported the modified form of Lamarckism, which is termed as Neo-Lamarckism. Some important observations in relation to Neo-Lamarckism are given below

- **William Lawrence Tower** observed the direct effect of environment on germ cells when he treated potato beetles to very high temperature and humidity during the development of their reproductive organs.
- **John William Heslop Harrison** observed the effect of environment on germ cells. The effect was perceived through the somatic cells, when he found a dark variety of peppered moth in manganese polluted localities whose ancestors were pale in colour.
- Sudden heritable variations or mutations were obtained by **Auerbach *et. al.*** on the exposure of *Drosophila* to high energy radiations like UV-rays, X-rays, γ-rays and mustard gas, etc.

Postulates of neo-Lamarckism

The postulates of neo-Lamarckism are given below

- There is no role of internal vital forces in evolution.
- Environment does influence an organism and change its heredity.
- Some of the variations acquired by an individual can be transmitted to its offsprings.
- Only those variations are inherited, which are associated with the germ cells or where, the somatic cells give rise to germ cells.

Major differences between Lamarckism and Neo-Lamarckism are given below

Table 12.2 Differences between Lamarckism and Neo-Lamarckism

Lamarckism	Neo-Lamarckism
Lamarckism was proposed by Lamarck originally.	It is the modification of Lamarckism proposed by a group of scientists.
Theory emphasises on the internal vital forces.	Concept of internal vital force was discarded.
It gives importance to use and disuse of organs.	It does not give any importance to the concept of use and disuse of organs.
According to this theory, change in environment brings about a conscious reaction in animals.	According to this theory, changed environment affects directly the organism.
It states that all the acquired characters are inherited by the offsprings.	It explains that only those acquired characters are inherited by the offsprings, which influence the germplasm or germ cells.

CHECK POINT 12.1

1. What is Lamarck credited with?
   (a) Natural selection as a mechanism of evolution
   (b) The observation of mass extinction
   (c) A mechanism to explain evolution
   (d) The discovery of giraffe
2. According to Lamarckism, long necked giraffes evolved because
   (a) nature selected only long-necked ones
   (b) short necks suddenly changed into long necks
   (c) human preferred only long-necked ones
   (d) change in climate
3. Which of the following is not a concept of Lamarckian theory?
   (a) Environmental pressure causes variation
   (b) Rate and survival of organism is different due to variation
   (c) Inheritance of acquired characters
   (d) If an organ is used constantly it will continuously increase its size
4. Which of the following evidences does not favour the Lamarckian concept of inheritance of acquired characters?
   (a) Lack of pigments in cave-dwelling animals
   (b) Melanisation in peppered moth
   (c) Absence of limbs in snakes
   (d) Presence of webbed toes in aquatic birds
5. Lamarckism fails to explain which of the following phenomenon?
   (a) Absence of all the four limbs amongst amphibians
   (b) Exceptionally long neck of giraffe
   (c) An intellectual having a dull son
   (d) Loss of vision in cave-dwelling mammals
6. According to Neo-Darwinism, variations which are the raw material of evolution occur
   (a) in an individual and remain restricted to him
   (b) in gene pool of a population
   (c) in all the members of one species
   (d) in all the members of all species

DARWINISM OR DARWIN'S THEORY OF EVOLUTION

- Charles Darwin was born in 1809. In 1831, he accepted an unpaid post of naturalist on the survey ship, called **HMS Beagle**. In his voyage, he spent five years in sea charting the East Coast of South America. The Beagle returned to Falmouth in October, 1836 *via* the coast of Chile, the Galapagos islands, Tahiti, New Zealand, Tasmania and South Africa.
- During a five week stay on the Galapagos islands, he was struck by the similarities shown by the flora and fauna of the islands and mainland. In particular, he was intrigued by the characteristic distribution of species of tortoises and finches.
- Darwin formulated his theory of evolution with natural selection as its foundation. His work was inspired by **Thomas R Malthus**, who wrote an essay on the principles of population. This essay was published in 1778.
  He highlighted the 'consequences of reproductive potential' in this essay.
- In the meantime, another naturalist **Alfred Russel Wallace**, came to the same conclusions as Darwin, regarding natural selection. In 1858, Darwin and Wallace presented papers on their ideas at a meeting of the Linnean Society in London.
- In November 1859, Darwin published his thoughts on evolution in *'Origin of Species'* by the name of Natural Selection.

- An overview of his thoughts is given below

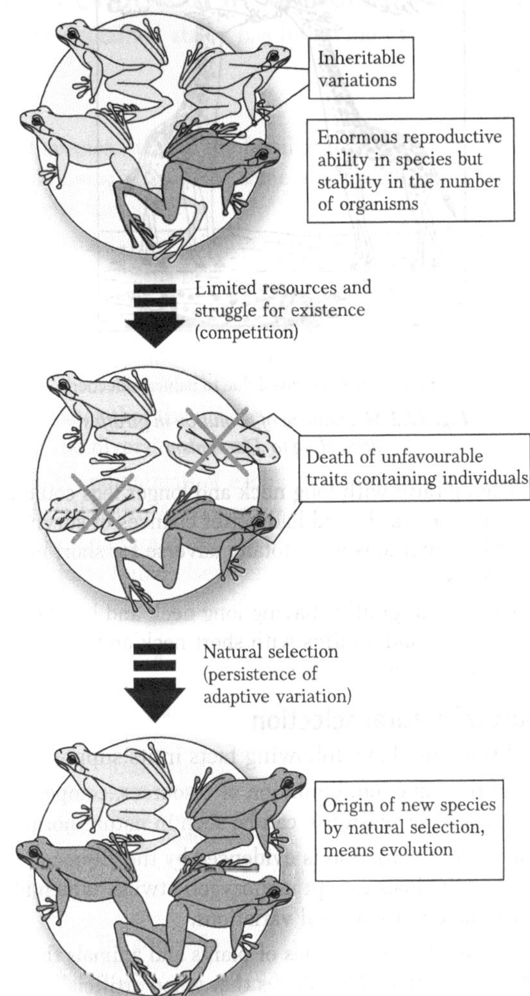

Fig. 12.1 Schematic arrangement of the Wallace's chart showing origin of new species

Postulates of Darwinism

The main postulates of Darwin's theory of natural selection are as follows

1. Overproduction (Rapid multiplication)

- All organism possess enormous fertility. They multiply in a geometric proportion with some organisms producing very large number of individuals. Despite of this high rate of reproduction of a species, its number remains constant under fairly stable environment.
- The production of more offsprings by some organisms and fewer by others is termed as **differential reproduction**.
- Some examples of overproduction of some animals are given below

Organisms	Eggs/Young ones (whole number)
Female Salmon	28000000 eggs/season
Oyster	60-80 million eggs/yrs
Cod fish (Ovaries)	10 million eggs
Elephant	6 offspring/entire life
Rabbit	24 offspring/yrs

2. Limited resources

The resources like food, space, etc., remain limited inspite of rapid multiplication of the individuals of all the species.

3. Struggle for existence

The limited resources present in the environment are the main cause of struggle for existence, which may occur at following three levels.

(i) **Intraspecific struggle** It is the struggle among the individuals of same species for their common requirements like food, shelter, mate, breeding places, etc. Intraspecific struggle is very severe because the individuals of a species are closest to each other.

(ii) **Interspecific struggle** It is the struggle between the individuals of different species for their similar requirements like food and space. For example, a frog feeds on insects and is prayed upon by snakes. A kite on the other hand, feeds on both frogs as well as snakes. It is comparatively less intense struggle.

(iii) **Environmental struggle** It is the struggle of living forms against the environmental conditions like extreme heat, cold, drought, earthquakes, storms, disease, volcanic eruption, etc.

4. Appearance of variations

- All individuals are dissimilar in some of their characters except the identical twins. Technically, this dissimilarity is called **variations.** These differences may be small or large and allow better adjustment with the environment.
- Variations can be categorised into the following types

(i) **Somatic variations** These variations affect the somatic cells of an organism. These are also called **modifications** or **acquired** characters because these are aquired by an individual during its lifetime.

These variations arose due to various environmental factors, use and disuse of organs and conscious efforts, etc.

Drawbacks of Darwinism

The Darwinian theory had following drawbacks

- Darwin could not explain the basis of variation and mode of transmission of these variations to the next generation, i.e. heredity.
- **Theory of pangenesis** have been proposed by Darwin to explain the inheritance of characteristics from the parents to their offsprings. It was refuted by August Weismann's **theory of continuity of germplasm.**

Criticism of Darwin's natural selection theory

Darwin's theory was widely accepted, but **Sir Richard Owen** and **Adam Sedgewick** criticised it due to following reasons

- Darwin emphasised on inheritance of useful variation. However, sometimes inheritance of small variations, which are not useful to individuals are also seen.
- He could not explain the presence of vestigial organs and effect of their use and disuse.
- Darwinism failed to explain the arrival of the fittest.
- Darwinism failed to differentiate between the somatic and germinal variations and considered all types of variations as heritable.
- Darwinism failed to explain over specialisation of some organs such as elephant's tusk of Jefferson mammoth, antlers of iris deer, which led to the extinction of their possessors.
- His natural selection was failed in explaining the evolution of terrestrial animals from the aquatic organisms.
- His natural selection was failed in explaining some adaptations such as electric organs of fish (*Torpedo*), mimicry in Karama butterfly, etc.
- The explanation of coordinated development and co-adaptation was not under the perview of natural selection.
- Darwinism does not account for the degeneration of certain animal organs.

Note *Darwin's theory was rejected by neo-Lamarckism, theory of orthogenesis and mutation theory. The term 'orthogenesis' was introduced by* ***Wilhelm Haacke*** *in 1893.*

Theory of orthogenesis

According to this theory, it was told that variations are directed towards fixed goals, so that species evolve in predetermined direction without the aid of natural selection. That's why, it is also called **progressive evolution** or **progressionism**.

Neo-Darwinism

Ronald Fisher, Haldane and **Sewall Wright** combined the ideas of natural selection and Mendelian genetics to form neo-Darwinism. This concept explained evolution on the basis of genetics, molecular biology, palaeontology, ecology and ethology, i.e. the study of behaviour.

Postulates of Neo-Darwinism

Following postulates are given under neo-Darwinism

- There is a clear cut difference between the germplasm and somatoplasm.
- The adaptations result from the multiple forces and natural selection is one of them.
- As per neo-Darwinism, characters are not inherited as such, instead there are character determiner's (genes), which control the development.
- The origin and evolution of new characters are the result of changes in genes of organisms and the environment during its development.

The key differences between Darwinism and neo-Darwinism are given below

Darwinism	Neo-Darwinism
Darwinism is an original theory explained by Darwin (1859).	Neo-Darwinism is a modification of Darwinism proposed by a group of scientists to remove the drawbacks of original theory.
New species are formed as a result of continuous variations.	Mutation becomes more effective than continuous variations during new species formation.
Variations are accumulated in individuals.	Variations are accumulated in the gene pool.
Darwin thought that the adaptations result mainly due to a single source, i.e. natural selection.	Neo-Darwinians thought that the adaptations result from the multiple forces along with natural selection.
Darwinism does not believe in isolation.	Isolation is a significant component of evolution in neo-Darwinism.

MUTATION THEORY OF HUGO de VRIES

- **Hugo de Vries** (1848-1935) was a Dutch botanist who proposed the mutation theory in order to explain the mechanism of evolution. His results were based on the observations of the wild variety of evening primrose, *Oenothera lamarckiana.*
- Mutation theory was published in 1901, in his book entitled *'Die Mutation Theorie'.*

- Hugo de Vries stated that new species arise due to the jerky, discontinuous variations or **saltatory variations** which were named by him as **mutations**. He rejected the idea of accumulation of minor and continuous variations in speciation.

Salient features of mutation theory

- Mutations are large and sudden changes in contrast to small, directional fluctuating variations as explained by Darwin.
- These act as raw material for evolution.
- Mutations are heritable and are subjected to natural selection.
- These mutations may occur in any direction and may be useful or harmful. The harmful mutations are usually eliminated, while useful mutations are selected by the nature.
- Mutations are recurring, so that the same mutants appear again and again, thereby increasing the chance of selection by nature.

Criticism against mutation theory

BM Davis claimed that the *Oenothera lamarckiana* was a hybrid plant, which could be obtained by the hybridisation of two wild species and it is not a normal plant. So, he criticised mutation theory with the following facts

- Natural mutations are not common phenomenon.
- Most of the mutations are recessive and retrogressive.
- de Vries mutations were mainly chromosomal aberrations, which are unstable.
- Mutation theory failed to explain the role of nature.

MODERN SYNTHETIC THEORY OF EVOLUTION

- The modern theory of origin of species or evolution is also known as the modern synthetic theory of evolution. The basic concept of this theory is based on Dobzhansky's book '*Genetics and the Origin of Species*'. This book was published in 1937.
- Other scientists who contributed to this theory are **Julian Huxley** (1942), **Ernst Mayr** (1970), **RA Fisher** (1958), **JBS Haldane**, **Sewall Wright** (1968) and **GL Stebbins** (1971). Stebbins in his book '*Process of Organic Evolution*' discussed the modern synthetic theory.

Main postulates of modern synthetic theory of evolution

- This theory recognises following five basic processes
  - Gene mutation
  - Changes in chromosome structure and number
  - Genetic recombination
  - Natural selection
  - Reproductive isolation by various means like migration, hybridisation, chance, etc.
- Out of these, the first three processes provide the genetic variability without which changes cannot take place. Natural selection and reproductive isolation guide populations of organisms for adaptation.
  Besides these, three accessory processes affect the working of above five basic processes. These include
  - **Migration** of individuals from one population to another, increases genetic variability.
  - **Hybridisation** between races or closely related species also increase the genetic variability.
  - The **effect of chance**, acts on small population. This may alter the way in which natural selection guides the course of evolution.
- All sexually reproducing organisms contain a large gene pool of genetic variability which maintain a dynamic equilibrium between inflow and outflow of genes.
- Genes may be added to gene pool by immigration from other gene pool and mutation.
- Genes are removed from the gene pool by natural selection and chance elimination of alleles, which take place in small population (Genetic drift) or during reduction of population size.
- **Genetic recombination** is the constant reshuffling of the genes in the gene pool.
- **Natural selection** may either stabilise gene composition by eliminating most immigrants and mutants or change it in various ways.
- Evolution takes place through alterations of the frequency of genes and gene combinations in the population.
- **Reproductive isolation** includes all the barriers to gene exchange between two populations. The populations that are reproductively isolated evolve in different directions, while those that are not so isolated will evolve in the same direction because of genic exchanges.

CHECK POINT 12.2

1. Darwin in his 'Natural Selection Theory' did not believe in any role of which one of the following in organic evolution?
(a) Parasites and predators as natural enemies
(b) Survival of the fittest
(c) Struggle for existence
(d) Discontinuous variations

2. The phrase 'Survival of the fittest' was first used by Herbert Spencer. The same phrase was used by Darwin as
(a) inheritance of acquired characters
(b) natural selection
(c) differential reproduction
(d) struggle for existence

3. The best description of natural selection is
(a) the survival of the fittest
(b) the struggle for existence
(c) the reproductive success of the members of a population best adapted to the environment
(d) a change in the proportion of variations within a population

4. 'Darwin's finches' refers to
(a) fossils of birds collected by Darwin at Galapagos islands
(b) a type of birds present on Galapagos islands
(c) migratory birds collected by Darwin at Galapagos islands
(d) fossils of reptiles collected by Darwin at Galapagos islands

5. Hugo de Vries experimental material, *Oenothera lamarckiana* was a
(a) complex heterozygote with anomalous chromosome behaviour
(b) homozygous with fragile chromosomes
(c) heterozygote which developed gene mutations
(d) homozygous with stable chromosomes

6. The process which is not associated with modern synthetic theory is
(a) genetic recombination
(b) chromosomal mutation
(c) point mutation
(d) gene splicing

EXAM POINTS

- The concept of inheritance of acquired chracter in support of evolution was proposed by Lamarck. **[J&K CET 2011]**
- Lamarckism could not explain weak muscle in the some of a wrestler. **[UP CPMT 2013]**
- According to theory of germplasm every cell of the body contributes gemmules to the germ cells and so shares in the transmission of inherited characters. **[JCECE 2011]**
- Malthus theory of human population states that human population grow exponentially while food production grows at an arithmetic rate, leading to overpopulation and social problem. **[Chhattisgarh PMT 2015]**
- Darwin published his work in a famous book called *'Origin of Species'*. **[WB JEE 2013]**
- According to Darwin, the organic evolution is due to intraspecific competition. **[NEET 2013]**
- Darwin held that small favourable variations formed raw material for evolutions. Darwin did not study the factors which produce variations. **[AIIMS 2017]**
- Natural selection is evident in the reproductive success of the members of a population best adapted to the environment. **[AIIMS 2017]**
- The term 'Darwin fitness' means the ability to survive and reproduce. **[DUMET 2011]**
- Darwin judged the fitness of an individual by number of offspring. **[DUMET 2011]**
- Darwin's finches represent geographical isolation. They provide an excellent evidence in favour of organic evolution. These are related to embryology. **[Manipal 2012, JCECE 2012]**
- Hugo de Vries pioneered the theory of mutation to explain the mechanism of evolution. According to him, evolution is discontinuous and jerky process. **[NEET 2019, AFMC 2013]**
- Hugo de Vries gave the term saltation, Thomas Malthus is known for his studies on population, Charles Darwin explained branching descent and Lamarck gave the use and disuse theory. **[Kerala CEE 2014]**

Chapter Exercises

(A) Topical Exercise

History of Evolutionary Thoughts

1 Who claimed that the *Oenothera lamarckiana* was a hybrid plant, which could be obtained by hybridisation of two wild species and it is not a normal plant?

(a) Theodosius (b) Julian
(c) BM Davis (d) TR Malthus

2 Consider the following statements.

I. The term 'Evolution' was used by Spencer.
II. Theory of evolution is based on mutation, reproductive isolation and sexual reproduction.

Choose the correct option.

(a) Statement I is true, but II is false
(b) Statement I is false, but II is true
(c) Both statements I and II are true
(d) Both statements I and II are false

3 Which of the following pairs are not correctly matched?

(a) Cuvier – Continuous fossil record with no breaks
(b) Darwin – Natural selection as a mechanism for evolution
(c) James Hutton – Theory of uniformitarianism
(d) Lamarck – Characters acquired during an organism's lifetime are passed on to offsprings

4 Who opposes the theory of catastrophism?

(a) Hugo de Vries (b) HJ Muller
(c) Charles Darwin (d) William Smith

5 Find the mismatch pair.

(a) Concept of Biological species - E Mayr
(b) Recapitulation theory - Watson
(c) Theory of origin of isolation - Dobzhansky
(d) All of the above

6 Which one is linked to evolution?

(a) Extinction
(b) Competition
(c) Variation
(d) Reproduction

7 Whose bicentenary is the year 2009?

(a) Lamarck (b) Darwin
(c) Mendel (d) Hugo de Vries

8 The first step attempt to solve the problem of organic evolution is related to

(a) E Darwin (b) JB Lamarck
(c) G Cuvier (d) W Smith

Lamarckism and Neo-Lamarckism

9 '*Philosophie Zoologique*' book written by

(a) Wallace (b) Charles Darwin
(c) Lamarck (d) de Vries

10 According to Lamarck, well-developed auricle muscles of rabbit have evolved due to

(a) continuous use (b) internal vital force
(c) increasing need (d) All of these

11 The present giraffe has a long neck as compared to its ancestors. Lamarck believed it could be due to

(a) natural selection
(b) isolation
(c) inheritance of acquired characters
(d) speciation

12 Which of the following statements about Lamarck is true?

(a) He was a French botanist, who later became zoologist
(b) He was an English naturalist who gave the theory of evolution
(c) He was a Polish scientist and gave the law of inheritance
(d) He was a French scientist, who gave the concept of inheritance of acquired characters

13 Which of the following two papers on evolution were submitted by Lamarck in 1801 and 1802?

(a) *Systeme des Animauxe Sans Vertebras* and *Recharches Surl Organisation des Crops Vivans*
(b) *Animauxe Sans des Systeme Vertebras* and *Surl des Recharches Crops Vivans Organization*
(c) *Philosophie Zoologique* and *Principles* of *Populations*
(d) *Proceedings* of the *Linnean Society* and *Origin* of *Species*

14 Consider the following statements.

I. Lamarck stressed on adaptation as a means of evolutionary modification.
II. Lamarck said, when an organ is used it will develop and if it is not used, it weakens to become vestigial.

Choose the correct option.

(a) Statement I is true, but II is false
(b) Statement II is true, but I is false
(c) Both statements I and II are true
(d) Both statements I and II are false

15 Which of the following examples supports the Lamarckism?

(a) Well-developed biceps muscles of blacksmith as an effect of much efforts
(b) Well-developed muscles in pinna of rabbits for receiving sound waves from different directions
(c) Flightlessness of kiwi
(d) All of the above

16 According to August Weismann, change in ...*A*... are inherited whereas change in ...*B*... are not transmitted.

	A	B
(a)	somatoplasm,	germplasm
(b)	tissue,	somatoplasm
(c)	germplasm,	somatoplasm
(d)	somatoplasm,	tissue

17 Which of the following statement is correct?

(a) Theory of germplasm was proposed in 1892
(b) Germplasm theory against Lamarck's principle, was given by Weismann
(c) Weismann cut the till of mice for 22 generation
(d) All of the above

18 In a famous experiment, A Weismann cut off the tails of newborn mice generation after generation. At the end of experiment, tails of mice neither disappeared nor shortened. This experiment

(a) supported Darwin's theory of natural selection
(b) proved that the tail is an essential organ of vertebrates
(c) disproved de Vries mutation theory
(d) showed that Lamarck was wrong in his theory of inheritance of acquired characters

19 On an average, each female of species X leaves 10 female offsprings in her lifetime. If all offsprings survive to reproduce, then how many female descendants will a single female leave after 10 generations?

(a) 100
(b) 100000
(c) 10000000
(d) 10000000000

20 Which of the following evidence proved that Lamarck's theory of evolution is not reliable?

(a) Indian women have been getting their ears pierced for thousands of years, but not a single baby with pierced ears is born
(b) Giraffes have long necks because they have to eat leaves from the tall trees on their habitat
(c) Deers have the capacity to escape from agile enemies because these can run very fast
(d) None of the above

21 Today, again the faith in Lamarck's theory has been revived by some people due to the fact that

(a) if the environment influences the genes of the organisms, the acquired change will be transmitted to the next generation
(b) genetic studies refuted the Darwinism
(c) mutation theory supports the Lamarckism
(d) germplasm theory supports the Lamarckism

Darwinism and Neo-Darwinism

22 On the voyage of the Beagle, Charles Darwin (1809-1882) found that the plants and animals of temperate South America are most similar to plants and animals of

(a) Tropical South America
(b) Australia
(c) Asia
(d) Europe

23 TR Malthus is famous for his book on

(a) geography (b) mathematics
(c) population (d) genetics

24 Which one of the following sequences was proposed by Darwin and Wallace for organic evolution?

(a) Overproduction, variations, constancy of population size, natural selection
(b) Variations, constancy of population size, over production, natural selection
(c) Overproduction, constancy of population size, variations, natural selection
(d) Variations, natural selection, overproduction, constancy of population size

25 When was Darwin's '*Origin of Species*' published?

(a) July, 1858 (b) July, 1859
(c) November, 1859 (d) December, 1859

26 Darwin proposed the theory of origin of species by

(a) hybridisation
(b) natural selection
(c) mutation
(d) acquired characters

27 Consider the following statements.

I. In postulating the theory of evolution by natural selection, Darwin was greatly influenced by Lamarck's theory of acquired characters.
II. According to Charles Darwin, evolution is descent with modification.

Choose the correct option.

(a) Statement I is true, but II is false
(b) Statement I is false, but II is true
(c) Both statements I and II are true
(d) Both statements I and II are false

28 Darwin proposed that the new species evolve from ancestral forms by
(a) the gradual accumulation of adaptations to changing environment
(b) the inheritance of acquired adaptation to the environment
(c) the struggle for limited resources
(d) the accumulation of mutations

29 Natural selection is based on
(a) natural resources are limited
(b) members of a population vary in characteristics
(c) populations are stable in size except seasonal fluctuation
(d) All of the above

30 The idea of natural selection as the fundamental process for evolutionary change was reached
(a) independently by Charles Darwin and Alfred Russel Wallace in 1900
(b) by Charles Darwin in 1866
(c) by Alfred Russel Wallace in 1901
(d) independently by Charles Darwin and Alfred Russel Wallace in 1859

31 Alfred Wallace (1823-1913) was a naturalist from Dutch East Indies, who was working on Malaya Archipelago. Today, Malaya Archipelago is situated in
(a) India (b) China
(c) Indonesia (d) Sri Lanka

32 Both C Darwin and AR Wallace developed independently the theory of evolution by natural selection. Yet, Darwin was given credit for the theory because he
(a) published it first
(b) had travelled outside Europe for his evidence
(c) was older and more respected
(d) presented more evidence

33 Which of the following described the process of natural selection?
(a) Change from simple to more complex organisms
(b) Differential reproduction success between genotypes
(c) Increase in the size of the population
(d) Occurrence of new mutations

34 Three forms of the peppered moth (*Biston betularia*), namely the melanic form, the pale form and a form intermediate between these two, are found in Britain today. The melanic form was first observed in 1848 and its frequency subsequently increased, this is thought to be the result of
(a) adaptive radiation (b) convergent evolution
(c) divergent evolution (d) natural selection

35 The Darwinian fitness of an organism is a measure of
(a) its ability, relative to others in the population, to pass its genes to the next generation
(b) the number of offsprings it produces
(c) its lifespan
(d) its physical vigour

36 Which one of the following phenomena supports Darwin's concept of natural selection in organic evolution?
(a) Development of transgenic animals
(b) Production of 'Dolly' the sheep by cloning
(c) Prevalence of pesticide resistant insects
(d) Development of organs from 'stem cells' for organ transplantation

37 In which type of evolution similar sequences of morphological modifications appear successively from the basic stock?
(a) Divergent evolution (b) Coevolution
(c) Iterative evolution (d) Parallel evolution

38 Evolutionary changes do not come about at the level of individual, but at the level of
(a) two persons (b) ten persons
(c) population (d) small group

39 Darwin believed that the giraffe has the long neck because
(a) the creator designed it that way
(b) the catastrophes eliminated short-necked forms
(c) its ancestors stretched their necks to get food
(d) ancestral giraffes with slightly longer necks than others got more food and left more surviving adapted offsprings

40 According to Wallace's chart, the main points of Darwin's theory of natural selection were
I. high rate of reproduction and variation
II. survival of the fittest and struggle for existence
III. total number almost constant and natural selection
Choose the correct option.
(a) I and II (b) Only III (c) I, II and III (d) II and III

41 According to Darwin, two different areas within a continent have different species because they have different
(a) evolutionary mechanisms (b) ancestors
(c) environments (d) evolutionary times

42 Darwin found that South American fossils are most similar to the
(a) Australian fossils
(b) Asian fossils
(c) living species of South America
(d) living species of North America

43 The name Galapagos islands has been given on the basis of occurrence of
(a) black cooled lava (b) giant tortoises
(c) giant iguanas (d) All of these

44 Ancestor finches that colonised the Galapagos islands were from
(a) Australia (b) South-East America
(c) North America (d) South America

45 An adaptive radiation, which involves major changes as in organisation plane resulting in the formation of new families, orders, classes and phyla is
(a) microevolution
(b) macroevolution
(c) megaevolution
(d) intraspecific evolution

46 Which types of birds were absent on Galapagos Islands when they were surveyed by Darwin?
(a) Warblers and wood peckers
(b) Carnivores
(c) Cactus feeding
(d) Seed eating

47 Which one cannot be explained by Darwinism?
I. Over specialisation
II. Persistence of vestigial organs
III. Occurrence of unchanged forms
Choose the correct option.
(a) I and III (b) Only II
(c) Only I (d) I, II and III

48 Which of the following are the objections to Darwin's theory of natural selection?
(a) The type of variations that provide the raw material for the natural selection are generally non-inheritable
(b) It fails to explain the role of discontinuous variation
(c) It fails to explain the possible reasons behind speciation
(d) All of the above

49 Darwin in his 'Natural Selection Theory' did not considered the role of which one of the following in organic evolution?
(a) Parasites and predators as natural enemies
(b) Survival of the fittest
(c) Struggle for existence
(d) Discontinuous variations

50 Which one of the following was not explained by the Darwinism?
(a) Natural selection
(b) Struggle for existence
(c) Arrival of the fittest
(d) Origin of species

51 Darwinism explains all the following except
(a) within each species, there are variations
(b) organisms tend to produce more number of offspring that can survive
(c) offspring with better traits that overcome competition are best suited for the environment
(d) variations are inherited from parents to offspring through genes

52 Choose the incorrect match.
(a) *Geospiza* fortis - Ground finch
(b) *Certhidea olivacea* - Warbler - Finch
(c) Uses twig to prise out insects - Woodpecker finch
(d) Takes insects in the air and - Ground finch on the ground

53 Theory of pangenesis given by Darwin is connected with
(a) continuity of germplasm (b) origin of variations
(c) inheritance of characters (d) struggle for existence

54 Darwin's theory of pangenesis shows similarity with the theory of inheritance of acquired characters then what shall be correct according to it?
(a) Useful organs become strong and developed while useless organs become extinct
(b) Size of organs increases with aging
(c) Development of organs is due to will power
(d) There should be some physical basis of inheritance

55 Weismann's theory of germplasm rejected
(a) mutation theory
(b) Darwin's theory of natural selection
(c) Darwin's theory pangenesis
(d) Neo-darwinism

56 Neo-Darwinism believes that new species develops through
(a) mutation with natural selections
(b) continuous variations with natural selection
(c) hybridisation
(d) mutations

57 According to Neo-Darwinism, natural selection operates through
(a) fighting between organisms
(b) killing the weaker organism
(c) differential reproduction
(d) variations

58 Darwin's theory of natural selection is objected because it
(a) stresses upon slow and small variations
(b) explains the adaptations of certain inherited characters
(c) stresses on interspecific competition
(d) explains that natural calamities take a heavy annual toll of lives

Mutation Theory of Hugo de Vries and Modern Synthetic Theory of Evolution

59 Mutation theory was published in which of the following book?
(a) *Origin of Species*
(b) *Theory of Mutation*
(c) *Die Mutation Theory*
(d) *Genetics and Origin of Species*

60 Consider the following statements about mutation.
I. Mutation causes speciation.
II. Mutation is more common when it is in dominant condition.
Choose the correct option.
(a) Statement I is true, but II is false
(b) Statement I is false, but II is true
(c) Both statements I and II are true
(d) Both statements I and II are false

61 According to de Vries, mutations are
(a) random and directionless
(b) raw material for evolution
(c) heritable and recurring
(d) All of the above

62 Which of the following is not true about mutation theory of Hugo de Vries?
(a) It emphasised on the adaptive nature of variation
(b) It focused on abrupt and drastic changes as a cause of speciation
(c) Speciation is the result of saltation
(d) None of the above

63 The modern synthetic theory of evolution is based on
(a) genetic and chromosomal mutation
(b) genetic recombination and natural selection
(c) reproductive isolation
(d) All of the above

64 Forthcoming generations are less adaptive than the parental generation due to
(a) natural selection (b) mutation
(c) genetic drift (d) adaptation

65 The species of *Oenothera* absent from the reterogressive group of Hugo de Vries was
(a) *O. nuttallii* (b) *O. laevifolia*
(c) *O. gigas* (d) *O. brevistylis*

66 Which of the following variations are temporary and have nothing to do with the last or next generation?
(a) Hereditary variations
(b) Discontinuous variations
(c) Environmental variations
(d) None of the above

67 The most accepted and recent theory of organic evolution is
(a) Lamarck's theory of acquired characters
(b) Darwin's theory of natural selection
(c) Theory of isolation
(d) Modern synthetic theory

68 Modern synthetic theory of evolution is not involved in
(a) gene mutation (b) gene recombination
(c) natural selection (d) increase in size

(B) Cumulative Exercise

(Assorted Questions of the Chapter for Advanced Level Practice)

1 The correct statements about the survival of the fittest are
I. the term survival of the fittest was coined by Herbert Spencer.
II. natural selection tends to favour fittest organisms.
III. fittest means more healthy, but sterile.
IV. survival means less healthy, but sterile.
Codes
(a) I and II (b) Only IV
(c) III and IV (d) I, II, III and IV

2 Which of the following is correct about Neo-Darwinism?
I. Neo-Darwinism distinguished between germplasm and somatoplasm.
II. Neo-Darwinism explains that adaptations result from multiple forces and natural selection is one of them.
III. Variations accumulate in individuals.
IV. Accepted the inheritance of acquired characters.
Codes
(a) I and II
(b) III and IV
(c) I and III
(d) II and IV

3. Which of the following is correct about Darwin?
I. Darwin started travelling in 1831 by HMS Beagle.
II. Darwin found a living laboratory of evolution in Galapagos island.
III. Darwin wrote the book '*Origin of Species*'.
IV. Darwin's work was published with TR Malthus.
Codes
(a) I and II (b) III and IV
(c) II and IV (d) I, II and III

4 Match the following columns.

Column I	Column II
A. August Weismann	1. Developed concept of species
B. John Ray	2. Theory of continuity of germplasm
C. George Cuvier	3. Life originated from water
D. William Smith	4. Father of palaeontology
E. Thales	5. Opposed theory of catastrophism

Codes **[NCERT Exemplar]**

	A	B	C	D	E
(a)	2	1	4	5	3
(b)	1	5	3	2	4
(c)	4	1	3	2	5
(d)	5	2	4	1	3

5 Which of the following statements is correct?

I. Accumulation of useful mutations through ages has led to the creation of new species of living beings.
II. Genetic variability provides raw material for the operation of natural selection and reproductive isolation.
III. Genetic variability is produced by gene mutations.
IV. Darwin called discontinuous variations as sports.

(a) I and II (b) II and III
(c) I, III and IV (d) I, II, III and IV

6 Given, 1= natural selection, 2 = variations and their inheritance, 3 = survival of the fittest, 4 = struggle for existence. According to Darwinism, which of the following represents the correct sequence of events in the origin of a new species?

(a) 1, 2, 3, 4 (b) 2, 3, 1, 4
(c) 3, 4, 1, 2 (d) 4, 2, 3, 1

7 Match the following columns.

Column I	Column II
A. Survival of fittest	1. Termed as 'sports' by Darwin
B. Natural selection	2. Changes in a population's allele frequencies due to chance alone
C. Mutation	3. A term coined by Herbert Spencer
D. Discontinuous variation	4. Outcome of differences in survival, reproduction, among the individuals that vary in forms shared traits.

Codes

	A	B	C	D
(a)	2	1	4	3
(b)	3	4	2	1
(c)	1	2	3	4
(d)	4	3	2	1

8 Select the correct statement from the given options.

(a) Darwinism variations are small and directionless
(b) Fitness is the end result of the ability to adapt and gets selected by nature
(c) Hugo de Vries's mutation theory was published in 2001
(d) Mutations are random and directional

9 Which of the following statements are against lamarckism?

I. Blind parents do not produce blind offsprings.
II. Wounds of parents do not appear in children.
III. Deaf parents do not produce deaf baby.
IV. Flightless birds like ostrich develops from flying ancestors.

Codes

(a) I and IV (b) Only III
(c) III and IV (d) I, II and III

10 In what sequence, should these evolutionary events be placed to support Darwin's theory of evolution by natural selection?

I. Inherited variations, which are favoured in a particular environment are passed on.
II. There is a struggle for existence.
III. In time, favoured inherited variations may accumulate causing gradual changes in the species.
IV. Populations tend to overproduce, but they remain more or less constant in numbers from generation to generation.

Codes

(a) I, II, III, IV
(b) III, I, II, IV
(c) II, I, III, IV
(d) IV, II, I, III

11 Match the following columns. **[NCERT Exemplar]**

Column I	Column II
A. Darwin	1. Abiogenesis
B. Oparin	2. Use and disuse of organs
C. Lamarck	3. Continental drift theory
D. Wagner	4. Evolution by natural selection

Codes

	A	B	C	D
(a)	1	4	2	3
(b)	4	1	2	3
(c)	2	4	3	1
(d)	4	3	2	1

12 Galapagos islands are a group of volcanic Islands in the Eastern Pacific ocean, about 1000 km from South America. Thirteen species of finches are found on the Islands; they resemble each other closely but differ in their feeding habits and in the shape of their beaks. Assuming that an ancestral stock of finches came from the mainland, what is the most likely explanation for the existence of similar but distinct species of Galapagos finches?

(a) Finches developed different kinds of beaks in order to feed on different kinds of food
(b) Finches evolved separately according to the habitat in which they settled
(c) Finches from the mainland bred with a resident population of a related species and produced new genotypes
(d) Finches underwent convergent evolution to produce very similar species

13 In which situation would evolution be slowest for an interbreeding population?

	Migrations	Selection pressures	Variations due to mutation
(a)	Absent	High	High
(b)	Absent	Low	Low
(c)	High	High	Low
(d)	High	Low	High

14 Which of the following are examples of evolution?

(a) Different finch species found on different Galapagos Islands
(b) The rise of antibiotic resistant strains of bacteria
(c) Changes in guppy populations after the introduction of predators
(d) All of the above

15 Which of the following statements is correct about neo-lamarckism?

I. Some of the variations acquired by individuals can be transmitted to its offspring.
II. Characters of organism are the result of interaction of genes and the environmental conditions.
III. Theory emphasises on internal vital force.
IV. Theory gives importance to the use and disuse of organs.

Codes

(a) I and II (b) III and IV
(c) I, II and III (d) III and IV

16 Match the following columns.

Column I	Column II
A. Darwin	1. Evening primrose
B. Alfred Wallace	2. HMS Beagle
C. Hugo de Vries	3. Giraffe
D. Lamarck	4. Archipelago

Codes

	A	B	C	D		A	B	C	D
(a)	2	4	1	3	(b)	2	1	4	3
(c)	4	1	2	3	(d)	3	2	1	4

Assertion and Reason

Direction (Q. Nos. 17-23) *In each of the following questions, a statement of Assertion (A) is given followed by the corresponding statement of Reason (R). Of the statements, mark the correct answer as*

(a) Both A and R are true and R is the correct explanation of A
(b) Both A and R are true, but R is not the correct explanation of A
(c) A is true, but R is false
(d) A is false, but R is true
(e) Both A and R are false

17 **Assertion** (A) The theory of survival of the fittest is widely misunderstood.

Reason (R) Evolution does not always increase the chances of a species survival and species do not survive when such chances happen rapidly.

18 **Assertion** (A) Human ancestors never use their tails and so the tail expressing gene has disappeared in them.

Reason (R) Lamarck's theory of evolution is popularly called theory of continuity of germplasm.

19 **Assertion** (A) Gene flow increases genetic variations.

Reason (R) The random introduction of new alleles into recipient population and their removal from the donor population affects allele frequency.

20 **Assertion** (A) Genes are never added or removed from the gene pool.

Reason (R) Generation of a new species depends solely on the environment of the individual.

21 **Assertion** (A) Mutation theory was proposed by Hugo de Vries.

Reason (R) Mutations are heritable and subjected to natural selection.

22 **Assertion** (A) Darwin regarded discontinuous variations more important than continuous variations.

Reason (R) The survival of the fittest is a result of selection and proliferation of fittest organisms.

23 **Assertion** (A) Intraspecific competition is more common than interspecific competition.

Reason (R) Similar species have similar food and space requirements, thus competition between them is more severe.

(C) Medical Entrances' Gallery

(Collection of questions Asked in NEET & Various Medical Entrance Exams)

1 Variations caused by mutation, as proposed by Hugo de Vries are **[NEET 2019, AFMC 2013]**
(a) random and directionless
(b) small and directional
(c) small and directionless
(d) random and directional

2 The best description of natural selection is **[AIIMS 2017]**
(a) the survival of the fittest
(b) the struggle for existence
(c) the reproductive success of the members of a population best adapted to the environment
(d) a change in the proportion of variations within a population

3 **Assertion** (A) Darwin held that small favourable variations formed raw material for evolutions.

Reason (R) He did not study the factors which produce variations. **[AIIMS 2017]**
(a) Both A and R are true and R is the correct explanation of A
(b) Both A and R are true, but R is not the correct explanation of A
(c) A is true, but R is false
(d) Both A and R are false

4 Human population grow exponentially while food production grows at an arithmetic rate, leading to over population and social problem. This is **[Chhattisgarh PMT 2015]**
(a) Kenze theory population
(b) Malthus theory of human population
(c) Kenze theory modified by Malthus
(d) Malthus theory modified by Darwin

5 Match the following columns. **[Kerala CEE 2014]**

	Column I		Column II
A.	Thomas Malthus	1.	Branching descent
B.	Hugo de Vries	2.	Studies on populations
C.	Charles Darwin	3.	Use and disuse theory
D.	Lamarck	4.	Saltation

Codes

	A	B	C	D
(a)	4	1	3	2
(b)	2	4	1	3
(c)	2	4	3	1
(d)	3	2	1	4
(e)	2	1	3	4

6 The animal group, which does not exist in Galapagos island is **[AIIMS 2013]**
(a) Insects (b) Protozoa
(c) Crustacea (d) Amphibia

7 Lamarckism cannot explain **[UP CPMT 2013]**
(a) webbed toes in aquatic birds
(b) weak muscles in the son of a wrestler
(c) long narrow and limbless body of snakes
(d) heterophylly

8 According to Darwin, the organic evolution is due to **[NEET 2013]**
(a) interspecific competition
(b) competition within closely related species due to the presence of interfering species
(c) reduced feeding efficiency in one species
(d) intraspecific competition

9 According to Hugo do Vries theory, evolution is **[UP CPMT 2013]**
(a) discontinuous (b) jerky
(c) continuous and smooth (d) Both (a) and (b)

10 Who wrote the famous book *Origin of Species*? **[WB JEE 2013]**
(a) Lamarck (b) Darwin
(c) de Vries (d) Mendel

11 If Darwin's theory of pangenesis shows similarity with theory of inheritance of acquired characters then what shall be correct according to it? **[AIIMS 2013]**
(a) Useful organs become strong and developed while useless organs become extinct. These organs help in struggle for survival
(b) Size of organs increases with ageing
(c) Development of organs is due to will power
(d) There should be some physical basis of inheritance

12 Darwin's finches provide an excellent evidence in favour of organic evolution. These are related to which of the following evidences? **[JCECE 2012]**
(a) Embryology
(b) Palaeontology (fossils)
(c) Anatomy
(d) Biogeography (geographic distribution)

13 Darwin's finches represent **[Manipal 2012]**
(a) morphological variation
(b) geographical isolation
(c) climatic variation
(d) reproductive isolation

14 The concept of inheritance of acquired character in support of evolution was proposed by [J&K CET 2011]
(a) Darwin
(b) Cuvier
(c) Lamarck
(d) Hugo de Vries

15 What is meant by the term 'Darwin fitness'? [DUMET 2011]
(a) The ability to survive and reproduce
(b) High aggressiveness
(c) Healthy appearance
(d) Physical strength

16 'Every cell of the body contributes gemmules to the germ cells and so shares in the transmission of inherited characters', this theory is known as
(a) theory of inheritance of acquired characters [JCECE 2011]
(b) theory of germplasm
(c) Both (a) and (b)
(d) theory of natural selection

17 Darwin judged the fitness of an individual by
(a) ability to defend itself [DUMET 2011]
(b) strategy to obtain food
(c) number of offsprings
(d) dominance over other individuals

ANSWERS

Check Point 12.1

1. (c)	2. (d)	3. (b)	4. (b)	5. (c)	6. (b)

Check Point 12.2

1. (d)	2. (b)	3. (c)	4. (b)	5. (a)	6. (d)

(A) Topical Exercise

1. (c)	2. (c)	3. (a)	4. (d)	5. (b)	6. (c)	7. (b)	8. (b)	9. (c)	10. (d)
11. (c)	12. (d)	13. (a)	14. (c)	15. (d)	16. (c)	17. (d)	18. (d)	19. (d)	20. (a)
21. (a)	22. (a)	23. (c)	24. (a)	25. (c)	26. (b)	27. (c)	28. (a)	29. (d)	30. (d)
31. (c)	32. (d)	33. (b)	34. (d)	35. (a)	36. (c)	37. (c)	38. (c)	39. (d)	40. (c)
41. (c)	42. (d)	43. (b)	44. (d)	45. (c)	46. (b)	47. (d)	48. (d)	49. (d)	50. (c)
51. (d)	52. (d)	53. (c)	54. (d)	55. (c)	56. (a)	57. (c)	58. (a)	59. (c)	60. (c)
61. (d)	62. (a)	63. (a)	64. (b)	65. (c)	66. (c)	67. (d)	68. (d)		

(B) Cumulative Exercise

1. (a)	2. (a)	3. (d)	4. (a)	5. (d)	6. (d)	7. (b)	8. (b)	9. (d)	10. (d)
11. (b)	12. (a)	13. (b)	14. (d)	15. (a)	16. (a)	17. (b)	18. (c)	19. (b)	20. (e)
21. (b)	22. (d)	23. (b)							

(C) Medical Entrances' Gallery

1. (a)	2. (c)	3. (b)	4. (b)	5. (b)	6. (d)	7. (b)	8. (d)	9. (d)	10. (b)
11. (d)	12. (d)	13. (b)	14. (c)	15. (a)	16. (b)	17. (c)			

Explanations

(A) Topical Exercise

3 (*a*) Option (a) is not correctly matched pair and can be corrected as
George Cuvier established palaeontological evidences.
Rest options are correctly matched pairs.

4 (*d*) William Smith opposes the theory of catastrophism gives by Cuvier on the basis of connectivity of similar species is related strata.
Hence, option (d) is correct.

52 (*d*) Option (d) is not correctly matched pair and can be corrected as
Ground finch feed on large seeds on the ground while warble finch eats insects in the air and on the ground.

62 (*a*) Statement in option (a) is not true and can be corrected as
Darwin's theory of evolution emphasised on the adaptive nature of variation.

(B) Cumulative Exercise

2 (*a*) Statements I and II are correct, while III and IV are incorrect. Incorrect statements can be corrected as
- Variations accumulate in gene pool.
- Some of the variations acquired by an individual can be transmitted to its offspring.

3 (*d*) Statements I, II and III are correct about Darwin except statement IV. Incorrect statement can be corrected as
Darwin's work was published with Wallace in 1858.

8 (*b*) Statement in option (b) is correct, while others are incorrect. Incorrect statements can be corrected as
- Darwinism variations are small and directional.
- Hugo de Vries's Mutation theory was published in 1901, in his book '*Die Mutation Theories*'.
- According to mutation theory, mutations are large and sudden changes.

13 (*b*) In an inbreeding population, evolutions will be slow if there is no mutation of species from one place to another, selection pressure is low and variation due to mutation is also low. Thus, option (b) is correct.

17 (*b*) Both A and R are true, but R is not the correct explanation of A.
The theory of 'survival of fittest' is widely misunderstood. The phrase conjures up a violent struggle for survival although in reality, the word fittest can mean anything from best camouflaged or the most fecund. Evolution is usually thought to be a very slow process, something that happens over many generations in response to the change in environment. But if the change occurs rapidly, some of the organisms die due to their lack of characteristics that could accommodate that change, the species would become smaller over time and eventually die out.

18 (*c*) A is true, but R is false because.
If human shares ancestry with other primates such as prosimian, monkeys, etc., then remnants of that common ancestry should be present in our genes, e.g. tail in vertebrae. But human ancestors never used their tails, so the tail expressing gene has disappeared in them. The theory of continuity of germplasm was proposed by Weismann. Lamarck's theory of inheritance is commonly known as theory of inheritance of acquired characters.

19 (*b*) Both A and R are true, but R is not the correct explanation of A.
Gene flow is the movement of alleles from one population to another as a result of interbreeding between members of the two populations. The random introduction of new alleles into the recipient population and their removal from the donor population affect the allele frequency of both populations and leads to increase in genetic variations.

20 (*e*) Both A and R are false and can be corrected as
Genes may be added to gene pool by immigration from other gene pool and mutation. The genes may be removed from the gene pool by natural selection and chance elimination of alleles, which take place in small population or during reduction of the population size.

21 (*b*) Both A and R are true, but R is not the correct explanation of A.
Hugo de Vries, a Dutch botanist proposed the mutation theory after experiments on evening primrose (*Oenothera lamarckiana*). Mutations are sudden, heritable changes, which are subjected to natural selection.

22 (*d*) A is false, but R is true because.
The survival of the fittest is a result of selection and proliferation of only those organisms, which were most suitably adapted to the environment and most successful in mating. Darwin regarded continuous variations to be more important because discontinuous variations being most harmful would not be selected again.

23 (*b*) Both A and R are true, but R is not the correct explanation of A.
Struggle for existence may be interspecific (between individuals of different species) and intraspecific (between individual of same species). There is more competition for food, light and space between the two closely related species of same niche or similar animals of same niche.

(C) Medical Entrances' Gallery

1 (*a*) Hugo de Vries proposed that the variations caused by mutation are random and directionless. These are the sudden, heritable changes in the genetic material and these variations constitute the raw material for evolution. He also proposed that mutations play a key role in speciation and used the term saltation for single step large mutations.

2 (*c*) Natural selection is evident in the reproductive success of the members of a population best adapted to the environment. The organisms which adapt the useful variations can successfully survive in changing environment and reproduce further to increase their numbers.

3 (*b*) Both A and R are true, but R is not the correct explanation of A. Darwin proposed that small favourable variations led to evolution. According to Darwin, variations which are helpful in adaptation will be passed to next generation, while other disappears. However, he did not study the factors which actually cause such variation, i.e. mutation, which forms raw material for evolution.

4 (*b*) Malthus theory of human population explains how unchecked human population grows exponentially whereas food and other resources grow arithmetically, which leads to population explosion.

6 (*d*) Amphibians are absent in Galapagos islands as they could not leave the mainland and travel to the Island by crossing saline water.

9 (*d*) Hugo de Vries pioneered the theory of mutation to explain the mechanism of evolution. According to him, evolution is discontinuous and jerky process.

Frequency of a mutated gene in a population is expected to increase if that gene is selected by nature.

Thus, option (d) is correct.

10 (*b*) Darwin's work was published with R Wallace's paper in the *'Proceedings of Linnean Society'* in 1859. Later on, Darwin published his work in a famous book called *Origin of Species.*

11 (*d*) According to both the views, 'something' is passed from parent to offspring, which causes development of specific characters, i.e. all that has been acquired by the organism during its lifetime to offspring in form of pangenes.

Hence, there should be a physical way by which these pangenes are transferred from parents to offspring.

13 (*b*) Thus, option (d) is correct. Darwin's finches represent geographical isolation, because starting from a point in a geographical area, giving rise to new species depending upon habitat. Main Darwin's finches were in South America, some flew to Galapagos islands and same variations got selected and gave rise to new species.

14 (*c*) The concept of inheritance of acquired character in support of evolution was proposed by Lamarck. According to him, new traits are acquired by organism during their lifetime and are passed on to the next generation.

15 (*a*) Darwin proposed the theory of natural selection. According to him, the organisms with favourable variations would survive because they are fit to face their surroundings while unfits are destroyed originally, it was an idea of Herbert Spencer who used the term survival of the fittest while Darwin named it as Natural Selection.

17 (*c*) Darwin began to realise that under the intense competition among the members of a population, any variation which favours survival in a particular environment would increase that individual's ability to reproduce and produce fertile offspring. Less favourable variations would be at a disadvantage and organisms possessing them would therefore, have less chances of successful reproduction. So, the number of offspring is the parameter to judge the fitness of an individual. Favourable variations lead to increase in number of offspring.

CHAPTER 13

Mechanism of Evolution

Evolution is the end result of a number of factors working together. It is said to be complete when a new species is formed *via* speciation. It occurs through accumulation of genetic variations in the gene pool of a population followed by its transference from generation to generation. Thus, its the population that evolves and not its individual members. The individual's role in an evolutionary process is to pass its genetic variations to its offsprings. In this chapter, we will learn about the formation of new species, with procedures involved in the mechanism of evolution and factors affecting this process.

SPECIES CONCEPT

Species is the basic unit of classification. The term 'species' was coined by **John Ray** in 1686. Most evolutionary taxonomists define **species** as groups of actually or potentially interbreeding natural populations, which are reproductively isolated from other such groups.

However, technically a species is defined on following three basis

(i) Morphological species concept

- This concept was proposed by **Davis** and **Heywood** in 1963.
- According to it, a species is the smallest group of organisms that can be consistently distinguished by the presence or absence of body parts, their numbers, shapes and sizes.
- This concept is not suitable for *Opuntia* and *Ranunculus* like plants because *Opuntia* includes 400-1000 species due to great morphological diversity and *Ranunculus* shows two types of leaves based on the habitat.

Inside

(ii) Biological species concept

- This concept was proposed by evolutionary biologist **Ernst Mayr** in 1942.
- According to it, a species is sexually interbreeding or potentially interbreeding group of individuals, which are reproductively isolated from other such groups. Thus, genetic exchange is absent between any two such species.
- A species, therefore is a group of organisms that can mate among themselves to produce fertile offsprings.
- Many botanists have abandoned the biological species concept because of the problems seen when this concept was applied on plants.

(iii) Evolutionary species concept

- This concept was given by **George Simpson** (1961).
- He defined a species as the group of individuals having common evolutionary lineage.
- Evolutionary concept of species uses a wide variety of evidences including morphological, molecular, reproductive, ecological, genetic and geographic characteristics to distinguish one species from another.
- However, evolution does not work simultaneously on all the traits. Neither its rate nor direction (in which it is occurring) are the same.

Some special types of species

(i) **Polytypic species** A species having two or more varieties or subspecies.
(ii) **Sibling species** When the individuals of two species are morphologically almost identical, but do not normally interbreed.
(iii) **Endemic species** The species which is restricted to a specific area.
(iv) **Monotypic species** A species without any distinct subdivision or variety.
(v) **Morphospecies** A species in which individuals are distinguished from the others only by their morphology.

SPECIATION

- It is the process of formation of one or more new species from an existing species.
- In terms of population, a species is a collection of demes. The **deme** is a group of populations with common gene pool. The gene pool is defined as total collection of all genes and its allele in a population.
- The factors which influence speciation include mutation, recombination, natural selection, hybridisation, genetic drift, polyploidy and isolation.

Types of speciation

These are of following types

(i) **Allopatric speciation** (*Allos*-other, *patria*-native land) When two related populations occupy geographically or spatially separated areas, they are called as **allopatric species.** Formation of these species is called allopatric speciation. It is defined as the formation of a new species through geographical isolation, e.g. Darwin's finches that formed separate species in the Galapagos islands.

(ii) **Sympatric speciation** (*Sym*-together, *patria*-native land) Formation of these species is called sympatric speciation. It is defined as formation of two species within a single population by reproductive isolation or without geographical isolation, e.g. polyploids. When two related population occupy same geographical areas, they are called as **sympatric species.**

(iii) **Peripatric speciation** It is a subform of allopatric speciation. In this, new species are formed from isolated smaller peripheral populations that are prevented from exchanging genes with the main population, e.g. Australian bird, *Petroica multicolor.*

(iv) **Parapatric speciation** In this, the neighbouring populations become distinct species while maintaining contact along a common border. Here, reproductive isolation evolves when a segment of population enters a new niche or habitat, e.g. caucasian rock lizards, *Darevskia rudis.*

(v) **Multiplicative speciation** (Cladogenesis) It is the formation of two or more species from a single species, e.g. allopatric and sympatric speciation. This can be gradual or abrupt.

(vi) **Phyletic speciation** (Anagenesis) It is autogenous transformation of a species with passage of time due to piling up of variations.

On the other hand, **stasigenesis** is the condition in which lineage neither split nor change, but persist as such without any change, e.g. *Limulus, Coelocanth,* etc.

(vii) **Fusion species** It is an allogenous transformation. In some species, isolation mechanism may breakdown due to a mutation. Afterwards, the two species interbreed and merge to form a single new species.

Mechanism of speciation

There are certain mechanisms that allow the formation of new species from existing species. These mechanisms involve

(i) Agents of genetic variations in a population.

(ii) The separator of genetic variation, i.e. isolation.

A description of all these mechanisms is given below

I. Agents of genetic variations in a population

- A population may be defined as individuals of the same species occurring in the same area at a particular time.
- Natural populations are generally random mating. It means that each male of a population has equal chance of mating with any female of the population and *vice-versa*.
- In random mating populations, there occur various agents which bring about genetic variations. These are as follows

1. Mutation

- It is a sudden and heritable change in an organism. It generally occurs due to the change in base sequences of nucleic acid in the genome of an organism.
- Mutations are considered to be the ultimate source of variations. These have the ability to produce a new allele which was not present earlier in the population.
- Mutation can also change the frequency of existing alleles.
- Virtually, any characteristic of an organism can be changed by mutation. However, some mutations are selectable while others are not selectable.
- A selectable mutation provides a clear advantage to the individual having them under certain environmental conditions. So, the progeny of the mutant cell is able to outgrow and replace the parent cells.

Replica plate experiment to demonstrate significance of mutation

- The preadaptive significance of mutation was demonstrated by **Joshua Lederberg** and **Esther Lederberg** (1952) by replica plate experiment.
- In the experiment, the genetic basis of drug resistant mutation in the bacteria *Escherichia coli* was tested.

Procedure

- From a culture of *Escherichia coli* derived from a single cell, they spreaded cells onto a 'master agar plate'. Each cell had the ability to gave rise a distinct colony.
- Then, they placed a velvet cloth onto a wooden block and pressed it gently on master plate. As a result of this, replica plate of master agar plate was made.
- They later touched this replica plate to a new plate containing a medium of antibiotic penicillin.

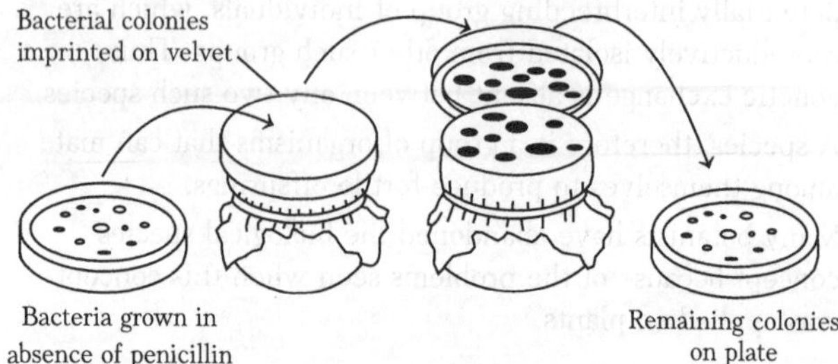

Fig. 13.1 Isolation and test of colonies

Result and conclusion

- As a result, most colonies found on the master plate died due to penicillin.
- However, a few colonies appeared on the replica plates. They were penicillin resistant.
- Later, all the colonies on the master plate were tested for penicillin resistance. Among these, only those colonies that had been the source of penicillin resistant cells of the replica plate displayed resistance.
- Thus, the experiment revealed that the drug resistant mutation in bacterial cells are not induced by the drug, but had been present prior to the exposure of bacteria to drug.
- The given experiment indicates that some bacterial cells had acquired drug resistant mutation even before they were exposed to penicillin.
- These mutations are actually preadaptive and advantageous. These occurred only after the exposure to new environment to which the organisms are to adapt themselves as shown below

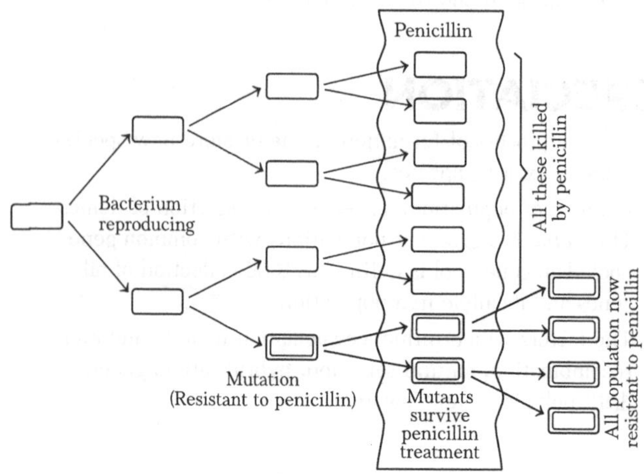

Fig. 13.2 Selection of penicillin resistant bacteria by natural selection

- Therefore, we can say that natural selection has selected and supported the progeny carrying the beneficial mutation.

Fast mutation in mosquitoes

- Mosquitoes bite infect millions causing lethal diseases, such as malaria, dengue and West Nile encephalitis.
- For centuries, humans are using insect repellents to counter these buzzing menace.
- DEET (N, N-diethyl-meta toluamide) is the world's most popular and efficacious repellent.
- Normally, it is seen that present day mosquitoes show early resistance to this compound.
- Mutation of **Orco** gene (heteromeric odour-gated ion channel) is one of such examples which is responsible for this kind of resistance.
- Now scientists are working to develop a new repellent which directly act on the other olfactory proteins of mosquitoes.

2. Recombination

- The non-parental arrangement of alleles in a progeny is called as recombination. It can result from independent assortment and crossing over.
- Recombination can occur not only between genes, but also within genes, resulting in the formation of new alleles in a population.

3. Gene flow (Gene migration)

- It is the physical movement of alleles into and out of a population. It can be a powerful agent of variation because in it, the members of two different populations may exchange their genetic materials. Sometimes, gene flow is obvious when an animal moves from one place to another.
- If the characteristics of newly arrived individual differ from those of the pre-existing ones and if the newcomer survive and successfully mate in new area, then the genetic composition of the receiving population may be altered.

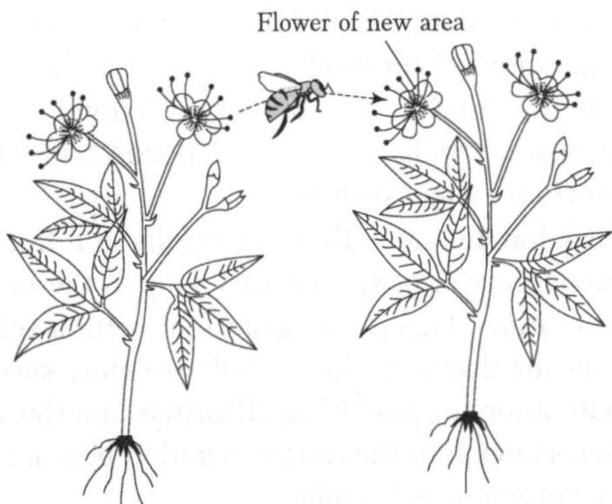

Fig. 13.3 Gene flow during cross-pollination

4. Non-random mating (Inbreeding)

- Individuals with certain genotypes sometimes mate with each other more commonly than would be expected on a random basis. This phenomenon is known as non-random mating.
- For example, **inbreeding** (mating with relatives) is a type of non-random mating that causes the frequencies of particular genotypes to differ greatly from those predicted by the Hardy-Weinberg equilibrium.
- It does not changes the frequency of the alleles, but rather increases the proportion of homozygous individuals.
- However, the relatives are likely to be genetically similar and thus, produce offsprings with two copies of the same allele.
- By increasing homozygosity in a population, inbreeding tends to increase the expression of recessive alleles. Due to this, marriages between close relatives are discouraged and to some degree outlawed.
- Inbreeding may also increase the possibility of producing children homozygous for an allele that might be associated with one or more recessive genetic disorders.

5. Random genetic drift

It was discovered by American geneticist **Sewall Wright**, hence also called **Sewall Wright effect**. It is described below

- In small population, frequencies of particular alleles may change drastically by chance alone.
- Such changes in allele frequencies occur randomly, as if the frequencies are drifting. This is known as **genetic drift.**
- It is usually rare in case of large populations. Thus, a population must be large enough to participate in the normal proceedings of evolution.
- Genetic drift fixes new alleles, genes that arise by mutation from time to time and eliminate the original gene, thereby changing the genetic makeup of small population as shown below

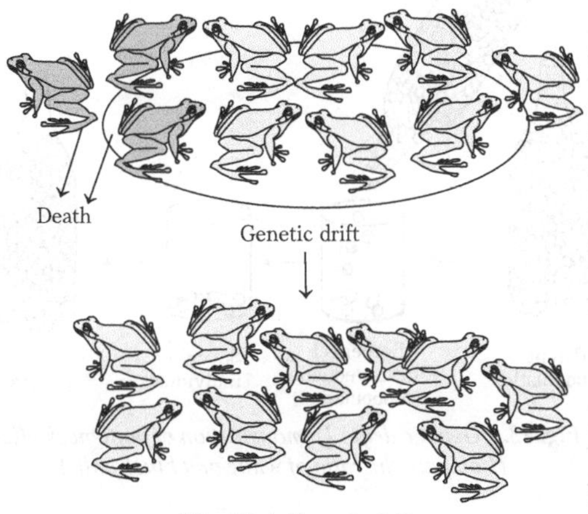

Fig. 13.4 Genetic drift

- As the result, the allele frequencies of the next generation's gene pool may be marked different from those of the previous generation.

Effects of genetic drifts

Genetic drifts have two principal effects on population of small size. In laboratory, a series of investigations were conducted by **WE Kera** and **S Wright** on several mutations in *Drosophila melanogaster.* Their results showed following effects

(i) Founder's effect

- This effect have been particularly important in the evolution of organisms on distant oceanic islands, such as the Hawaiian islands and the Galapagos islands visited by Darwin.
- Most of the organisms in such areas are probably derived from one or a few initial 'founders'.
- Factual details of this effect are given below
  - Sometimes, one or a few individuals disperse and become the founder of a new isolated population at some distance from their place of origin.
  - These pioneers are not likely to have all the alleles present in the source population.
  - In some cases, previously rare alleles in the source population, may form a significant fraction in the new population's gene pool.
  - This effect by which rare alleles and combinations of alleles may be enhanced in new populations is called the Founder's effect. It is a common phenomenon in nature.

(ii) Bottleneck effect

- Even if organisms do not move from place to place, yet occasionally, their populations may get drastically reduced in size.

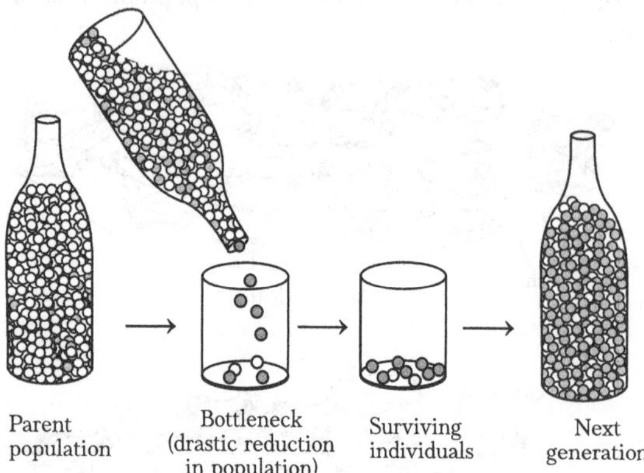

Fig. 13.5 Genetic drift : Demonstration of bottleneck effect (Compare the ratio of white and black balls)

- This may occur due to flooding, drought, epidemic disease and other natural forces or from progressive changes in the environment.
- The few surviving individuals may constitute a random genetic sample of the original population.
- The resultant alterations and loss of genetic variability has been termed as bottleneck effect.
- Some living species appear to be severely depleted genetically and have probably suffered from a bottleneck effect in the past. For example,
  - The Northern elephant seal, which breed on the Western coast of North America and nearby islands.
  - These were nearly hunted to extinction in the nineteenth century.
  - They got reduced to a single population containing about not more than 20 individuals on the island of Guadalupe off the coast of Baja, California.
  - As a result of bottleneck effect, even though the sealed populations have rebounded and now number remains in the tens of thousands. Now, this species has lost almost all of its genetic variations.

6. Natural selection

- Some genetic variability is always present in a population.
- Among these variabilities, some help in making the organism better adapted to the environment. This leads to their survival and continuous reproduction.
- The frequency of alleles associated with such variations, thus increases gradually in a population. This process is called **selection.**
- If the breeders select for the desired characteristic, it is **artificial selection** and if the environmental conditions operate in the natural population, it is said to be **natural selection.**

Conditions for natural selection

For natural selection to occur and result in evolutionary change, following three conditions must be met

(i) Variations must exist among individuals in a population. Natural selection works by favouring individuals with some traits over individuals with alternative traits. If no variation exists, natural selection cannot operate.

(ii) Variation among individuals results in differences in the number of offsprings surviving in the next generation. This is the essence of natural selection. It means that some individuals are more successful than others in producing offsprings and thus, pass their genes into the next generation because of their phenotype or behaviour.

(iii) Variations must be genetically inherited for natural selection to result in evolutionary change. It means that the selected variations must have a genetic basis. However, not all variations have a genetic basis, even genetically identical individuals may be phenotypically distinctive, if they grow in different environments.

Therefore, when phenotypically different individuals do not differ genetically, then no evolutionary change would occur.

Types of natural selection

Following three kinds of natural selection processes occur in nature

(i) Stabilising/Normalising selection

- This occurs when the environment does not change and favours the individuals possessing the mean character value.
- Thus, natural selection produce changes in favour of those individuals which possess intermediate forms of a trait, while eliminating extremes from the population. This is shown in figure given below

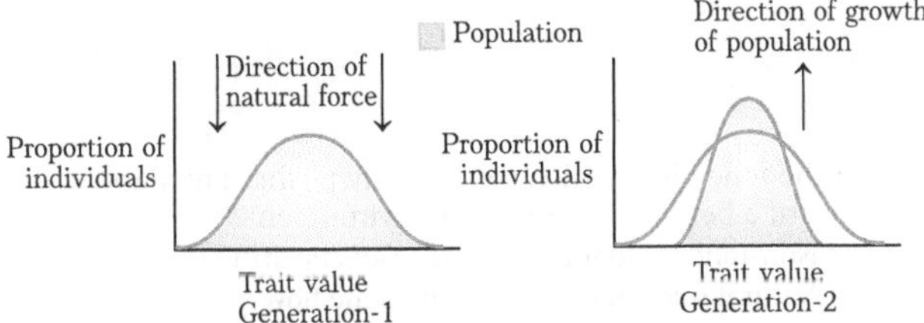

Fig. 13.6 Modes of stabilising selection

- The stabilising selection pressure does not promote evolutionary change, but tend to maintain phenotypic stability within the population from generation to generation.
- Fossil evidences suggest that many species remain unchanged for long periods of geological time.
- For example, *Coelacanth* (a fish species) was assumed to have been extinct for 70 million years until a living specimen was found in a trawler net of South Africa in 1938. So, with the passage of time no change was visible in this species.
- Another example of stabilising selection can be seen in the birth weight of humans. The heaviest and the lightest babies have the highest mortality and are less likely to survive. So, their alleles meet a dead end.

(ii) Directional selection

- This occurs whenever the environment show changes in a particular direction.
- Thus, natural selection produces change in favour of one extreme while eliminating the other extreme. This is shown in the figure given below

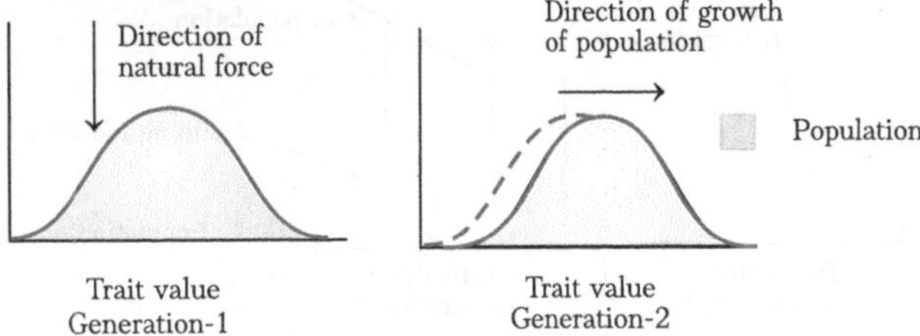

Fig. 13.7 Modes of directional selection

- Therefore, there is selective pressure for species to change in response to that environmental change, e.g. industrial melanism.

Industrial melanism

- The occurrence of this process is closely associated with the progress of the industrial revolution in Great Britain during the 19th century.
- It has occurred in several species of moths. Of these, peppered moth (*Biston betularia*) is the most intensely studied. These moth existed in two varieties, *viz*, light coloured (white) and dark coloured (black).
- Before the emergence of industrialisation, the white moth were numerous than dark moth in Britain.

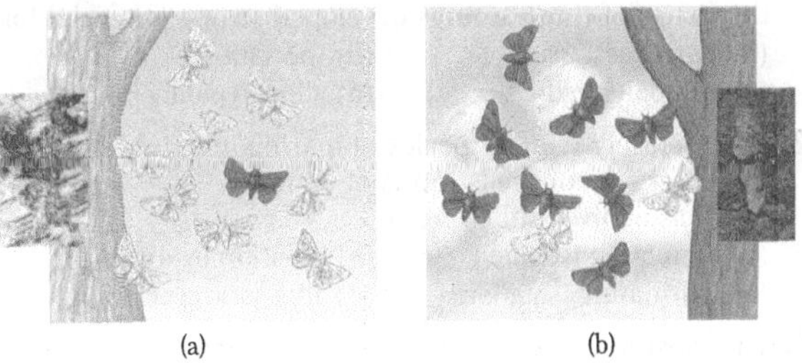

Fig. 13.8 (a) Original population; 10% dark-coloured phenotypes (b) Population after industrial revolution (Black moth in plenty)

- However, **after industrialisation**, i.e. in 1920, the condition was reversed. This was due to the fact that, white moth were easily spotted by predators (birds) on soot covered tree trunks, so there population decreased and the population of black moths increased.
- We can also say that black moths got naturally selected. But remember no variant was completely wiped out.

(iii) Disruptive/Diverging selection

- This occurs where an environmental change may produce selection pressure that favours two extreme characteristics.
- This results in the decline of average individuals of a population and increase in the population of extreme types as shown below

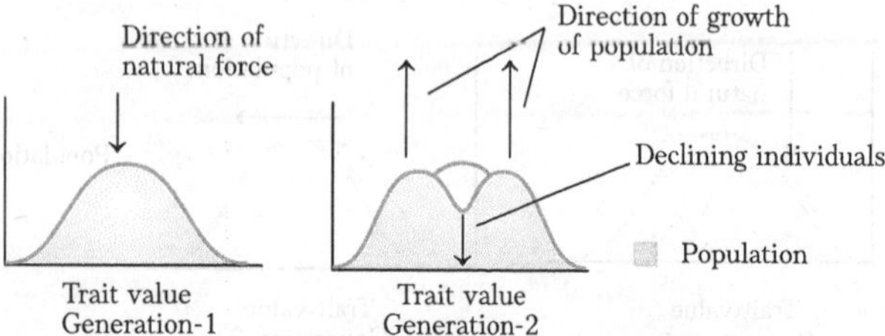

Fig. 13.9 Modes of disruptive selection

- Some of the examples of disruptive selection are given below
  (a) **Grass plants of Wales** (United Kingdom) copper mines grew in soil contaminated by copper, which was lethal to normal grass plants. However, a chance mutation allowed one plant to grow. This plant prospered and reproduced, but only on the contaminated soil. On normal soil, it grew more slowly than the normal plants and was easily out-competed. So, now there are two varieties of grass plants growing close together.
  (b) **Sickle-cell anaemia** People who are homozygous for this recessive allele, usually die before reproduction. People heterozygous for sickle-cell anaemia are more resistant to malaria than people homozygous for the normal allele because malarial parasite is not able to survive in sickle-shaped RBCs. Hence, where malaria is found, people with heterozygous alleles are at an advantage.

Raw materials for natural selection

The process of natural selection acts on phenotype, the physical, biochemical and behavioural traits of an organism. Thus, phenotypes are raw material for natural selection. It indirectly adapts a population to its environment by selecting and maintaining favourable genotypes in their gene pool.

Most variations that natural selection acts upon are **polygenic**, i.e. depend on quantitative characters, which are influenced by several gene loci. So, the selection acts on those organism which have integrated composition of many phenotypic features.

CHECK POINT 13.1

1. Since in the Pleistocene ice age, deserts have gradually formed in the South-Western United States. As the lakes and rivers of these areas shrunk into isolated springs. So, the fishes of these springs developed strong potential for
   (a) introgression (b) speciation
   (c) autopolyploidy (d) allopolyploidy
2. Many closely related species of marine invertebrates exist on either side of the isthmus of Panama.
   They probably resulted from
   (a) premating isolation (b) isolation by distance
   (c) postmating isolation (d) allopatric speciation
3. The most likely reason for the development of resistance against pesticides in insect is
   (a) Random mutations
   (b) Genetic recombination
   (c) Direct mutations
   (d) Acquired heritable changes
4. Of the following, which consistently pushes populations toward a better 'fit' with their environment?
   (a) Non-random mating (b) Genetic drift
   (c) Natural selection (d) Gene flow
5. If nature selects individuals acquiring value other than the mean character value, the type of natural selection is called
   (a) directional (b) disruptive
   (c) balancing (d) stabilising
6. The occurrence of large and small birds and the absence of medium-sized birds are an example of
   (a) stabilising selection
   (b) balancing selection
   (c) directional selection
   (d) disruptive selection

II. The separator of genetic variation: Reproductive isolation

- It is the prevention of mating amongst potential interbreeding groups as a result of physical barriers, (i.e. ecological, geographical, etc.) and biotic barriers like physiological, behavioural, mechanical, genetical, etc.
- It does not permit these populations to exchange genes.
- Thus, it isolates the gene pool of different species. It may also lead to the origin of new species (speciation).

Isolating mechanisms

According to **Mayr** (1942), these mechanisms are the biological properties of individuals, which prevent the interbreeding of naturally sympatric populations. These biological properties must be involved in the process of speciation. The list of isolation mechanisms described below are based on an original list by **Dobzhansky**.

1. Premating (Prezygotic) isolation mechanisms

These mechanisms usually prevent mating between species. Premating isolation is efficient because the resources and efforts in reproduction are not wasted to produce offsprings.

It is of following types

(i) **Geographical isolation** The separation of groups of related organisms by geographical barriers like mountains, valleys, glaciers, dense forests, water bodies, etc., is called geographical isolation.

(ii) **Ecological/Habitat/Niche isolation** In this there is difference in habitat or niche of organism which allow the species to be reproductively isolated. For example one living is freshwater while the other in sea.

(iii) **Behavioural/Sexual/Ethological isolation** Individuals choose members of their own species and reject other species as mates due to the differences in behavioural patterns, e.g. in courtship patterns, songs, etc.

(iv) **Temporal/Seasonal isolation** Different species mate at different times of the day or year.

(v) **Spatial isolation** Individuals present at the two ends of a wide range of population seldom interbreed, they develop different variations and ultimately become reproductively isolated.

This is due to different timings of maturity, body patterns, etc.

(vi) **Mechanical isolation** The difference in genitalia in animals or pollinia in plants prevent copulation or pollen transfer, respectively.

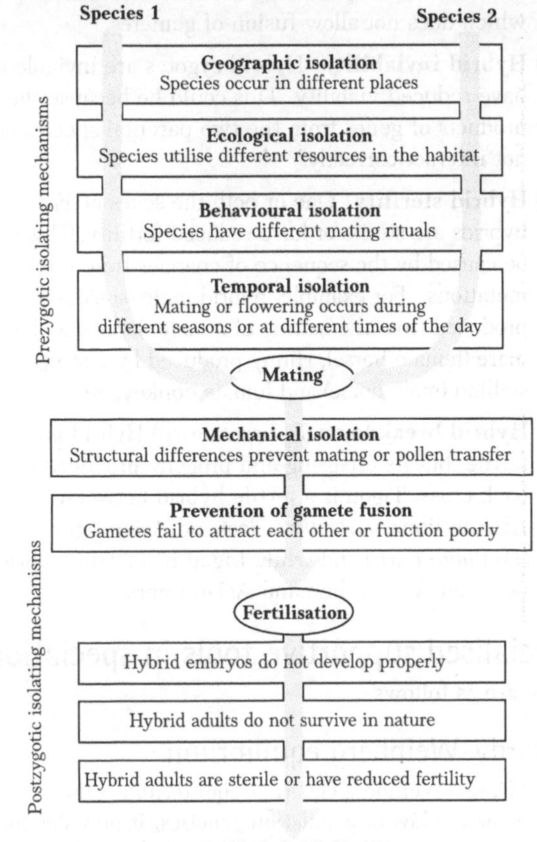

Fig. 13.10 *Reproductive isolation mechanisms: A variety of associated mechanisms can prevent successful reproduction between the individuals of different species.*

(vii) **Gametic isolation** In externally fertilised species, gametes show selective attraction and/or acceptance. Sperm may only swim towards eggs of their own species. In plants, styles may prevent entry of incompatible gametophytes. In internally fertilised species, the male gametes may not survive in the sex ducts of the other species.

2. Postmating (Postzygotic) isolation mechanisms

In these mechanisms, mating occurs but the offspring produced is sterile or infertile. Postmating mechanisms are very inefficient because reproductive effort is wasted in producing useless offsprings.

Different types of postmating isolation mechanisms are as follows

(i) **Gametic incompatibility** It is the mechanism which does not allow fusion of gametes.

(ii) **Hybrid inviability** Hybrid zygotes are inviable or have reduced viability. This could be because the products of genes from the two parental species do not interact correctly.

(iii) **Hybrid sterility** One or both the sexes of F_1 hybrids are sterile or have reduced fertility. This can be caused by the sequence of changes from random mutations. For example, hybrid mule (sterile) is produced from the mating of a male donkey and a mare (female horse), Hinny produced by mating stallion (male horse) and female donkey, etc.

(iv) **Hybrid breakdown** (F_2 breakdown) Hybrid is fertile, but its offspring and progeny produced from back cross. Tigon is a fertile hybrid between African lioness (*Panthera leo*) and Asian tiger (*Panthera tigris*) and while Ligon is a fertile hybrid between African lion and Asian tigers.

Specialised supportive tools in speciation

These are as follows

1. Hardy-Weinberg equilibrium

- The Hardy-Weinberg equation/equilibrium is the fundamental law of population genetics. It provides the basis for studying the Mendelian populations.
- This law was independently developed by **GH Hardy**, an English mathematician and **G Weinberg**, a German physician in 1908.
- 'The Hardy-Weinberg law states that the genes and genotypic frequencies in a Mendelian population remain constant generation after generation, if there is no selection, mutation, gene migration or gene flow and genetic drift.'
- Thus, the original population is said to be in genetic equilibrium, as long as the following assumptions are met.
  - The population size is very large.
  - Random mating is occurring.
  - No mutation takes place.
  - No genes are added from other sources, i.e. no immigration takes place.
  - No selection occur.

All these are depicted in the figure below

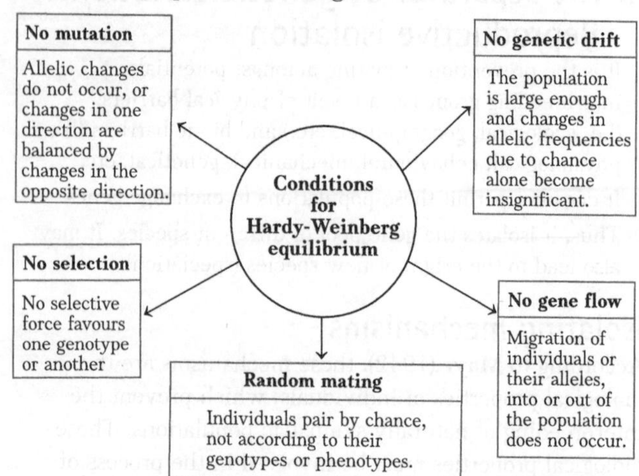

Fig. 13.11 Conditions for Hardy-Weinberg equilibrium

Use of Hardy-Weinberg equilibrium in evolution

- Genetic equilibrium means that the gene pool remains more or less constant.
- Hardy-Weinberg principle gives the geneticists a tool to determine whether the evolution is occurring or not.
- Population geneticists use Hardy-Weinberg principle to calculate allele frequency at a starting point and then compare it with the frequencies measured at some future time. This can be easily figured out from the mathematical explanation of Hardy-Weinberg law.

Mathematical explanation

Mathematically, it can be interpreted as a binomial expression $p^2 + 2pq + q^2$ or $(p+q)^2$ to calculate the genotypic and allele frequencies of a population

where, p = Frequency of dominant allele (A)

p^2 = % homozygous dominant (AA) individuals

q = Frequency of recessive allele (a)

q^2 = % homozygous recessive (aa) individuals

pq = Heterozygous or hybrid individual (Aa)

$2pq$ = % heterozygous individuals (2Aa)

Realise that $(p+q)^2 = 1$ (there are only 2 alleles)

$p^2 + 2pq + q^2 = 1$ (these are the only genotypes)

Hardy-Weinberg principle says that the sum total of all the allelic frequencies of a gene is 1. Any disturbance in Hardy-Weinberg equilibrium, i.e. change in frequency of alleles would be interpreted as the result of evolution.

Example An investigator has determined by the inspection that 16% of a human population has a recessive trait. Using this information, calculate all the genotypes and allele frequencies for the population, provided the conditions for Hardy-Weinberg equilibrium are met.

Solution

Given $q^2 = 16\% = 0.4 =$ frequency of recessive allele

$p = 1.0 - 0.4 = 0.6 =$ frequency of dominant allele

So, $p^2 = (0.6)(0.6) = 0.36 = 36\%$ individuals are homozygous dominant

Similarly,

$2pq = 2(0.6)(0.4) = 0.48 = 48\%$ individuals are heterozygous

This can be verified as

$$p^2 + 2pq + q^2 = 1$$

$$0.36 + 0.48 + 0.16 = 1$$ **Hence proved**

2. Polymorphism

It is defined as the existence of two or more forms or phenotypes of the same species within the same population. Polymorphism can apply to biochemical, morphological and behavioural characteristics. It also plays a significant role in the process of natural selection.

Polymorphism in population may develop due to the following reasons

- Changes in the environment.
- Superiority of heterozygotes.
- Mutation pressure, which may introduce a variety of alleles.
- Frequency dependent selection.

Types of polymorphism

It is of following two types

(i) Transient polymorphism

- This arises when different forms or morphs, exist in a population undergoing a strong selection pressure.
- The frequency of the phenotypic appearance of each form is determined by the intensity of the selection pressure, such as the melanic and non-melanic forms of the peppered moth.
- Transient polymorphism usually applies in following situations
  (a) When one form is gradually being replaced by another.
  (b) A newly arose mutation is found to be advantageous and is favoured by selection. It spreads through the population and becomes more and more abundant, while the wild type is becoming rare due to negative selection.
  (c) In a changed environment, a previously rare form may become advantageous and is favoured by selection. It spreads throughout the population.

(ii) Balanced (Stable) polymorphism

- This occurs when different forms coexist in the same population in a stable environment like the existence of the two sexes in animals and plants.
- The genotypic frequencies of the various polymorphic forms exhibit equilibrium since, each form has a selective advantage of equal intensity.
- Some examples of this type of polymorphism are
  (a) **ABO blood groups** In humans, the existence of the A, B, AB and O blood groups are the examples of balanced polymorphism.
    - However, their genotypic frequencies within different populations may vary, but they remain constant from generation to generation within that population. This is because none of them have selective advantage over the other.
    - Statistics reveal that the white men with blood group O have a greater life expectancy than those of other blood groups.
    - Interestingly, they also have an increased risk of developing duodenal ulcer, which may perforate and lead to death.

  (b) **Other examples** Red-green colour blindness in humans; existence of workers, drones and queen in social insect; pin-eyed and thrum-eyed forms in primroses; sickle-cell anaemia and Tay-Sachs disease, etc.

CHECK POINT 13.2

1. Population of Kaibab squirrels on the North rim of the Grand Canyon do not mate with the populations on South rim. They are isolated by a
   (a) sympatric barrier (b) autopatric barrier
   (c) geographic barrier (d) genetic barrier
2. If two species of a plant in the same pond do not interbreed because one blooms at night while the other blooms during day, this reproductive barrier between them is an example of
   (a) gametic isolation
   (b) mechanical isolation
   (c) temporal isolation
   (d) geographical isolation
3. Two organisms of different species mate and produce an offspring. This offspring cannot mate with its siblings, nor with the members of either parental species. This is an example of
   (a) hybrid sterility (b) gametic isolation
   (c) behavioural isolation (d) ecological isolation
4. Population is said to be non-evolving if all the following features exist, except
   (a) random mating
   (b) large population size
   (c) mutations are not taking place
   (d) new members migrate into this population form outside
5. Microevolution can be measured by comparing observed allelic frequencies with those predicted by
   (a) chance
   (b) the Hardy-Weinberg equilibrium
   (c) Mendelian ratios
   (d) All known environmental factors
6. The factor which is correct for transient polymorphism is
   (a) stable environment
   (b) selective advantage of equal intensity
   (c) strong selection pressure
   (d) equilibrium between forms

EXAM POINTS

- Stabilising selection eliminates individuals from both ends of a phenotypic distribution, hence maintains the same distribution average. **[NEET 2019]**
- Disruptive selection favours individuals at both extremes of the distribution. It eliminates the members with mean expression thus, producing two peaks in trait distribution. This leads to development of two different population. **[AIIMS 2017, JIPMER 2017]**
- The black coloured peppered moth (*Biston betularia*) became dominant over the light coloured moth in England during industrial revolution. This is an example of natural selection whereby the darker forms were selected. **[AIIMS 2018]**
- Industrial melanism is an example of natural selection. **[CBSE AIPMT 2015, WB JEE 2014]**
- Population are said to be allopatric when they are physically isolated by natural barriers. **[Karnataka CET 2013]**
- Related species which are reproductively isolated, but morphologically similar are called sibling. **[MHT CET 2011]**
- The tendency of population to remain in genetic equilibrium may be distributed by random mating. **[NEET 2013]**
- Biological concept of species is mainly based on reproductive isolations. **[Manipal 2012]**
- Geographic isolation is the first step in allopatric speciation. **[EAMCET 2014]**
- Gene mutation affects the genetic makeup in a population. **[J&K CET 2014]**
- Genetic drift operates in small isolated population. **[NEET 2016]**
- Variation in gene frequencies in population can occur by chance rather than by natural selection. This is referred to as genetic drift. **[JIPMER 2017]**
- Species are closely related interbreeding population. **[Manipal 2012]**
- A population will not exist in Hardy-Weinberg equilibrium if there are mutations. **[CBSE AIPMT 2015]**
- In Hardy-Weinberg equation, the frequency of heterozygous individual is represented by $2pq$. **[NEET 2016]**

Chapter Exercises

(A) Topical Exercise

Introduction and Species Concept

1 Study of frequency of different genes and trends of their change is
(a) gene pool
(b) population genetics
(c) gene flow
(d) Hardy-Weinberg genetic equilibrium

2 Which one is a raw material for evolutionary change?
(a) Reshuffling of gene combinations
(b) Variability of gene pool
(c) Unrestricted gene flow
(d) Balancing selection

3 A species as a group of individuals with common evolutionary lineage is a species concept proposed by
(a) George Simpson (b) Davis
(c) Heywood (d) Ernst Mayr

4 The possibilities of hereditary and evolutionary changes are greatest in species, which are reproduced by
(a) fission
(b) budding
(c) asexual means
(d) sexual means

5 Evolution of life shows that life forms had a trend of moving from
(a) land to water
(b) dryland to wetland
(c) freshwater to sea water
(d) water to land

6 Find the odd one out.
(a) John Ray – Morphological species concept
(b) Davis - Morphological species concept
(c) E. Mayr – Biological species concept
(d) George Simpson – Evolutionary species concept

Speciation

7 The kaibab squirrels and Darwin's finches are the example of ....
(a) sympatric speciation
(b) parasympatric speciation
(c) allopatric speciation
(d) fusion speciation

8 In the Galapagos finches, adaptive radiation occurred .... islands, while allopatric speciation occurred .... islands.
(a) within, on large (b) between, within
(c) on large, on small (d) within, between

9 Sympatric speciation develops reproductive isolation without
(a) barrier to mating (b) geographical barrier
(c) barrier to gene flow (d) genetic change

10 When populations of a plant species are located adjacent to one another because of abrupt changes in soil conditions, they are called
(a) allopolyploid (b) autopolyploid
(c) sympatric (d) parapatric

11 Consider the following statements.
I. Formation of true species from an ancestor is known as cladogenesis or divergent evolutions.
II. The formation of a new species through changes in a single lineage is known as anagenesis or phyletic evolution.

Choose the correct option.
(a) Statement I is true, but II is false
(b) Statement I is false, but II is true
(c) Both statements I and II are true
(d) Both statements I and II are false

12 Most often, the factor that initiates the speciation of two populations is
(a) geographic separation
(b) inability of gametes to fuse
(c) different courtship behaviours
(d) different copulatory organs

13 Single step large mutation leading to speciation is also called
(a) founder's effect (b) saltation
(c) branching descent (d) natural selection

14 Consider the following statements.
I. The genetic basis of adaptations was known by the experiment of Lederberg and Lederberg.
II. Their experiment is known as replica plating experiment.

Choose the correct option.
(a) Statement I is true, but II is false
(b) Statement I is false, but II is true
(c) Both statements I and II are true
(d) Both statements I and II are false

15 Appearance of antibiotic resistant bacteria is an example of
(a) adaptive radiation
(b) transduction
(c) pre-existing variation in the population
(d) divergent evolution

16 Which of the following increases the number of different alleles in a population?
(a) Crossing over
(b) Random fusion of gametes
(c) Gene mutation
(d) Reassortment of chromosomes in meiosis

17 Consider the following processes.
I. Gene flow
II. Non-random mating
III. Genetic drift
IV. Transduction

Which of these is an agent of evolutionary change?
(a) I and II (b) III and IV
(c) Only III (d) II and IV

18 Which of the following would cause phenotypic variation among the organisms of the same genotype?
(a) Continuous variation within the species
(b) Different varieties of the same species
(c) Different sexes
(d) Exposure to different environments

19 Random genetic drift in a population probably results from
(a) low genetically variable individuals
(b) interbreeding within a population
(c) small population size
(d) All of the above

20 Of the following possibilities, the best way to estimate an organism's evolutionary fitness, is to measure the
(a) size of its offspring
(b) number of eggs it produces
(c) number of eggs it produces over its lifetime
(d) number of offsprings it produces over its lifetime that survive to breed

21 In a random mating population in an equilibrium, which one of the following brings about a change in gene frequency in a non-directional manner?
(a) Mutation (b) Random drift
(c) Selection (d) Migration

22 Consider the following statements.
I. Genetic drift occurs when a few individuals colonise an island. It is called founder effect.
II. Founder effect results in large and rapid changes in gene frequencies.

Choose the correct option.
(a) Statement I is true, but II is false
(b) Statement I is false, but II is true
(c) Both statements I and II are true
(d) Both statements I and II are false

23 A change in the relative abundance of an allele (the allelic frequency) within a population, over a succession of generations is called
(a) microevolution or adaptive evolution
(b) macroevolution or speciation
(c) coevolution
(d) phylogenetic evolution

Natural Selection and its Types

24 Natural selection acts on an organism's
(a) dominant alleles
(b) recessive, homozygous alleles
(c) combined genotype
(d) phenotype

25 A potential danger to a population that has been greatly reduced in number is the
(a) loss of genetic variability
(b) tendency towards assortative mating
(c) reduced gene flow
(d) Hardy-Weinberg disequilibrium

26 Which type of natural selection favours intermediate form of traits?
(a) Disruptive
(b) Stabilising
(c) Directional
(d) Both (a) and (b)

27 All the members of a bird population have the same intermediate green colouration. What type of selection is likely to taking place?
(a) Disruptive (b) Directional
(c) Stabilising (d) Natural

28 After the demise of the dinosaurs, mammals evolved rapidly into many new forms because of
(a) the founder effect (b) a genetic bottleneck
(c) adaptive radiation (d) geological time

29 Directional selection usually acts to favour
(a) both extreme forms of a trait
(b) intermediate forms of a trait
(c) environmental differences
(d) one extreme form over the other extreme form and over intermediate forms of a trait

30 Which type of selection is industrial melanism observed in moth, *Biston betularia?*
(a) Stabilising (b) Disruptive
(c) Directional (d) Artificial

31 Consider the following statements.

I. Industrial melanism is an example of protective resemblance with the surrounding.

II. It is observed in peppered moth proves that the true black melanic forms arise by a recurring random mutation.

Choose the correct option.

(a) Statement I is true, but II is false
(b) Statement I is false, but II is true
(c) Both statements I and II are true
(d) Both statements I and II are false

32 Which of the following statements is supported by change in peppered moths?

(a) Natural selection acts on favourable variations, which appear among individuals
(b) Environment has a role in evolution
(c) Acquired characters during life of an individual are inherited
(d) Heritable variations arise due to the changes in the gene complex

33 People who carry an allele for normal haemoglobin and an allele for sickle-cell, are resistant to malaria. They are examples of the

(a) heterozygote advantage (b) extreme diploidy
(c) outbreeding (d) recessive superiority

Isolation Mechanism

34 Under the biological species concept, the main criterion for identifying a species is

(a) anatomical distinctiveness
(b) behavioural distinctiveness
(c) geographic isolation
(d) reproductive isolation

35 Which is related to premating reproductive isolation?

(a) Gametic isolation (b) Temporal isolation
(c) Behavioural isolation (d) All of these

36 When certain members of a population reproduce and pass on their genes to the next generation and the allele frequencies of the next generations gene pool are markedly different from those of the previous generation, then it is known as

(a) non-random mating (b) genetic drift
(c) selection (d) gene flow

37 Consider the following statements.

I. A postzygotic isolating mechanism prevents successful development, survival or reproduction of the hybrid.

II. It is efficient because the resource and effort are not wasted.

Choose the correct option.

(a) Statement I is true, but II is false
(b) Statement I is false, but II is true
(c) Both statements I and II are true
(d) Both statements I and II are false

38 Two species of garter snakes occur in the same geographic areas, but one lives mainly in water and the other mainly on land. Consequently, they do not encounter one another and so, do not interbreed. This is an example of prezygotic isolation caused by

(a) ecological isolation (b) temporal isolation
(c) behavioural isolation (d) mechanical isolation

39 When two related populations that have been geographically isolated come back into contact, retain their reproductive isolation and compete for the resources, there may be a divergence in traits known as

(a) character convergence (b) sibling speciation
(c) phyletic evolution (d) character displacement

40 The genus–*Rhagoletis* is a group of small, brightly coloured flies. Each species in the genus feeds, during its larval stage, on the fruit of just one plant family, and when the larvae hatch into adults, they court and mate on the same fruit. The species that feed on fruits from different plant families are reproductively isolated by

(a) ecological isolation (b) temporal isolation
(c) behavioural isolation (d) mechanical isolation

41 Eastern and Western meadowlarks look almost the same and inhabit the same areas of Prairie. They recognise mates of their own species by distinctive courtship songs. This is an example of prezygotic isolation by

(a) ecological isolation (b) behavioural isolation
(c) mechanical isolation (d) gametic isolation

42 Male fireflies attract mates by blinking their 'lights', each species does so, in a characteristic pattern recognised only by females of that species. This is an example of premating isolation by

(a) ecological isolation
(b) temporal isolation
(c) behavioural isolation
(d) mechanical isolation

43 Two individuals from different populations attempt to mate, but are unable to successfully coordinate the mating dance. This is an example of a/an .... isolating mechanism.

(a) ecological (b) temporal
(c) behavioural (d) mechanical

44 Different species of dragonflies do not mate with each other because the males of each species have appendages that can clasp and hold, for copulation, only females of their own species. This is an example of

(a) ecological isolation (b) temporal isolation
(c) behavioural isolation (d) mechanical isolation

45 When species mate at different times of the day or year. It is called

(a) temporal isolation (b) mechanical isolation
(c) spatial isolation (d) gametic isolation

46 Two species of pines, *Pinus radiata* and *Pinus muricata,* occur sympatrically in California and are capable of forming hybrids. They do not interbreed, because one releases pollen in February and the other in April. They are the example of prezygotic isolation by

(a) ecological isolation (b) temporal isolation
(c) gametic isolation (d) geographic isolation

47 Very similar species of fish release their eggs and sperms into the same water, but the sperms of one species cannot penetrate the eggs of another species. This is an example of prezygotic isolation by

(a) ecological isolation (b) behavioural isolation
(c) mechanical isolation (d) gametic isolation

48 Many hybrids are sterile because their chromosomes do not pair up correctly during meiosis. Why are not polyploid plants sterile?

(a) They backcross to the parental generation
(b) Most are triploid
(c) They cross-pollinate
(d) They self-fertilise, using their diploid gametes

49 Consider the following statements.

I. Mule is an example of hybrid sterility.
II. Mule is produced by the mating of male donkey and female horse.

Choose the correct option.

(a) Statement I is true, but II is false
(b) Statement I is false, but II is true
(c) Both statements I and II are true
(d) Both statements I and II are false

50 A horse has a karyotype of 64 chromosomes and a donkey has a karyotype of 62 chromosomes. The hybrid offspring of a horse-donkey cross is a mule, which has 63 chromosomes. A mule is sterile because it cannot successfully

(a) court other mules
(b) copulate with mules, donkeys or horses
(c) form gametes
(d) complete development of the zygote

51 Viviparity is considered to be more evolved because

(a) the young ones are left on their own
(b) the young ones are protected by a thick shell
(c) the young ones are protected inside the mother's body and looked after they are born leading to more chances of survival
(d) the embryo takes a long time to develop

Hardy-Weinberg Equilibrium and Polymorphism

52 $(p+q)^2 = p^2 + 2pq + q^2 = 1$, represents an equation used in

(a) population genetics (b) Mendelian genetics
(c) biometrics (d) molecular genetics

53 Hardy-Weinberg used the binomial expression $p^2 + 2pq + q^2$ to calculate the genotype and allele frequency of a population. In this equation, p is

(a) frequency of recessive allele
(b) frequency of dominant allele
(c) homozygous dominant individuals
(d) homozygous recessive individuals

54 Consider the following statements.

I. Hardy-Weinberg proposed that change of frequency of allele in a population results in evolution.
II. Hardy-Weinberg equation is used for knowing whether or not a population is evolving.

Choose the correct option.

(a) Statement I is true, but II is false
(b) Statement I is false, but II is true
(c) Both statements I and II are true
(d) Both statements I and II are false

55 Hardy-Weinberg equilibrium is known to be affected by gene flow, genetic drift, mutation, genetic recombination and

(a) evolution (b) limiting factors
(c) saltation (d) natural selection

56 Balancing selection is connected with the successful reproduction of

(a) homozygous recessives (b) homozygous dominants
(c) heterozygous individuals (d) All of the above

57 Human blood groups A, B, AB and O, are examples of

(a) gradualism (b) cline
(c) gradient of diploidy (d) polymorphism

58 For the MN-blood group system, the frequencies of M and N alleles are 0.7 and 0.3, respectively. The expanded frequency of MN-blood group bearing organisms is likely to be

(a) 42% (b) 49% (c) 9% (d) 50%

(B) Cumulative Exercise

(Assorted Questions of the Chapter for Advanced Level Practice)

1 Which of the following represents directional selection?

I. Industrial melanism
II. Bacterial resistance to antibiotics
III. Pesticide resistance
IV. Sickle-cell anaemia

Choose the correct option from the codes given below

(a) I and II (b) I, II and III
(c) III and IV (d) I, II, III and IV

2 An isolated population of humans, with approximately equal numbers of blue-eyes and brown-eyes individuals, was decimated by an earthquake. Only a few brown-eyes people remained to form the next generation. This kind of change in the gene pool is called a

(a) Hardy-Weinberg equilibrium
(b) blocked gene flow
(c) bottleneck effect
(d) founder effect

3 Match the following columns.

Column I	Column II
A. Mutation	1. A drastic reduction in population size brought about by severe pressure or a calamity.
B. Genetic drift	2. Individuals and their alleles, move into or out of populations.
C. Gene flow	3. A heritable change in DNA.
D. Bottleneck effect	4. Random fluctuation in allele over time due to chance occurrences alone.

Codes

	A	B	C	D		A	B	C	D
(a)	3	4	2	1	(b)	4	3	2	1
(c)	1	2	3	4	(d)	2	1	4	3

4 Most of the 700 species of fruitflies found in the Hawaiian archipelago, are each restricted to a single island. One hypothesis to explain this pattern is that each species diverged after a small number of flies, had colonised a new island. This mechanism is called

(a) sexual selection (b) genetic equilibrium
(c) disruptive selection (d) the founder effect

5 What is the consequence of genetic drift?

I. Improvement of the population
II. Increase in strength of a population
III. Increase in IQ of a population
IV. Unpredictable effects on characters in a population

Choose the correct option from the codes given below.

(a) I and II (b) II and III
(c) III and IV (d) I, II, III and IV

6 Match the following columns.

Column I	Column II
A. Ford	1. Stabilising selection in land snails
B. Weldon	2. Observed stabilising selection in sparrows
C. Bumpus	3. Defined polymorphism
D. Hardy	4. An English mathematician

Codes

	A	B	C	D		A	B	C	D
(a)	3	2	4	1	(b)	3	1	2	4
(c)	2	3	4	1	(d)	1	4	3	2

7 In a population of land snails, some have dark shells and others have light shells. Each morph produces 100 offsprings per year, but the dark-shelled morphs live long enough to reproduce for five seasons, whereas the light-shelled morphs, which are easily seen by bird predators, live to reproduce for only one season. The Darwinian fitness of the light-shelled morphs is

(a) 0.0 (b) 0.20 (c) 5.00 (d) 100.00

8 In a population of large and small flowered daisies, those with large flowers leave an average of 1000 surviving offsprings, whereas those with small flowers leave an average of only 250 offsprings. The Darwinian fitness of the large-flowered daisies is

(a) 1000.00 (b) 4.00 (c) 1.00 (d) 0.25

9 Which of the following is correct about genetic drift?

I. It is called as Sewall Wright effect.
II. It is a random change in gene frequency due to sampling error.
III. It increases genetic variability within a small population.
IV. It is more effective in large population.

Choose the correct option from the codes given below.

(a) I and II (b) II and III
(c) III and IV (d) I and IV

10 Which of the following is correct?

I. Migration is the movement of individuals from a population to another population.
II. Emigration is the migration of individuals out of an area.

III. Immigration is the migration of individuals into an area.
IV. Gene flow cannot alter the genetic characteristics of populations.

Choose the correct option from the codes given below.

(a) I and II (b) III and IV
(c) I, II and III (d) II, III and IV

11 You are studying leaf size in a natural population of plants. The second season is particularly dry and the following year the average leaf size in the population is smaller than the year before. But the amount of overall variation is the same and the population size has not changed. Also, you have done experiments that show that small leaves are better adapted to dry conditions than are large leaves. Which of the following has occurred?

(a) Genetic drift
(b) Directional selection
(c) Stabilising selection
(d) Disruptive selection

12 Match the following columns.

Column I	Column II
A. Polymorphism	1. Relating to groups of similar organisms that could interbreed but do not, because they are geographically isolated.
B. Speciation	2. Organisms whose range overlap or are even identical so that they occur together at least in some places.
C. Sympatry	3. The existence of two or more distinctly different forms within a plant or animal species.
D Allopatry	4. A genetically distinct geographic variety population or race within species which is adapted to specific environmental conditions.
E. Ecotypes	5. The development of one or more species from an existing species.

Codes

	A	B	C	D	E
(a)	1	2	3	4	5
(b)	5	4	3	2	1
(c)	3	5	2	4	1
(d)	4	3	5	1	2

13 Which of the following is correct about random mating population?

I. The pattern of transmission of individual genes can not be determined.
II. Gene pool and gene frequencies are two main attributes.
III. There is no control over mating.
IV. There is no free mating.

Choose the correct option from the codes given below.

(a) I, II and III (b) II, III and IV
(c) III and IV (d) Only IV

14 In the absence of which of the following the gene frequencies in a Mendelian population remain constant generation after generation.

I. Photosynthesis and respiration.
II. Selection and mutation.
III. Growth and development.
IV. Migration and random drift.

Choose the correct option from the codes given below.

(a) I and II (b) II and III
(c) I and III (d) II and IV

15 Match the following columns.

Column I	Column II
A. Phenotype	1. The appearance or behaviour of an organism.
B. Founder effect	2. A limit imposed on allelic variation caused by the limited representation of alleles in the population that migrates into a new region.
C. Adaptation	3. The change in an appearance or behaviour over time in response to environmental pressure.
D. Non-random mating	4. The situation where not all members of a population have an equally likely chance to mate and reproduce.

Codes

	A	B	C	D
(a)	1	2	3	4
(b)	4	3	2	1
(c)	3	4	1	2
(d)	2	1	4	3

16 Match the following columns.

Column I	Column II
A. Favours the extreme range of a phenotype	1. Directional selection
B. The total alleles existing in a population	2. Gene pool
C. Relative measure of the ability to reproduce	3. Microevolution
D. Genetic change in population causing new phenotypes to appear	4. Fitness

Codes

	A	B	C	D
(a)	1	2	4	3
(b)	1	2	3	4
(c)	2	1	4	3
(d)	2	1	3	4

Assertion and Reason

Direction (Q. Nos. 17-28) *In each of the following questions, a statement of Assertion (A) is given followed by corresponding statement of Reason (R). Of the statements, mark the correct answer as*

(a) Both A and R are true and R is the correct explanation of A
(b) Both A and R are true, but R is not the correct explanation of A
(c) A is true, but R is false
(d) A is false, but R is true
(e) Both A and R are false

17 **Assertion** (A) Hardy-Weinberg equilibrium is not applicable for large population size.

Reason (R) Non-random mating is necessary for Hardy-Weinberg equilibrium.

18 **Assertion** (A) Genetic drift is also called Sewall Wright effect.

Reason (R) It was discovered by American geneticist Sewall Wright.

19 **Assertion** (A) Mating in most natural population is random.

Reason (R) Hardy-Weinberg equilibrium is successful in non-random population.

20 **Assertion** (A) Founder principle is associated with the genetic drift.

Reason (R) Genetic drift is significant in small populations.

21 **Assertion** (A) Gene flow increases genetic variations.

Reason (R) The random introduction of new alleles into recipient population and their removal from the donor population affects allele frequency.

22 **Assertion** (A) Dominant alleles are selected more frequently than recessive alleles.

Reason (R) They appear in phenotype more frequently.

23 **Assertion** (A) Directional selection operates in response to gradual changes in environmental conditions.

Reason (R) Stabilising selection operates when phenotypic features coincide with the optimal environmental conditions.

24 **Assertion** (A) Disruptive selection is the rarest form of selection.

Reason (R) It leads to speciation.

25 **Assertion** (A) Inbreeding is the reproduction between closely related organisms.

Reason (R) Intensive inbreeding reduces the variability of the genome.

26 **Assertion** (A) Industrial melanism is an example of disruptive selection.

Reason (R) Evolutionary change in moth is provided by the response of moth species to the directional selection pressure produced by the atmospheric pollution.

27 **Assertion** (A) Polymorphism is the existence of two or more forms of the same species within the same population.

Reason (R) Balanced polymorphism occurs when different forms co-exist in the same population in a stable environment.

28 **Assertion** (A) In intraspecific speciation, a single species may give rise to new species.

Reason (R) Gene flow within the populations must be interrupted.

(C) Medical Entrances' Gallery

(Collection of questions Asked in NEET & Various Medical Entrance Exams)

1 A gene locus has two alleles A, a. If the frequency of dominant allele A is 0.4, then what will be the frequency of homozygous dominant, heterozygous and homozygous recessive individuals in the population? **[NEET 2019]**

(a) 0.16 (AA), 0.24 (Aa), 0.36 (aa)
(b) 0.16 (AA), 0.48 (Aa), 0.36 (aa)
(c) 0.16 (AA), 0.36 (Aa), 0.48 (aa)
(d) 0.36 (AA), 0.48 (Aa), 0.16 (aa)

2 In a species, the weight of newborn ranges from 2-5 kg. 97% of the newborn with an average weight between 3 to 3.3 kg survive whereas 99% of the infants born with weights from 2 to 2.5 kg or 4.5 to 5 kg die. Which type of selection process is taking place? **[NEET 2019]**

(a) Stabilising selection
(b) Disruptive selection
(c) Cyclical selection
(d) Directional selection

3 The peppered moth (*Biston betularia*), the black coloured form became dominant over the light coloured form of moth in England during industrial revolution. This is an example of **[AIIMS 2018]**
(a) appearance of the darker coloured individuals due to very poor sunlight
(b) protective mimicry
(c) inheritance of darker colour character acquired due to the darker environment
(d) natural selection whereby the darker forms were selected

4 From the statements given below, which one most likely represents an example of disruptive selection? **[AIIMS 2017]**
I. Industrial melanism in peppered moth.
II. Population of butterflies that are either all yellow or all blue.
III. Population of rabbits that evolve more body fat in response to a cold climate.
IV. Population of wrens that evolve to be smaller at sexual maturity in response to predation pressure.
V. Very tall and very short pine trees being removed from a population by herbivores.
Choose the correct option.
(a) Only II (b) II and III (c) Only IV (d) III and IV

5 Variation in gene frequencies within population can occur by chance rather than by natural selection. This is referred to as **[JIPMER 2017, NEET 2013]**
(a) genetic flow (b) genetic drift
(c) random mating (d) genetic load

6 Which one of the following graphs correctly describes disruptive selection, when studying fitness level associated with body size? **[JIPMER 2017]**

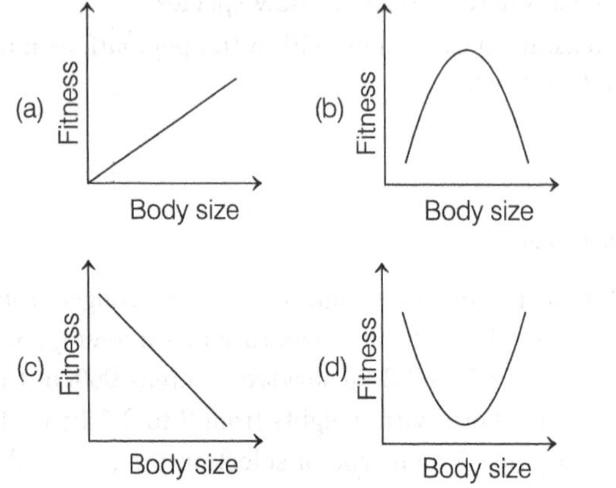

7 Genetic drift operates in **[NEET-II 2016]**
(a) small isolated population
(b) large isolated population
(c) non-reproductive population
(d) slow reproductive population

8 In Hardy-Weinberg equation, the frequency of heterozygous individual is represented by **[NEET-II 2016]**
(a) P^2 (b) $2pq$
(c) pq (d) q^2

9 According to Hardy-Weinberg equilibrium, the allelic frequencies in a population will remain constant from generation to generation under which of these two conditions?
I. Large population size.
II. Non-random mating.
III. There should be differential success among the organisms of the population.
IV. There should be no mutations or large scale migrations.
Choose the correct option from the codes given below. **[EAMCET 2016]**
(a) I and III (b) I and IV
(c) I and II (d) II and III

10 Allopatric speciation is **[EAMCET 2016]**
(a) appearance of a new species in the same area as the parent population
(b) initiated by the appearance of a geographical isolation
(c) the emergence of many species from a single ancestor
(d) seen only in species exhibiting sexual dimorphism

11 Industrial melanism is an example of **[CBSE AIPMT 2015; WB JEE 2014]**
(a) neo-Darwinism (b) natural selection
(c) mutation (d) neo-Lamarckism

12 A population will not exist in Hardy-Weinberg equilibrium if **[CBSE AIPMT 2015]**
(a) individuals mate selectively
(b) there are mutations
(c) there is no migration
(d) the population is large

13 Which mechanism of evolution affects the genetic makeup in a population? **[J&K CET 2014]**
(a) Natural selection (b) Adaptation
(c) Genetic drift (d) Gene mutation

14 In a population of 1000 individuals, 360 belongs to genotypes AA, 480 to Aa and the remaining 160 to aa. Based on this data, the frequency of allele A in the population is **[CBSE AIPMT 2014]**
(a) 0.4 (b) 0.5
(c) 0.6 (d) 0.7

15 Which one of the following is the first in allopatric speciation? **[EAMCET 2014]**
(a) Geographic isolation (b) Hybridisation
(c) Genetic drift (d) Polyploidy

16 The tendency of population to remain in genetic equilibrium may be disturbed by **[NEET 2013]**
(a) random mating (b) lack of migration
(c) lack of mutations (d) lack of random mating

17 Which of the following species are restricted to an area? **[AFMC 2013, Manipal 2013]**
(a) Sibling species (b) Endemic species
(c) Allopatric species (d) Sympatric species

18 Population are said to be allopatric when **[Karnataka CET 2013]**
(a) they are physically isolated by natural barriers
(b) they are sharing the same area, but cannot interbreed
(c) they live together and breed freely to produce viable offspring
(d) they are isolated, but often come together for breeding

19 Biological concept of species is mainly based on **[Manipal 2013]**
(a) reproductive isolation
(b) morphological feature only
(c) methods of reproduction only
(d) morphology and methods of reproduction

20 The process by which organisms with different evolutionary history evolve similar phenotypic adaptations in response to a common environmental challenge, is called **[NEET 2013]**
(a) natural selection (b) convergent evolution
(c) non-random evolution (d) adaptive radiation

21 Species is a **[Manipal 2012]**
(a) group immediately below a phylum
(b) closely related interbreeding population
(c) taxonomic division of similar genera
(d) closely related non-breeding population

22 Read the following statements and choose the correct option.
I. Increase in melanised moths after industrialisation in Great Britain is a proof for natural selection.
II. When more individuals of a population acquire a mean character value, it is called disruption.
III. Changes in allelic frequency in a population will lead to Hardy-Weinberg equilibrium.
IV. Genetic drift changes the existing gene or allelic frequency in future generations.

Choose the correct option from the codes given below. **[Kerala CEE 2012]**
(a) Only II (b) Only IV (c) I and IV (d) I and III

23 Related species which are reproductively isolated, but morphologically similar are called **[MHT CET 2011]**
(a) sibling (b) sympatric
(c) allopatric (d) morphospecies

24 The theory of random genetic drift was proposed by **[J&K CET 2011]**
(a) Sewall Wright (b) Hardy Weinberg
(c) RA Fisher (d) Mayr

ANSWERS

Check Point 13.1

1. (b)	2. (d)	3. (a)	4. (c)	5. (a)	6. (d)

Check Point 13.2

1. (c)	2. (c)	3. (a)	4. (d)	5. (b)	6. (c)

(A) Topical Exercise

1. (b)	2. (b)	3. (a)	4. (d)	5. (d)	6. (a)	7. (c)	8. (d)	9. (b)	10. (d)
11. (c)	12. (a)	13. (b)	14. (c)	15. (c)	16. (c)	17. (a)	18. (b)	19. (d)	20. (d)
21. (b)	22. (c)	23. (a)	24. (d)	25. (a)	26. (b)	27. (c)	28. (c)	29. (d)	30. (c)
31. (c)	32. (a)	33. (a)	34. (d)	35. (d)	36. (c)	37. (c)	38. (a)	39. (d)	40. (c)
41. (b)	42. (c)	43. (c)	44. (d)	45. (a)	46. (b)	47. (d)	48. (d)	49. (c)	50. (c)
51. (c)	52. (a)	53. (b)	54. (c)	55. (d)	56. (c)	57. (d)	58. (a)		

(B) Cumulative Exercise

1. (b)	2. (c)	3. (a)	4. (d)	5. (d)	6. (b)	7. (b)	8. (b)	9. (a)	10. (c)
11. (b)	12. (c)	13. (a)	14. (d)	15. (a)	16. (a)	17. (d)	18. (a)	19. (e)	20. (b)
21. (a)	22. (a)	23. (b)	24. (b)	25. (b)	26. (d)	27. (b)	28. (b)		

(C) Medical Entrances' Gallery

1. (b)	2. (a)	3. (d)	4. (a)	5. (b)	6. (d)	7. (a)	8. (b)	9. (b)	10. (b)
11. (b)	12. (b)	13. (d)	14. (c)	15. (a)	16. (a)	17. (b)	18. (a)	19. (a)	20. (b)
21. (b)	22. (c)	23. (a)	24. (a)						

Explanations

(B) Cumulative Exercise

1 (*b*) Industrial melanism, bacterial resistance to antibiotics and pesticide resistance represents directional selection while sickle-cell anaemia shows disruptive or diverging selection.

9 (*a*) Statements I and II are correct while III and IV are incorrect and can be corrected as
Genetic drift is a random change in gene frequency. It decreases genetic variability within a population. It is more effective in small population.

13 (*a*) Statements I, II and III are correct while statement IV is incorrect and can be corrected as
In random mating population these is no control over mating. Free mating occur.
Rest statements are correct.

17 (*d*) A is false, but R is true because
As per Hardy-Weinberg equilibrium, the frequency of dominant and recessive alleles in a population will remain constant from generation to generation provided that certain conditions exist, i.e. population should be large, mating should be random, no mutation occurs, no natural selection occurs, generations do not overlap and there is no immigration or emigration or gene flow between populations, etc.

18 (*a*) Both A and R are true and R is the correct explanation of A.
Random genetic drift or the Sewall Wright effect named after the American geneticist, who realised its evolutionary significance may be an important mechanism in evolutionary change in small or isolated populations.

19 (*e*) Both A and R are false because
Mating in most natural populations is non-random. Sexual selection occurs whenever the presence of one or more inherited characteristics increase the likelihood of bringing about successful fertilisation of gametes. There are many structural and behavioural mechanisms in both plants and animals which prevent mating from being random.
Hardy-Weinberg equilibrium is successful in random mating, large population in which there is no mutation, selection, random drift and gene flow.

20 (*b*) Both A and R are true, but R is not the correct explanation of A.
Founder principle is a phenomenon associated with genetic drift. This refers that when a small population splits off from the parent population, it may not be truly representative, in terms of alleles, of the parent population. Some alleles may be absent and others may be disproportionally represented. Continuous breeding, within the pioneer population will produce a gene pool with allele frequencies different from that of the original parent population. Genetic drift is significant in small populations. It tends to reduce the amount of genetic variation within the population, mainly as a result of the loss of those alleles, which have low frequency.

21 (*a*) Both A and R are true and R is the correct explanation of A.
Gene flow is the movement of alleles from one population to another as a result of interbreeding between the members of two populations. The random introduction of new alleles into the recipient population and their removal from the donor population affects the allele frequency of both populations and leads to increased genetic variation.

22 (*a*) Both A and R are true and R is the correct explanation of A.
Major changes in genotypes of organisms arise from the mutant alleles through the gene pool. If the allele is dominant, it will appear in the phenotype, more frequently and be selected for or against more rapidly. If the allele is recessive and has no effect in the heterozygous state, will not undergo selection until it appears in the homozygous state.

23 (*b*) Both A and R are true, but R is not the correct explanation of A.
Directional selection operates in response to gradual changes in environmental conditions. It operates on the range of phenotypes existing within the population and exerts selection pressure which moves the mean phenotype towards one phenotypic extreme. Stabilising selection operates when phenotypic features coincide with the optimal environmental conditions and competition is not severe. It occurs in all populations and tends to eliminate extremes from the population.

24 (*b*) Both A and R are true, but R is not the correct explanation of A.
Disruptive selection is the rarest form of selection which can be very important in bringing about evolutionary changes. Fluctuating conditions in environment such as season and climate, may favour the presence of more than one phenotype within a population.
This can split a population into two subpopulations. If gene flow between the subpopulations is prevented, each population may give rise to a new species (speciation). In some cases, disruptive selection can give rise to the appearance of different phenotypes within a population.

25 (*b*) Both A and R are true, but R is not the correct explanation of A.
Inbreeding involves selective reproduction between the closely related organisms. Intensive breeding reduces the variability of the genome by increasing the number of heterozygous genotypes. In order to overcome these problems, breeders resort to outbreeding after several generations of inbreeding.

26 (*d*) A is false, but R is true because
Upto 1848, all reported forms of the peppered moth (*Biston betularia*) appeared creamy white with black dots and dark shaded areas. In 1848, a black form of moth was recorded in Manchester and by 1895, 98% of peppered moth population in Manchester was black within the last 100 years.

Darkened forms of about 80 species of moths have appeared in varying frequencies throughout the United Kingdom. This is a phenomenon known as industrial melanism. It is an example of directional selection in which evolutionary change is provided by the response of moth species to the directional selection pressure produced by the atmospheric pollution, which accompanied the industrial revolution.

27 (*b*) Both A and R are true, but R is not the correct explanation of A.

Polymorphism is the existence of two or more forms of same species within the same population and can apply to biochemical, morphological and behavioural characteristics.

There are two forms of polymorphism

(i) **Balanced polymorphism** This occurs, when different forms co-exist in the same population in a stable environment.

For example, existence of two sexes in animals and plants. Existence of A, B, AB and O blood groups. Red-green ± colour blindness.

Existence of workers, drones and queens in social insects.

(ii) **Transient polymorphism** This arises, when different forms or morphs exist in a population undergoing a strong selection pressure.

The frequency of the phenotypic appearance of each form is determined by the intensity of the selection pressure. Transient polymorphism usually applies in those situations where one form is gradually being replaced by the another, e.g. melanic and non-melanic forms of the peppered moth.

28 (*b*) Both A and R are true, but R is not the correct explanation of A.

A single species may give rise to new species (i.e. intraspecific speciation) or two different species may give rise to a new species (i.e. interspecific hybridisation). If intraspecific speciation occurs in geographically separated population, it is termed as allopatric speciation. If intraspecific speciation occurs in the population occupying the same geographical area, it is called sympatric speciation. There are several factors involved in intraspecific speciation, but in all cases, gene flow within the populations must be interrupted.

(C) Medical Entrances' Gallery

1 (*b*) The frequency of homozygous dominant, heterozygous and homozygous recessive individuals would be 0.16 (AA), 0.48 (Aa), 0.36 (aa). The frequencies are calculated as follows

Frequency of dominant allele (p) = 0.4 (given)

Frequency of recessive allele (q) $= 1 - 0.4 = 0.6$

Frequency of homozygous dominant individuals (AA)

$= p^2 = 0.16$

Frequency of heterozygous individual (Aa) $= 2pq$

$= 2\,(0.4)\,(0.6) = 0.48$

Frequency of homozygous recessive individual (aa)

$= q \;= (0.6)^2 = 0.36$

2 (*a*) The given data represent stabilising selection. It eliminates individuals from both ends of a phenotypic distribution and hence, maintains the same distribution average. In the given situation, most of the newborn of average weight 3 to 3.3 kg survive. Babies having more or less weight had low survival rate. Disruptive selection favours both extremes of continuous variation.

Directional selection favours one extreme of continuous variation. Cyclical selection is regarded as a source of polymorphism.

3 (*d*) In peppered moth (*Biston betularia*), the black coloured form become dominant over the light coloured form of moth in England during industrial revolution. This is an example of natural selection whereby the darker forms were selected. It can be explained as, before industrialisation, light-coloured moths remain unnoticed by predatory birds due to whitish lichens on the bark of trees.

After industrialisation, the barks became dark due to smoke so the white moths were more evidently visible and thus, picked up by predators. But, black moths escaped unnoticed so they managed to survive resulting in more population of black moths and less population of white moths.

4 (*a*) Statement II is correct because

The disruptive selection favours individuals at both extremes of the distribution. It eliminates the members with mean expression, thus producing two peaks in trait distribution. This may lead to the development of two different populations. Thus, statement II, i.e. population of butterflies that are either all yellow or all blue, is most suited example of disruptive selection.

5 (*b*) Variation in gene (allele) frequencies within small populations can occur drastically by chance. Such changes in allele frequencies occur randomly and is called as genetic drift.

6 (*d*) The option (d) is correct. Disruptive selection occurs when an environmental change may produce selection pressure that favours two extreme characteristics.

It produces two peaks in the distribution of a trait. Selection acts on the phenotype, physical, biochemical and behavioural traits of an organism. It indirectly adapts a population to its environment by selecting and maintaining favourable genotypes in their gene pool.

7 (*a*) The genetic drift is a drastic change in allele frequency when population size is very small. Its effects are more marked in a small isolated population.

8 (*b*) Hardy-Weinberg principle states that the allele frequencies in a population are stable and remain constant from generation to generation.

This can be expressed by the equation

$$p^2 + 2pq + q^2 = 1$$

or

$$(p+q)^2 = 1$$

where, p^2 represents frequency of homozygous dominant genotype, $2pq$ represents the frequency of heterozygous genotype and p^2 represents the frequency of homozygous recessive genotype.

Hence, option (b) is correct.

9 (*b*) Statements I and IV are correct because

According to Hardy-Weinberg equilibrium, allele frequency in a population will remain constant from generation to generation if the population size is large, random mating occurs and selection mutation and migration do not occur.

10 (*b*) Allopatric speciation is initiated by the appearance of a geographical isolation when two different species will be formed after long time when species formation takes place in same habitat then this mode of speciation is known as sympatric speciation. Parapatric speciation occurs in geographically adjacent areas.

12 (*b*) Hardy-Weinberg equilibrium exists in population only when following conditions are present.

- Large population size
- No mutation
- No gene flow
- No genetic recombination
- Random mating occurs
- No natural selection pressure.

If the individuals in the population mate selectively, it will have mutation thus shifting the Hardy-Weinberg equilibrium.

14 (*c*) According to Hardy-Weinberg principle

$(p+q)^2 = p^2 + 2pq + q^2 = 1$

Where, $p =$ The frequency of allele 'A'

$q =$ The frequency of allele 'a'

$p^2 =$ The frequency of individual 'AA'

$q^2 =$ The frequency of individual 'aa'

$2pq =$ The frequency of individual 'Aa'

(AA) $p^2 = 360$ out of 1000 individual

or $p^2 = 36$ out of 100.

$q^2 = 160$ out of 1000 or $q^2 = 16$ out of 100.

So, $q = \sqrt{0.16} = 0.4$

As $p + q = 1$

So, p is 0.6

15 (*a*) In allopatric speciation (*Allos*-other; *patria*-native land), a part of the population becomes geographically isolated from the main population. The population becomes entirely separated and finally constitutes a new species.

16 (*a*) According to Hardy-Weinberg principle, allele frequencies in a population are stable and constant from generation to generation. In a population, it will remain constant over generation only if the following conditions are met.

(i) There is no mutation, no gene flow and all mating is random.

(ii) All genotypes reproduce equally well, i.e. no natural selection. But all these conditions rarely occur in nature.

17 (*b*) Endemic species are species which are restricted geographically in a particular area at a given time.

Other options are explained as

Sibling species are species produced from same parents, but they are reproductively isolated from each other.

Allopatric species are species, which share different geographical area, i.e. these are geographically separated from one another.

Sympatric species are species, which share the same geographical area.

19 (*a*) Species is a natural inbreeding population which have essentially similar morphological traits, are genetically distinct and reproductively isolated from others.

Reproductive isolation or absence of interbreeding maintains the identity of species. Thus, biological concept of species is mainly based on reproductive isolation.

24 (*a*) Sewall Wright was an American geneticist known for his influential work on evolutionary theory. The theory of random, genetic drift was proposed by him. Genetic drift is the change in the frequency of a gene variant in a population due to random sampling. The effect of genetic drift is larger in small population and smaller in large population.

CHAPTER 14

Evolution of Human

Human is the wisest creature on the earth. Biologists explain human as just another animal based on their body structure and working.

Carolus Linnaeus placed humans among the monkeys and apes. He coined scientific name, *Homo sapiens* for humans.

Charles Darwin stated that origin and evolution of human could be traced just like that of any other species. His ideas about human ancestry were published in the book '*Descent of Man*' and '*Selection in Relation to Sex*'. He suggested that man, apes and monkeys have a common ancestor.

TH Huxley explained the origin of humans scientifically in his book *'Man's Place in Nature'*.

The unique qualities of human are language, advanced thoughts and culture which have evolved through the natural selection. The course of human phylogeny like other mammals, can be followed only from the fossil records. The stages of human evolution or **anthropogenesis** have been studied by following means

- Comparative morphology of fossils.
- Comparative anatomy of fossils.
- Comparative biochemistry of present day human, apes and primates.
- Similarities in the sequences of proteins and nucleic acids.
- Later stages in human evolution are based on stone tools, pottery and the fossils of other animals along with human.

Table 14.1 Classification of human

Kingdom	—	Animalia	Absence of chlorophyll, cell wall, presence of locomotion and intake of complex food.
Phylum	—	Chordata	Presence of notochord and dorsal hollow central nervous system.
Subphylum	—	Vertebrata (Craniata)	Presence of vertebral column and cranium (brain box).
Section	—	Gnathostomata	Jaws are present.
Superclass	—	Tetrapoda	Four limbs are present.

Table 14.3 Differences between apes and man

Characters	Apes	Man
Habitat	Mainly arboreal	Terrestrial
Posture	Less erect	Fully erect
Eyebrow ridges	Very prominent	Less prominent
Feeding nature	Herbivorous	Omnivorous
Chin	Round or absent	Prominent chin
Locomotion	Mainly quadrupedal	Bipedal
Jaws	Protruded	Not protruded
Teeth	Incisor and canine are large, canines are projecting	Incisor and canine are comparatively small and not projecting
Anterior premolar in lower jaw	Strong and pointed	Small and bicuspid
Language spoken and written	Not used	Used
Body hair	Long and coarse	Short and sparse
Brain box	Small size	Large size
Cranial capacity	450 cc	1450 cc
Vertebral column	One curve	Four curves
Toe (hallux)	Opposable	Non-opposable
Pelvic girdle	Narrow and elongated	Broad and flattened
Arms	Longer than legs	Smaller than legs
Neck	Very short	Comparatively long
Neck muscles	Allow very little movement of head on the neck	Allow more movement of head on the neck
Face	Prognathous	Orthognathous
Foramen magnum	Backward	Forward
Dental arrangement	U-shaped	Semicircular

CHECK POINT 14.1

1. Choose the incorrect match pair.
(a) Lemuroidea – Shrews
(b) Anthropoidea – Rhesus monkey
(c) Ceboidea – Spider monkey
(d) Tarsioidea – Gibbon

2. A feature presents in old world monkeys, but absent in new world monkeys.
(a) More number of teeth (b) Longer prehensile tail
(c) Resemblance to man (d) No cheek pouches

3. Choose the correct synonyms.
(a) Anthropoidea – Simians
(b) Catarrhini – Ceboidea
(c) Cercopithecoidea – Platyrrhini
(d) Hominoidea – Prosimians

4. What do you understand by orthognathous face in humans?
(a) There are 36 teeth in the jaws
(b) Elongated face with or directed eyes
(c) Face with protruding canines in the lower jaw
(d) None of the above

5. Humans do not have
(a) bipedal locomotion (b) stereoscopic vision
(c) large cerebral hemisphere (d) All of these

6. The feature(s) present in apes is/are
(a) T-shaped dental arrangement
(b) opposable thumb and non-opposable toe
(c) round or absent chin
(d) All of the above

HUMAN EVOLUTION

- It is the aspect of evolution which is concerned with emergence of human as distinct species. Various evidences support that humans and apes have descended from common ancestors.
- The beginning of primates evolution is presumed in Eocene of Tertiary Period (75-60 million years ago) in evergreen forests and later in Oligocene (25-30 million years ago).
- Ancestral human returned to the ground from trees due to replacement of evergreen forests into dried Savanna grassland.
- Thus, the evolution of apes and man started together from tree dwelling common ancestors approximately 25-30 million years ago.
- The place of origin of human is a great controversial matter.
- The fossils of ancestral human forms are obtained from widely diverse regions of Africa, Asia and Europe, but origin of human probably occurred in Central Asia, China, Java and India (Shivalik hills).
- Many fossils have been discovered from East Africa (Olduvai Gorge, Lake Victoria and Lake Natron in Tanzania and Lake Turkana in Kenya) which indicate a significant role of Africa in regard to the site of origin of human.

Changes during human evolution

Some changes that took place during human evolution are given below

- **Skull and brain** Increased in size, complexity and intelligence.
- **Bipedal locomotion** Due to bipedal locomotion, forelimbs became free.
- **Forelimbs** They modified into organs of manipulation and accompanied by lengthening of hindlimbs and shortening of forelimbs.
- **Thumb** Perfection of thumb opposability in forelimbs.
- **Toe** Loss of opposability of great toe in hindlimbs.
- **Upright posture** Because of the development of lumbar curve.
- **Jaw** Power reduced.
- **Teeth** Due to omnivorous food habit, the size of incisors and canines is reduced.
- **Chin** Development of chin.
- **Pelvic girdle** Development and broadening of iliac bones of pelvic girdle.
- **Social organisation** and cultural evolution.

History of human evolution

The study of living and fossil primates (including monkey and man) shows that they had descended from a common ancestor and separated from the main stock (of a homonisation) during Oligocene period.

The evolutionary history of man can be divided into following three steps, only for the convenience of study.

1. **Prior to ape man.**
2. **Ape man** (including prehistoric man).
3. **True man** (including the living modern man).

Table 14.4 Prior to ape man

Propliopithecus	**Discovery** • Fossils obtained from Faiyum deposits of Egypt. • Fossils have jaws and teeth. • They lived about 35-30 million years ago in Oligocene epoch. **Characteristics** • They were more or less ape like. • These were short statured with monkey like teeth. • Their dental formula was 2, 1, 2, 3, i.e. both jaws had 8 incisors, 4 canines, 8 premolars and 12 molars like modern man. • Their incisor teeth were vertical rather than directed forward. • Their molars had five cusps each. • There are two views regarding the ancestry. One says that *Propliopithecus* directly gave rise to *Ramapithecus*, while as per the other view *Propliopithecus* gave rise to *Dryopithecus*, which in turn, evolved into apes and humans.
Aegyptopithecus (also called Egyptian monkey)	**Discovery** Fossils found from Faiyum province of Egypt in 1980 by **E Simon**. **Characteristics** • These were similar to *Propliopithecus*. • These lived between 35-33 million years ago in the early part of the Oligocene epoch. • They existed before the divergence between hominoids (apes and humans) and old world monkeys.
Limnopithecus* and *Pliopithecus	**Discovery** Fossils found from Faiyum deposits of Africa. **Characteristics** • They existed in Miocene and Pliocene periods. • They had a short tail and 7 lumbar vertebrae. • They represent altogether a different line of evolution which diverged from the hominid line quite early and became extinct during the late Pliocene.

Proconsul
(intermediate between apes and man)

Discovery

- Fossils of *Proconsul africanus* or *D. africanus* were described by **Louis SB Leakey** (1948).
- The fossils were obtained from the rocks of East Africa near Victoria Lake in Kenya.
- They lived in early Miocene epoch.

Characteristics

- Face was prognathous.
- *Proconsul* walked on its four legs.
- Its molars had five cusps each.
- *Proconsul* had long, pointed ape-like canines.
- It had man like forehead.
- *Proconsul* is not considered as base ancestor of man because it walked on its four legs.
- About 4 million years ago, during Pliocene, *Proconsul* gave rise to the ancestors of chimpanzee and gorilla.
- Diversion of chimpanzee and gorilla took place during Pleistocene epoch about 2.3 million years ago.

Dryopithecus
(*common ancestor of man and apes*)

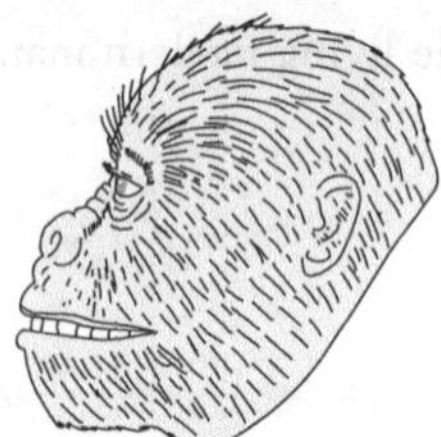

Dryopithecus

Discovery

- Fossil of *Dryopithecus africans* was obtained from the rocks of Africa and Europe.
- Recently, a lower jaw of *Dryopithecus* was found from Haritalyangar in Bilaspur district of Himachal Pradesh, India.
- Several members of Dryopithecine have been discovered from Shivalik hills as well.

Characteristics

- It lived about 15 million years ago during the Miocene.
- *Dryopithecus africans* shows close similarity to chimpanzee.
- *Dryopithecus* is considered to be a common ancestor of man and apes (gibbon, orangutan, chimpanzee and gorilla).
- *Dryopithecus* was ape-like with same length of arms and legs.
- Legs and heels in its feet indicate that *Dryopithecus* was of a semi-erect posture and Knuckle walker.
- *Dryopithecus* was arboreal and herbivorous, which ate soft fruits and leaves.
- *Dryopithecus* had large canines and incisors.

Shivapithecus

Discovery

- Fossils of *Shivapithecus* were discovered from middle and late Pliocene rocks of **Shivalik hills** of India, hence named *Sivapithecus.*

Characteristics

- Its forelimbs, skull and brain resembled with those of monkeys.
- Its face, jaws and teeth had resemblance with those of apes.

Ramapithecus (earliest man like primate or oldest of man's ancestor or first hominoid)

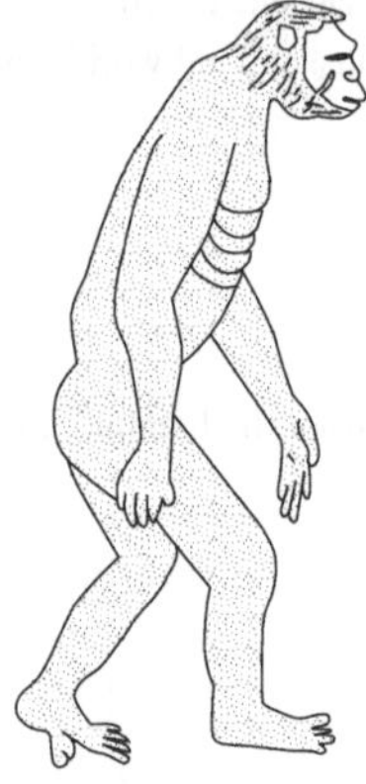

Ramapithecus

Discovery

- **Edward Lewis** (1932) obtained fossil of *Ramapithecus* from Pliocene rocks of Shivalik hills of India.
- Fossil was represented by few teeth and some fragments of jaw.
- ***Kenyapithecus*** (*Kenyapithecus wickeri*) similar to *Ramapithecus* was discovered by **LSB. Leakey** (1955) from Pliocene rocks of Kenya in Africa. But *Ramapithecus* was older than *Kenyapithecus.*

Characteristics

- *Ramapithecus* survived about 14-15 million years ago during late Miocene to Pliocene.
- *Ramapithecus* walked erect on its hindlegs.
- It was similar to ape, which lived on the tree tops, but also walked on the ground.
- It ate hard nuts and seeds like modern man. Its jaws and teeth were similar to humans.
- Its canine teeth were small, but molar teeth were broad and flattened with thicker enamel.
- *Dryopithecus* gave rise to *Ramapithecus,* which is on direct line of human evolution.
- *Ramapithecus* became extinct about 7-8 million years back.
- There is a fossil gap of about 9-10 million years in *Ramapithecus* and *Australopithecus.* The fossil records of man's ancestor from Pliocene are completely blank and once again reappeared in Pleistocene.

Table 14.5 Ape man (including prehistoric man)

Australopithecus (first ape-man)

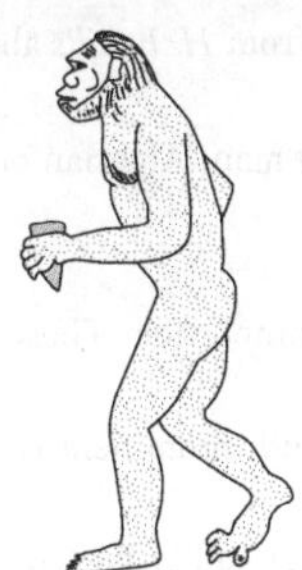

Australopithecus

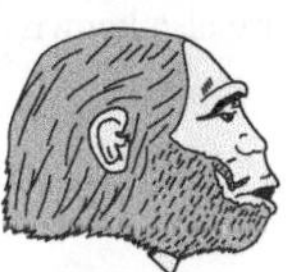

A. afarensis

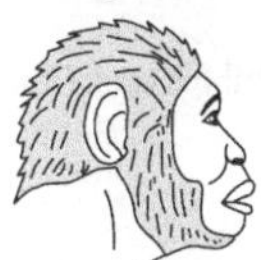

A. robustus

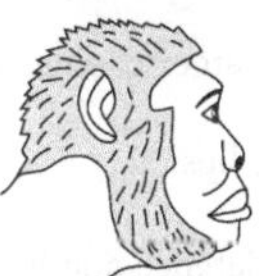

A. boisei

Discovery

- Prof. **Raymond Dart** (1924), a South African anthropologist discovered the skull of 5-6 year old baby which was about 5 million years old near Taung river in Africa. This baby fossil is termed as *Australopithecus africanus* (**African ape man** or **Taung baby**).
- The 3.8 million years old fossils of a new species *Australopithecus afarensis* was first discovered by **Mary Leakey** from the volcanic ash of Lateoli. He named it **Lucy**. Later on **Donald Johanson** and **Timorthy D White** established it as a new species. They named it **Lucy**.
- *Zinjanthropus* (the oldowan tool maker) was discovered by **Mary Leakey** and **LBS Leakey** (1959) from Tanzania (East Africa) which has been named as *Australopithecus boisei* by Leakey.
- *A. africanus* (African ape man or Southern ape man or Taung baby), *A. boisei* (Olduvain tool man), *A. afarensis* (Lucy), *A ramidus, A. aethiopicus* and *A. robustus* are six known species of *Australopithecus.*

So, we can say that *Australopithecus* had two main types

(i) **Gracile type** *A. afarensis* (Johanson) represented by fossil, Lucy (*A. afarensis*) with small brain, small molar teeth, pelvic girdle and short fingers like human.

(ii) **Robust type** *A. robustus* had heavier body structure and massive cheek tooth (also called originally Paranthropus) cranial capacity 600 cc.

Characteristics

- Its height was 1.5 m and had both human and ape's characters.
- It was fully bipedal hominid.
- It lived from 4-1.5 million years ago in caves during Pleistocene period.
- Evidence show they hunted with stone weapons but essentially ate fruits (i.e. had omnivorous diet).
- Its cranial capacity volume (brain size) was 500-700 cc, i.e. equivalent to modern gorilla.
- Brow ridges projected over the eyes and lack chin.
- Distinct lumbar curve was present in vertebral column.
- Its thighs and hips were adapted for erect standing, walking and running.
- Its arms were somewhat less mobile than humans and pelvis was broad.
- Its ankle bone was intermediate between human and ape.
- It had protruding jaws (i.e. prognathous face) and modern man like teeth.
- *Australopithecus africanus* gave rise to *Homo habilis* approximately 2 million years ago, also separate lines, gave rise to *Australopithecus robustus* and *Australopithecus boisei.*

Homo habilis (handy man or able man or skillful man or the tool maker)

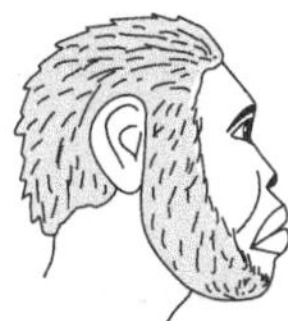

Homo habilis

Discovery

- **Louis SB Leakey** and his wife **Mary Leakey** (1961) obtained the fossils of *Homo habilis* from Pleistocene rocks of Olduvi Gorge in East Africa.
- **Richard Leakey** (1972) also obtained fossils of *Homo habilis* from East side of Lake Turkana in Kenya.

Characteristics

- *Homo habilis* was the **first tool maker**. They used tools of chipped stones extensively. It is also called **handy man** because heaps of tools made up of sharpened stones were found with their fossils. This indicates they were capable of making tools.
- *Homo habilis* man was about 1.2-1.5 m tall.
- It had bipedal locomotion and moved erect.
- It had teeth like that of modern man.
- Its cranial capacity was 700-800 cc, which lived in Africa about 2 million years ago.
- *Homo habilis* was carnivorous and had begun hunting for meat.
- *Homo habilis* lived in small community or groups in caves. They greatly cared for the young ones.
- Perhaps they showed sexual division of labour and communicated with visual signals and simple audible sounds.

Homo erectus* (erect man)** 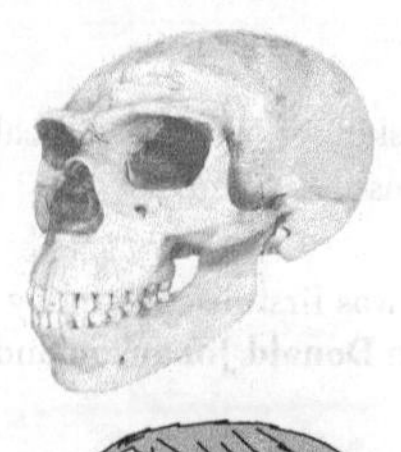 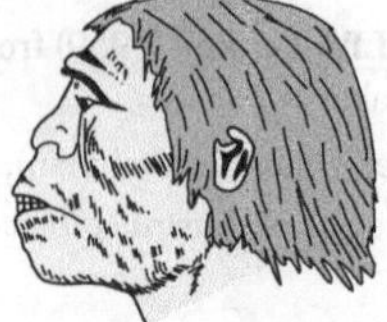 ***Homo erectus	**Discovery** • Fossils of *Homo erectus* were obtained from diverse sites from Olduvai Gorge in Africa to Java, Algeria, Germany, Hungary and China. • Fossils were 8,00,000 to 30,000 years old. • *Homo erectus* is considered as the direct ancestor of modern man. It evolved from *H. habilis* about 1.7 million years ago in the Pleistocene. • *Homo erectus* species include the fossils of Java man, Peking man, Heidelberg man, Algerian or Atlantic man. **Characteristics** • They were the oldest known early human to have modern human like body proportion. These males were taller than females. • They were the first human species to have fleshy nose. They had flat skull with prominent ridges over the brow. • They had short arm and long legs. The short arms depict that the tree climbing ability was lost completely in them. The long legs depict that they are better suited for long distance migrations. • They were the first one to walk upright and stood erect thus, named so. They are also known as *Homo ergaster.* • They were the first hominid to live in hunter-gatherer society.
Java man or *Pithecanthropus erectus* or *Homo erectus erectus* (ape man that walks erect) 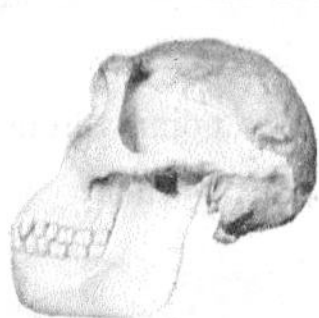 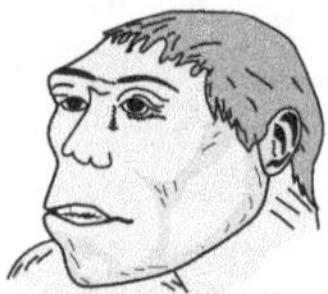 ***Java man***	**Discovery** • In 1891, **Eugene Dubois** obtained fossils (some teeth, skull cap and femur bone) from Pleistocene deposits (5,00,000-1,50,0000 years back) in Central Java (an island of Indonesia). • It was named *Pithecanthropus erectus* (ape man that can walk erect) by Eugene Dubois and *Homo erectus erectus* by **Mayer** (1950). **Characteristics** • Java man was more than 1.65-1.75 m tall and had weight about 70 kg. • Its legs were long and erect, but body slightly bent during movement. • The face of Java man was prognathous, whereas forehead was low and slanting. • Its jaws were large and heavy, but quite similar to those of modern man, except larger canines of the lower jaw. • Its nose was flattened and chin was inconspicuous along with thick and protruding lips. • Java man was omnivorous and cannibal. • Java man was the first pre-historic man, who began the use of fire for cooking, defence and hunting. • Its cranial cavity was 940 cc, which is about intermediate between *Australopithecus* (600-700 cc) and modern man (1400-1600 cc).
Peking man (*Homo erectus pekinensis* or *Pithecanthropus pekinensis* or *Sinanthropus pekinensis*) 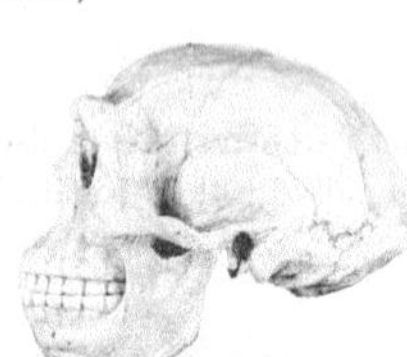 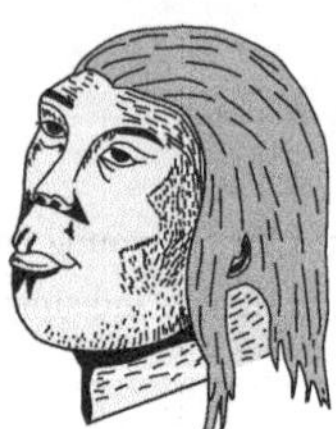 ***Peking man***	**Discovery** • The fossils (skulls, jaws and post cranial bony fragments) of peking man were discovered by **WC Pai** (1924) from the lime stone caves of Choukoutien near Peking (Peking is the former name of China's capital Beijing). • **WC Pai** named Java man *Sinanthropus*, whereas **Davison Black** (1927) named it *Sinanthropus pekinensis* and **Mayer** (1950) called it *Homo erectus pekinensis.* • These fossils of Peking man were about six lakh years old. **Characteristics** • Peking man was 1.55-1.60 m tall, i.e. slightly shorter, lighter and weaker than Java man. • The cranial cavity of Peking man was 850 -1200 cc that is more than Java man. • Morphology was similar to Java man with heavy bony eyebrow ridges, low slanting forehead and chinless face. • The Peking ape man was omnivorous and cannibal. • Clear evidences have been obtained from Hungary and China in support of use of fire by Peking man. These were hunters and food gatherers. • Like Java man, Peking man also lived in caves in small groups or tribes or communities. • Peking man was the first to begin with the use of clothes (made from animal skins), rudimentary languages and tools made with wood and bones. • In tool making, it was more expert than java man and tools were relatively more sophisticated. • Their tools included chopping tools, hand axes, flakes, scrapers paints, etc. • They used these stone tools for hunting and butchering deers, antelopes, bears, wild oxen and even elephants.

Heidelberg man
(*Homo erectus heidelbergensis*)

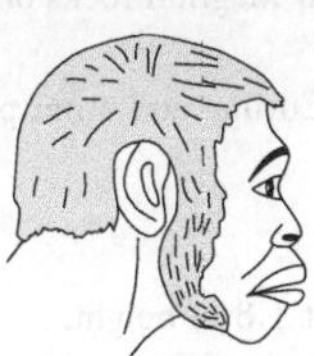

Heidelberg man

Discovery

- The fossil of Heidelberg man is represented by lower jaw, which was found from the middle Pleistocene rocks of Heidelberg (Germany).
- Credit for the discovery of Heidelberg man goes to **Otto Schoetensack**.

Characteristics

- It had ape like lower jaw with all the teeth. The teeth were human like.
- The jaw was large, heavy and lack a chin.
- Its cranial cavity was probably about 1300 cc, intermediate between erect man (*H. erectus*) and Neanderthal man (*H. sapiens neanderthalensis*).
- Heidelberg man is regarded as an ancestor of Neanderthal man and contemporary to *Homo erectus*.

True man (including living modern man)

Homo erectus gave rise to *Homo sapiens* during late Pleistocene period. In support of this evolution, some transitional forms connecting *Homo erectus* with *Homo sapiens* have been discovered, which are given below

Steinheim skull	—	Germany
Swanscombe skull	—	England
Fhringsdorf skull	—	Germany
Neanderthal skull	—	Germany
Solo	—	Java
Rhodesian	—	Africa
Cro-Magnon	—	Europe

Piltdown man fossil was discovered in 1912. It was thought to be a missing link for over 50 years.

Table 14.6 True man (including living modern man)

Neanderthal man (*Homo sapiens neanderthalensis*)

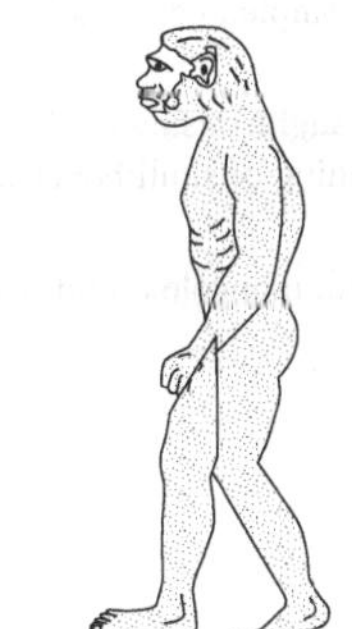

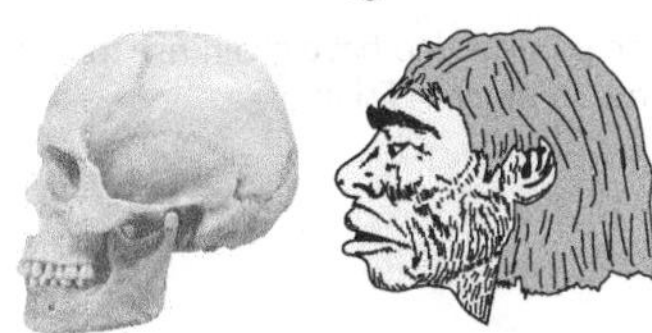

Neanderthal man

Discovery

- Fossils of Neanderthal man were discovered by **C Fuhlrott** (1856) from Neander valley in Germany.
- Neanderthal man arose about 1,50,000 years ago and flourished in Asia, Europe and North Africa. Neanderthal man extinct about 25,000 years ago.

Characteristics

- Neanderthal man existed in the late Pleistocene period.
- Neanderthal walked upright with bipedal movement.
- The face was slightly prognathous and had low brows, receding jaws and high domed heads.
- The cranial cavity of Neanderthal man was 1300-1600 cc average 1450 cc.
- The jaw was deep with no chin and skull bones were thick.
- Culturally, these were more advanced than Java and Peking man.
- They used to kill the large animals by group attack and used knives to butcher.
- Neanderthal man was omnivorous and cannibal, which used fire for cooking and warmth. They used animal skin as clothing to protect themselves against cold environment and got adapted to cold environment.
- It is believed that Neanderthal man had the concept of life and death and followed rituals. It is also believed that they buried dead bodies with flowers and tools. They may have had a religion.

Cro-Magnon man (*Homo sapiens fossilis*) or fossil man closest to modern man or direct ancestor of living modern man.

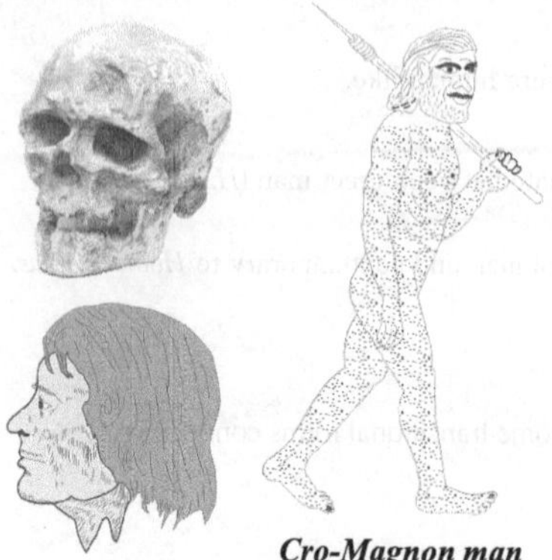

Cro-Magnon man

Discovery

- **Mac Gregor** discovered the fossil of Cro-Magnon man from Cro-Magnon rocks of France in 1868.
- Cro-Magnon man arose about 3,40,000 years ago and lived in Europe and other parts of world, which became extinct about 10,000-11,000 years ago.

Characteristics

- Cro-Magnon man was almost similar to modern man with about 1.8 m height. orthognathous face, broad and arched forehead, strong jaws, elevated nose and well-developed chin as well as dentition.
- Cranial capacity was about 1650 cc, i.e. much more than modern man (1450 cc).
- They were intelligent, hard worker, swift footed and cave dweller hunters.
- They could run fast and lived in families.
- They used spears, bows and arrows as tools, which were made up of stones, bones or elephant tusks.
- They were omnivorous and wore skin clothes.
- Probably they succeeded from Neanderthal man and distributed in Africa, Europe and Middle East.
- They used to made **cave paintings** on the cave walls. Paintings that represented reindeer, bison and wild bear have been discovered.
- Cro-Magnon lived during old stone age which is also known as **Palaeolithic** (began more than 2 million years ago)

Living Modern man (*Homo sapiens sapiens*)

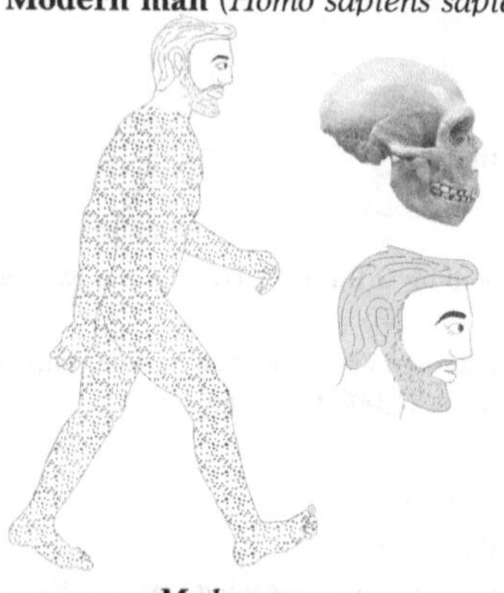

Modern man

Discovery

- It is believed that living modern men first appeared about 10,000 years ago in the regions of Caspian sea and Mediterranean sea.

Characteristics

- Its cranial capacity is average 1450 cc, which is lesser than Cro-Magnon.
- Its limbs are straight and arms are shorter than legs.
- It shows erect posture with upright head with complex cerebral hemispheres and cerebellum.
- It is distinguished from Cro-Magnon merely by slight raising of skull cap, reduction in volume of cranial capacity (1300-1600 cc), thinning of skull bones and formation of four curves in the vertebral column.
- Human species (*sapiens*) have white or caucasoid, mongoloid and black or negroid races.

Recently discovered fossils

Grimaldi : From the caves in village Grimaldi on the Mediterranean coast, cranial capacity 1655 cc is belived to have given rise to Negroid stock.
Chancelade In rock shetter near Chancelade in Dordogne France, cranial capacity 1450 cc gave rise to modern Eskimos.

Table 14.7 Time line related to human evolution

Human evolution	Time scale
Apes (hominoids) diverged from monkeys.	25 million years ago
Gibbons diverged from other apes.	10 million years ago
Orangutan diverged from other apes.	8 million years ago
Ancestral ape population divided into three lineages, which would separately give rise to bipedal humans, chimpanzees and massive vegetarian gorillas.	4 million years ago
Most famous fossil 'Lucy' (40% complete female skeleton obtained by Mary Leakey from Hadar).	3.6-3.8 million years old
Australopithecus obtained by Raymond Dart (1924).	2.8 million years old
Robust *Australopithecus* co-existed with early human ancestors.	2.0-1.5 million years ago
The oldest stone tools associated with *Homo habilis.*	2.5 million years old
Homo habilis replaced by *Homo erectus.*	1.5 million years ago
Homo erectus migrated from Africa and had colonised the accessible world.	7,00,000 years ago
African population continued to evolve and gave rise to modern human (*Homo sapiens*).	1,00,000-2,00,000 years ago
Neanderthal people lived.	1,20,000-35,000 years ago
Cro-Magnon man was present in middle East.	40,000 years ago
Cro-Magnon man who replaced the Neanderthal man spread through Europe.	35,000 years ago
Cro-Magnon man became extinct.	10,000 years ago
Living modern man (*Homo sapiens sapiens*) spread all over the world.	About 10,000 years ago

Table 14.8 Cranial cavity volume of different hominoids

Hominoids	Cranial cavity volumes
Gibbon (*Hylobates hoolock*)	100 cc
Orangutan (*Pongo pigmaeus*)	400 cc
Chimpanzee (*Anthropithecus satyrus*)	400 cc
Gorilla (*Gorilla*)	550 cc
Dryopithecus (Common ancestor of man and ape)	400 cc
Australopithecus africans (First ape man)	450-700 cc
Zinjanthropus man (*Australopithecus boisei*)	615 cc
Homo habilis (Handy man)	680 cc
Homo erectus (Erect man)	680 cc
(a) Java man (*Homo erectus erectus*)	750-900 cc
(b) Peking man (*Homo erectus pekinensis*)	1075 cc
Neanderthal man (*Homo neanderthalensis*)	1400-1450 cc
Cro-Magnon man (*Homo sapiens fossilis*)	1600 cc (highest)
Modern man (*Homo sapiens sapiens*)	1450 cc

CULTURAL EVOLUTION OF HUMAN

Cultural evolution of *Homo sapiens* in the upper Pleistocene period took place through following revolutions

- Cultural revolution, i.e. living in groups with protected life.
- Tool making revolution, i.e. the use of fine tools for hunting.
- Agricultural revolution, i.e. use of agricultural practices, settled life and domestication about 6,000 years ago.
- Scientific industrial revolution, i.e. the use of improved techniques of food production, industrialisation and medicine about 300 years ago.

The first population explosion occurred during tool making revolution and second and third during agricultural and scientific industrial evolution, reoccurred spectively.

The most prominent feature of humans is their mental ability. Human beigns are capable of learning from experiences. This is the reason human beings exhibit adaptive behaviour which is not present in anyone else.

Human can acquire and transmit practices and behaviour through social exchange which involves language or teaching. This forms the base of cultural evolution.

Table 14.9 Some events of cultural evolution

Age	Years ago	Events of cultural evolution
Palaeolithic	> 2,00,0000	Production of tools and cave drawings.
Mesolithic	12,000	Domestication of animals (dog first) and development of water transport.
Neolithic	7,000	Change from hunting and gathering to agriculture.
Bronze age	5,000	Use of copper and tin, origin of urbanisation.
Iron age	3,500	Use of iron.
Industrial	150	Industrial revolution.
Atomic	30	Use of nuclear energy.

Future man (*Homo futuris*)

The organic evolution is a continuous process of nature. It is still continued and probably will continue to do so in future as well. It is believed that in future, human could be changed as a result of the factors like gene mutation, gene recombination and natural selection. According to the forecasting of **HL Shapiro**, an American anthropologist, the future man (named *Homo futuris*) will possess following characteristics

- Height will be higher.
- Hair will reduced and skull may become dome-shaped.
- Body and cranium will be more developed.
- The fifth finger probably may get reduced.
- The age will increase.

Out of Africa Again

The origin of humans race is a much-debated point among scientists studying human evolution. Many argue that the diffrent transitional forms connecting *Homo erectus* with *Homo sapiens* have been uncovered from Europe. These are Steinheim skull (Germany), Swanscombe skull (second interglacial period), Fontechvade skulls (France, third interglacial period) and Ehringsdorf skull. All of these are called early *Homo sapiens*.

Other believe that the same species would be unlikely to evolve more than once and argue that human races appeared after *Homo sapiens* evolved from *H. erectus*. Recently, scientists studying mitochondrial DNA from living humans all over the world have argued. Their research shows that all human races originated from one *Homo sapiens* ancestor in Africa.

As the time passed the *Homo sapiens* born in Africa spread to all parts of the world, retracting the path taken by *Homo erectus* half millon years before.

CHECK POINT 14.2

1. The study of human evolution is based on fossil records found all over the world. Out of these, fossil of which of the following were found in Egypt?
(a) *Propliopithecus* and *Proconsul*
(b) *Limnopithecus* and *Pliopithecus*
(c) *Aegyptopithecus* and *Propiopithecus*
(d) All of the abvoe

2. Which is considered as the common ancestor of gibbon, orangutan, chimpanzee, gorilla and man?
(a) *Proconsul* (b) *Dryopithecus*
(c) *Shivapithecus* (d) *Pliopithecus*

3. Tool making is one of the important evolutionary aspect seen in humans. Out of the given option, which of the following did not used tool for their survival?
(a) *Homo habilis*
(b) Peking man
(c) Java man
(d) *Australopithecus*

4. A difference between handy man and erect man is that former
(a) lived in small community in caves
(b) had fleshy nose
(c) had short arm and long legs
(d) had cranial capacity of 700-800 cc

5. Which of the following hominoid does not have a cranial capacity between 400 cc to 700 cc?
(a) Java man
(b) Handy man
(c) Erect man
(d) Ape man

6. Where were the signals of first living modern man appeared?
(a) Caspian sea
(b) Mediterranean sea
(c) Arabian sea
(d) Both (a) and (b)

EXAM POINTS

- The rise of Ist primates occurred in Paleocene epoch. **[MHT CET 2014]**
- DNA of both autosomes and sex chromosomes suggest that the chimpanzee is more closely related to humans than other hominoid apes. **[CBSE AIPMT 2012]**
- About 15 mya, primates called *Dryopithecus* and *Ramapithecus* were existing. They were hairy and walked like gorillas and chimpanzees. **[NEET 2019]**
- The first fossil of *Australopithecus* was discovered in Taung in South Africa. **[MHT CET 2015]**
- *Ramapithecus* is the name given to fossil hominid of Shivalik hills in India. **[WB JEE 2013]**
- The primate, which existed 15 million years ago was *Ramapithecus.* **[Kerala CEE 2011, 2010]**
- *Ramapithecus punjabicus* is the most primitive ancestor of man. **[WB JEE 2011]**
- The scientific name of Java man is *Homo erectus erectus.* **[WB JEE 2013]**
- *Homo erectus* evolved during Pleistocene and had brain capacity of 900 cc. **[WB JEE 2012]**
- *Homo erectus* probably ate meat. **[NEET 2019]**
- *Homo erectus* fossil was the hominid fossil discovered in Java in 1891 now extinct having cranial capacity of about 900 cc. **[NEET 2020]**
- The hominid fossils discovered in Java in 1891 revealed a stage in human evolution which was called *Homo erectus.* **[Kerala CEE 2014]**
- The extinct human who lived 1,00,000-40,000 years ago in Europe, Asia and parts of Africa, with short stature, heavy eyebrows, retreating foreheads, large jaws with heavy teeth, stocky bodies, lumbering gait and stoped posture was Neanderthal human. **[CBSE AIPMT 2012]**
- Neanderthal men lived in Asia between 1,00,000 and 40,000 year back. **[NEET 2019]**
- *Homo neanderthalensis* shows similarity with first man. **[EAMCET 2015]**
- Agriculture came around 10,000 years back. **[NEET 2019]**
- *Homo habilis* brain size is 650- 800 cc, *Homo neanderthalensis* brain size is 1400 cc, *Homo erectus* brain size is 900 cc and *Homo sapiens* brain size is 1350 cc. **[NEET 2019]**
- The correct sequence of man taxonomically starting from superfamily to subfamily is
  Hominoidea $\rightarrow$ Hominidae $\rightarrow$ Homininae **[EAMCET 2015]**
- The cranial capacity of modern man is about 1200-1600 cc. **[AFMC 2013, UP CPMT 2011]**
- Increasing brain capacity is the most significant trend in the evolution of modern man (*Homo sapiens*) from his ancestors. **[CBSE AIPMT 2012]**
- *Dryopithecus* $\rightarrow$ *Ramapithecus* $\rightarrow$ *Australopithecus* $\rightarrow$ *Homo habilis* $\rightarrow$ *Homo erectus* $\rightarrow$ *Homo neanderthalensis*
  The above given sequence represents the origin and evolution of man. **[NEET 2016]**

Chapter Exercises

(A) Topical Exercise

Primates

1 Who gave the concept of placing man among apes?
(a) TH Huxley (b) C Darwin
(c) C Linnaeus (d) E Darwin

2 Which of the following statements is incorrect for *Homo sapiens.*
(a) The term *Homo sapiens* was coined by C Linnaeus
(b) *Homo sapiens* belongs to the class-Mammalia
(c) *Homo sapiens* belongs to the order-Primates
(d) The scientific explanation of human evolution was given by C Linnaeus

3 Which of the following is correct in taxonomical and evolution point of view?
(a) Bat — Monkey — Man
(b) Bat — Pigeon — Man
(c) Monkey — Chimpanzee — Man
(d) Monkey — Bat — Man

4 Which of the following is considered to be a trend in primate evolution?
(a) Development of non-prehensile hands
(b) Development of monocular vision
(c) Elimination of the clavicle
(d) Decreased dependence on smell

5 First mammal occurred in which era/period?
(a) Permian-Palaeozoic (b) Triassic-Mesozoic
(c) Tertiary-Cenozoic (d) None of these

6 The primates were originated from
(a) tree shrew (b) tarsiers
(c) apes (d) monkey

7 The period in which lemurs were evolved
(a) Miocene epoch
(b) Paleocene period
(c) Both (a) and (b)
(d) None of the above

8 The cranial capacity is minimum in
(a) rhesus monkey (b) gorilla
(c) chimpanzee (d) cebus monkey

9 The suborder-Prosimians of class-Mammalia includes
(a) lemurs (b) tarsiers
(c) monkey (d) Both (a) and (b)

10 Which primate group (groups) existed during the first half of the Eocene epoch (53-38 million years ago)?
(a) prosimians
(b) prosimians and monkeys
(c) prosimians, monkeys and apes
(d) prosimians, monkeys, apes and hominids

11 Which of the following is not an adaptation in prosimians for life in the trees (i.e. an arboreal existence)?
(a) Flat, sensitive pads at the ends of fingers and toes
(b) Forward facing eyes
(c) Prehensile tails
(d) Flat nails on most digits rather than claws

12 Which of the following was the second group to appear in primate evolution, with fossil remains dated to the early Oligocene epoch (over 31 million years ago)?
(a) Prosimians (b) Anthropoids
(c) Great apes (d) Hominids

13 The suborder-Anthropoidea of class-Mammalia includes
(a) *Homo sapiens* (b) Apes
(c) Both (a) and (b) (d) None of these

14 Which of the following is a Catarrhine primate?
(a) Humans (b) Lemur
(c) Rhesus monkeys (d) Loris

15 The most obvious and consistent difference between the old world monkey and new world monkey lies in the form of
(a) hands (b) legs (c) nose (d) colour

16 Which of the following is correct for old world monkey?
(a) Narrow nose (b) Non-prehensile tail
(c) 32 teeth (d) All of these

17 Which of the following is true of new world monkeys?
(a) Most have prehensile tails
(b) Most have ischial callosities on their buttocks
(c) Includes langurs, guenons and mandrills
(d) Forward and downward, rather than lateral, orientation of nostrils

18 The new world monkeys belong to the superfamily
(a) Catarrhini (b) Cercopithecoidea
(c) Platyrrhini (d) Hominoids

19 Which of these represent *Pongo*?
(a) Gibbon (b) Chimpanzee
(c) Gorilla (d) Orangutan

20 Orangutan is found in
(a) Sumatra and Borneo
(b) India and Pakistan
(c) West Indies and America
(d) Australia and Sri Lanka

21 The three apes included in family-Pongidae are
(a) chimpanzee, gorilla and monkey
(b) chimpanzee, monkey and tarsiers
(c) chimpanzee, gorilla and tarsiers
(d) orangutan, gibbon and chimpanzee

22 Among the primates, knuckle walkers are
(a) man and gorilla (b) monkey and tarsiers
(c) gibbons and orangutans (d) gorilla and chimpanzee

23 The Brachial style of locomotion is related to the evolution of erect body posture. This type of locomotion is observed in
(a) gorilla (b) chimpanzee
(c) gibbons (d) monkey

24 Consider the following statements.
I. The most intelligent ape is chimpanzee.
II. Chimpanzee is called the cousin of modern man.
Choose the correct option.
(a) Statement I is true, but II is false
(b) Statement I is false, but I is true
(c) Both statements I and II are true
(d) Both statements I and II are false

25 The largest ape is
(a) chimpanzee (b) gibbon
(c) gorilla (d) orangutan

26 Tail is absent in
(a) lorises (b) tarsiers (c) simians (d) *Homo erectus*

27 The common relationship between chimpanzee and man is shown by
(a) binocular vision
(b) bipedal locomotion
(c) dental formula
(d) banding pattern in chromosomes

28 The banding pattern study of chromosomes of human and chimpanzee shows great similarity on chromosome numbers.
(a) 2 and 4 (b) 6 and 9 (c) 3 and 6 (d) 6 and 6

29 On the basis of banding pattern study of chromosome, apes chromosomes are similar to human chromosomes about
(a) 50% (b) 70% (c) 90% (d) 99%

30 The percentage of homology between haemoglobin, a protein of man and chimpanzee is
(a) 10% (b) 30%
(c) 75% (d) 100%

31 Which of the following is not the characteristic of apes?
(a) Movement in the trees by the brachiation
(b) Movement on the ground by knuckle walking
(c) Wrists that bend backward
(d) Highly mobile shoulder joints

32 The most important character of man from evolution point of view is
(a) erect posture and bipedal locomotion
(b) opposable thumb
(c) larger size of brain with creative intelligence
(d) All of the above

33 Simian shelf is a characteristic of apes, which connects the
(a) posterior part of the mandibles
(b) anterior part of the mandibles
(c) brains and limbs
(d) limbs and girdle

34 Genus-*Homo* is included in family-Hominidae, has following common characters except one
(a) excellent monocular vision
(b) bipedal locomotion
(c) erect posture
(d) arms shorter than legs

35 Dexterity in man means that he has
(a) his thumb opposite to fingers
(b) more brain volume
(c) binocular vision
(d) an erect posture

36 The evolution of man was possible because our ape like ancestors had
(a) migratory habits (b) binocular vision
(c) omnivorous diet (d) quadrupedal locomotion

37 The modern man differs from the apes in
(a) protruding eyes (b) spare body hair
(c) wearing of clothes (d) arms shorter than legs

38 Which of the following is not in the direction of evolution of human species?
(a) Erect posture (b) Opposable thumb
(c) Binocular vision (d) Raised eyebrow ridges

39 Which of the following changes have taken place from apes to man?
(a) Canine become short
(b) Pelvis became short and wide
(c) Foot became short and small
(d) All of the above

Human Evolution

40 The evolution of man has started during
(a) Oligocene and Miocene period
(b) Eocene and Oligocene period
(c) Paleocene and Eocene period
(d) Miocene and Pliocene period

41 According to fossils discovered upto present time origin and evolution of man was started from which country?
(a) France (b) Java (c) Africa (d) China

42 Hominisation is a
(a) process of development of human characteristics that differentiate them from their ancestors
(b) fossil formation of man
(c) process of becoming caves
(d) process of soil formation

43 Where were the fossils for *Pliopithecus* obtained?
(a) Faiyum deposits of Egypt
(b) Victoria lake, Kenya
(c) Faiyum deposits of Africa
(d) Rocks in Europe

44 The characteristic feature of *Dryopithecus* is
(a) semierect posture (b) rounded skull
(c) large canine (d) All of these

45 The age of fossil of *Dryopithecus* on the geological time scale is
(a) 25×10^6 years ago (b) 50×10^6 years ago
(c) 90×10^6 years ago (d) 95×10^6 years ago

46 Choose the correct option about *Ramapithecus.*
(a) They were the first hominids
(b) Edward Lewis obtained their fossils from Shivalik hills
(c) Arched palate, uniformed sized teeth were found in them
(d) All of the above

47 A female fossil skeleton named 'Lucy' is a popular name in human evolution. It refers to
(a) *A. afarensis* (b) *A. africanus*
(c) *A. ramidus* (d) *A. robustus*

48 The ancestor of man, who showed first bipedal form and entirely erect posture was
(a) *Australopithecus* (b) Neanderthal man
(c) Java ape man (d) Cro-Magnon man

49 *Australopithecus* is also known as Southern ape, because it had
(a) man like characters (b) ape like characters
(c) monkey like characters (d) Both (a) and (b)

50 Consider the following statements for *Homo habilis.*
I. They used tools for the first time in evolution.
II. Their cranial capacity is 680 cc.
Choose the correct option.
(a) Statement I is true, but II is false
(b) Statement I is false, but II is true
(c) Both statements I and II are true
(d) Both statements I and II are false

51 Which of the following is considered to be the members of the species *Homo erectus?*
(a) Peking man (b) Java man
(c) Neanderthal man (d) Both (a) and (b)

52 Which of these is believed to have first made use of fire for hunting, cooking and protection?
(a) Java man (b) Peking man
(c) Neanderthal man (d) Cro-Magnon man

53 Which of these presumably possessed a cranial capacity almost equal to or even a bit larger than of today's man?
(a) Neanderthal man (b) Java man
(c) Peking man (d) *Australopithecus*

54 The fossils of Peking man were found in caves near Peking in China. The Peking man was also named as
(a) *Pithecanthropus chinensis* (b) *Homo pekinensis*
(c) *Sinanthropus pekinensis* (d) *Pithecanthropus erectus*

55 Which of the following became extinct in competition with *Homo sapiens* and also inbreed with *Homo sapiens?*
(a) Cro-Magnon man (b) Neanderthal man
(c) *Australopithecus* (d) *Ramapithecus*

56 First evidences of religious feeling of worship and ceremonials burial of dead have been found with fossils of
(a) Cro-Magnon man (b) Neanderthal man
(c) Peking man (d) Java man

57 The primitive form of *Homo sapiens,* who made tools, cover his body with hides and built huts was
(a) *Homo sapiens neanderthalensis*
(b) *Homo habilis*
(c) *Homo pekinensis*
(d) *Homo sapiens sapiens*

58 Neanderthal man have
(a) equal cranial cavity than Cro-Magnon
(b) more cranial cavity than Cro-Magnon
(c) more cranial cavity than modern man
(d) less cranial cavity than modern man

59 Match the Column I with Column II. Select the correct option from the codes given below.

Column I (Primates)	Column I (Cranial capacities in cubic centimetres)
A. Chimpanzee and gorilla	1. 325 -510 cc
B. *Australopithecus*	2. 500 cc
C. *Homo habilis*	3. 700 cc
D. Java ape man	4. 800-1000 cc

Codes

	A	B	C	D		A	B	C	D
(a)	4	3	2	1	(b)	2	3	4	1
(c)	1	2	3	4	(d)	3	2	1	4

60 Consider the following statements.

I. Most of the cave paintings discovered are associated with Cro-Magnon man.
II. The discovery of fossils of Cro-Magnon man was done by Mac Gregor.

Choose the correct option.
(a) Statement I is true, but II is false
(b) Statement I is false, but II is true
(c) Both statements I and II are true
(d) Both statements I and II are false

61 The false statement about Cro-Magnon man is
(a) his cranial cavity was less than *Homo sapiens*
(b) he walked erect and was swift
(c) he was intelligent and cultured
(d) he started metal work, painting and farming

62 Which one is called a man with ape brain?
(a) *Australopithecus* (b) *Dryopithecus*
(c) *Sinanthropus* (d) *Pithecanthropus*

63 There was a cultural evolution rather than structural evolution after
(a) *Homo erectus* stage
(b) Cro-Magnon stage
(c) *Australopithecus* stage
(d) Neanderthal man stage

64 The Latin meaning of *Homo sapiens* is
(a) man, who is wise
(b) man with lower cranial capacity
(c) man, who appears same as ape
(d) man, who thinks same

65 *Homo sapiens sapiens* first appeared about
(a) 5 thousand years ago (b) 1 lakh years ago
(c) 2 lakh years ago (d) 10 thousand years ago

66 The difference between *Homo sapiens* and *Homo erectus* was
(a) *Homo sapiens* originated in Africa, while *Homo erectus* originated in Asia
(b) *Homo erectus* states much smaller in size than *Homo sapiens*
(c) *Homo erectus* states in Africa, while *Homo sapiens* did not
(d) the size of the brain of *Homo erectus* was smaller than that of *Homo sapiens*

67 The major advantage of bipedal locomotion is that it
(a) increases speed
(b) reduces body weight
(c) releases the forelimbs for other better functions
(d) provides better body support

68 The diagram given here shows the skull of two different mammals. Choose the most appropriate difference between *A* and *B*.

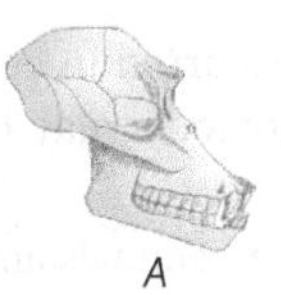

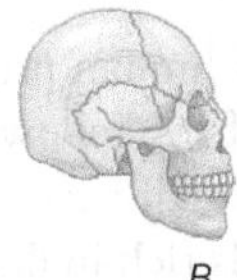

(a) Skull *A* has more teeth than skull *B*
(b) Skull *A* has more brain capacity than skull *B*
(c) Skull *A* is of a human and skull *B* is of an ape
(d) Skull *A* is of an ape and skull *B* is of human

69 The earliest site where human civilisation and crop cultivation started, was presumably
(a) around river Nile
(b) around Caspian and Mediterranean seas
(c) Chinese river valley
(d) Indus river valley

70 The domestication of first animal (dog) and development of water transport have taken place about 12000 years ago in
(a) Neolithic age (b) Mesolithic age
(c) Palaeolithic age (d) Atomic age

71 Which of the following revolution is characterised by living in groups and leading a protected life which enabled a large number of individuals to survive?
(a) Industrial revolution (b) Tool making revolution
(c) Cultural revolution (d) Agricultural revolution

72 Which of the following change in evolution of man is irrelevant?
(a) Development of opposable thumb
(b) Development of erect posture
(c) Loss of tail
(d) Excellent stereoscopic vision

73 The evidence from molecular biology, such as comparisons of DNA base-pair sequences in genes, indicates that hominids diverged from the African apes sometime between
(a) 5,00,000 and 1 million year ago
(b) 5 million and 10 million years ago
(c) 15 million and 20 million years ago
(d) 50 million and 60 million years ago

(B) Cumulative Exercise

(Assorted Questions of the Chapter for Advanced Level Practice)

1 Which of the following statements is correct?

I. *Homo erectus* is the ancestor of man.
II. Cro-Magnon fossils were found in Germany.
III. *Australopithecus* is the real ancestor of modern man.
IV. Neanderthal man is almost a direct ancestor of modern man.

Codes
(a) I and II (b) II, III and IV
(c) Only III (d) Only IV

2 Origin of human probably occurred in central Asia. Which of the following statements may be a reason for this?

I. Asia is rich in domesticated animals and plants.
II. Climatic conditions of Asian places were most favourable for human evolution.
III. The oldest known fossils have been originated from Asia.
IV. Human fossils are found only at these places.

Codes
(a) I, II and III (b) I and IV
(c) I and II (d) II, III and IV

3 Read the given statements regarding *Homo erectus*?

I. Fossils of *Homo erectus* obtained from diverse sites of Africa, Java and China.
II. *Homo erectus* survived about 14-15 million years ago during late Miocene to Pliocene.
III. *Homo erectus* species include Java man, Peking man, Heidelberg man, Algerian and Atlantic man.
IV. The forelimbs, skull and brain of *Homo erectus* resembled with monkeys.

Codes
(a) I and II (b) III and IV (c) I and IV (d) I and III

4 Human blood, when mixed with antibodies of human blood, will give maximum precipitation. If another animal's blood is mixed with antibodies of human blood, the percentage of precipitation indicates how similar the animal is to a human. The following experimental results were obtained.

Species : H 100%; M 37%; N 75%; O 79%; P 17%,
Which phylogeny would fit these results?

(a)
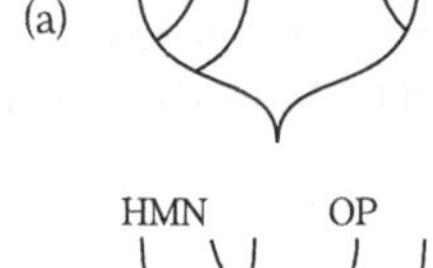

(b)
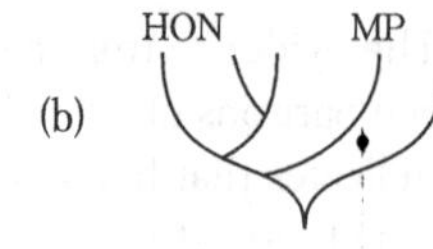

(c)
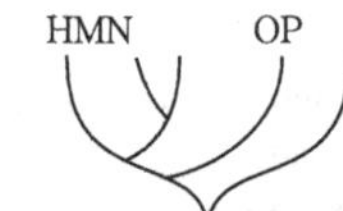

(d)
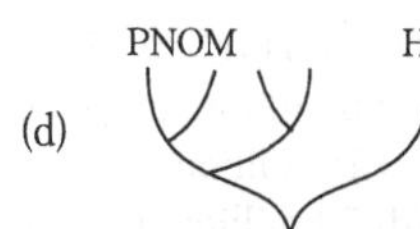

5 The correct sequence of human evolution is

(a) *Australopithecus* → Neanderthal man → Cro-Magnon man → *Homo sapiens*
(b) *Homo erectus* → *Ramapithecus* → Java man → Cro-Magnon man → *Homo sapiens*
(c) *Australopithecus* → *Homo erectus* → Neanderthal man → Cro-Magnon man → *Homo sapiens*
(d) *Australopithecus* → Neanderthal man → Cro-Magnon man → *Homo erectus* → *Homo sapiens*

6 Match the following columns.

Column I	Column II
A. *Homo habilis*	1. Fossil found in lime stone caves of Choukoutien
B. Gibbon	2. Fossils found in Pleistocene rock
C. Peking man	3. Diverged from apes 10 million year ago
D. Heidelberg man	4. Begun hunting for meat

Codes

	A	B	C	D		A	B	C	D
(a)	2	1	3	4	(b)	4	3	1	2
(c)	4	2	3	1	(d)	1	4	2	3

7 Consider the following evolutionary changes regarding human evolution.

I. Perfection of thumb opposability in forelimbs.
II. Loss of opposability of great toe in hindlimbs.
III. Erect posture of the development of lumbar curve.
IV. Presence of tail in human babies.

Choose the correct evolutionary changes.
(a) I, II and III (b) Only II
(c) Only III (d) II, III and IV

8 Go through the given statements.

I. First primates were tree shrews.
II. First primates were the group of prosimians.
III. First primates were having front eyes with colour vision, flat padded digits with claws or nails, etc.
IV. First primates were evolved from ancestral arthropods.

Choose the option containing correct statements.
(a) I and II (b) III and IV
(c) I, II and IV (d) Only III

9 Apes differ from hominids as

I. Hominids became bipedal, walking upright, while the apes evolved knuckle walking.
II. Human is with S-shaped spine whereas apes have C-shaped spine.
III. Hominids have mobile shoulder joints.
IV. Only apes have broadened chest due to flattening of sternum.

Choose the option containing correct statements.
(a) III and IV
(b) II and III
(c) I and II
(d) I, II, III and IV

10 Match the following columns.

Column I	Column II
A. Pliocene	1. *Sinanthropus pekinensis*
B. Richard Leakey	2. *Australopithecus*
C. Middle Pleistocene	3. *Homo neanderthalensis*
D. Fuhlrott	3. *Homo habilis*
E. Raymond Dart	4. *Oreopithecus*

Codes

	A	B	C	D	E
(a)	5	1	4	3	2
(b)	5	4	1	2	3
(c)	5	4	3	1	2
(d)	5	4	1	3	2

11 Consider the following statements about *Proconsul*?
I. It is the intermediate between apes and man.
II. Its canine teeth were small, but molar teeth were broad and flattened.
III. It had man like forehead and face was prognathous.
IV. It walked erect on its hind legs.
Choose the option containing incorrect statements.
(a) II and IV (b) I and II
(c) III and IV (d) Only I

12 The living modern man is characterised by
I. the average cranial capacity of about 1450 cc.
II. arms are shorter than legs.
III. erect posture and upright head with complex cerebral hemispheres and cerebellum.
IV. deep jaws with no chin.
Codes
(a) I, II and IV
(b) III and IV
(c) I, II and III
(d) I and IV

13 Consider the following statements regarding *Australopithecus.*
I. They were the first ape man and were omnivorous.
II. These were intelligent, hard worker, swift footed and cave dweller hunters.
III. It had prognathous face and high domed heads.
IV. It lived during old stone (Palaeolithic) age and made extraordinary painting on the cave walls.
V. Their body weight is 100-110 pound in males.
Choose the option containing incorrect statements.
(a) I and II (b) I, II and V
(c) III and IV (d) II and III

14 HL Shapiro, an American anthropologist, forecasted about the future man (*Homo futuris*) that
I. their hair will be reduced and body and cranium will be more developed.
II. the age will decrease.
III. height will be higher and the fifth finger probably will reduced.
IV. the skull will become rounded.
Codes
(a) Only I (b) I and II (c) I and III (d) III and IV

15 The new world monkeys use their tails for grasping the branches of trees due to
I. the presence of a long tail.
II. non-opposable thumbs.
III. short and weak hands.
IV. mostly clawed digits.
Codes
(a) I and IV (b) II and III (c) I and II (d) II and IV

16 Find out the incorrect statements about *Homo habilis.*
I. Also called able or skillful man.
II. Also called tool maker.
III. Fossil discovered from East Africa.
IV. 500 cc was its cranial capacity.
V. Have teeth like modern man.
VI. Lived nearly 2 million years ago.
Codes
(a) IV and V (b) Only IV
(c) II, III and VI (d) I, II, III, IV and VI

Assertion and Reason

Direction (Q. Nos. 17-23) *In each of the following questions, a statement of Assertion (A) is given followed by the corresponding statements of Reason (R). Of the statements, mark the correct answer as*
(a) Both A and R are true and R is the correct explanation of A
(b) Both A and R are true, but R is not the correct explanation of A
(c) A is true, but R is false
(d) A is false, but R is true
(e) Both A and R are false

17 **Assertion** (A) Among primates, chimpanzee is closest relative to the present day humans.
Reason (R) The banding pattern of autosomes 3 and 6 of humans and chimpanzee is remarkably similar.

18 **Assertion** (A) The immediate ancestor of present day humans was *Australopithecus.*
Reason (R) *Australopithecus* was discovered from Australia and its cranial capacity was 1150-1300 cm^2, which is very close to that of human 1400-1450 cm^3.

19 Assertion (A) Cro-Magnon man has more intelligence than the man of present time.

Reason (R) He is regarded as most recent ancestor of today's man.

20 Assertion (A) *mt*DNA of Africans shows about twice as much genetic variation as *mt*DNA among non-Africans.

Reason (R) *mt*DNA study supports the African hypothesis.

21 Assertion (A) Cranial capacity of Cro-Magnon man was 1600 cc.

Reason (R) Modern man has higher cranial capacity than Cro-Magnon man.

22 Assertion (A) *Dryopithecus africanus* is a common ancestor of man and great apes.

Reason (R) It gave rise to *Ramapithecus.*

23 Assertion (A) *Homo habilis* was the first tool maker.

Reason (R) He was a cave dweller.

(C) Medical Entrances' Gallery

(Collection of questions Asked in NEET & Various Medical Entrance Exams)

1 A hominid fossil discovered in Java in 1891 now extinct having cranial capacity of about 900 cc was **[NEET 2020]**

(a) *Homo erectus* (b) Neanderthal man
(c) *Homo sapiens* (d) *Australopithecus*

2 Match the Column I in hominids with Column II in their correct brain size. **[NEET 2019]**

Column I	Column II
A. *Homo habilis*	1. 900 cc
B. *Homo neanderthalensis*	2. 1350 cc
C. *Homo erectus*	3. 650-800 cc
D. *Homo sapiens*	4. 1400 cc

Codes

	A	B	C	D
(a)	3	2	1	4
(b)	3	4	1	2
(c)	4	3	1	2
(d)	3	1	4	2

3 Which of the following statements is correct about the origin and evolution of men? **[NEET 2016]**

(a) Agriculture came around 50,000 years back
(b) The *Dryopithecus* and *Ramapithecus* primates existing 15 million years ago, walked like men
(c) *Homo habilis* probably ate meat
(d) Neanderthal men lived in Asia between 1,00,000 and 40,000 years back

4 Identify the correct sequence with regard to the origin and evolution of *Homo sapiens.*

I. *Australopithecus* II. *Ramapithecus*
III. *Dryopithecus* IV. *Homo erectus*
V. *Homo neanderthalensis* VI. *Homo habilis*

Codes **[EAMCET 2016, NEET 2016]**

(a) II → III → I → IV → VI → V
(b) III → I → II → IV → VI → V
(c) II → III → I → IV → V → VI
(d) III → II → I → VI → IV → V

5 Which of the following shows similarity with first man? **[EAMCET 2015]**

(a) *Homo neanderthalensis* (b) *Australopithecus*
(c) *Homo erectus* (d) *Homo habilis*

6 What is correct sequence of man, taxonomically starting from superfamily to subfamily **[EAMCET 2015]**

(a) Hominoidea, Hominidae, Homininae
(b) Homininae, Hominoidea, Hominidae
(c) Hominidae, Homininae, Hominoidea
(d) Hominoidea, Homininae, Hominidae

7 The first fossil of *Australopithecus* was discovered in **[MHT CET 2015]**

(a) Olduvai Gorge, Tanzania
(b) Fayum deposits of Egypt
(c) Shivalik hills in India
(d) Taung in South Africa

8 Which of the following had the smallest brain capacity? **[CBSE AIPMT 2015]**

(a) *Homo erectus* (b) *Homo sapiens*
(c) *Homo neanderthalensis* (d) *Homo habilis*

9 The hominid fossils discovered in Java in 1891 revealed a stage in human evolution which was called **[Kerala CEE 2014]**

(a) *Homo erectus* (b) *Dryopithecus*
(c) *Australopithecus* (d) *Homo habilis*
(e) *Ramapithecus*

10 The rise of Ist primates occurred in .... epoch. **[MHT CET 2014]**

(a) Paleocene (b) Oligocene
(c) Miocene (d) Eocene

11 Name given to fossil hominid of Shivalik hills in India is **[WB JEE 2013]**

(a) *Ramapithecus*
(b) *Australopithecus*
(c) *Pithecanthropus*
(d) *Neanderthalensis*

12 The cranial capacity of modern man is **[AFMC 2013; UP CPMT 2011]**
(a) 430-650 cc^3
(b) 600-1000 cc^3
(c) 900-1100 cc^3
(d) 1200-1600 cc^3

13 The scientific name of Java man is **[WB JEE 2013]**
(a) *Homo habilis*
(b) *Homo sapiens neanderthalensis*
(c) *Homo erectus erectus*
(d) *Australopithecus boisei*

14 What was the most significant trend in the evolution of modern man (*Homo sapiens*) from his ancestors? **[CBSE AIPMT 2012]**
(a) Shortening of jaws
(b) Binocular vision
(c) Increasing brain capacity
(d) Upright posture

15 What evidence suggests that the chimpanzee is more closely related to humans than other hominoid apes? **[CBSE AIPMT 2012]**
(a) DNA from sex chromosomes only
(b) Chromosomes morphology only
(c) Fossil remains
(d) DNA of both autosomes and sex chromosomes

16 The extinct human who lived 1,00,000-40,000 years ago, in Europe, Asia and parts of Africa, with short stature, heavy eyebrows, retreating foreheads, large jaws with heavy teeth, stocky bodies, a lumbering gait and stooped posture was **[CBSE-AIPMT 2012]**
(a) *Homo habilis* (b) Neanderthal human
(c) Cro-Magnon human (d) *Ramapithecus*

17 *Homo erectus* evolved during **[WB JEE 2012]**
(a) Oligocene (b) Pliocene
(c) Pleistocene (d) Miocene

18 The brain capacity of *Homo erectus* was about **[Kerala CEE 2011]**
(a) 650 cc (b) 900 cc (c) 1200 cc (d) 1400 cc
(e) 1600 cc

19 The primate, which existed 15 million years ago, among these was **[Kerala CEE 2011, 10]**
(a) *Homo habilis* (b) *Australopithecus*
(c) *Ramapithecus* (d) *Homo erectus*
(e) Neanderthal man

20 Which one of the following is the most primitive ancestor of man? **[WB JEE 2011]**
(a) *Homo habilis* (b) *Australopithecus*
(c) *Ramapithecus punjabicus* (d) *Homo neanderthalensis*

ANSWERS

Check Point 14.1

1. (d)	2. (c)	3. (a)	4. (c)	5. (b)	6. (c)

Check Point 14.2

1. (c)	2. (b)	3. (d)	4. (d)	5. (a)	6. (d)

(A) Topical Exercise

1. (c)	2. (d)	3. (c)	4. (d)	5. (b)	6. (a)	7. (b)	8. (a)	9. (d)	10. (a)
11. (c)	12. (b)	13. (c)	14. (c)	15. (c)	16. (d)	17. (a)	18. (c)	19. (d)	20. (a)
21. (d)	22. (d)	23. (c)	24. (c)	25. (c)	26. (d)	27. (d)	28. (c)	29. (d)	30. (d)
31. (c)	32. (d)	33. (b)	34. (a)	35. (a)	36. (a)	37. (d)	38. (d)	39. (d)	40. (a)
41. (c)	42. (a)	43. (a)	44. (d)	45. (a)	46. (d)	47. (a)	48. (a)	49. (d)	50. (c)
51. (d)	52. (a)	53. (a)	54. (c)	55. (b)	56. (b)	57. (a)	58. (c)	59. (c)	60. (c)
61. (a)	62. (a)	63. (b)	64. (a)	65. (d)	66. (d)	67. (c)	68. (d)	69. (b)	70. (b)
71. (c)	72. (c)	73. (b)							

(B) Cumulative Exercise

1. (d)	2. (a)	3. (d)	4. (d)	5. (c)	6. (b)	7. (a)	8. (c)	9. (d)	10. (d)
11. (a)	12. (c)	13. (c)	14. (c)	15. (c)	16. (b)	17. (a)	18. (e)	19. (b)	20. (b)
21. (c)	22. (b)	23. (b)							

(C) Medical Entrances' Gallery

1. (a)	2. (b)	3. (d)	4. (d)	5. (a)	6. (a)	7. (d)	8. (d)	9. (a)	10. (a)
11. (a)	12. (d)	13. (c)	14. (c)	15. (d)	16. (b)	17. (c)	18. (b)	19. (c)	20. (c)

Explanations

(A) Topical Exercise

2 (*d*) Statement in option (d) is incorrect and can be corrected as
The scientific explanation of human evolution was given by Charles Darwin.
Rest statements are correct from *Homo sapiens.*

17 (*a*) Option (a) is true of new world monkeys. Rest options are incorrect and can be corrected as
- Old world monkeys have ischial callosities (i.e. sitting pads) on their buttocks.
- Old world monkeys include langurs, guenons and mandrills.
- Old world monkeys have forward and downward, rather than lateral, orientation of nostrils.

31 (*c*) Statement in option (c) is not the characteristic of apes and can be corrected as
Chimpanzees have wrists that bend backward.
Rest options are the characteristics of apes.

61 (*a*) Statement in option (a) is false and can be corrected as
The cranial cavity of Cro-Magnon man is 1600 cc which is more than *Homo sapiens*, i.e. 1400 cc.
Rest statements are correct about Cro-Magnon man.

(B) Cumulative Exercise

3 (*d*) Statements I and III are correct regarding *Homo erectus.* Statements II and IV are incorrect regarding *Homo erectus* and can be corrected as
- *Homo erectus* survived about 1.7 million years ago in the Pleistocene.
- *Homo erectus* resembled modern man not monkeys.

7 (*a*) Statements I, II and III are correct evolutionary changes regarding human evolution. Statement IV does not evolutionary changes regarding human evolution and can be corrected as
There is absence of tail in human babies.

8 (*c*) Statements I, II and IV are correct. Statement III is incorrect and can be corrected as
First primates had rods only in their eyes. Thus, had black and white vision.

11 (*a*) Statements II and IV are incorrect and can be corrected as
- *Proconsul* had long, pointed ape like canines.
- *Proconsul* walked on its four legs.

Rest statements are correct about *Proconsul.*

12 (*c*) Statements I, II and III are the characteristic of living modern man. Statement IV is not the characteristic of living modern man and can be corrected as
Living modern man has chin.

13 (*c*) Statements III and IV are incorrect for *Australopithecus* and can be corrected as
- Neanderthal man had prognathous face.
- Cro-Magnon man made cave paintings.

Rest statements are correct regarding *Australopithecus.*

14 (*c*) According to HL Shapiro, an Anthropologist the future man will have reduced hair, more developed body and cranium, higher height, reduced 5th finger, dome-shaped skull and their age will increase. Hence, option (c) is correct.

16 (*b*) Statement IV is incorrect about *Homo habilis* and can be corrected as
- *Homo habilis* cranial capacity of is 700-800 cc.

Rest statements are correct about *Homo habilis.*

17 (*a*) Both A and R are true and R is the correct explanation of A.
Among the primates, chimpanzee is the closest relative to the present day humans, because banding pattern in the autosome number 3 and 6 of both are similar, RNA content of diploid set is similar and DNA of man shows more than 90% similarity with chimpanzees.

18 (*e*) Both A and R are false and can be corrected as
The immediate ancestor of present day humans is *Homo sapiens fossilis*, i.e. Cro-Magnon man. They lived about 3,40,000 years ago. *Australopithecus* was first discovered in Taung Africa. Its cranial capacity is 500-700 cc, which is equivalent to modern gorilla.

19 (*b*) Both A and R are true, but R is not the correct explanation of A.
The Cro-Magnon man were more intelligent than modern man as their cranial capacity was about 1650 cc, i.e. much more than modern man (1450 cc). He is the most recent ancestor of modern day man.

20 (*b*) Both A and R are true, but R is not the correct explanation of A.
Mitochondrial DNA study supports the African hypothesis according to which modern human (*Homo sapiens*) evolved from *Homo erectus* only in Africa. *mt*DNA of Africans shows about twice as much genetic variation as *mt*DNA of non-Africans.

21 (*c*) A is true, but R is false because
The cranial capacity of Cro-Magnon man was about 1600 cc, whereas cranial capacity of modern man is 1450 cc, which is less than Cro-Magnon man.

22 (*b*) Both A and R are true, but R is not the correct explanation of A.
Dryopithecus africanus had broadened jaws semi-erect posture and large canines. It is considered as a common ancestor of man and great apes. It gave rise to *Ramapithecus* in late Miocene epoch.

23 (*b*) Both A and R are true, but R is not the correct explanation of A.
Homo habilis is called the first hominid tool maker because it had developed the most primitive stone tools.
It is also known as handy man or able man or skillful man. It lived in small groups or communities in caves, i.e. cave dweller.

(C) Medical Entrances' Gallery

1 (*a*) A hominid fossil discovered in Java in 1891 now extinct having cranial capacity of about 900 cc was *Homo erectus*. It probably ate meat.

3 (*d*) Statement in option (d) is correct about the origin and evolution of men.
Neanderthal men lived in Asia between 1,00,000 and 40,000 years back.

Rest statements are incorrect and can be corrected as

- Agriculture came around 10,000 years back.
- About 15 mya , primates called *Dryopithecus* and *Ramapithecus* were existing. They were hairy and walked like gorillas and chimpanzees.
- *Homo habilis* probably did not eat meat while *Homo erectus* probably ate meat.

8 (*d*) *Homo habilis* had the smallest brain capacity. *Homo habilis* also called the tool maker of handy man had a brain capacity of 700 cc.

Other options are explained as
Homo erectus had a brain or cranial capacity of 800-1300 cc.
Homo neanderthalensis had the brain or cranial capacity of 1300-1600 cc.
Homo sapiens or modern man showed a slight reduction in brain/cranial capacity, i.e. 1300-1600 cc will an average of 1450 cc.

9 (*a*) *Homo erectus* was known as Java man and reveal a stage in human evolution. In 1891, Eugene Dubois discovered fossil (some teeth, skull cap and femur bone) from Pleistocene deposits (5,00,000-15,00,000) years back in Central Java (an island Indonesia). It was named *Pithecanthropus erectus* (ape man that can walk erect) by him and *Homo erectus* by Mayr (1950).

10 (*a*) The first primate like mammals or protoprimates, evolved in the early Paleocene epoch (655-558 million years ago) at the beginning of the Cenozoic era. They were roughly similar to squirrels and tree shrews in size and appearance. The existing very fragmentary fossil evidence (from Asia, Europe, North Africa and especially Western North America) indicates an arboreal way of life in warm moist climates.

11 (*a*) *Ramapithecus* was first man like primate. The first fossil of *Ramapithecus* was fragment of upper jaw from Shivalik hills of India.

Other options are explained as
Australopithecus is intermediate between *Ramapithecus* and *Homo erectus* or *Pithecanthropus* and its fossils were described by Raymond Dart in 1925 from South America.
Fossils of Neanderthal man was discovered from Neander valley in Germany.

12 (*d*) The cranial capacity of a modern man is 1200-1600 cc^3, average about 1450 cc. *Homo sapiens sapiens* appeared about 25,000 years ago in Holocene epoch.

13 (*c*) Java man is the name given to fossils discovered in 1891 on the banks of the Solo river in East Java in Indonesia, one of the first known specimens of *Homo erectus erectus*. Its discoverer, gave it the scientific name *Pithecanthropus erectus*, a name derived from Greek and Latin roots meaning upright ape man.

14 (*c*) Modern man (*Homo sapiens sapiens*) is most evolved. The most significant trend in the evolution of modern man from his ancestors is the gradual increase in the cranial capacity. Cranial capacity of modern man is an average of 1450 cc.

15 (*d*) Chimpanzee is more closely related to man than other hominoids. It is evidenced by chromosome banding pattern, DNA extracted from sex chromosomes, autosomes and mitochondria.

Molecular clock based on mitochondrial DNA are used to date recent events because this DNA mutates 5-10 times faster than nuclear DNA.

Some similarities between human and chimpanzee are

- DNA matching shows that similarity of human with chimpanzee is 100%.
- There is a little difference in banding pattern in chromosomes 3 and 6 in human and chimpanzee.
- Serum test indicates maximum homology between human and chimpanzee.

16. (*b*) Neanderthal man with a brain size of 1400 cc lived near East and Central Asia, Europe and North Africa between 1,00,000 to 40,000 years ago. It had slightly prognathous face, retreating forehead, eyebrow ridges, no chin, large receding jaws with heavy teeth, thick boned skull and high domed head stocky bodies and stooped posture. They used hides to protect their body and buried their dead.

17. (*c*) *Homo erectus* (upright man or straight man) appeared about 1.3-4.8 million years ago in middle Pleistocene. This species originated in Africa and spread as far as India, China and Java. It walked erect over long legs height 0.5-1.79 m, brain size (cranial capacity) 775-1225 cm^3, (prognathous) face with prominent, brow ridges, no chin, massive jaws and large teeth use of tools made up of bones and stones, fire, acheulean hand axes and some primitive type of speech had developed.

18. (*b*) The brain capacity of *Homo erectus* was about 800-1100 cc. 900 cc comes in this range hence, option (b) is correct.

19. (*c*) *Ramapithecus* survived about 14-15 million years ago during late Miocene to Pliocene. Edward Lewis (1932) obtained fossil of *Ramapithecus* from Pliocene rocks of Shivalik hills of India. *Ramapithecus* became extinct about 1-8 million years ago.

20. (*c*) *Ramapithecus punjabicus* was the most primitive ancestor of man.

CHAPTER 15

Human Health and Diseases

Human health is related to overall fitness of the body. This fitness of the body sometimes gets altered due to some factors. These factors include bacteria, viruses, environmental contamination and improper lifestyle. In this chapter, we are dealing with human health and diseases associated with it.

Health

According to World Health Organisation (WHO), 'health is a state of complete physical, mental and social well-being and not merely an absence of disease'. Some basic factors, which contribute to our good health are balanced diet, personal hygiene and regular exercise. Good health increases longevity and reduces mortality rate of a population.

Diseases

Any change from normal state of the body which causes discomfort or disability in the body is called **disease.** In this condition, normal physiological functions of the body or an organ gets disturbed. This disturbance is mostly caused by disease causing organisms called **pathogens**. Various microorganisms responsible for causing infectious diseases are bacteria, viruses, fungi, protozoans, worm, etc.

Types of disease

Various types of pathogens enter our body, multiply and disturb the normal metabolic activities. They shatter the major organ systems that result in major diseases. The study of all factors that contribute to the appearance of a particular disease is called **epidemiology**. Diseases can be classified in the following ways

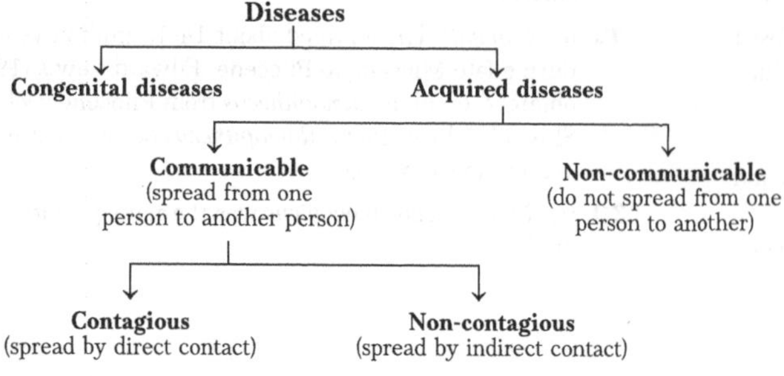

Inside

1. Communicable diseases or infectious diseases
2. Non-communicable diseases or Non-infectious diseases
3. Community health

Congenital diseases These diseases are present in the human beings since birth and may occur due to

- **Mutation**, e.g. alkaptonuria, phenylketonuria, albinism, sickle-cell anaemia, haemophilia, colour blindness, etc.
- **Chromosomal aberration,** e.g. Down's syndrome, Klinefelter's syndrome, Turner's syndrome, etc.
- **Environmental factors**, e.g. cleft palate, harelip cleft, etc.

Acquired diseases These diseases develop after birth. These are not inherited from parents to offspring. These can be communicable and non-communicable diseases. Some communicable diseases are described below

COMMUNICABLE OR INFECTIOUS DISEASES

These diseases are transferred from one diseased person to a normal person. Depending on the causative agent (pathogen), communicable diseases are of following types

(i) **Viral diseases** AIDS, measles, chicken pox, rabies, mumps, polio, smallpox, influenza, common cold, hepatitis, dengue, chikungunya, etc.
(ii) **Bacterial diseases** Typhoid, diphtheria, tetanus, cholera, tuberculosis, pertussis, meningitis, anthrax, syphilis, etc.
(iii) **Protozoan diseases** Kala-azar, malaria, sleeping sickness, amoebiasis, etc.
(iv) **Helminthic diseases** Filariasis, taeniasis, liver rot, ascariasis, trichinosis, etc.
(v) **Fungal diseases** Athlete's foot, ringworm, etc.
(vi) **Rickettsial diseases** Trench fever, Q-fever, typhus fever, rocky mountain spotted fever, etc.

Communicable diseases are further of two subtypes on the basis of mode of infection.

(i) **Contagious diseases** These diseases are transferred through simple contact with infected person.
For example, smallpox, ringworm, chickenpox, influenza, measles, leprosy, etc.
(ii) **Non-contagious diseases** These diseases are transferred in two ways
- Through **abiotic physical carriers** such as air, water, food, etc.
For example, cholera, taeniasis, ascariasis, typhoid, etc.
- Through **biotic carrier** or **vectors** such as flies mosquitoes, etc.
For example, plague, AIDS, malaria, hepatitis, etc.

Common communicable diseases

The common communicable diseases, which affect human health are described below

Viral diseases

Some of the viral diseases are as follows

1. Hepatitis

It is an infectious inflammation of the liver. There are five different viruses (HAV-HEV) which cause hepatitis. Other viruses such as **Epstein Barr Virus** (EBV) or **Cytomegalo Virus** (CMV), some drugs and chemical toxicity can also cause acute hepatitis.

Severity of hepatitis infection ranges from subclinical infections to acute liver necrosis. Hepatitis can be of following types

(i) Hepatitis-A

- It is caused by **Hepatitis-A Virus** (HAV). Hepatitis-A is also known as **infectious epidemic hepatitis** or **epidemic jaundice**. This virus contains a non-enveloped single-stranded RNA.
- **Transmission of HAV** It gains entrance *via* the oral route. It can multiply within epithelial lining of the intestinal tract. It finally reaches the liver, kidneys and spleen.
- **Incubation period** It ranges from 2-6 weeks.
- **Symptoms** These include nausea, malaria, diarrhoea, abnormal discomfort, fever and chills. These symptoms generally appear in adults. Other symptoms include yellowing of the skin, pale eyes and dark urine.
- The acute infection of HAV can be diagnosed by the detection of IgM anti-HAV.
- **Prevention** Avoid faecal contamination of food and water.
- **Treatment** Immunoglobulin is used as post-exposure prophylaxis. No antiviral agents are currently available for treating infections.

(ii) Hepatitis-B

- It is caused by **Hepatitis-B Virus** (HBV). Hepatitis-B is also called **transfusion hepatitis** or **serum hepatitis.**
- The virion of HBV is referred to as the **dane particle**. It consists of a circular double-stranded DNA molecule surrounded by an envelope.
- **Transmission of HBV** It takes place through the semen, saliva, vaginal secretion of infected person to healthy persons. Mother's milk can also be a source of infection in suckling babies.
HBV is most frequently contracted by adults through sexual intercourse. Fully differentiated hepatocytes are the primary cell to get infected by HBV.

- **Incubation period** It ranges from 4-26 weeks.
- **Symptoms** It includes loss of appetite, low grade fever and joint pain. Jaundice usually appears in the later stages.
- **Prevention** Infants should be protected from infection by giving them **Hepatitis-B Immunoglobulin** (HBIG) and first dose of hepatitis-B vaccine. Use of barriers should be encouraged during sexual intercourse. Donated blood and semen should be used only after testing.
- **Treatment** Prolonged treatment with α-interferon, which is an antiviral protein is effective. Antiviral analogs used in HIV therapy tests can be used.

(iii) Hepatitis-C

- It is caused by a **Hepatitis-C Virus** (HCV). This virus was discovered while scientists were searching the cause of non-A, non-B hepatitis. It has a linear single-stranded positive-sense RNA genome. It is an enveloped virus.
- **Incubation period** It generally lasts for 2-22 weeks.
- **Transmission of HCV** It occurs through cuts, injury, use of contaminated syringes, dental instruments, sexual contact, contaminated blood, etc.
- **Symptoms** It involve liver cirrhosis and possibly liver cancer.
- **Treatment** It includes the use of α-interferon and ribavirin.

(iv) Hepatitis-D

- This is caused by a **Hepatitis-D Virus** (HDV). It occurs only as a co-infection with HBV. This virus has a single-stranded RNA genome. It is negatively polarised and codes only for one protein. The **delta antigen** molecules of this protein are associated with RNA genome and form the virion.
- **Transmission of HDV** With the simultaneous infection of HBV is known as **backing**.
- **Symptoms** Liver damage is essentially the same as in other cases of hepatitis. But the presence of HDV usually increases the severity.

(v) Hepatitis-E

- It is caused by **Hepatitis-E Virus** (HEV). It is a linear, single-stranded, positive-sense RNA containing virus. It do not have an envelope. Hepatitis-E is another form of NANB (Non-A and Non-B) hepatitis. It resembles HAV in being a naked virus with a single-strand of RNA.
- **Incubation period** It ranges from 2-8 weeks.
- **Transmission of HEV** It spreads through faecal-oral contamination, much like hepatitis-A. HEV is a major cause of enterically transmitted water borne hepatitis.
- **Symptoms of hepatitis-E** are similar to that of hepatitis-A. The disease is especially severe in pregnant women.

2. Common cold/Rhinitis

- It is caused by rhinoviruses. It infects nose and respiratory passage, but not the lungs.
- **Transmission** It occurs through inhalation of droplets released during cough or sneezes.
- **Incubation period** It generally lasts for 3-7 days.
- **Symptoms** are nasal congestion, sore throat, nasal secretion, cough and headache.

3. Influenza

- It is commonly known as **'Flu'** and is highly infectious. This is caused by various types of influenza viruses, e.g. Orthomyxo and Paramyxo viruses. It is RNA virus. The mode of infection is same as common cold.
- **Incubation period** It lasts for about 1-4 days.
- **Symptoms** include sore throat, fever, sneezing and bodyache.

4. Chickenpox

- It is caused by *Varicella zoster virus.* It is passed out as droplets in the discharges of respiratory tract of an infected person.
- **Symptoms** are high fever and rashes. The rash comes out in crops. These appear first on trunk region. These undergo change to form pustules and finally shed as dark scabs.
- **Treatment** It can be prevented by *Varicella* vaccine.

5. Poliomyelitis

- It is caused by enterovirus (*ss*RNA).
- **Transmission** It occurs through contaminated food or water, flies or other insects that may contaminate food and water.
- There are three serotypes of poliovirus, PV-1, PV-2 and PV-3. Each of them have slightly different capsid protein. PV-I is most common and infectious form among them.
- This disease was initially called **infantile paralysis**. But it is now known that the disease may occur at any stage. Approximately 70% of all polio infections are asymptomatic.
- **Incubation period** It ranges from 7-14 days.
- **Symptoms** Poliovirus (picornavirus) causes inflammation of nervous system. Stiffness of neck is an important sign. Paralysis attack begins with high fever, headache, chills and pain all over the body.
- **Treatment** Polio vaccine is available in both injectable (Salk vaccine) and oral (Sabin vaccine) forms.
- However in 2014, India was officially declared polio free by WHO.

6. Rabies

- It is caused by Rabies virus (*Rhabdovirus*).
- **Transmission** It occurs through the bite of rabid (mad) dogs.
- **Symptoms** Fear of water (hydrophobia) is the most important symptom of this disease. Other symptoms include severe headache, excessive salivation and inability to swallow. The virus destroys the brain and spinal cord. Rabies is 100% fatal, once established.
- **Prevention** The bitten person should be vaccinated. September 28th is observed as World Rabies Day. Lakshdweep is the non-rabies zone of India.

7. Dengue fever

- Dengue or break-bone fever is caused by a RNA containing Arbovirus of *Flavivirus* group.
- **Transmission** Its vector is *Aedes aegypti* (yellow fever) mosquito. Dengue fever is of two types, i.e. classical dengue fever and haemorrhagic dengue fever.
- **Symptoms of classical dengue fever** It includes severe frontal headache, muscles or joint pain, loss of appetite, rashes, sudden onset of high fever.
- **Symptoms of dengue haemorrhagic fever** It includes bleeding from nose, mouth or gum, stomach pain, frequent vomiting, excessive thirst, weak pulse and difficulty in breathing.
- **Treatment** It can be done by taking proper rest and adequate amount of liquid diet. Paracetamol can be given on the advice of doctor. Aspirin and disprin must be avoided. There is no vaccine for dengue.

8. AIDS

Acquired Immuno Deficiency Syndrome (AIDS) is a disorder caused by **Human Immunodeficiency Virus** (HIV). This virus is pathogenic to human beings as it damages the immune system of human body. It results in the loss of natural defence of body.

> **History**
> - The first AIDS case was reported from California, USA in 1981.
> - In India, AIDS infection was detected in 1986.
> - HIV was first isolated by Montagnier *et. al.* (1983) of the Pasteur Institute of Paris.
> - **1st December** is recalled as **World AIDS Day** every year. It aims at creating awareness among people regarding AIDS.

Various names given to AIDS causing agent are as follows

- LAV-II (Lymphadenopathy Associated Virus-II) by Montagnier *et. al.* HTLV-III (Human T-Lymphotropic Virus-III) by Gallo *et. al.*
- WHO has redesignated LAV-II and HTLV-III as HIV.

Structure of HIV

HIV virus belongs to a group of virus called **retrovirus.**

The structural features of HIV are given below

(i) **Envelope** It has an envelope consisting of a lipid bilayer. It is derived from host cell membrane. It has projecting knob-like glycoprotein spikes, GP120 and GP41 with pedicel formed of virus coded glycoprotein.

(ii) **Genetic material** This envelope encloses the RNA genome (single-stranded RNA filament is segmented into two identical filaments and associated with a reverse transcriptase enzyme). HIV consists of a core RNA with **reverse transcriptase** surrounded by a protein coat. The protein coat around the core consists of a protein called **P24.**

Outside this protein coat is a layer composed of another protein called **P17.**

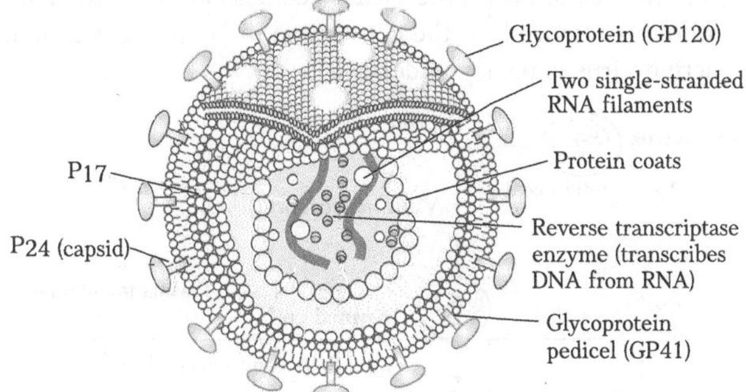

Fig. 15.1 Diagrammatic representation of HIV

Transmission of HIV

There are three main routes for the transmission of HIV

(i) **Through sexual act** It is a common route of HIV transmission from an infected partner to his/her unaffected partner. About 65% of HIV infection takes place through this route.

(ii) **Through blood transfusion, blood products and contaminated equipments** These includes the use of contaminated razors, dental instruments, unsterilised needles and blood products.

Contaminated needles and syringes are frequently shared among the intravenous drug users. About 10% of HIV transmission takes place through this route.

(iii) **Transmission from mother to baby** About 25% transmission of HIV takes place through this route. In this, pregnant woman can transfer HIV to her baby through placenta, before birth and through breast milk after birth.

Note *HIV is not transmitted through mosquito bites, shaking hands, sharing meals, towels, toilets of AIDS patients, hugging, dry kissing with patient.*

HIV infection in body cells

Following are the steps of HIV infection in human body after the exposure to virus

- HIV enters the T-cells (host cell) by the process of endocytosis. The major cell infected by HIV is the **Helper T-lymphocyte** that bears the **CD4 receptors site**. The attachment of virus to CD4 receptor site occurs by the help of GP 120 on the protein coat of the virus.
- The viral RNA is released into the cytoplasm of the host cell together with the enzyme reverse transcriptase.
- HIV makes double-stranded copy of DNA from RNA by the use of enzyme reverse transcriptase.
- This copy of viral DNA enters the nucleus of host cell and integrates with the host DNA. This viral DNA increases their number (replicates) when the host DNA multiplies.
- The viral DNA remains dormant for some years. This is known as **latency** or **latent period**. On an average, it lasts for five years. Later, the virus becomes active again. The stimulus required for the conversion of latent virus into an active virus is poorly understood.

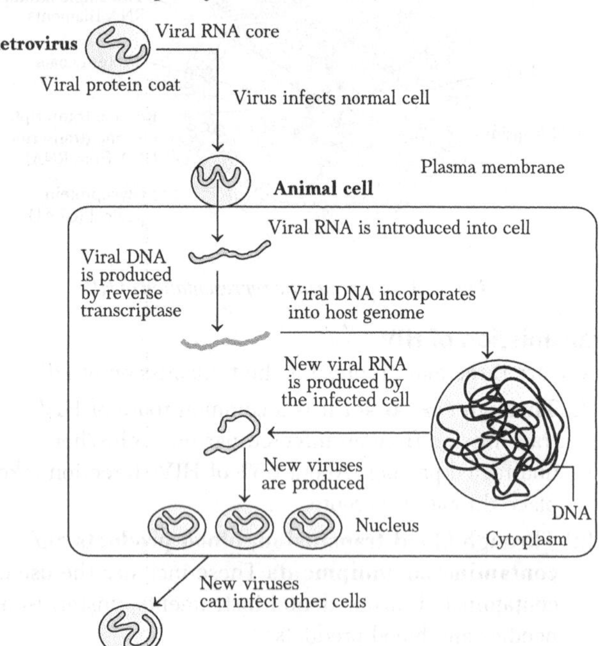

Fig. 15.2 Replication of retrovirus

- Through the process of transcription, new RNA molecules are formed. By the process of translation, viral proteins are formed. During protein synthesis, host protein synthesising machinery is used by virus.
- Now, newly formed elements of virus are assembled.
- Through the process of exocytosis, newly formed virus particles emerge from host cells.
- The final stage of this process is marked by a low helper T-cells. The person becomes susceptible to opportunistic diseases due to deficient cell mediated immune response.

Diagnosis of HIV infection

There are several methods for the diagnosis of HIV infection such as viral culture, ELISA, PCR test, Western blot test, etc. Out of these, ELISA (Enzyme Linked Immunosorbent Assay) and Western blot test are widely used

Prevention of AIDS

AIDS can be prevented by keeping following points in mind

- A barrier should be used during sexual act with the suspected partner.
- Restriction to one sexual partner.
- Use of sterilised needles and syringes.
- Before donating blood, HIV test should be done.
- Education and awareness about AIDS should be given to people.
- Blades, razors and dental equipments should be sterilised.
- Controlling drug abuse.

Treatment of AIDS

- **Azidothymidine** (AZT) or **retroni** is the most commonly used drug to treat AIDS.
- Other drugs include Stavudine (D4T), **Dideoxycytidine** (DDC) and **Dideoxyinosine** (DDI). These drugs block the conversion of retroviral RNA to gene.
- Drugs belonging to protease inhibitor category interfere with the protein proccessing steps used in HIV capsid. They include ritonavir, saquinavir (invirase) and indinavir (crisivan).

Note *Four AIDS reference centres have been established in India. They are*

- *National Institute of Virology, Pune.*
- *All India Institute of Medical Science (AIIMS), New Delhi.*
- *Centre for Advance Research on Virology, Vellore (Maharashtra).*
- *National Institute of Communicable Disease, New Delhi.*

CHECK POINT 15.1

1. The term 'Health' is defined in many ways. The most accurate definition of the health would be
   (a) health is the state of body and mind in a balanced condition
   (b) health is the reflection of a smiling face
   (c) health is a state of complete physical, mental and social well-being
   (d) health is the symbol of economic prosperity
2. Mark the incorrect statement regarding hepatitis-A virus.
   (a) Its genetic material is single-stranded RNA
   (b) IgM anti HAV confirm the infection
   (c) Infected person has pale skin and yellow eyes
   (d) None of the above
3. Hepatitis-A is also known as
   (a) dane particle
   (b) NANB
   (c) epidemic jaundice
   (d) rhinitis
4. Which of the following option is incorrect with respect to poliovirus?
   (a) It is transmitted by faecal oral route
   (b) Asymptomatic infections are common in children
   (c) There is only single serotype which causes infection
   (d) None of the above
5. Which of the following is incorrect for AIDS?
   (a) It is a congenital disease
   (b) It was first reported in 1981 in USA
   (c) It is caused by HIV
   (d) It may result in opportunistic infection
6. Treatment of AIDS with antiretroviral drugs
   (a) is fully effective
   (b) can only prolong life of the patient, but cannot prevent death
   (c) is ineffective
   (d) can eliminate the HIV totally from the body if treatment starts just after the infection gets confirmed

Bacterial diseases

Various types of bacterial diseases are as follows

1. Typhoid (Enteric fever)

- It is caused by Gram negative bacteria, *Salmonella typhi* and *S. paratyphi* (the flagellate bacilli bacteria).
- **Transmission** This bacterium is transferred by flies, faeces and fomites. Humans are the only host.
- The **incubation period** of the disease is 1-3 weeks.
- Pathogens mainly infect blood and intestine. The lysed bacteria release toxin that causes high fever periodically.
- **Symptoms** include severe headache, fever, loss of appetite, constipation and often delirium. It is diagnosed by Widal test.
- **Treatment** Ceftriaxone antibiotic is effective. Initially ampicillin and chloramphenicol were the drugs of choice for typhoid.

2. Pneumonia

- It is caused by *Pneumococcus* bacteria and *Streptococcus pneumoniae.*
- This is a disease of lungs which causes difficulty in breathing. It can occur as primary infection in healthy people or as a secondary complication due to some infection or disease. Infection is limited to one or more lung lobes rather than the entire lung.
- **Transmission** It is transmitted from one person to another by airborne droplets from cough or sneeze.
- **Symptoms** High fever, fast pulse and rapid shallow breathing with cough. It is dry in early stage disease, but later blood mixed with sputum is seen. It may lead to pleurisy and septicemia.

3. Diphtheria

- It is a dreaded disease caused by *Corynebacterium diphtheriae.*
- Diphtheria is an infection of pharynx. The bacterium produces an exotoxin. It enters the blood circulation and damages the heart, nervous system, liver, kidneys, etc.
- **Transmission** Disease is spread through coughing, sneezing, talking and kissing, etc.
- **Symptoms** include mild fever, sore throat and headache.
- **Treatment** Antitoxin can be given within 12 hrs and the treatment with antibiotics provide relief. Air passage has to be surgically cleared.
- **Prevention** involves vaccinating children with DPT in first six weeks of birth. Injection of antitoxin or toxoid serum is given to patient to prevent diphtheria.

4. Tetanus

- It is caused by *Clostridium tetani.* The bacterium occurs in the intestines of horse and other animals.
- **Transmission** It is contracted through wounds, accidents and by the use of improperly sterilised surgical instruments. Spores released from animal faeces remain viable in the dust or air for several years. Once the

bacterial spores enter a human body, bacteria are released and multiply. They secrete toxin, tetanospasmin.

- **Incubation period** It varies from 4 days to 3 weeks.
- **Symptoms** It includes headache, followed by back pain, muscular rigidity and painful muscular spasms. The spasm of jaw muscles locks the jaws and hence, it is also called **lock jaw**. Heart failure and death may occur if proper treatment is not available. All wounds should be cleaned with iodine solution.
- **Treatment** Antitetanus Serum (ATS) should be administered in case of an injury.

5. Cholera

- It is a highly infectious disease caused by *Vibrio cholerae.* The causative agent was first isolated by **Robert Koch** in 1884.
- **Transmission** This is a waterborne infection. It is commonly acquired by drinking water contaminated with faeces from infected persons. The bacteria produce a toxin in the intestine of the host.
- **Symptoms** Frequent watery stools (diarrhoea) and repeated vomiting.
- **Treatment** The patient is given Oral Rehydration Solution (ORS). It is a solution of electrolytes and glucose. It helps to replenish the loss of nutrients and water from the body. A cholera vaccine is available, which provides immunity for a few months (short-term vaccine).

6. Tuberculosis (TB)

- It is caused by *Mycobacterium tuberculosis.* This is commonly called **Koch's infection**, since the causative agent was first identified by **Robert Koch.**
- On the basis of pattern of infection, tuberculosis is divided into two types
  - (i) **Primary tuberculosis** is seen as initial infection, usually in children.
  - (ii) **Secondary tuberculosis** is observed in adults as a reactivation of previous infection when immunity declines.
- **Transmission** The disease spreads by droplet infection through coughing or sneezing.
- **Incubation period** It varies from a few days to few months.
- **Symptoms** are high fever, sweating, loss of weight, cough, difficulty in breathing, blood in sputum and acute pain. Sputum is laden with the bacteria in case of pulmonary TB.
  It is diagnosed by X-ray, sputum, tuberculin (Montoux) and gastric analysis.
- **Treatment** Antituberculosis drugs like streptomycin, isomazid, thiacetazone, ethambatol, pyrazinamide, rifampicin have proved to be effective.
  The treatment generally lasts for 6 months which should not be stopped because the bacteria develop resistance to the drugs.
  Vaccination with **Bacillus Calmette Guerin** (BCG) provides immunity against TB.

Note **DOTS** *(Directly Observed Treatment– Short-course) is the new strategy to combat the disease. It ensures that the patient takes the full course of the treatment and does not stop it midway.*

7. Leprosy

- It is also called **Hansen's disease.** It is caused by rod-shaped bacterium, *Mycobacterium leprae.* This pathogen was first isolated and identified by **GA Hansen** in 1870.
- There are two main types of leprosy
  - (i) **Tuberculoid leprosy** It is characterised by lesions in the skin (specially nose and outer areas) and in superficial nerve endings. It can be observed by skin test with **lepromin.**
  - (ii) **Lepromatous leprosy** In this, skin cells get infected and disfiguring nodules are formed all over the body.
- **Transmission** It occurs from person to person through prolonged contact. The infectivity of *Mycobacterium leprae* is slow. Most people acquire the infection, when secretions containing the pathogen contact their nasal mucosa.
- **Incubation period** It lasts upto 5 yrs.
- **Symptoms** The affected sites of the body are mucous membrane, skin and nervous system. Leprosy is characterised by scaly and nodulated skin, formation of ulcers, hypopigmentation of skin, deformity of fingers and toes. Infected areas show loss of nervous sensation.
- **Treatment** Rifampicin and clofazimine are often used along with sulfodrug dapsone. It is also seen that the vaccine BCG, which provides protection against tuberculosis is somewhat protective against leprosy also.

8. Pertussis (Whooping cough)

- It is caused by *Bordetella pertussis.*
- **Transmission** It is an airborne infection. The site of infection is mucosa of the trachea, bronchi, bronchioles.
- **Incubation period** It is of 1-3 weeks.
- **Symptoms** are cold, cough and mild fever in early stages, convulsions and pneumonia may also occur. A violent attack of cough forces air out of the lungs. It is followed by the typical inspiratory whooping cough. This may be

followed by vomiting, cyanosis and hemorrhage in nose, eyes, brain, etc.

- **Prevention** DPT is a triple vaccine for diphtheria, pertussis and tetanus. It should be given to infants three times at monthly intervals. It has considerably reduced the disease among children.

9. Plague

- This was once a dreaded disease and called as the **black death of the middle ages**. It is caused by a rod-shaped bacterium, *Yersinia pestis*. It is a flea-borne pathogen of rats and other rodents in which it causes heavy mortality.
- **Transmission** to man occurs through infected rat flea (*Xenopsylla cheopis*). When a rat dies of plague, the flea leaves the dead rats. If humans are around, flea begin to feed on human blood and inject plague germ in human's blood.
- **Incubation period** It is of 2-6 days.
- **Symptoms** include fever, malaria, headache and swelling of lymph nodes into the painfull bubos, hence it is called **bubonic plague**.
  The rare but severe form of bacterial septicemia caused by *Yersinia pestis* is called **pneumonic plague**. The septicemia of bubonic plague may lead to pulmonary infection, which results in high mortality.
  The patient of pneumonic plague is a source of droplet infection that spreads infection to healthy humans by inhalation.
- **Treatment** Antibiotics particularly injectable streptomycin or oral tetracycline are effective, but it should be given under the supervision of a doctor.

10. Syphilis

- The disease is caused by *Treponema pallidum.*
- **Transmission** It is a sexually transmitted disease. Intercourse with multiple partners (unsafe sex) and intrauterine infection are the modes of its transmission.
- **Symptoms** These appear in three phases as follows
  (i) The first sign of infection are painless lesions called **primary syphilis**. It appears on skin or mucosa of genitalia.
  (ii) It is followed by **secondary syphilis.** It is characterised by red skin lesions, mouth and throat ulcers, fever and general enlargement of lymph nodes.
  (iii) **Tertiary syphilis** is evident and characterised by the presence of lesions both superficially and beneath the tissue. They are capable of causing serious damage to cardiovascular and central nervous system.
  Treatment Penicillin is used for the treatment of syphilis.

CHECK POINT 15.2

1. The antibiotic used for treatment of typhoid is
(a) Ceftrioxone
(b) DPT
(c) Rifampicin
(d) None of the above

2. Injection of antitoxin or toxoid serum is given to prevent
(a) diphtheria
(b) smallpox
(c) chickenpox
(d) chronic headache

3. Different species of *Mycobacterium* cause
(a) syphilis and diphtheria
(b) whooping cough and leprosy
(c) tuberculosis and leprosy
(d) syphilis and gonorrhoea

4. Leprosy is diagnosed by which of the following set of symptoms?
(a) Fever, loss of pigmentation
(b) Deformity of fingers, scales, ulcers, loss of pigmentation, wasting of body parts
(c) Frequent watery stools and deformities in fingers and toes
(d) White spots on the skin without any scares or ulcer

5. Choose the incorrectly matched pair.
(a) Tetanus – Lock jaw
(b) Plague – Bubos
(c) Cholera – TAB vaccine
(d) Tuberculosis – DOTS

6. Choose the odd one out.
(a) Malaria (b) Diphtheria
(c) Pertussis (d) Pneumonia

Protozoan diseases

Some common protozoan diseases are described below

1. Malaria

It is caused by a tiny protozoan, called *Plasmodium.* Female *Anopheles* mosquito is the vector of this protozoan. Four different species of *Plasmodium, viz. P. vivax, P. ovale, P. malariae* and *P. falciparum* are responsible for causing different types of malaria.

(i) ***P. falciparum*** infection is the most serious as it affects the brain and can be fatal.

It causes malignant tertian or subtertian malaria, characterised by fever cycles every 36-48 hrs.

(ii) ***Plasmodium vivax*** causes benign tertiary malaria. Incubation period is 13-15 days. Fever occurs after 48 hrs.

(iii) ***Plasmodium malariae*** causes quartan malaria. Incubation period is 28-30 days, fever occurs after 72 hrs.

(iv) ***Plasmodium ovale*** causes mild tertiary malaria. Incubation period is 14 days. The life cycle of *Plasmodium* is discussed in brief below, as we have discussed it in detail in Exploring Biology volume-I.

Life cycle of *Plasmodium*

- The life history of malaria parasite in female *Anopheles* was studied by **B Grassi** (1917). Erythrocytic schizogony in human RBC was studied by **Golgi** (1885).
- The host of protozoan parasite are typically distinguished into two types
  - (i) **Intermediate host** (Human)
    - In which asexual reproduction occurs.
    - In which the immature form harbors.
  - (ii) **Definitive host** (Mosquito)
    - In which sexual reproduction occurs.
    - It harbors the mature form.
- To understand infection by *Plasmodium*, study of its life cycle is important. The infective stage of *Plasmodium* is a minute sickle-shaped, **sporozoite**.

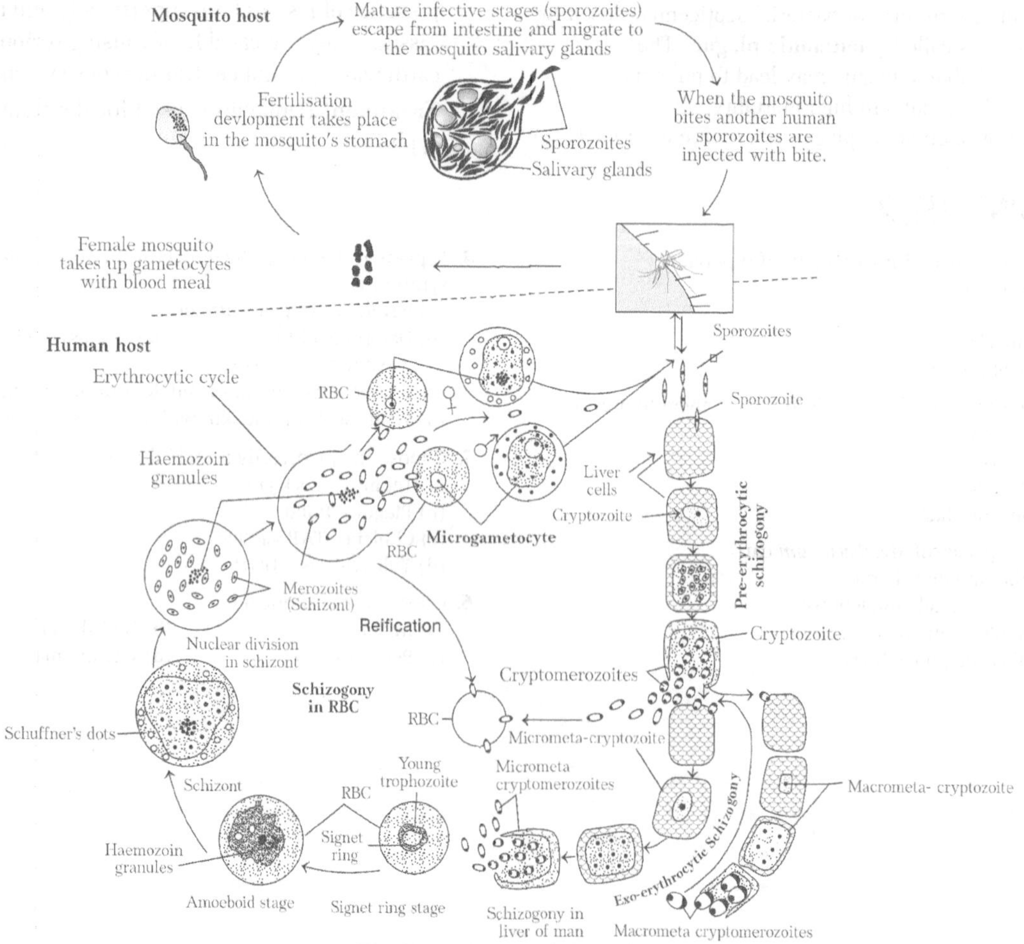

Fig. 15.3 Life cycle of Plasmodium

- The sporozoites of *Plasmodium* are injected into human blood through the bite of its vector, a female *Anopheles* mosquito.
- These sporozoites enter in liver cells from blood. They multiply asexually and rupture the liver cells to release **merozoites** into the blood.
- Inside the RBCs, merozoites develop through a ring stage to form a schizont (trophozoite). When the schizont gets matured, the RBCs burst to release merozoites into the blood.
- They invade more red cells and repeat the erythrocytic cycle. The rupture of RBCs is associated with the release of a toxic substance called **haemozoin.**
- Some merozoites develop into immature sexual stages called **gametocytes**. These forms are taken up by the female *Anopheles* when it bites infected human.
- The male and female gametocytes fertilise and develop in the mosquito's stomach to form zygote, followed by oocysts.
- The oocysts develop into sporonts which further develop into mature sporozoite.
- The sporozoites escape from intestine and moves to the salivary glands of the mosquito.
- When infected mosquito bites another human, sporozoites are injected into the blood through the saliva and they start the liver and RBCs cycle again.
- **Treatment** is available and should be taken at the earliest. **Chloroquine** is the most commonly used drug to treat malaria. Artemisinin-based combination therapy is recommended for the treatment of *P. falciparum* malaria.

2. Amoebiasis

- *Entamoeba histolytica* is the causative organism of amoebiasis (amoebic dysentery) in man. This parasitises found in the lumen of upper part of large intestine, i.e. colon. It occurs worldwide wherever sanitation and hygiene are poor.
- **Transmission** and **life cycle** Houseflies are the mechanical carriers of this disease. They transmit the parasite from the faeces of the infected person to the food items and contaminate them.
- Through contaminated food, trophozoite enters the human body. It invades mucosa and submucosa of intestinal wall by secreting histolysins.
- **Trophozoite** is the parasitic stage and it reproduces asexually by binary fission. These trophozoites form cysts which pass in the faeces. These can survive for 2-3 weeks in adverse conditions and upto four weeks in water.
- Cysts transform into 4-nucleus stage which is capable of infecting a new person.
- Inside the new host, this tetranucleated cyst undergoes encystment. The four daughter amoebae (trophozoites) start to grow, multiply and cause disease.
- **Symptoms** are constipation, abdominal pain, cramps, stools with mucus and blood.
  The faeces of infected person contain white, stone-shaped charcot leyden crystals.
- **Treatment** Emetine (an alkaloid) provides temporary relief. Etronidazole and tinidazole are effective amoebicides.

3. Kala-azar

- Kala-azar or **dum-dum fever** is caused by a protozoan, *Leishmania donovani*, hence it is called **leishmaniasis.**
- **Transmission** The infection to man is caused by the bite of infected sandflies, *Phlebotomus papatasi* and *P. argentipus.* When a sandfly bites an infected host, it picks protozoan parasite along with the blood meal. Spleen, liver and sometimes bone marrow are the target organs.
- **Symptoms** Weight loss, anaemia, constant fever and darkening of skin. Spleen and liver become enlarged. The infection is severe and sometimes can be fatal, particularly in children.
  This may become a chronic infection that may last a year or more. It is characterised by dry cutaneous lesions or sores in hand, feet, legs and face. Lesions heal, but leave scars.
- **Treatment** includes administration of sodium antimony gluconate (pentahexonate), pentamidine isethionate, etc.
- **Prevention** from sandfly bite is important, because these flies are very tiny, hence cannot be observed easily by the naked eye.

4. Sleeping sickness

- It is caused by a flagellate protozoan parasite. It belongs to the class—Mastigophora and genus—*Trypanosoma* and hence, the disease is also called **trypanosomiasis.** *Trypanosoma gambiense* causes Central African sleeping sickness or gambian fever.
- It is a chronic form of sleeping sickness in which death results in 12-18 months if proper treatment is not available.
- **Transmission** It is spread by blood sucking tse-tse flies of the genus-*Glossina palpalis* and *Glossina tachicnoids.* *Trypanosoma rhodesiense* is transmitted by the tse-tse fly, *G. marsitans. T. rhodesiense* infects cattle and antelope which serve as reservoir host.
- **Symptoms** Headache, fever, lethargy, anaemia and loss of appetite. It affects nervous system and the patient feels lethargic, sleepy and cannot respond to any stimuli. There is also disturbance in coordination and reflexes.
- **Treatment** It includes a course of injections of suramin, pentamidine isethionate or melarsoprol, tryporasamide and nitrofurazone (furacin).

5. Chagas' disease

- It is caused by *T. cruzi*. It is a common disease in South and Central America and Mexico.
- **Transmission** It is transmitted mainly by the blood sucking reduviid bugs or kissing bugs, *Panstrongylum megistus*, in South America. Thus, it is also known as **South America trypanosomiasis**. These bugs are also called **assassin bugs.**

  Trypomastigotes of trypanosome forms are taken up by the bug along with the blood meal. They multiply and develop in the insect's intestine. The infection to man occurs when infective trypomastigote forms are rubbed into the site of bite.

  The conjunctiva is a common site of infection. Children and young adults are commonly affected.
- **Common symptoms** are continuous fever, anaemia, oedema and disorders of nervous system.
- **Prevention** Better hygienic conditions and use of insecticides helps in controlling the number of insects.
- **Treatment** Benznidazole and nifurtimox are given to kill the parasite.

6. Giardiasis

- It is caused by a flagellate protozoan parasite, *Giardia intestinalis* (*G. lamblia*) of intestinal tract.

  It is a worldwide zoonotic disease, i.e. it can spread from animals to man who come in contact with animals very often.
- **Transmission** It occurs by faecal-oral route. The trophozoite of *Giardia* multiplies and attaches to the walls of intestines. Rapid multiplication results in the formation of layer of parasite on the intestinal walls.

  In the lumen of intestine, the trophozoites form oval cysts which are passed in faeces. Also, intestinal epithelial cells are damaged as a result of heavy infection.
- **Symptoms** are abdominal pain, loss of appetite, headache. diarrhoea, fever, etc.
- **Treatment** Metronidazole, mepacrine, etc., help in controlling the disease.

Helminthic infections

Some common diseases caused by helminthes are as follows

1. Ascariasis

- It is a common helminthic infection caused by *Ascaris lumbricoides.* It is an endoparasite of small intestine of human beings. It also infects pigs and cattle.
- **Transmission and life cycle** The eggs of adult *Ascaris* are excreted along with the faeces of infected person and contaminate soil, water and plants, etc.

  A healthy person is infected by these eggs through water, food, raw vegetables, fruits, etc.

  The eggs hatch and release worms. These worms penetrate the wall of the intestine and reach the lungs *via* the bloodstream.

  In the lungs, they break into alveolar spaces. They get matured as they migrate to the respiratory route.

  They are coughed into the oesophagus and swallowed into the intestine again where they mature in about 10 weeks. They may live for 1-2 yrs.
- **Symptoms** The disease is characterised by internal bleeding, muscular pain, fever, anaemia and blockage of intestinal passage.
- **Treatment** Antihelminthic drugs like albendazole and mebendazole are helpful in the countering ascariasis.

2. Filariasis

- It is caused by filarial nematodes, *Wuchereria bancrofti* and *Wuchereria malayi.*
- **Transmission** Filarial infection is caused by different species of mosquitoes, e.g. *Culex*, *Aedes*, etc. The immature larvae called **microfilariae** are inoculated in human when these mosquitoes suck the blood. The larvae enter the body through the puncture in the skin made by mosquito.

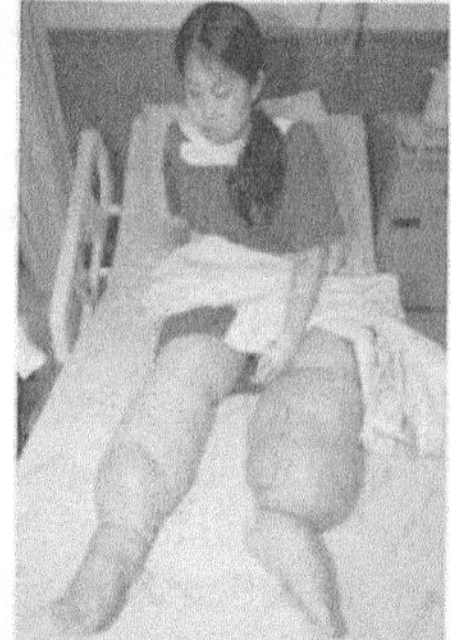

Fig. 15.4 Elephantiasis in human

The larvae migrate to the peripheral lymphatic system and then to lymph nodes and large lymph vessels.

The larvae develop into adults which obstruct the flow in the lymph vessels. It results in the oedema (accumulation of fluid) in the affected area.

The lower extremities swell and resemble the feet of elephant. Due to this resemblance, the disease is also called **elephantiasis**. The genital organs are also often affected and get deformed.

- **Treatment** The useful drugs are heterozan, MSF and diethylcarbamazine.

3. Taeniasis

- It is caused by the two species of *Taenia*, i.e. *T. solium* and *T. saginata.* Their larvae are found in pig and cattle, respectively.

- **Transmission and life cycle** Infection to man occurs by eating raw or improperly cooked pork, cattle's meat or foods contaminated with infective larval stages called **cysticercus**. These are the cysts in which larvae is embedded.
  The cysticercus excysts in the human intestine. The scolex (head) of *Taenia* attaches to the intestinal wall. Their body consists of a chain of segments called **proglottids**. These are full of fertilised eggs in adults. These eggs pass out in the faeces. If these eggs are ingested by pigs (*T. solium*) or cattle (*T. saginata*), the embryo hatches from the eggs in their gut.
  The embryo then bores through the gut wall and migrates upto the muscles. It then transforms into a cysticercus larva.
  Eggs of *T. solium* develop into cysticercus in humans and cause **cysticercosis.** The larvae or cysticerci may be found in most tissues, liver and brain. If present in brain, they can cause much damage such as blindness.
- **Treatment** Niclosamide is used to control taeniasis.

Fungal diseases

Most of the fungal infections are superficial and cause no serious threat to health, but they cause inconvenience.

1. *Tinea* or Ringworm

- *Tinea* is the most common skin disease of humans.
- It is caused by dermatophytes that include three genera
  (i) ***Trichophyton*** It infects skin, hair and nails.
  (ii) ***Microsporum*** It infects skin and hair, but not nails.
  (iii) ***Epidermophyton*** It infects skin and nails, but not hair
- **Transmission** The infection is generally acquired from soil, using towels, clothes and comb of the infected persons. Warmth and moisture help in the growth of fungal organisms, especially in skin folds.
- **Symptoms** It is characterised by dry scaly lesions on the outer parts of the body such as skin, nails and scalp.
- **Treatment** It involves griseofulvin (orally) and miconazole (topically).

2. Candidiasis

- The causative agent is yeast like fungi of the genus-*Candida.* Superficial candidiasis affects mucous membranes or skin.
- Various species may cause oral candidiasis or **thrush**, e.g. *Candida oesophagitis, Vulvovaginaitis* (vaginal thrush), dermatitis, chronic mucocutaneous candidiasis, etc.
- **Treatment** Antifungal agents like **imidazole** or all other azole derivatives.

Dermatophytes

These do not attack deeper tissues. The diseases caused by various species of dermatophytes are termed according to the site they infect.

Some of these are given in the table below

Table 15.1 Some species of dermatophytes

Organisms	Sites of infection	Dermatophytes
Tinea pedis	Foot (athlete's foot)	*Trichophyton rubrum, Epidermophyton floccosum* and *E. cruris*
Tinea capitis	Hair and scalp skin	*Microsporum canis, M. andoninii, T. tonurans* and *T. violaceum*
Tinea cruris	Groin	*T. rubrum, E. floccosum* and *E. cruris*
Tinea corporis	Body	*T. mentagrophytes, E. floccosum, E. cruris* and *M. canis*
Tinea barbae	Beard (barber's itch)	*T. mentagrophytes*
Tinea anguium (onychomylosis)	Nails and finger	*T. rubrum* and *T. mentagrophytes*

Deep mycoses

This fungi invades deeper tissues of the body. It produces a spectrum of disease resembling to TB.

Such diseases and their causative fungal agents are as follows

(i) **Blastomycosis** *Blastomyces dermatidis* may affect lungs, skin, bone, viscera and meninges.

(ii) **Histoplasmosis** *Histoplasma capsulatum* may affect lungs, lymph, etc.

Treatment Amphotericin-B is an effective treatment.

Rickettsial diseases

Members of ricketssiae bear resemblance to both bacteria and viruses. Rickettsiae are intestinal parasites of ticks, mites, rat fleas and lice. These are blood sucking arthropods.

They do not cause any harm to their hosts, but are harmful to man. Human beings get infected by direct bite of blood sucking arthropods or inhalation of dried arthropod faeces.

Rickettsial diseases are of two types as follows

1. Typhus fever

- Epidemic typhus is also called as **classical** or **European typhus**. It is purely a human disease caused by *Rickettsiae prowazeki* and transmitted by louse.
- **Transmission** Once ingested by the louse during blood sucking, the rickettsiae multiply in its intestine and leave it

along with faeces in large numbers. The next victim gets the infection by another louse bite or the scratches inflicted as a result of louse bite.

- **Symptoms** Severe illness followed by fever, cerebral disturbances and rashes in axillary folds. If antibiotic treatment is not given, death may result, especially in elderly people.

Epidemic typhus

Endemic typhus also called **murine typhus**, is a disease of rats. It is caused by *R. typhale*. It is transmitted by the rat flea and rat louse.

Stray cases of infection occur, where there is a high population of rats. This is an urban disease and is less severe than epidemic typhus. The rash when present, affects the chest and abdomen.

Note **Rickettsiae** *which cause typhus and related diseases are named after Dr. HT Ricketts. He died of typhus while investigating its causes and transmission.*

2. Spotted fever

It is also referred as **Rocky Mountain Spotted Fever** (RMSF). It is caused by *Rickettsiae rickettsi.* It is commonly found in North and South America. The dog ticks and wood ticks are vectors of this disease.

This disease is of following types

(i) **Boutonneuse fever** It is a relatively mild form of tick typhus which is transmitted by dog tick. The causative agent is *Rickettsiae conori.*

(ii) **Rickettsial pox** It is a mite-borne disease caused by *R. akari.* It is transmitted to man from rodents. The disease is mild. The vescicular rash that resembles chickenpox appears in it.

(iii) **Q-fever** The name of Q-fever is derived from the query of its etiology and not from its place of origin, i.e. queensland. The causative agent is rickettsia like organism, *Coxiella burneti.* Ticks cause the infections in birds and animals.

- **Transmission** Human infection is generally caused by inhalation of dust or droplets contaminated by the excreta of infected animals or ingestion of contaminated milk.
- **Symptoms** Infection with Q-fever causes an influenza like illness with high fever, headache and pneumonia. In acute infection, hepatitis also occurs.
- **Treatment** Tetracyclines are the most useful antibiotics for its treatment.

CHECK POINT 15.3

1. Recurrence of high fever in malaria occurs due to the completion of
   (a) sporogony
   (b) erythrocytic schizogony
   (c) exoerythrocytic schizogony
   (d) gamogony
2. Artemisinin based Combination Therapies (ACTs) prescribed for malaria include
   (a) artesunate, sulfadoxine, pyrimethamine
   (b) artesunate, diethylcarbamazine, levamisole
   (c) piperazine, mebendazole, pyrantel
   (d) penicillin, ampicillin and chloramphenicol
3. A person is showing the following symptoms; constipation, abdominal pain and cramps, stools with excess mucus and blood. This person is most likely to be suffering from
   (a) amoebiasis (b) typhoid
   (c) ringworm (d) ascariasis
4. Modes of prevention of ascariasis include the following except
   (a) avoid detection in open spaces
   (b) washing hands with water and soap
   (c) washing vegetables throughly
   (d) use of *Gambusia* fish to prevent larvae
5. Ringworm infection cannot be prevented by
   (a) avoiding sharing of clothes, sports equipment and towels
   (b) washing clothes in hot water with fungicidal soap after suspected exposure to ringworm
   (c) avoiding barefooted walking
   (d) using handkerchief while sneezing
6. Endemic typhus is transmitted by following agents except
   (a) by rat flea
   (b) by rat louse
   (c) ticks
   (d) Both (a) and (b)

NON-COMMUNICABLE DISEASES OR NON-INFECTIOUS DISEASES

These diseases are not transferred from an affected person to a normal healthy person. There are various kinds of non-communicable disease, which affect the health of human beings.

These are of following types

(i) **Deficiency diseases** These are related to deficiency of nutrients in our diet. For example,

- kwashiorkor and marasmus are caused due to protein deficiency.
- pellagra, scurvy, rickets are caused due to vitamin deficiency.
- mineral deficiency such as calcium and phosphorus deficiency causes rickets.
- iodine deficiency causes thyroid problems like goitre.

(ii) **Ageing and degenerative diseases** Degeneration of body tissues results in various diseases.
For example, arteriosclerosis, i.e. hardening of the arteries and arthritis (joint and bone disease), etc.

(iii) **Mental illness** Mental disorders, e.g. schizophrenia, etc.

(iv) **Malfunctioning diseases** Various diseases caused by malfunctioning of organs are as follows

- Improper functioning of heart, i.e. cardiac failure.
- Improper functioning of kidney, i.e. kidney failure.
- Weakening of bones, i.e. osteoporosis.
- Improper functioning of eyes, i.e. myopia, hypermetropia and cataract.
- Uncontrolled growth of cells in body causes cancer.

(v) **Allergic diseases** The unfavourable response of the body to certain substances like dust, serum, drugs, fabrics and pollen, etc., is called **allergy**.

Sneezing, irritation of throat, itching and skin rashes, etc., are the main symptoms.

(vi) **Diseases caused by addictive substances** Some addictive substances and their resultant diseases are as follows

- **Alcohol** Reduces alertness of mind and causes liver damage or cirrhosis.
- **Narcotic drugs** These include morphine, cocaine, heroin, hashish, ganja, opium, marijuana, barbiturates and LSD (Lysergic Acid Diethylamide).

  Use of drugs causes serious damage to nervous system and various organs of body alongwith bad effect on vision (eyes), ear and respiratory tract.
- **Tobacco** Chewing of tobacco leads to mouth disease, cancer and smoking leads to lung disease and cancer.
- **Psychological factors** Cause hypertension, peptic ulcers, mental illness and depression.

(vii) **Hormonal diseases** These diseases occur due to the defect in production of hormones. These are as follows

- **Cretinism** In children, the deficiency of thyroxine makes a child mentally retarded.
- **Diabetes mellitus** It is caused due to the deficiency of insulin.
- **Dwarfism** It is caused due to the sluggish activity of the pituitary gland. The affected person has diminished growth of the bones.
- **Gigantism** It is caused due to the excessive activity of the pituitary gland. The affected person shows excessive growth of the bones.

Common non-communicable diseases

These are as follows

Cancer

It is an abnormal growth and uncontrolled division of cells. **Contact inhibition** is the property shown by normal cells. Due to this, uncontrolled growth of cells is inhibited by contact with other cells. Cancerous cells have lost this property due to which they show uncontrolled growth (**hyperplasia**).

Cancerous cells keep on dividing and produce more cells even when it is not required. The cells which show rapid, abnormal and uncontrolled growth are called **neoplastic cells.** As a result, mass of tissue forms and this extra mass of tissue is called **tumour.**

Tumours are of two types

(i) **Benign tumours** Cells of benign tumours stay together and do not spread to other parts of the body. Hence, they cause little damage to body.

(ii) **Malignant tumours** Cells of malignant tumour break away from the original site. These can spread to the other parts of the body through the blood stream and lymphatic system. The spread of cancer to other sites or organ in the body is called **metastasis**. It is the most feared property of malignant tumours.

Malignant tumours generally can be classified as

(i) **Carcinoma** type of cancers originate in epithelium.

(ii) **Sarcomas** are the cancers of connective tissue.

(iii) **Leukemias** are the cancers of blood and their precursors in bone marrow.

Other types of cancers are

- **Melanoma,** i.e. cancer of pigment cells of the skin.
- **Adenoma,** i.e. cancer of gland .
- **Lymphoma,** i.e. cancer of lymphatic tissue.
- **Glioma,** i.e. cancer of glial cells of CNS.

Causes of cancer

Cancers are induced by physical, chemical and biological factors or agents. These are called **carcinogens** or **cancer causing agents.** These agents are discussed below

- **Radiations** include both ionising radiations such as X-rays, γ-rays and non-ionising radiations such as ultraviolet (UV) rays. They damage the DNA, leading to neoplastic transformation.
- **Viruses** also cause cancer. These are called **oncogenic virus** as they have genes called **viral oncogenes.** These are present in all nucleated cells.
- These genes code for proteins that are necessary for the cell's growth and are normally called **proto-oncogenes** or **cellular oncogenes** (c-onc). Mutation in proto-oncogenes lead to the uncontrol growth and division of cells.
- Many chemicals are responsible for cancerous growth. Such chemicals are found in tobacco, artificial sweetners etc.

Table 15.2 Major factors that increase the risk of cancer

Factors	Examples of implicated cancers
Heredity	Retinoblastoma (childhood eye cancer), osteosarcoma (childhood bone cancer)
Tumour viruses	Liver cancer, adult T-cell leukaemia/lymphoma, Epstein-Barr virus causes Burkitt's lymphoma, genital herpes infection causes cervical cancer.
Tobacco use	Lung cancer, cancers of the oral cavity, oesophagus and larynx, cancer of the kidney and bladder.
Alcohol consumption	Cancer of oral cavity, oesophagus, larynx and breast.
Industrial hazards	Lung cancer
Ultraviolet radiation from the sun	Skin cancer
Ionising radiation	Related to location and type of exposure.
Hormones (oestrogen and possibly testosterone)	Breast, endometrial, ovarian and prostate cancer.
Diet	Colon and rectum, breast (weak association), endometrium and prostate cancer (fat), stomach and oesophageal cancer (nitrites).

Cancer detection and diagnosis

Detection of cancer at early stages is important to treat it successfully.

The techniques of detecting different cancers are as follows

- Leukaemias are detected by biopsy, histopathological studies of the tissue and blood tests.
- Cancers of internal organs are detected by radiography, Computed Tomography (CT) and Magnetic Resonance Imaging (MRI).
- CT scan generates a 3-D image of the internal organs by using X-rays.
- MRI is the most accurate method to detect pathological and physiological changes in the living tissue by the use of strong magnetic field and non-ionising radiations.
- Cancer can also be detected by antibodies formed against cancer specific antigens.

Treatment of cancer

The most widely used approaches for the treatment of cancer are as follows

(i) **Surgery** It involves the removal of the whole cancerous tissue from the body.

(ii) **Radiation therapy** It involves the use of radiations (X-rays, γ-rays) to destroy growing cancerous cells. It targets the cancerous tissue without damaging surrounding tissues. **Radon** (Rn-220), **Cobalt** (Co-60) and **Iodine** (I-131) are commonly used radio isotopes for radiation therapy.

(iii) **Immunotherapy** It involves the use of anti-cancer immunological defence mechanism. Substances such as α-interferon are given to activate immune system and destroy tumours.

(iv) **Chemotherapy** In this, anticancer drugs are administered in the body. Some of the anticancer drugs are specific for particular tumour, e.g. two anticancer drugs, i.e. **vincristine** and **vinblastin** are used in the treatment of leukaemia. They keep a check on cancerous cell division.

Chemotherapeutic drugs kill cancerous cells but most of them have side effects like anaemia, hair loss, etc.

Cardiovascular diseases

These diseases involve the heart and the blood vascular system. Various harmful products of metabolism are carried through blood circulation, to be expelled from the body.

Some of these diseases are described below

1. Arteriosclerosis

- It is a chronic disease associated with abnormal thickening and hardening of the walls of arteries. This results in the loss of elasticity.
- It occurs when there is too much pressure on the arterial walls throughout the body.
- It affect the blood vessels of brain, interfere with blood flow in it and causes stroke. This may lead to a loss of consciousness followed by some degree of paralysis. This condition is called **Transient Ischaemic Attack** (TIA).
- TIA results in heart attack and in limbs, it causes Deep Vein Thrombosis (DVT).
- The loss of elasticity of the blood vessels can also lead to the development of high blood pressure (hypertension) and impotence (erectile dysfunction).
- **Treatment** involves lowering the blood pressure and thinning the blood. Drugs are used to reduce the blood pressure and platelet count. It inhibits the ability of blood to clot.

2. Atherosclerosis

- It is most common form of arteriosclerosis.
- It occurs when fatty material (cholesterol) carrying lipoproteins in the circulating blood gets deposited on the inner linings of arterial wall.
- This increases the formation of plaques or blood clots (thrombus) and atheromas. It causes narrowing of the arteries and obstruct the flow of blood through them.
- Atherosclerosis in coronary arteries decreases the blood flow to the heart itself and the oxygen supply to heart muscles also decreases.
- Narrowing of the vessels can affect any part of the body, i.e. eyes, kidneys and legs. It results in blindness, kidney failure, peripheral vascular disease, etc.
- Other coronary artery associated diseases are heart blockage, heart failure and ischemia. Together, they are called **ischaemic heart diseases**. Their treatment include coronary bypass surgery and balloon angioplasty.

3. Hypertension

- High blood pressure or hypertension is a condition in which blood pressure in blood vessels (arteries and veins) is abnormally high. The normal blood pressure of a healthy adult is considered close to 120/80 mm Hg.
- Sometimes, the heart pumps more forcefully to move some amount of blood through the narrowed blood vessels into the capillaries. This results in increased blood pressure or high blood pressure.
- This high blood pressure can damage the arterioles of liver, kidney or brain and even the overworked heart.
- Thus, hypertension presents an increased risk of death from congestive heart failure, kidney failure or stroke.
- It is further divided into two types as follows
  (i) **Essential or idiopathic hypertension** It is the most common form of hypertension. It is caused due to smoking, alcohol consumption, emotional and physical stress, lifestyle and diabetes.
  (ii) **Mild hypertension** It is caused due to excess secretion of epinephrine by adrenal medulla, aldosterone by cortex and renin by kidney.
- **Treatment** involves the use of vasodilator drugs (to dilate the arteries) to lower the blood pressure. The medical therapy for essential hypertension once started must continue for the rest of life.

Diabetes mellitus

(Gk. *Diabainein*—to pass through; *mellitus*—sweetened with honey)

- It is a disorder of carbohydrate metabolism. Glucose is the main carbohydrate that yield instant energy in the body.
- Diabetes is caused when glucose is not properly utilised by the cells of the body. Thus, the concentration of glucose increases in the blood.
- The increase in blood sugar levels is termed as **hyperglycemia**. It leads to accumulation of more glucose in the blood. The extra sugar (glucose) is excreted in urine and this condition is called **glycosuria**.
- The increased level of glucose in blood is characterised by increased frequency and volume of urine, excessive thirst, hunger, weight loss and weakness.
- Diabetes is of two types
  (i) **Type I** is Insulin Dependent Diabetes Mellitus (IDDM). Insulin injections are required to control this type of diabetes. Pancreas does not secrete insulin, hence it must be taken from an outside source. It is also called **juvenile diabetes**.
  (ii) **Type II** is a Non-Insulin Dependent Diabetes Mellitus (NIDDM). It occurs due to insulin resistance in the liver and skeletal muscles. In contrast to type I, it is also called adult onset diabetes.
- Untreated diabetes leads to ketosis, followed by acidosis, nausea and vomiting. Other serious complications include retinopathy, kidney disease and frequent infections.
- **Treatment** aimed in controlling diabetes is highly successful. A diet suited to the patient maintains normal body weight and limits intake of carbohydrates and fats. Mild regular exercise can help a diabetic person to lead a normal life.

Arthritis

It is an autoimmune disease in which there is an inflammation of joints. **Acute arthritis** is characterised by pain, inflammation, redness and swelling of joints. Arthritis can be classified into three groups

1. Osteoarthritis

- It is a degenerative joint disease that affects majority of persons in the age group of 65-70 or above. There is excessive joint inflammation in this disease.
- Gradually, there is an increase in the stiffness and inflammation of joints that bear the weight of the body.
- Genetic factors also contribute to the degenerative process.
- **Treatment** Hip or knee replacements or joint debridement are the surgical procedures employed to relieve pain and improve joint function.

2. Rheumatoid arthritis

- It is an inflammatory disease of connective tissues of the body. Synovial membranes are the sacs, filled with fluid that lubricate the joints.
- Inflammation and thickening of synovial membranes results in the red and swollen joints. It is followed by scar tissue that protrudes over the surface of cartilage. The cartilage gets eroded and gets destroyed by this scar tissue.
- The bands of adhesion make the joints fixed (ankylosed), displaced and deformed. There is atrophy of skin, bones and muscles adjacent to the joint.
- There is a characteristic auto-antibody, called the rheumatoid factor in the blood of persons with rheumatoid arthritis. It is used to diagnose the disease.
- **Treatment** The drugs which are used to relieve the pain are aspirin, ibuprofen, etc.
    - If these anti-inflammatory drugs fail to relieve the pain, small doses of corticosteroids, such as prednisone may be used.
    - Physical therapy also helps in relieving pain and reducing swelling in affected joints.
    - Surgical replacement of destroyed hip, knee or finger joints with artificial substitutes is recommended in severe disability.

3. Septic arthritis

- It is the acute inflammation of one or more joints caused by infectious agents. Septic arthritis is of two types

  (i) **Suppurative arthritis** It is caused by bacteria, e.g. *Streptococcus haemolyticus*, *Staphylococcus aureus*, *Pneumococcus* or *Meningococcus*.

  Symptoms It is characterised by swollen pus-filled joints and fever. Pus is the result of infection and causes erosion of cartilage.

  Treatment Antibiotic treatment, drainage of swollen joints and rest provide relief.

  (ii) **Non-suppurative arthritis** It may occur along with diseases such as tuberculosis, typhoid, German measles, gonorrhea, syphilis, fungal infections or rheumatic fever.
- **Symptoms** include stiffness, swelling and pain on movements, etc.
- **Treatment** includes drug therapy and orthopedic care.

Gout

- It is characterised by repeated attacks of burning pain and stiffness. The joints become red, tender, hot and swollen. Hyperuricemia, i.e. increased levels of uric acid in blood is the underlying cause of gout.
- It results due to decreased excretion of uric acid through kidneys. Genetics also plays a role in the development of gout.
- It generally occurs in combination with other medical problems. For example, abdominal obesity, hypertension, insulin resistance and abnormal lipid levels, renal failure, haemolytic anaemia, psoriasis. Gout diagnosis is confirmed by the presence of characteristic crystals in the joint fluid.
- **Treatment** involves the steroids, colchicine and non-steroidal anti-inflammatory drugs.

Osteoporosis

- It is a bone disorder in which the bones become porous, which may increase the risk of fracture. The porosity of bones occurs due to the reduction of Bone Mineral Density (BMD).
- It is of two types

  (i) **Primary type 1** or **Postmenopausal osteoporosis** It occurs due to oestrogen deficiency in menopausal females.

  (ii) **Primary type 2** or **Senile osteoporosis** It occurs due to ageing and calcium deficiency.
- This may be the result of chronic disease or use of medicines such as glucocorticoids. The overuse of steroids and glucocorticoids also induces osteoporosis.
- Osteoporosis itself has no symptoms, but the bones become fragile, weak and are at greater risk of fractures.
- Advance oestrogen deficiency following menopause in women and testosterone deficiency in male, family history of fracture, etc., are non-modifiable risk factors.
- The modifiable risk factors are excessive alcohol intake, vitamin-D deficiency, tobacco smoking, malnutrition, high protein diet, under weight, etc.

- **Treatment** Antiresorptive or bone anabolic agents are used to treat osteoporosis. Antiresorptive drugs are biophosphonates oestrogen analogs, selective oestrogen receptor modulators, calcitonin, etc. Bone anabolic drugs are teriparatide, calcium salts and sodium fluoride, vitamin-D, vitamin-K.

Schizophrenia

- The term 'Schizophrenia' was coined by **Eugene Bieuler** from Greek *Skhizeinto*–split.
- It is a mental disorder characterised by hallucinations, delusions and disorganised thinking and speech.
- Important contributing factors are genetic, environmental, neurobiological, psychological and use of some recreational drugs. Some prescription drugs may cause or worsen the symptoms.
- **Symptoms** Schizophrenia mainly affects cognition and also contributes to chronic problems of behaviour and emotion. Major depression and anxiety disorders are additional conditions in person affected by schizophrenia. Associated social problems such as unemployment, poverty, homelessness and non-cooperation from near ones aggravate the condition.
- **Treatment** Antipsychotic drugs such as closapine, quetiapine, risperidone, perphenazine are given under guidance of qualified psychiatrist.

COMMUNITY HEALTH

This is the sum total of all the programmes, which help in protection, maintenance and improvement of health of people. It is also defined as the branch of science that helps in promoting physical and mental health. It helps to prevent diseases and prolong lifespan through the organised community attempts.

The major community health services are

1. Health centres
2. National programmes
3. Blood banks

Health centres

These are the centres run by the governments to take care of the health of the people in cities, town and villages. Health centres provide following activities

(i) **Environmental sanitation** These are as follows

- Treatment of domestic sewage by chemicals.
- Prevention of air pollution.
- Proper waste disposal through soak pits, composite pits, kitchen garden and smokeless chullah.
- Providing supply of germ free and safe drinking water.
- Elimination of breeding of insect vectors.

(ii) **Control of communicable diseases** These are as follows

- Vaccination against the communicable diseases such as TB, measles, smallpox, whooping cough, diphtheria, polio, tetanus and cholera.
- Careful treatment of diseased person.
- Malaria eradication.
- Regular supervision of food and trade.
- Eradication of disease spreading vectors.
- Inoculation of water storing reservoirs by larvicidal fishes, plants, bacteria, etc.
- Isolation of patients from contagious disease.

(iii) **Health education** People should be provided education regarding transmission, prevention and mechanism of control of communicable diseases. It can be achieved through personal contact, posters, pamphlets, audio-visual aids, seminars, newspapers, TV, radio, etc.

(iv) **School dealt services** These include

- Checkup of children should be done before admission. Regular medical checkup at definite interval of time should be organised at school.
- Education regarding health should be included in syllabus.
- Immunisation of the students from communicable diseases.
- Clean classroom and fresh drinking water should be provided to all children.

(v) **Maternity and child health services** These are as follows

- Routine checking of pregnant women.
- Care should be taken during delivery of child.
- Training of midwife.
- Prophylaxis against deficiency of vitamins and anaemia disease.
- Proper family planning.

(vi) **Nutrition education** These are as follows

- Educate the people about the balanced diet.
- Educate people about the various deficiency diseases, importance of green and yellow vegetation, availability of nutrients in common food, etc.

(vii) **Mental health** It includes guidance to mentally ill persons.

(viii) **Collection and cross checking of statistics** Accurate picture of health conditions in an area should be obtained by accurate data of birth, death and infectious diseases.

(ix) **Family planning** These provide free family planning advices to newly wedded couples. It also provides guidance and facilities in having a small family.

Chapter Exercises

(A) Topical Exercise

Communicable Diseases

1 Health is a combination of
(a) physical fitness
(b) presence of disease
(c) mental and social well-being
(d) Both (a) and (c)

2 Necessary steps for achieving good health are
(a) awareness about diseases
(b) vaccination
(c) proper disposal of wastes
(d) All of the above

3 Vehicle borne transmission of a disease is the transmission occurring through
(a) certain vectors like arthropods
(b) agencies like water, food blood, etc.
(c) through infectious clothes
(d) unhygienic conditions

4 One of the following diseases, where the thymus produced lymphocytes decreases to less than half, is
(a) gonorrhoea (b) *Salmonella* (c) hepatitis (d) anthrax

5 Consider the following statements with respect to common cold.
I. It is characterised by nasal congestion and discharge, sore throat, hoarseness, cough, headache and tiredness.
II. It usually lasts for 3-7 days.
Choose the correct option.
(a) Statement I is true, but II is false
(b) Statement I is false, but II is true
(c) Both statements I and II are true
(d) Both statements I and II are false

6 HIV/AIDS
(a) symptoms always appear within a month of infection
(b) can spread by mere touch or physical contact
(c) spreads when a infected person's body fluid comes in contact with the body fluid of a healthy person
(d) is related to all of the above options

7 HIV, the AIDS causing virus is also known as
(a) HTLV-III (b) HLV-II (c) HTV (d) HTLV-II

8 HIV, the Human Immunodeficiency Virus belongs to which of the following viral groups?
(a) Reoviruses
(b) Retroviruses
(c) Rhabdoviruses
(d) None of the above

9 In 1981, the first case of AIDS was recognised by
(a) Robert Gallo
(b) Luc Montagnier
(c) Luc Montagnier and Robert Gallo
(d) George Kohler and Cesar Milstein

10 Asymptomatic carrier state of HIV
(a) occurs usually 2-8 weeks after infection
(b) shows fatigue, shortness of breath, etc.
(c) is characterised by opportunistic infections
(d) has an incubation period ranging from 6 month to 10 years

11 HIV causes a complete breakdown of immune system by
(a) binding to T-cells and destroying them
(b) binding to B-cells and destroying them
(c) binding to T_4-lymphocytes through CD4 antigen and destroying them
(d) destroying B-cells and T-cells of immune system

12 Consider the following statements.
I. There is always a time lag between the infection and appearance of AIDS symptoms.
II. The time period for the AIDS symptoms may vary from a few months to many years, usually 5-10 years.
Choose the correct option.
(a) Statement I is true, but II is false
(b) Statement I is false, but II is true
(c) Both statements I and II are true
(d) Both statements I and II are false

13 AIDS is caused by HIV. Among the following, which one is not a mode of transmission of HIV **[NCERT]**
(a) transfusion of contaminated blood
(b) sharing the infected needles
(c) shaking hands with infected persons
(d) sexual contact with infected persons

14 Match the following columns with respect to HIV enzymes and their functions.

	Column I		Column II
A.	Reverse transcriptase	1.	Integrates the DNA produced by reverse transcription into host's genome
B.	Protease	2.	Performs teminism
C.	Integrase	3.	Cleaves large proteins in functional forms

Codes

	A	B	C
(a)	1	3	2
(b)	2	3	1
(c)	2	1	3
(d)	3	1	2

15 AIDS does not transmit from one person to other through
(a) sexual contacts
(b) blood transfusion
(c) placental contacts (in foetus)
(d) mosquito bites

16 Which of the following individuals are at high risk of HIV infection?
(a) Individuals having multiple partners
(b) Individuals who require repeated blood transfusion
(c) Drug addicts who take drugs intravenously
(d) All of the above

17 Symptom of AIDS Related Complex (ARC) is
(a) weight loss and diarrhoea
(b) swollen lymph nodes and fever
(c) loss of appetite and night sweating
(d) All of the above

18 Azidothymidine (AZT) is a/an
(a) biocatalyst (b) antibiotic
(c) anti-AIDS drug (d) anabolic hormone

19 Antiretroviral drugs of AIDS include
(a) Efavirenz, Lamivudine, Tenofovir
(b) Penicillin, Chloramphenicol, Ampicillin
(c) Chloromycetin, Diethylcarbamazine, Nystatin
(d) Fluconazole, Itraconazole, Nystatin

20 James Phipps and Ali Marvow are related to which viral disease that has disappeared?
(a) Cowpox (b) Smallpox
(c) Chickenpox (d) Tuberculosis

21 Severe Acute Respiratory Syndrome (SARS)
(a) is caused by a variant of *Pneumococcus*
(b) is caused by a variant of the common cold virus (corona virus)
(c) is an acute form of asthma
(d) affects non-vegetarians much faster than the vegetarians

22 Typhoid fever could be confirmed by
(a) Widal test (b) Mantoux test
(b) Schick test (d) Dick test

23 In which of the following disorders, the alveoli get filled with fluid leading to severe problems in respiration?
(a) Common cold (b) Whooping cough
(c) Diphtheria (d) Pneumonia

24 Match the following columns.

	Column I (Causative agents of pneumonia)		Column II (Species)
A.	Viral	1.	*S. pneumoniae*
B.	Bacterial	2.	*P. jirovecii, P. carinii*
C.	Fungal	3.	RSV, adenovirus, para influenza

Codes

	A	B	C		A	B	C
(a)	3	2	1	(b)	2	1	3
(c)	1	2	3	(d)	3	1	2

25 Pneumonia is an infection of the ...*A*... . The most common cause of pneumonia is a type of bacteria known as ...*B*... and ...*C*... .
Most suitable combination to fill the blanks is
(a) *A*-liver, *B*-*Salmonella typhi*, *C*-*Streptococcus pneumoniae*
(b) A-lungs, *B*-*Streptococcus pneumoniae* , *C*-*Haemophilus influenzae*
(c) A-blood, *B*-*Salmonella pneumoniae*, *C*-*Haemophilus influenzae*
(d) A-heart, *B*-*Salmonella typhi*, *C*-*Haemophilus influenzae*

26 Many diseases can be diagnosed by observing the symptoms in the patient. Which group of symptoms are indicative of pneumonia?
(a) Difficulty in respiration, fever, chills, cough, headache
(b) Constipation, abdominal pain, cramps, blood clots
(c) Nasal congestion and discharge, cough, sore throat, headache
(d) High fever, weakness, stomach pain, loss of appetite and constipation

27 Choose the incorrectly matched pair.
(a) Leprosy — Hansen's disease
(b) Syphilis — Sexually transmitted disease
(c) Cholera — Water borne infection
(d) Tuberculosis — Black death disease

28 Out of the following diseases which are caused due to bacterial infection?
I. Typhoid II. Elephantiasis
III. Cholera
IV. Tuberculosis
(a) I and II only (b) II and III only
(c) I, III and IV only (d) I, II, III and IV

29 Which of the following statements is not correct regarding malarial infection?
(a) Gametocytes are formed by the transformation of sporozoites in salivary gland of *Anopheles*
(b) High fever recurring every three to four days
(c) Sporozoites initially multiply within the liver cells and then attack the RBCs resulting in their rupture
(d) When a female *Anopheles* mosquito bites an infected person, these parasites enter the mosquito's body and undergo further development

30 Match the following columns.

	Column I		Column II
A.	*Plasmodium ovale*	1.	Benign tertiary malaria
B.	*Plasmodium malariae*	2.	Mild tertiary malaria
C.	*Plasmodium vivax*	3.	Malignant tertiary malaria
D.	*Plasmodium falciparum*	4.	Quartan malaria

Codes

	A	B	C	D
(a)	1	2	3	4
(b)	3	1	2	4
(c)	2	1	3	4
(d)	2	4	1	3

31 Match the following columns.

	Column I (Species of *Plasmodium*)		Column II (Incubation period)
A.	*P. vivax*	1.	28 days
B.	*P. malariae*	2.	12 days
C.	*P. ovale*	3.	17 days
D.	*P. falciparum*	4.	14 days

	A	B	C	D
(a)	3	2	1	4
(b)	4	1	3	2
(c)	1	2	3	4
(d)	3	1	4	2

32 Malarial parasite (*Plasmodium*)
(a) requires both human and male *Anopheles* to complete its life cycle
(b) is digenetic
(c) Both (a) and (b)
(d) performs the sexual cycle called schizogony in liver and RBC of humans

33 The most serious type of malaria is ...*A*... . as it affects ...*B*... and can be fatal.

	A	*B*
(a)	Malignant malaria	Brain
(b)	Quartan malaria	Liver
(c)	Benign tertian malaria	Brain
(d)	Mild tertian malaria	Kidney

34 The sporozoites of the malarial parasite are found in
(a) RBCs of humans suffering from malaria
(b) spleen of infected person
(c) salivary glands of freshly moulted male *Anopheles* mosquito
(d) saliva of infected female *Anopheles* mosquito

35 Which of the following toxic substance is responsible for the chill and high fever recurring every three to four days in malaria?
(a) Haemotoxin (b) Haemoglobin
(c) Haemozoin (d) Sporozoites

36 During the erythrocytic schizogony of *Plasmodium vivax*, fine granules appear in the cytoplasm of infected RBC. They are known as
(a) maurer's dots (b) hemozoin granules
(c) ferritin (d) None of these

37 Consider the following statements with respect to Schuffner's dots.
I. Represent granules on RBC of a malaria infected human.
II. Are red or red-yellow dots in erythrocytes of human infected with *Plasmodium vivax.*

Choose the correct option.
(a) Statement I is true, but II is false
(b) Statement I is false, but II is true
(c) Both statements I and II are true
(d) Both statements I and II are false

38 Mark the incorrect statement with respect to infection of *Entamoeba histolytica*.
(a) It is a protozoan parasite of human
(b) It is characterised by constipation and abdominal pain
(c) It is a parasite in small intestine of man
(d) Houseflies act as mechanical carriers and serve to transmit the parasite from faeces of infected person to food and food products

39 Cysts transform in .... stage are capable of infecting healthy person.
(a) 2-nuclei (b) 3-nuclei
(c) 4-nuclei (d) 6-nuclei

40 Amoebiasis is treated by
(a) Metronidazole and Tinidazole
(b) Sulfadoxine and Pyrimethamine
(c) Piperazine and Mebendazole
(d) Penicillin and Ampicillin

41 Choose the incorrectly matched pair.
(a) Kala-azar – Treated with pentahexonate
(b) Chagas' disease – Transmitted by contaminated water
(c) Giardiasis – Cause diarrhoea
(d) Sleeping sickness – Treated with suramin

42 Match the following columns.

Column I	Column II
A. Lymphatic filariasis	1. *Mansonella* sp.
B. Subcutaneous filariasis	2. *Loa loa, Mansonella* sp.
C. Serous filariasis	3. *W. bancrofti, B. malayi, B. timori*

Codes

	A	B	C		A	B	C
(a)	3	2	1	(b)	2	1	3
(c)	1	2	3	(d)	3	1	2

43 In filariasis, hydrocele is characterised by
(a) enlarged testis due to accumulation of lymphatic fluids
(b) inflammation in alveolar wall
(c) liver enlargement
(d) joint pain

44 Internal bleeding, muscular pain, fever, anaemia and blockage of the intestinal passage are the common symptoms of
(a) amoebiasis (b) elephantiasis
(c) ascariasis (d) typhoid

45 The most prominent symptom of elephantiasis is
(a) hepatomegaly
(b) edema with thickening of the skin and underlying tissue
(c) gastrointestinal discomfort
(d) rose coloured spots on the skin

46 Give the name of two helminths, which cause ascariasis and filariasis, respectively.
(a) *Ascaris* and *Wuchereria*
(b) *Wuchereria* and *Ascaris*
(c) Roundworm and Flatworm
(d) *Plasmodium* and *Wuchereria*

47 The larval stage of *Taenia solium* also called bladder worm and commonly found in muscle tissue in humans is known as
(a) hydatid cyst (b) hexacanth
(c) oncosphere (d) Cysticercus

48 The features which go in favour of haemolytic anaemia are
(a) increased serum bilirubin level
(b) jaundice
(c) increased breakdown of Hb
(d) All of the above

49 Which of the following is correct for ringworm disease?
(a) Heat and dry conditions help the causative organism to grow fast
(b) The causative agents thrive in skin folds of groin and toes
(c) The causative microorganisms are acquired from soil or by using towels, clothes and comb of infected individuals
(d) Both (b) and (c)

50 Which of the following are viral and mosquito borne diseases?
(a) Filaria and typhus
(b) Kala-azar and diphtheria
(c) Malaria and chagas disease
(d) Yellow fever and dengue

51 Mildest rickettsial disease of man is
(a) scrub typhus
(b) rocky mountain spotted fever
(c) Q-fever
(d) rickettsial pox

52 Match the following columns.

Column I	Column II
A. Oral candidiasis	1. *R. prowazeki*
B. Typhus fever	2. *R. conori*
C. Spotted fever	3. *R. rikettsi*
D. Boutonneuse fever	4. *Vulvovaginaitis*

Codes

	A	B	C	D
(a)	4	3	2	1
(b)	2	1	3	4
(c)	4	1	3	2
(d)	2	3	1	4

53 Which of the following is used for the treatment of Q-fever?
(a) Tetracyclines
(b) Metronidazole
(c) Niclosamide
(d) Benznidazole

Non-Communicable Diseases and Community Health

54 Which of the following is associated with cancer?
(a) Oncogene (b) Proto-oncogenes
(c) Loss of contact inhibition (d) Both (a) and (c)

55 Identify the incorrectly matched pair.
(a) Skin cancer – UV radiation
(b) Breast cancer – Hormones
(c) Mouth cancer – Tobacco
(d) Liver cancer – HPV

56 Among the non-infectious diseases, which of the following is most common fatal diseases of human beings?
(a) AIDS (b) Cancer
(c) Cystic fibrosis (d) Cholera

57 Match the following columns.

	Column I		Column II
A.	Cartilage cancer	1.	Myosarcoma
B.	Muscle tumour	2.	Liposarcoma
C.	Bone tumour	3.	Chondrosarcoma
D.	Adipose tissue tumour	4.	Osteosarcoma

Codes

	A	B	C	D
(a)	1	3	2	4
(b)	3	1	4	2
(c)	2	3	1	4
(d)	4	2	3	1

58 Identify the incorrect statement about benign tumour.
(a) It grows slowly and can attain a large size
(b) Benign brain tumours are dangerous
(c) Benign tumours can become malignant in some cases
(d) They can spread through blood or lymph

59 Which of the following is not correctly matched?
(a) Carcinomas—Cartilage
(b) Sarcomas – Connective tissue
(c) Lymphomas – Lymph node
(d) Adenomas – Thyroid gland

60 Match the following columns.

	Column I		Column II
A.	Glioma	1.	Cancer of pigment cells of skin
B.	Lymphoma	2.	Cancer of glands
C.	Melanoma	3.	Cancer of lymphatic tissue
D.	Adenoma	4	Cancer of glial cells of central nervous system

Codes

	A	B	C	D
(a)	4	3	1	2
(b)	1	2	3	4
(c)	1	4	3	2
(d)	2	1	4	3

61 Which of the following is incorrect ?
(a) Leukaemia results in uncontrolled proliferation of WBCs
(b) Carcinomas are malignant growths of the epithelial tissues
(c) Sarcoma is a malignant tumour of connective tissues and lymph nodes
(d) None of the above

62 Identify the incorrect match.
(a) Diethylstilbestrol - Vagina
(b) Vinyl chloride - Liver
(c) Mustard gas, nickel chromium - Lungs
(d) Coal tar - Prostrate

63 Consider the following statements.
I. Most cancer are treatment by combination of surgery, radio therapy and chemotherapy.
II. Molecular biology techniques are being applied to detect gene in individual with inherited susceptibility to certain cancer.

Choose the correct option.
(a) Statement I is true, but II is false
(b) Statement I is false, but II is true
(c) Both statements I and II are true
(d) Both statements I and II are false

64 The bombardment of cancerous tissue with rays from radioactive material like cobalt, iridium and iodine is called
(a) immunotherapy
(b) chemotherapy
(c) radiotherapy
(d) supportive therapy

65 Ionising radiations like ...*A*... and ...*B*... and non-ionising radiations like ...*C*... cause DNA damage leading to neoplastic transformation.

	A	*B*	*C*
(a)	X-rays	Gamma rays	UV rays
(b)	X-rays	UV rays	Gamma rays
(c)	X-rays	Gamma rays	Infrared rays
(d)	Infrared rays	X-rays	UV rays

66 Computed Tomography (CT) uses
(a) X-rays to generate 3D image of areas inside the body
(b) Gamma rays to generate 3D image of areas inside the body
(c) Either (a) or (b)
(d) Ultrasound to generate 2D image of the areas inside the body

67 National Programme for Leprosy Eradication is
(a) NLEP (b) NLCP (c) NCCP (d) NMEP

(B) Cumulative Exercise

(Assorted Questions of the Chapter for Advanced Level Practice)

1 Which of the following are acquired diseases in humans?

I. Kala-azar II. Haemophilia
III. AIDS IV. Albinism

Codes
(a) Only I (b) I and III (c) III and IV (d) II and IV

2 Arrange the following steps of life cycle of HIV in sequence.

I. The progeny viruses released in the blood attack other helper T-lymphocytes.
II. RNA genome of virus replicates to form viral DNA with the help of reverse transcriptase.
III. The viral DNA gets incorporated into host cell's (macrophages and helper T-lymphocytes) DNA and directs the infected cells to produce virus DNA.
IV. Progressive decrease in the number of helper T-lymphocytes in the body of infected person.

(a) II → I → III → IV (b) II → III → I → IV
(c) II → I → III → IV (d) II → IV → III → I

3 Find out whether the given statements are true (T)/ false (F) and choose the correct option.

I. Cancer causing viruses called oncogenic viruses modify the host's genome.
II. Cancer detection is based on biopsy, bone marrow tests and histopathological studies of the tissue and blood.
III. Techniques likes radiography (X-rays), Computed Tomography (CT) and Magnetic Resonance Imaging (MRI) are very useful to defect cancers of internal organs.
IV. Antibodies against cancer-specific antigens are used for the detection of certain cancers.

	I	II	III	IV
(a)	T	T	T	F
(b)	T	F	F	T
(c)	T	T	T	T
(d)	F	F	F	T

4 Sandflies play significant role in spreading kala-azar because they

I. suck blood only from the patients suffering from kala-azar.
II. covert amastigote into promastigote.
III. engulf amastigote at the time of blood sucking from the infected persons.
IV. inject promastigote into the body of non-infected persons at the time of blood sucking.

Codes
(a) I and II (b) II and III
(c) II, III and IV (d) III and IV

5 Match the following columns.

	Column I		Column II
A.	*Glossina* sp.	1.	Tse-tse fly
B.	*Panstrongylus* sp.	2.	Chagas' disease
C.	*Coxiella burnetii*	3.	Q-fever
D.	*Clostridium* sp.	4.	Tetanospasmin

Codes

	A	B	C	D
(a)	2	3	1	4
(b)	4	3	2	1
(c)	3	4	1	2
(d)	1	2	3	4

6 In the given figure of HIV virus, identify *A*, *B* and *C*.

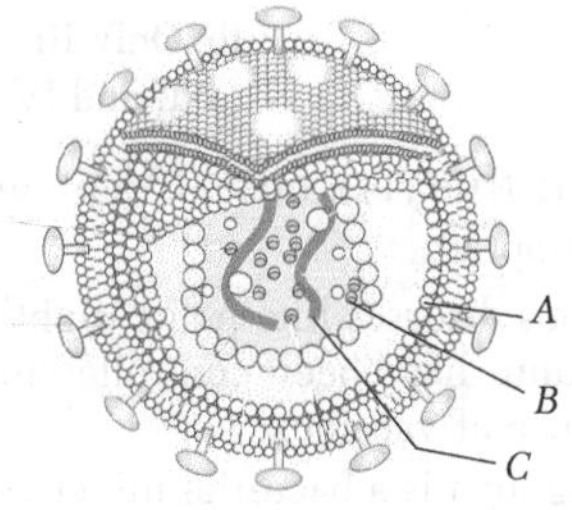

(a) *A*-Lipid coat; *B*-capsid protein; *C*-*ds*RNA
(b) *A*-Protein coat; *B*-Capsid protein; *C*-*ss*RNA
(c) *A*-Lipid coat; *B*-Capsid protein; *C*-*ss*RNA
(d) *A*-Glycoprotein; *B*-Capsid protein; *C*-*ds*RNA

7 Consider the following statements about cancer.

I. Cancer is unusual and untimely proliferation of cells.
II. Benign tumour is not as serious as malignant tumour.
III. Malignant tumour causes overcrowding and disruption of normal cells.
IV. Malignant tumour spreads to other organs through metastasis.

Choose the option containing correct group of statements.

(a) I, II, III and IV (b) I and II
(c) I, II and III (d) III and IV

8 Identify the incorrect statement with respect to filariasis.

(a) Larvae enter skin when mosquito takes a blood meal
(b) Mosquito ingests microfilariae when it takes a blood meal
(c) Microfilariae penetrate mosquito's midgut and migrate to thoracic muscles
(d) L3 larvae migrate to the' head and proboscis of mosquito

9 Diseases are broadly grouped into infectious and non-infectious diseases. In the list given below, identify the infectious diseases.

I. Cancer
II. Influenza
III. Allergy
IV. Smallpox

Choose the correct option.

(a) I and II (b) II and III (c) III and IV (d) II and IV

10 Which of the following statements regarding treatment of cancer is false?

I. Chemotherapy has side effects like hair loss and anaemia.
II. Radon (Rn-220) is the most commonly used isotope for radiation therapy.
III. α-interferon are used as immunological substances which activate the immune system.
IV. Isotope of carbon is widely used for radiation therapy.

Codes

(a) I and II (b) Only III
(c) Only IV (d) II and IV

11 Find out the true (T) / false (F) statements and choose the correct option.

I. Infectious diseases like polio, diphtheria, pneumonia and tetanus have been controlled to a large extent by the use of vaccines.
II. Chikungunya is a bacterial infectious disease.
III. *Mycobacterium* causes leprosy and tuberculosis.
IV. Smallpox has been eradicated from the world by the use of vaccines.

	I	II	III	IV
(a)	T	F	T	F
(b)	F	F	T	T
(c)	T	F	F	T
(d)	T	F	T	T

12 Identify the stage marked as *A*, *B*, *C* and *D* in the life cycle of *Plasmodium*.

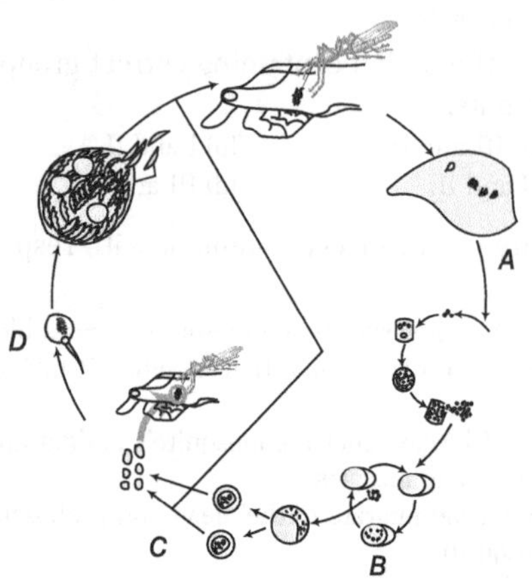

	A	*B*	*C*	*D*
(a)	Sporozoites in spleen	Sexual reproduction of *Plasmodium* in RBC	Gametocytes in RBC	Fertilisation of gametocytes in mosquito's intestine
(b)	Sporozoites in liver	Asexual reproduction of *Plasmodium* in RBC	Gametocytes in RBC	Fertilisation of gametocytes in mosquito's intestine
(c)	Sporozoites in liver	Asexual reproduction of *Plasmodium* in RBC	Gametocytes in RBC	Fertilisation of gametocytes in mosquito's salivary glands
(d)	Sporozoites in kidney	Sexual reproduction of *Plasmodium* in RBC	Gametocytes in RBC	Fertilisation of gametocytes in mosquito's intestine

13 Which of the statements are correct?

I. Gout is a type of arthritis.
II. Non-suppurative arthritis is caused by *Pneumococcus* bacteria.
III. Diabetes mellitus is a communicable disease characterised by high blood sugar level.
IV. Senile osteoporosis occurs due to ageing.

Codes

(a) I and II (b) I and IV
(c) II, III and IV (d) Only I

14 Match the diseases in Column I with the appropriate items (pathogen/prevention/treatment) in Column II.

Column I	Column II
A. Amoebiasis	1. *Treponema pallidum*
B. Diphtheria	2. Use only sterilised food and water
C. Cholera	3. DPT vaccine
D. Syphilis	4. Use of oral rehydration therapy

Codes

	A	B	C	D		A	B	C	D
(a)	1	2	3	4	(b)	2	4	1	3
(c)	2	1	3	4	(d)	2	3	4	1

15 Read the following statements.

I. Ronald Ross received Nobel Prize for physiology or medicine (1902) for this work on the transmission of malaria.
II. Malaria means 'Bad air'.
III. Asexual cycle called schizogony (of *Plasmodium*) is a type of binary fission.
IV. Pernicious malaria or 'black-water fever' is caused by *Plasmodium falciparum*.
V. The incubation period of all the species of *Plasmodium* is same.

Which of the above statements are correct?

(a) III and V (b) I, II and IV
(c) I, II and III (d) IV and V

16. Match the following columns.

Column I (Diseases)	Column II (Causative organisms)
A. Dysentery	1. *Entamoeba histolytica*
B. Malignant malaria	2. *Plasmodium falciparum*
C. Common cold	3. Rhinovirus
D. Ringworm	4. *Trichophyton*

Codes

	A	B	C	D
(a)	1	2	3	4
(b)	2	3	4	1
(c)	3	4	1	2
(d)	4	1	2	3

17 Read the given statements carefully.

I. In India NACO and other NGOs are making efforts to educate people about AIDS.

II. To prevent HIV infections, use of disposable needles and syringes in hospitals, use of condoms during sex, control of drug abuse, etc., is necessary.

III. 1st December is celebrated as World AIDS Day.

IV. AIDS is characterised by decrease in the number of killer T-cells.

Which of the above statements are correct?

Codes

(a) I, II and IV (b) I, II, III and IV

(c) I and III (d) I and IV

18 HIV is a ...*A*... and has genetic material composed of ...*B*..., HIV replicates inside the host cells. It is considered a retrovirus because it uses an enzyme, ...*C*..., to convert ...*D*... into ...*E*... . Here, *A* to *E* refers to

(a) *A*-retrovirus, *B*-RNA, *C*-reverse transcriptase, *D*-RNA, *E*-DNA

(b) *A*-retroviral, B-DNA, *C*-reverse transcriptase, *D*-DNA, *E*-RNA

(c) *A*-rhinovirus, B-DNA, *C*-reverse transcriptase, *D*-DNA, *E*-RNA

(d) *A*-adenovirus, *B*-RNA, *C*-reverse transcriptase, *D*-RNA, *E*-DNA

19 Match the following columns.

Column I	Column II
A. Ascariasis	1. Inflammation of lymphatic vessels of lower limbs and genital organs
B. Filariasis	2. Internal bleeding, muscular pain, fever, anaemia, blockage of intestinal passage
C. Amoebiasis	3. Dry, scaly lesions on various body parts like skin, nail and scalp with intense itching
D. Ringworm	4. Abdominal pain, stools with excess mucus and blood clots

Codes

	A	B	C	D
(a)	2	4	3	1
(b)	2	1	4	3
(c)	1	2	3	4
(d)	4	2	1	3

20 Select the correct statements.

I. The word AIDS stands for Acquired Immuno Deficiency Syndrome. This means deficiency of immune system, acquired during the lifetime of an individual.

II. AIDS was first reported in 1981 and the word 'syndrome' in this, means a group of symptoms.

III. There is always a time-lag between the infection and appearance of AIDS symptoms, i.e. vary from a few months to many years (usually 5-10 years).

IV. During HIV infection, the macrophages cells of body continues produce virus and in this way acts like a HIV factory.

Codes

(a) I, II and III (b) III and IV

(c) I and IV (d) I, II, III and IV

21 Which of the following are the reasons for rheumatoid arthritis?

I. The ability to differentiate pathogens or foreign molecules from self cells increases.

II. Body attacks self cells.

III. More antibodies are produced in the body.

IV. The ability to differentiate pathogens or foreign molecules from self cells is lost.

Codes

(a) I and II (b) II and IV (c) III and IV (d) I and III

22 Read the following statements and select the incorrect one.

(a) When the functioning of one or more organs or systems of the body is adversely affected, characterised by appearance of various signs and symptoms, i.e. we have disease

(b) Some of the infectious diseases like AIDS are fatal

(c) Pathogens cause harm to the host by living in (or on) them

(d) None of the above

23 Identify *A*, *B*, *C* and *D* in the diagram of HIV.

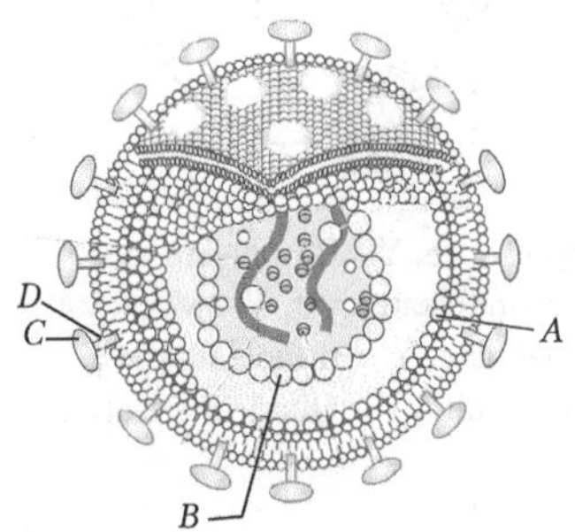

	A	B	C	D
(a)	p 17	gp 120	gp 41	p 24
(b)	p 24	gp 41	gp 120	p 17
(c)	p 17	p 24	gp 120	gp 41
(d)	gp 120	gp 41	p 17	p 24

24 Normal cell have genes called ...*A*... which are present in inactivated state but under certain conditions like ....*B*... they get transformed to ...*C*... . Here *A*, *B* and *C* refer to

(a) *A*-cellular oncogenes, *B*-mutation, *C*-cancer causing oncogenes
(b) *A*-viral oncogenes, *B*-mutation, *C*-disease causing genes
(c) *A*-viral oncogenes, *B*-mutation, *C*-tumour causing gene
(d) None of the above

25 Arrange the stages of life cycle of *Plasmodium* starting from human host and ending in mosquito host.

I. RBC releases the toxic haemozoin.
II. Parasite reproduces asexually in liver cells.
III. Parasites attack RBC.
IV. Sporozoites enter human body through the mosquito bite.
V. Mature sporozoites escape from intestine and migrate to the mosquito's salivary gland.
VI. Fertilisation of gametocytes occurs in mosquito's intestine.
VII. Mosquito takes up gametocytes while sucking blood of an infected-person.

(a) IV → II → I → III → VII → V → VI
(b) I → II → III → V → VI → IV → VII
(c) IV → II → III → I → VII → VI → V
(d) III → IV → II → I → V → VII → VI

26 Identify the stages labelled as 'X' and 'Y' in the life cycle of *Entamoeba histolytica.*

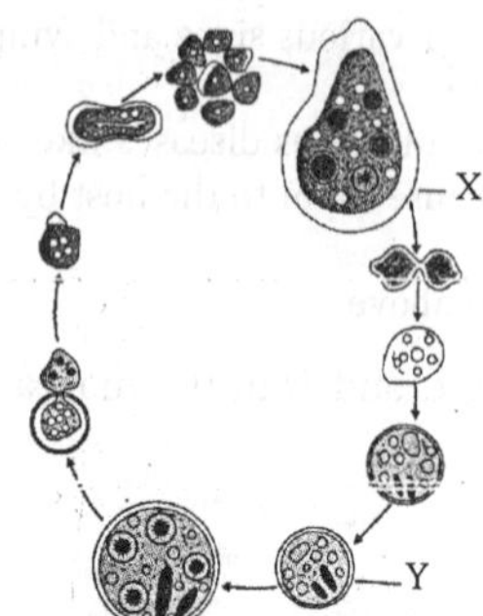

(a) X - Trophozoite, Y - Binucleate cyst
(b) X - Quadrinucleate cyst, Y - Metacystic *Amoeba*
(c) X - Amoebulae, Y - Binucleate cyst
(d) X - Trophozoite, Y - Quadrinucleate cyst

27 Match the following columns.

	Column I (Carcinogens)		Column II (Organ affected)
A.	Aflatoxin	1.	Urinary bladder
B.	Diethylstilbestrol	2.	Liver
C.	N-nitrosodimethylamine	3.	Vagina
D.	4-aminobiphenyl	4.	Lungs

Codes

	A	B	C	D
(a)	1	3	2	4
(b)	3	1	4	2
(c)	2	3	4	1
(d)	4	2	3	1

28 Match the following columns.

	Column I		Column II
A.	HIV infection	1.	Widal test
B.	Typhoid	2.	Biopsy
C.	Cancer	3.	Tuberculin analysis
D.	Tuberculosis	4.	ELISA

Codes

	A	B	C	D
(a)	1	3	4	2
(b)	3	2	4	1
(c)	4	1	2	3
(d)	2	4	3	1

29 Which of the following statements is incorrect regarding carcinogens?

(a) Tobacco smoke contains chemical carcinogens which can cause lung cancer
(b) They are physical, chemical and biological agents
(c) Radiations like X-rays and UV-rays can cause damage to RNA which leads to neoplastic transformation
(d) When proto-oncogenes gets activated in normal conditions, they lead to oncogenic transformation of the cells

30 Match the following columns.

	Column I		Column II
A.	African sleeping sickness	1.	*Sacculina*
B.	Dumdum fever	2.	*Haemophilus influenzae*
C.	Pneumonia	3.	*Leishmania donovani*
D.	Parasitic castration	4.	*Trypanosoma gambiense*
		5.	*Leishmania tropica*

Codes

	A	B	C	D
(a)	4	3	2	1
(b)	3	4	1	2
(c)	3	1	2	4
(d)	4	3	1	5

31 Choose the incorrect statement regarding AIDS.
(a) AIDS is an immunodeficiency disease
(b) It is caused by a retrovirus, HIV
(c) HIV selectively infects and kill B-lymphocytes
(d) Retroviruses have RNA genomes that replicate *via* DNA intermediate
(e) Viral RNA genome is converted into DNA copy by reverse transcriptase

Assertion and Reason

Direction (Q. Nos. 32-37) *In each of the following questions, a statement of Assertion (A) is given followed by corresponding statement of Reason (R). Of the statements, mark the correct answer as*
(a) Both A and R are true and R is the correct explanation of A
(b) Both A and R are true, but R is not the correct explanation of A
(c) A is true, but R is false
(d) A is false, but R is true
(e) Both A and R are false

32 **Assertion** (A) Rickettsiae should be regarded as bacteria.
Reason (R) It contains both RNA and DNA and respond to antibiotics.

33 **Assertion** (A) Q-fever is an influenza like illness with fever.
Reason (R) It was first recognised as a disease in 1935 in Queensland and Australia.

34 **Assertion** (A) AIDS is a disorder caused by HIV.
Reason (R) HIV is a virus that damages the immune system of its host.

35 **Assertion** (A) Virus multiplies only, inside the living cells.
Reasons (R) Viruses help host cells in growth and development.

36 **Assertion** (A) Pneumonia affects brain and causes dizziness.
Reason (R) It is mainly viral zoonotic disease.

37 **Assertion** (A) Pertussis is caused by a bacterium, *Bordetella pertussis*.
Reason (R) It is also called whooping cough.

(C) Medical Entrances' Gallery

(Collection of questions asked in NEET & Various Medical Entrance Exams)

1 Match the following columns and select the correct option from the codes given below.

	Column I		Column II
A.	Typhoid	1.	*Haemophilus influenzae*
B.	Malaria	2.	*Wuchereria bancrofti*
C.	Pneumonia	3.	*Plasmodium vivax*
D.	Filariasis	4.	*Salmonella typhi*

Codes **[JIPMER 2019, NEET 2019]**

	A	B	C	D
(a)	4	3	1	2
(b)	3	4	2	1
(c)	1	3	2	4
(d)	1	2	4	3

2 The infectious stage of *Plasmodium* that enters the human body is **[NEET 2019]**
(a) trophozoite (b) sporozoite
(c) female gametocyte (d) male gametocyte

3 Carcinogen present in cigarette smoke is **[JIPMER 2019]**
(a) benzopyrene (b) nicotine
(c) carbon monoxide (d) All of these

4 In which disease does mosquito transmitted pathogen cause chronic inflammation of lymphatic vessels?
(a) Ringworm disease (b) Ascariasis **[NEET 2018]**
(c) Elephantiasis (d) Amoebiasis

5 Which of the following is not an autoimmune disease? **[NEET 2018]**
(a) Alzheimer's disease
(b) Rheumatoid arthritis
(c) Psoriasis
(d) Vitiligo

6 Adults of *Wuchereria bancrofti* attack **[AIIMS 2018]**
(a) excretory system (b) digestive system
(c) lymphatic system (d) nervous system

7 Person 'A' cannot step out of his house. He has to spend his entire life in sterile isolation otherwise, he would quickly contract a fatal infection. This person has almost no effective immune system. This disease is also called as baby in a bubble syndrome. Identify the disease, this person 'A' is suffering from.
(a) Cystic fibrosis (b) Diabetes **[AIIMS 2018]**
(c) AIDS (d) SCID

8 Characteristics of cancer are **[AIIMS 2018]**

(a) all viruses are oncogenic
(b) all tumours are cancers
(c) cancerous cells show property of contact inhibition
(d) cancer cells show metastasis

9 Match the following sexually transmitted diseases in Column I with their causative agent in Column II and select the correct option. **[NEET 2017]**

Column I	Column II
A. Gonorrhoea	1. HIV
B. Syphilis	2. *Neisseria*
C. Genital warts	3. *Treponema*
D. AIDS	4. Human papilloma virus

Codes

	A	B	C	D
(a)	2	3	4	1
(b)	3	4	1	2
(c)	4	2	3	1
(d)	4	3	2	1

10 Note the following features and choose the ones applicable to *Wuchereria bancrofti*.

I. Coelozoic parasite
II. Histozoic parasite
III. Monogenetic parasite
IV. Digenetic parasite
V. Monomorphic, acoelomate parasite
VI. Dimorphic, pseudocoelomate parasite **[JIPMER 2017]**

Choose the correct option.

(a) II, III and V
(b) II, III and VI
(c) II, IV and VI
(d) I, III and VI

11 Which of the following factors is incorrect for the low levels of immune response during *Plasmodium* infection? **[AIIMS 2017]**

(a) Different types of antigens are expressed at varying stages of *Plasmodium* life cycle
(b) The stages during its life cycle are mostly intracellular
(c) The sporozoites of *Plasmodium* are rapidly cleared from blood circulation
(d) *Plasmodium* infection primarily destroys the macrophages and dendritic cells present in blood

12 Which of the following diseases is caused by a protozoan? **[CBSE AIPMT 2015]**

(a) Syphilis
(b) Influenza
(c) Babesiosis
(d) Blastomycosis

13 Which of the following sets of diseases is caused by bacteria? **[NEET-II 2016]**

(a) Cholera and tetanus
(b) Typhoid and smallpox
(c) Tetanus and mumps
(d) Herpes and influenza

14 Which of the following statements is not correct with respect to malaria? **[Karnataka CET 2015]**

(a) RBC's rupture and release haemozoin which causes chills
(b) Sporozoites multiply in blood
(c) Female *Anopheles* mosquito is the vector
(d) Malignant malaria is caused by *Plasmodium falciparum*

15 Which of the following is correct regarding AIDS causative agent HIV? **[NEET-II 2016]**

(a) HIV is enveloped virus containing one molecule of single-stranded RNA and one molecule of reverse transcriptase
(b) HIV is enveloped virus that contains two identical molecules of single-stranded RNA and two molecule of reverse transcriptase
(c) HIV is unenveloped retrovirus
(d) HIV does not escape, but attacks the acquired immune response

16 Which one of the following statements is correct? **[EAMCET 2015]**

(a) Benign tumours show the property of metastasis
(b) Heroin accelerates body functions
(c) Malignant tumour exhibits metastasis
(d) Patients who have undergone surgery are given cannabinoids

17 Match the following columns. **[EAMCET 2015]**

Column I	Column II
A. HIV	1. Ghost
B. Pilus	2. Prophage
C. Virus penetration	3. Retroviridae
D. Lysogeny	4. Donor
	5. Polyhedral virus

Codes

	A	B	C	D
(a)	1	2	3	4
(b)	5	4	3	2
(c)	5	3	2	1
(d)	3	4	1	2

18 Select the incorrect combination(s) from followings. **[WB JEE 2015]**

(a) Encephalitis — Viral disease
(b) Kala-azar — *Phlebotomus*
(c) Rhabditiform larvae — *Ascaris*
(d) *Entamoeba* — Sporogony

19 World AIDS day is celebrated on **[J&K CET 2015]**

(a) 1st May
(b) 1st December
(c) 20th December
(d) 1st June

20 AIDS is caused by **[J&K CET 2015]**

(a) blood cancer
(b) TMV
(c) bacterium
(d) Human Immunodeficiency Virus (HIV)

21 Choose the correct set of disease transmitting arthropods. **[Chhattisgarh PMT 2015]**

(a) Tse-tse fly, housefly, rat flea, sand fly
(b) *Anopheles*, louse, housefly, termite
(c) Cockroach, louse, termite, housefly
(d) Rat flea, butterfly, housefly, tse-tse fly

22 Which one of the following is not a property of cancerous cells? **[Chhattisgarh PMT 2015]**

(a) They compete with normal cells for vital nutrients
(b) They may not remain confined in the area of formation
(c) They divide in an uncontrolled manner
(d) They show contact inhibition

23 Identify the wrong statements.

I. The tumour of haematopoietic cell is called leukemia.
II. Cancer arising from the epithelial tissues of internal organs and glands is referred as melanoma.
III. Sarcoma is type of cancer where bone and cartilage are involved.
IV. Only benign tumours are called as true cancer or neoplasm. **[Chhattisgarh PMT 2015]**

Codes

(a) I and II (b) II and IV
(c) II and III (d) I and III

24 Which of the following virus is not transferred through semen of an infected male? **[CBSE AIPMT 2015]**

(a) Hepatitis-B virus
(b) Human Immunodeficiency virus
(c) Chikungunya virus
(d) Ebola virus

25 HIV that causes AIDS, first starts destroying **[CBSE AIPMT 2015]**

(a) B-lymphocytes (b) leucocytes
(c) helper T-lymphocytes (d) thrombocytes

26 Match each disease with its correct type of vaccine.

	Column I		Column II
A.	Tuberculosis	1.	Harmless virus
B.	Whooping cough	2.	Inactivated toxin
C.	Diphtheria	3.	Killed bacteria
D.	Polio	4.	Harmless bacteria

Codes **[CBSE AIPMT 2015]**

	A	B	C	D
(a)	2	1	3	4
(b)	3	2	4	1
(c)	4	3	2	1
(d)	1	2	3	4

27 Infection of *Ascaris* usually occurs by **[NEET 2013]**

(a) eating imperfectly cooked pork
(b) tse-tse fly
(c) mosquito bite
(d) drinking water containing eggs of *Ascaris*

28 It is a disease which mainly affects mucous membrane of urinogenital tract. In males, burning feeling on passing urine, after a yellow discharge occurs, that is accompanied by fever, headache and feeling of illness

(a) syphilis (b) gonorrhoea **[AMU 2012]**
(c) AIDS (d) None of these

29 Schizogony occurs in **[BHU 2012]**

(a) RBC of human (b) intestine of parasite
(c) liver of human (d) liver of parasite

30 Which one of the following is not a property of cancerous cells whereas, the remaining three are? **[CBSE AIPMT 2012]**

(a) They compete with normal cells for vital nutrients
(b) They do not remain confined in the area of formation
(c) They divide in an uncontrolled manner
(d) They show contact inhibition

31 The pair of disease caused by virus is **[BHU 2012]**

(a) typhoid and tetanus (b) rabies and mumps
(c) cholera and tuberculosis (d) AIDS and syphilis

32 Motile zygote of *Plasmodium* occurs in

(a) gut of female *Anopheles* **[CBSE AIPMT 2012]**
(b) salivary glands of *Anopheles*
(c) human RBCs
(d) human liver

33 Hepatitis-B virus is **[AMU 2012]**

(a) hepadnavirus (b) variola virus
(c) retrovirus (d) picornavirus

34 Which one of the following is not a characteristic feature of malignant tumour? **[AFMC 2012]**

(a) Invasiveness
(b) Metastasis
(c) Lack of differentiation of cells
(d) None of the above

35 At which stage of HIV infection does one usually shows symptoms of AIDS? **[CBSE AIPMT 2011]**

(a) When viral DNA is produced by reverse transcriptase
(b) When HIV replicates rapidly in helper T-lymphocytes and damages large number of these cells
(c) With 15 days of sexual contact with an infected person
(d) When the infecting retrovirus enters host cells

36 Match the following columns.

	Column I		Column II
A.	*Haemophilus influenzae*	1.	Malignant malaria
B.	*Entamoeba histolytica*	2.	Elephantiasis
C.	*Plasmodium falciparum*	3.	Pneumonia
D.	*Wuchereria bancrofti*	4.	Typhoid
E.	*Salmonella typhi*	5.	Amoebiasis

Codes **[Kerala CEE 2011]**

	A	B	C	D	E
(a)	1	5	3	2	4
(b)	3	5	1	2	4
(c)	5	1	3	4	2
(d)	1	3	2	5	4
(e)	1	3	5	2	4

37 Which one of the following diseases is caused by virus? **[MHT CET 2011]**
(a) Cholera (b) Diphtheria
(c) Measles (d) Whooping cough

38 With regard to the transmission of the Human Immunodeficiency Virus (HIV), which one of the following statements is not correct? **[MHT CET 2011]**
(a) The chances of transmission from female to male are twice as likely as from male to female
(b) The chances of transmission are more if a person suffers from other sexually transmitted infections
(c) An infected mother can transmit the infection to her baby during pregnancy at childbirth and by breastfeeding
(d) The risk of contracting infection from transfusion of infected blood is much higher than an exposure to contaminate needle

39 The group of disease carried by insects is **[MHT CET 2011]**
(a) typhoid, jaundice, dysentery
(b) mumps, measles, smallpox
(c) scabies, ringworm, scarlet fever
(d) malaria, filaria, yellow fever

40 Food poisoning is caused by **[UP CPMT 2011]**
(a) *Nitrosomonas* (b) *Lactobacillus*
(c) *Escherichia coli* (d) None of these

41 Vaccine for tuberculosis is known as **[J&K CET 2011]**
(a) PAS vaccine (b) BCG vaccine
(c) OPV (d) DPT

42 Which of the following is STD? **[Gujarat CET 2011]**
(a) Cancer (b) Malaria
(c) Pneumonia (d) Trichomoniasis

ANSWERS

Check Point 15.1

1. (c)	2. (d)	3. (c)	4. (c)	5. (a)	6. (b)

Check Point 15.2

1. (a)	2. (a)	3. (c)	4. (b)	5. (c)	6. (a)

Check Point 15.3

1. (b)	2. (a)	3. (a)	4. (d)	5. (d)	6. (c)

Check Point 15.4

1. (c)	2. (c)	3. (d)	4. (d)	5. (d)

(A) Topical Exercise

1. (d)	2. (d)	3. (b)	4. (c)	5. (c)	6. (c)	7. (a)	8. (b)	9. (c)	10. (d)
11. (c)	12. (c)	13. (c)	14. (a)	15. (d)	16. (d)	17. (d)	18. (c)	19. (a)	20. (b)
21. (b)	22. (a)	23. (d)	24. (d)	25. (b)	26. (a)	27. (d)	28. (c)	29. (a)	30. (d)
31. (b)	32. (b)	33. (a)	34. (d)	35. (c)	36. (a)	37. (c)	38. (c)	39. (c)	40. (a)
41. (b)	42. (a)	43. (a)	44. (c)	45. (b)	46. (a)	47. (d)	48. (d)	49. (d)	50. (d)
51. (c)	52. (c)	53. (a)	54. (d)	55. (d)	56. (b)	57. (b)	58. (d)	59. (a)	60. (a)
61. (d)	62. (d)	63. (c)	64. (c)	65. (a)	66. (a)	67. (a)			

(B) Cumulative Exercise

1. (a)	2. (b)	3. (c)	4. (c)	5. (d)	6. (b)	7. (a)	8. (c)	9. (d)	10. (c)
11. (d)	12. (b)	13. (b)	14. (d)	15. (b)	16. (a)	17. (b)	18. (a)	19. (b)	20. (d)
21. (b)	22. (d)	23. (c)	24. (a)	25. (c)	26. (a)	27. (c)	28. (c)	29. (c)	30. (a)
31. (c)	32. (a)	33. (b)	34. (a)	35. (c)	36. (e)	37. (b)			

(C) Medical Entrances' Gallery

1. (a)	2. (b)	3. (a)	4. (c)	5. (a)	6. (c)	7. (d)	8. (d)	9. (a)	10. (c)
11. (d)	12. (c)	13. (a)	14. (b)	15. (b)	16. (c)	17. (d)	18. (d)	19. (b)	20. (d)
21. (a)	22. (d)	23. (b)	24. (c)	25. (c)	26. (c)	27. (d)	28. (b)	29. (a)	30. (d)
31. (b)	32. (a)	33. (a)	34. (d)	35. (b)	36. (b)	37. (c)	38. (a)	39. (d)	40. (c)
41. (b)	42. (d)								

Explanations

(A) Topical Exercise

15 (*d*) AIDS does not transmitted from one person to another through mosquito bite because HIV is unable to replicate in mosquito's gut as T-cell are not persent in mosquito's gut. Therefore, HIV particles get digested by mosquito along with blood meal.

27 (*d*) Option (d) is incorrectly matched pair and can be corrected as

Tuberculosis is not a black death disease. The latter is used for plague. Tuberculosis is called as Koch's disease.
Rest options are correctly matched pairs.

29 (*a*) Statement in option (a) is incorrect and can be corrected as

Gametocytes are formed by the transformation of merozoites in the blood of human host.

Rest statements are correct.

32 (*b*) Malarial parasite is digenetic, i.e. it needs true host to complete its life cycle, primary host female *Anophelese* for sexual reproduction and human as secondary or intermediate host for asexual reproduction.

38 (*c*) Statement in options (c) is incorrect and can be corrected as

Entamoeba histolytica is a parasite of large intestine in man.

Rest statements are correct.

41 (*b*) Option (b) is incorrectly matched pair and can be corrected as

Chagas' disease is transmitted by reduviid bugs called *Panstrongylus megistus.*

Rest options are correctly matched pairs.

55 (*d*) Option (d) represents incorrectly matched pair and can be corrected as

HPV or Human Papillomavirus causes genital warts. It is a transmitted through skin to skin contact or by sexual contact.

Rest options are correctly matched pairs.

58 (*d*) Statement in option (d) is incorrect and can be corrected as

Benign tumour do not invade or spread to other sites or organs. While malignant tumours can spread to the other parts of the body through blood and lymphatic system.

Rest statements are correct.

59 (*a*) Option (a) is not correctly matched pair and can be corrected as

Carcinomas are the cancer of epithelial tissue.
Rest options are correctly matched pairs.

62 (*d*) Option (d) is incorrect match and can be corrected as

Factor responsible for prostrate cancer is hormones like oestrogen and testosterones.

(B) Cumulative Exercise

10 (*c*) All given statements are true except statement IV regarding treatment of cancer. Incorrect statement can be corrected as

For radiation therapy radio isotopes, i.e. X-rays, γ-rays, etc., are used which destory growing cancerous cell.

11 (*d*) Only statement II is false and can be corrected as

Chikungunya is a viral disease, which spreads through *Aedes* mosquito. Rest statements are true.

15 (*b*) Statements I, II and IV are correct, while III and V are incorrect. Incorrect statements can be corrected as

Asexual cycle called schizogony (of *Plasmodium*) is a type of multiple fission.
The incubation period of all the species of *Plasmodium* is different, i.e. incubation period for *P. oval* is 17 days, for *P. vivax* is 14 days. *P. malariae* is 28 days, etc.

32 (*a*) Both A and R are true and R is the correct explanation of A.
Rickettsiae should be regarded as bacteria because of the presence of both RNA and DNA. These are primarily intestinal parasites of ticks, mites, rat fleas and lice which are blood sucking arthropods.

33 (*b*) Both A and R are true, but R is not the correct explanation of A.
Q-fever is an influenza like illness with high fever, headache and typical pneumonia. In acute infection, hepatitis also occurs.

34 (*a*) Both A and R are true and R is the correct explanation of A.
HIV or Human Immunodeficiency Virus is a causative agent of AIDS. It damages the immune system of the human body. HIV virus belongs to the family of retroviruses.

35 (*c*) A is true, but R is false because
Viruses belong to both living and non-living category. As non-living, virus cannot multiply on their own. They require living cells for their growth and multiplication which causes damage to their host cells.

36 (*e*) Both A and R are false and can be corrected as
Pneumonia is a disease of lungs in which difficulty in breathing occurs. It is caused by *Pneumococcus* bacteria, i.e. *Streptococcus pneumoniae.*

37 (*b*) Both A and R are true, but R is not the correct explanation of A.
Pertussis or whooping cough is an airborne infection caused by the bacteria, *Bordetella pertussis.* In this diseases, cough forces air out of the lungs. It is followed by a typical inspiratory whooping cough in which air is drawn into the lungs in a massive inflow.

(C) Medical Entrances' Gallery

3 (*a*) Benzopyrene is a polycyclic aromatic hydrocarbon formed as a result of incomplete combustion of organic matter such as coal tar, tobacco, etc.

It is potential carcinogenic compound listed as Group 1 carcinogen by IARC, i.e. International Agency for Research on Cancer. It reacts and binds to DNA, resulting in mutation and eventually cancer.

4 (*c*) Elephantiasis is a helminthic disease caused by *Wuchereria bancrofti.* The infestation is transmitted by female *Culex* mosquitoes from one individual to the others. The worms live in the lymphatic system. Other options are explained as

- Ascariasis is caused by *Ascaris lumbricoides.* It is an endoparasite of the small intestine of human beings. Amoebiasis is caused by *Entamoeba histolytica.* It lives in the large intestine of humans.
- Ringworm is a fungal skin disease.

5 (*a*) Alzheimer's disease is not an autoimmune disease. It is caused due to the destruction of vast number of neurons in the hippocampus of brain. It occurs due to a combination of genetic factors, environmental or lifestyle factors and the ageing process.
There is loss of neurotransmitter acetylcholine. Individuals with this disease have trouble remembering recent events.
Rheumatoid arthritis, vitiligo and psoriasis, all are autoimmune diseases. In rheumatoid arthritis, antibodies are produced against the synovial membrane and cartilage. Vitiligo causes white patches on skin, while psoriasis causes itchy-skin.

7 (*d*) Severe Combined Immunodeficiency Disease (SCID) is a rare genetic disease that affects the immune system of the person. This disease can be treated by either bone marrow transplant or by enzyme replacement therapy but neither of the two are completely curative. Thus, gene therapy has been attempted to cure it permanently.

8 (*d*) In cancer, the cells break away from the original site and can spread to the other parts of the body through bloodstream and lymphatic system, thus forming malignant tumours.
The spread of cancer to other sites or organs in the body is called metastasis. Other statements are incorrect as cancer cells do not exhibit the property of contact inhibition, all tumours are not cancerous, e.g. benign tumour and also not all viruses are oncogenic.

10 (*c*) Features II, IV and VI are correct.
Wuchereria bancrofti commonly called filarial worm is a digenetic, dimorphic, pseudocoelomate, histozoic and pathogenic parasite. It is digenetic because it has two stages of multiplication in two different hosts, one sexual in the mature form and the other asexual in larval stages. It is a histozoic parasite as it lives in the tissue outside of a cell body.

11 (*d*) The statement in option (d) is incorrect for the low levels of immune response during *Plasmodium* infection. It can be corrected as

Plasmodium infection primarily destroys the liver cells, where the sporozoites immediately multiply asexually and rupture the liver cells. These are released into the blood where they attack fresh red blood cells. They invade further red blood cells and repeat the erythrocyte cycle.
Rest other statements are correct.

12 (*c*) Babesiosis is a malaria like parasitic disease caused by *Babesia bigemina,* a genus of Protozoa piroplasms.
Other given diseases and their causative agents are as follows
Syphilis – *Treponema pallidum* (bacterium)
Influenza – Influenza virus
Blastomycosis – *Blastomyces dermatitidis* (fungus)

13 (*a*) Cholera and tetanus are diseases caused by bacteria. Cholera is caused by a bacterium *Vibrio cholerae* and tetanus is caused by a bacterium *Clostridium tetani.* Mumps, influenza, herpes and smallpox are viral diseases. Typhoid is a bacterial disease but, it is not paired with a bacterial disease. Hence, option (a) is correct.

16 (*c*) Statement in option (c) is correct. Tumours that metastasis are considered 'malignant'. However, benign does not show such character. Other statements are incorrect and can be corrected as
The effects of heroin are felt throughout the whole body as it slow down physical, mental and emotional responses.

Cannabinoids help to manage postoperative pain. There are several types of medication that are used to provide anesthesia for patients having surgery. To keep patients calm immediately before the procedure, these may be used, e.g. isoflurane, nitrous oxide, pancuronium, propofol. succinylcholine and vecuronium.

18 (*d*) Option (d) represents incorrect combination and can be corrected as

Sporogony is found in the life cycle of *Plasmodium* that causes malaria.

Rest other options are correct combinations.

22 (*d*) Option (d) represents not a property of cancerous cells because

These cells do not possess the property of contact inhibition. Thus, they divide indefinitely even after coming in contact with other cells.

Rest other options represent properties of cancerous cells.

23 (*b*) Statements II and IV are wrong and can be corrected as

- Cancer arising from the epithelial tissues of internal organs and glands is called carcinoma.
- True cancer or neoplasm are malignant tumours.

Rest other statements are correct.

27 (*d*) *Ascaris* is an intestinal parasite that causes ascariasis. Symptoms of these disease include internal bleeding, muscular pain, fever, anaemia and blockage of the intestinal passage.

The eggs of the parasite are excreted along with the faeces of infected persons which contaminate soil, water, plants, etc. A healthy person acquires this infection through contaminated water, vegetables, fruits, etc.

28 (*b*) Gonorrhoea is a bacterial disease caused by *Neisseria gonorrhoeae*. It spreads through sexual contact, common toilets, under garments and also from infected mother to the newborn. The bacterium lives in genital tubes, produces pus-containing yellow discharge, pain around genitalia and burning sensation during urination.

29 (*a*) Schizogony is an asexual reproduction of *Plasmodium* (malarial parasite) in which schizont is formed from the human blood (RBCs) sporozoites.

It then enters the liver cells. The sporozoite grows in size to become a rounded schizont called cryptozoite. The latter divides to form cryptomerozoites (merozoites). The merozoites are asexual haploid forms. The host liver cells rupture to liberate the cryptomerozoites into the liver sinusoids.

34 (*d*) Malignant tumour shows metastasis and such type of tumour cells have lost the ability to differentiate.

35 (*b*) HIV enters into T-lymphocytes, replicates and produces progeny viruses. The progeny viruses release in the blood and damages other helper T-lymphocytes. This is repeated leading to a progressive decrease in the number of T-lymphocytes in the body of the infected person.

During this period, the person suffers from bouts of fever diarrhoea and weight loss. The person starts suffering from infections.

Thus, options (b) is correct.

38 (*a*) Statement in option (a) is not correct.

Human Immunodeficiency Virus (HIV) is transmitted in following ways

- Through sexual intercourse (65%).
- Transmission through blood transfusion, blood products and contaminated equipment (10%).
- Transmission from mother to baby (25%).

40 (*c*) Food poisoning is caused by consuming contaminated food and water. The most common pathogens responsible for causing food poisoning are *E. coli*, *Salmonella*, etc.

42 (*d*) Trichomoniasis is a sexually transmitted disease. It is caused by *Trichomonas vaginalis* on the other hand.

Malaria is caused by *Plasmodium* sp.

Cancer is a large and complex family of malignancies. It usually develops from normal cells that has changed or mutated. Pneumonia is caused by *Diplococcus pneumoniae*.

CHAPTER 16

Basic Concepts of Immunology

Human body is frequently exposed to disease causing organisms such as bacteria, fungi, virus, helminthes, protozoans, etc. However, only a few of these exposures result in diseases. Our immune system has the ability to defend us from these diseases causing microorganisms. The branch of science which deals with components of immune system is called **immunology**. Before discussing the various aspects of immunology, let us understand the concept of antigen first.

ANTIGENS

These are the substances which stimulate the production of antibodies in the body. Technically, antigen and immunogen are not the same.

- **Antigens** are the foreign molecules, which have ability to bind with the components of immune system.
- **Immunogen**, not only binds with the components of immune system, but also induces immune response.

Various characteristics of antigens are listed below

- Majority of antigens are proteins or polysaccharides. Some are also carbohydrates, lipids or nucleic acids.
- **Antigenic determinants** or **epitopes** are the sites on antigens, which are recognised by antibodies and receptors present on B and T-cells.
- The smallest units of antigen are antigenic determinants. Each determinant can stimulate the formation of a particular kind of antibody or effector cell. Thus, a single antigen may give rise to several distinct antibodies and effector cells.
- Antigens which are present on the body's own cell are self antigen, e.g. antigen related to blood group.

Based upon the ability of the antigens to carryout their functions, these are of two types

(i) **Complete antigen** It is capable of inducing antibody formation. It produces a specific and observable reaction with the antibody thus, produced.

(ii) **Hapten** (Partial or Incomplete antigens) It is incapable of inducing antibody formation by themselves. But, they can induce antibody formation on combining with larger molecules (generally proteins). The latter serve as carriers.

Inside

IMMUNITY

The ability of an organism to fight against disease causing agents is called immunity. It may be grouped into two categories, *viz* innate or non-specific immunity and acquired or adaptive immunity.

Innate immunity or Non-specific immunity

It includes all the defence elements with which an individual is born. It is present at the time of birth and passed down genetically from parents to children. It is also called as non-specific immunity because it does not differentiate between different type of pathogens.
It respond to each foreign substance using same mechanism.

The various barriers of innate immunity are discussed below

1. Physical (Anatomic) barriers

- **Skin** It is formed by outer tough layer of the body called **stratum corneum.** It prevents the entry of bacteria and viruses.
- **Mucous membrane** Mucus secreted by mucous membrane traps the microorganisms and immobilises them. The trapped microorganisms and debris are propelled out of the body by synchronous movement of cilia.

2. Physiological barriers

- It includes acid in stomach (hydrochloric acid), bile, saliva in mouth, cerumen (ear wax), tears from eyes, etc.
- Oil ond sweat make the surface of skin acidic. It prevents the growth of microorganisms on skin.
- Tears and saliva contain lysozymes which destroy bacterial pathogens.

3. Cellular barriers

- They include certain types of phagocytic blood cells. These are called **leucocytes** (WBC), e.g. Polymorpho-Nuclear Leucocytes (PMNLs), neutrophils, monocytes, natural killer cells (type of lymphocytes) and macrophages.
- The macrophages are large irregular-shaped cells. They engulf microbes, viruses, cellular debris, etc.
- In response to an infection, monocytes are released at the site of infection and are converted into macrophages.

Table 16.1 Phagocytic cells and their locations

Phagocytic cells	Locations
Neutrophils	Blood and all tissues
Monocytes	Blood
Macrophages (histiocytes)	All tissues (including spleen, lymph nodes, bone marrow)
Kupffer's cells	Liver
Alveolar macrophages	Lungs
Microglial cells	Central nervous system

4. Cytokine barriers

Certain kinds of cells, when infected with a virus, release a glycoprotein called **interferons** (IFNs). These IFNs inhibit the viral replication by stimulating the synthesis of an enzyme. It inhibits the synthesis of proteins required for viral replication. So, they are used to control viral diseases, but they do not kill the virus.

5. Inflammatory barriers

An infection or tissue injury usually causes redness (**rubor**), swelling (**tumour**), pain (**dolor**) and production of heat (**calor**) that may result in fever. Such localised expressions are called **inflammatory responses**.

The mechanisms of inflammatory response are discussed below

- It starts by the release of certain chemicals such as histamines and prostaglandins by the damaged mast cells.
- The vascular fluid also comes out of the blood vessels. This fluid contains serum proteins which kill bacteria.
- Phagocytic cells, i.e. monocytes and neutrophils also move towards affected area.
- First, they form a barrier that prevents the microbes from invading other parts of the body.
- Then, they engulf and digest the microbes by phagocytosis.
- The dead white cells, microbes and fragments of damaged body cells accumulate during this process.
- They form the whitish fluid called **pus**. This oozes out from the infected area and should be removed.
- All these responses inhibit and destroy the invading pathogenic microorganisms.
- Fever may occur due to
  (a) **Toxins** produced by the pathogens.
  (b) **Protein** called **endogenous pyrogens** (fever producing substance), also called **interleukins** (released by macrophages).

- When enough pyrogens reach the brain, the body's thermostat is reset to a higher temperature.
- It allows the temperature of the entire body to rise.
- A very high temperature may prove dangerous.
- It must be quickly brought down by giving antipyretics (fever reducing drugs-like aspirin).

Note *The phenomenon of phagocytosis was discovered by* ***Metchnikoff*** *(1883). Metchnikoff and Paul Ehrlich got the Nobel Prize in 1908 for their work on body resistance.*

Host defence mechanism

The barriers of immunity can be grouped into three main categories on the basis of their mechanism of action. These are as follows

(i) First line of defence (Non-specific)

This defence comprises of physical and chemical barriers. It prevents the entry of pathogens in the body.

The components of first line of defence are as follows

- It is formed by skin and mucous membranes. The infectious microbes rarely penetrate through these layers.
- The membrane lining the respiratory, digestive, urinary and genital tracts are covered with hair-like projections called **cilia**. It also has a layer of mucous membrane that secretes sticky fluid, **mucus**. Cilia and mucus work together to trap microbes and move them out of the body.
- The stomach and vagina are so acidic that very few microbes can pass through these areas.
- Perspiration, saliva and tears contain an enzyme, lysozyme. It digests bacterial cell walls, thereby causing the bacterial cell to burst.
- Oil glands and sweat glands secrete acidic fluids with a pH between 3-5. It creates an environment that interferes with bacterial activity.

(ii) Second line of defence (Non-specific)

When the first line of defence fails to prevent the access of pathogen, second line of defences become active.

It is primarily dependent upon neutrophils, macrophages, interferon and complement proteins.

Natural Killer (NK) cells

- These are large granular lymphocytes that kill virus-infected cells and some tumour cells.
- They release g-interferon which stimulates their cytolytic activity.
- NK cells produce **perforins**. They create pores in the plasma membrane of the target cells. These pores allow the entry of water into the target cells, which then swell and burst.
- NK cells attack cells that do not display Major Histocompatibility Complex (MHC) antigens.
- NK cells are present in spleen, lymph nodes, red bone marrow and blood. Their number is very less in AIDS and cancer patients.

Complement system

- It is a set of 30 different protein molecules found in the blood. There are no cells in this system.
- With an infection, this system of molecules gets activated.
- It leads to a sequence of events on the surface of the pathogen. It helps to destroy the pathogen and eliminates the infection.
- A complement system can be activated in two main ways as follows
  (a) The first and most potent way is known as **classical pathway**. It occurs when IgG or IgM binds to the antigen at the surface of a cell. This exposes the Fc region of the antibody such that the first complement protein (C_1) binds.
  (b) The second mean of activation is known as **alternate pathway**. It is a part of the natural (innate) immune response (i.e. neither antibodies nor T-cells receptors are involved).
  Here, certain polysaccharides found on the surface of bacteria activate the system. These are known as Membrane Attack Complex (MAC).
  This can occur immediately and does not require prior exposure to the molecules.
  Different components of complement system work in following manner to kill microbes
    - Complement proteins create pores in the plasma membrane of microbes. Through these pores, water enters the microbial cells and causes them to burst and die.
    - Some components of the complement system form a coat around the invading microbes. This coating attracts phagocytes (neutrophils and macrophages) for engulfing them.
    - The complement system also causes agglutination of microbes, neutralisation of viruses, activation of mast cells and basophils and has some inflammatory effects too.

The process involved in second line of defence include fever and inflammatory response.

- **Inflammatory responses** increase capillary permeability at infected sites, recruite WBCs and lead to localised swelling. Antimicrobial proteins (such as cytokinins and complement proteins) regulate immune activity within the body.
- **Fever** increases body temperature to activate heat shock proteins and suppresses microbial growth and propagation.

(iii) Third line of defence (Specific)

The final lines of defence against infection are the lymphocytes. They produce antibodies specific to antigenic fragment. It is a part of the adaptive or acquired immune response.

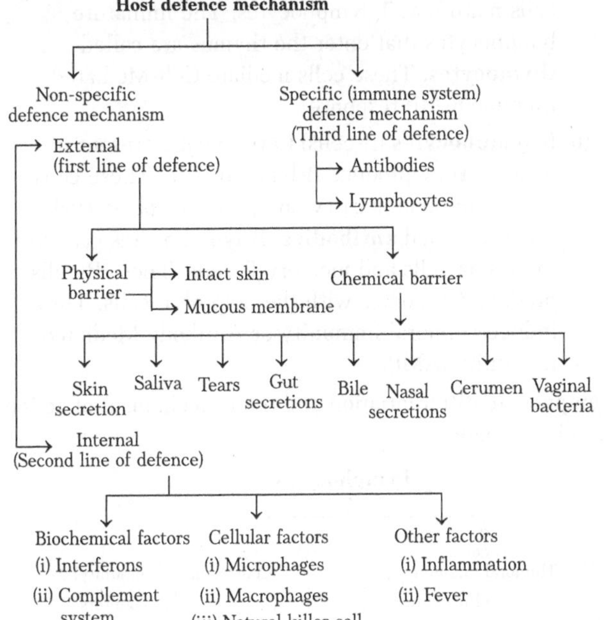

Fig. 16.1 Types of host defence mechanism

Acquired immunity

It is also known as **adaptive** or **specific immunity**. It is found in vertebrates only.

It supplements the protection provided by innate immunity. It is generated in response to an exposure to the microorganisms or a pathogen.

Important features of acquired immunity are as follows

(i) **Specificity** It has the ability to distinguish among various kinds of foreign molecules/particles.

(ii) **Diversity** It can recognise a large variety of foreign molecules.

(iii) **Discrimination between self and non-self** It is able to recognise and respond to molecules that are foreign or non-self. At the same time, it can avoid response to those molecules which are present within the body (self) of animals.

Note *Major Histocompatibility Complex (MHC) is a tightly linked cluster of genes present in every vertebrate species. It plays important roles in intercellular recognition and discrimination between self and non-self.*

(iv) **Memory** When the immune system encounters a specific foreign agent for the first time, it generates an immune response. It helps to eliminate the invader but immune system retains the memory of this encounter. As a result, a second encounter with the same microbe evokes a heightened immune response.

Types of acquired immunity

Acquired immunity or adaptive immunity are further categorised as follows

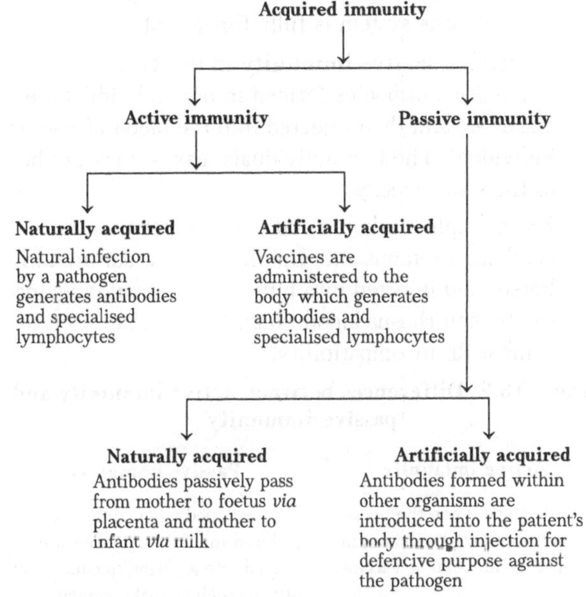

Active immunity

It involves the active functioning of the person's own immune system. It leads to the synthesis of antibodies and production of immunologically active cells. It takes a few days or weeks to buildup.

Types of active immunity are as follows

(i) **Natural active immunity** In this, body's own cells develop antibodies after the onset of certain kind of disease or infection for that particular disease, e.g. measles.

(ii) **Artificial active immunity** In this, immunity resistance is induced by vaccines. They are prepared from microorganisms or their products. These are used for immunisation, e.g. BCG, TAB, MMR vaccine, etc. In response, body forms antibodies and memory cells.

Passive immunity

In this type of immunity, antibodies from one individual are passed into another individual. They give immediate protection. However, they are short-lived. The antibodies are broken down by the body's natural processes. Thus, their number slowly falls and protection is lost.

Types of passive immunity are as follows

(i) **Natural passive immunity** This immunity is gained naturally. For example, antibodies from a mother can cross the placenta and enter her foetus. In this way, antibodies provide protection to the baby until its own immune system is fully functional.

(ii) **Artificial passive immunity** In this type of immunity, antibodies formed in one individual are extracted and then injected into the blood of another individual. The two individuals may or may not be of the same species.

For example, earlier specific antibodies used for combating tetanus and diphtheria were cultured in horses and injected into humans. Antibodies against the human rhesus blood groups antigen are used to combat Rh incompatibility.

Table 16.2 Differences between active immunity and passive immunity

Active immunity	Passive immunity
It is developed when the person's own cells produce antibodies in response to infection or vaccine.	It is developed when antibodies produced in other organisms are injected into a person to counteract antigens such as snake venom.
It provides relief only after long period.	It provides immediate relief.
It has no side effects.	It may cause reaction.
It is long lasting.	It is not long lasting.

Cells involved in acquired immunity

The cells involved in acquired immunity forms the third line of defence in the body. These are as follows

(i) Lymphocytes

These are the main cells of immune system in human body. These are T-lymphocytes (T-cells) and B-lymphocytes (B-cells). These cells are produced in bone marrow. The process of their production is called **haematopoiesis**. The primary and secondary immune responses are carried out with the help of these cells only.

(a) **T-lymphocytes** (T-cells) Stem cells present in bone marrow give rise to immature lymphocytes. These migrate *via* the blood to the thymus where these cells mature as T-lymphocytes. The immature lymphocytes that enter the thymus are called **thymocytes.** These cells mediate Cell-Mediated Immune (CMI) response.

(b) **B-lymphocytes** (B-cells) Certain cells present in bone marrow produce B-lymphocytes. These cells mature in bone marrow and produce specialised proteins called **antibodies.** B-lymphocytes give rise to plasma cells and memory B-cells. These B-cells produce antibodies with the help of T-cells. They induce Humoral immunity or Antibody Mediated Immunity (AMI).

Lymphocyte differentiation and their mechanism of action are given below

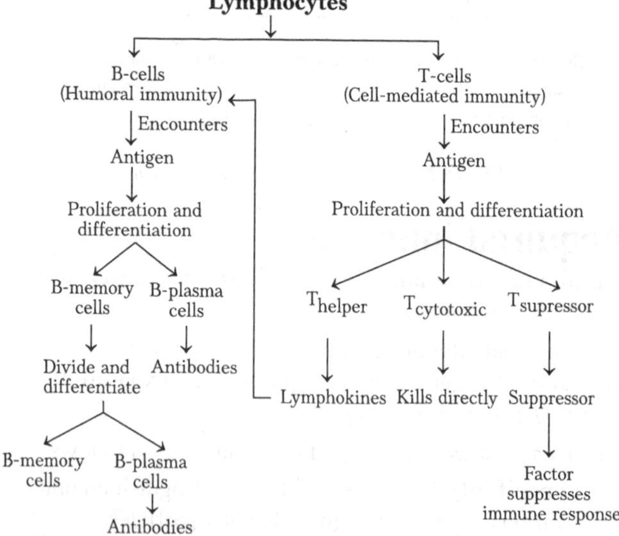

(ii) Antigens presenting cell

These are special types of cells involved in acquired immunity. They include macrophages, B-lymphocytes and dendritic cells (e.g. Langerhans cells of epidermis of skin). These cells engulf and destroy invading pathogen present on their surface.

CHECK POINT 16.1

1. Which of the following statements is true?
   (a) All immunogens are antigens, but all antigens are not immunogens
   (b) All immunogens are antigens and all antigens are immunogens
   (c) All immunogens are not antigens, but all antigens are immunogens
   (d) All immunogens are proteins and all proteins are immunogens.

2. A person suffering from a very high fever
   (a) will have interleukins in body
   (b) can be given antipyretics
   (c) might have a pathogen in body
   (d) All of the above

3. One principle function of complement system is to
   (a) phagocytise antigens
   (b) inactivate perforins
   (c) mediate the release of histamine
   (d) enhance the ability of antibodies and perform cell lysis

4. The immune system retains the memory of first encounter with that microbe and evokes a heightened immune response in second encounter. The type of immune response is called
   (a) active immunity (b) passive immunity
   (c) acquired immunity (d) cell-mediated immunity

5. Transfusing a person with blood plasma proteins from a person or animal that has been actively immunised against a specific antigen provides
   (a) active immunity
   (b) passive immunity
   (c) autoimmunity
   (d) anti-immunity

6. Choose the incorrectly matched pair.
   (a) Thymocyte – Mature lymphocyte
   (b) Antigen presenting cells – Dendritic cell
   (c) B-cells – Memory cells
   (d) Active immunity – No side effects

ANTIBODIES/ IMMUNOGLOBULINS (Ig)

- An antibody is a protein molecule generated in the living body by plasma membrane. It specifically inactivates an antigen.
- Antibodies belong to a class of serum proteins called **γ-globulins**. These form about 17-20% of the total protein in the blood serum. That is why, antibodies are also known as **immunoglobulins** (Ig).
- The antibodies produced in our body are IgA, IgM, IgE, IgD and IgG. As these antibodies are produced in blood, the immune response is called **humoral** (fluid) **immune response.**
- The antibodies are generated by **B-lymphocytes** and **plasma cells.** Infact, B-lymphocytes get transformed into plasma cells. The mature plasma cell produces antibodies at extremely rapid rate, i.e. about 2000 molecules/second. An antibody does not usually destroy an antigen directly, but targets it for elimination by complement system or phagocytes.

Structure of immunoglobulins

- Each antibody molecule is a Y-shaped protein molecule having two identical halves. Each half contains
  (i) A heavy (H) chain (molecular weight 50,000 Da).
  (ii) A light (L) chain (molecular weight 2500 Da).
- These are connected to each other by disulphide bonds. Hence, an antibody is represented as H_2L_2.
- It has a flexible hinge region. The stalk of this structure is called **crystallisable fragment** (Fc). This fragment contains the site which binds to the cell.
- The top of 'Y' structure contains two antigen binding fragments (Fab), which bind with specific antigens.
- The two chains contain two distinct regions
  (i) **Constant region** It has amino acid sequences, which do not vary significantly.
  (ii) **Variable region** It has distinct sequence of amino acid molecules. The antigen binding sites (paratopes) are located on the variable regions of the antibody. Small variations in the variable regions make each antibody highly specific for a particular antigen. The variable region enables the antibody to recognise the specific antigen.

- The isotype of an Ig is determined by the constant region. Since disulphide bonds are present in Ig, sulphur is thus, a very important element to maintain the structure of Igs.

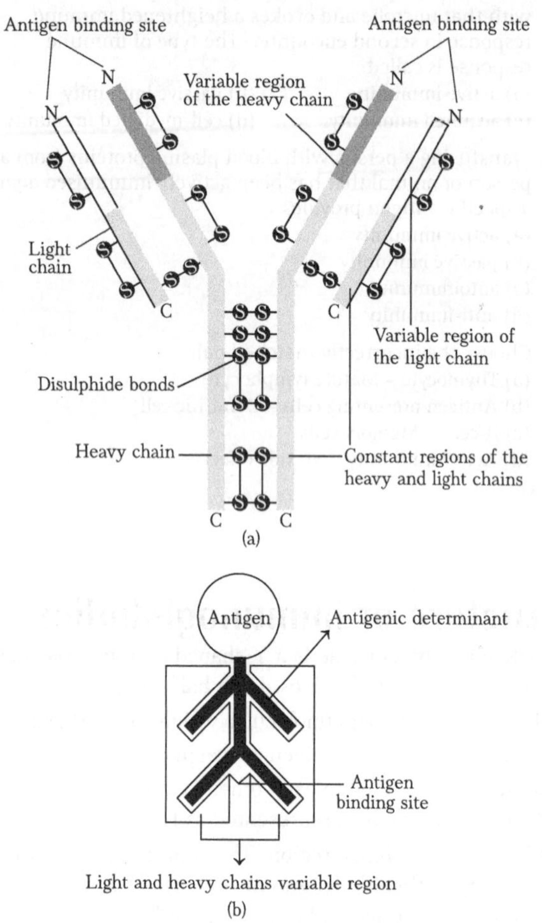

Fig. 16.2 Immunoglobulins : (a) Structure, (b) Antigen binding site

Table 16.3 Differences between antibody and antigen

Antibody (Immunoglobulins)	**Antigen** (Immunogens)
It is a protein molecule.	It is a protein or polysaccharide molecule.
It is synthesised by an animal to combat foreign material.	It is usually a foreign material that stimulates antibody formation.
It occurs on the surface of a plasma cell and also in body fluids.	It may occur on the surface of a microbe or as a free molecule.
It directly joins to an antigen to destroy it.	It binds to a macrophage to reach a helper T-cell to initiate immune response.

Classes of immunoglobulins

The immunoglobulins are classified on the basis of size, charge, amino acid composition, sequence and carbohydrate contents. They behave differently in similar physiological systems.

Various types of immunoglobulins along with their characteristics are discussed in the table given below

Table 16.4 Immunoglobulins are classified into following five types

Classes	Locations	Percentage of serum	Functions
IgG	Blood, lymph, intestine	75%	It stimulates phagocytes and complement system. It binds with neutrophils. It can opsonises and can neutralise toxins. It protects the developing foetus by providing natural passive immunity. It has two paratopes.
IgM (Largest)	Blood, lymph, B-cell surface	7-10%	It activates complement system. It exists as pentamer, where five molecules are linked by J-chain. It has high number of antigen binding sites (10). Thus, it is an effective agglutinator of antigen. It generates immune response against organisms like virus and bacteria.
IgA	Seromucous secretions such as saliva, tear, colostrum milk, tracheo-branc-hial and genital-urinary secretions.	15-20%	It protects newborn babies from infections (component of colostrum and provides passive immunity). It protects the surface of body from inhaled and ingested pathogens. Dimeric IgA has four paratopes. The link between monomers are made by a J-chain of polypeptide.
IgE	Surface membrane of basophils and mast cells.	Less than 1%	It acts as mediator in allergic response. It mediates hypersensitivity reactions. It plays an important role against helminth parasites. It has two paratopes.
IgD	B-cell surface, blood, lymph.	Less than 1%	It activates B-cells to secrete antibodies. It plays an important role in antigen recognition by B-cells. It has two paratopes.

Antigen-immunoglobulin interaction

Study of antigen-antibody interaction is called **serology**. Each antibody is specific for a particular antigen. Binding sites of antigen, called antigenic determinants (**epitopes**) react with the corresponding antigen binding sites of antibodies called **paratopes**.

They bind in a lock and key manner to form an antigen-antibody complex.

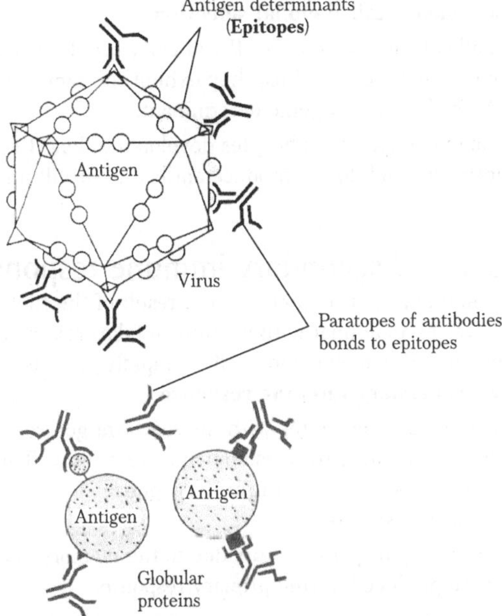

Fig. 16.3 Formation of antigen-antibody complex

Antibodies bind with antigen *via* non-covalent bonds like hydrogen bonds, van der waal interactions, etc. They can inactivate the foreign agent in the following ways

(i) **Agglutination** Clumping of microorganism typically due to an antigen binding reaction. The antibodies that cause agglutination of cells are called **agglutinins**.

(ii) **Opsonisation** or **Adherence** Antibodies (especially IgG) called **opsonins** coats or get attached to the surface of antigen containing pathogen. This enhances recognition of microbes by phagocytes.

(iii) **Precipitation** In this, an antibody binds with a soluble antigen, so that antigen becomes insoluble and precipitates. It permits easy phagocytosis of antigen.

(iv) **Neutralisation** Antibodies cover the toxic sites of antigen. This converts virulent form into non-virulent form. Some antibodies neutralise toxins by acting as antitoxin.

(v) **Lysis** It involves rupturing of plasma membrane of antigen by antibodies.

Polyclonal and monoclonal antibodies

Antibodies used for research and diagnostic purposes are often obtained by injecting specific antigen in lab animal like rabbit or a goat. Within a few weeks, the animal's immune system produces high levels of antibodies specific for that antigen. These antibodies can be obtained from **antisera** (sign. antiserum). It is whole serum collected from an animal following exposure to an antigen.

On the basis their presence in antisera, the antibodies are of following types

(i) **Monoclonal antibodies** These are produced by the same clone of plasma B-cells. Thus, these are homogeneous population of antibodies.

They recognise a single epitope of the antigen. The production of monoclonal antibody requires both animals and hybridoma cells. These cells were originated by the fusion of spleen cells and myeloma cells. Monoclonal antibodies have been called **magic bullets**, since they can directly attack the target antigen when injected into the body.

(ii) **Polyclonal antibodies** These are produced by different clones of plasma B-cells. Thus, these are heterogeneous population of antibodies. They recognise multiple epitopes in the antigen. The production of polyclonal antibodies is carried out by immunising an animal with immunogen bearing the antigen of interest. The humoral response thus produced in animal result in the formation of antibodies.

IMMUNE RESPONSES

It is a specific reactivity induced in a host by an antigenic stimulus. The immune responses are of following types

1. Humoral immunity

In humoral immunity, B-cells secrete soluble substances called **antibodies** into the body fluids. Antibodies interact with circulating antigens such as bacteria, toxic molecules and complement proteins. The antibodies then clear the antigen by binding and forming complexes with them.

2. Cell-mediated immunity

It is mediated by a subgroup of T-cells, called **T-cytotoxic** cells. An activated T-cytotoxic cell is specific to a target cell which is infected. It kills the target cell by a variety of mechanisms. It also prevents the completion of life cycle of the pathogen. T-cells do not release antibodies. Since, the complete cell is involved in attack, it is described as cell-mediated immunity.

The different cells of cell-mediated immunity are as follows

Table 16.5 Cells involved in cell-mediated immune responses

Cells	Immune responses
Cytotoxic T-cells or Killer T-cells	Destroy infected body cells or cancerous body cells. They secrete perforins which create pores on the infected cell membrane from which water enter to cause lysis of cell.
Helper T-cells	Stimulate immune responses by both B-cells and killer T-cells.
Suppressor T-cells	Inhibit immune responses by other lymphocytes.
Memory T-cells	A subset of the offspring of B-cells that are long-lived. They provide immunity against a second invasion by the same antigen.

The diagram showing humoral and cell-mediated response is given below

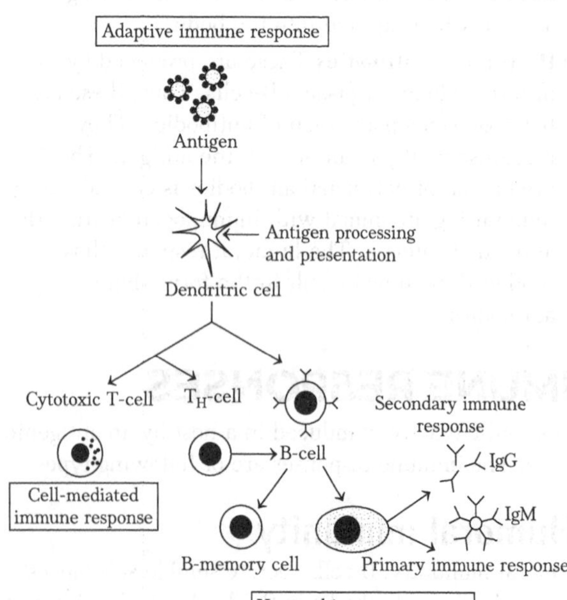

Clonal selection

- Both B-cells and T-cells display a specific receptor on their surface. The number of cells expressing a given receptor is rather small.
- In case of a B-lymphocyte, this receptor is the antibody produced by that cells.
- This receptor interacts with the antigenic determinant specific to it. Thus, the lymphocyte becomes activated and divides to form a clone of cells.
- These cells are also transformed into the effector cells, i.e. antibody producing B-cells and T-cytotoxic cells. This phenomenon is called **clonal selection.**
- Here, all cells in a given T or B-cell clone are derived from a single parental cells. Thus, they exhibit the same specificity for the antigenic determinant.
- But some activated lymphocytes develop into long-lived memory cells and do not produce antibodies or kill infected cells.

Primary and secondary immune responses

- The immune response mounted as a result of the first encounter of an animal with an antigen takes relatively longer time. It is feeble and declines rapidly. This is known as **primary immune response.**
- The subsequent encounter with the same antigen results in a hightened immune response much more rapidly. This is referred to as **secondary immune response** or **anamnestic response.**
- The secondary response occurs due to the memory cells that were produced during primary response.
- It lasts much longer than primary response. This is why, a person surviving a disease such as chicken pox or measles becomes immune to subsequent attacks by the same pathogen.

Table 16.6 Differences between primary and secondary immune responses

Primary immune response	Secondary immune response
The immune response occurs as a result of the first contact of the animal with an antigen.	This immune response occurs at the second and subsequent exposure of the same host to same antigen.
It takes longer time to establish immunity.	It is more rapid.
It declines rapidly.	It lasts for longer periods.

CHECK POINT 16.2

1. Which of the following elements is important to maintain structure of immunoglobulin?
   (a) P
   (b) Fe
   (c) S
   (d) Ca
2. Which of the following provides immunity in newborn babies against antigen?
   (a) IgA
   (b) IgD
   (c) IgM
   (d) IgE
3. Which Ig is produced in primary immune response against viruses and bacteria?
   (a) IgA (b) IgE (c) IgD (d) IgM
4. The process, in which antibody comes in contact with antigen and convert them into harmless insoluble matter is called
   (a) activation (b) agglutination
   (c) neutralisation (d) opsonisaton
5. Opsonisation refers to
   (a) adherence to mucosal epithelial cells
   (b) antibody mediated viral inactivation
   (c) Coating of microorganisms or other particles by antibody
   (d) Parasitic lysosomal degranulation

IMMUNE SYSTEM IN THE BODY

Immune system of human beings consists of lymphoid organs, tissues, cells and soluble protein molecules such as antibodies. The role of immune system is to recognise and respond to foreign antigens and memorise them.

Lymphoid organs

These are the organs where the maturation and proliferation of lymphocytes take place.

There are two types of lymphoid organs as follows

1. Primary lymphoid organs (Central lymphoid organs)

These organs comprise bone marrow and thymus gland. T-lymphocytes and B-lymphocytes mature and acquire their antigen-specific receptors in these sites. They are responsible for cellular and humoral immune responses, respectively.

(i) **Bone marrow** It is main organ of immune system in human body. It is the site of blood cell production including lymphocytes. Maturation of B-lymphocytes takes place in bone marrow.

(ii) **Thymus** T-lymphocytes produced by stem cells of bone marrow pass through thymus before they become fully functional. These are called **thymocytes** and some of them mature into T-cells. Rest of them learn to recognise self antigens, so that body does not attack itself later. Thymus gland reduces in size with ageing. Thus, immunity also decreases as age progresses.

Note *Bursa of fabricius is the primary lymphoid organ in birds.*

2. Secondary lymphoid organs (Peripheral lymphoid organs)

- After maturation, B and T-lymphocytes migrate *via* blood vascular and lymphatic system to the secondary lymphoid organs. Here, they undergo proliferation and differentiation.
- Acquired immune response to antigens develops in these organs.
- Once differentiated in the secondary lymphoid tissues, the lymphocytes do not remain there. They move from lymphoid organs to other organs through blood and lymph.
- They comprise of lymph nodes, spleen and Mucosa Associated Lymphoid Tissues (MALT), such as tonsils and Peyer's patches of small intestine.
- Some of these are discussed below

(i) **MALT** These are located within the lining of major tracts like digestive, respiratory, etc. It constitutes about 50% of lymphoid tissue in human body.

(ii) **Spleen** It is an immunogenic filter of blood. It contains B-cells, T-cells, macrophages, NK-cells and RBCs. B-cells become activated and produce antibodies in it. Spleen acts as a graveyard of RBCs.

(iii) **Lymph nodes** These are found throughout the body. It helps to filter the antigens out of the lymph.

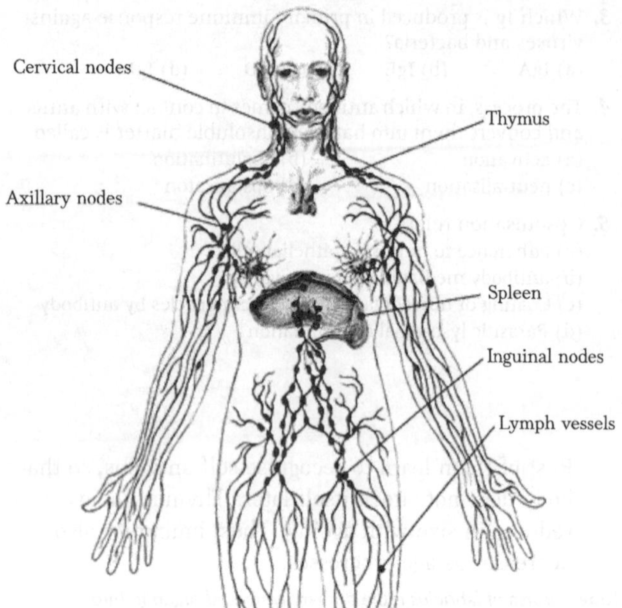

Fig. 16.4 Human lymphatic system

Table 16.7 Differences between primary and secondary lymphoid organs

Primary lymphoid organs	Secondary lymphoid organs
These are the organs, where T and B-cells mature and acquire their antigen-specific receptors.	These are the organs, where the lymphocytes undergo proliferation and differentiation in response to specific antigens.
e.g. Bone marrow (site of B-cell maturation) and thymus (site of T-cell maturation).	e.g. Lymph nodes, spleen and Mucosa Associated Lymphoid Tissues (MALT), such as tonsils.

VACCINATION OR IMMUNISATION

The introduction of harmless antigenic material into healthy person for providing acquired immunity against the disease is known as immunisation or vaccination.

A vaccine is either a cell suspension or a byproduct secreted by the cell. When introduced into the body, it stimulates the production of antibodies. Serum is used for obtaining antibodies.

The principles of immunisation are as follows

- The principle of immunisation or vaccination is based on the property of 'memory' of the immune system.
- A preparation of antigenic proteins of pathogens or inactivated/weakened pathogens (vaccine) is introduced into the body.
- These antigens generate the primary immune response and the memory B and T-cells.
- When the vaccinated person is attacked by the same pathogen, the existing memory T or B-cells recognise that antigen quickly.
- They counter the invaders with a massive production of lymphocytes and antibodics.

Table 16.8 Principal vaccines used to prevent bacterial/viral diseases in human

Diseases	Vaccines	Recommendations	Boosters
Bacterial			
Cholera	Crude fraction of *Vibrio cholerae*	For people who work and live in endemic areas	Every 6 months as needed
Diphtheria	Purified diphtheria toxoid	For children 2 months to 16 yrs	Every 10 yrs for adults
Meningococcal meningitis	Purified polysaccaride from *Neisseria meningitidis*	For people with substantial risk of infection	Need not to be established
Pertussis (whooping cough)	Killed whole or fragments of *Bordetella pertussis*	Children prior to school age (3-4 yrs)	For high risk adults
Plague	Crude fraction of *Yersinia pestis*	For people who come in regular contact with wild rodents in endemic areas	Every 6-13 months for continuing exposure
Pneumococcal pneumonia	Purified polysaccharide from *Streptococcus pneumoniae*	For adults with certain chronic diseases, people over 65 yrs old	Normally not recommended
Tetanus	Purified tetanus toxoid	For both children and adults	Every 10 yrs for adults
Typhoid fever	Killed or attenuated *Salmonella typhi*	For people in endemic areas or areas having outbreak	Every 3 yrs with killed, every 5 yrs with attenuated
Viral			
Influenza	Killed	For chronically ill people, especially with respiratory diseases or for healthy people over 65 yrs old	Annual
Measles	Attenuated virus	For infants 15 months old	At high risk condition

Diseases	Vaccines	Recommendations	Boosters
Mumps	Attenuated virus	For infants 15 months old	(Duration of immunity not known)
Rubella	Attenuated virus	For infants, 15 months old baby, females of child bearing age who are not pregnant	(Duration of immunity not known)
Poliomyelitis	Attenuated or killed virus (enhanced potency type)	For children, adults, as risk to exposure warrants	(Duration of immunity not known)
Rabies	Killed virus	For field biologists in contact with wildlife in endemic areas, veterinaries	Every 2 yrs
Yellow fever	Attenuated virus	For people travelling to endemic areas, military personnel	Every 10 yrs
Hepatitis-B	Antigenic fragments of virus	For children, for adults, especially health care workers, homosexual males, injecting drug users, heterosexual persons with multiple partners and household contacts of hepatitis-B carriers	Duration of protection at least 7 yrs, need for boosters uncertain

Types of vaccines

These are of following types

(i) **Toxoids** The toxins produced by certain organisms are inactivated. These are used in the preparation of vaccines. These vaccines provide short-lived passive immunity, e.g. tetanus, diphtheria vaccines.

(ii) **Live vaccines or Attenuated vaccines** These vaccines are prepared from attenuated pathogen. The pathogen is weakened to make it non-virulent organisms.
For example, OPV (Oral Polio Vaccine) developed by **J Sack** in 1952, BCG (Bacillus Calmette Guerin), tuberculosis, smallpox, yellow fever and influenza vaccines. These vaccines provide long-lived active immunity.

(iii) **Killed vaccines or Inactivated vaccines** Such vaccines are prepared by killing the pathogenic organisms. It is carried out using heat, ultraviolet rays, alcohol/formalin or phenol.
For example, typhoid vaccine, polio vaccine, typhus vaccine, cholera vaccine, rabies vaccine, plague vaccine.

(iv) **Combinations** If more than one kind of immunising agent is included in the vaccine, it is called a mixed or combined vaccine. Some of the well-known combinations are as follows
- DPT [Diphtheria + Pertussis (whooping cough) + Tetanus]
- DT (Diphtheria + Tetanus)
- DP (Diphtheria + Pertussis)
- Tetanus + Influenza, typhoid vaccine
- MMR (Measles + Mumps + Rubella), etc.

Classification of vaccines

Vaccines are classified under following categories

(i) **First generation vaccines** These vaccines are produced by conventional ways in which whole microorganisms are used. These are not of uniform quality and produce side effects.

(ii) **Second generation vaccines** These vaccines do not contain the whole microorganism, but their subunits are present.
For example, hepatitis-B virus vaccine, herpes virus vaccine, pneumonia vaccine, tetanus, etc.

(iii) **Third generation vaccines** These vaccines are DNA vaccines, produced by genetic engineering. These are chemically synthesised multivalent vaccines. They have one or two specific proteins (antigens) of a pathogen.
The DNA vaccine is injected into the cell of the body. The host cell reads the DNA and synthesises the pathogen protein. Because these proteins are recognised as foreign, a range of immune responses are triggered.
For example, third generation hepatitis-B vaccines has been developed. These vaccines have high purity.

Note *The first vaccination was carried out by a British physician, Edward Jenner (1796) to protect people from smallpox. The first true vaccine against chicken cholera was developed in 1880 by Louis Pasteur.*

Immunisation and pregnancy

Some of the important points related to immunisation during pregnancy are as follows

(i) In pregnant woman, immunisation should be performed before gestation because some vaccines are not perfectly safe during pregnancy. Pregnant women are often vaccinated either because they

(ii) During pregnancy, vaccines like oral poliomyelitis and rubella should be avoided.

(iii) The safe vaccines for immunisation during pregnancy are tetanus, influenza, inactivated poliomyelitis, cholera and hepatitis-B.

ORGAN TRANSPLANTATION

In this procedure, an organ is removed from the body of donor and placed in the body of recipient. It is performed to replace a damaged or missing organ. Most commonly transplanted organs are heart, kidneys, lungs, liver, intestine, pancreas. Kidneys are most frequent transplanted organ. Brain is one of the organ, which cannot be transplanted.

Most commonly transplanted tissues are bones, tendons, cornea, skin, heart valves, etc.

Types of transplant

The following terms are used for the different kinds of transplant

(i) **Autograft** Tissue grafted from one place to another, within the same individual.

For example, skin grafting, rotation plasty (foot or ankle joint is used to replace knee joint), etc.

(ii) **Allograft** Tissue or an organ transplant between two individuals of same species. It is further of two types

- In most of the cases, it occurs between two genetically non-identical individuals. This is the condition of normal **allograft**.
- Within a very few cases, it occurs between genetically identical individual, i.e. between twins. This condition is named as **isograft**. In isograft, immune response is not triggered.

(iii) **Xenograft** The transplantation of organs or tissue from one species to another, e.g. heart valve transplant.

Graft rejection

- A transplant may be rejected by the recipient's body. It is one of the major problem with organ transplant. This can be explained by simplest case of blood transfusion.
- Blood of different groups can be regarded as an allograft. Here, rejection may occur and results in agglutination of the donor's red cells within the recipient body.
- Finding a suitable donor for blood transfusion is relatively easy because there are only two antigens involved in it.
- However, all other cells in the body have many possible antigens. Thus, organ transplantation is a complex process.

Prevention of graft rejection

There are several means of preventing graft rejection. These are as follows

(i) **Tissue matching** is an obvious and necessary precaution to be taken before any surgery. The major histocompatibility complex is relevant here. Tissue matching is much more likely to occur between close relatives than between non-relatives.

(ii) **Exposure of bone marrow** and **lymph tissues** to radiation like X-rays tend to inhibit production of white blood cells. Therefore, it slows down rejection. Unpleasant side-effects and an increased risk of infection during the treatment might occur in it.

(iii) **Immunosuppression** is based on the principle of using chemicals which inhibit the entire activity of the immune system. When this occurs, graft rejection is delayed.

The main problem with this technique is that the patient becomes susceptible to all kind of infections. It has also been shown that immunosuppression may make the patients more prone to develop cancer.

IMMUNE DISORDERS AND DEFICIENCY

The immune system is a multicomponent interactive system. It effectively protects the host from various infections. But an improper functioning of the immune system can cause discomfort, disease or even death.

Major groups of immune disorder are as follows

Allergy or Hypersensitivity

This is an inappropriate, over-reaction of the immune system. It occurs when the immune system reacts vigorously to substances normally recognised as foreign. Substances that cause allergies are called **allergens**. It includes dust, moulds, pollen, certain food and some medicines such as penicillin. The responses to the foreign substance are of two types

(i) **Immediate allergic responses** These include cold like symptoms, due to the activity of antibodies.

(ii) **Delayed allergic responses** These are produced due to the activity of T-cells such as contact dermatitis. Common allergies seen in humans are hives, hay fever, asthma and eczema.

Allergic response is produced in body in following manner

- Antibodies belonging to the IgE class trigger the allergic reaction.

- Antibodies belonging to the IgE class trigger the allergic reaction.
- They combine with both the antigen and the surfaces of mast cells.
- They cause the release of large amounts of histamine and serotonin into the blood stream.
- **Histamine** is an initiator of the inflammatory response. It stimulates the dilation of arteries and increases permeability of capillaries.
- It results in fluid buildup in the interstitial areas of the affected tissues.
- Sneezing, coughing, itching, difficulty in breathing and rashes are the symptoms of an inflammatory response.
- **Anaphylactic shock** occurs when large amount of histamine is suddenly released by the mast cells.
- Due to this, all the peripheral arteries dilate at once.
- It causes a precipitous drop in blood pressure or shock. It is fatal, if not treated immediately.

Treatment

(i) In case of normal allergic reactions, drugs that cause vasoconstriction or antihistamines are used.

(ii) In case of anaphylactic shock, epinephrine is used.

Autoimmune diseases

These diseases occur when immune system fails to recognise 'self' molecules and starts destroying body's own proteins. This condition may cause chronic and serious diseases.

For examples, insulin-dependent diabetes, multiple sclerosis, rheumatoid arthritis, etc.

Table 16.9 Some autoimmune diseases and their antigens

Diseases	Antigens
Post-vaccinal and post-infectious encephalomyelities	Myelin, cross-reactive
Aspermatogenesis	Sperm
Sympathetic ophthalmia	Uvea
Hashimoto's disease	Thyroglobulin
Graves' disease	Receptor proteins for TSH
Autoimmune haemolytic disease	Rh and others on surface of RBCs
Thrombocytopenic purpura	Hapten-platelet or hapten-absorbed antigen complex
Myasthenia gravis	Acetylcholine receptors
Rheumatic fever	Streptococcal, cross-reactive with heart valves
Glomerulonephritis	Streptococcal, cross-reactive with kidney
Rheumatoid arthritis	IgG
Systemic lupus erythematosus	DNA, nucleoprotein RNA, etc.
Diabetes mellitus (type-1)	β-cells in pancreatic islets
Multiple sclerosis	Components of myelin sheaths

Immunodeficiency diseases

These diseases result due to the defect in one or more components of the innate or acquired immunity. Affected individuals are susceptible to diseases, which normally would not bother most people.

Immunodeficiency may result from gene mutations, infections, malnutrition or accidents. Some immunodeficiency diseases are given below

1. Severe Combined Immuno-Deficiency (SCID)

It results due to one of many genetic defects. One such genetic defect leads to adenosine deaminase deficiency.

Various characteristics of SCID are as follows

- SCID is characterised by a very low number of circulating lymphocytes.
- The affected individuals usually die at an early age.
- It is a rare genetic disorder characterised by disturbed development of T-cells and B-cells.
- It involves defective antibody response.

2. Congenital immunodeficiency

It is found since birth due to defective immune system. The absence or defect in a number of inherited genes may result in such congential immunodeficiencies. It is also called **primary immunodeficiency**. This disorder can affect anyone regardless of age or gender. It can affect single or multiple part of the immune system.

3. Acquired immunodeficiency

These are acquired after birth due to a wide variety of drugs, cancer or infectious agents. It depletes the cell-mediated immune response, e.g. Hodgekin's disease (cancer), AIDS, etc.

Table 16.10 Description of some immunodeficiency diseases

Diseases	Cells affected	Comments
Acquired Immuno Deficiency Syndrome (AIDS)	T-cells, virus destroys T_H CD_4	Promotes cancer and various bacterial, viral, fungal, protozoan diseases.
Selective IgA immunodeficiency	B, T-cells	Affects about 1 in 700, cause frequent mucosal infections.
Common variable hypogammaglobulinemia	B, T-cells (decreased immunoglobulins)	Frequent viral and bacterial infections, second most common immune deficiency disease, affects about 1 in 70000.
Reticular dysgenesis	B, T and stem cells (a combined immunodeficiency, deficiencies in B and T-cells and neutrophils)	Usually fatal in early infancy, very rare, bone marrow transplant is a possible treatment.
Severe Combined Immuno Deficiency (SCID)	B, T and stem cells (deficiency of both B and T-cells)	Occurs in several forms, affect about 1 in 100000; allows severe viral, fungal infections; treated with transplanation of bone marrow.
Thymic hypoplasia (Di-George syndrome)	T-cells (defective thymus causes deficiency of T-cells)	Lack of cell-mediated immunity; usually fatal in infancy from *Pneumocystis,* cause pneumonia or viral or fungal infections.
Wiskott-Aidrich syndrome	T-cells (few platelets in blood, abnormal T-cells)	Frequent infections by viruses, fungi, protozoan; eczema, defective blood clotting; usually causes death in childhood.
X-linked infantile (Bruton's) agammaglobulinemia	B-cells (decreased immunoglobulins)	Frequent extracellular bacterial infections; occurs in about 1 in 200000; the first immunodeficiency disorder recognised in (1952); usually affects males.

CHECK POINT 16.3

1. The modern idea about ageing is that our body slowly loses the power of defence against the invasion of germs and pathogens. This process starts by the disappearance of which organ?
   (a) Pituitary gland (b) Spleen
   (c) Thymus (d) Adrenal gland
2. Which of the following statement is true regarding vaccination?
   (a) Vaccination is a method of active immunisation
   (b) Vaccination is a method of passive immunisation
   (c) Vaccination is a method of artificial passive immunisation
   (d) Vaccination is a method of natural passive immunisation
3. Vaccines produced from ...*A*... provides long term immunisation whereas vaccines produced by ...*B*... provides short term immunisation.
   (a) *A* – combination vaccine, *B* – live vaccines
   (b) *A* – toxoids, *B* – live vaccines
   (c) *A* – attenuated pathogen, *B* – toxoids
   (d) *A* – toxoids, *B* – combination vaccine
4. Skin grafting within one organism is an example of
   (a) allograft
   (b) autograft
   (c) isograft
   (d) xenograft
5. Mast cells secrete a protein, which causes the dilation of blood vessels. The protein is
   (a) pyrogens
   (b) histamine
   (c) interferon
   (d) None of the above
6. When one goes to a new place and suddenly starts sneezing and wheezing for no explained reason and then these symptoms disappear when on returns.
   This condition is called
   (a) autoimmunity
   (b) allergy
   (c) passive immunisation
   (d) vaccination

EXAM POINTS

- Tears act as physiological barrier of immunity. [AIIMS 2012]
- PMNL and monocytes act as cellular barrier of immunity. [CBSE AIPMT 2012]
- Interferons are antiviral substances. [AFMC 2012]
- The main function of Kupffer's cells is phagocytosis. [JIPMER 2018]
- Humans have acquired immune system that produces antibodies to neutralise pathogens. Still innate immune system is present at the time of birth because it has natural killer cells which can phagocytose and destroy microbes. [NEET 2019]
- Active immunity is slow and takes time to give full effective response in comparison to passive immunity. [NEET 2020]
- When exposed to antigen (living or dead), antibodies are produced in the host's body. It is called active immunity. [NEET 2020]
- When readymade antibodies are directly given, it is called passive immunity. [NEET 2020]
- The yellowish fluid 'colostrum' secreted by mammary glands of mother during the initial days of lactation has abundant antibodies (IgA) to protect the infant. This type of immunity is called as natural passive immunity. [NEET 2020]
- Immunity acquired after smallpox infection is natural active immunity. [EAMCET 2014]
- Antirabies serum is an example of artificial passive immunity. [EAMCET 2014]
- To treat the bite of viper snake, preformed antibodies are injected in body. [CBSE AIPMT 2012]
- Foetus receives some antibodies from mother throgh placenta, it is an example of passive immunity. [NEET 2020]
- Immunity tolerance is developed by interaction with antigen. [AIIMS 2019]
- IgG can cross the placenta, IgA provides localised protection from pathogens, IgE is involved in hypersensitive reactions and IgM exists as pentamer. [JIPMER 2019]
- IgG is most abundant immunoglobulin in human body. [OJEE 2013]
- IgE is an antiallergic immunoglobulin. [JIPMER 2018]
- IgA is involved in passive immunity. [JIPMER 2018]
- Monoclonal antibodies and polyclonal antibodies are produced by plasma cells of B-lymphocytes. [JIPMER 2017]
- Humoral immunity is mediated by plasma cells. [JIPMER 2019]
- Thymus is primary lymphoid organ. [MHT CET 2014]
- Spleen is secondary lymphoid organ and it also acts as graveyard of RBCs. [UK PMT 2014]
- MA3LT constitutes about 50% of the lymphoid tissue in human body. [NEET 2017]
- Cell-mediated immune response is responsible for rejection of kidney graft. [NEET 2019, 2017]
- The term vaccine was introduced by Jenner. [RPMT 2011]
- Vaccine for tuberculosis is BCG vaccine. [J&K CET 2011]

Chapter Exercises

(A) Topical Exercise

Immunity and Innate Immunity

1 A portion of the antigen, the antigenic determinant, which can bind to the antigen binding site of the antibody is

(a) opsonin (b) antigen-antibody complex
(c) epitope (d) paratope

2 Consider the following statements.

I. The substance that stimulates the production of antibodies in the body are antigens.
II. The substances which are incapable of inducing antibody formation by themselves are called partial antigens.

Choose the correct option.

(a) Statement I is true, but II is false
(b) Statement I is false, but II is true
(c) Both statements I and II are true
(d) Both statements I and II are false

3 The term 'immunity' refers to

(a) the combined actions of all white blood cells
(b) events that occur within the lymphatic system
(c) general defences against all microorganisms
(d) specific defences against microbes encountered during an earlier exposure

4 Innate immunity includes all the defences with which a person is born. It includes

I. PMNL–neutrophils II. T-lymphocytes
III. B-lymphocytes IV. Mucous membrane
V. Natural killer cells
VI. Interferons

Choose the correct option from the codes given below.

(a) I, II, III and IV (b) I, IV, V and VI
(c) III, IV, V and VI (d) II, III and IV

5 The anatomic barrier is formed by

(a) skin and cilia (d) mucous membrane
(c) bile and enzymes (d) Both (a) and (b)

6 Most bacteria ingested with food are killed by

(a) cilia and mucus on the linings of the tract
(b) stomach acids
(c) the intrinsic factor in the stomach
(d) bile in the small intestine

7 Which of the following is involved in defence mechanism of the body?

(a) Lymphocytes (b) Neutrophils
(c) Macrophages (d) All of these

8 Find the incorrect matched pair.

(a) HCl Physiological barrier
(b) Kupffer cell – Liver
(c) Microglial cell – Kidney
(d) Alveolar macrophages – Lungs

9 Consider the following statements.

I. Phagocytosis was discovered by Metchnikoff.
II. Macrophages engulf and digest other cells and perform phagocytosis.

Choose the correct option.

(a) Statement I is true, but II is false
(b) Statement I is false, but II is true
(c) Both statements I and II are true
(d) Both statements I and II are false

10 Which of the following is correct for immuno-modulators?

(a) They always suppress immune system
(b) They never suppress immune system
(c) They always stimulate immune system
(d) Specific immuno-modulators stimulate the immunoresponse of immune system, whereas some other immuno-modulators inhibit it

11 Match the following columns.

Column I	Column II
A. Physiological barriers	1. Interferons
B. Cellular barriers	2. Histamines
C. Cytokine barriers	3. Cerumen
D. Inflammatory barriers	4. Neutrophils

Codes

	A	B	C	D
(a)	1	3	2	4
(b)	3	4	1	2
(c)	4	2	3	1
(d)	2	4	3	1

12 Sensitivity to any allergen is related to

(a) deviation from the process of immunity
(b) age of the person
(c) eating habit
(d) rise in environmental temperature

13 A localised inflammatory response appears at the site of infection causes redness, swelling, pain and heat due to certain chemicals, they are
(a) histamine and prostaglandins
(b) cerumen and mucus
(c) histamine and cerumen
(d) prostaglandins and cerumen

14 Certain compounds are released by the WBC, which raise the body temperature. These compounds are known as
(a) pyrogens (b) histamines
(c) toxigens (d) pathogens

15 Messenger molecules, secreted by helper T-cells that recruit other white blood cells are called
(a) interferons (b) antibiotics
(c) cytotoxins (d) lymphokines

16 Choose the correct statement(s).
(a) Perspiration, saliva and tears contain an enzyme lysozyme that kills bacteria
(b) Lysozyme kills bacteria by destroying their cell walls
(c) White blood cells that are non-specific killer of microbes are phagocytes
(d) All of the above

17 The thick and yellow exudate from an inflamed tissue containing large number of leucocytes is called
(a) lymph (b) pus (c) serum (d) plasma

18 Which of the following components of natural killer cell is responsible for creating pores in plasma membrane?
(a) Histamine (b) Serum (c) Perforins (d) Interleukin

19 A chemical substance produced by a microorganism for inhibiting the growth of another is
(a) antibody (b) antibiotic (c) aflatoxin (d) antiallergic

20 Messenger molecules released by virus-infected cells that bind to the surface of healthy cells and stimulate them to synthesise proteins that prevent viral reproduction are called
(a) interferons (b) antibiotics
(c) cytotoxins (d) lymphokines

21 If the person shows the production of interferons in his body, chances are that he is suffering from
(a) anthrax (b) malaria
(c) measles (d) tetanus

22 Choose the incorrectly matched pair.
(a) Histiocytes – All tissues
(b) Rubor – Pain due to infection
(c) NK cells – Reduced in AIDS patients
(d) Cytokinins – Antimicrobial protein

23 Consider the following statements.
I. Complement system causes activation of mast cells and basophils.
II. Complement system is formed of various phagocytic cells.

Choose the correct option.
(a) Statement I is true, but II is false
(b) Statement I is false, but II is true
(c) Both statements I and II are true
(d) Both statements I and II are false

24 Which one of the following statements is incorrect?
(a) Body's first line of defence is skin
(b) Second line of defence is skin and phagocytic cells
(c) Third line of defence is immune system
(d) Lines of body defence are skin, phagocytic cells and immune system

Acquired Immunity

25 Characters of acquired immunity are
(a) specificity
(b) difference between self and non-self
(c) retains memory
(d) All of the above

26 Active immunity is
(a) borrowed from an active disease case
(b) developed in direct response to a disease agent
(c) the product of borrowed antibodies
(d) passive immunity that is activated

27 Short-lived immunity acquired from mother to foetus across placenta or through mother's milk to the infant is categorised as
(a) active immunity
(b) passive immunity
(c) cellular immunity
(d) innate or non-specific immunity

28 Passive immunity is defined as immunity
(a) genetically inherited from the parents
(b) achieved through vaccination
(c) acquired through first exposure to the disease
(d) achieved through the serum of other animals enriched in antibodies

29 Antibodies from a mother can be used for the protection of baby. It is an example of
(a) natural passive immunity
(b) natural active immunity
(c) artificial passive immunity
(d) artificial active immunity

30 Both B and T-cells are formed from
(a) lymph nodes (b) thymus gland
(c) pituitary gland (d) bone marrow

31 The basic difference between B and T-cells is
(a) their origin is different
(b) their maturation and storage is different
(c) they are found at different places in the lymphoid pool
(d) they do not show any difference

32 Which one of these does not pertain to B-cells?
(a) Have passed through the thymus
(b) Have specific receptors
(c) Are responsible for antibody mediated immunity
(d) Synthesise and liberate antibodies

33 Certain children are immune to certain diseases due to
(a) T-cells immune system (b) plasma B-cells
(c) memory B-cells (d) phagocyte antigen reactions

34 Which of these pertains to T-cells?
(a) Have specific receptors
(b) Are more than one type
(c) Are responsible for cell-mediated immunity
(d) All of the above

35 Which of the following is not true for T-lymphocytes?
(a) They cannot release antibodies
(b) They attain maturity in thymus
(c) They comprise 10-15% of lymphocytes
(d) They are short-lived and live for 5-10 days

36 The cells, which suppress the entire immune system from its attack in the same body, are known as
(a) helper T-cells (b) killer B-cells
(c) suppressor cells (d) suppressor T-cells

37 The cells which directly attack and destroy the antigens, are known as
(a) helper T-cells (b) killer T-cells
(c) helper B-cells (d) killer B-cells

38 In the cell-mediated immune response, T-lymphocytes divide and secrete
(a) antigens (b) plasmalogens
(c) collagens (d) cytokines

39 Consider the following statements.
I. Active immunity provides immediate relief.
II. An Antigen Presenting Cell (APC) includes macrophages and dendritic cells.
Choose the correct option.
(a) Statement I is true, but II is false
(b) Statement I is false, but II is true
(c) Both statements I and II are true
(d) Both statements I and II are false

40 Deficiency of B-cells and T-cells is known as
(a) pathogenicity
(b) autoimmunity
(c) cytotoxicity
(d) immune deficiency

41 Plasma cells are
(a) the same as memory cells
(b) formed from blood plasma
(c) B-cells that are actively secreting antibody
(d) inactive T-cells carried in the plasma

Antibodies

42 Antibodies are
(a) also called immunoglobulins
(b) foreign bodies in a cell
(c) molecules synthesised in response to foreign structures
(d) Both (a) and (c)

43 Which of the following statements is/are correct?
(a) Antibodies belong to the class of γ-globulins
(b) Antibodies combine with antigens at variable regions
(c) Antibody production is assisted by lymphocytes
(d) All statements are correct

44 Antigen binding site in an antibody is found between
(a) two light chains
(b) two heavy chains
(c) one heavy and one light chain
(d) either between two light chains or between one heavy and one light chain depending upon the nature of antigen

45 Which of the following statements is incorrect?
(a) Crystallisable region of antibody is Fc
(b) A flexible region in antibody is hinge region
(c) The immunoglobulin abundant in colostrum is IgA
(d) The maximum amount of serum immunoglobulins present in blood is IgD

46 The function of IgE is
(a) mediate in allergic response
(b) activation of B-cells
(c) protection from inhaled and ingested pathogens
(d) stimulation of complement system, passive immunity to foetus

47 Match the following columns.

	Column I		Column II
A.	IgM	1.	Complement system
B.	IgA	2.	Protect developing foetus
C.	IgD	3.	Protection of newborn babies
D.	IgG	4.	Activates B-cells

Codes

	A	B	C	D		A	B	C	D
(a)	1	3	4	2	(b)	4	1	3	2
(c)	2	1	3	4	(d)	2	3	4	1

48 During blood typing, agglutination indicates that the
(a) plasma contains antibodies
(b) red blood cells carry certain antigens
(c) plasma contains certain antigens
(d) red blood cells carry certain antibodies

49 Recognition and digestion by the phagocytes due to the coated surface of antigens by the antibodies, is known as
(a) opsonisation
(b) immunisation
(c) T-cells immunisation reaction
(d) B-cells immunisation reaction

50 Consider the following statements.
I. Antiserum is rich in antigens.
II. Antiserum is obtained by the exposure to antibodies.
Choose the correct option
(a) Statement I is true, but II is false
(b) Statement I is false, but II is true
(c) Both statements I and II are true
(d) Both statements I and II are false

51 .... are produced by same clone of plasma B-cells and are homogeneous.
(a) Polyclonal antibodies (b) B-cells
(c) Monoclonal antibodies (d) Leucocytes

52 Hybridomas are the fusion product of
(a) normal antibody producing cell with myeloma
(b) abnormal antibody producing cell with myeloma
(c) sex cells with myeloma
(d) bone cells with myeloma

53 If you suspect major deficiency of antibodies in a person, to which of the following would you look for confirmatory evidence?
(a) Serum albumins (b) Serum globulins
(c) Fibrinogen in the plasma (d) Haemocytes

54 Choose the incorrectly matched pair.
(a) Monoclonal antibody - Homogeneous antibodies
(b) Polyclonal antibody - Magic bullet
(c) Helper T-cells - Stimulate B-cells to produce antibodies
(d) None of the above

Immune Responses

55 The immune system of body made up of specific antibodies present in blood plasma and lymph defending against foreign bodies entering the body fluid, is called
(a) humoral immune system
(b) antibody system
(c) cell-mediated immune system
(d) lymphocyte system

56 What is the major benefit of the specific defence system?
(a) Specific defence systems act as barriers to foreign invaders
(b) Specific defences provide a quicker response than non-specific defences
(c) Specific responses are generated no matter what the situation is
(d) Specific defences can produce immunity

57 Humoral immunity is associated with
(a) T-cells
(b) B-cells
(c) Macrophages
(d) Both (a) and (b)

58 Choose the incorrect matched pair.
(a) Killer T-cells - Destroy infected cells
(b) Helper T-cells - Stimulates immune response by B-cells only
(c) Suppressor T-cells -Inhibit immune response
(d) Memory T-cells - Subset of the offspring of B-cells

59 Choose the incorrect statement.
(a) Immunogenicity and specificity are two characteristics of an antigen
(b) The specific immune responses consist of humoral and cellular immunity
(c) B-cells are responsible for humoral immunity and T-cells for cellular immunity
(d) Humoral immunity is mediated by immunoglobulins

60 Which of the following would not be a participant in cell-mediated immune responses?
(a) Helper T-cells (b) Macrophages
(c) Cytokines (d) Plasma cells

61 Which of the following immune responses is more potent and long-lived?
(a) Primary immune response only
(b) Secondary immune response only
(c) Tertiary immune response only
(d) Both (a) and (b)

Immune System and Lymphoid Organs

62 The immune system is involved in
(a) destruction of abnormal or mutant cell types that arise within the body
(b) allergic reactions
(c) rejections of organ transplants
(d) All of the above

63 The odd one out in the following is
I. Spleen and Peyer's patches
II. Spleen and thymus
III. Liver and spleen
IV. Thymus and Peyer's patches
Codes
(a) I and IV (b) II and III (c) Only III (d) Only II

64 Which of the following organs is primarily concerned with immunity?
(a) Liver (b) Lymphatic tissue
(c) Kidney (d) Thyroid

65 The primary lymphoid organ is ...*A*.... and secondary lymphoid organ is ...*B*... .
(a) *A*-tonsils, *B*-thymus
(b) *A*-Peyer's patches, *B*-lymph nodes
(c) *A*-thymus, *B*-tonsils
(d) *A*-lymph nodes, *B*-Peyer's patches

66 Choose the incorrect statement.
(a) In birds, the lymphocytes mature in Bursa of fabricius
(b) The primary lymphoid organs are those where B-cells and T-cells mature and activate
(c) The secondary lymphoid organs are those where B-cells and T-cells proliferate and differentiate after maturation
(d) Cortisol helps in differentiation of cells of immune system

67 Which of the following glands is large-sized at birth, but reduces in size with ageing? **[NCERT Exemplar]**
(a) Pineal (b) Pituitary
(c) Thymus (d) Thyroid

68 Removal or absence of thymus in early life shall bring about
(a) lack of lymphocytes (b) lack of macrophages
(c) death of organism (d) All of these

69 'Mammalian thymus' is mainly concerned with
(a) regulation of body temperature
(b) regulation of body growth
(c) immunological functions
(d) secretion of thyrotropin

70 The spleen does not
(a) house lymphocytes
(b) filter foreign particles, damaged red blood cells and cellular debris from the blood
(c) contain phagocytes
(d) change undifferentiated lymphocytes into T-lymphocytes

71 Damage to thymus in a child may lead to
(a) loss of cell-mediated immunity
(b) a reduction in the haemoglobin content in blood
(c) a reduction in the amount of plasma proteins
(d) loss of antibody-mediated immunity

72 Choose correctly matched pair. **[NCERT Exemplar]**
(a) MHC- Minor Histamine Complex
(b) MALT - Mucosa Associated Lymphoid Thymocyte
(c) PMNLs - Poly-Morpho Nuclear Leucocytes
(d) SCID - Somatic Combined Immuno Deficiency

73 Choose the odd one out.
(a) Tonsils (b) Spleen
(c) Peyer's patches (d) Pancreas

Vaccination and Immunisation

74 Consider the following statements.
I. Artificial immunity can be acquired from a vaccine.
II. Vaccines are extracted from lymph.
Choose the correct option.
(a) Statement I is true, but II is false
(b) Statement I is false, but II is true
(c) Both statements I and II are true
(d) Both statements I and II are false

75 Vaccination protects a person from disease because it
(a) helps in better digestion
(b) increases RBC count
(c) produces antibodies
(d) corrects body heating system

76 Vaccines are
(a) the same as monoclonal antibodies
(b) treated bacteria or viruses or one of their proteins
(c) short-lived
(d) MHC proteins

77 Choose the incorrect statement.
(a) The first vaccine against cholera was developed by Edward Jenner
(b) Weak living bacteria unable to cause a disease are called attenuated organism
(c) Vaccines produced from inactivated organisms are called toxoids
(d) Toxoid is purified toxin

78 Vaccination against smallpox means the introduction of
(a) leucocytes obtained from animal
(b) antibodies produced in other animals
(c) antibodies
(d) actual weakened germs or attenuated smallpox virus

79 Vaccine against rabies was first developed by
(a) Jenner (b) Shull
(c) Pasteur (d) Goror

80 DPT vaccination is given for
(a) Diphtheria, Pneumonia, Tetanus
(b) Diphtheria, Pertussis, Tetanus
(c) Diphtheria, Polio, Tetanus
(d) Diphtheria, Pertussis, Tuberculosis

81 Which vaccine is effective against poliomyelitis?
(a) Salk vaccine administered orally
(b) Sabin vaccine administered by injection
(c) Salk vaccine administered by injection and Sabin vaccine administered orally
(d) All of the above

82 A living attenuated bovine strain of *Mycobacterium tuberculosis* is used as a vaccine to protect human tuberculosis is
(a) Anti-tuberculosis
(b) Rifampicin
(c) Bacillus Calmette-Guerin
(d) None of the above

83 Choose the incorrect match pair.
(a) Tetanus - Purified tetanus toxoid
(b) Cholera - Crude fraction of *Vibrio cholerae*
(c) Whooping cough - Killed whole or fragments of *Bordetella pertussis*
(d) Rabies - Crude fraction of virus

Organ Transplantation

84 Transplantation of tissues/organs to save certain patients often fails due to rejection of such tissues/ organs by the patient. Which type of immune response is responsible for such rejection?
(a) Autoimmune response
(b) Humoral immune response
(c) Physiological immune response
(d) Cell-mediated immune response

85 Which of the following is a method of preventing graft rejection?
(a) Tissue matching
(b) Exposure of bone marrow
(c) Immunosuppression
(d) All of the above

86 Cyclosporin and endosporins are the drugs that are used as
(a) antiretroviral drugs (b) immunosuppressants
(c) immunomodulators (d) immunovaccines

87 Choose the correctly matched pair.
(a) Autograft - Skin graft in a person
(b) Allograft - Between twins
(c) Xenograft - Heart transplant
(d) All of the above

Immune Disorders and Deficiencies

88 During an allergic reaction, the binding of antigens to IgE antibodies initiates a response, in which chemicals cause the dilation of blood vessels. Such chemicals are
(a) interferons (b) hormones
(c) histamines (d) acetylamine

89 Consider the following statements.
I. Hypersensitivity to an allergen is caused due to over-reaction of immune system.
II. Pollen like agents which produce allergy are known as globulins.

Choose the correct option.
(a) Statement I is true, but II is false
(b) Statement I is false, but II is true
(c) Both statements I and II are true
(d) Both statements I and II are false

90 Which among the following is an example of allergy?
(a) Hives (b) Hay fever
(c) Asthma (d) All of these

91 The condition caused due to release of large amounts of histamine is
(a) anaphylactic shock (b) eczema
(c) pertussis (d) immune side effects

92 When body starts producing antibodies against its own RBCs, the disease is known as
(a) chronic disease (b) immunity control disease
(c) autoimmune disease (d) acute anaemia

93 Which of the following are immunity related diseases?
I. AIDS II. Addison's disease
III. SCID IV. Smallpox
V. Multiple sclerosis VI. Cancer
Codes
(a) I, II and VI (b) I, II, III and V
(c) II and VI (d) III, IV, V and VI

94 Someone with severe combined immunodeficiency has no
(a) interferons (b) macrophages
(c) T or B-cells (d) functioning lymph nodes

95 Which of the following is not the example of an autoimmune disease?
(a) Multiple sclerosis
(b) Rheumatic fever
(c) Haemolytic disease of the newborn
(d) Rheumatoid arthritis

96 Allergy condition caused by pollen grains of certain flowers causing inflammation of the nose is called
(a) pharyngitis (b) laryngitis
(c) bronchitis (d) rhinitis

97 An autoimmune disease where the body's own antibodies attack the cells of the thyroid gland is
(a) Hyperthyroidism (b) Hashimoto's disease
(c) Graves' disease (d) Turner's syndrome

98 Which of the following acts as antigen in rheumatoid arthritis?
(a) Sperm (b) Myelin
(c) IgG (d) Thyroglobulin

99 Thymic hypoplasis is also known as
(a) Reticular syndrome (b) Di-George syndrome
(c) Wiskott-Aldrich syndrome (d) Bruton's syndrome

(B) Cumulative Exercise

(Assorted Questions of the Chapter for Advanced Level Practice)

1 Autoimmunity is caused due to
I. ability of immune cells to damage self-cells.
II. ability of immune cells to discriminate between self-cells and non-self-cells.
III. inability of immune cells to damage self-cells which represent antigens.
IV. inability of cells to distinguish self-cell and non-self cells.

Codes
(a) I and II (b) II and III (c) III and IV (d) I and IV

2 Which of the following statements are correct?
I. Bone marrow and spleen are primary lymphoid organs.
II. Mucosa Associated Lymphoid Tissue (MALT) forms about 50% of the lymphoid tissue.
III. MHC are the molecules responsible for recognition and labelling.
IV. Innate immunity shows primary and secondary responses.

Codes
(a) I, III and IV (b) I and II (c) II and III (d) II and IV

3 Which of the following statements are correct for innate immunity?
I. Bacteria enter through a break in the skin.
II. Resident phagocytic cells engulf the bacteria.
III. B-cells are stimulated to produce specific antibodies.
IV. Diapedesis allows new phagocytic leucocytes to invade the infected area.

Codes
(a) III and IV (b) I and II (c) I and III (d) II and IV

4 Match the following columns.

Column I		Column II
A. Active natural	1.	Vaccination D
B. Second line of defence	2.	Direct contact with pathogens
C. First line of defence	3.	Surface barriers
D. Louis Pasteur	4.	Complement proteins

Codes

	A	B	C	D		A	B	C	D
(a)	1	2	3	4	(b)	2	4	3	1
(c)	3	2	1	4	(d)	1	4	3	2

5 Which of the following statements are correct?
I. IgM is the first immunoglobulin produced in a primary response to an antigen.
II. IgD protects the body fluids and also stimulates phagocytes and complement system.
III. IgE acts as a mediator in allergic response.
IV. IgE protects from inhaled and ingested pathogens thus, it protects the body surface.

Codes
(a) Only I (b) Only III (c) I and II (d) I and III

6 Antibody
I. is a protein molecule.
II. is synthesised by an animal to combat foreign material.
III. occurs on the surface of a plasma cell and also in the body fluids.
IV. binds to a macrophage to reach a helper T-cell to initiate immune response.

Codes
(a) II, III and IV (b) I, II and III
(c) II and III (d) I and IV

7 B-lymphocytes
I. form humoral or antibody-mediated immune system.
II. are formed by the division of erythroblasts.
III. defend against viruses and bacteria that enter the blood and lymph.
IV. move to the site of infection.

Codes
(a) I and IV (b) I and III (c) II and IV (d) I and II

8 Match the following columns.

	Column I		Column II
A.	T-lymphocytes	1.	Sites on antigens recognised by antibodies
B.	B-lymphocytes	2.	Cell-mediated immune response
C.	Haptens	3.	Antibody mediated immunity
D.	Epitopes	4.	Incapable of inducing antibodies formation by themselves

Codes

	A	B	C	D		A	B	C	D
(a)	2	3	4	1	(b)	1	2	3	4
(c)	4	3	2	1	(d)	3	4	1	2

9 Match the following columns.

	Column I	Column II
A.	Interferon	1. Treatment of rickets
B.	Calcitonin	2. Treatment of infertility
C.	Interleukin	3. Formation of erythrocytes
D.	Erythropoietin	4. Treatment of viral infections
E.	Gonadotropin	5. Enhancement of immune action

Codes

	A	B	C	D	E
(a)	3	1	4	2	5
(b)	3	2	1	5	4
(c)	4	3	2	1	5
(d)	4	1	5	3	2

10 Which of the following statements are correct?

I. Inflammatory response in allergy is caused by the release of histamine by mast cells.

II. An insect bite may result in inflammation triggered by the chemicals histamine and kinins.

III. Second line of defence is formed by antibodies.

IV. The regions of an antibody that make it distinct from all other kinds of antibodies are its variable (V) regions. Diapedesis allows new phagocytic leucocytes to invade the infected area.

Codes

(a) I and II (b) II and IV
(c) I and III (d) I, II, III and IV

11 Which of the following statement(s) is/are incorrect?

I. Globulins contained in human blood plasma are primarily involved in defence mechanisms of body.

II. Antigen binds to antibody as a result of electrostatic interactions.

III. Six polypeptide chains are present in gamma immunoglobulin.

IV. The protein which helps in making antigen susceptible for phagocytosis is perforin and opsonin.

Codes

(a) I and II (b) III and IV (c) I and IV (d) II and III

12 Which of the following statements are correct?

I. The most commonly transplanted tissue is cornea.

II. The role of helper T-cells is to stimulate immune response.

III. After infection by germs, immunity acquired is active immunity.

IV. Memory cells are responsible for immunogenic memory.

Codes

(a) I and II (b) III and IV
(c) II and III (d) I, II, III and IV

13 Choose the incorrect statement.

I. Sabin vaccine for polio is a live oral vaccine.

II. After vaccination, the body builds up antibodies.

III. Genetically engineered vaccines are also called as second generation vaccine.

IV. A disease on the verge of extinction in India is Poliomyelitis.

Codes

(a) I and III (b) III and IV (c) I and IV (d) Only III

14 Consider the following matches.

I. SCID – B and T-cells are absent

II. Graft refection – Carried out by $CD4^+$ and $CD8^+$ cells

III. Addison's disease – Autoimmunity

Choose the option containing correctly matched pairs.

(a) Only I (b) I and II
(c) I, II and III (d) Only III

15 Which is the proper order of events in cell-mediated immunity?

(a) Antigen enters tissue, macrophages engulf antigen, antigen presented to members of a clone of lymphocytes, sensitised T-lymphocytes attack antigen-bearing agents

(b) Antigen enters tissues, passed to members of a clone of lymphocytes, lymphocytes sensitised, macrophages engulf antigen, T-lymphocytes attack antigen- bearing agents

(c) Antigen enters tissues, macrophages engulf antigen, antigen passed to members of a clone of lymphocytes, lymphocytes sensitised, B-lymphocytes secrete antibodies that react with antigen-bearing agents

(d) Antigen enters tissues, lymphocytes sensitised, antigen passed to members of a clone of lymphocytes, macrophages engulf antigen, T-lymphocytes attack antigen-bearing agents

Assertion and Reason

Direction (Q. Nos. 16-23) *In each of the following questions, a statement of Assertion (A) is given followed by corresponding statement of Reason (R). Of the statements, mark the correct answer as*

(a) Both A and R are true and R is the correct explanation of A

(b) Both A and R are true, but R is not the correct explanation of A

(c) A is true, but R is false

(d) A is false, but R is true

(e) Both A and R are false

16 **Assertion** (A) The antibodies separated from serum are homogeneous.

Reason (R) Monoclonal antibodies are homogeneous immunological reagents.

17 **Assertion** (A) Second generation vaccines are safer to use.

Reason (R) They are produced by genetic engineering.

18 **Assertion** (A) Interferons are effective against viruses.

Reason (R) Proteins which can be synthesised only by genetic engineering are effective against viruses.

19 **Assertion** (A) The most successful transplants are autografts.

Reason (R) In autograft, antigens encoded by Major Histocompatibility Complex (MHC) are properly matched.

20 **Assertion** (A) Xenograft is a transplant between animals of the same species.

Reason (R) Allograft is a transplant between different individuals of same species.

21 Assertion (A) Interferons are a type of antibodies produced by body cells infected by bacteria.

Reason (R) They stimulate inflammation at the site of injury.

22 Assertion (A) Mast cells in the human body release excessive amounts of inflammatory chemicals, which cause allergic reactions.

Reason (R) Allergens in the environment on reaching human body stimulate mast cells in certain individuals.

23 Assertion (A) A person who has received a cut and is bleeding need to be given anti-tetanus treatment.

Reason (R) Anti-tetanus injection provides immunity by producing antibodies for tetanus.

(C) Medical Entrances' Gallery

(Collection of questions asked in NEET & Various Medical Entrance Exams)

1 Identify the incorrect statement with reference to immunity. **[NEET 2020]**

(a) When readymade antibodies are directly given, it is called passive immunity
(b) Active immunity is quick and gives full response
(c) Foetus receives some antibodies from mother, it is an example for passive immunity
(d) When exposed to antigen (living or dead), antibodies are produced in the host's body. It is called active immunity

2 The yellowish fluid 'colostrum' secreted by mammary glands of mother during the initial days of lactation has abundant antibodies (IgA) to protect the infant. This type of immunity is called as **[NEET 2020]**

(a) passive immunity (b) active immunity
(c) acquired immunity (d) autoimmunity

3 Humans have acquired immune system that produces antibodies to neutralise pathogens. Still innate immune system is present at the time of birth because it **[NEET 2019]**

(a) is very specific and uses different macrophages
(b) produces memory cells for mounting fast secondary response
(c) has natural killer cells which can phagocytose and destroy microbes
(d) provides passive immunity

4 Immunity tolerance is developed by **[AIIMS 2019]**

(a) interaction with the antigen (b) giving antibodies
(c) present by birth (d) giving antibiotics

5 Which of the following immune responses is responsible for rejection of kidney graft?

(a) Humoral immune response **[NEET 2019, NEET-I 2016]**
(b) Inflammatory immune response
(c) Cell-mediated immune response
(d) Autoimmune response

6 Choose the correct match pair regarding antibodies. **[JIPMER 2019, NEET-I 2016]**

(a) IgA - helps in allergic reaction
(b) IgG - crosses placenta
(c) IgE - found in secretions
(d) IgM - exists as dimer

7 What is the function of Kupffer's cells? **[JIPMER 2018]**

(a) Bile secretion (b) Digestion of lipid
(c) Phagocytosis (d) Digestion of protein

8 Which one is an antiallergic antibody? **[JIPMER 2018]**

(a) IgA (b) IgG (c) IgE (d) IgD

9 Which of the following is involved in passive immunity? **[JIPMER 2018]**

(a) IgA (b) IgE (c) IgM (d) IgD

10 MALT constitutes about .... per cent of the lymphoid tissue in human body. **[NEET 2017]**

(a) 50% (b) 20% (c) 70% (d) 10%

11 Transplantation of tissues/organs fails often due to non-acceptance by the patient's body. Which type of immune response is responsible for such rejections?

(a) Autoimmune response **[NEET 2017]**
(b) Cell-mediated immune response
(c) Hormonal immune response
(d) Physiological immune response

12 Monoclonal antibodies and polyclonal antibodies are produced by **[JIPMER 2017]**

(a) T-memory cells
(b) NK-cells
(c) plasma cells of B-lymphocytes
(d) memory cells of B-lymphocytes

13 Humoral immunity is mediated by **[JIPMER 2017, WB JEE 2012]**

(a) R-cells (b) T-cells
(c) NK-cells (d) plasma cells

14 Asthma may be attributed to **[NEET-I 2016]**

(a) allergic reaction of the mast cells in the lungs
(b) inflammation of the trachea
(c) accumulation of fluid in the lungs
(d) bacterial infection of the lungs

15 Helper T-cells : Lymphokines as killer T-cells. **[MHT CET 2015]**

(a) Interferons (b) Lysozymes
(c) Perforins (d) Prostaglandins

16 Plasma cells are derived from **[MHT CET 2015]**
(a) cytotoxic T-cells (b) helper T-cells
(c) memory B-cells (d) memory T-cells

17 Natural killer lymphocytes are an example of **[Karnataka CET 2015]**
(a) physiological barrier (b) cellular barrier
(c) cytokine barrier (d) physical barrier

18 Identify the set of secondary lymphoid organs from the following. **[EAMCET 2015]**
(a) Bone marrow and lymph nodes
(b) Spleen and bone marrow
(c) Bone marrow and thymus gland
(d) Spleen and lymph nodes

19 Antigen binds to this part of antibody **[EAMCET 2015]**
(a) Paratope (b) Epitope
(c) Fc fragment (d) Fab fragment

20 The cytokine barrier among these is **[Kerala CEE 2015]**
(a) polymorphonuclear neutrophil
(b) monocyte (c) interferon
(e) macrophage (d) None of these

21 Read the following statements and find the correct ones.
I. IgE antibodies are produced in an allergic reaction.
II. B-lymphocytes mediate cell-mediated immunity.
III. The yellow fluid colostrum has abundant IgE antibodies.
IV. Spleen is a secondary lymphoid organ.
Codes **[Kerala CEE 2015]**
(a) Only I (b) I and II
(c) II and III (d) I and IV
(e) III and IV

22 The colostrum provides **[MHT CET 2014]**
(a) naturally acquired active immunity
(b) naturally acquired passive immunity
(c) artificially acquired active immunity
(d) artificially acquired passive immunity

23 The primary lymphoid organ is **[MHT CET 2014]**
(a) tonsils (b) Peyer's patches
(c) lymph nodes (d) thymus

24 Immunity that develops in the foetus after receiving antibodies from mother's blood through placenta is
(a) naturally acquired active immunity **[WB JEE 2014]**
(b) artificially acquired active immunity
(c) naturally acquired passive immunity
(d) artificially acquired passive immunity

25 Which of the following statements (s) is/are true?
I. Antibiotics can kill bacteria, but disinfectants do not.
II. Disinfectants have better bactericidal efficiency than antibiotics.
III. Antibiotics are of microbial origin, but disinfectants are chemical compounds.
IV Antibiotics can be injected into the patients, whereas disinfectants are not. **[WB JEE 2014]**
Codes
(a) Only I (b) Only II (c) Only III (d) II, III and IV

26 Passive immunity is **[J&K CET 2014]**
(a) inherited from parents
(b) acquired through first exposure to the disease
(c) achieved directly through readymade antibodies
(d) achieved through vaccination

27 Which of the following organ is called graveyard of RBCs? **[UK PMT 2014]**
(a) Spleen (b) Liver (c) Kidney (d) Heart

28 Match the following columns.

Column I	Column II
A. Natural active immunity	1. Develops due to vaccination
B. Natural passive immunity	2. Anti-rabies serum
C. Artificial active immunity	3. Acquired after smallpox infection
D. Artificial passive immunity	4. Transferred from mother to child

Codes **[EAMCET 2014]**

	A	B	C	D		A	B	C	D
(a)	4	3	1	2	(b)	3	1	4	2
(c)	3	4	1	2	(d)	3	4	2	1

29 The secondary stem cells that produce neutrophils is
(a) granulocyte monocyte progenitor **[EAMCET 2014]**
(b) B-cell committed progenitor
(c) megakaryoblast
(d) erythrocyte committed progenitor

30 The cell mediated immunity inside the human body is carried out by **[NEET 2013]**
(a) T-lymphocytes (b) B-lymphocytes
(c) thrombocytes (d) erythrocytes

31 The most abundant immunoglobulin found in human body is **[Odisha JEE 2013]**
(a) IgM (b) IgG (c) IgD (d) IgA

32 Match the following columns.

Column I	Column II
A. Natural active	1. Immunity developed by heredity.
B. Artificial passive	2. From mother to foetus through placenta.
C. Artificial active	3. Injection of antiserum to travellers.
D. Natural passive	4. Fighting infections naturally.
	5. Induced by vaccination.

Codes **[Karnataka CET 2013]**

	A	B	C	D		A	B	C	D
(a)	1	2	3	5	(b)	4	3	5	2
(c)	4	5	2	3	(d)	5	4	3	1

33 In which one of the following options, the two examples are correctly matched with their particular type of immunity? **[CBSE AIPMT 2012]**

	Examples	Types of immunity
(a)	Polymorphonuclear leucocytes and monocytes	Cellular barriers
(b)	Anti-tetanus and anti-snake bite injection	Active immunity
(c)	Saliva in mouth and tears in eyes	Physical barriers
(d)	Mucus coating of epithelium lining the urinogenital tract and the HCl in stomach	Physiological barriers

34 Which one of the following statements is correct with respect to immunity? **[CBSE AIPMT 2012]**
(a) Preformed antibodies need to be injected to treat the bite by a viper snake
(b) The antibodies against smallpox pathogen are produced by T-lymphocytes
(c) Antibodies are protein molecules, each of which has four light chains
(d) Rejection of a kidney graft is the function of B-lymphocytes

35 Which one of the following acts as physiological barrier to the entry of microorganism in human body? **[AIIMS 2012]**
(a) Tears (b) Monocytes
(c) Skin (d) Epithelium of urogenital tract

36 Antiviral substances are **[AFMC 2012]**
(a) antibody antigen
(b) antigen
(c) interferon
(d) All of the above

37 Lymphoid tissues are found in **[AFMC 2012]**
(a) thymus (b) tonsils
(c) lymph nodes (d) All of these

38 Your immune system helps to protect you against viruses and bacteria that can cause sickness. Which cells are part of the immune system? **[MHT CET 2011]**
(a) White blood cells (b) Red blood cells
(c) Nerve cells (d) None of these

39 The term 'vaccine' was introduced by **[Rajasthan PMT 2011]**
(a) Jenner
(b) Koch
(c) Pasteur
(d) Jointly by Koch and Pasteur

40 The immune system is made up of **[Rajasthan PMT 2011]**
(a) humoral system
(b) humoral and cell-mediated system
(c) humoral and fibrous system
(d) antigen induced antibodies

41 Vaccine for tuberculosis is known as **[J&K CET 2011]**
(a) PAS vaccine (b) BCG vaccine
(c) OPV (d) DPT

ANSWERS

Check Point 16.1

1. (a)	2. (d)	3. (d)	4. (c)	5. (b)	6. (a)

Check Point 16.2

1. (c)	2. (a)	3. (d)	4. (c)	5. (c)

Check point 16.3

1. (c)	2. (a)	3. (c)	4. (b)	5. (b)	6. (b)

(A) Topical Exercise

1. (c)	2. (c)	3. (c)	4. (b)	5. (d)	6. (b)	7. (d)	8. (c)	9. (c)	10. (d)
11. (b)	12. (a)	13. (a)	14. (a)	15. (d)	16. (d)	17. (b)	18. (c)	19. (b)	20. (a)
21. (c)	22. (b)	23. (a)	24. (b)	25. (d)	26. (b)	27. (b)	28. (d)	29. (a)	30. (d)
31. (b)	32. (a)	33. (c)	34. (d)	35. (d)	36. (d)	37. (b)	38. (d)	39. (b)	40. (d)
41. (c)	42. (d)	43. (d)	44. (c)	45. (d)	46. (a)	47. (a)	48. (b)	49. (a)	50. (d)
51. (c)	52. (a)	53. (b)	54. (b)	55. (a)	56. (d)	57. (b)	58. (b)	59. (a)	60. (d)
61. (b)	62. (d)	63. (c)	64. (b)	65. (c)	66. (d)	67. (c)	68. (a)	69. (c)	70. (d)
71. (a)	72. (c)	73. (d)	74. (a)	75. (c)	76. (b)	77. (a)	78. (d)	79. (c)	80. (b)
81. (c)	82. (c)	83. (d)	84. (d)	85. (d)	86. (b)	87. (d)	88. (c)	89. (a)	90. (d)
91. (a)	92. (c)	93. (b)	94. (c)	95. (c)	96. (d)	97. (b)	98. (c)	99. (b)	

(B) Cumulative Exercise

1. (d)	2. (c)	3. (b)	4. (b)	5. (d)	6. (b)	7. (b)	8. (a)	9. (d)	10. (d)
11. (b)	12. (d)	13. (d)	14. (c)	15. (b)	16. (d)	17. (b)	18. (c)	19. (a)	20. (d)
21. (e)	22. (a)	23. (a)							

(C) Medical Entrances' Gallery

1. (b)	2. (a)	3. (c)	4. (a)	5. (c)	6. (b)	7. (c)	8. (c)	9. (a)	10. (a)
11. (b)	12. (c)	13. (d)	14. (a)	15. (c)	16. (c)	17. (b)	18. (d)	19. (a)	20. (c)
21. (d)	22. (b)	23. (d)	24. (c)	25. (d)	26. (c)	27. (a)	28. (c)	29. (a)	30. (a)
31. (b)	32. (b)	33. (a)	34. (a)	35. (a)	36. (c)	37. (d)	38. (a)	39. (a)	40. (b)
41. (b)									

Explanations

(A) Topical Exercise

8 (*c*) Option (c) is incorrect matched pair and can be corrected as
Microglial cells are the phagocytic cells in brain.
Rest options are correct matched pairs.

22 (*b*) Option (b) represents incorrectly matched pair and can be corrected as
The term rubber signifies redness due to an infection. The term dolor is used for pain.
Rest options are correctly matched pairs.

23 (*a*) Statement I is true, but II is false. Incorrect statement can be corrected as
Complement system does not have any cell. Rather, it is formed of 30 different proteins only.

24 (*b*) Statement in option (b) is incorrect and can be corrected as
Second line of defence is formed by cellular components only skin forms the first line of defence.
Rest statements are correct.

35 (*d*) Statement in option (d) is not true. Incorrect statement can be corrected as
T-cells are long lived cells. They live for about 4-5 years or even longer.
Rest statements are true for T-lymphocytes.

39 (*b*) Statement I is false, but II is true. Incorrect statement can be corrected as
Active immunity provides relief after a long period. Immediate relief is provided by passive immunity.

45 (*d*) Statement in option (d) is incorrect and can be corrected as
The abundant serum immunoglobulin in blood is IgG.
Rest statements are correct.

50 (*d*) Both statements are incorrect and can be corrected as
Antiserum is rich in antibodies. It is obtained from an animal following the exposure to an antigen.

54 (*b*) Option (b) is incorrectly matched pair and can be corrected as
The term magic bullet is used for monoclonal antibody because of target specificity.
Rest options are correctly matched pairs.

59 (*a*) Statement in option (a) is incorrect and can be corrected as
Immunogenicity and specificity are the characters of antibody.

66 (*d*) Statement in options (d) is incorrect and can be corrected as
Cortisol is a steroid hormone. It has no role in differentiation of cells of immune system. Rather, thymosin aids in this function.
Rest statements are correct.

74 (*a*) Statement I is true, but II is false. Incorrect statement can be corrected as
Vaccine is either a cell suspension or a byproduct secreted by the cell.

77 (*a*) Statement in option (a) is incorrect and can be corrected as
The first vaccine against chicken pox, cholera was developed by Louis Pasteur.

83 (*d*) Option (d) is incorrectly matched pair and can be corrected as
Rabies vaccine contains killed virus.
Rest options are correctly matched pairs.

89 (*a*) Statement I is true, but II is false. Incorrect statement can be corrected as
Allergy causing agents are known as allergens, e.g. pollens.

(B) Cumulative Exercise

2 (*c*) Statements II and III are correct, while I and IV are incorrect. Incorrect statements can be corrected as

- Bone marrow and thymus are primary lymphoid organs.
- Innate immunity shows inflammatory responses and phagocytosis.

11 (*b*) Statements III and IV are incorrect and can be corrected as
- Four polypeptide chains are present in gamma immunoglobin.
- The protein which helps in making antigen susceptible for phagocytosis is preforin and opsonin.

Rest statements are correct.

13 (*d*) Only statement III is inocrrect and can be corrected as Genetically engineered vaccines are also called as third generation vaccine.
Rest statements are correct.

16 (*d*) A is false, but R is true. A can be corrected as
For the purpose of research and use in medicine, antibodies are often isolated by sacrificing animals after hyper immunising them with antigens. From such hyperimmunised animals, the blood serum may be taken and the antibodies may be isolated from the serum. However, the antibodies, whenever separated from the serum after induction due to an antigen, are usually heterogeneous, since the cells keep on producing a variety of antibodies. Monoclonal antibodies, on the other hand are homogeneous immunological reagents of defined specificity so that these can be utilised for diagnosis and screening with ease and certainty.

17 (*b*) Both A and R are true, but R is not the correct explanation of A.
Second generation vaccines consist of a few antigens present on the surface of the infecting agents rather than the whole inactivated organisms. The surface antigens are produced in huge quantities with the help of recombinant, DNA technique or genetic engineering. Then, they are injected in safer dose to healthy individuals for development of immunity. Second generation vaccines are simple, safer and more potent.

18 (*c*) A is true, but R is false because
Interferons are the proteins that are effective against most viruses. They are naturally produced by virus infected cells. The proteins interact with adjacent cells and make them resistant to virus attack.

Now-a-days interferons are also being manufactured through genetic engineering.

Two mechanisms for the control of virus interferons have been suggested *viz.*

(i) the interferons affect the cellular membranes, so that the virus particles are not disseminated to the other cells.

(ii) interferons control the multiplication of virus particles by inhibiting their protein synthesis.

19 (*a*) Both A and R are true and R is the correct explanation of A.
Replacement of injured, diseased-tissue or organ by grafting a healthy tissue or organ, e.g. skin, cornea, heart, lungs, kidney, bone marrow, liver, pancreas, etc., is now known as transplantation and tissue or organ being grafted is called transplant. Autograft is the most successful transplant, because it involves transplantation of a tissue from one part of body to another part, e.g. skin. Success of any transplantation depends upon the matching of Major Histocompatibility Complex (MHC) or Human Leucocyte Antigen (HLA). In case of autograft, antigens encoded by MHC, are perfectly matched.

20 (*d*) A is false, but R is true. A can be corrected as Xenograft is a transplantation of tissue or organ between two different species. Allograft is a transplantation of organ or tissue between the same species that is from one man to other.

21 (*e*) Both A and R are false and can be corrected as Interferon is a glycoprotein, production of which is induced in virally infected cells. It induces adjacent cells to make them resistant against viral attack.

22 (*a*) Both A and R are true and R is the correct explanation of A
The symptoms of an allergic reaction develop in response to histamine. Mast cells on being stimulated due to the presence of allergens, release a large amount of histamine into the bloodstream and it also acts as initiator of the inflammatory response. This aids in the arrival of leucocytes at the site of infection. Histamine stimulates capillary dilation, increased capillary permeability, closure of bronchial tubes, mucus secretion, pain and swelling.

23 (*a*) Both A and R are true and R is the correct explanation of A.
Tetanus is a bacterial disease caused by exotoxin, produced by *Clostridium tetani* (motile, anaerobic, endospore forming rod-shaped bacterium).
In the wound, anoxic conditions allow the germination of endospores and growth of the organism. *C. tetani* produces a potent exotoxin, the tetanus toxin. The organism is non-invasive and so its sole method of causing disease is through the direct action of tetanus toxin on host cells.
Anti-tetanus injection or antitoxin is a preparation of antibodies to tetanus. It is usually made in horses and takes part in neutralisation of tetanus toxins produced by *C. tetani.*

(C) Medical Entrances' Gallery

1 (*b*) Statement in option (b) is incorrect and can be corrected as Active immunity is slow and takes time to give its full effective response in comparison to passive immunity where preformed antibodies are administered.

2 (*a*) In passive immunity, readymade antibodies are directly given to protect the body against foreign agents.
For example, the yellowish fluid colostrum secreted by mother during the initial days of lactation has abundant antibodies (IgA) to protect the infant. Also the foetus receives some antibodies from their mother through the placenta during pregnancy.

3 (*c*) Innate immunity is non-specific type of defence that is present at the time of birth because it has natural killer cells (lymphocytes and macrophages). These can phagocytose and destroy microbes (cellular barriers). Other forms of innate immunity are physical barriers, physiological barriers and cytokine barriers.

4 (*a*) Immunity tolerance is developed by interaction with the antigen. It is the state of unresponsiveness of immune system to a substance/tissue/pathogen that has the capacity to induce immune response in a given organism.
It can be induced by prior exposure to that specific antigen.

5 (*c*) Cell-mediated immune response is responsible for the rejection of kidney graft. It is mediated by T-lymphocytes which confer a long term memory. They are able to discriminate between self and non-self cells.

These cells sometimes consider graft as non-self and attack the same which causes its rejection.

6 (*b*) Option (b) is correct match.
IgG antibody can cross placenta and provides natural passive immunity to the developing foetus. Other options represent incorrect matches and can be corrected as

- IgA is found in body secretions like sweat, tears, saliva, mucus, colostrum , etc. It provides localised protections from pathogens.
- IgE is involved in hypersensitive reactions and is present in mast cells and basophil cells.
- IgM is found in pentamer form, not as dimer.

7 (*c*) The main function of Kupffer's cells is phagocytosis. They are specialised macrophages located in the liver, lining the walls of the sinusoids. Kupffer's cell activation is responsible for early ethanol induced liver injury, common in chronic alcoholics.

8 (*c*) IgE is an antiallergic antibody. It plays a vital role in response to allergens such as anaphylactic drugs, bee stings, etc. It is synthesised by plasma cells and found only in mammals.

9 (*a*) IgA antibody is involved in passive immunity. In this type of immunity, antibodies from one individual are passed into another individual. It is short-lived. Human colostrum (mother's first milk) is rich in IgA antibodies. It provides natural passive immunity to the infant till the age of three months.

10 (*a*) The MALT constitutes about 50% of the lymphoid tissue in human body. It is Mucosal Associated Lymphoid Tissue located within the lining of the major tracts in the body like respiratory, digestive and urinogenital tracts.

12 (*c*) Monoclonal and polyclonal antibodies are particularly produced by plasma cells of B-lymphocytes when combined with myeloma cells on specific medium. These cells play a key role in specific immunological reactions. Antibodies are produced by B-lymphocytes.

13 (*d*) Humoral immunity activates the secretion of various antibodies against specific antigens entering the body by stimulating the B-cells (also called as plasma cells).

15 (*c*) Helper T-cells promote immune response by secreting lymphokines. Perforin is a cytolytic protein found in killer T-cells. These help to create pore in target cell's plasma membrane.

21 (*d*) Statements I and IV are correct whereas II and III are incorrect. Incorrect statements can be corrected as

- B-lymphocytes mediate humoral immunity.
- Colostrum contains abundant IgA antibodies.

22 (*b*) Colostrum is the first mother/milk which oozes out of the mammary glands of female body after parturition.

It acts as natural defence system for a newborn baby as it provides naturally acquired passive immunity to the newborn baby.

25 (*d*) All given statements are true except I because
Antibiotics are the agent used by living beings to kill or inhibit the growth of microorganisms in them. They are of microbial origin and can be injected into the patients. While, disinfectants are the substances that are applied to the non-living objects to destroy microorganisms living on the objects. They do not necessarily kill the microorganisms but are more potent bactericidal agents and have better bactericidal effect than antibiotics. They are chemical compounds that cannot be injected into the living being or patients.

26 (*c*) Passive immunity is the transfer of active humoral immunity in the form of readymade antibodies from one individual to another. It can occur naturally when maternal antibodies are transferred to the foetus through the placenta and can also be induced artificially to a non-immune individuals.

29 (*a*) The granulocyte monocyte progenitor cells are secondary stem cells that produce neutrophils. Leucocyte development starts with myeloid and lymphoid stem cells in the bone marrow.

34 (*a*) Statement in option (a) is correct.

In artificially acquired passive immunity, preformed antibody in an immune serum is introduced into the body, as the antivenom used to treat snake bites. In this case, the body does not produce any antibodies by itself.
Rest other statements are incorrect and can be corrected as

Antibody is a protein molecule having two light chains and two heavy chains. B-cells recognise and bind antigens and may differentiate to memory cell or plasma cells (produce antibody as in smallpox infection), T-cells causes transplant rejection.

35 (*a*) Physiological barriers inhibit the entry of microorganisms in human body as tears in eyes, saliva in mouth and HCl in stomach. The enzyme called lysozyme is found in tears and saliva that inhibits the synthesis of peptidoglycan present in the cell wall of microorganism especially in bacteria.

CHAPTER 17

Adolescence and Drug/Alcohol Abuse

Adolescence (Latin *Adolescere* – to grow up) is the period of psychological, social and physical transition from childhood to adulthood. A person undergoing adolescence is known as an **adolescent**. Adolescence is marked by rapid physical growth and development of reproductive organs. It also includes changes in the functioning of neuroendocrine system.

During this phase, there are greater chances of adolescents to come in contact with psychoactive substances such as drugs, alcohol, tobacco, etc. It is mainly due to the fact that adolescents are prone to error of judgement.

In this chapter, we will study about adolescence and the factors associated with increasing drug and alcohol abuse among adolescents.

ADOLESCENCE

The World Health Organisation (WHO) defines adolescence as the period of life between 12-19 yrs of age.

It is considered as the preparatory phase for the adult life. Thus, a healthy adolescence is essential for a healthy adulthood.

Characteristics of adolescene

Some characteristics of adolescents are given below

- During adolescence, synaptic pruning occurs. In this process, the overall number of neurons and synapses reduces in brain. It helps to provide more efficient synaptic configuration.
- The adolescents start believing in imaginary audience. They are intensely interested in their appearance and assume that everyone judge their every move. It is in fact, a false belief.
- Adolescents believe that they are highly special and destined to live a heroic or legendary life.
- Adolescents have their own thought process and understanding regarding different things or activities. Thus, metacognitive abilities develop during this time.
- Egocentrism develops in a person during adolescence. Its effects on behaviour can be unpleasant. However in adolescence, it promotes healthy cognitive and psychosocial outcomes.

Common problems during adolescence

Adolescents of both sexes, i.e. male and female face various problems due to different factors. Some important problems are as follows

(i) **Acne** It is the most common problem of almost all adolescents of both the sexes. It results from clogged pores in skin due to the influx of sex hormones, particularly testosterone. It increases self-consciousness, especially if it appears on the face.

(ii) **Hypochondria** It is undue concern about health. Adolescents, especially 'late developers' often suffer from anxiety and psychosomatic disorders.

(iii) **Mood swings** Adolescents may experience alternate periods of loneliness (withdrawal from social surroundings) and gregariousness (a tendency to be with the social surroundings).

(iv) **Irregular food habits** Some adolescents do not consume proper food as they may develop feeling to 'control' weight.
Some others, may have an irresistible craving for food, leading to overeating.

(v) **Irregular menstruation** In females, physiological aberrations, such as absence of monthly periods or perceptual disturbances may also occur.

(vi) **Addiction** to drugs, alcohol, tobacco chewing and smoking are also common among adolescents.

Among all the listed problems, addiction to drugs and other addictive substances is a major social evil. Further in this chapter, we will discuss about these topics only.

DRUGS

Comprehensive definition of drug given by WHO is as follows

- 'Drug is any substance used or intended to be used to modify or explore physiological or pathological states for the benefits of the recepient'.
- It is a single active chemical entity present in a medicine.
It is used for diagnosis, prevention and treatment (cure) of a disease.
- People usually become dependent on drugs because of their action on the brain. Such drugs are known as **addictive** or **habituating** drugs. They can be of two types, i.e. **psychotropic** or **psychedelic drugs**.

Psychotropic drugs

- These drugs act on the brain. They change behaviour, consciousness and capacity of perception of the addict. They are also called **mood altering drugs**.
- The repeated use of these drugs makes the body dependent on them.
- Psychotropic drugs are classified into five major groups, i.e. tranquilisers, sedatives, stimulants, opiates and antidepressants.

These categories are described below

1. Tranquilisers

These drugs decrease tension and anxiety by producing a feeling of calmness without inducing sleep. They are of following two types

(i) **Minor tranquiliser** These are antianxiety drugs used in anxiety and phobic conditions. They produce skeletal muscle relaxation without disturbing voluntary activity.
e.g. Benzodiazepines (BZDs), midazolam, temazepam, clonazepam, diazepam, oxazepam, etc.

(ii) **Major tranquiliser** These are antipsychotic drugs. These have good effect in all types of psychoses, especially schizophrenia. They are chemically phenothiazines. In a psychotic patient, these drugs reduce aggressiveness, relieve anxiety and gradually normalise the thoughts as well as behaviour,
e.g. reserpine (hyposensitive drug obtained from roots *Rauwolfia serpentina*), phenothiazines, butyrophenones, pimozide, etc.

2. Sedative-hypnotics

These drugs are **CNS depressants**. They reduce excitement and lower intensity of pain. They also lower the physiological or functional activity, leading to drowsiness or sleep. Hypnotics are also the drugs that induce sleep (sedative). Sedative-hypnotic drugs are of two types

(i) **Barbiturates** These are synthetic drugs that are derivatives of barbituric acid. They are general depressants for all excitable cells, but CNS is most sensitive to these drugs. They reduce anxiety and induce sleep thus, used as sleeping pills. If taken in excess amount, they result in permanent damage to brain. Sudden withdrawal of these drugs causes epilepsy, e.g. pentobarbitone, mephobarbitone phenobarbitone, thiopentone, etc.

(ii) **Benzodiazepines** These are antianxiety (anxiolytic), muscle relaxant as well as sedative drugs,
e.g. alprazolam, estazolam, valium, etc.

3. Opiates/Opioid narcotics

These are derived from opium alongwith their synthetic relatives. Opium is the dried latex of unripe capsular fruits of poppy plant, *Papaver somniferum* (family-Papaveraceae). It has a strong smell and bitter taste. It contains a number of alkaloids and it is the king of narcotics. They are smoked or chewed.

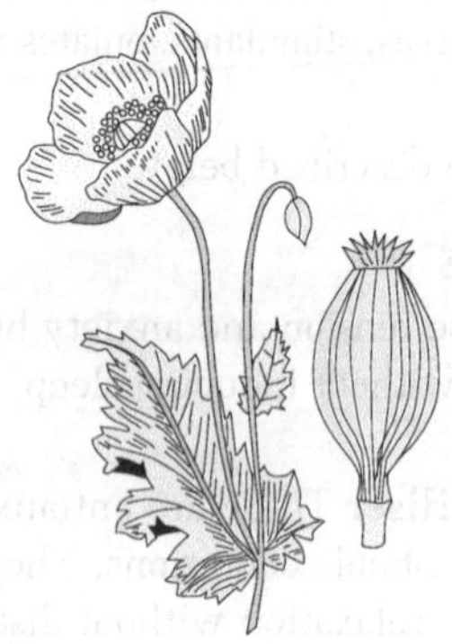

Fig. 17.1 Flowering branch of Papaver somniferum

Effect of Opiates

- They have narcotic, analgesic (painkiller), sedative and astringent (that cause contraction of body parts) effects.
- They slow down respiratory activity, cause constriction of pupil of eye, decrease glandular secretions, impair digestion, produce nausea, vomiting and sterility.
- Opium addicts lose weight, fertility and interest in work.

Note *A drug called **naloxone** is used as an antidote for the overdose of opium.*

Types of opiates

Opiates are of following three types

(i) **Natural opiates**

- **Morphine** It is the main opium alkaloid with molecular formula ($C_{17}H_{19}O_3N$). It is a strong sedative and analgesic thus, useful for patients who have undergone surgery. It causes addiction, bradycardia (slow heartbeat), hyperglycaemia, reduction in urine output, constipation, etc.

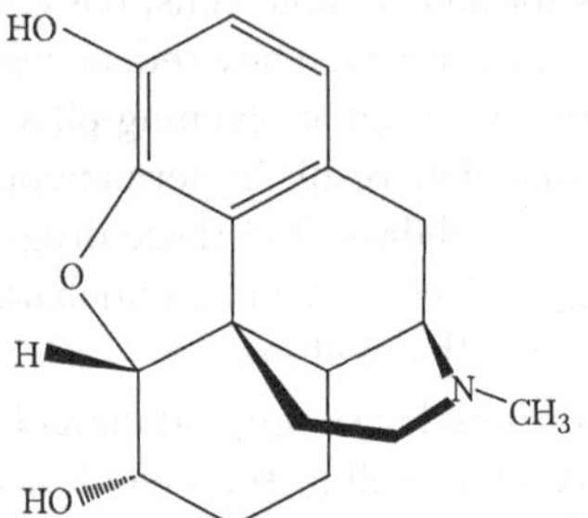

Fig. 17.2 Chemical structure of morphine

- **Diacetyl morphine hydrochloride** It is commonly called **brown sugar/smack.** It is a more powerful analgesic.
- **Codeine** (C_3-Methoxy morphine) It is a naturally occurring derivative of opium. It gets converted to morphine in body. It is mild analgesic and does not cause addiction. It is an ingredient of many cough syrups. Its prominent side effect is constipation.

(ii) **Semisynthetic opiates**

- **Heroin** [diacetylmorphine—$C_{17}H_{17}(OC_2H_3O)_2ON$] It is white, odourless, bitter crystalline compound. It is three times more potent than morphine. It causes indigestion, reduced vision, decreased weight, sterility, epilepsy, etc. It is also called **H-smack.** It is obtained by the acetylation of morphine.

(iii) **Synthetic opiates**

- **Pethidine** (Meperidime) It is less similar to morphine and acts as sedative and euphoriant. It causes less histamine release. It has local anaesthetic action and is metabolised in liver.
- **Methadone** Pharmacologically, it is similar to morphine. It has analgesic, respiratory depressant actions.

4. Stimulants

These drugs stimulate the nervous system. This makes a person more wakeful, alert, active and causes excitement. Sudden withdrawal of a stimulant may cause depression, anxiety and restlessness. Some examples of stimulants are caffeine, cocaine, amphetamines, etc.

Types of stimulants

These are of following two types.

(i) **Natural stimulants**

- **Caffeine** (1,3,7-trimethylxanthine) ($C_8H_{10}N_4O_2$) It is found in non-alcoholic beverages, e.g. tea, coffee, cola, etc. It is obtained from the leaves of tea plant (*Thea sinensis*), seeds of coffee (*Coffee arabica*) and seeds of cocoa plant (*Theobroma*).
  Effects It is white, crystalline and a bitter alkaloid that acts as a CNS stimulant. It is mild diuretic (increases urine output), increases contractile power of skeletal muscle, high doses cause renal dysfunctioning, nervousness, etc.
- **Cocaine or Coca alkaloid** ($C_{17}H_{21}NO_4$) It is obtained from dried leaves and young twigs of coca plant, *Erythroxylum coca*. It is also known as coke, crack, snow, sniff or Big C.
  Effects It interferes with the transport of dopamine and inhibits the release of histamine. It is a good local anaesthetic, delays fatigue and excessive dosage causes hallucinations.

(ii) **Synthetic stimulants**

- **Amphetamines** [$C_6H_5CH_2CH(NH_2)CH_3$] It is commonly called **pep pills, antisleep drugs** or **speed uppers.** These are structurally very similar to adrenaline and are included in **dope test** for athletes.
  Effects They cause alertness, increase self-confidence, talkativeness, suppress hunger, etc. High doses cause euphoria, sleeplessness, vomiting, etc. Due to slow metabolism, they are found in urine for several days. Benzedrine, methedrine and dexedrine, all are prototypes of synthetic drugs. They help to remove fatigue and stimulate respiratory centre.

5. Antidepressants

Depression is a mood disorder characterised by hopelessness, sadness, decline in interest, energy, concentration, etc. It is treated with the help of antidepressants. These drugs elevate mood in depressive illness and phobic states.

Monoamine Oxidase Inhibitors (MAO) form the major class of antidepressants, e.g. phenelzine, isocarboxazid, hydrazines, non-hydrazine, clorgilline, moclobemide, selegilline (deprenyl) and tranylcypromine.

Psychedelic drugs or Hallucinogens

- These drugs change mood, behaviour, thoughts and perceptions without any actual sensory stimulus.
- They generally produce a dream-like state with disorientation and loss of contact with reality.
- They usually make users see colour and hear sound. Thus, they are also called **vision producing drugs**.
- These produce false imaginations or extreme feeling of either despair or euphoria by affecting cerebrum and sense organs.

Types of hallucinogens

These are of following types

(i) **Natural hallucinogens**

(a) **Lysergic Acid Diethylamide** (LSD) It is the most powerful psychedelic compound. It is obtained from ergot fungus present on rye plant. It causes horrible dreams, hallucination, etc., and results in chromosomal and foetal abnormalities.

(b) **Cannabinoids** These are the products of hemp plant, *Cannabis* sp. They interact with cannabinoid receptors present in brain and affect cardiovascular system. These are mostly abused by sport persons.

Some of the products of hemp plant are as follows

- **Bhang** is obtained from fresh/dried leaves and flowering shoots of both male and female plants.
- **Ganja** is obtained from unfertilised female inflorescence.
- **Charas** is obtained from flowering tops of female plants.
- **Marijuana** is obtained from dried flowering plants.

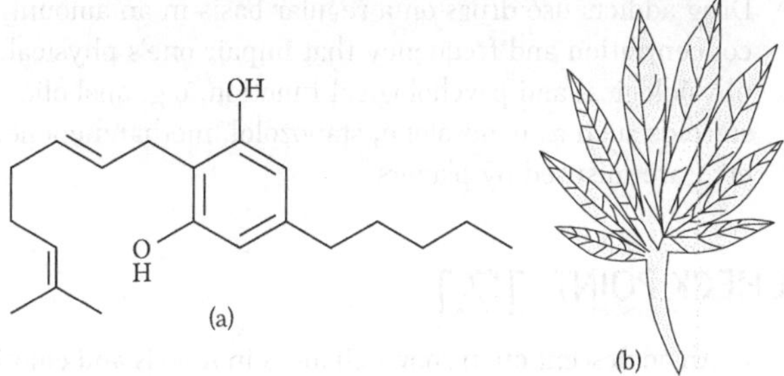

Fig. 17.3 (a) Skeletal structure of cannabinoid molecule, (b) Leaves of Cannabis sativa

(c) **Mescaline** It is a white powdery alkaloid obtained from the tops of a spineless cactus, *Lophophora williamsii.* It is known for its hallucinogenic effects. Other side effects include anxiety, rapid heart beat tremeox, etc.

(d) **Psilocybin** It is obtained from a mushroom, *Psilocybe mexicana.* Psilocybin is a crystalline solid that is used in psychological medicine. Its effects are similar to mescaline. Other side effects includes dizziness, distorted thinking, drowsiness, etc.

- **Atropine** Seed of *Datura* and arial parts of *Atropa belladonna* have hallucinogenic properties. It is due to the presence of alkaloid atropine, hyoscyamine and scopolamine. Stromonium drug is extracted from *Datura.*

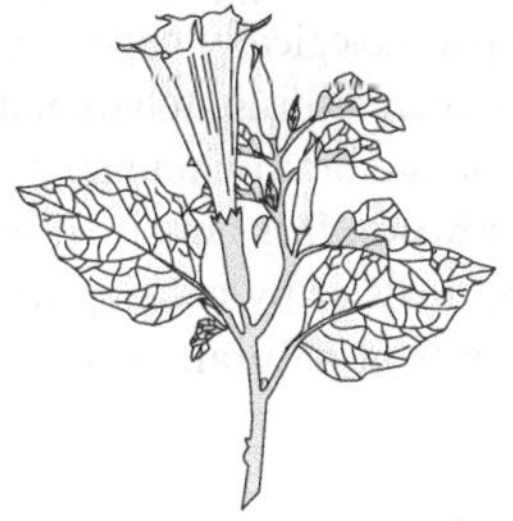

Fig. 17.4 Flowering branch of Datura

(ii) **Synthetic hallucinogens**

- **Phencyclidine Piperidine** (PCP) It has analgesic and hallucinogenic properties.
- It is widely used in veterinary medicine to immobilise large animals. High doses cause hypersalivation, fever, coma, etc.
- It is available to addicts as angel dust (white granular powder).
- Other examples of synthetic hallucinogens include Dimethyl Tryptamine (DMT), Dimethoxymethylamphetamine (DOM) and Dimethoxyamphetamine (DMA).

Drug abuse

- Most of the drugs are developed for clinical purposes.
- Drug abuse involves the use of drugs for a purpose other than clinical use.
- Drug addicts use drugs on a regular basis in an amount, concentration and frequency that impair one's physical, physiological and psychological function, e.g. anabolic steroids such as nandrolone, stanozolol, methandienone, etc., are misused by players.
- The term abuse denotes the following three points
  - Non-medical use
  - Not prescribed by doctors
  - Use for experiencing pleasure and excitement
- Drug abuse plays a major role in many social, biological and psychological problems.
- Commonly abused drugs include amphetamines, anabolic steroids, cocaine, heroin, marijuana, etc.

CHECK POINT 17.1

1. An adolescent often shows changes in moods and emotions due to
(a) Difficulty in social adjustments
(b) Hormone flushes
(c) Search for self identity
(d) Egocentrism

2. Alprazolam belongs to same category of drugs as
(a) valium (b) pimozide (c) methadone (d) cocaine

3. Opium addictions lead to
(a) cardiovascular diseases
(b) loss of weight and interest in work
(c) gastritis
(d) induce deep sleep

4. Drug that is commonly abused by sports person is
(a) Amphetamine
(b) Benzodiazepines
(c) Psilocybin
(d) Pimozide

5. All of these are the prototypes of amphetamine except
(a) benzedrine
(b) dexedrine
(c) methedrine
(d) pethidine

6. Choose the odd one out.
(a) Psilocybin (b) Mescaline
(c) Methadone (d) LSD

ADDICTIVE SUBSTANCES AND THEIR ADDICTION

Addiction is a state of becoming physically, physiologically and psychologically dependent on an addictive substances such as drug, tobacco, alcohol, etc. These substances change brain chemistry by flooding the brain with **dopamine**. It is acheived by either imitating brain chemicals or by causing the brain to release larger amounts of naturally occurring chemicals.

Drug addiction

It is a state of periodic or chronic intoxication produced by repeated consumption of a drug (natural or synthetic). The initial stage of drug addiction is called **habituation.** Characteristics of drug addiction include

- An overpowering desire or need (compulsion) to continue taking the drug and to obtain it by any means.
- A tendency to increase the dose.
- A psychic (psychological) and physical dependence on the drug.
- Detrimental effects on the individual and society.

Reasons of drug addiction

There are various reasons that cause drug addiction. These are as follows

(i) **Peer pressure** Inspiration from friends and peer groups acts as a pressure to start drugs consumption.

(ii) **To overcome frustration and depression** The desire to get relief from personal problems may initiate the use of drugs.

(iii) **Excitement and adventure** It is natural for the young generation to look for some excitement in life. The intake of drug being illegal, satisfies that feeling of excitement and adventure.

(iv) **Desire to do more physical or Mental work** Some people use drugs to increase their working power. Many students use drugs to work whole night before examinations. This leads to mental breakdown.

(v) **Apathy** The lack of interest in day to day activities of an individual may lead to drug addiction.

(vi) **Family history** Consumption of drugs by parents or other members of the family, act as the most natural stimulant.

(vii) **Availability of drugs** Over prescribing and relative decline in price of drugs has added to the availability of various drugs.

Effects of drug addiction

Drug addiction is a sign of disgrace in society. The drug addicts are neither liked by friends or colleagues, nor by family members.

People avoid company of drug addicts. In addition to various physical and psychological problems, dependence on drugs can create a number of other disruptions in the addict's life. It can affect one's life in the following ways

(i) **Family** Behavioural changes may cause conflicts with friends and family.

(ii) **Work** It may decline work efficiency.

(iii) **Social** Addict may lose contact with family, relative, long time friends, etc.

(iv) **School** Academic performance may suffer.

(v) **Corrupt practices** In order to meet expenses, an addict may steal or resort to corrupt practices.

(vi) **Financial** Spending money to support one's habit takes away money from other important needs. It could create financial crisis and poverty.

(vii) **Health** Using drugs may make a person more likely to participate in other unsafe behaviours. These include sharing needles or having unprotected sex. These can increase the chances of HIV or hepatitis infection. Overdose of drugs may cause impaired memory, lethargy, passivity, acute anxiety, depression, profuse sweating, etc.

Some drug addicts use mixtures of drugs to have an immediate effect. Such combinations worsen the health. Some of these combinations and their effects are given in the table below

Table 17.1 Combinations of drugs and their effects

Combinations of drugs	Effects
Alcohol + Antihistamines	Marked drowsiness (normally little or no sedative effect).
Alcohol and other depressants, e.g. barbiturates	Dramatically increased depressant effect.
Alcohol + Aspirin	Increased risk of damage to gastric mucosa.
Alcohol + Marijuana or hashish	Decreased coordination, increased reaction time, impaired judgement.
Alcohol + Benzodiazepines	Rapid increase in sedative effect
Benzodiazapines + Barbiturates	Increased sedation.
Nicotine + Cocaine (speed ball)	Increased cardiovascular effects.
Amphetamine + Insulin	Decreased insulin effect.
Cocaine + Antidepressants	Hypertension

Alcohol addiction

Alcohol addiction or alcoholism is the dependency of a person on regular consumption of alcohol (ethyl alcohol). The person who suffers from alcoholism is called an **alcoholic.**

Reasons for alcohol addiction

There may be several reasons of drinking alcohol. Some of them are given below

- Friend's or social pressure
- Overcoming frustration due to loss or failure
- Desire to overcome the hardships of daily life
- Relief from pain
- Desire for excitement
- Liking of taste
- Desire to do more work
- Feeling of independence
- Family history

Effects of alcohol addiction

Various effects of alcohol addiction are as follows

(i) **Effects on liver** Alcohol is directly absorbed by the mucous membrane of alimentary canal. This absorbed alcohol changes into acetaldehyde (a toxic substance) by aldehyde dehydrogenase and alcohol dehydrogenase in the liver.

(a) **Alcoholic fatty liver** The liver becomes enlarged, yellow greasy and firm. Due to this, fat synthesis is increased in liver and causes **fatty liver syndrome**.

(b) **Alcoholic hepatitis** In this disease, the hepatocytes are degenerated. This stage acts as a precursor of cirrhosis.

(c) **Alcoholic cirrhosis** Continued alochol intake causes hepatocyte destruction and collagen fibre stimulation. Due to this, liver shrinks and acquires a nodular appearance. It becomes hard and this condition is called cirrhosis.

(d) **Cholestasis** In this condition, bile flow stops. It is accompanied by jaundice, intense pain in abdomen and enlargement of liver.

(ii) **Effects on nervous system** Will power, judgement power and self-control gets reduced. Similarly control on emotions and moral sense declines.

Cerebellum is affected which results in the loss of muscle coordination. As a result, affected person shows staggering gait.

Incoherent speech is observed due to damage to cerebrum. Inflammation of axons of neurons leads to neuritis.

Note *Wernicke's and Korsakoff's syndrome related to thiamine deficiency are caused by excessive alcohol intake.*

(iii) **Effects on stomach** High doses of alcohol cause ill effect on gastric glands of stomach.

These glands secrete gastric juices in excess which causes the inflammation of gastric mucosa. This condition is known as **gastritis**. It may also result into gastric carcinoma and peptic ulcer.

Heavy drinking lead to severe vomiting and it may cause **Mallory-Weiss syndrome.** In this disease, a longitudinal cut is produced in mucosa at gastrointestinal junction.

(iv) **Effects on heart and blood** Due to the deposition of alcoholic fat in the wall of blood vessels, the lumen of blood vessels becomes reduced. This increases the blood pressure hence, impacts the activity of heart. The size of RBCs increases, but the number of RBCs, WBCs and platelets gets reduced.

(v) **Effects on kidneys** Alcohol reduces the release of hormone ADH (Antidiuretic Hormone). Due to this, excess amount of water is released from the body (diuresis). So, alcoholism results in rapid dehydration.

(vi) **Effects on immunity** Alcoholism causes decrease in resistance to infection. The alcoholics, in most cases, are victims of malnutrition. They are also susceptible to diseases like pneumonia.

(vii) **Effect on blood sugar level** Alcoholism reduces the blood sugar level by inhibiting the formation of glycogen. Thus, the nutrient supply to other different tissues gets reduced.

(viii) **Effect on behaviour** Alcohol dulls the senses and acts as a depressant of almost all body functions. It inhibits the learned social behaviour.

Tobacco addiction

- Tobacco (tambaku) can be obtained from dried and cured leaves of young branches of two species of tobacco plant, i.e. *Nicotiana tobaccum* and *N. rustica.* Tobacco plant belongs to angiospermic family–Solanaceae.
- The use of tobacco started in America where Red Indians started to use it.
- It is consumed in many forms and through a number of methods. Some methods of tobacco usage are beedi (tobacco wrapped in tendu leaves), cigars, cigarettes, gutka, hookah, kreteks, pipe smoking, snuff, tobacco chewing, tobacco paste and tobacco water, etc.

Note *Cotinine is an alkaloid found in tobacco and it is a predominant metabolite of nicotine.*

Various toxic substances of tobacco and their effects are tabulated below

Table 17.2 Toxic substances of tobacco and their effects

Particulate constituents	Effects	Gaseous constituents	Effects
Nicotine	Ganglionic stimulant and depressant, cocarcinogenic, causes addiction	–	–
Tar	Carcinogenic, immobilisation of cilia in respiratory tract	Carbon monoxide (CO)	Impairs haemoglobin functioning
Polynuclear, aromatic hydrocarbons	Carcinogenic	Nitrosamines, hydrazine, vinyl chloride	Carcinogens
Phenol, cresol	Carcinogenic, irritants	HCN, acrolein, formaldehyde, nitrogen oxides, acetaldehyde	Ciliotoxins and irritants.
Benzopyrene, trace metals (e.g. polonium-210, nickel, arsenic)	Carcinogen	–	–
β-Naphthylamine	Carcinogenic	–	–
N-Nitrosononicotine	Carcinogenic	–	–

Effects of tobacco addiction

Various ill effects tobacco are as follows

- About 90% of victims of lung cancer are associated with smoking. Mouth cancer is caused due to chewing of tobacco.
- Immunity weakens due to regular use of tobacco.
- It might cause male infertility.
- Adrenaline release increases which also increases blood pressure and rate of heartbeat. It may lead to cardiovascular diseases.
- Nicotine alkaloid causes reduced foetal growth and development.
- Carbon monoxide present in tobacco smoke combines with haemoglobin present in blood and forms carboxyhaemoglobin. It greatly reduces the oxygen carrying capacity of blood.
- Premature wrinkling might occur.
- It increases the susceptibility of pulmonary tuberculosis.
- Smoking causes inflammation of lung alveoli. It decreases surface area for the gaseous exchange and leads to emphysema.
- Smoking causes irritation and inflammation of mucosa of throat and bronchi. It causes coughing and bronchitis.
- Smoking accelerates the secretion of gastric juices. It causes gastric and duodenal ulcers.

DE-ADDICTION

Treatment of addiction of any addictive substance is called **de-addiction.** It varies widely according to the type, amount, duration of the addiction, medical complications and the social needs of the individual.

The following four ways are usually used for curing addicts

- Addiction treatment is a methodical and slow process. For example, if an addict smoke fifteen cigarettes a day, during treatment, it reduces to three cigarettes by the end of the month. This is because his body would not be able to bear the strain of more cigarettes. This may also lead to serious complications.
- Addiction rehabilitation centre can provide a temporary relief to the addict problems. For example, **Alcohol Anonymous** (AA) is an international organisation that provides group support and counselling to alcoholics.
- Active interest of friends and family members in de-addiction process can help the addicts tremendously by means of counselling.
- There are many natural therapies available to cure the patient. These therapies are permanent. These therapies work well in the mindset of an addict. Once the patient's mindset is changed, he can take control of his life without any external assistance.
- Medically, addicts are prescribed clinical drugs to treat addiction. Disulfuram or tetraethylthiuram sulphate is used as an aversion drug for treating alcoholics.

Note *It is believed that when the drug is denied to an addict, the level of a chemical called **C-amp** in the brain shoots up. It results in withdrawal symptoms. But vitamin-C prevents the C-amp from rising and thus, it averts the withdrawal symptoms.*

TERATOGENS

- Some substances cause foetal abnormalities if consumed by a pregnant woman, e.g. drugs, alcohol, etc. Such substances are called teratogens and their ability is called **teratogenicity**.
- The teratogens can cross the placenta to a greater or lesser extent. The most well-known synthetic teratogen is **thalidomide**. It resulted in thousands of babies being born with **phocomelia** (seal-like limbs) in 1958-61.
- Drugs can affect the foetus at the following three stages
  - (i) **Fertilisation and implantation** It occurs from conception to 17 days of pregnancy. There are chances of failure of pregnancy.
  - (ii) **Organogenesis** It occurs from 18-55 days of gestation. It is the most vulnerable period of pregnancy and may cause organ deformity.
  - (iii) **Growth and development** It occurs from 56 days onwards. Developmental and functional abnormalities can occur at this stage.

Foetal Alcohol Syndrome (FAS) is an abnormal pattern of growth and development which occurs in children born to chronically alcoholic women. These children are under weight, under sized and have deformed facial appearance and suffer from mental retardation.

Table 17.3 Some important teratogenic drugs and abnormalities

Drugs	Abnormalities
Androgens	Virilisation limb, oesophageal and cardiac defects.
Stilbesterol	Vaginal carcinoma in teenage female offspring.
Anticancer drugs (Methotrexate)	Multiple defects.
Antithyroid drugs	Foetal goitre and hypothyroidism.
Tetracycline	Affects bone development.
LSD	Fragmented chromosome.
Morphine	Neonatal hypoxia.
Warfarin	Nose, eye and hand defects, growth retardation.
Corticosteriods	Discoloured and deformed teeth, retarded bone growth.

CHECK POINT 17.2

1. Narcotics are those drugs which
(a) increase the activity of central nervous system
(b) increase the blood circulation and the general metabolism of the body
(c) block the normal inhibitory activities of certain nerves
(d) depress the activities of CNS

2. In which of the following diseases, liver becomes enlarged, yellow, greasy and firm?
(a) Alcoholic fatty liver (b) Alcoholic hepatitis
(c) Alcoholic cirrhosis (d) Cholestasis

3. Sedative effect is increased in all these combinations, except
(a) Alcohol + Antihistamine
(b) Alcohol + Benzodiazepines
(c) Cocaine + Antidepressant
(d) Benzodiazepines + Barbiturates

4. All these diseases affect the liver of alcoholics except
(a) cholestasis
(b) Mallory-Weiss syndrome
(c) cirrhosis
(d) hepatitis

5. The drug used for treating alcoholism is
(a) 3-methoxy morphine
(b) thalidomide
(c) disulfurum
(d) Both (b) and (c)

6. Which among the following teratogenic drugs causes vaginal carcinoma in teenage females?
(a) Tetracycline
(b) Warfarine
(c) Stilbesterol
(d) LSD

EXAM POINTS

- Barbiturate is a sedative drug that induces calmness, relaxation and drowsiness. **[J&K CET 2014]**
- Heroin is synthesised by acetylation of morphine. **[NEET 2019]**
- Heroin is diacetyl morphine. **[KCET 2014]**
- Heroin is sedative which depresses body functions. **[MHT CET 2015]**
- Smack is obtained from the latex of poppy plant. **[NEET 2018]**
- Morphine is a sedative and it is obtained from *Papaver somniferum*. **[CBSE AIPMT 2012]**
- Morphine is useful analgesic in patients undergoing surgery **[Uttrakhand CET 2014]**
- Morphine is an alkaloid. **[BHU 2008]**
- *Erythroxylum* is used to obtain traditional anesthesia. **[JIPMER 2019]**
- Cocaine or Crack is obtained from *Erythroxylum coca*. **[NEET 2019]**
- Cocaine interferes with the transport of neurotransmitter dopamine. **[COMEDK 2013]**
- *Cannabis sativa* is the source of marijuana. **[J&K CET 2011]**
- *Atropa belladonna* is used to obtain hallucinogen atropine. **[AMU 2015]**
- Alcohol consumption leads to acetaldehyde accumulation and fat synthesis in liver. **[AMU 2013]**
- Korsakoff's syndrome is related to alcohol abuse. **[Chhattisgarh PMT 2015]**
- Alcohol affects cerebellum due to which alcoholic walks clumsily. **[MHT CET 2011]**
- Dipsomania is severe addiction to alcohol. **[J&K CET 2011]**
- Addiction to tobacco is caused due to nicotine in it. **[OJEE 2013]**

Chapter Exercises

(A) Topical Exercise

Adolescence and Drugs

1 During adolescence, the brain may lose many of the connections between neurons by a process called .... which lead to more efficient and focused information processing.

(a) myelination (b) synapses
(c) pruning (d) modularity

2 Some adolescents become so absorbed in their own unique thoughts and experiences that they are special and no one else has ever had these feelings and experiences. This condition is known as

(a) imaginary audience (b) interpersonal vanity
(c) personal fable (d) adolescent egocentrism

3 Consider the following statements.

I. Adolescence is a very vulnerable phase of mental and psychological developments of individual.
II. Adolescence is marked by accelerated physical growth, development of reproductive organs and changes in functioning of reproductive organs and changes in functioning of the neuroendocrine system.

Choose the correct option.

(a) Statement I is true, but II is false
(b) Statement I is false, but II is true
(c) Both statements I and II are true
(d) Both statements I and II are false

4 Psychotropic drugs are

(a) vision producing (b) mood altering
(c) cannabinoids (d) All of these

5 Which of the following statements is correct?

(a) Tranquilisers are antianxiety drugs
(b) Tranquilisers increase aggressiveness
(c) Tranquilisers are chemical compounds that do not affect thoughts and behaviour
(d) Tranquilisers are chemical compounds that can relieve pain and fever

6 All the listed drugs are tranquilisers except

(a) reserpine (b) alprazolam
(c) diazepam (d) midazolam

7 Consider the following compounds

I. lorazepam II. pentobarbitone
III. diazepam IV. thiopentone

Which of the following are barbiturates?

(a) Only I (b) II and III (c) II and IV (d) I, II and III

8 Effect of the combination of benzodiazepines and barbiturates is

(a) hypertension
(b) drowsiness
(c) impaired judgement
(d) increased sedation

9 .... is an effective painkiller and a natural opiate.

(a) Amphetamine (b) Morphine
(c) Cocaine (d) Benzodiazepines

10 Which of the following drug gets partly converted to morphine in the body?

(a) Mescaline (b) Benzedrine
(c) Psilocybin (d) Codeine

11 Identify the wrong statement.

(a) Opiate narcotic drugs are analgesics
(b) Excessive alcohol intake causes fatty liver
(c) Dipsomania refers to craving for alcohol due to severe addiction
(d) Heroin is commonly called coke or crack

12 Which of the following is incorrect with respect to drug heroin?

(a) It is commonly called smack
(b) It is chemically dimethylmorphine
(c) It is a white, odourless, bitter crystalline compound
(d) It is a depressant and slows down body functions

13 Consider the following statements.

I. Heroin is obtained by the acetylation of morphine which is extracted from the latex of *Papaver somniferum.*
II. Pethidine is synthetic opiate.

Choose the correct option.

(a) Statement I is true, but II is false
(b) Statement I is false, but II is true
(c) Both statements I and II are true
(d) Both statements I and II are false

14 Smack is a drug obtained from **[NCERT Exemplar]**

(a) latex of *Papaver somniferum*
(b) leaves of *Cannabis sativa*
(c) flowers of *Datura pinata*
(d) fruits of *Erythroxylon coca*

15 Choose the opiates from the following set of drugs.

(a) Hashish, morphine and heroin
(b) Hashish, codeine, pethidine, morphine and methadone
(c) Codeine, pethidine, methadone, morphine and heroin
(d) Codeine, pethidine, methadone and cocaine

16 Which of the following is an incorrect statement with respect to opioids?
(a) Opioids bind to specific receptors presents in our central nervous system
(b) They are obtained from *Papaver somniferum*
(c) Methadone is a poisonous drug
(d) Codeine is chemically methylmorphine and used to suppress cough

17 Identify the wrong statement.
(a) Cocaine is obtained from coca plant *Erythroxylum coca*
(b) Cocaine is a potent depressant for CNS
(c) Excessive dosage of cocaine causes hallucinations
(d) It interferes with transport of neurotransmitter dopamine

18 Which one of the following is incorrect matching pair of a drug and its category?
(a) Amphetamines – Depressant
(b) Lysergic acid diethylamide – Psychodelic
(c) Heroin – Psychotropic drug
(d) Benzodiazepines – Muscle relaxant

19 The effects of opiates are
(a) numbing of pain causing drowsiness, lethargy, etc
(b) reduction in anxiety and tension
(c) lowering of blood pressure and breathing rate
(d) All of the above

20 Marijuana is extracted from
(a) dried flowers of hemp plant (b) ergot fungus
(c) roots of hemp plant (d) cocoa plant

21 Identify the psychedelic drug amongst the following.
(a) Lysergic Acid Diethylamide (b) Barbiturate
(c) Cocaine
(d) Monoamine oxidase

22 Which of the following drugs are obtained from the same source?
(a) Morphine and Charas (b) Charas and Marijuana
(c) Charas and Cocaine (d) Morphine and Marijuana

23 All of the following are correct match between the drug and its source, except.
(a) Lysergic acid diethylamide – *Claviceps purpurea*
(b) Coke – *Erythroxylum coca*
(c) Mescaline – *Lophophora williamsii*
(d) Marijuana – *Psilocybe mexicana*

24 Which of the following statements given below is/are correct?
I. Large number of people take LSD and other drugs like barbiturates and amphetamines to cope with mental illness.
II. Several plants, fruits and seeds having hallucinogenic properties have been used in folk-medicine.
(a) Statement I is true, but II is false
(b) Statement I is false, but II is true
(c) Both statements I and II are true
(d) Both statements I and II are false

25 Identify the leaf whose diagram is given below.

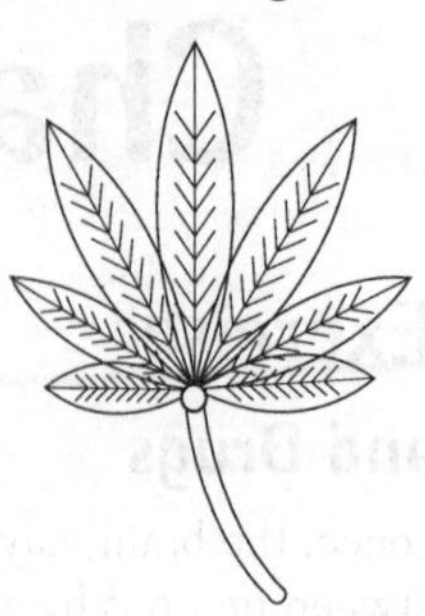

(a) *Papaver somniferum* (b) *Atropa belladonna*
(c) *Cannabis sativa* (d) *Datura*

26 Psilocybin, mescaline and LSD are categorised under
(a) hallucinogenic drug (b) opiate drug
(c) stimulants (d) All of these

27 Match the following columns.

Column I		Column II	
A.	Hashish	1.	Dried unfertilised female inflorescence
B.	Ganja	2.	Dried leaves and flowering shoots
C.	Marijuana	3.	Resinous exudate from the flowering tops of female plant
D.	Bhang	4.	Dried flowers and top leaves of female *Cannabis* plant

Codes

	A	B	C	D		A	B	C	D
(a)	1	2	4	3	(b)	2	1	4	3
(c)	3	1	4	2	(d)	4	3	2	1

28 Psilocybin is obtained from
(a) dried tops of plant (b) dried leaves of plant
(c) dried seeds of plant (d) fruiting bodies of plant

29 The given diagram shows flowering branch of

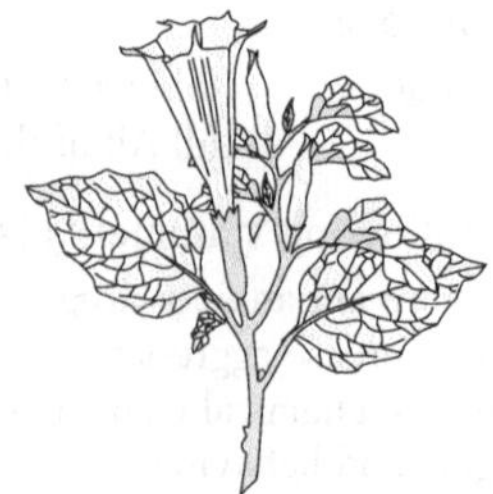

(a) *Datura* (b) *Cannabis sativa*
(c) Poppy plant (d) *Atropa belladonna*

30 Mark the wrong statement.
(a) Marijuana is obtained from hemp plant
(b) Psilocybin is a hallucinogen obtained from *Claviceps purpurea*
(c) Cocaine has a potent stimulating action on CNS, producing sense of euphoria and increased energy
(d) These days cannabinoids are used by some sports persons

31 Identify the given structure.

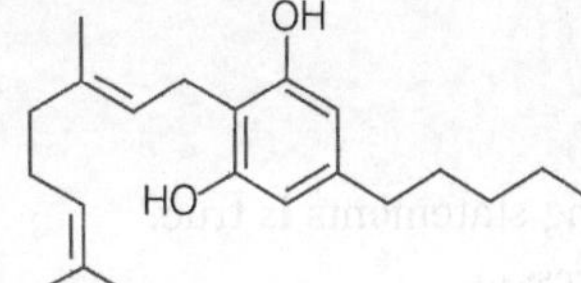

(a) Morphine (b) Cannabinoid molecule
(c) Aspirin (d) Cholesterol

32 Cannabinoids are obtained from
(a) inflorescence of the plant *Cannabis sativa*
(b) fruits of the plant *Papaver somniferum*
(c) latex of the plant *Cannabis sativa*
(d) plant *Papaver somniferum* inflorescence

33 Choose the odd one out.
(a) Mescaline (b) Psilocybin
(c) LSD (d) Phencyclidine piperidine

Addiction, De-addiction and Teratogens

34 Warning signs of drug and alcohol abuse include
I. drop in academic performance.
II. excellent performance in school/college.
III. lack of interest in personal hygiene.
IV. isolation, depression, fatigue, aggressive and rebellious behaviour.
Which of the statements given above are correct?
(a) I, II and III (b) I, III and IV
(c) II, III and IV (d) I, II, III and IV

35 Impaired memory, lethargy, passivity, acute anxiety, depression and profuse sweating are symptoms associated with
(a) alcoholism (b) drug addiction
(c) mental illness (d) All of these

36 Heavy drinking leads to severe vomiting and causes
(a) Wernicke's syndrome
(b) Mallory-Weiss syndrome
(c) Korsakoff's syndrome
(d) Foetal alcohol syndrome

37 Speed ball is a mixture of
(a) Nicotine + Cocaine
(b) Cocaine + Heroin
(c) Heroin + Hashish
(d) Hashish + Afeem

38 Consider the following statements.
I. Alcohol normally consumed is ethyl alcohol.
II. About 90% of the absorbed alcohol is eliminated by body through urine.
Choose the correct option.
(a) Statement I is true, but II is false
(b) Statement I is false, but II is true
(c) Both statements I and II are true
(d) Both statements I and II are false

39 The body organs markedly affected by alcohol are ...*A*... and ...*B*....

	A	*B*
(a)	respiratory	circulatory
(b)	skeletal	nervous
(c)	nervous	digestive
(d)	reproductive	circulatory

40 In chronic alcoholism, the liver is damaged due to
(a) liver destruction (b) degradation of metabolites
(c) more urea formation (d) deposition of fats

41 Anaemia in alcoholism may be caused due to the deficiency of
(a) vitamin-A (b) vitamin-B_{12}
(c) folic acid and vitamin-B_{12} (d) vitamin-C

42 Consider the following statements with respect to effects of alcoholism in an individual.
I. Decreases the release of antidiuretic hormone.
II. Increased number of WBCs and platelets.
Choose the correct option.
(a) Statement I is true, but II is false
(b) Statement I is false, but II is true
(c) Both statements I and II are true
(d) Both statements I and II are false

43 Alcohol addiction is harmful because it causes
(a) deposition of protein in liver
(b) deposition of fat in liver
(c) rise in blood sugar level
(d) cancer growth

44 Addiction to smoking is harmful because it produces polycyclic hydrocarbons which causes
(a) retardation in foetal growth
(b) reduction in oxygen transport
(c) increase in blood sugar level
(d) cancer

45 Which among the following particulate constituents of tobacco causes immobilisation of cilia in respiratory tract?
(a) Tar (b) Nicotine (c) Phenol (d) Cresol

46 Which of the following is an incorrect statement?
(a) Tobacco contains number of chemical substances including nicotine, an alkaloid
(b) Nicotine stimulates adrenal gland to release adrenaline and nor-adrenaline, which increase blood pressure and heart rate
(c) Tobacco chewing is associated with increase risk of cancer of the oral cavity
(d) Smoking reduces carbon monoxide content in blood and increases the concentration of haem-bound oxygen

47 Drugs that cause malformation in embryo during pregnancy are called
(a) tranquilisers (b) teratogens
(c) alcoholic beverages (d) nicotine

(B) Cumulative Exercise

(Assorted Questions of the Chapter for Advanced Level Practice)

1 Which one of the following statements is false?
(a) Psychoactive drugs have the ability to alter the activity of the nervous system
(b) Adolescence is marked by accelerated physical growth, development of reproductive organs and changes in functioning of the neuroendocrine system
(c) Hallucinogen can alter a person's thoughts, feelings and perceptions
(d) Mescaline is a stimulant

2 Identify the molecule (*A*) shown below and select the right option regarding it.

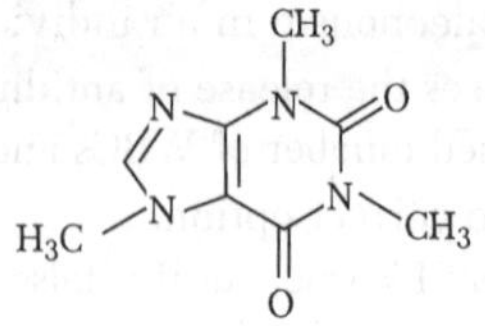

A

	Molecules	Sources	Uses
(a)	LSD	Ergot fungus of wheat	Powerful anaesthetic
(b)	Caffeine	Leaves of tea plant	CNS stimulant
(c)	Cocaine	Spineless cactus	Mild analgesic
(d)	Morphine	Hemp plant	Strong analgesic

3 Side effects of anabolic steroids in females include
I. masculinisation.
II. aggressiveness.
III. mood swings, depression.
IV. abnormal menstrual cycle.
V. excessive facial and body hair.
Choose the correct option.
(a) I, II and III (b) I, II, III and IV
(c) II, III, IV and V (d) I, II, III, IV and V

4 Nicotine intake stimulates the ....*A*... to release ...*B*.... and ....*C*.... into blood circulation. This leads to increase in ...*D*... and an increase ....*E* .... . Identify *A* to *E*.
(a) *A*-adrenal gland, *B*-adrenaline, *C*-nor-adrenaline, *D*-blood pressure, *E*-heart rate
(b) *A*-thyroid gland, *B*-thyroxine, *C*-parathyroxine, *D*-blood pressure, *E*-heart rate
(c) *A*-adrenal gland, *B*-thyroxine, *C*-nor-adrenaline, *D*-blood pressure, *E*-heart rate
(d) *A*-gonads *B*-adrenaline, *C*-nor-adrenaline, *D*-blood pressure, *E*-heart rate

5 Which of the following statements is true?
(a) Cocaine is CNS depressant
(b) Barbiturates cause memory impairment and slurred speech
(c) No tobacco day is observed on 1st December
(d) None of the above

6 Tobacco inhalation causes
(a) stimulation of nerve induction and cough depressant
(b) heart diseases and low blood pressure
(c) inhibits the oxygen carrying capacity and destroy haemoglobin structure
(d) heart diseases, decrease in O_2 carrying capacity, lung cancer, chronic bronchitis, etc

7 Find out the true (T)/false (F) statements and choose the correct option.
I. Addiction is a psychological attachment to certain effects such as euphoria and a temporary feeling of well-being associated with drugs and alcohol.
II. Hepatitis-B infection does not spread by infected needles and syringes among drug abusers but AIDS can.
III. The chronic use of alcohol causes cirrhosis.
IV. Tobacco chewing is associated with the increased risk of oral cancer.

	I	II	III	IV
(a)	T	T	T	T
(b)	T	F	T	T
(c)	F	F	T	F
(d)	T	T	T	F

8 Which one of the following is correct statement regarding the particular psychotropic drug specified?
(a) Barbiturates cause relaxation and temporary euphoria
(b) Hashish causes after thought perceptions and hallucinations
(c) Opium stimulates nervous system and causes hallucinations
(d) Morphine leads to delusions and disturbed emotions

9 Choose the correct statement from the following.
(a) Cocaine is given to patients after surgery as it stimulates recovery
(b) Barbiturates when given to criminals make them tell the truth
(c) Morphine is often given to persons who have undergone surgery as a painkiller
(d) Chewing tobacco lowers blood pressure and heart rate

10 Read the following statements about a drug and identify the drug.

I. These are known for their effects on cardiovascular system of the body.
II. These interact with the receptors present principally in brain.
III. Generally taken by inhalation and oral ingestion.
IV. These are obtained from a variety of hemp plant.

(a) *Papaver somniferum* (b) *Erythroxylon coca*
(c) *Atropa belladonna* (d) *Cannabis sativa*

11 Read the following statements.

I. Psychoactive drugs have the ability to alter the activity of the nervous system.
II. *Theobroma* is a form of caffeine obtained from the seeds of cocoa plant.
III. When the drugs are taken for a purpose other than medicinal use or in amounts/frequency that impairs one's physical, physiological or psychological functions, it is called drug abuse.
IV. Smoking increases carbon monoxide content in blood and reduces the concentration of oxygen.

Choose the option containing correct statements.

(a) I and II (b) III and IV
(c) I, II and IV (d) I, II, III and IV

12 Withdrawal symptoms of drug addiction are

(a) showed during epilepsy
(b) unpleasant symptoms showed due to non-availability of addicted drugs
(c) unpleasant symptoms showed due to alcoholism
(d) unpleasant symptoms showed due to narcotic drugs

13 Match the following columns.

	Column I		Column II
A.	LSD and cannabinoids	1.	Synthetic stimulant
B.	Amphetamines	2.	Hallucinogen
C.	Barbiturates and benzodiazepines	3.	Interferes with transport of dopamine
D.	Cocaine	4.	Sedative

Codes

	A	B	C	D		A	B	C	D
(a)	1	3	2	4	(b)	1	2	3	4
(c)	2	1	4	3	(d)	3	2	4	1

14 Observe the molecules *A* and *B* given below and select the right option giving their use and source.

A *B*

	Molecules	Uses	Taken by
(a)	*A*-Morphine	Sedative and pain killer	Snorting and injection
(b)	*B*-Morphine	Product marijuana	Oral ingestion
(c)	*A*-Cannabinoid	Produces hallucinations	Inhalation
(d)	*B*-Cannabinoid	Accelerates the transport of dopamine	Injection

15 Fill up the blanks.

I. The period between ....*A*....years of age may be thought of as adolescence period.
II. Adolescence is a bridge linking ....*B* .... and ....*C*... .
III. The chronic use of drug and alcohol damages ...*D*... and ...*E*... .
IV. Alcoholism during ....*F*.... adversely affects the foetus.

(a) *A*-12-18, *B*-childhood, *C*-adulthood, *D*-nervous system, *E*-liver, *F*-pregnancy
(b) *A*-10-15, *B*-adulthood, *C*-childhood, *D*-heart, *E*-stomach, *F*-adulthood
(c) *A*-15-20, *B*-adulthood, *C*-childhood, *D*-liver, *E*-kidney, *F*-pregnancy
(d) *A*-20-28, *B*-adulthood, *C*-childhood, *D*-liver, *E*-nervous system, *F*-pregnancy

16 Reasons for alcohol abuse in adolescents are

I. social pressure.
II. curiosity and need for adventure, excitement and experiment.
III. to escape from stress, depression and frustration.
IV. to overcome hardships of daily life.

Which of the statements given above are correct?

(a) I, II and III (b) I, III and IV
(c) II, III and IV (d) I, II, III and IV

17 Identify the plant *A*, *B* and *C* which yield the popular drugs.

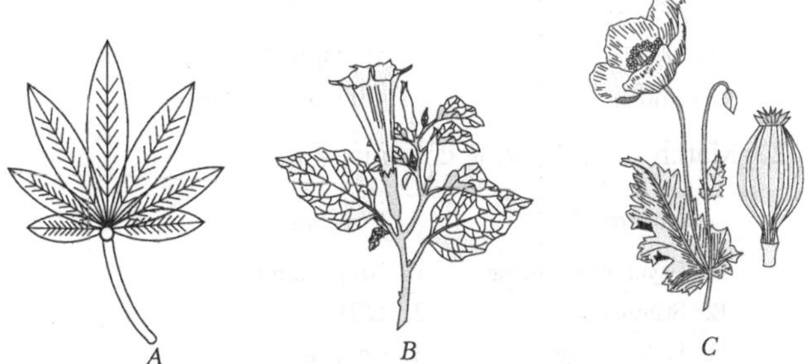

A	Drug	B	Drug	C	Drug
(a) *Cannabis*	Cannabinoid	*Datura*	Morphine	*Papaver*	Hallucinogen
(b) *Cannabis*	Morphine	*Datura*	Cannabinoid	*Papaver*	Hallucinogen
(c) *Cannabis*	Cocaine	*Datura*	Hallucinogen	*Papaver*	Morphine
(d) *Cannabis*	Cannabinoid	*Datura*	Hallucinogen	*Papaver*	Morphine

18 Match the following columns.

Column I	Column II
A. Alcohol	1. Emphysema
B. Nicotine	2. Fatty acid syndrome
C. Thalidomide	3. Phocomelia
D. Smoking	4. Ganglionic stimulant

Codes

	A	B	C	D		A	B	C	D
(a)	4	3	1	2	(b)	1	3	2	4
(c)	2	4	3	1	(d)	2	1	3	4

19 Consider the following statements.

I. Dependence is the tendency of the body to manifest a characteristic and unpleasant withdrawal syndrome if regular dose of drugs/alcohol is abruptly discontinued.
II. Excessive doses of drugs may lead to coma and death due to respiratory failure, heart failure or cerebral haemorrhage.
III. Education about harmful effects of drugs and alcohol, counselling professional and medical help would relive the individuals from the drug and alcohol abuse.
IV. Sports persons often misuse drugs to enhance their performance.

Choose the correct option.

(a) I and II (b) II and IV
(c) I, II and III (d) I, II, III and IV

20 Consider the following statements.

I. LSD is a crystalline alkaloid obtained from ergot of fungus, *Claviceps purpurea.*
II. LSD causes hallucination and foetal abnormalities.
III. LSD is a low potency hallucinogen.
IV. LSD is widely used in veterinary medicine to briefly immobilise large animals.

Choose the option with containing correct statement(s).

(a) Only I (b) Only II
(c) I and II (d) None of these

21 Match the following columns.

Column I	Column II
A. Psychotropic drug	1. Amphetamines
B. Stimulants	2. LSD
C. Hallucinogens	3. Codeine
D. Opiates	4. Temazepam
E. Sedatives	5. Barbiturate

Codes

	A	B	C	D	E
(a)	1	3	5	2	4
(b)	4	1	2	3	5
(c)	2	3	1	4	5
(d)	5	4	3	1	2

22 Find out the true (T) or false (F) statements.

I. With the repeated use of drugs/alcohol, the tolerance level of the receptors in our body increase. Thus, these receptors respond to higher doses of drugs/alcohol only.
II. Alcohol gets converted into acetaldehyde by aldehyde dehydrogenase in the liver.
III. Amphetamines and marijuana are commonly abused drugs among human population.
IV. The adverse effects of drugs and alcohol abuse are manifested in the form of reckless behaviour, vandalism and violence.

Choose the correct option.

	I	II	III	IV
(a)	T	T	T	F
(b)	T	T	T	T
(c)	F	T	T	T
(d)	T	T	F	T

Assertion and Reason

Direction (Q.Nos. 23-35) *In each of the following questions, a statement of Assertion* (A), *is given followed by the corresponding statement of Reason* (R). *Of the statements, mark the correct answer as*

(a) Both A and R are true and R is the correct explanation of A
(b) Both A and R are true, but R is not the correct explanation of A
(c) A is true, but R is false
(d) A is false, but R is true
(e) Both A and R are false

23 **Assertion** (A) Pregnant ladies should not take alcohol.

Reason (R) Alcohol intake may result in foetal alcohol syndrome.

24 **Assertion** (A) Alcohol along with other stimulants or narcotic drugs is extremely harmful.

Reason (R) It damages only digestive system.

25 **Assertion** (A) Alcoholics may show deficiency symptoms of Wernicke's and Korsakoff's syndromes.

Reason (R) Alcohol acts as depressant.

26 **Assertion** (A) Sometimes non-smokers are prone to lung cancer.

Reason (R) Non-smokers are also called passive smokers.

27 **Assertion** (A) Charas is a psychoactive drug.

Reason (R) It contains THC of 25-60%.

28 **Assertion** (A) LSD is the most powerful psychedelic.

Reason (R) Phychedelic drugs cause hallucination.

29 **Assertion** (A) Brown sugar is morphine derivative.
Reason (R) Morphine is the principal opium alkaloid.

30 **Assertion** (A) Hypnotic drugs induce sleep.
Reason (R) Central nervous system is sensitive to hypnotic drugs.

31 **Assertion** (A) LSD and charas are hallucinogenic drugs.
Reason (R) These drugs alter thought, feelings and perceptions.

32 **Assertion** (A) Caffeine is a stimulant.
Reason (R) Barbiturate is a depressant.

33 **Assertion** (A) Alcohol is not digested in human body.
Reason (R) Alimentary canal absorbs alcohol directly.

34 **Assertion** (A) Fatty liver syndrome occurs by alcoholism.
Reason (R) Alcoholics have a rate of carcinoma ten times higher than that expected in the general population.

35 **Assertion** (A) Nicotine is an alkaloid found in tobacco.
Reason (R) It is used in the preparation of niacin vitamin.

(C) Medical Entrances' Gallery

(Collection of questions Asked in NEET & Various Medical Entrance Exams)

1 Traditional anesthesia is obtained from **[JIPMER 2019]**
(a) *Datura* (b) Poppy
(c) *Cannabis* (d) *Erythroxylum*

2 Drug called heroin is synthesised by **[NEET 2019]**
(a) acetylation of morphine
(b) glycosylation of morphine
(c) nitration of morphine
(d) methylation of morphine

3 Coca alkaloid or cocaine is obtained from **[NEET 2019]**
(a) *Papaver somniferum* (b) *Atropa belladonna*
(c) *Erythroxylum coca* (d) *Datura*

4 Which part of poppy plant is used to obtain the drug smack? **[NEET 2018]**
(a) Roots (b) Latex
(c) Flowers (d) Leaves

5 Korsakoff's syndrome is related to **[Chhattisgarh PMT 2015]**
(a) alcohol abuse (b) Drug abuse
(c) smoking abuse (d) None of these

6 Match the following columns and choose the correct option form the codes given below.

Column I	Column II
A. Phobia	1. Maladaptive habit
B. Neurosis	2. Undue concern about health
C. Hypochondria	3. Lack of sleep
D. Insomnia	4. Intense fear

Codes **[Chhattisgarh PMT 2015]**

	A	B	C	D
(a)	2	1	4	3
(b)	2	1	3	4
(c)	3	1	4	2
(d)	4	1	2	3

7 Smack and Crack are produced from **[KCET 2015]**
(a) *Papaver somniferum* and *Erythroxylum coca*
(b) *Erthroxylum coca* and *Atropa belladonna*
(c) *Cannabis sativa* and *Atropa belladonna*
(d) *Cannabis sativa* and *Papaver somniferum*

8 Which of the following options are correct?

I. Heroin	—	Stimulant
II. Marijuana	—	Cardiovascular diseases
III. Cocaine	—	Hallucination
IV. Morphine	—	Sedative

[MHT CET 2015]
(a) I, II and III (b) I, III and IV
(c) II, III and IV (d) I, II and IV

9 Which drug pair is incorrect? **[AMU 2015]**
(a) *Papaver somniferum* — Morphine
(b) *Cannabis sativa* — Marijuana
(c) *Erythroxylum coca* — Cocaine
(d) *Atropa belladona* — Hashish

10 Name the drug which is useful analgesic in patients undergoing surgery **[Uttarakhand CET 2014]**
(a) Chloropromazine (b) Barbiturate
(c) Amphetamine (d) Morphine

11 Heroin is **[KCET 2014]**
(a) a cannabinoid
(b) diacetyl morphine
(c) commonly called 'coke' or 'crack'
(d) used to treat mental illnesses like depression and insomnia

12 Excessive consumption of alcohol results in **[COMEDK 2014]**
(a) fatty liver syndrome
(b) fixity of facial expression
(c) twitching of face
(d) atrophy of cerebral cortex

13 Which is the particular type of drug that is obtained from the plant? **[CBSE AIPMT 2014]**

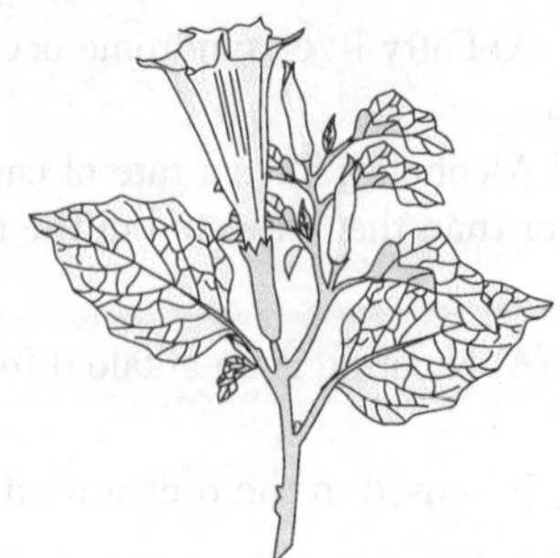

(a) Depressant (b) Stimulant
(c) Painkiller (d) Hallucinogen

14 Which is a sedative drug that gives feeling of calmness, relaxation and drowsiness? **[J&K CET 2014]**
(a) Heroin (b) Cocaine
(c) Barbiturate (d) Opium

15 Consumption of alcohol leads to **[AMU 2013]**
(a) acetaldehyde accumulation in liver
(b) fat synthesis in liver
(c) lowering of blood glucose level
(d) All of the above

16 Addiction to tobacco is caused by **[Odisha JEE 2013]**
(a) cocaine
(b) nicotine
(c) caffeine
(d) histamine

17 The drug that interferes with transport of neurotransmitter dopamine is **[COMEDK 2013]**
(a) cocaine (b) marijuana
(c) charas (d) heroin
(e) benzodiazepines

18 Identify the molecules '*A*' and '*B*' shown below and select the right option regarding them.

A

B **[CBSE AIPMT 2012]**

	Molecules	**Sources**	**Uses**
(a) *A*	Cocaine	*Erythroxylum coca*	Accelerates the transport of dopamine
(b) *B*	Heroin	*Cannabis sativa*	Depressant and slow down body functions
(c) *B*	Cannabinoid	*Atropa belladonna*	Produces hallucination
(d) *A*	Morphine	*Papaver somniferum*	Sedative and painkiller

19 After drinking alcohol, a person walks clumsily because, the alcohol affects his **[MHT CET 2011]**
(a) cerebellum (b) cerebrum
(c) medulla oblongata (d) spinal cord

20 *Cannabis sativa* is the source of **[J&K CET 2011]**
(a) opium (b) LSD
(c) marijuana (d) cocaine

21 Alcoholism may lead to **[J&K CET 2011]**
(a) skin cancer (b) liver cirrhosis
(c) viral disease (d) eye infections

22 Dipsomania is **[J&K CET 2011]**
(a) a type of depression
(b) insanity due to psychosis
(c) a condition involving severe addiction to alcohol
(d) tendency to take much water

23 Everytime when the dosage of a drug has to be increased to achieve the same kick that initially occurred in response to a smallest dose, the condition is known as **[KCET 2010]**
(a) withdrawal symptoms (b) addiction
(c) rebound effect (d) tolerance

24 Morphine obtained from opium is a/an **[BHU 2008]**
(a) latex (b) pome
(c) alkaloid (d) tannin

25 The stimulant present in tea, cocoa and coffee is **[AMU 2008]**
(a) cocaine (b) tannin
(c) astringent (d) caffeine

26 **Assertion** (A) Dope test is used to estimate the level of blood alcohol by analysing the breath of person drinking alcohol.

Reason (R) A drunken person usually feels tense and less talkative. **[AIIMS 2008]**
(a) Both A and R are true and R is the correct explanation of A
(b) Both A and R are true, but R is not the correct explanation of A
(c) A is true, but R is false
(d) Both A and R are false

ANSWERS

Check Point 17.1

1. (b)	2. (a)	3. (b)	4. (a)	5. (d)	6. (c)

Check Point 17.2

1. (d)	2. (a)	3. (c)	4. (b)	5. (c)	6. (c)

(A) Topical Exercise

1. (c)	2. (c)	3. (c)	4. (b)	5. (a)	6. (b)	7. (c)	8. (d)	9. (b)	10. (d)
11. (d)	12. (b)	13. (c)	14. (a)	15. (c)	16. (c)	17. (b)	18. (a)	19. (d)	20. (a)
21. (a)	22. (b)	23. (d)	24. (c)	25. (c)	26. (a)	27. (c)	28. (d)	29. (a)	30. (b)
31. (b)	32. (a)	33. (d)	34. (b)	35. (d)	36. (b)	37. (a)	38. (c)	39. (c)	40. (d)
41. (c)	42. (a)	43. (b)	44. (d)	45. (a)	46. (d)	47. (b)			

(B) Cumulative Exercise

1. (d)	2. (b)	3. (d)	4. (a)	5. (b)	6. (d)	7. (b)	8. (b)	9. (c)	10. (d)
11. (d)	12. (b)	13. (c)	14. (a)	15. (a)	16. (d)	17. (d)	18. (c)	19. (d)	20. (c)
21. (b)	22. (b)	23. (a)	24. (c)	25. (b)	26. (b)	27. (a)	28. (a)	29. (b)	30. (a)
31. (a)	32. (b)	33. (a)	34. (b)	35. (b)					

(C) Medical Entrances' Gallery

1. (d)	2. (a)	3. (c)	4. (b)	5. (a)	6. (d)	7. (a)	8. (c)	9. (d)	10. (d)
11. (b)	12. (a)	13. (d)	14. (c)	15. (d)	16. (b)	17. (a)	18. (d)	19. (a)	20. (c)
21. (b)	22. (c)	23. (d)	24. (c)	25. (d)	26. (d)				

Explanations

(A) Topical Exercise

5 (*a*) Statement in option (a) is correct while other three are incorrect. Incorrect statements can be corrected as

Tranquilisers decrease aggressiveness, normalise thoughts and behaviour and relive anxiety, not pain or fever.

11 (*d*) Statement in option (d) is wrong and can be corrected as

Heroin is commonly called smack. Crack is the common name of cocaine.

Rest statements are correct.

12 (*b*) Statement in option (b) is incorrect and can be corrected as

Heroin is diacetylmorphine.

Rest statements are correct.

16 (*c*) Statement in option (c) is incorrect and can be corrected as

Methadone is pharmacologically similar to morphine and it is used as an analgesic.

Rest statements are correct.

17 (*b*) Statement in option (b) is incorrect and can be corrected as

Cocaine is a potent stimulant for CNS.

Rest statements are correct.

18 (*a*) Option (a) represents incorrectly matched pair and can be corrected as

Amphetamine is a synthetic stimulant.

All options are correct match between the drug and its source except option (d).

Rest options are correct matching pair of a drug and its category.

23 (*d*) All options are correct match between the drug and its source except option (d).

Incorrect match can be corrected as

Marijuana is obtained from the dried *Cannabis sativa.*

30 (*b*) Statement in option (b) is wrong and can be corrected as

Psilocybin is a hallucinogen obtained from *Psilocybe mexicana.*

42 (*a*) Statement I is true, but II is false. Incorrect statement can be corrected as

The number of WBCs and platelets decreases in an alcoholic individual.

46 (*d*) Statement in option (d) is incorrect and can be corrected as

Smoking increases carbon monoxide content in blood due to which concentration of O_2 decreases in body.

(B) Cumulative Exercise

1 (*d*) Statement in option (d) is false and can be corrected as Mescaline is a hallucinogen and not a stimulant.

3 (*d*) The side effects of the use of anabolic steroids in females include masculinisation (features like males), increases aggressiveness, mood swings, depression, abnormal menstrual cycle, excessive facial and body hair, etc. In males, the side effects include acne, increased aggressiveness, mood swings, decreased sperm production, etc. These effects may be permanent with prolonged use.

Thus, option (d) is correct.

5 (*b*) Statement in option (b) is true. Rest others are false and can be corrected as

- Cocaine is CNS stimulant.
- No tobacco day is observed on 31st May.

8 (*b*) Statement in option (b) is correct while others are incorrect. Incorrect statements can be corrected as

- Opium is depressant of nervous system and has sedative, analgesic and narcotic effects.
- Morphine is strong sedative and analgesic which act of central nervous system.
- Barbiturates are sedative hypnotics that have a calming effect and induce sleep.

9 (*c*) Statement in option (c) is correct.

Morphine is a strong sedative and analgesic (painkiller). It acts on CNS. It is useful for patients who have undergone surgery.

Other statements are incorrect and can be corrected as

- Cocaine is a natural stimulant. It stimulates nervous system and delays fatigue.
- Tobacco increases the release of adrenaline due to which blood pressure and heart rate in increased.
- Barbiturates are sedative-hypnotics which means they have sleep inducing effect.

20 (*c*) Statements I and II are correct whereas III and IV are incorrect. Incorrect statements can be corrected as

LSD is a powerful psychedelic drug. It is not used in veterinary medicines.

23 (*a*) Both A and R are true and R is the correct explanation of A.

Heavy drinking in pregnancy results in the rapid placental transfer of both ethanol and acetaldehyde which may have serious consequences during foetal development. The Foetal Alcohol Syndrome (FAS) includes facial changes, small teeth with faulty enamel, defects in atria and ventricles of heart, limitation in joint movement and mental retardation.

24 (*c*) A is true, but R is false because

Effect of alcohol is enhanced by taking some other substances, e.g. tobacco, hashish, etc. Exhaustion or hunger also make alcohol more dangerous. The nervous system and digestive system are most markedly affected.

25 (*b*) Both A and R are true, but R is not the correct explanation of A.

Alcohol acts as a depressant of nervous system and acts as sedative and reduces the efficiency of body organs by reducing blood supply. Deficiency of nutrients such as minerals, proteins and vitamins are found in alcoholics. Thiamine (B_1) deficiency causes Wernicke's and Korsakoff syndromes. Wernicke's syndrome is characterised by mental disturbance, paralysis of eye movements and ataxia or gait. Korsakoff's syndrome is characterised by confusion and severe impairment of memory.

26 (*b*) Both A and R are true, but R is not the correct explanation of A.

Indoor atmospheres and other confined spaces are often contaminated by tobacco smoke which is inhaled involuntarily by both smokers and non-smokers. It is called involunary smoke inhalation or passive smoking. It is now recognised as a cause of lung cancer in non-smokers.

27 (*a*) Both A and R are true and R is the correct explanation of A.

Charas is the dried resinous extract from the flowering tops and leaves of *Cannabis sativa*. In some countries like America, charas is called hashish. Liquid hashish is called hash oil, which may contain 25-60%, THC (Tetra hydrocannabinol).

28 (*a*) Both A and R are true and R is the correct explanation of A.

Psychedelic drugs changes ones mood, behaviour, thoughts, feeling and perceptions, without any true sensory stimulus. They cause hallucinations, a sense perception (sight, touch sound, smell or taste) that has no basis in external stimulation. LSD causes horrible dreams, emotional outbursts, hallucination, chronic psychosis and severe damage to the central nervous system. It also brings about chromosomal and foetal abnormalities. An LSD addict can be easily recognised from incoherence in writing and drawing.

29 (*b*) Both A and R are true, but R is not the correct explanation of A.

Morphine is a derivative of the opium. It is the principal opium alkaloid and a strong analgesic. Diacetylmorphine hydrochloride is brown sugar/smack and is more powerful analgesic than morphine.

30 (*a*) Both A and R are true and R is the correct explanation of A.

Hypnotic drug induces sleep. They are more or less general depressants of central nervous system. They are used as antianxiety drugs.

31 (*a*) Both A and R are true and R is the correct explanation of A.

Hallucinogens are the drugs, which can alter a person's thoughts, feelings and perceptions. The sensations may be pleasant or more usually unpleasant, e.g. LSD, mescaline, psilocybin, charas, hashish, marijuana (bhang), etc.

32 (*b*) Both A and R are true, but R is not the correct explanation of A.

Stimulant increases alertness and activity and may produce excitement, e.g., caffeine, cocaine, etc., whereas depressants depress brain activity and produce a feeling of calmness, e.g. barbiturates.

33 (*a*) Both A and R are true and R is the correct explanation of A.

Alcohol is absorbed from mucous membranes of mouth, oesophagus, small intestine and large intestine. As alcohol is absorbed directly by the alimentary canal, there is no need of digestion within the body.

34 (*b*) Both A and R are true, but R is not the correct explanation of A.

Fatty liver syndrome is a condition of permanent damage to the structure and functioning of liver cells. It is the result of alcoholism. Alcoholics have ten times higher rate of carcinoma than that expected in the general population.

35. (*b*) Both A and R are true, but R is not the correct explanation of A.

Tobacco contains an alkaloid nicotine which can be used as raw material for the preparation of a niacin vitamin or nicotinic acid or antipellagra vitamin.

(C) Medical Entrances' Gallery

1 (*d*) Before stronger anesthetics were available, *Erythroxylum* (cocaine) was used as an anesthetic and analgesic to relieve the pain of headache, rheumatism, wounds and sores, etc. It was also used in case of broken bones, childbirth and performing trepanning operations on the skull.

2 (*a*) Drug 'heroin' is synthesised by the acetylation of morphine. Chemically, heroin is diacetylmorphine and commonly it is called smack. It is an opium derivative which is used as medicine. Excessive use of heroin causes addiction.

3 (*c*) Coca alkaloid or cocaine is obtained from the coca plant *Erythroxylum coca* which is native to South America. It is a natural stimulant and interferes with the transport of the neurotransmitter dopamine.

4 (*b*) The latex of poppy plant (*Papaver somniferum*) is used to obtain 'smack'. It is a white, crystalline, odourless, bitter compound, which acts as a depressant and slows down the body functions.

5 (*a*) Korsakoff's syndrome is caused when there is deficiency of vitamin-B due to severe alcoholism, i.e. alcohol abuse.

8 (*c*) Matching pairs II, III and IV are correct, whereas statement I is incorrect. Incorrect pair can be corrected as

Heroin is an opiate which depresses the body functions.

9 (*d*) Option (d) is incorrect pair and can be corrected as

Hashish is a product of hemp plant, i.e. *Cannabis sativa*. *Atropa belladonna* is used to yield a drug called atropine.

13 (*d*) The given twig is of *Datura* plant. This plant yields hallucinogens.

18 (*d*) Morphine (*A*) is a natural opiate which is obtained from the unripe fruits of *Papaver somniferum*. It is sedative and painkiller.

Cannabinoids (*B*) are natural hallucinogens obtained from the leaves and flowers of *Cannabis sativa*.

19 (*a*) Alcoholism is dependency of a person on regular consumption of alcohol. In this, cerebellum is affected which results in the loss of muscle coordination. Therefore, affected person shows staggering gait and walks clumsily.

20 (*c*) The flower tops, leaves and the resin of the plant *Cannabis sativa* are used in various combinations to produce marijuana, hashish, charas and ganja. Generally taken by inhalation and oral ingestion, these are known for their effect on cardiovascular system of the body. A group of chemicals called cannabinoids interact with cannabinoid receptors present principally in the brain. Natural cannabinoids are obtained from the inflorescence of the plant *Cannabis sativa*.

21 (*b*) Alcoholism is a chronic often progressive disease in which a person craves for alcohol and drinks it despite of knowing about alcohol related problems. It involves a physical dependence on alcohol. It may lead to liver cirrhosis. Cirrhosis is build up of scar tissue that changes the structure of the liver and blocks the blood flow.

22 (*c*) Dipsomania is a term describing a medical condition involving severe addiction to alcohol. The term was coined by the German Physician CW Hufeland in 1819.

23 (*d*) Tolerance is a state in which an organism no longer responds to a drug. A higher dose is required to achieve the same effect.

24 (*c*) Morphine is the main opium alkaloid, which is a strong analgesic and also has sedative and calming effect.

25 (*d*) Tea, cocoa and coffee are obtained from dried leaves and seeds of different plants. All these contain caffeine.

26 (*d*) Both A and R are false and can be corrected as

Dope test is a blood test to know whether a person taking part in a competition used any drug (like anabolic steroids) to make their performance better. This test is not related with alcohol, also a drunken person feels confident and become talkative.

CHAPTER 18

Animal Husbandry

Animals have long been used by man for various purposes, e.g. transport, wars, agriculture, etc. These are also used for various products like milk, eggs, meat, wool, silk, honey, etc. As the population and living standard are increasing, demand for milk, egg and meat is also going up.

To meet these demands, man had started the management of domestic affair, i.e. **husbandry**. This term is mostly used in connection with **animal husbandry** or **livestock**.

Animal husbandry is the science of rearing, caring, feeding, breeding, improvement and utilisation of domesticated animals or livestock. It also deals with poultry farming, fisheries, sericulture, lac culture and apiculture. In this chapter, we will discuss all these topics in detail.

Inside

LIVESTOCK

- The term 'Livestock' is used for domesticated animals. These animals are kept by humans for commercial purposes, including agriculture, transport, dairy, industry, food, etc. The most common livestock include cattle, horse, pig, camel, sheep, goat, etc.
- According to a survey, about 70% of world livestock population is found in India and China. However, India's contribution to the world farm produce is only 25%. This reflects that the productivity per unit area is very low in India. It is mainly because the practices to domesticate animals have always remained conventional. Therefore, new and latest technologies need to be applied in order to obtain sufficient productivity and quality improvement in livestock.
- Different types of livestock are used for different purposes. On the basis of utility, livestock can be categorised into the following categories
  - (i) **Milk yielding animals** Cows, buffaloes and goats.
  - (ii) **Meat and egg yielding animals** Sheep, goats, pigs, ducks and fowls.
  - (iii) **Animals utilised as motive power** Buffaloes, horses, donkeys, bullocks, camels and elephants are used in transport and ploughing the fields.
  - (iv) **Wool giving animals** Sheep and goats.
  - (v) **Miscellaneous** Honeybees, silkworm, lac insect, fishes, etc.

Domesticated animals

Commonly used breeds of domesticated animals are as follows

Cattle

The family of domestic cattle is Bovidae. It includes two main groups

(i) ***Bos indicus*** It is also called **zebu** or humped cattle, found in India and Africa.

(ii) ***Bos taurus*** It is non-humped cattle, found in Europe and North America.

Cow (*Bos indicus*)

It is one of the most important milk yielding cow in our country. Its various uses are as follows

- Cows produce yellow coloured milk due to the presence of carotene.
- Their bullocks, i.e. castrated males are used in farm practices and drawing carts.
- Hide of cows is used for preparing leather articles.
- Their excreta is used as manure and to produce biogas.
- Their bones, horns and hoofs yield glue and gelatin.

The important Indian breeds of cow and their distribution are given in the following table

Table 18.1 Breeds of Indian cows

Breeds	Distributions
Milch breeds (Yield milk)	
Sahiwal	Punjab, Haryana and Uttar Pradesh
Deoni	Andhra Pradesh and Maharashtra
Gir	Gujarat, Rajasthan and Maharashtra
Red Sindhi	Andhra Pradesh
Vechur (smallest breed)	Kerala
Rathi	Rajasthan
Drought breeds (For doing labour in field)	
Nageri	Delhi, Haryana, Uttar Pradesh
Kangayam	Tamil Nadu and other parts of South India
Malvi	Rajasthan and Madhya Pradesh
Hallikar	Karnataka
General utility breeds (For both milching and labour)	
Ongole	Andhra Pradesh, Gujarat
Tharparkar	Gujarat, Rajasthan, Haryana
Haryana	Haryana, Punjab, Bihar and Madhya Pradesh
Kankrej	Gujarat, Rajasthan
Exotic breeds (Foreign breeds)	
Jersey	Island of Jersey
Holstein-Friesian (best milk yielding breed)	Holland
Ayrshire	Scotland
Brown Swiss	Switzerland

Note
- *There are about 75 breeds of zebu, split evenly between Africa and South Asia.*
- *Lactation in sterile cow is induced by stilbestrol.*
- *The gestation period in cows is 9 months.*

Cross breeds

Some of the cross breed cows are as follows

(i) **Karan Swiss** This breed was developed at National Dairy Research Institute, Karnal, by the breeding of Sahiwal cows with Brown Swiss bulls imported from USA.

(ii) **Sunandini** This breed originated in Kerala by crossing the local non-descript cattle with Jersey, Brown Swiss and Holstein-Friesian breeds.

(iii) **Karan Fries** This breed was developed at the National Dairy Research Institute, Karnal by the crossing between Tharparkar and Holstein-Friesian.

Buffalo (*Bubalus bubalis*)

It is mainly raised for milk production. Number of breeds of Indian buffalo are 26 which differ in their body colour, horns and shape of forehead. Various uses of buffalo are as follows

- The buffaloes are about three times better milk producer than cows.
- They live longer the cows.
- Their milk has high fat content, calcium and phosphorus.
- They are more resistant to diseases.
- Their bulls are used for agricultural practices and driving carts.

The important Indian breeds of buffaloes and their distributions are tabulated below

Table 18.2 Breeds of Indian buffaloes

Breeds	Distributions
Jaffrabadi	Gujarat
Mehsana	Gujarat
Nili Ravi	Punjab and Haryana
Murrah (most demanded)	Punjab, Haryana and Uttar Pradesh
Surti	Rajasthan and Gujarat
Bhadawari	Uttar Pradesh and Madhya Pradesh
Nagpuri or Ellichpur (Milch breed)	Central and South India

Note
- *Water buffalo is an Asian breed of buffalo that prefers living in water for most of the day.*
- *Buffalo milk is almost free from carotenoids due to its conversion into vitamin-A inside the liver cells.*
- *The gestation period in buffaloes is 10 months.*

Horse (*Equus caballus*)

- It is mainly used for transporting goods and recreation purposes such as polo, racing, etc.
- Horses are kept in well-ventilated places with straw or grass spread on the floors.
- These are fed on oats, barley, gram and hay.
- Better varieties are reared for racing and polo as they require fast running horses with more stamina.
- Breeding rate of horses is very low. The gestation period in horse is 11-12 months.
- The important breeds of Indian horses and their distributions are given below

Table 18.3 Breeds of Indian horses

Breeds	Distributions	Breeds	Distributions
Manipuri	North-Eastern mountains	Kathiawari	Rajasthan and Gujarat
Marwari	Rajasthan	Bhutia	Punjab and Bhutan
Zanskari	Ladakh	Spiti	Himachal Pradesh

Pigs (*Sus scrofa*)

Pigs (swine or hog) are the most economical meat yielding animal. They are mainly reared for pork, hide and fat. Their fat can be used in soap making and some other industries. Rearing of pigs is comparatively easy due to the following reasons

- These are quick growers among the domestic animals.
- They feed upon kitchen wastes, farm byproducts and human faeces.
- The life cycle of a pig from conception to birth, growth and then slaughter is upto 310 days.
- Pigs breed all around the year, regardless of the season.

Some important breeds of pigs and their distributions are as follows

Table 18.4 Breeds of pigs

Domesticated and indigenous pigs	Distributions
Ghori	Manipur, Assam, Meghalaya and Arunachal Pradesh
Desi	Uttar Pradesh, Bihar, Punjab and Madhya Pradesh
Exotic pigs	**Distributions**
Landrace	Switzerland and Denmark
Large white yorkshire	United Kingdom
Berkshire	United Kingdom

Sheep (*Ovis aries*)

- It is reared for wool and mutton. It is herbivore and feed upon farm waste, oil cake and other cattle feed.
- Some of the **exotic breeds** are Merino (most popular fine wool breed), Dorset Horn and Suffolk- Corriedale.

Important Indian sheep breeds are as follows

Table 18.5 Breeds of Indian sheep

Breeds	Distributions	Uses
Bhakarwal	Jammu and Kashmir	Under coat used for high quality woollen shawls
Lohi	Punjab, Rajasthan	Good quality wool, milk
Deccani	Karnataka	Mutton, no wool
Rampur-Bushair	Uttar Pradesh, Himachal Pradesh	Brown coloured wool
Marwari	Gujarat	Coarse wool
Nali	Haryana, Punjab, Rajasthan	Superior carpet wool
Patanwadi	Gujarat	Wool for army hosiery
Nellore	Maharashtra	Mutton, no wool

Goat (*Capra capra*)

- It is also called **poor man's cow** because it produces a little amount of milk.
- Goat milk contains a protein Lectoperoxide (LP), which is effective against a number of bacterial diseases.
- It is reared for meat (mutton), skin and Pashmina wool (in case of Kashmiri goat).
- Angora wool is also obtained from a goat in addition to Angora rabbit.
- Most of the domestic breeds of goats have been derived from the wild goat (*Capra hircus*). It is found in Balochistan and Western parts of Sindh.

Important goat breeds and their distributions are as follows

Table 18.6 Breeds of Indian goat

Breeds	Distributions	Breeds	Distributions
Beetal	Punjab	Jamunapari	Uttar Pradesh and Madhya Pradesh
Gaddi	Himachal Pradesh	Marwari	Rajasthan
Bengal	Bihar and Odisha	Kashmiri Pashmina	Hills of Kashmir, Tibet and Himachal Pradesh
Berari	Maharashtra	Malabari	Kerala

Donkey (*Equus asinus*) and mule

- In India, two types of donkeys are found. The smaller one is grey and the larger is white in colour. The larger one is also called **wild ass** and it is found in the Rann of Kutch in Gujarat.
- Donkeys are hardy animals and can withstand adverse weather conditions without requiring much care. They are mainly used for transporting goods.
- **Mule** is a sterile hybrid breed of male donkey (jack) and female horse (mare).
- **Hinny** is the reciprocal cross hybrid of male horse and female donkey.
- Hybrids are stronger than either of its parents.

Elephant

- It is the largest land animal and becomes sexually mature at the age of 8-16 years.
- Its reproduction rate is very low.
- Its gestation period is 22 months.
- The two main species of elephants are *Elephas maximus* (Indian elephant) and *Loxodonta africana.*
- There is another species *Elephas cyclotis*, which is also called **pygmy African elephant.**
- It is mainly used for transport, hunting, circus, etc.
- Its tusks, i.e. upper incisor teeth are used to get ivory.

Camel

- It is mostly used in deserts and are commonly known as **ship of deserts.**
- The main uses of camel are transport, ploughing, drawing water, etc.
- It is also reared to get milk, meat, hide and hair.
- Camel's hair are used for preparing brushes. Some of the species of camel are
  (i) ***Camelus dromidarius*** (Arabian camel) It is one humped and it is found in India.
  (ii) ***Camelus bactrianus*** (Bactrian camel) It is dual humped and has thick coat.
  (iii) The indigenous breeds of camel are **Bikaneri** (good height and strong inbuilt) **Kutchi, Sindhi** and **Jaisalmeri.**

CHECK POINT 18.1

1. Animal husbandry is
   (a) agricultural practice of breeding and raising livestock
   (b) dealing with care and breeding of livestock such as buffaloes, cow, pigs, horses, sheep and goat
   (c) poultry farming and fisheries
   (d) All of the above
2. All the given animals yield meat except
   (a) sheep (b) pig
   (c) Horse (d) goat
3. The most important livestocks of India are
   (a) cattle and cat (b) cattle and elephant
   (c) cattle and dog (d) cattle and buffalo
4. Choose the odd one out.
   (a) Gir (b) Deoni
   (c) Sahiwal (d) Malvi
5. Following breeds are found in Punjab, except
   (a) Sahiwal (b) Mehsana
   (c) Murrah (d) Nili Ravi

ANIMAL BREEDING : IMPROVEMENT OF ANIMALS

A breed is a group of animals related by common descent. It is similar in most of the characteristics such as general appearance, features, size, configuration, etc.
Animal breeding involves the production of improved breeds of domesticated animals by improving their genotype through selective mating.

Objectives of animal breeding

The main objectives of animal breeding are as follows

- Increased production of milk, meat, egg, wool, etc.
- Superior quality of milk, meat, egg, wool, etc.
- Resistance to various diseases.
- Increased or atleast acceptable reproduction rate.
- Increased productive life.
- Improved growth rate.

Methods of animal breeding

Some scientific methods, which are used for animal breeding are given below

1. Inbreeding

- It refers to the mating of more closely related individuals within a breed for 4-6 generations. In this type of breeding, superior male and superior female are identified and mated.
- It may help in the accumulation of superior genes and elimination of less desirable genes also. It increases the

homozygosity which leads to the reduction in the variation within a group. It leads to stabilisation of a particular type (i.e. pureline). Thus, inbreeding is necessary if we want to develop a **pureline**.

- At genetic level, inbreeding may expose harmful recessive genes that are usually eliminated by selection.
- Continued inbreeding may reduce the fertility of animals and even their productivity. This condition is called **inbreeding depression**. Thus, to overcome the effects of inbreeding depression, outbreeding is carried out.

2. Outbreeding

It refers to the mating of unrelated animals. It can be done by following ways

(i) **Outcrossing** It refers to mating between unrelated members of same breed, having no common ancestor on either side of their pedigree upto 4-6 generations. The offspring of such a mating is known as an **outcross**.
It is the best breeding method for animals suffering from inbreeding depression and having poor productivity of milk with reduced growth rate (beef and cattle), etc.

(ii) **Cross breeding** It refers to the mating of superior males of one breed with superior females of another breed. It helps to accumulate the desirable genes of the two breeds into a progeny.
The hybrid progeny may be used directly for commercial production. For example, *Hisardale* (sheep) was developed in Punjab by crossing Bikaneri ewes and Merino rams for wool.

(iii) **Interspecific hybridisation** It refers to the mating between male and female animals of two different species. The progeny obtained from such a mating is usually different from both the parental species, i.e. Mule and Hinny.

Controlled breeding experiments

These are carried out in following ways

1. Artificial insemination

- In this method, firstly semen is collected from the selected male parent. It is then injected into the reproductive tract of the selective female by the breeder. The semen is usually injected either deep in the cervix or within the uterus.
- The first ever artificial insemination in India was performed at the **Indian Veterinary Research Institute, Uttar Pradesh.**

Advantages of artificial insemination are listed below

(i) Collected semen can be frozen for later use or can be transported in frozen form.
(ii) It helps to overcome several problems of normal mating.
(iii) The semen collected from a single superior bull can be used to fertilise many cows.
(iv) Fewer sperms are required to achieve conception when semen is deposited artificially.

2. Multiple Ovulation Embryo Transfer (MOET)

- In this method, hormones (FSH) are injected in cow for inducing follicular maturation and superovulation.
- Thus, instead of one egg, cow produces 6-8 eggs per cycle. The cow is now either bred with a superior bull or artificially inseminated. After fertilisation, the embryo at 8-32 cell stage are collected and transplanted into a carrier cow (surrogate cow).
- By deep freezing (–196° C), it is possible to preserve 7 day old foetuses for several years to be used when needed.
- It has been done in cattle, sheep, rabbits, buffaloes, mares, etc., mainly for herd improvement.
- The calf produced by this method may grow into a super milch cow or a high quality bull.
- This method is also used for obtaining high quality soft wool (shahtoosh) from chiru (*Pantholops hodgsonii*).

3. Transgenesis

- It involves the transfer of genes into special cells or embryos.
- In this method, the unfertilised egg is enucleated by treating it with **cytochalasin B** and then blastula stage nuclei are obtained from the embryo donor. These two are incubated together in the presence of **Polyethylene Glycol** (PEG) and later transferred into surrogate mother for fusion.
- The foetus thus, develops into a transgenic animal.
- Various products like α-antitrypsin, haemoglobin, lactoferrin, iron binding protein, etc., are obtained from transgenic animals.

Note *In Japan, gynogenesis is being used to improve fish size.*

LIVESTOCK DISEASES

Infectious diseases in animals are caused by pathogens (like viruses, bacteria, protozoans, fungi) and parasitic animals (like worms).
Some of these are discussed below

Diseases caused by viruses

Animals suffer from a large variety of viral diseases. Some viral diseases are given below

Foot and mouth diseases

- **Disease-causing agent** *ss*RNA, *Aphthovirus.*
- **Hosts** Cattle, sheep, goats, pigs and other mammals.
- **Transmission** These diseases spread by direct or indirect contact.
- **Symptoms** Eruption of vesicles over the lips, inside buccal cavity, pharynx, overfeet, udder and even teats; fever and loss of appetite, dribbling of saliva, lameness etc.
- **Prevention and control** The infected animal should be separated and the animal house should be thoroughly disinfected. Antiseptic solution should be applied regularly, except over lips or inside mouth.
  Vaccination prevents the occurrence of the disease.

Rinderpest (Cattle plague)

- **Disease-causing agent** Rinderpest Virus (RPV).
- **Hosts** It is a contagious disease of cattle, domestic buffaloes, antelopes, giraffes, sheep, goats, *Hippopotamus*, etc. This disease is rare among camels.
  There is no report of RPV infection in human beings.
- **Transmission** Spread of Rinderpest Virus (RPV) occurs by the direct and indirect (contaminated feed, water, equipment, clothing) contact with infected animals.
- **Incubation period** The incubation period ranges from 3-15 days.
- **Symptoms** Body temperature upto 40-42.2°C, congested mucous membranes, ocular and nasal discharge, leukopenia (fall in WBC count), oral erosions, diarrhoea, dehydration and death in 6-12 days after the onset of illness.
  Rinderpest predominantly affects animals between 4 and 24 months of age.
- **Diagnosis** The samples should be collected from live animals, such as ocular and nasal secretions, necrotic tissue from the oral cavity.
- **Treatment** Injection of sulphamethazine sodium is often effective. The injection of rinderpest antiserum is highly effective, especially when combined with sulphamethazine sodium.
- **Prevention and control** This can be described under two separate heads
  (i) **Sanitary prophylaxis** Prophylaxis means prevention of disease. Sanitary prophylaxis includes
    - Isolation of sick animals.
    - Disinfection
    - Destruction of dead bodies of animals died due to rinderpest.
    - Protection of free zones.

  (ii) **Medical prophylaxis** Attenuated virus vaccines are highly effective for the prevention and control of the disease.

Cowpox

- **Disease-causing agent** Cowpox virus.
- **Hosts** It mainly affects cows, but cowpox may spread to humans accidentally during milking of infected animals.
- **Transmission** It is a contagious disease and spreads by direct contact with infected animal.
- **Symptoms** Blisters with pus, rupture and spread to hands, but heal without scarring. Local oedema with or without fever also occurs.
- **Prevention and control** The infected animals should be isolated and the animal house should be thoroughly disinfected.

Note *Inoculum from cowpox lesions was used by Edward Jenner in 1798 as vaccine against smallpox.*

Diseases caused by bacteria

Animals suffer from many bacterial diseases. Some of the bacterial diseases in animals are given below

Anthrax (Splenic fever)

It is a disease of domestic animals like cattle, sheep, goats, camels, etc.

- **Disease-causing agent** The disease is caused by *Bacillus anthracis.*
- **Transmission** In animals, anthrax spreads *via* contaminated feed, water and pastures.
- **Incubation period** It is usually 1-3 days.
- **Symptoms** Increased respiration and blood-mixed foamy discharge from mouth, nose and anus. The infected animals may die within 2-3 days. The anthrax bacterium creates hypoxic conditions in body and the animals die due to the lack of oxygen.
- **Diagnosis** The disease can be diagnosed by microscopic observation of the bacterium in the blood of the patient or by culturing it.

- **Treatment** In cattle, ciprofloxacin is effective only in chronic cases. Anthrax antiserum can also be used for the treatment.
- **Prevention and control** The healthy animals should be vaccinated. The animals coming in contact with the diseased animals should be given anthrax antiserum to protect them from the disease.

Mastitis

- **Disease causing agent** Mastitis often occurs in dry cows and it is caused by *Corynebacterium pyogenes.*
- **Symptoms** The disease is characterised by inflammation of the udder. It leads to watery milk and hardness of udder. It occurs when white blood cells are released into the mammary glands.

Diseases caused by protozoans

Several diseases in animals are caused by protozoan parasites. Some examples of protozoan diseases are tick fever, coccidiosis, etc.

Coccidiosis

- **Disease causing agent** It is caused by protozoans like *Eimeria, Isospora,* etc.
- **Symptoms** The disease is characterised by the erosion of intestinal mucosa, which leads to intestinal haemorrhage and blood stained diarrhoea.
- **Prevention and control** It is highly infective in young poultry birds. Infected birds should be isolated.

Tick fever

- **Disease causing agent** This disease is caused by a protozoan, *Babesia bigemina* in India. The parasite enters the Red Blood Cells (RBCs) and destroys them.
- **Host and vector** Tick fever occurs in cattle and domestic buffaloes. The parasite is transmitted by the ticks of the genus—*Hyalomma.*
- **Symptoms** Increase in body temperature, upto 41.1-41.7°C, lacrimation, nasal discharge, enlargement of lymph nodes. In the later stage, haemolytic anaemia and jaundice occur within the host.
- **Diagnosis** A clear diagnostic feature of tick fever is the presence of pear-shaped protozoan parasite within the RBCs.
- **Treatment** Injections of trypan blue, caprin or berenil are administered. Naphthaquinone compounds and halofuginone are the drugs of choice.
- **Prevention and control** The control of *Babesia* is based on tick control measures. Ticks should be removed and killed immediately. Vaccination also supports better control of tick fever.

Diseases caused by parasites

A large number of parasitic animals such as tapeworm, fluke, roundworms and a number of arthropods, may also cause diseases in animals. The parasites are of two types

(i) **Ectoparasites**, which live on the skin and suck the blood, e.g. ticks.

(ii) **Endoparasites**, which live within the animal body, e.g. tapeworms, liverflukes, roundworms, etc.

Both types of parasites feed on animal fluids like blood, etc., and interfere with their normal growth and development.

Some common parasitic diseases are given below

Fascioliasis (Liver rot)

- **Disease causing agent** *Fasciola hepatica, Fasciola gigantica* (liver fluke). In India, fascioliasis is caused by *F. gigantica.*
- **Hosts** *F. hepatica* and *F. gigantica* live in the bile ducts of sheep, goats and cattle. These may also require certain snails (e.g. *Lymnaea*) to complete their life cycle.
- **Symptoms** The parasites *Fasciola hepatica* and *F. gigantica* cause inflammation of bile duct, anaemia, diarrhoea, loss of appetite, eosinophilia and liver rot that may lead to the death of animal.
- **Treatment** It is treated by certain antihelminth drugs like hexachloroethane, emetine, folcin, phenothiazine, tetrachloroethane, carbon tetrachloride, etc.
- **Prevention** It indudes

  (i) Killing of heavily infected sheep and cattle.

  (ii) Breeding of snails can be checked by removing vegetation from the ponds.

  (iii) Sterilisation of cattle food or feedings with salt and dry food.

  (iv) Destroying manure of infected sheep and cattle.

  (iv) Proper drainage of grazing grounds.

CHECK POINT 18.2

1. The term 'breed' refers to
   (a) a group of animals not related by decent but similar in few characteristics
   (b) a group of animals related by decent and similar in most characteristics
   (c) a group of animals not related by decent but similar in most characteristics
   (d) a group of animals related by decent but have almost different characteristics
2. Inbreeding is carried out in animal husbandry because it
   (a) increases vigour (b) improves the breed
   (c) increases homozygosity (d) increases heterozygosity
3. In MOET, the animal is either mated with an elite bull or artifically inseminated. The fertilised eggs are collected to transfer to surrogate mothers. Which among these statements is correct?
   (a) Fertilised egg is collected at 8-32 cell stage and no need of surgery
   (b) Fertilised egg is collected at only 4 celled stage and it is done by surgery
   (c) Fertilised egg is collected at 8-32 cells stage and surgery is done for it
   (d) Fertilised egg is collected at 64 celled stage and surgery is done for it
4. Choose the odd one out.
   (a) Rinderpest (b) Anthrax
   (c) Mastitis (d) Splenic fever
5. Which livestock disease can be controlled by destroying *Hyalomma*?
   (a) Coccidiosis (b) Tick fever
   (c) Cattle plague (d) Anthrax

LIVESTOCK MANAGEMENT

It is a professional approach to provide a much needed boost or improvement in food production. The measures taken for managing livestock differ depending upon the livestock.

Some livestock managements are discussed below

Dairy farm management

- Dairying is the management of animals for milk and its production for human consumption.
- Dairy animals include cows, buffaloes, goats, etc. Cows and buffaloes generally give more milk than goats and sheep.
- Some dairy farms have cats to keep the barn, free of rodents.
- Dairy products indude milk, cream, curd, buttermilk, ghee, condensed milk, powdered milk and cheese.
- In dairy farm management, we deal with processes and systems that increase yield and improve quality of milk.
- These processes are as follows

(i) **Selection of Breed** Milk yield depends on the breed quality. Thus, good breeds with following characteristics are selected.
- High-yielding potential under the climatic conditions of the area.
- Resistance to diseases in breed.

(ii) **Housing** The cattles are kept in well built houses with adequate water and disease free conditions.

(iii) **Feed** The feeding of cattle is done in scientific manner with special emphasis on quality and quantity of fodder.

The feed is of two types
- **Roughages** They include fodder, silage, hay and straw. It has high fibre content.
- **Concenterates** They include cereals, millets, forage crops, leaves, oil cake, oil seeds and animal by products. It has high nutrient content.

(iv) **Cleanliness** Proper hygiene is maintained for both the cattle and the handler.

(v) **Vaccination** Regular visits by veterinary doctor is mandatory and regular vaccination should be done.

(vi) **Breeding** Mature cattle more than 3 yrs of age should be used for breeding. An average cow or buffalo produces 8-10 calves during its productive lifetime. Cattle breeders select and mate best type of cattle.

Note
- *India has lowest milk yield per cow.*
- *Cows and buffaloes remain in heat for 24-36 hours.*
- *Infertility in local breeds of cattle can be overcome by the use of gonadotropin.*

COMMERCIAL MANAGEMENT OF OTHER ANIMALS

Pisciculture

- It can be defined as the process of breeding, rearing and management of fish in water bodies under controlled conditions. It is also known as **fish farming** or **culture fishery**.
- Most common fish species raised by pisciculture are salmon, carp and cod. In India, Rohu and Catla are extensively reared.
- Fishes are generally captured from natural water bodies like river, lake, pond, sea, etc. For large scale production, **culture fishery** is practiced in small water bodies. In this, fishes are first reared and then harvested.
- In India, premier institutes like **Central Inland Capture Fisheries Research Institute** (CICFRI) Barrackpore (WB) **Central Marine Fisheries Research Institute** (CMFRI) Kochi Kerala, **Central Institute of Freshwater Aquaculture** (CIFA), Bhubaneshwar (Odisha) are engaged in the field of fisheries.

Note
- *In culture fishery, pituitary hormone extract is injected into male and female breeder fish. Two males and one female are then kept in a breeding happa, a bamboo and cloth contain spawning take place in 3-6 hours. The fertilised eggs are removed and kept in hatchery, where they hatch in 15-18 hours and further processes take place.*
- ***Capture fishery** is the management of catching of fish without raising them.*

Qualities of culturable fishes

These are as follows

- Able to feed on natural as well as artificial food diet.
- Fast growing.
- Able to tolerate sudden changes in climatic conditions.
- Able to resist different diseases.
- The taste of meat should be pleasing and nutritive.

Some of the culturable exotic and marine fishes are tabulated below

Table 18.7 Some exotic fishes

Zoological names	Common names	Native places
Osphronemus goramy	Gourami	Indonesia
Tinca tinca	Tench	England
Carassius carassius	Crucian carp	Central Europe
Cyprinus carpio	Common carp	China

Table 18.8 Some marine water fishes

Zoological names	Common names	Areas of availability
Sardinella	Sardine	West and South Coast
Stromateus	Pomphret	Indo-Pacific Coast
Anguilla sp.	Eel	Coastal India
Eleutheronema	Salmon	East and West Coast
Harpodon	Bombay duck	Coastal Maharashtra
Hilsa ilisha	Hilsa	Coastal India
Chanos chanos	Milk fish	Indian ocean and across the Pacific ocean

Steps used in pisciculture

The various steps of fish farming or pisciculture are as follows

(i) **Breeding** It is the first step in pisciculture. It can be divided into two types on the basis of mode of breeding.

(a) **Natural breeding** In this process, the fishes are allowed to breed naturally and the eggs are collected manually.

(b) **Induced breeding** This method of breeding is used to obtain desirable eggs. The ova from the desired female and sperms from the desired male are obtained by artificial mechanical processes. Later, the ova are fertilised by the collected sperms.

Note *Many carps do not breed in ponds due to environmental factors. The pituitary extract can be utilised successfully in inducing spawnings of major carp.*

(ii) **Hatching** The fertilised eggs are kept into the hatching pits. In this process, small-sized fish called **fish fry** come out after few days. These have a size of about 4.5 mm.

(iii) **Nursery ponds** Fish fry are transferred to nursery ponds. These ponds contain natural zooplanktons and phytoplanktons. Here, fish fry are allowed to feed for about 15-30 days. Now, these fish fry are called **fingerlings**.

(iv) **Rearing ponds** The fingerlings are transferred to bigger tanks called **rearing ponds**. Here, fingerlings are allowed to grow for about 2-3 months till they attain a length of 20 cm. Nutrients like phosphorus and calcium are essential for the fish growth.

(v) **Stocking ponds** These are deep and large-sized ponds. Fishes are kept in these ponds until they attain maturity.

(vi) **Harvesting** Big-sized fishes are taken out for marketing. Smaller once are again released into the stocking ponds for their proper growth.

Note • *Aquaculture is farming of freshwater and saltwater organisms like molluscs, crustaceans and aquatic plants.*
• *Pisciculture is a principal form of aquaculture.*

Economic importance of fishes

These are as follows

(i) **Food source** Fishes are used as food as they are good source of protein, vitamin and rich in iodine.

Table 18.9 Some edible freshwater fishes

Zoological names	Common names	Areas of availability
Heteropneustes heteropneustes	Singhi	All over India
Clarias batrachus	Magur	All over India
Catla catla	Catla	All over India
Labeo rohita (carp family)	Rohu	North, East and South India
Mystus singhara	Singhara	All over India
Wallago attu	Lachi or Malii	North, East and South India
Labeo calbasu	Calbasu	All over India

(ii) **Disease control** Certain carnivorous fishes like *Macropodus, Trichogaster* and *Gambusia affinis* (feed on mosquito larva), etc., help in controlling diseases.

(iii) **Ornamental purpose** A large number of fishes like *Pterophyllum* (angel fish) and *Carasinus* (gold fish) are nurtured in aquarium.

(iv) **Fish byproducts** These include
- Fish oil — from liver of sharks used as a source of vitamin-A and D
- Fish manure — used as fertiliser for coffee, tea and tobacco plant.
- Fish glue — from skin of cod fish
- Shagreen — sharp placoid scales on sharks are used for polishing wood, etc.
- Leather — skin of sharks.
- Artificial pearls — manfactured from silvery bony scales of cyprinid
- Isinglass — obtained from the dried swim bladders of fish. It is a form of collagen, used mainly for clarification of vinegar, wine and beer.
- Gelatin — used for the preparation of photographic emulsion.

(v) **Fish meal** It is used as major food of domestic animals like pig, poultry and cattle.

Fish diseases

Many bacterial, viral and parasitic diseases are found in the fishes, e.g. abdominal dropsy of carps, furunculosis of salmons, viral haemorrhage, septicaemia, fish leech, etc.

Poultry

- The term 'Poultry' means rearing of fowls, ducks, geese, turkeys and some varieties of pigeons. More often, it is used for fowl rearing.
- Fowls are reared for eggs and meats.
- *Cockerel* is a young male fowl and *Rooster* is the mature male fowl.
- The fowls may be categorised into two breeds

1. Indigenous breeds

Various indigenous breeds of poultry are as follows
- The major indigenous breeds are Aseel (best table bird), Chittagong and Ghagus.
- Malay or Chittagong bird grows faster. It is ideal for eating purposes as its flesh is excellent in taste.
- Ghagus is a big and hardy breed found in Andhra Pradesh and Karnataka.
- Bustra, a minor breed of desi class is found in small numbers in Gujarat and Maharashtra.

2. Exotic breeds

The term 'Improved' is applied generally to the exotic and comparatively modern breeds of chickens. Various exotic breeds are as follows
- **American breeds** Polymouth rock, Wyandotte, New Hampshire, Rhode Island Red and White leghorn.
- **Asian breeds** Brahma, Cochin, Langshan
- **English breeds** Sussex, Cornish, Dorking, Redcap
- Some important improved, high yielding breeds developed in India by cross breeding are ILS-82, B-77, HH-260.

Other poultry birds

- Ducks comprise 6% of the total poultry population in India. There are 20 breeds of ducks. Muscori, Pekin, Aylesbury and compbell are popular **exotic breeds**, while **indigenous breeds** include Indian punner, Sylhelt Meta, etc.
- Some important breeds of turkeys in India are Narfolk, British white, Broad breasted bronze and Beltsville small white.

Poultry feed

- It includes bajra, jowar, barley, maize, wheat, rice bran, oil, cake, fish meal, bread, green residue of vegetables, salt, vitamins and minerals.
- Minerals that should be present in poultry diets are calcium, phosphorus, sodium, copper, iodine, iron, zinc, etc.

Poultry products

The fowls are reared to obtain following useful products for human. These include

(i) **Egg layers** are female fowls raised for egg production. These are the rich source of easily digestable animal protein. Eggs are the good sources of calcium, protein, iron, vitamins and a moderate amount of fat. Each egg consists of shell and shell membranes (12%), albumin and chalaza (56%) and yolk (32%).

The hens normally start laying eggs from February and continue till August with some intervals. The average production of an Indian breed is about 60 eggs per annum.

(ii) **Poultry meat** It is a good source of nutritive food for non-vegetarians. Poultry birds reared for meat are called **broilers**.

(iii) **Feathers** They are used for commercial purposes such as for making pillows and quilts.

(iv) **Manure** It is obtained from the dropping of poultry birds. It is highly valuable for field crops.

Diseases of poultry

Poultry animals suffer from a number of diseases as follows

(i) **Ranikhet** (New castle disease) is caused by paramyxovirus of the genus-*Rubulavirus.* It affects the respiratory and nervous system. In this disease, bird opens the beak, becomes thirsty, suffer from fever and yellowish white diarrhoea occurs.

(ii) **Bird flu** is caused by H_5N_1 virus. The virus infects the man through chicken.

(iii) **Marck's disease** is primarily a disease of the young fowls caused by DNA virus. Paralysis is one of the major clinical symptom.

(iv) **Spirochaetosis** (tick fever) is caused by a parasite tick which feeds on the blood of fowls in night. It is a bacterial disease caused by *Borrelia anserina.*

(v) **Aspergillosis** is caused by fungus *Aspergillus* and occurs through food and litter. Due to this disease, breeding becomes difficult.

Note *Broodiness in layer and birds can be rectified by giving a hormonal injection of adrenaline.*

(vi) **Fowl pox** is a viral disease in which blisters appear on the body, nose, mouth and over comb.

(vii) **Infectious coryza** is caused by bacterium *Haemophilus gallinarum.* Infected birds show discharge from eyes and nostrils.

(viii) **Peroses** is caused due to manganese deficiency in poultry birds. There is enlargement of tibiometatarsal joints in it.

(ix) **Thrush disease** is a disease of alimentary canal, caused by fungal yeast, *Candida albicans.*

(x) **Black head disease** is caused by protozoan parasite *Histomonas meleagridis.* It leads to yellow watery dropping.

(xi) **Pullorum disease** is caused by bacteria *(Salmonella).* Heart, spleen, kidney and lungs are affected.

(xii) **Mycosis** is caused by a yeast, *Candida albicans.* It affects the upper portion of digestive tract (crop gizzard, etc.)

(xiii) **Fowl cholera** is caused by bacterium, *Pasteurella.*

(xiv) **Diarrhoea** is caused due to overfeeding and dirty water.

Treatment The administration of sulpha drugs and broad spectrum antibiotic treatments help in curing several diseases.

Sericulture

- The word 'sericulture' is derived from latin word *Sericus* – silk; *culturare* – cultivation.
- It is the production of raw silk on a commercial scale by rearing practices of silkworm.
- It is believed that the technique of cloth preparation from the cultivated silk had originated from China. Later, it was introduced to a number of countries like Japan, India, Russia, Brazil, Italy and France.
- India is the second largest producer of silk in the world.

Species of silkworm

- Some species of silkworm are as follows

(i) **Mulberry or Cultivated silkworm** (*Bombyx mori*) It belongs to family–Bombycidae. It is native to China, however now it has been introduced in different countries. The natural food of this worm is mulberry plant leaves. The silk produced by this worm is yellow or white in colour. It is known as **mulberry silk** (best silk).

(ii) **Tussar or Kosa silkworm** (*Antheraea paphia*) It belongs to the family–Saturniidae. It is found in China, India and Sri Lanka. Caterpillars of this silkworm feed on oak, sal and fig plants. Tussar silk is mainly used for furnishings and interiors.

(iii) **Muga silkworm** (*Antheraea assama*) It belongs to family—Saturniidae. Native to Assam (India), Caterpillars feed on *Machilus, Cinnamon* plants. Silk produced by this moth is known as **muga silk**. It is superior to tussar silk in gloss and is excellent material for embroidery.

(iv) **Eri or Arundi silkworm** (*Attacus ricinii*) It belongs to the family—Saturniidae. It feeds on castor leaf. Life history of this worm resembles with that of mulberry worm.

(v) **Oak silkworm** (*Antheraea pernyi*) It belongs to the family—Saturniidae. Oak silkworm is found in Japan and China and feeds on oak plant.

(vi) **Giant silkworm** (*Attacus altas*) This worm is found in India and Malaysia. It is the largest living insect.

- The percentage of production of different silk in India is Mulberry silk (contributes about 91.7%), eri silk (contributes about 6.4%), tussar silk (contributes about 1.4%) and muga silk (contributes about 0.5%).

Life cycle of mulberry silkworm *(Bombyx mori)*

It is a unisexual organism. It reproduces *via* sexual reproduction and fertilisation is internal.

The life cycle of silkworms proceeds as follows

- One female moth lays about 400-500 fertilised eggs.
- The eggs are glued to the under surface of the leaves of the host plant i.e. mulberry tree.
- After 10 days of incubation, the eggs hatch into the caterpillar larvae.
- The larvae pass through five stages. **Moulting** takes place after each stage and the larval skin is cast off. These larvae are voracious feeder.
- Each caterpillar larva has well-developed mandibulate type of mouth parts. These are adapated to feed easily on the mulberry leaves.
- A fully grown larva stops feeding and develops salivary glands and undergoes **pupation**.
- During pupation, the larva secretes a sticky fluid through a narrow pore situated on the hypopharynx. This secreted fluid, when comes in contact with air, becomes solidified.
- It is wrapped around the body of the caterpiller in the form of a covering called as **cocoon.**
- Each cocoon contains about 1000-1200 m long continuous silk thread.
- Through practical applications, it has been estimated that one pound of silk can be obtained from 2500 cocoons.
- The pupal period lasts for about 10-12 days and the larva cuts the cocoon and emerges into an adult moth.

Note *Cocoon is formed by two pairs of glands called **spinneret**. One secretes proteinaceous material-fibroin and other secretes gummy material-sericin.*

Process of sericulture

- The cocoon is a whitish or yellowish-coloured, 2.5× 1.5 cm and oval-shaped structure.
- A good quality of cocoon is judged by the quantity of raw silk, filament length, strength and splitting power.
- The process to obtain silk from cocoon is called **post-cocoon** processing.
- Grainage is the centre where silkworm eggs are produced and supplied.
- The process of sericulture includes following steps

(i) **Stifling**, i.e. killing of cocoons. 8-10 days old cocoons are selected for stifling. This can be done through hot water, dry heat, sun exposure for three days or fumigation.

(ii) **Reeling** It means removal of silk threads from the killed cocoon. 4-5 threads are passed through eyelets and twisted into one thread. This thread is wound round on a large wheel and it is transferred to spools. This is called **raw silk** or **reeled silk** (it contains sericin).

(iii) **Spinning** For attaining lustre and to remove excess of natural gum, the raw silk is further boiled, stretched and purified by acid or fermentation. It is then thoroughly washed (degumming of silk).

Several such silk threads are twisted to get fibre silk through the process of spinning. The waste out layers or damaged cocoon are separated, teared and then the filaments are spun. Such silk is known as **spun silk**. It is soft, estrous and light in weight.

Note ***Ahimsa silk** or **non-violence silk** is made by deriving silk from cocoon only on completion of worm's natural life cycle without killing the worm. Ahimsa silk is procured through piercing of cocoons. The process is more laborious and requires more cocoons than regular silk. As a result, Ahimsa silk is more expensive than other silk.*

Silk

- It is a paste-like secretion of silkworm caterpillar during cocoon formation.
- The silk is secreted from the salivary glands for larva. These glands extend from the 4-8th segments of the abdomen.
- Silk becomes hard and changes into strong and flexible silk fibres.
- Silk is composed of following two types of proteins
  (i) **Fibroin** It constitutes 80% of the silk thread (inner part of the thread).
  (ii) **Sericin** It constitutes 20% of the silk thread (outer envelope of the thread).

Economic importance of silk

The economic importances of silk are as follows

- Raw silk threads are used in the manufacturing of sarees, kurtas, jackets, shawls, blouses and other garments.
- The remaining part of the cocoon is used to prepare a kind of cloth called **matka**.
- Special type of tyres for car, parachute, the outer covering of telephone wire, etc., are prepared using silk threads.
- Now-a-days, the intestine of the silk moth is being utilised to form a substance, known as **gut**. It is useful in fishing and surgical works.

Diseases related to sericulture

These are as follows

(i) **Powdery mildew** It is a fungal disease of mulberry plant.
(ii) **Flacherie** It is a viral disease in silkworm.
(iii) **Pebrine** It is caused by *Nosema bombycis*. It infects the eggs of silkworm. It is transmitted from one generation to other.
(iv) **Muscardine** It is caused by fungus *Spicaria* and *Botrytis*.

Apiculture

- It is the rearing of honeybees for obtaining bee wax and honey on commercial scale. For apiculture, large places, called **apiaries** or **bee farms** are established scientifically.
- The Khadi and Village Industries Commission (KVIC) and the Indian Council of Agricultural Research (ICAR) are making efforts to raise the commercial production of honeybee products.
- Honeybee is one of the most important pollinators in agriculture and in flowering plants like sunflower, guava, etc., also.

Species of honeybees

Four species of honeybees are reported in different parts of India. These are as follows

- ***Apis florea F.*** (Little bee) It rarely stings and can be easily used for honey extraction.
- ***Apis indica F.*** (Indian bee) It can be easily domesticated and most commonly used for honey production. Therefore, it is reared in artificial hives.
- ***Apis dorsata F.*** (Rock bee) It is a giant bee that yields maximum honey.
- ***Apis mellifera F.*** (European bee) Best species from commercial point of view.

Social organisation of honeybees

Honeybees are social and polymorphic insects. They live in highly organised colonies. An ordinary colony has about 40-50 thousand individuals. These are of following three main types

(i) Queen

- It is a well-developed fertile female.
- Generally, only one queen is found in each hive.
- Sting is curved, modified as egg laying organ called **ovipositor**.
- She lays both fertilised and unfertilised eggs.
- Queen feeds on **Royal Jelly** which is secreted by worker. It includes digested honey, pollen and secretion of maxillary gland.
- Queen develops from the fertilised egg of the mother queen bee.

(ii) Drones

- These are haploid and fertile males. Drones are called **king of colony**.
- They develop parthenogenetically and have lifespan of about 5 weeks. Their main funtion is to fertilise the queen. They die after copulation.

(iii) Workers

- They are diploid and sterile female.
- Worker bees are of three types, i.e. scavenger bees, nurse bees and scout bees.
- They are developed from the fertilised eggs laid by queen. They live in a chamber called **worker cell**. Lifespan of a worker is about 6 weeks.

- Total indoor and outdoor activities are performed by workers only. For this purpose, they have been provided with some specific features such as
  (a) They have a powerful sting for defence.
  (b) They have long proboscis for sucking the nectar.
  (c) They have strong wings for fanning.
  (d) For collection of pollens, they have **pollen baskets.**
  (e) They have **wax secreting glands** on ventral surface of second to fifth abdominal segment.

Note *Honeybees show different types of behaviour such as*

- *Swarming, i.e. honeybees come out of the hive in large number.*
- *Supersedure, i.e. new young and vigorous queen takes the position of the old queen.*
- *Absconding, i.e. migration of complete colony from one place to another due to unfavourable conditions.*

Bee enemies

A number of bee enemies harm the bee colony in different ways.

These include wasps (*Vespa* sp. and *Palarus* sp.), black ants (*Componotus compressus*), bee eaters (*Merops orientalis*), wax moths (*Galleria mellonella, Achroia grisella*) and kingcrow (*Dicrurus macrocercus*).

Life history of honeybee

After mating, the queen lays down two types of eggs, i.e.

(i) **Fertilised** (diploid with 32 chromosomes) Larvae coming out from fertilised eggs develop into a female queen or sterile workers. One of the larvae from fertilised egg feed on royal jelly and becomes queen.

(ii) **Unfertilised** (haploid with 16 chromosomes) Larvae coming out from unfertilised eggs develop into drones. About 14, 16 and 21 days are required for the development of drones, queen and workers, respectively.

Note ***Nuptial or Marriage flight*** *The new queen takes her first aerial flight followed by a swarm of drones. The queen flies very high and drones gradually drop out of the race. The last drone left in the race, mates with her. Mating occurs in the mid air and it is known as nuptial flight.*

Methods of bee-keeping

Indigenous methods of bee-keeping were very crude, cruel and unplanned. These are now replaced by modern scientific methods. In these methods, bees are reared in artificial hives having following features

- Indian standard institute has standardised the hives of small and big sized frames of 21 × 14.5 and 31 × 20.4 cm, respectively.
- The modern beehive is made up of a series of square or oblong boxes without tops or bottoms, set one above the other.
- This hive has the floor at the bottom and a crown board at the top and a roof over all.
- Inside these boxes, wooden frames are vertically hung, parallel to each other.
- The wooden frames are filled with sheets of wax foundation on which the combs are built by the bee.
- The only entrance to the hive is below the large bottom box (brood chamber).
- The queen is usually confined to the brood chamber.
- The boxes termed as supers are used for the storage of honey.
- The queen is prevented from going to the supers by the queen excluder that allow only the workers to move.

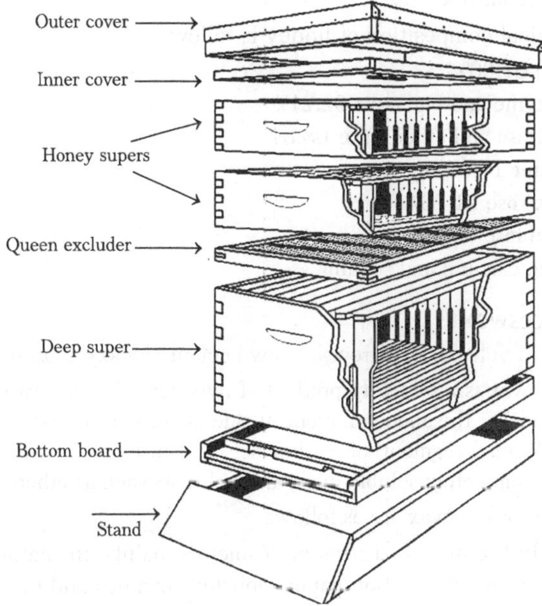

***Fig. 18.1** Typical movable beehive*

- Collected swarm is transferred to the hive to buildup the colony and produce honey. Honey is stored in combs of super frames. It is extracted from the comb by a simple machine called **honey extractor.**

Products of bees

Bees are raised to obtain the following products

(i) Honey

It is golden brown in colour and very sweet in taste. The smell of honey is variable depending upon juices collected by bees from different flowers.

Various benefits of honey are as follows

- 2.1 g honey provides about 68 kcal energy. About 200 g of honey provides as much energy as 11.6 L of milk.
- In illness, honey is preferred over milk.

- Honey contains many kinds of acids (both organic and amino) and vitamin-B_1, B_2, nicotinic acid (B_3), pantothenic acid (B_5).
- A number of ayurvedic medicines are taken with honey.
- Honey is a good blood purifier.
- It works as a curative for ulcers on tongue and alimentary canal.
- It is also used in making bread cake and biscuits.

Honey is prepared in presence of enzyme invertase which convert sucrose of nectar into glucose and fructose.

Nectar is stored in the crop and extra amount of water is evapored by the fanners bees. Honey is a concentrated product. The average pH of honey is 3.9, but can change range from 3.4-6.1.

Chemical composition of honey is follows

- Ash 01.00%
- Enzyme and pigments 02.21%
- Maltose and other sugar 08.81
- Water 17.20%
- Dextrose 21.28%
- Levulose 38.90%
- Iron, calcium and sodium

(ii) Beeswax

- It is a yellowish to greyish-brown coloured waxy substance.
- Bee wax is a secretory product of hypodermal glands (wax glands) of the abdomen (ventral side of second to fifth abdominal segment) of worker bee. It is insoluble in water, but completely soluble in organic solvents such as ether.
- Uses of beeswax are as follows
  (a) In the manufacturing of cosmetics, paints, insulators, ointments, carbon paper, polishes, candles and many other lubricants.
  (b) In biology lab, for block preparation, for microtome sectioning, etc.

(iii) Bee venom

It is used in the treatment of arthritis and snake bite.

Bee diseases

Bees suffer from following diseases

(i) **Acarine disease** It is caused by parasitic mite, *Acarapis woodi.*

(ii) **Nosema disease** It is caused by protozoan, *Nosema apis.*

Lac culture

- Lac is obtained from the Indian lac insect *Laccifer* (*Tachardia lacca*). It is a type of scale insect found in thick forests of India, Burma and other South Asian countries. It lives on trees such as *Ficus glomerata, Ficus benghalensis* (banyan), *Acacia arabica* (kikar), *Zizyphus jujuba* (beri), *Shorea robusta* (sal) and *Butea frondosa* (palash).
- The lac insects feed on the sap of the host tree. The distinct features of male and female lac insects are as follows
  (i) The female insects are dark red and without wings, legs and eyes. Thus, the females are motionless and have a body like an insect.
  (ii) The males are active and are like insect. During unfavourable season, lac is secreted as a protective covering around the twigs of trees, mostly by the females. Lac is scrapped from the twigs and processed to get shell-lac. The lac or shell lac is a resinous substance.

  The Indian Institute of Natural Resin and Gum (IINRG), Namkum (Ranchi) is engaged in the research and extension programmes to promote and improve the lac culture.

Uses of lac

Various uses of shell lac are as follows

- **Shell lac** is used in the preparation of varnishes, paints and polishes.
- It is used in making gramophone records, printing ink, buttons and pots. It is used in filling ornaments such as bangles and bracelets.
- It is also used as insulating material.
- India is a major lac producing country and exports more than two crore kilograms of lac each year.

Chemical composition of lac

These are as follows

Resin	68-90%
Dye	2-10%
Wax	6%
Albuminous matter	5-10%
Mineral matter	3-7%
Water	3%

CHECK POINT 18.3

1. The young ones which hatches from the eggs of a fish are known as
(a) hatchings (b) fingerlings (c) fry (d) nymph

2. Which pair is essential for the growth of fish in water?
(a) Nitrates and sulphates (b) Sulphate and carbonates
(c) Calcium and phosphorus (d) Carbonate and phosphates

3. Exotic breeds of poultry are
(a) White leghorn and Rhode Island Red
(b) Rhode Island Red and Aseel
(c) Plymouth and Aseel
(d) White leghorn and Aseel

4. In silkworm, silk is the product of
(a) culticle of the adult
(b) cuticle of the larva
(c) salivary gland of the adult
(d) salivary gland of the larva

5. Apiculture is associated with which of the following groups of plants?
(a) Grapes, maize, potato
(b) Sugarcane, paddy, banana
(c) Guava, sunflower, strawberry
(d) Pineapple, sugarcane, strawberry

6. Honeybees exhibit following behaviour except
(a) swarming
(b) supersedure
(c) abscending
(d) stifling

7. Lac is produced as
(a) faces of lac insect
(b) secretion from body
(c) excretion from body
(d) excess food oozing out of body

EXAM POINTS

- One of the breeding techniques useful to eliminate harmful recessive gene by selection is inbreeding. **[JIPMER 2017]**
- Homozygous purelines in cattle can be obtained by mating of related individuals of same breed. **[NEET 2017]**
- Inbreeding depression decreases productivity due to continued inbreeding. **[NEET 2020, 2019]**
- Inbreeding depression can be overcome by outcrossing **[NEET 2019]**
- Making two varieties of a cattle breed like Red dane which have no common ancestors on either sides of their pedigree upto 4-6 generations is an example for outcrossing. **[Karnataka CET 2014]**
- Homozygosity leads to reduction in variation within a group. It is a process of mating of related individuals of same breed. **[NEET 2017]**
- Interspecific hybridisation is the mating of two different related species. **[NEET 2016]**
- Interspecific hybridisation is the method of animal breeding of two different species of male and female animals. **[J&K CET 2014]**
- Late maturity is not selected for culture practices and does not possess any feature to make culture profitable. **[EAMCET 2016]**
- Obtaining fishes from random water bodies is capture fishery. **[Chst PMT 2015]**
- Sussex, Australorp and Orpington are poultry birds and are English breed. **[WB JEE 2012]**
- The red jungle fowl is *Gallus gallus*. **[AMU 2015]**
- Ayrshire is a breed of cattle. **[AMU 2012]**
- Silk is the product of salivary gland of larva of silkworm. **[Chst. PMT 2015]**
- Percentage composition of fibroin and sericin in silk is 80:20. **[WB JEE 2010]**
- *Nosema* is a protozoan which is threat to apiculture and sericulture. **[AIIMS 2013]**
- Kokichi Mikimoto is referred as Father of Pearl Industry. **[AMU 2015]**

Chapter Exercises

(A) Topical Exercise

Livestock and Domesticated Animals Breeds

1 Rearing, caring and feeding of domesticated animals is known as
(a) breeding
(b) animal husbandry
(c) artificial insemination
(d) None of the above

2 Find the odd one out.
(a) Gir (b) Rathi
(c) Kangayam (d) Vechur

3 Which of the following statement(s) is incorrect?
(a) Deoni is a milch breeds
(b) Drought breed used for labour
(c) Milch breed used for milk
(d) Nageri is a milch breeds

4 Sunandini breed originates from crossing between
(a) Local breed, Jersey and Holstein
(b) Local breed and Holstein
(c) Tharparkar and Holstein
(d) Sahiwal and Brown Swiss bull

5 Water buffalo is
(a) Asian breed of buffalo that prefers living in water for most of the day
(b) buffalo-like animal living in rivers
(c) llama
(d) Bison

6 Consider the following statements.
I. The buffaloes are better than cows, because they are disease resistant.
II. Murrah breeds of buffaloes are mostly demanded.
Choose the correct option.
(a) Statement I is true, but II is false
(b) Statement I is false, but II is true
(c) Both statements I and II are true
(d) Both statements I and II are false

7 Merino sheep has been imported for
(a) increasing wool output through Merino farms
(b) increasing mutton availability
(c) improving indigenous breeds
(d) developing hybrid between sheep and goat

8 Consider the following statements.
I. Lohi is a breed of sheep.
II. Famous Angora wool is obtained from sheep.
Choose the correct option.
(a) Statement I is true, but II is false
(b) Statement I is false, but II is true
(c) Both statements I and II are true
(d) Both statements I and II are false

9 Long neck of camel is due to
(a) number of neck vertebrae
(b) length of each neck vertebrae
(c) development of extra bony plates between successive neck vertebrae
(d) development of muscular pads between successive neck vertebrae

10 Bactrian camel is characterised by
(a) two humps and long neck
(b) two humps and long limbs
(c) two humps and thick coat
(d) single hump and thick coat

11 Match the following columns.

Column I	Column II
A. Camel	1. *Capra*
B. Goat	2. *Bos indicus*
C. Buffalo	3. *Bubalus*
D. Cow	4. *Camelus*

Codes

	A	B	C	D
(a)	1	4	2	3
(b)	4	1	3	2
(c)	2	4	1	3
(d)	4	1	2	3

12 Match the following columns.

Column I (Utilities)	Column II (Livestocks)
A. Milk, butter and driving carts	1. Goat
B. Milk and flesh	2. Horse
C. Transport and recreation	3. Sheep
D. Wool and mutton	4. Buffalo

Codes

	A	B	C	D
(a)	4	1	2	3
(b)	1	3	2	4
(c)	1	2	4	3
(d)	3	2	1	4

13 The following figure shown improved breed of animal and bird. Identify *A* and *B*.

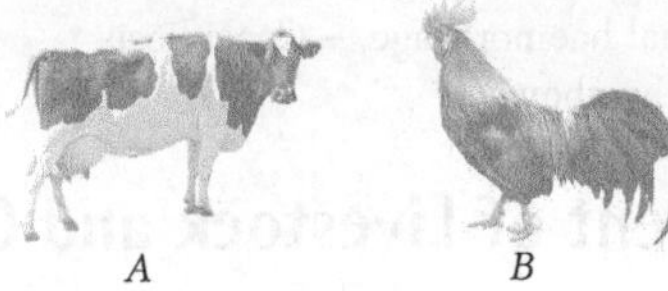

(a) *A* - Beetal, *B*- Jamunapari
(b) *A* - Marwari, *B* - Sirohi
(c) *A* - Surti, *B* - Sangammeri
(d) *A* - Jersey, *B* - Leghorn

Animal Breeding and Diseases

14 Which of the following is not the objective of animal breeding?
(a) Resistance to various diseases
(b) Increased productive live
(c) Improved growth rate
(d) Low quality of milk

15 Inbreeding is carried out in animal husbandry because it **[NCERT Exemplar]**
(a) increases vigour
(b) improves the breed
(c) increases heterozygosity
(d) increases homozygosity

16 Consider the following statements.
I. Animals which are similar in characters, general appearance, features, size, etc., belong to different breed.
II. Pureline can be obtained by outbreeding.
Choose the correct option.
(a) Statement I is true, but II is false
(b) Statement I is false, but II is true
(c) Both statements I and II are true
(d) Both statements I and II are false

17 .... refers to the mating of superior males of one breed with superior female of another breed.
(a) Outbreeding (b) Inbreeding
(c) Cross breeding (d) Interspecific hybridisation

18 The process of breeding of unrelated animals belonging to the same species, but is from different breeds or the breeding between two genetically distant groups or population to obtain offspring can be done by
(a) cross breeding (b) outcrossing
(c) interspecific hybridisation (d) All of these

19 The mating between male and female animals of two different species is called
(a) cross breeding (b) outcrossing
(c) lose breeding (d) Interspecific hybridisation

20 Which of the following hormone is provided for follicular maturation?
(a) Oxytocin (b) FSH
(c) LH (d) Both (a) and (c)

21 Semen from the selected male parent is injected into the reproductive tract of the female parent artificially with the help of a process known as
(a) MOET (b) outcrossing
(c) artificial insemination (d) inbreeding

22 Consider the following statements.
I. Bull semen for the purpose of artificial insemination is stored in liquid oxygen.
II. Multiple ovulation embryo transfer is a method of hybridisation of cattle.
Choose the correct option.
(a) Statement I is true, but II is false
(b) Statement I is false, but II is true
(c) Both statements I and II are true
(d) Both statements I and II are false

23 Artificial insemination was first introduced in India at
(a) Veterinary College
(b) Indian Veterinary Research Institute
(c) Animal and Fisheries Science University
(d) None of the above

24 Consider the following statements.
I. Artificial insemination is better than natural insemination in cattle because there is no likelihood of contagious disease.
II. Hinny is a hybrid of male donkey and female horse.
Choose the correct option.
(a) Statement I is true, but II is false
(b) Statement I is false, but II is true
(c) Both statements I and II are true
(d) Both statements I and II are false

25 Infertility of local breeds of cattle can be overcome by the use of
(a) cross breeding with exotic breeds
(b) good nourishment
(c) stilbesterol
(d) gonadotropin

26 What will you conclude, when a cow is crossed to a bull and the female progeny is yielding more milk than its mother?
(a) More number of genes for high yielding milk are inherited only from the female parent
(b) More number of genes for high yielding milk are inherited only from the male parent
(c) More number of genes for high yielding milk are inherited from both the parents
(d) The progeny through mutation achieved more number of genes for high yielding milk

27 Consider the following statements.
I. The unfertilised egg is enucleated by cytochalasin B.
II. Transgenic animals are used for the production of haemoglobin and lactoferrin.

Choose the correct option.
(a) Statement I is true, but II is false
(b) Statement I is false, but II is true
(c) Both statements I and II are true
(d) Both statements I and II are false

28 Blisters with pus present on hand is when cattle is infected with
(a) *Streptococcus* (b) Cowpox virus
(c) *Bacillus* (d) RNA *Aphthovirus*

29 Consider the following statements.
I. The disease rinderpest is also called blue tongue.
II. Aspergillosis is a fungal disease of poultry.

Choose the correct option.
(a) Statement I is true, but II is false
(b) Statement I is false, but II is true
(c) Both statements I and II are true
(d) Both statements I and II are false

30 Which one of these diseases in animals is caused by *Babesia bigemina*?
(a) Rinderpest (b) Tick fever
(c) Anthrax (d) Diarrhoea

31 Study the following pathogens.
I. *Yersinia pestis* II. *Borrelia* sp.
III. *Odium albicans* IV. *Mycobacterium leprae*
V. *Haemophilus gallinarum*

Which of the above cause damage to poultry industry?
(a) I and IV (b) II, III and V
(c) II and V (d) IV and V

32 In poultry birds, nasal and eye discharges with foul smell, acute respiratory problem and inflammed and swollen eyes are the symptoms of
(a) chronic respiratory disease
(b) infectious coryza disease
(c) brooder pneumonia disease
(d) Marck's disease

33 An uncommon illness in cattle, usually mild, that can spread from a cow to human *via* sores on the cow, vaccine against the disease was first used by
(a) Odum (b) Flemming (c) Jenner (d) None of these

34 Mastitis is caused by
(a) *Corynebacterium pyogenes*
(b) *Eimeria*
(c) *F. gigantica*
(d) *Aphthovirus*

35 Choose the correct match.
(a) *Bacillus anthracis* – Anthrax
(b) *Corynebacterium pyogenes* – Mastitis
(c) Intestinal haemorrhage – Coccidiosis
(d) All of the above

Management of Livestock and Other

36 Cattle fed with spoilt hay of sweet clover which contains dicumarol
(a) are healthier due to a good diet
(b) catch infections easily
(c) may suffer vitamin-K deficiency and prolonged bleeding
(d) may suffer from beri-beri due to deficiency of vitamin-B

37 Consider the following statements.
I. Pisciculture is commercial raising and production of fishes.
II. Gelatin, a raw material for the preparation of photographic emulsion is a byproduct of fish.

Choose the correct option.
(a) Statement I is true, but II is false
(b) Statement I is false, but II is true
(c) Both statements I and II are true
(d) Both statements I and II are false

38 Isinglass, a type of byproduct of fish industry, is principally used for
(a) feeding cattle, pigs and poultry
(b) preparation of paints and varnishes
(c) clarification of vinegar, wines and beer
(d) production of insulin

39 Fish rohu widely used for high biological value is rich in
(a) thymine, creatine and tyrosine
(b) lecithin and cholesterol
(c) vitamins-B, C, D and E
(d) All of the above

40 Exotic breeds of poultry are
(a) White Leghorn and Rhode Island Red
(b) Rhode Island Red and Andalusian
(c) plymouth and Andalusian
(d) White Leghorn and Andalusian

41 Which culture is performed to obtain feed for silkworm
(a) culture silkworm (b) culture of honeybee
(c) culture of mulberry plant (d) culture of fish

42 The process of cultivating worms and extracting a strong thread from them is the practice of
(a) rearing silkworm for silk
(b) rearing of honeybee for honey
(c) rearing lac insects for lac
(d) All of the above

43 A fine, strong soft lustrous fibre produced by silkworms in making cocoons and collected to make thread and fibre is composed of

(a) trypsin and amylopsin
(b) creatine and fibrin
(c) fibroin and sericin
(d) fibrin and fibrinogen

44 Consider the following statements.

I. In honeybee, swarming is found.
II. Royal jelly, honey is the only product of insects.

Choose the correct option.

(a) Statement I is true, but II is false
(b) Statement I is false, but II is true
(c) Both statements I and II are true
(d) Both statements I and II are false

45 Secretion of silk gland comes through a small pore. This pore is situated on

(a) exopodite of second maxilla
(b) endopodite of first maxilla
(c) prostheca of mandible
(d) anterior part of hypopharynx

46 Which one of the following statements is correct?

(a) *Apis dorsata* is most commonly used for honey production
(b) Karl von Fritsch discovered bee dance
(c) Honey is rich in glucose and maltose sugars
(d) All of the above

47 Honey that has a high concentration of sugar, does not decay because

(a) it contains natural antioxidant that prevents bacterial attack
(b) bacteria cannot survive in an active state in a solution of high osmotic strength as water is drawn out of honey
(c) in honey, bacteria are totally deprived of oxygen
(d) None of the above

48 Silk and lac are

(a) secretory products of animals
(b) secretory products of plants
(c) synthetic chemicals
(d) Both (a) and (c)

49 Which is a product of insect body?

(a) Honey, wax and silk (b) Silk, lac and wax
(c) Royal jelly, wax and lac (d) All of these

50 Match the following columns.

Column I (Terms)	Column II (Features)
A. Pisciculture	1. Rearing of fishes
B. Aquaculture	2. Rearing and management of economically useful aquatic plants and animals
C. Apiculture	3. Concerned with maintenance of honeybees

Codes

	A	B	C		A	B	C
(a)	3	2	1	(b)	2	3	1
(c)	2	1	3	(d)	1	2	3

(B) Cumulative Exercise

(Assorted Questions of the Chapter for Advanced Level Practice)

1 In poultry industry, production of hatching eggs is more expensive than the production of market eggs. Read the given statements regarding this

I. cost of males and their depreciation value is high.
II. mortality among females is usually lower when they are mated with males.
III. number of eggs produced by hatchery flock are to be sold only as market eggs.
IV. some of the eggs produced by hatchery flocks are not acceptable for incubation.

Which of the above statements are incorrect.

(a) I, II and III (b) II, III and IV
(c) I, III and IV (d) I, II and IV

2 Match the following columns.

Column I	Column II
A. *Bombyx mori*	1. Disease of mulberry
B. *Morus alba*	2. Centre where silkworm eggs are produced and supplied
C. Grainage	3. Silk moth
D. Powdery mildew	4. Mulberry plant
	5. Freshly hatched silkworm

Codes

	A	B	C	D		A	B	C	D
(a)	2	3	4	5	(b)	3	4	2	1
(c)	3	2	5	4	(d)	4	3	2	5

3 The parameters carried out for managing dairy farm are

I. selection of both the male and female animals having high yielding potential and resistance to diseases
II. regular visits by a veterinary doctor.
III. each animal should be fed with a balance diet.
IV. pay attention to good animal management and general supervision.

Which of the above statements are correct?

(a) I and II (b) I, II and III
(c) II, III and IV (d) I, II, III and IV

4 Read the given statements.

I. Cross breeding refers to the cross of superior males of one breed with superior females of another breed.
II. Artificial insemination is a method of controlled breeding in which semen from the selected male parent is injected into the reproductive tract of the selected female parent.
III. MOET refers to crossing between male and female animals of two different species.
IV. Interspecific hybridisation is a programme for herd improvement in animals like cattle, sheep, buffaloes, etc.

Which of the given statements are incorrect?

(a) Only III (b) Only IV (c) III and IV (d) None of these

5 Strategic steps for inbreeding are

I. identify superior male and superior female of the same breed.
II. identified animals are then mated in pairs.
III. evaluate the progeny obtained from the mating to identify superior males and females.
IV. in cattle, superior female is the cow or buffalo that produce more milk per lactation and superior male is the bull that gives rise to superior progenies.
V. superior progenies obtained are further mated.

Arrange the above given steps in correct sequence and select the correct answer.

(a) I → III → II → IV → V (b) I → II → III → IV → V
(c) III → I → II → IV → V (d) III → II → I → V → IV

6 Read the given statements.

I. The progeny of cross breeding may be used for commercial production.
II. In case of artificial insemination, the semen can be used immediately or can be frozen for later use.
III. Controlled breeding experiments are carried out using artificial insemination only.
IV. Cattle breeds can be improved by superovulation and embryo transplantation.

Which of the following statements are correct?

(a) I and II (b) I, II and III
(c) I, III and IV (d) III and IV

7 Which of the following procedures is/are followed in poultry farm management?

I. Regular inspections and visits by veterinary doctors.
II. Usage of manure to increase crop yields.
III. Adequate environmental condition is provided.
IV. Weeding away unproductive and harmful plants from the brood house.

Codes

(a) I and II are correct
(b) I and III are correct
(c) III and IV are correct
(d) All procedures are correct

8 The following flowchart shows methodology which has been for cattle, sheep, buffaloes, etc. Identify missing steps (*A*, *B* and *C*).

Cow is administrated with (*A*) hormone
↓
(*B*)
↓
6-8 eggs per cycle are derived
↓
Artificially inseminated
↓
Fertilised eggs at 8-32 cells are recovered
↓
(*C*)

(a) *A*-Oestrogen, *B*-Superovulation due to induced follicular maturation, *C*-Transfer to surrogate mother
(b) *A*-origesteribe, *B*-Superovulation due to induced follicular maturation, *C*-Transfer to surrogate mother
(c) *A*-LH, *B*-Superovulation due to induced follicular maturation, *C*-Transfer to surrogate mother
(d) *A*-FSH, *B*-Superovulation due to induced follicular maturation, *C*-Transfer to surrogate mother

9 Match the breeds of cattle given under Column I with place of their origin listed under Column II.

	Column I (Cattle breeds)		Column II (Place of origin)
A	Amrit mahal	1.	Hassan and Tumkur Districts
B	Ongole	3.	Coimbatore District
C	Khillari	3.	Nellore and Guntur Districts
D	Hallikar	4.	Chikmagalur and Chitradurga Districts
		5.	Satara and Sholapur Districts

Codes

	A	B	C	D		A	B	C	D
(a)	4	3	5	1	(b)	2	4	5	1
(c)	4	5	2	3	(d)	2	4	1	5

10 Which of the following points should be kept into considering for successful bee-keeping?

I. Selection of suitable location for keeping the beehives.
II. Light management according to the habits of honey bees.
III. Knowledge of the behaviour of honeybees.
IV Handling and collection of honey and bee wax.

Codes

(a) I, II and III (b) I, III and IV
(c) I, II, III and IV (d) None of these

11 Given below are four statements (I-IV) which two of the following statements are correct?

I. It is estimated that more than 70% of the world livestock population is in India and China.
II. Maintaining cleanliness and hygiene (both of the cattle and the handlers) is important while milking, storage and transport of the milk and its products
III. Outbreeding is the breeding between animal of the same breed only.
IV Crosses between different breeds are called inbreeding.

Choose the correct option.

(a) I and II (b) III and IV (c) I and IV (d) II and III

12 Match the following columns.

Column I (Breeding types)	Column II (Features)
A. Outcrossing	1. Exposes harmful recessive genes that are usually eliminated by selection
B. Cross breeding	2. Mating of animals belonging to different breeds
C. Interspecific hybridisation	3. Mating of animals of same breed but having no common ancestor on either side of their pedigree for 4-6 generations
D. Inbreeding	4. Mating of animals of different species

Codes

	A	B	C	D		A	B	C	D
(a)	1	2	3	4	(b)	4	3	2	1
(c)	3	2	4	1	(d)	2	4	3	1

13 Which of the following statements represents the qualities of culturable fishes?

I. Ability to feed on natural as well as artificial food diet.
II. Ability to tolerate a sudden change in climatic condition.
III. Omnivorous in nature.
IV. Slow growing.

Choose the correct option.

(a) II and III (b) II and IV (c) I and II (d) III and IV

Assertion and Reason

Direction (Q. Nos. 14-21) *In each of the following questions, a statement of Assertion (A) is given followed by the corresponding statement of Reason (R). Of the statement, mark the correct answer as*

(a) Both A and R are true and R is the correct explanation of A
(b) Both A and R are true, but R is not the correct explanation of A
(c) A is true, but R is false
(d) A is false, but R is true
(e) Both A and R are false

14 **Assertion** (A) Honey is an animal product produced by honeybee.

Reason (R) Honey contains only sugar nothing else.

15 **Assertion** (A) India ranks fifth in the world in cattle population, but figures poorly in milk production.

Reason (R) Buffaloes give more milk with higher fat and mineral contents than cows.

16 **Assertion** (A) Techniques called superovulation and embryo transplantation are used for cattle improvement.

Reason (R) Gonadotropin injection releases more than one ova (superovulation) in high yielding cows.

17 **Assertion** (A) An interspecific hybrid of the male ass and the mare is a sterile mule.

Reason (R) Mule is inferior to the parents as a beast of burden.

18 **Assertion** (A) The honeybee queen copulates only once in life.

Reason (R) It can lay both fertilised and unfertilised eggs.

19 **Assertion** (A) Fish meal is a rich source of protein for cattle and poultry.

Reason (R) It is produced from non-edible parts of fishes like fins and tail.

20 **Assertion** (A) Ranikhet disease is the disease of poultry.

Reason (R) It is caused by a virus.

21 **Assertion** (A) Cattle breeds can be improved by superovulation and embryo transplantation.

Reason (R) Superovulation in high milk-yielding cows is induced by hormonal injection.

(C) Medical Entrances' Gallery

(Collection of Questions Asked in NEET & in Various Medical Entrance Exams)

1 By which method was a new breed 'Hisardale' of sheep formed by using Bikaneri ewes and Marino rams? **[UK PMT 2014, NEET 2020]**
(a) Mutational breeding (b) Cross breeding
(c) Inbreeding (d) Outcrossing

2 Inbreeding depression is **[NEET 2020, 2019]**
(a) reduced motility and immunity due to close inbreeding
(b) decreased productivity due to mating of superior male and inferior female
(c) decrease in body mass of progeny due to continued close inbreeding
(d) reduced fertility and productivity due to continued close breeding

3 Select the incorrect statement regarding inbreeding. **[NEET 2019]**
(a) Inbreeding helps in the elimination of deleterious alleles from the population
(b) Inbreeding is necessary to evolve a pureline in any animal
(c) Continued inbreeding reduces fertility and leads to inbreeding depression
(d) Inbreeding depression cannot be overcome by outcrossing

4 Homozygous purelines in cattle can be obtained by
(a) mating of related individuals of same breed **[NEET 2017]**
(b) mating of unrelated individuals of same breed
(c) mating of individuals of different breeds
(d) mating of individuals of different species

5 One of the breeding techniques useful to eliminate harmful recessive genes by selection is **[JIPMER 2017]**
(a) artificial insemination (b) outbreeding
(c) inbreeding (d) MOET

6 Interspecific hybridisation is the mating of **[NEET 2016]**
(a) animals within same breed without having common ancestors
(b) two different related species
(c) superior males and females of different breeds
(d) more closely related individuals within same breed for 4-6 generations

7 Choose the set of bacterial diseases in poultry.
(a) Ranikhet and Marek's **[EAMCET 2016]**
(b) Ranikhet and Fowl cholera
(c) Fowl cholera and infectious coryza
(d) Aflatoxicosis and Trush

8 Fish selected for culture practices must possess some features to make culture profitable. Identify the wrong one. **[EAMCET 2016]**
(a) Fast growth rate (b) Late maturity
(b) Disease resistance (d) High nutritious value

9 The red jungle fowl is **[AMU 2015]**
(a) *Gallus gallus* (b) *Pavo cristatus*
(c) *Choriotis nigriceps* (d) *Raja hamsa*

10 Silk is the product of **[Chhattisgarh PMT 2015]**
(a) salivary gland of larva (b) cuticle of the adult
(c) cuticle of the larva (d) salivary gland of the adult

11 Who is referred as Father of Pearl Industry? **[AMU 2015]**
(a) Ivanovsky (b) Louis Pasteur
(c) Kokichi Mikimoto (d) Harvey

12 Obtaining fishes from random water bodies is **[Chhattisgarh PMT 2015]**
(a) culture fishery (b) capture fishery
(c) pisciculture (d) ichthyology

13 In which method of animal breeding, two different species of male and female animals are mated? **[J&K CET 2014]**
(a) Cross breeding (b) Interspecific hybridisation
(c) Outbreeding (d) Outcrossing

14 Making two varieties of a cattle breed like red dane which have no common ancestors on either sides of their pedigree upto 4-6 generations is an example for **[KCET 2014**
(a) inbreeding
(b) cross breeding
(c) outcrossing
(d) interspecific hybridisation

15 One of these protozoans is threat to apiculture and sericulture. **[AIIMS 2013]**
(a) *Eimeria* (b) *Ceratium*
(c) *Nosema* (d) *Monocystis*

16 Which one of the following is a breed of cattle? **[AMU 2012]**
(a) Ayrshire (b) Ghagus (c) Kadaknath (d) Scampi

17 Which of the following pairs is mismatched? **[UP CPMT 2012]**
(a) *Pila globosa* - Pearl (b) *Apis indica* - Honey
(c) *Kenia lacca* - Lac (d) *Bombyx mori* - Silk

18 Which one of the following poultry birds is not an English breed? **[WB JEE 2012]**
(a) Sussex (b) Australorp
(c) Orpington (d) Aseel

19 Percentage composition of fibrin and sericin in silk is **[WB JEE 2010]**
(a) 50 : 40 (b) 80 : 20
(c) 30 : 70 (d) 40 : 60

ANSWERS

Check Point 18.1

1. (d)	2. (c)	3. (d)	4. (d)	5. (b)

Check Point 18.2

1. (b)	2. (c)	3. (a)	4. (a)	5. (b)

Check Point 18.3

1. (c)	2. (c)	3. (a)	4. (d)	5. (c)	6. (d)	7. (b)

(A) Topical Exercise

1. (b)	2. (c)	3. (d)	4. (a)	5. (a)	6. (c)	7. (c)	8. (a)	9. (c)	10. (c)
11. (b)	12. (a)	13. (d)	14. (d)	15. (d)	16. (d)	17. (c)	18. (a)	19. (d)	20. (b)
21. (c)	22. (b)	23. (b)	24. (a)	25. (d)	26. (c)	27. (c)	28. (b)	29. (b)	30. (b)
31. (b)	32. (b)	33. (c)	34. (a)	35. (d)	36. (c)	37. (a)	38. (c)	39. (d)	40. (a)
41. (c)	42. (a)	43. (c)	44. (a)	45. (d)	46. (d)	47. (a)	48. (a)	49. (d)	50. (d)

(B) Cumulative Exercise

1. (a)	2. (b)	3. (d)	4. (c)	5. (b)	6. (a)	7. (b)	8. (d)	9. (a)	10. (b)
11. (a)	12. (c)	13. (c)	14. (c)	15. (b)	16. (b)	17. (c)	18. (b)	19. (b)	20. (a)
21. (b)									

(C) Medical Entrances' Gallery

1. (b)	2. (d)	3. (d)	4. (a)	5. (c)	6. (b)	7. (c)	8. (b)	9. (a)	10. (a)
11. (c)	12. (b)	13. (b)	14. (c)	15. (c)	16. (a)	17. (a)	18. (d)	19. (b)	

Explanations

(A) Topical Exercise

1 (*b*) Animal husbandry is a branch of agriscience. It is the science of breeding, feeding and tending domestic animals.

2 (*c*) Whereas Gir, Rathi and Vechur are Milch breeds (yield milk) of cow.

Option (c) is odd one out because

Kangayam is a drought breed (labour in field) of cows.

3 (*d*) Statement in option (d) is incorrect and can be corrected as

Milch breeds also known as milk breeds of cows which produce high milk. The examples of Indian Milch breeds are Sahiwal, Gir, Deoni and Red Sindhi. Nageri is not a Milch breed, it is Drought breed of cows.

Rest statements are correct.

6 (*c*) Both statements I and II are true.

Buffaloes are considered better than cows because they are more resistant to diseases, they give more milk. Their milk has more protein and fat content than cow. They also live longer having average age of about 25 years whereas cow has average age of 20 years. Murrah breeds of buffaloes are mostly in demand.

7 (*c*) The Merino sheep have been imported for improving indigenous breeds. The merino sheep are the most economically influenced breeds. This breed is originated from Spain.

8 (*a*) Statement I is true, but II is false. Incorrect statement can be corrected as

Famous Angora wool is obtained from Angora goat known as Mohair.

9 (*c*) Long neck of camel is due to development of extra bony plates between successive neck vertebrae. Their long necks are excellent adaptations, so as to help them reach out for their food and water sources without bending their body or legs much.

15 (*d*) Inbreeding increases homozygosity, i.e. state of possessing two identical alleles, one inherited from each parent. It is necessary if we want to evolve a pureline in any animal. Inbreeding exposes harmful recessive genes that are eliminated by selection. It also helps in accumulation of superior genes and elimination of less desirable genes.

16 (*d*) Both statements I and II are false and can be corrected as

- Animals which are similar in characters, general appearance, features, etc., belong to same breed.
- Pureline can be obtained by inbreeding.

20 (*b*) FSH hormone is provided for follicular maturation.

22 (*b*) Statement I is false, but II is true. Incorrect statement can be corrected as

- Bull semen for the purpose of artificial insemination is stored in liquid nitrogen at -196°C.

24 (*a*) Statement I is true, but II is false. Incorrect statement can be corrected as

- Hinny is the reciprocal cross hybrid, i.e. male horse and female donkey.

26 (*c*) In this case, more number of genes for high yielding milk are inherited from both the parents. It is practiced under outcrossing and cross breeding.

29 (*b*) Statement I is false, but II is true. Incorrect statement can be corrected as

- Rinderpest is also known as cattle plague.

30 (*b*) Babesiosis is a tick borne disease of cattle caused by *Babesia bigemina* and *Babesia bovis* and is transmitted by the tick vector *Boophilus microplus.*

31 (*b*) Pathogens mentioned in points II, III and V cause damage to poultry industry.

Infectious coryza - *Haemophilus gallinarum*

Moniliasis - *Odium albicans*

Tick fever - Borrelia

Thus, option (b) is correct.

32 (*b*) All the given symptoms are of infectious coryza disease of poultry birds. It is caused by a bacterium, *Haemophilus gallinarum.*

37 (*a*) Statement I is true, but II is false because

Fish farming or Pisciculture consist raising fish commercially in tanks or enclosures like fish ponds. Gelatin or gelatine is derived from collagen obtained from various animals byproducts. It is usually obtained from cows or pigs.

42 (*a*) Sericulture is the practice of rearing silkworms for production of raw silk. The entire practice from silk to silk, can be classified into four interdependent agro-industrial activities.

Mulberry forming for leaf production. Silkworms rearing and cocoon production.

44 (*a*) Statement I is true, but II is false. Swarming is found in honeybee. Royal jelly is a substance, produced by honeybees to feed to developing larvae.

(B) Cumulative Exercise

1 (*a*) All the statements are incorrect except IV. These can be corrected as

In the poultry industry, production of hatching egg is more expensive because it requires optimum temperature for incubation, but the major factor is the weight of the hatching egg and chick weight. Under optimal egg storage and incubation conditions, chick weight is 67-69 per cent of egg weight at setting.

Therefore, the more uniform the egg weight, the more uniform the chick weight. Breeder uniformity determines uniformity in the hatching eggs produced, the more uniform the breeder flock, the more uniform the egg weights. Hence, some of the eggs produced by hatchery flocks are not acceptable for incubation and is rejected.

4 (*c*) Statements III and IV are incorrect and can be corrected as

- MOET is for herd improvement in animals like cattle, sheep, buffaloes, etc.
- Interspecific hybridisation refers to crossing between male and female animals of two different species.

Rest of the statements are correct.

5 (*b*) Inbreeding involves

- Identification of superior males and superior females of the same breed.
- Mating of the superior animals.
- Progeny obtained from such mating are evaluated and assessed for the desirable traits.
- It should be kept in mind that a superior cow or buffalo is that which gives more milk per lactation. Similarly, a superior bull is that which gives rise to superior progeny as compared to those of other bulls.
- This process of mating of superior progenies is continued for 4-6 generations.

Thus, option (b) is correct.

6 (*a*) Statements I and II are correct, while III and IV are incorrect. Incorrect statements can be corrected as

- Controlled breeding experiments are carried out by artificial insemination, multiple ovulation embryo transfer, transgenesis, etc.
- Cattle breeds can be improved by outbreeding.

7 (*b*) Statements I and III are correct, while II and IV are incorrect. Incorrect statements can be corrected as

- Manure is not in dairy management. It is used in plant breeding.
- Weeding is also a procedure of plant breeding.

10 (*b*) Statements I, III and IV are correct, while II is incorrect. Incorrect statement can be corrected as

Light management is not related to bee-keeping.

11 (*a*) Statements I and II are correct, while III and IV are incorrect. Incorrect statements can be corrected as

- Outbreeding is the breeding between the animals of the same breed, but no common ancestors or different breeds or different species.
- Crosses between the same breeds are called inbreeding.

13 (*c*) Statements I and II are correct, while III and IV are incorrect. Incorrect statements can be corrected as

- Culturable fishes are herbivorous.
- They are also fast growing.

14 (*c*) A is true, but R is false because

Honey is a viscous sugary fluid formed by the nectar within the stomach of the honeybee. The bee visits flowers, sucks the nectar, stores it in the stomach and returns to hive. Honey contains many different substances of importance to human beings. These are levulose, dextrose, maltose and other sugars, enzyme , pigments, ash, water, vitamins, minerals, etc.

15 (*b*) Both A and R are true, but R is not the correct explanation of A.

The best Indian breeds are found in dried part of the country. There are 26 breeds of cattle, but the milk production is very poor. Number of buffaloes is one third of cows, but their milk yield is better. Buffalo milk is superior to cow's milk in fat content as well as minerals, etc.

16 (*b*) Both A and R are true, but R is not the correct explanation of A.

Superovulation (more ova and hence, more embryos), help in improving the improve breeds. Artificial breeding is done through artificial insemination. It involves the introduction of semen of selected bull artificially, when the cow is in its heat period. The gonadotropin injection is an effective method for artificial insemination.

17 (*c*) A is true, but R is false because

A mule is a hybrid of male donkey (jack) and a female horse (mare). The hybrid from the reciprocal cross is called Hinny. Mule shows hybrid vigour. They are sterile, larger than the donkeys and sturdier than the horses.

18 (*b*) Both A and R are true, but R is not the correct explanation of A.

It is said that the queen gets mated only once in her life, but in a single chance of mating it lays about 1500-2000 eggs in a day. After mating the queen lays eggs in one brood cell. The larvae emerge out from both the fertilised as well as unfertilised eggs. Thus, the larvae from the unfertilised eggs form the drones while the worker is developed from the larvae of fertilised eggs.

19 (*b*) Both A and R are true, but R is not the correct explanation of A.

Fish meal is prepared from the wastes of fish oil or canning industry or from the whole fish of non-oil-type. Wastes of cod industry are known as white 'fish meal'. The protein content of this meal is highly digestible, nutritive and is of biological importance. This fish meal also contains calcium, phospholipids and iodine, fish meal is also used as major food of domestic animals like pigs, poultry and cattle.

20 (*a*) Both A and R are true and R is the correct explanation of A.

The most common disease amongst fowls (poultry) is Ranikhet disease, which is caused by a filter passing virus. In this disease, bird opens the beak, becomes thirsty, suffer from fever and yellowish diarrhoea occurs.

21 (*b*) Both A and R are true, but R is not the correct explanation of A.

Superovulation is induced by hormone injection. Superovulation and embryo transplantation techniques have been used in India for cattle improvement.

(C) Medical Entrances' Gallery

1 (*b*) Hisardale is a new breed and of sheep developed in Punjab by crossing Bikaneri ewes and Marino rams. In cross-breeding, superior male of one breed is mated with superior female of another breed.

2 (*d*) Inbreeding depression is continued inbreeding, especially close breeding which reduces fertility and even productivity in animals. This problem is usually overcome by outbreeding.

3 (*d*) The statement in option (d) is incorrect regarding inbreeding and can be corrected as

Inbreeding depression can be overcome by outcrossing.
As continuous inbreeding among cattle causes inbreeding depression. It decreases the fertility and even productivity of an animal. In this, mating is done between different breeds or individuals of the same breed but having no common ancestors upto 4-6 generations.

4 (*a*) When closely related species of same breed are crossed continuously for few successive generations (inbreeding), it increases the homozygosity and purelines can be obtained. This leads to the reduction in the variation within a group and stabilisation of a particular type (i.e. pureline).

5 (*c*) When breeding is done between animals of the same breed for 4-6 generations, it is called inbreeding. Inbreeding is necessary if we want to develop a pureline of any animal. It exposes harmful recessive genes that are eliminated by selection. It also helps in accumulation of superior genes and elimination of less desirable genes.

6 (*b*) The process of interspecific hybridisation is the mating or cross between two different related species belonging to the same genus, e.g. mule is the result of cross between female horse and male donkey.

7 (*c*) Fowl cholera and infectious coryza are bacterial diseases of poultry.

Whereas Ranikhet is a viral disease. Aflatoxicosis is a fungal disease. Marek's disease, coccidiosis and scaly legs are other diseases found in poultry.

8 (*b*) Fishes selected for culture practices should have a fast growth rate, high nutrition value, disease resistance and ability to mature early. Thus, option (b) is wrong one.

13 (*b*) Interspecific hybridisation is the practice of animal breeding in which male of one species is mated with the female of another species, e.g. mule is the result of cross between female horse and male donkey.

14 (*c*) Outcrossing is the phenomenon of mating of two animals within the same breed having no common ancestors on either sides of their pedigree upto 4-6 generations, while inbreeding is the crossing of closely related animals within the same breed for 4-6 generations. Cross breeding is the breeding of superior males of one breed with superior female of another breed, e.g. Hisardale and interspecific hybridisation is the mating of animals of two different species.

15 (*c*) *Nosema,* a protozoan, a threat to apiculture and sericulture, was discovered by Pasteur (1865). It causes chronic disease pebrine.

17 (*a*) Pair in option (a) is incorrectly matched and can be corrected as

Pinctada vulgaris is a bivalve from which pearl is obtained. A pearl due to its delicate appearance and shine has retained its position as a costly ornamented object.

Rest pairs are correctly matched.

CHAPTER 19

Microbes in Human Welfare

Microorganisms are the major components of biological system on earth. They are present everywhere, i.e. in soil, water, air, inside our bodies and in that of other living organisms. They even exist on sites where no other lifeform could possibly exist. For example, highly saline or highly acidic atmosphere, under layers of snow and even deep inside the thermal vents.

Microbes play an important role in various chemical reactions and help human beings in various ways. In this chapter, we will discuss about the varied roles of microbes in different fields.

Inside

MICROBES IN HOUSEHOLD PRODUCTS

For thousands of years, the microorganisms have been used to make products such as curd, cheese, butter, vinegar and alcohol, etc.

Some important products produced by microorganisms are given below

Curd

- It is prepared by the action of *Lactobacillus*, which is commonly called **Lactic Acid Bacteria** (LAB). It grows in milk and convert it into curd.
- LAB produces some enzymes (e.g. lactase) that coagulate and partially digest the milk proteins. It helps to improve the nutritional quality of curd by increasing vitamin-B_{12} and organic acid content in it.
- LAB also plays a beneficial role in checking the growth of disease causing microbes in our stomach.

Yoghurt

- It is produced by fermenting whole milk with a mixture of *Streptococcus thermophilus* and *Lactobacillus bulgaricus* at 40-46° C.
- It has the flavour of lactic acid and acetaldehyde. It is rich in protein, calcium, riboflavin, vitamin-B_6 and vitamin-B_{12}.

Cheese

It is one of the oldest food items in which microbes are used. This is formed by coagulation of the milk protein, casein.

Different microbes impart different properties in cheese are as follows

- The large holes in '**Swiss cheese**' are due to the production of a large amount of CO_2 by a bacterium, *Propionibacterium shermanii.*
- The '**Roquefort cheese**' is ripened by growing *Penicillium roqueforti* on them. It gives them a particular flavour.
- In order to prepare special cheese, such as **blue Roquefort** and **soft Camembert**, the blue mould *Penicillium* is commonly used.

Bread

- *Saccharomyces cerevisiae*, the common yeast is used in baking bread. It converts the sugars present in dough into carbon dioxide.
- During the bread making process, yeast is mixed with flour, salt and warm water or milk. The dough is kneaded and left to swell up. Swelling of dough during bread making is called **leavening.**
- Yeast acts as a leavening agent by secreting enzymes such as amylase, maltase and zymase.

Butter

- The microorganisms such as *Streptococcus lactis* and *Leuconostoc citrivorum* are used to prepare butter by churning sweet or sour cream.
- The characteristic butter aroma develops due to a volatile substance–diacetyl.
- It is produced by the action of *Streptococcus* on pasteurised milk.

Other food products

Various food products of daily life are prepared using microbes. These include:

- A number of traditional drinks and foods are made through fermentation by the microbes. For example, '**toddy**', a traditional drink in some parts of Southern India is made by fermenting sap from unopened spadices of *Caryota urens* (palms).
- Dosa and idli are fermented by bacteria like *Leuconostoc* and *Streptococcus* species.
- Microbes are also used to ferment fish, soybean and bamboo shoots to make food items. For example, soju and tofu are cheese-like products of soybean. These are obtained after fermentation by *Mucor* species. Similarly, **tempeh** is an Indonesian food formed by fermentation.

MICROBES IN SEWAGE TREATMENT

- A large quantity of wastewater is generated every day in cities and towns. The major component of this wastewater is human excreta. It also contains large amounts of organic matter and pathogenic microbes.
- This huge quantity of sewage or urban wastewater is not discharged directly into natural water bodies like rivers and streams. It is first treated and made less polluted by passing it through **Sewage Treatment Plants** (STPs).
- In this, treatment of wastewater is done by the heterotrophic microbes which is naturally present in the sewage.
- The treatment of sewage is carried out in following stages

Primary treatment

- It is a **physical** process that involves physical removal of large as well as small particles from the sewage. It is done through filtration and sedimentation in primary settling tanks.
- Initially, the floating debris is removed by sequential filtration. Then, soil and small pebbles are removed by sedimentation.
- The primary treatment generates primary sludge and effluent.
- All solids undergo sedimentation and settle down to constitute the **primary sludge**. It is treated *via* sludge digestion. This sludge can also be disposed by several ways. It can be used to produce biogas also.
- The supernatant left after removing primary sludge, constitutes the effluent. This effluent is taken out for secondary treatment.

Secondary or Biological treatment

It involves microbial degradation of organic matter.

It is carried out in following steps

- The primary effluent is passed into large **aeration tanks**, where it is constantly agitated mechanically.
- Air is constantly pumped into the effluent. This allows a vigorous growth of aerobic microbes into **flocs**. These are the masses of bacteria associated with fungal filaments to form mesh-like structures.
- While growing, these microbes consume the major part of the organic matter present in the effluent. It significantly reduces the **BOD** (Biochemical Oxygen Demand) of effluent.

Note
- *BOD refers to the amount of oxygen that would be consumed if all the organic matter in one litre of water is oxidised by bacteria.*
- *The BOD test measures the rate of uptake of oxygen by the microorganisms in a sample of water. It helps to measure the amount of organic matter present in the water. The greater the BOD of wastewater, more is its polluting potential.*

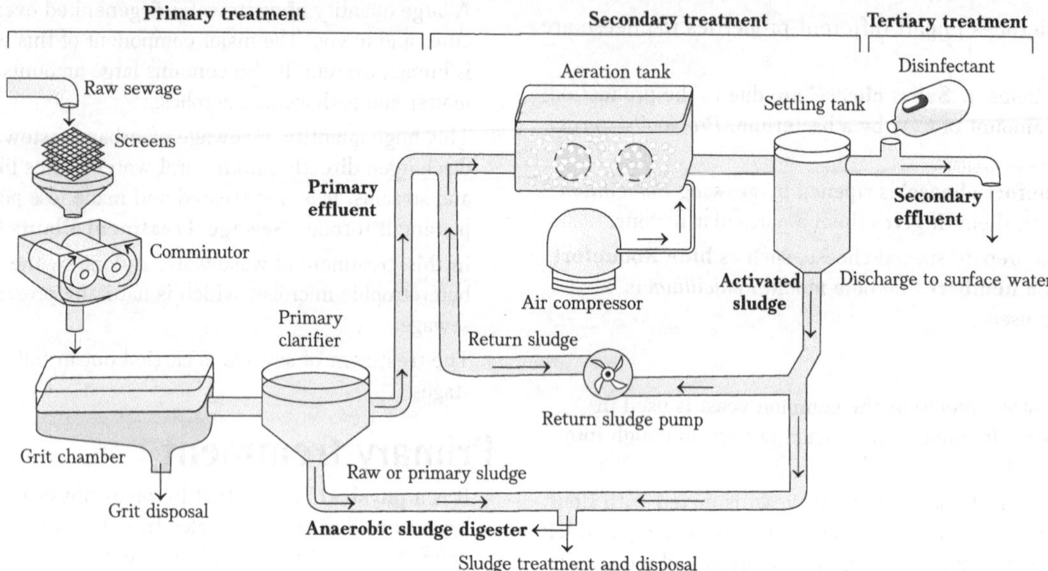

Fig. 19.1 Sewage treatment plant

- The sewage water is further treated till the BOD reduces significantly.
- Then, the effluent of aeration tank is passed into a settling tank, where the bacterial 'flocs' are allowed to sediment. This sediment is called **activated sludge**.
- A small part of the activated sludge is pumped back into the aeration tank to serve as bacterial inoculum.
- The remaining major part of the sludge is pumped into large tanks called **anaerobic sludge digesters**. Here, methanogenic bacteria, which grow anaerobically, digest the bacteria and fungi present in the sludge.

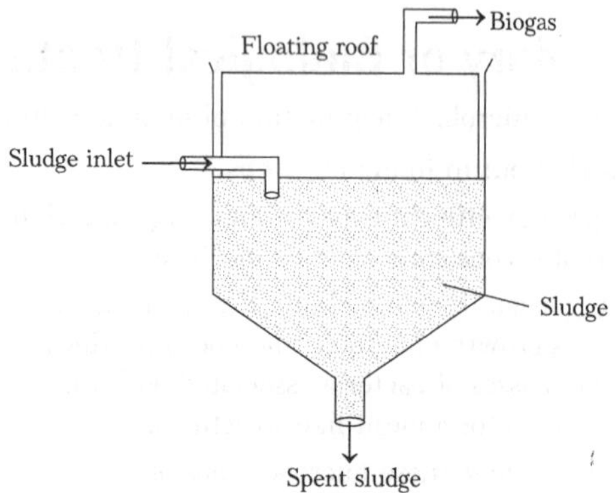

Fig. 19.2 Anaerobic sludge digester

- During this digestion, bacteria produce a mixture of gases such as methane, hydrogen sulphide and carbon dioxide. These gases form biogas which can be used as a source of energy as it is inflammable.
- The effluent from the secondary treatment plant is generally released into natural water bodies like rivers and streams.

Tertiary treatment

It is a physico-chemical process. It involves disinfecting the water if it is to be used for domestic purposes. It is done by various methods such as reverse osmosis, treating with chlorine, ozone gas or perchlorate salts.

Note *The Ministry of Environment and Forests has initiated Ganga Action Plan (GAP, 1986) and Yamuna Action Plan (YAP, 1993) to save the major rivers of our country from pollution. Under these plans, it is proposed to build a large number of sewage treatment plants so that only treated sewage may be discharged in the rivers.*

Biogas or Gobar gas

- Biogas is a methane rich fuel gas. It is produced by the anaerobic breakdown or digestion of biomass with the help of methanogenic bacteria, *Methanobacterium.*
- **Composition** It is predominantly composed of methane (50-70%), carbon dioxide (30-40%), traces of hydrogen sulphide, nitrogen and hydrogen (10%).
  The energy released from biogas depends upon the proportion of methane present in it. If biogas contains 50% methane, its calorific value is 4430 Kcal/m3

Production of biogas

- The biogas production was first started in India by the joint efforts of **Indian Agricultural Research Institute** (IARI) and **Khadi** and **Village Industries Commission** (KVIC).
- **Biogas plant** It is a large concrete airtight cylindrical tank containing digester. It is povided with the inlet and outlet holders.

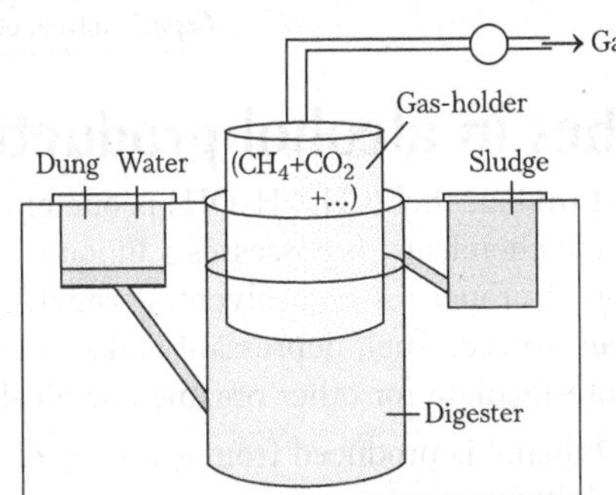

- **Raw material** Biogas is produced using animal and plant wastes. These contain a large amount of glucose in the form of cellulose. It is utilised by the microbes to produce methane gas. Cattle dung is the most important substrate for biogas production as it contains cellulose as well as *Methanobacterium* and other methanogens.

The process of biogas production

(i) **Solubilisation** Lipids, proteins, cellulose, hemicellulose, etc., present in organic matter are decomposed into monomers. It is done by the action of hydrolytic enzymes like lipases, cellulases, proteases, peptidases, etc., secreted by microorganisms.

(ii) **Acidogenesis** Conversion of monomers to organic acids with the help of fermentative microbes, e.g. *Propionibacterium, Acetovibrio,* etc. The most common organic acid produced by these microbes is acetic acid.

(iii) **Methanogenesis** Biogas production by the action of methanogens, e.g. *Methanococcus, Methanobacillus,* etc.

Chemical reactions involved in the above described proceses are as follows

(i) $CO_2 + H_2O \longrightarrow CO_2 + H_2$

(ii) $CO_2 + 4H_2 \longrightarrow \underset{\text{Methane}}{CH_4} + 2H_2O$

(iii) $\underset{\text{Acetic acid}}{CH_3COOH} \longrightarrow CH_4 + CO_2$

CHECK POINT 19.1

1. Which of the following is true?
   (a) Viruses can be grown on artificial culture medium
   (b) Cheese can be ripened using *Penicillium* strain
   (c) Curd is made with the help of *Mucor*
   (d) All of the above
2. *Streptococcus lactis* perform same function as
   (a) *Saccharomyces*
   (b) *Leuconostoc citrivorum*
   (c) *Bacillus licheniformis*
   (d) *Trichoderma reesei*
3. A sewage treatment process in which a part of decomposer bacteria present in the wastes is recycled into the starting of the process is called
   (a) cyclic treatment
   (b) activated sludge treatment
   (c) primary treatment
   (d) tertiary treatment
4. Formation of biogas is a three step sequential anaerobic processes involving
   (a) Solubilisation → Acidogenesis → Methanogenesis
   (b) Acidogenesis → Methanogenesis → Abiogenesis
   (c) Methanogenesis → Solubilisation → Acidogenesis
   (d) Solubilisation → Methanogenesis → Acidogenesis
5. *Methanobacterium* acts anaerobically on cellulose to produce
   (a) $H_2 + CO_2$ (b) $CH_4 + CO_2 + H_2$
   (c) $CH_4 + H_2$ (d) $CH_4 + NH_3$

MICROBES IN INDUSTRY

The fermentative ability of microbes is used on industrial scale to produce a number of products such as enzymes, antibiotics, beverages, medicines, etc.

For the large scale production of these products, large vessels called **fermentors** are used.

An account of these products is discussed below

Microbes in biofuels production

- Biofuels are fuels of biological origin, which are used for the production of heat and other forms of energy. The energy derived from the biofuels is called **bioenergy**.
- Biologically generated hydrogen, methane, ethanol, butanol and diesel are referred as biohydrogen, biomethane, bioethanol, biobutanol and biodiesel, respectively. All of these are considered as **biofuels**.
- Various microorganisms used in the production of biofuels are listed below

Table 19.1 Biofuels and related microorganisms

Biofuels	Substrates	Microorganism(s)
Bioethanol	Starch, sugar crops	*Bacillus licheniformis* (amylase activity)
	Cellulosic wastes	*Saccharomyces cerevisiae*, *Zymomonas* (sugar fermentation)
	(a) Enzyme hydrolysis	*Trichoderma reesei* (cellulase)
		S. cerevisiae (hexose fermentation)
		Recombinant *E. coli* (pentose fermentation)
		Clostridium sp., *Fusarium oxysporum* (consolidated processing)
	(b) Acid hydrolysis	*S. cerevisiae*, *Zymomonas* (for fermentation) *Clostridium ljungdahlii*
Biomethane	Farm and human wastes, municipal solid wastes, effluents from food and dairy industries, etc.	A group of anaerobic microorganisms
Biobutanol	Soluble carbohydrates	*Clostridium acetobutylicum*, *C. beijerinckii*
Biohydrogen	Sunlight and water sugars and fatty acids (from starch, cellulose)	*Chlamydomonas reinhardtii*, *C. moewusii*, anerobic bacteria like *Clostridium*
Biodiesel	Sunlight and carbon dioxide	*Monoraphidium minutum*, *Cyclotella cryptica*, *Euphorbia* plants, *Copaifera* tree, etc.

Microbes in alcohol production

Ethanol or Ethyl alcohol (CH_3CH_2OH) is one of the most exotic organic chemicals. It possesses a unique combination of properties as a solvent, germicide, beverage, antifreeze, fuel, depressant and as a versatile chemical intermediate for other organic chemicals.

Alcohol or ethanol is produced from a variety of raw material as follows

- Agricultural products such as grain, molasses, fruit, whey and sulphite waste liquor.
- The most widely used sugar for ethanol fermentation is blackstrap molasses. It contain about 35-40% sucrose, 15-20% invert sugars such as glucose and fructose and 28-35% of non-sugar solids.
- Ethanol (alcohol) production in industries is carried out by both yeasts as well as bacteria.

Alcohol production by yeasts

Various species of yeast are used for the fermentation of carbohydrate. These are *Saccharomyces cerevisiae* (Brewer's yeast and Baker's yeast), *S. uvarum*, *Kluyveromyces marxianus*, *S. ellipsoideus* (wine yeast), *S. sake* (sake yeast) *S. pireformis* (ginger yeast), etc.

The steps in alcohol production are as follows

- Yeast is grown in very large vessels called **fermenters**.
- The fermenter is filled with a nutrient solution such as sugars (e.g. sugarcane, sugarbeets), starches (e.g. grains, potatoes) and cellulose (e.g. wood and paper mill).
- It is then inoculated with a pure culture of yeast.
- Temperature and pH of the media are adjusted and alcohol is produced along with CO_2 and energy.
- The whole process of breakdown of carbohydrates by yeast into carbon dioxide and alcohol in the absence of oxygen is summarised as follows

$$C_6H_{12}O_6 + \text{Yeast} \longrightarrow 2C_2H_5OH + CO_2 + \text{Energy}$$

Alcohol production by bacteria

- Great number of bacteria are capable of ethanol fermentation. The important ethanol producing bacteria are *Clostridium sporogenes, Clostridium indolis, Clostridium sphenoides, Zygomonas mobilis, Spirochaeta stenostrepta, Leuconostoc mesenteroides, Spirochaeta litoralis* and *Erwinia amylovora.*
- When fermentation is over, the microbial mass (cells, mycelia and conidia) is separated from the fluid. The fluid contains the mixture of ethanol, water and small amount of alcohols and ether.
- Ethanol is recovered by **distillation** process, i.e. vapourisation of ethanol/water mixture.
- Different types of alcoholic drinks can be obtained, depending upon the type of raw material used for fermentation and the type of processing, i.e. with or without distillation.
- Wine and beer are produced without distillation, whereas whisky, brandy and rum are produced by distillation. The table given below gives an account of alcoholic drinks and concentration of alcohol in them.

Table 19.2 Some fermented beverages their sources and alcohol content

Beverages	Produced from	Alcohol contents
Beer	*Hordeum vulgare* (barley) malt	4-8%
Wine	Grapes	10-20%
Gin	European rye, i.e. *Secale cereale*	30%
Rum	Molasses of sugarcane	40%
Whisky	Fermented cereal	50%
Vodka	Potato	60-80%
Brandy	Fruit juices	60-70%

Microbes in organic acid production

Certain microbes possess the ability to convert carbohydrates into organic acids. Thus, these microbes can be used in the industrial production of organic acids.

Various types of organic acids produced by microorganisms are given below

Lactic acid

- The first organic acid produced by fermentation was lactic acid. It is produced by the action of bacteria, (e.g. *Streptococcus lactis, Lactobacillus delbreckii, L. bulgaricus*) and fungus (*Rhizopus*) on hydrolysed corn, potato starch, molasses and sulphite liquor, etc.
- Lactic acid is commercially produced from pasteurised whey (the watery part of milk).
- **Use** It may be used in various industries such as confectionary, soft drinks, pickles and preservation of fruits/vegetables, canned fish, curing of meat, tannery, dye industry and medicines, etc.

Citric acid

- It was first isolated in 1784 by the Swedish chemist **Carl Wilhelm Scheele**. He crystallised citric acid from lemon juice. Industrially, citric acid is produced by fungus *Aspergillus niger* by the fermentation of sucrose or glucose containing medium.
- **Use** It is naturally present in citrus fruits and acts as a natural preservative for food. It adds acidic or sour taste to food and soft drinks.

Acetic acid

- Vinegar or acetic acid is an early microbial product used by man. It is a liquid substance consisting mainly of acetic acid and water.
- This is obtained by the microbial fermentation of sugary solution.
- It is prepared in two steps
  (i) Conversion of sugars into alcohols by yeast (*Saccharomyces cerevisiae*).
  (ii) Conversion of alcohol to acetic acid by the action of bacteria, *Acetobacter* (*A. orieansis, A. acetii* and *A. schuizenbachi*, etc).
- The process of vinegar formation is represented by the following equation

$$C_6H_{12}O_6 \xrightarrow{\text{Zymase (yeast)}} 2C_2H_5OH + 2H_2O$$

$$C_2H_5OH + O_2 \xrightarrow{\textit{Acetobacter}} \underset{\text{Acetic acid}}{CH_3COOH} + H_2O$$

- **Use** Vinegar is commonly used in food preparation such as mustard sauce, ketchups, mayonnaise, pickles condiment, etc. It is used for flavouring potato chips and as a preservative for meat and vegetables.
- The vinegar produced from the jamun (or rose apple) fruit in India is considered to be medicinally valuable for stomach, spleen and diabetic ailments.

Kojic acid

- It is produced as a result of fermentation carried out by *Aspergillus oryzae.*
- **Use** The acid is used for skin whitening and as a precursor for the synthesis of flavour enhancers.

Gluconic acid

- *Aspergillus niger* and *Penicillium chrysogenum* has been used in industrial production of gluconic acid.
- **Use** It is used as an additive in certain metal cleaning applications. It is also used in the therapy for calcium and iron deficiencies.

Table 19.3 Some other organic acids synthesised by various microbes

Organic acids	Microorganisms
Propionic acid	*Bacterium propioni*
Butyric acid	*Clostridium acetobutyricum*
Oxalic acid	*Aspergillus* sp.
Gallic acid	*Aspergillus niger*
Itaconic acid	*A. terreus*
Some amino acids	*Escherichia coli*

Microbes in enzyme production

Microbes synthesise enzymes that can be extracted from their culture media for commercial uses.

Some of these enzymes are discussed below

Amylase

- The starch digestive enzyme or amylase is synthesised by
  - Bacteria, e.g. *Bacillus diastaticus*, *B. subtilis*.
  - Fungi, e.g. *Aspergillus oryzae*, *A. niger* and *Rhizopus oryzae*.
- **Use** This enzyme is used in cleansing starch stains, desizing fibres, softening and sweetening bread and making alcoholic beverages from starchy substances.

Lipase

- The lipid digestive enzyme lipase is synthesised by microbial fungi such as *Candida lipolytica* (a kind of yeast), *Geotrichum candidum*, *Aspergillus niger* and *Mucor javanicus*, etc.
- **Use** This is used in soap industry for hydrolysing oil stains and in detergents for cleansing fat stains.

Protease

- The protein digestive enzymes is synthesised by
  - Bacteria such as *Bacillus subtilis* and *B. licheniformis*.
  - Fungi such as *Aspergillus oryzae*, *Penicillium roqueforti* and *Mortierella renispora*, etc.
- **Use** This enzyme is used in extracting fish liver oil, meat industry, alcoholic industry, cheese and bread industry, tannary and in glue and detergent making. In detergents, they act by removing proteinaceous spots. Bottled juices are also clarified using proteases.

Pectinase

- Pectin is a carbohydrate found in ripe fruits. Pectinase is a digestive enzyme that is synthesised by fungi, growing on pectin containing media.
- These fungi include *Aspergillus niger* and *Byssochlamys fulvo*.
- **Use** It is used in fruit-pulp juice industry, retting of fibres and fermentation or green coffee.

Streptokinase

- This enzyme is obtained from bacterium *Streptococcus*. The enzyme is also called **Tissue Plasminogen Activator** (TPA).
- **Use** It is used to remove blood clots from the blood vessels of the patients who have suffered myocardial infarction.

Glucose oxidase

- It is extracted from *Aspergillus niger* and *Penicillium notatum*.
- **Use** It is used in diagnostic technique to check blood glucose level and in food industry.

Rennin/Rennet

- It is obtained from fungi *Mucor pusillus* and *Endothia parasitica*.
- **Use** It is used for manufacture of cheese.

Table 19.4 Some other important products of microorganisms

Products	Microorganisms
Cyclosporin-A	
It is an 11-membered cyclic oligopeptide It acts as an immunosuppressive agent that inhibits activation of T-cell response to transplanted organs.	*Trichoderma polysporum* and *Tolypocladium inflatum.*
Statins	
Inhibitor of enzyme HMG Co-A reductase of liver. It lowers LDL cholesterol level.	Yeast—*Monascus purpureus*

Microbes in antibiotic production

Antibiotics are chemical substances that are produced by microorganisms and can kill or inhibit the growth of other disease causing microorganisms. These mainly act by inhibiting the metabolic activities of other microorganisms (mainly bacteria).

Various facts related to antibiotic discovery are as follows

- The term 'antibiotic' was defined by **Waksman** in 1942. A microorganism, which produces an antimicrobial substance is called an **antibiont**.

- The first antibiotic was penicillin (wonder drug). It is a product of the moulds *Penicillium notatum* and *P. chrysogenum.* It was discovered by **Fleming** in 1928.
- **Sir Alexander Fleming** noticed a halo (a plaque or zone of inhibition) of bacterial growth around a contaminant blue-green mould on a *Staphylococcus* culture plate. According to him, the mould released a substance that inhibited bacterial growth. He then grew a pure culture of the mould. Later, discovered that it was *Penicillium notatum,* which secreted this growth inhibitor known as **penicillin**.
- *P. chrysogenum* is a strain previously known as *Penicillium notatum.*
- *P. chrysogenum* has been used in industrially area to produce **penicillin** and **xanthocillin X**. These are used to treat pulp mill waste and to produce the enzymes polyamine oxidase, phosphogluconate dehydrogenase and glucose oxidase.

Till now, a number of antibiotics have been isolated from microorganisms. Some of these antibiotics and their sources are listed below

Table 19.5 Antibiotics and their sources

Antibiotics	Sources	Actions
Penicillin	*Penicillium chrysogenum, P. notatum.*	Tonsilitis, sore throat, gonorrhoea.
Streptomycin	*Streptomyces griseus*	Pneumonia, tuberculosis and local infections
Erythromycin	*Streptomyces erythreus*	Typhoid, diphtheria, whooping cough
Terramycin	*Streptomyces rimosus*	Intestinal and urinary infections
Tetracyclines	*Streptomyces aureofaciens*	Eye infections
Polymixin	*Bacillus polymyxa*	Antifungal

Microbes in healthcare

Microbes have therapeutic properties that are helpful in the treatment of certain diseases such as cancer. They produce insulin, growth hormones and antibodies too. Some of them are described below

(i) ***Clostridium*** selectively targets cancer cells. Various strains of non-pathogenic *Clostridium* have been shown to infiltrate and replicate within solid tumours. *Clostridium,* therefore have the potential to deliver therapeutic proteins to tumours.

(ii) ***Lactobacillus*** species and other lactic acid bacteria possess numerous potential therapeutic properties including anti-inflammatory and anticancer activities. These bacteria are used in the preparation of serum and vaccines.

Serums are effective against diphtheria, pneumonia, etc. Vaccines are effective against typhoid, smallpox, cholera, etc.

(iii) ***Claviceps purpurea*** is a fungus that causes the disease 'Ergot of rye' and yields a drug called **ergot**.

The ergot contains an alkaloid, ergotinine. It also contain many other substances like ergostetrine, ergotonic acid, cornutine, etc.

This drug stimulates muscles of uterus and used to assist childbirth. It is also used to increase blood pressure, control uterine haemorrhage and in many other uterine disturbances.

(iv) ***Acetobacter*** can be used to obtain vitamin-C, i.e. L-ascorbic acid.

(v) **Bacteria** such as *Propionibacterium freudenreichii, Pseudomonas denitrificans, Bacillus megaterium* and *Streptomyces olivaecus* are used to obtain vitamin-B_{12}, i.e. cobalamin.

(vi) ***Ashyba gossypii*** (mould) and *Clostridium butyricum* (bacteria) yields vitamin-B_2, i.e. riboflavin.

Microbes as nutritional supplements

- *Saccharomyces cerevisiae,* which is a deactivated yeast is known as **nutritional supplement organism.**
- It is an excellent source of protein and vitamins, especially B complex.
- The latter is required for metabolism and as cofactor of various enzymes thus, it is essential for growth.
- Nutritional yeast is low in fat and sodium and fortified with vitamin-B_{12}.
- It has a nutty, cheesy flavour that makes it popular as an ingredient in cheese substitutes. It is also used as topping for popcorn, in mashed and fried potatoes, scrambled eggs, etc.
- *Chlorella* (green algae) and *Spirulina* (simple, one-celled organism) are also referred as **sources of protein.**

Note *Probiotics are microorganism, which when administrated in adequate amount confer a health benefit in host, specifically by enhancing digestion.*

CHECK POINT 19.2

1. Brandy is generally a product of
   (a) cider wine (b) larger beer
   (c) grape wine (d) champagne
2. Vinegar is produced by acetic acid bacteria through
   (a) reduction of alcohol
   (b) oxidation of acetic acid
   (c) oxidation of alcohol
   (d) safe antibiotics
3. For the manufacture of gluconic acid and citric acid, which of the following microorganisms is used?
   (a) *Lactobacillus bulgaricus*
   (b) *Acetobacter* sp.
   (c) *Aspergillus niger*
   (d) *Gluconobacter* sp.
4. Proteases can be derived from all these microorganisms except
   (a) *Bacillus subtilis*
   (b) *Penicillium rogueforti*
   (c) *Penicillium chrysogenum*
   (d) *Mortierella reinspora*
5. The enzyme used in retting of fibres is
   (a) pectinase (b) protease
   (c) streptokinase (d) glucose oxidase
6. Which of the following microbes have the potential of deliver therapeutic protiens to tumours?
   (a) *S. cerevisiae* (b) *Claviceps*
   (c) *Clostridium* (d) Both (a) and (c)

MICROBES AS BIOFERTILISERS AND BIOCONTROL AGENTS

Environmental pollution is a major concern in present scenario. The use of chemical fertilisers, herbicides, pesticides, etc., seems to be the major causative factors in it.

Therefore, various products that involve the use of microorganisms are used for sustainable agriculture.

A few of these products are listed below

Biofertilisers

Biofertilisers or biological fertilisers are organisms that have the ability to enrich the nutrient quality of soil. They help crop plants in the uptake of nutrients.

These may also accelerate the microbial process in rhizosphere. It augment the extent of availability of nutrients.

Different groups of organisms are used as biofertilisers. These are given below

Bacteria as biofertiliser

(i) **Free-living nitrogen-fixing bacteria** are found in high concentrations in rhizosphere. They may be aerobic, facultative or anaerobic. These add about 10-25 kg of nitrogen per hectare per annum, e.g. *Azospirillum* and *Azotobacter. Clostridium* is free-living, anaerobic nitrogen-fixing bacteria.

(ii) **Symbiotic nitrogen-fixing bacteria** contain enzyme complex nitrogenase. It reduces atmospheric nitrogen into ammonia for the uptake by plants. They are present in the roots of leguminous plants, e.g. *Rhizobium.*

(iii) **Nitrogen-fixing Actinomycetes** which fix nitrogen in non-leguminous plants such as *Alder*, *Frankia*, *Purshia*, etc.

Cyanobacteria as biofertiliser

- They fix about 20-30 kg of nitrogen per hectare of soil and water. *Anabaena*, *Nostoc*, *Aulosira* are free, living nitrogen-fixing cyanobacteria.
- The water fern, *Azolla* has *Anabaena azollae* as symbiont, which fixes nitrogen within the fronds.

Mycorrhiza as biofertilisers

- Mycorrhizae are the mutualistic association of a fungus and the roots of higher plants. These are found in most of the vascular plants.
- Mycorrhizae absorb phosphorus from the soil and pass it to plants. Plants having mycorrhiza may also show resistance to root borne pathogens, tolerance to salinity and overall growth and development.

Biocontrol agents

- Conventional farming practices implement the use of chemical pesticides including herbicides and insecticides. These are extremely toxic and harmful to human beings as well as environment. Thus, farmers are now moving towards biocontrol agents.
- Biocontrol refers to the use of biological methods for controlling plant diseases and pests. This method of control is dependent on natural predation rather than introduced chemicals.

Biopesticides

Microbes such as bacteria, fungi, viruses, protozoan, etc., and their products are used for pest control. These are known as **biopesticides.**

They are further categorised as follows

1. Bioherbicides

They are organisms, which destroy weeds without harming the useful plants.

Biological control of weed may involve either

- Utilisation of insects - feed selectively on a weed
- Use of certain microorganisms - produce disease in weeds and eliminate them.

Bioherbicides can be further categorised as follows

(i) **Mycoherbicides** These were the first bioherbicides. **Devine** and **Collego** are fungal spores, which are sprayed over weeds for their elimination. These are ideal for marketing because they can tolerate adverse conditions and can remain viable for long periods.

Collego is made up of spores of *Collectotrichum gloeosorioides* and it controls *Aeschynomene virginica* disease in rice and soybean fields.

Devine is made up of spores of *Phytophthora palmivora* and it controls the growth of milk weed in citrus orchards.

(ii) **Predator herbivores** In India and Australia, cochineal insect (*Cactoblastis cactorum*) was used for the control of cacti (*Opuntia*).

Similarly in USA, *Chrysolina* beetles were used to control *Hypericum perforatum* (Kalmath weed). Beetle *Zygogramma bicolorata* is used for controlling *Parthenium hysterophorus* (the Congress grass).

(iii) **Transgenic plants** They are genetically engineered plants, which develop resistance against pests. They contain genes of smoother crops, pest and herbicide resistance. For example, transgenic tomato is resistant to horn worm larva and tobacco.

Other than microbes, some plants are also used as bioherbicides. These are given below

(i) **Smoother crops** The crops which do not allow the weeds to grow nearby are called **smoother crops**. For example, sweet clover, soybean, alfalfa, sunflower, rye, *Sorghum*, etc. These crops eliminate weeds through the chemicals. Therefore, crop rotation with these smoother crops can reduce the incidence of weeds.

(ii) **Vegetables** Certain weeds such as *Amaranthus*, *Chenopodium*, etc., can be eliminated or made useful by using them as vegetable or fodder.

2. Bioinsecticides

Living organisms or their products used for insect control are called bioinsecticides. These include pathogens, parasites, predators, etc.

Some of the important bioinsecticides are given below

(i) **Sporeine** was the first commercial bioinsecticide. It was developed in France in 1940s from the soil bacterium, *Bacillus thuringiensis israelensis* (*Bti*).

This bacterium carries a gene coding for ***Bt*-toxin proteins** (the toxic crystals). This toxin can damage the intestinal tract of insect by inhibiting ion transport in the midgut. For example, heavy destruction of coffee plantation by insects, *Prophantis smaragdina* is controlled by thurioside.

(ii) **Doom** is a mixture of *Bacillus papillae* and *Bacillus lentimorbus.* It has been commercially used for controlling Japanese beetles, *Popillia.*

(iii) **Ladybug** (ladybird beetle) and praying mantis can control scale insect or aphid pests of vegetables, cotton and apple.

(iv) **Vedalian beetle** (*Radiola cardinalis*) has been found effective against cottony cushion scale (*Icerya purchasi*).

(v) **Mycar** is a product obtained from the fungus, *Hirsutella thompsonii.* It is used to control citrus rust mite.

(vi) **Predator bug** (*Cyrtorhinus mundulus*) has been successfully used to control sugarcane leafhopper in Hawaii.

(vii) **Baculoviruses** are viral pathogens which mainly attack insect pests. For example, Nuclear Polyhedrosis Virus (NPV) can eliminate bollworms from cotton crop.

(viii) ***Trichoderma*** is a free-living fungi commonly present in rhizosphere. It helps in controlling several plant pathogens.

(ix) ***Bacillus sphaericus*** is toxic to larva of *Anopheles* mosquito.

(x) **Boverin** is obtained from a fungus, *Beauveria bassiana*. It is used for controlling colorado potato beetle (*Leptinotarsa decemlineata*).

(xi) **Pheromones** are chemical messengers secreted by female insects. These help in communication, sending alarm signals or attracting males. The traps containing pheromones are placed in infected fields so, they are unavailable for reproduction.

(xii) **Molting hormone**, ecdysone results in early death of insect pests.

Note • *DCMU is a herbicide that acts by blocking electron flow at the quinone acceptors of photosystem-II.*
• *Paraquat is a herbicide used on marijuana crops. It acts by reacting with oxygen to form superoxide, O_2^-. It very damaging to the chloroplast components, especially lipids.*

3. Natural insecticides

They are obtained mostly from the plants and occasionally from the microbes. Some of these are listed below

Natural insecticides	Sources
Rotenone	Roots of *Derris elliptica* and *Lonchocarpus*
Nicotine	From tobacco (*Nicotiana tabacum*)
Salanin, Azadirachtin, Meliantiol	From neem (*Azadirachta indica*)
Pyrethrin and cineria	From capitulum of pyrethrum (*Chrysanthemum cinerariaefolium*, *C. coccineum* and *C. marshalli*)
Ryania	Roots and stem of *Ryania speciosa*

Integrated Pest Management (IPM)

- The overall objective of the IPM is to create and maintain situations in which insects are prevented from causing damage to crops.
- It involves integration of tactics to control a single pest on one or more crops.

CHECK POINT 19.3

1. Which of the following is not a symbiotic nitrogen-fixing bacterium?
(a) *Clostridium*
(b) *Rhizobium leguminosarum*
(c) *Frankia*
(d) *Alder*

2. A non-symbiotic biofertiliser is
(a) *Rhizobium* and *Frankia*
(b) *Azospirillum* and *Azotobacter*
(c) *Rhizobium* and *Azospirillum*
(d) *Frankia* and *Azotobacter*

3. Which of the following is included in biopesticide?
(a) Viruses and bacteria only
(b) Viruses, bacteria and fungi only
(c) Viruses, bacteria, fungi and protozoan
(d) Viruses and protozoan only

4. The first bioinsecticide was
(a) sporeine based on *Bacillus thuringiensis*
(b) sporeine based on yeasts
(c) sporeine based on *Collectotrichum*
(d) sporeine based on *Phytophthora palmivora*

5. Ladybird beetle is useful in the control of
(a) citrus rust mite
(b) mosquito larvae
(c) aphid pests of vegetable
(d) sugarcane leafhopper

6. Which of the following is involved in early death of insects?
(a) Ecdysone
(b) *Bacillus*
(c) Vedalian
(d) Mycor

EXAM POINTS

- *Lactobacillus* also called Lactic Acid Bacteria (LAB) convert milk into curd. **[NEET 2019]**
- Conversion of milk to curd improves its nutritional value by increasing the amount of vitamin-B_{12}. **[NEET 2018]**
- Yeast is used in the production of bread and beer. **[J&K CET 2015]**
- Roquefort cheese is ripened by using a fungus, *Penicillium roqueforti*. **[JIPMER 2017]**
- Primary sewage treatment removes suspended solids. **[NEET 2017]**
- During wastewater treatment, trickling filter is used for secondary aerobic treatment. **[WB JEE 2015]**
- Biogas produced during sevage treatment include methane, hydrogen sulphide and carbon dioxide. **[NEET 2013]**
- Activated sludge is put into anaerobic sludge digester for further sewage treatment. **[NEET 2020]**
- BOD may not be the good index for water bodies that receive effluents from petroleum industry. **[NEET-II 2016]**
- BOD characterise the polluting strength of sewage. **[J&K CET 2015]**
- High BOD indicate polluted water. **[CBSE AIPMT 2015]**
- Ethanol is commercially produced through species of *Saccharomyces*. **[CBSE AIPMT 2011]**
- *Aspergillus niger* is used for the commercial and industrial production of citric acid. **[NEET 2019]**
- *Acetobacter aceti* is used for the commercial and industrial production of acetic acid. **[NEET 2019]**
- Statin is a commercial blood cholesterol lowering agent. **[NEET 2019]**
- Cyclosporin-A used as immunosuppression agent is produced from *Trichoderma polysporum*. **[NEET 2020]**
- Ther term 'antibiotics' was given by Waksman. **[Chhattishgarh PMT 2015]**
- Bioreactor is essentially required for growing microbes on a large scale for industrial production of enzymes. **[NEET 2019]**
- Cyanobacteria and *Rhizobium* are the microbes that can be used as biofertilisers. **[NEET 2019]**
- *Rhizobium* is used as biofertiliser in soybean crop. **[CBSE AIPMT 2011]**
- *Azolla* is used as a biofertiliser because it has association of nitrogen-fixing cyanobacteria. **[AIIMS 2018]**
- The biological control of agricultural pests is self-perpetuating non-polluting and less expensive. **[J&K CET 2015]**
- A biocontrol agent to be a part of an integrated pest management should be species-specific and inactive on non-target organisms. **[NEET 2019]**
- *Trichoderma*, baculovirus, *Bacillus thuringiensis* are group of biocontrol agents. **[NEET 2019]**
- *Trichoderma* can be used as a biocontrol agent in the treatment of plant disease. **[NEET 2019]**
- Retenone is an insecticide of plant origin. **[WB JEE 2015]**

Chapter Exercises

(A) Topical Exercise

Microbes in Household Products

1 Microbes are likely to be found in
(a) deep inside the geysers (thermal vents) where the temperature may be high as 100°C
(b) deep in the soil and under the layers of several meters thick snow
(c) highly acidic environment
(d) All of the above

2 *Lactobacillus* mediated change of milk to curd occurs due to
(a) coagulation and partial digestion of milk fats
(b) coagulation and partial digestion of milk proteins
(c) coagulation of milk proteins and complete digestion of milk fats
(d) coagulation and complete digestion of milk proteins

3 Which group is responsible for the formation and flavour of yoghurt?
(a) *Bacillus megaterium* and *Xanthomonas* sp.
(b) *Bacillus subtilis* and *E. coli*
(c) *Rhizobium meliloti* and *Azotobacter*
(d) *Lactobacillus bulgaricus* and *Streptococcus thermophilus*

4 Dough kept overnight in warm weather becomes soft and spongy because of
(a) osmosis (b) CO_2 absorption
(c) fermentation (d) cohesion

5 Consider the following statements.
I. Lactic acid bacteria produce acids that coagulate and partially digest the milk protein during curd making.
II. Curd is less nutritious than milk.
Choose the correct option.
(a) Statement I is true, but II is false
(b) Statement I is false, but II is true
(c) Both statements I and II are true
(d) Both statements I and II are false

6 Match the following columns.

	Column I		Column II
A.	Curd	1.	LAB
B.	Yoghurt	2.	*Penicillium*
C.	Butter milk	3.	*Lactobacillus bulgaricus*
D.	Cheese	4.	LAB and *Streptococcus cremoris*

Codes

	A	B	C	D		A	B	C	D
(a)	1	3	4	2	(b)	1	4	2	3
(c)	4	2	1	3	(d)	2	4	3	1

7 Consider the following statements.
I. Cheese is partially degraded concentrate of milk fat and casein.
II. Large holed swiss cheese is prepared by *Propionibacterium shermanii.*
Choose the correct option.
(a) Statement I is true, but II is false
(b) Statement I is false, but II is true
(c) Both statements I and II are true
(d) Both statements I and II are false

8 The bread becomes soft and porous, when the yeast cells are mixed in the lump of dough of wheat flour, because
(a) yeast is soft and flour also becomes soft
(b) yeast produces acetic acid and alcohol, which gives softness to the bread
(c) evolution of CO_2 makes the bread spongy
(d) yeast produces benzoic acid

9 *Streptococcus lactis* is responsible for the
(a) conversion of curd into lactic acid
(b) making of butter
(c) conversion of milk into curd
(d) flavouring of tea

Microbes in Sewage Treatment

10 The primary treatment of wastewater involves the removal of **[NCERT Exemplar]**
(a) dissolved impurities (b) stable particles
(c) toxic substances (d) harmful bacteria

11 Primary treatment of sewage is
(a) physical process (b) biological process
(c) chemical process (d) biochemical process

12 Primary sludge is used for
(a) preparation of compost (b) preparation of manure
(c) biogas production (d) All of these

13 During primary treatment, all solids that settle forms ...*A*... and the supplement forms ...*B*... .

	A	*B*
(a)	primary sludge	effluent
(b)	primary sludge	secondary effluent
(c)	activated sludge	clarified effluent
(d)	activated sludge	effluent

14 The effluent is passed into oxidation tank for
(a) primary treatment (b) secondary treatment
(c) Both (a) and (b) (d) tertiary treatment

15 Wastewater treatment generates a large quantity of sludge, which can be treated by **[NCERT Exemplar]**
(a) anaerobic digesters (b) floc
(c) chemicals (d) oxidation pond

16 Activated sludge should have the ability to settle quickly so that it can **[NCERT Exemplar]**
(a) be rapidly pumped back from sedimentation tank to aeration tank
(b) absorb pathogenic bacteria present in wastewater while sinking to the bottom of the settling tank
(c) be discarded and anaerobically digested
(d) absorb colloidal organic matter

17 Consider the following statements.
I. In a sewage treatment plant, the primary sludge is obtained by sequential filtration and sedimentation.
II. Methanogenic bacteria are found in anaerobic sludge digesters.
Choose the correct option.
(a) Statement I is true, but II is false
(b) Statement I is false, but II is true
(c) Both statements I and II are true
(d) Both statements I and II are false

18 Select the correct statement from the following.
(a) Activated sludge in settlement tanks of sewage treatment plant is a rich source of aerobic bacteria
(b) Biogas is produced by the activity of aerobic bacteria on animal waste (dung)
(c) *Methanobacterium* is an aerobic bacterium found in rumen of cattle
(d) Biogas commonly called gobar gas, is pure methane

19 Treatment of wastewater is done by the
(a) photoautotrophic microbes, naturally present in sewage
(b) chemoautotrophic microbes, naturally present in sewage
(c) heterotrophic microbes naturally present in sewage
(d) heterotrophic microbes inoculated in the swage from outside only

20 In a STP, the sewage water is treated till
(a) BOD of sewage water rises significantly at the end of secondary treatment
(b) BOD of sewage water is reduced significantly at the end of secondary treatment
(c) anaerobic oxidation becomes very fast
(d) reduction of organic wastes becomes complete

21 Consider the following statements with respect to BOD (Biochemical Oxygen Demand).
I. It refers to the amount of oxygen that would be consumed of all the organic matter in one litre of water were oxidised by bacteria.
II. The BOD test is a measure of the organic matter present in the water.
Choose the correct option.
(a) Statement I is true, but II is false
(b) Statement I is false, but II is true
(c) Both statements I and II are true
(d) Both statements I and II are false

22 Match the following columns.

Column I	Column II
A. Tertiary treatment	1. Action of methane producing bacteria on component of microbial fermentation
B. Biocontrol agents	2. Physical removal of particles
C. Methanogenesis	3. It involves disinfecting water from STP for domestic use
D. Primary treatment	4. Use of biological methods for pest control

Codes

	A	B	C	D		A	B	C	D
(a)	2	1	3	4	(b)	1	4	3	2
(c)	3	2	1	4	(d)	3	4	1	2

23 The following figure shows.

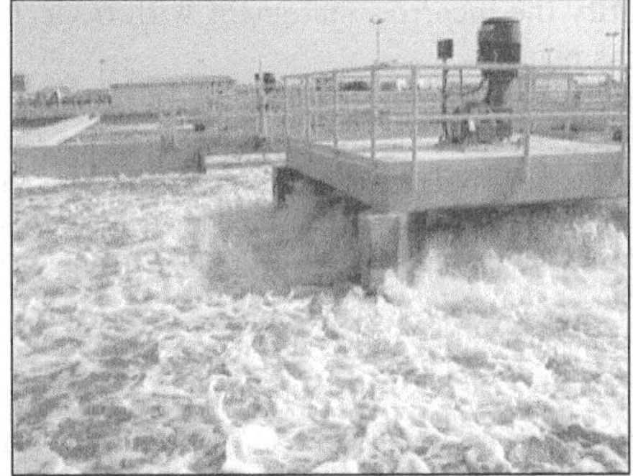

(a) Primary treatment (b) Secondary treatment
(c) Biological treatment (d) Both (b) and (c)

24 Sewage or municipal waste should not be directly passed into rivers, streams and other water bodies because
I. it contains human excreta and other organic waste.
II. it contains a number of pathogenic microbes.
Which of the statement(s) given above is/are correct?
(a) Only I (b) Only II (c) I and II (d) None of these

25 The ministry of environment and forests has initiated .... and .... to save our rivers from water pollution.

(a) Ganga Action Plan	Yamuna Action Plan
(b) Biogas Plant Setup	Chemical Insecticide
(c) Air Pollution Act	Sound Pollution Act
(d) Jhum Action Plan	Brahmaputra Action Plan

Biogas or Gobar gas

26 The technology of biogas production was developed in India mainly by the contribution of ...*A*... and ...*B*... .

	A	*B*
(a)	KVIC	IARI
(b)	NEERI	RRI
(c)	KVIC	NEERI
(d)	IARI	NEERI

27 Calorific value of biogas is .... kcal/m^3 at 50% methane content.
(a) 3000 (b) 4430
(c) 429 (d) 300

28 Biogas contains
(a) 30%-40% methane
(b) 50%-70% CO_2
(c) 50%-70% methane
(d) 20% methane

29 Identify the incorrect statement with respect to biogas plant.
(a) It consists of a concrete tank, 10-15 feet deep in which bio-waste are collected and a slurry of dung is fed
(b) A floating cover is placed over the slurry, which keeps on rising as the gas is consumed in the tank
(c) It has an outlet, which is connected to pipe to supply biogas to nearby houses
(d) The spent slurry is removed and may be used as fertiliser

30 Identify the parts labelled as *A*, *B* and *C* with respect to biogas plant.

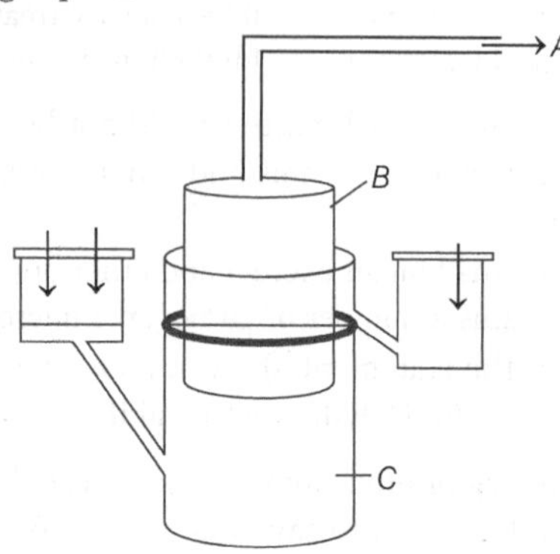

	A	*B*	*C*
(a)	Gas	Sludge	Dung water
(b)	Gas	Gas holder	Digester
(c)	Gas holder	Sludge	Dung water
(d)	Gas holder	Digester	Dung water

Microbes in Industry

31 Choose the incorrectly matched pair.
(a) Bioethanol - Amylase activity by *S. cerevisiae*
(b) Biobutanol - Soluble carbohydrates used as substrate
(c) Biodiesel - *Euphorbia* plants
(d) None of the above

32 During alcoholic fermentation, conversion of sugar into alcohol is due to direct action of
(a) temperature
(b) pH
(c) concentrate of sugar solution
(d) zymase enzyme

33 Anaerobic respiration of yeast produces
(a) alcohol
(b) carbon dioxide
(c) alcohol, carbon dioxide and energy
(d) None of the above

34 Types of the alcoholic drinks are depend on the
I. Type of raw material used
II. Type of processing
III. Type of fermentors
IV. Type of weather

Codes
(a) I, II and III (b) II, III and IV
(c) I, II and IV (d) I and II

35 Brewer's yeast is used for ...*A*... of malted cereals and fruit juices to produce ...*B*... .
(a) *A*-distillation, *B*-CO_2
(b) *A*-distillation, *B*-organic acid
(c) *A*-fermentation, *B*-CO
(d) *A*-fermentation, *B*-alcohol

36 Correctly identify the enzymes *A*, *B* and *C* of yeast during leavening process of bread making.

$$\text{Wheat flour starch} \xrightarrow{A} \text{Maltose} \xrightarrow{B} \text{Glucose} \xrightarrow{C} \text{Ethyl alcohol} + CO_2$$

	A	*B*	*C*
(a)	Zymase	Amylase	Maltase
(b)	Zymase	Maltase	Amylase
(c)	Amylase	Maltase	Zymase
(d)	Maltase	Amylase	Zymase

37 Yeasts are economically important because they
(a) spread plant diseases
(b) spread animal diseases
(c) are used in tea and tobacco industry
(d) are used in wine and baking industry

38 Select the incorrect statement.

(a) Lactic acid was the first organic acid produced by fermentation
(b) Kojic acid is produced by *Streptococcus lactis*
(c) Citric acid was crystallised from lemon juice
(d) None of the above

39 Match the following columns.

Column I		Column II
A. *Aspergillus niger*	1.	Lactic acid
B. *Acetobacter aceti*	2.	Butyric acid
C. *Clostridium butylicum*	3.	Acetic acid
D. *Lactobacillus*	4.	Citric acid

Codes **[NCERT Exemplar]**

	A	B	C	D
(a)	2	3	4	1
(b)	2	4	3	1
(c)	4	3	2	1
(d)	4	1	3	2

40 Fill in the blanks.

I. Lipases are obtained from ......*A*...... .
II. Pectinases are obtained from ......*B*...... .
III. Proteases are obtained from ......*C*...... .
IV. Statins are obtained from ......*D*...... .

	A	*B*	*C*	*D*
(a)	*Aspergillus niger*	*Monascus purpureus*	*Candida lipolytica*	*Mortierella renispora*
(b)	*Mortierella renispora*	*Candida lipolytica*	*Monascus purpureus*	*Aspergillus niger*
(c)	*Candida lipolytica*	*Mortierella renispora*	*Monascus purpureus*	*Aspergillus niger*
(d)	*Candida lipolytica*	*Aspergillus niger*	*Mortierella renispora*	*Monascus purpureus*

41 Identify *A*, *B*, *C* and *D* in the table given below.

Organisms	Biological names	Commercial products
A	*Saccharomyces*	Ethanol
Bacteria	*B*	Butyric acid
Fungi	*Trichoderma polysporum*	*C*
Bacteria	*Streptococcus*	*D*

(a) *A*—Multicellular fungi, *B*—*Clostridium butylicum*, *C*—Cyclosporin-A, *D*—Streptokinase
(b) *A*—Bacteria, *B*—*Clostridium butylicum*, *C*—Cyclosporin-A, *D*—Streptokinase
(c) *A*—Fungi, *B*—*Bacillus*, *C*—Ethanol, *D*—Penicillin
(d) *A*—Unicellular fungi, *B*—*Clostridium butylicum*, *C*—Cyclosporin-A, *D*—Streptokinase

42 ...*A*... enzyme is used to remove clots from the blood vessels of patients who have undergone ...*B*... leading to heart attack.

	A	*B*
(a)	Streptokinase	Myocardial infarction
(b)	Lipases	Arteriosclerosis
(c)	Proteases	Myocardial infarction
(d)	Pectinases	Atherosclerosis

43 Consider the following statements.

I. Statins are produce by some yeasts.
II. Statins are competitive inhibitors of β-hydroxy-β-methyl glutaryl Co-A reductase (HMG Co-A).

Choose the correct option.

(a) Statement I is true, but II is false
(b) Statement I is false, but II is true
(c) Both statements I and II are true
(d) Both statements I and II are false

44 Antibiotics are

(a) drug to kill viruses
(b) toxins produced by bacteria
(c) products of bacterial metabolism
(d) Both (b) and (c)

45 Consider the following statements with respect to antibiotics.

I. Fleming, Chain and Florey were awarded the Nobel Prize in 1945.
II. Antibiotics have greatly improved our capacity to treat deadly disease.

Choose the correct option.

(a) Statement I is true, but II is false
(b) Statement I is false, but II is true
(c) Both statements I and II are true
(d) Both statements I and II are false

46 Which is false about antibiotics?

(a) The term was coined by Waksman in 1942
(b) Antibiotics are capable of curing any disease
(c) Some persons develop allergy to antibiotics
(d) Antibiotics are produced by microorganisms

47 Waksman and Woodruff (1941) were responsible for the isolation of

(a) streptomycin (b) penicillin
(c) actinomycin (d) neomycin

48 In 1928, a scientist discovered the first effective antibiotic. Choose the correct option.

(a) Fleming — Streptomycin
(b) Fleming — Penicillin
(c) Waksman — Penicillin
(d) Waksman — Streptomycin

49 Presently, the source of 'wonder drug' is
(a) *Penicillium notatum* (b) *Penicillium chrysogenum*
(c) *Penicillium camemberti* (d) *Penicillium roqueforti*

50 The antibiotic flavicin is obtained by the activity of
(a) *Aspergillus fumigatus* (b) *A. clavatus*
(c) *A. niger* (d) *Streptomyces fradiae*

51 polymyxin is prepared from
(a) *Streptomyces griseus* (b) *Streptomyces nodosus*
(c) *Bacillus polymyxa* (d) *Streptomyces rimosus*

52 Match the following columns.

Column I	Column II
A. Neomycin	1. *Streptomyces fradiae*
B. Terramycin	2. *Penicillium notatum*
C. Viridin	3. *Streptomyces rimosus*
D. Penicillin	4. *Gliocladium virens*

Codes

	A	B	C	D
(a)	3	1	4	2
(b)	4	3	1	2
(c)	1	3	4	2
(d)	4	1	3	2

53 Consider the following statements.
I. Non-pathogenic *Clostridium* replicate within tumours and cure them.
II. Nutritional yeast contains less amount of fat and sodium.

Choose the correct option.
(a) Statement I is true, but II is false
(b) Statement I is false, but II is true
(c) Both statements I and II are true
(d) Both statements I and II are false

Microbes as Biofertilisers and Biocontrol Agents

54 Biofertilisers
(a) increase dependence on chemical fertilisers
(b) are organisms that enrich the nutrient quality of soil
(c) include potash, phosphatic and nitrogenous organic and chemical compounds
(d) are used regularly in the fields to deplete soil nutrients

55 Which one is a biofertiliser?
(a) NPK mixture
(b) Rhizobia in legume roots
(c) Rhizobia in farmyard manure
(d) Green manure

56 Which of the following is a free-living nitrogen-fixing bioifertiliser?
(a) *Rhizobium* (b) *Microphos*
(c) *Pyrethrin* (d) *Azotobacter*

57 Biofertilisers give better yield when added along with
(a) phosphate (b) calcium
(c) nitrogen (d) urea

58 Which of the following is not an advantage of mycorrhiza?
(a) Nitrogen-fixation
(b) Resistance to root borne pathogens
(c) Tolerance to salinity and drought
(d) Phosphorus absorption

59 If wheat field is inoculated with *Rhizobium*,
(a) soil will become nitrogen rich
(b) no effect on soil nitrogen
(c) soil will be depleted of nitrogen
(d) soil will become rich in calcium

60 Farmers have reported 50% higher yield of rice by using biofertiliser
(a) *Azolla pinnata*
(b) Legume – *Rhizobium symbiosis*
(c) *Glomus*
(d) Mycorrhiza

61 The symbiotic association of fungi with plant is known as ...*A*... which is formed by many members of the fungal genus ...*B*... .

	A	B
(a)	Mycorrhiza	*Glomus*
(b)	Mycorrhiza	*Penicillium*
(c)	Lichen	*Trebouxia*
(d)	Lichen	*Rhizocarpon*

62 Which of the following is one of the advantage of application of viruses as bioinsecticides?
(a) They are not used in IPM
(b) They are less effective
(c) They are species specific
(d) They have negative impact on humans

63 Which of the following are natural insecticides?
I. Rotenone II. Pyrethrin
III. Nicotine IV. Azadirachtin
Codes
(a) I, II and III only (b) I, III and IV only
(c) I and II only (d) I, II, III and IV

64 The first mycoherbicide called 'Devine' is obtained from the fungus
(a) *Phytophthora palmivora* (b) *Colletotrichum*
(c) *Cercospora* (d) *Penicillium*

65 Consider the following statements.
I. *Trichoderma* is a symbiotic alga which is common in root ecosystem and effective against several plant pathogens.
II. *Nucleopolyhedrovirus* (NPV) have species specific, broad spectrum insecticidal applications.

Choose the correct option.
(a) Statement I is true, but II is false
(b) Statement I is false, but II is true
(c) Both statements I and II are true
(d) Both statements I and II are false

66 Consider the following statements.
I. *Bacillus thuringiensis* are available in sachets as dried spores which are mixed with kerosene and sprayed on to vulnerable plants.
II. The toxin of *B. thuringiensis* is released in the blood of larvae and the larvae get killed.

Choose the correct option.
(a) Statement I is true, but II is false
(b) Statement I is false, but II is true
(c) Both statements I and II are true
(d) Both statements I and II are false

67 Mark the mismatched pair.
(a) Dragonfly – Biocontrol agent
(b) Mycar – *Rodolia cardinalis*
(c) Anaerobic sludge digester – Biogas
(d) VAM – Biofertiliser

68 The ladybird beetle and dragonflies are useful to get rid of ...*A*... and ...*B*..., respectively.

	A	*B*
(a)	Caterpillars	Mosquitoes
(b)	Mosquitoes	Fruit borer
(c)	Mosquitoes	Aphids
(d)	Aphids	Mosquitoes

69 The majority of baculoviruses are used as biological control agents as
(a) they are species specific
(b) they have no negative impact on non-targets
(c) beneficial insects are being conserved
(d) All of the above

70 Which of the following statement (s) is/are correct with regard to biocontrol agents?
(a) Ladybird beetles and dragonflies are used to get rid of aphids and mosquitoes, respectively
(b) *Bacillus thuringiensis* bacteria are used to control butterfly and caterpillars
(c) *Trichoderma* species are used to control several plant pathogens
(d) All of the above

71 Match the following columns.

Column I	Column II
A. Rotenone	1. *Chrysanthemum Cinerariifolium*
B. Nicotine	2. *Derris elliptica*
C. Azadirachtin	3. *Azadirachta indica*
D. Pyrethrum and cinerin	4. *Nicotiana tabacum*

Codes

	A	B	C	D
(a)	2	4	1	3
(b)	2	4	3	1
(c)	3	4	1	2
(d)	1	2	4	3

(B) Cumulative Exercise

(Assorted Questions of the Chapter for Advanced Level Practice)

1 Consider the following statements.
I. Toddy, the traditional drink from South India is made by fermenting sap from *Caryota urens.*
II. Waksman and Albert discovered lactic acid.
III. The term antibiotic was given by Waksman.
IV. *Frankia* is the symbiont for non-leguminous trees and shrubs.

Choose the option containing correct statements.
(a) III and IV
(b) I, II, III and IV
(c) II and IV
(d) I, III and IV

2 Match the following columns.

Column I	Column II
A. Ladybird	1. *Methanobacterium*
B. Mycorrhiza	2. *Trichoderma*
C. Biological control	3. Aphids
D. Biogas	4. *Glomus*

[NCERT Exemplar]

Codes

	A	B	C	D		A	B	C	D
(a)	2	4	3	1	(b)	3	4	2	1
(c)	4	1	2	3	(d)	3	2	1	4

3 Consider the following microorganisms and choose which one is used for the production of acetic acid?
I. *Acetobacter aceti*
II. *Caryota urens*
III. *Aspergillus niger*
IV. *Clostridium butylicum*

Codes
(a) I and II (b) III and IV (c) Only I (d) Only II

4 The technology of biogas production from cow dung was developed in India largely due to the efforts of **[NCERT Exemplar]**
(a) Gas Authority of India
(b) Oil and Natural Gas Commission
(c) Indian Agricultural Research Institute, Khadi and Village Industries Commission
(d) Indian Oil Corporation

5 Identify *A, B, C* and *D* with respect to a Sewage Treatment Plant (STP).

Primary treatment	Secondary treatment
Physical process	*A*
B	Removes small-sized organic matter
Aeration is not required	*C*
D	Involves microbial digestion

(a) *A*–Biological process, *B*–Removes grit and large organic pieces, *C*–Aeration is required, *D*–Involves sequential filtration and sedimentation
(b) *A*–Physico-chemical process, *B*–Removes grit and large organic pieces, *C*–Aeration is required, *D*–Involves sequential filtration and sedimentation
(c) *A*–Biological process, *B*–Removes grit and large organic pieces, *C*–Aeration is not required, *D*–Involves sequential filtration and sedimentation
(d) *A*–Physical process, *B*–Removes grit and large organic pieces, *C*–Aeration is required, *D*–Involves sequential filtration and sedimentation

6 Match the following columns.

Column I	Column II
A. Free-living nitrogen-fixing bacteria	1. *Cyrtorhinus mundulus*
B. Predator bug	2. Roots of *Derris elliptica*
C. Rotenones	3. *Nostoc*
D. Boverin	4. *Beauveria bassiana*

Codes

	A	B	C	D		A	B	C	D
(a)	1	2	3	4	(b)	3	1	2	4
(c)	3	4	2	1	(d)	2	3	1	4

7 Consider the following diseases and choose the ones that can be treated by antibiotics.

I. Whooping cough II. Diphtheria
III. Myocardial infarction IV. Pneumonia

Codes
(a) I, II and III
(b) III and IV
(c) II and III
(d) I, II and IV

8 Consider the following statements.

I. After primary treatment of sewage, all solids that settle down forms the primary sludge and the supernatant form the effluent.
II. Spent slurry of biogas plant is used as fertiliser.

Which of the statements given above are correct?
(a) Only I (b) I and II
(c) Only II (d) None of these

9 Read the following statements.

I. Smother crops do not allow weeds to grow nearby.
II. Bhindi/Okra is a type of catch trap crop.
III. *Bt* cotton is a transgenic crop.
IV. *Aulosira* is the most abundant free-living nitrogen fixer in rhizosphere.
V. *Azolla*, a blue-green alga, fix nitrogen in non-leguminous plants.

Which of the above statements are correct?
(a) I, II and III (b) IV and V
(c) III, IV and V (d) I, IV and V

10 Which of the following is correct?
(a) *Aulosira* is the most active, non-symbiotic nitrogen fixer in the rice fields
(b) *Trichoderma* is a free-living fungi common in root ecosystems and effective against several plant pathogens to prevent fungal diseases
(c) Both (a) and (b)
(d) 'Collego' is obtained from a blue-green algae

11 Match the following columns.

Column I	Column II
A. *B. propioni*	1. Gallic acid
B. *Aspergillus* sp.	2. Propionic acid
C. *E. coli*	3. Butyric acid
D. *C. acetobutylicum*	4. Oxalic acid

Codes **[NCERT Exemplar]**

	A	B	C	D		A	B	C	D
(a)	1	2	4	3	(b)	4	1	2	3
(c)	2	4	1	3	(d)	2	1	4	3

12 Under the Ganga and Yamuna action plans,
(a) it is proposed to build a large number of sewage treatment plants, so that only treated sewage may be discharged in the rivers
(b) the river water is treated with potassium permanganate and bleaching powder, so that it is cleaned of microbes
(c) the river water to be considered sacred, so that bathing and adding pollutants is not allowed
(d) addition of effluents is banned in rivers

13 Observe the flow depicting a Sewage Treatment Plant (STP) and identify the components/steps *A, B, C, D* and *E*.

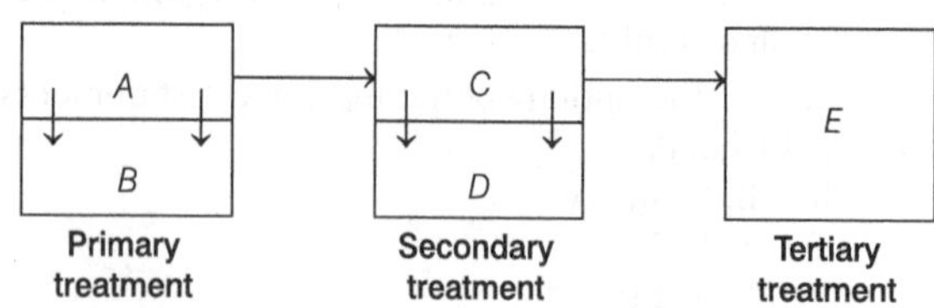

(a) *A*–Primary sludge, *B*–Primary effluent, *C*–Secondary effluent, *D*–Activated sludge, *E*–Physico-chemical treatment
(b) *A*–Primary effluent, *B*–Primary sludge, *C*–Secondary effluent, *D*–Activated sludge, *E*–Physico-chemical treatment
(c) *A*–Activated sludge, *B*–Primary sludge, *C*–Secondary sludge, *D*–Primary effluent, *E*–Secondary effluent
(d) *A*–Activated sludge, *B*–Secondary sludge, *C*–Primary sludge, *D*–Secondary effluent, *E*–Primary effluent

14 Match the following columns.

Column I	Column II
A. *Nitrobacter*	1. Free-living aerobic nitrogen fixer
B. *Clostridium*	2. Converts ammonia to nitrate
C. *Nitrosococcus*	3. Changes nitrite to nitrate
D. *Azotobacter*	4. Free-living anaerobic nitrogen fixer

Codes

	A	B	C	D		A	B	C	D
(a)	2	4	3	1	(b)	3	4	2	1
(c)	4	2	1	3	(d)	1	2	3	4

15 Which of the following is not the belief of an organic farmer?

(a) The more variety a landscape has, the more sustainable it is
(b) The insects that are sometimes called pests are not eradicated, but instead are kept at manageable levels by a complex system of checks and balances within a living and vibrant ecosystem
(c) For controlling plant diseases and pests, chemicals like insecticides and pesticides should be used extensively
(d) Eradication of the pests is undesirable because they act as food or hosts for beneficial predatory and parasitic insects

16 Which of the following statements is/are correct?

I. The dough, which is used for making bread, is fermented using Baker's yeast, i.e. *Saccharomyces cerevisiae*.
II. Production on an industrial scale requires growing microbes in very large vessels called fermentors.
III. The municipal wastewater is also called sewage.
IV. It is necessary to treat sewage in Sewage Treatment Plants (STPs) to make it less polluting.

Codes

(a) I and II (b) Only III
(c) I, II and IV (d) I, II, III and IV

17 Match the following columns.

Column I	Column II
A. Ascorbic acid	1. *Acetobacter*
B. Glucose oxidase	2. *Propionibacterium*
C. Propionic acid	3. *Aspergillus oryzae*
D. Protease	4. *Aspergillus niger*

Codes

	A	B	C	D		A	B	C	D
(a)	2	3	4	1	(b)	4	3	1	2
(c)	1	4	2	3	(d)	1	4	3	2

18 Mycorrhiza do not help the host plant in

I. enhancing its phosphorus uptake capacity
II. increasing its tolerance to drought
III. enhancing its resistance to root pathogens
IV. increasing its resistance to insects

Codes

(a) II and III (b) Only III (c) I and IV (d) Only IV

19 Match the Column I and Column II and choose the correct combination from the options given below

Column I	Column II
A. 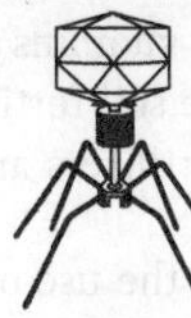	1. Adenovirus
B. 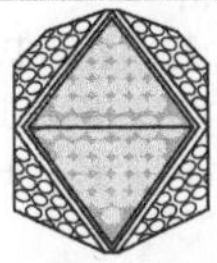	2. Bacteriophage
C. 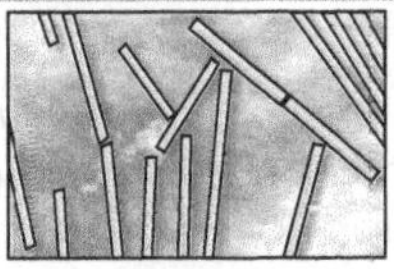	3. TMV

Codes

	A	B	C		A	B	C
(a)	1	2	3	(b)	2	3	1
(c)	2	1	3	(d)	3	2	1

20 In which of the following examples, CO_2 gas is produced?

I. Fermentation of dough
II. Cheese making
III. Production of beverages
IV. Biogas production
V. Alcoholic fermentation
VI. Lactic acid fermentation

Codes

(a) I, II, III and V (b) I, II, III and IV
(c) I, II, III, IV and V (d) I, II, III, IV, V and VI

21 Consider the following pairs.

I. Ethanol – *Spirochaeta litroales*
II. Itaconic acid – *A. terreus*
III. Statins – *Trichoderma polysporum*
IV. Amylase – *A. niger*

Choose the incorrect match pair.

(a) I and III (b) Only III
(c) II, III and IV (d) II and IV

22 Consider the following statements.

I. Antibiotics are chemical substances produced by some microorganisms which can kill or retard the growth of other disease-causing microorganisms.
II. Penicillin was the first antibiotic discovered by Alexander Fleming (1928), while working on bacterium *Staphylococcus aureus.*
III. *Ashbya gossypii* is used to yield vitamin-B_{12}.

Which of the statements given above are correct?

(a) I and II (b) I and III
(c) II and III (d) I, II and III

23 Consider the following four statements (I-IV) related to organic farming and select the correct option stating which ones are true (T) and which ones are false (F) statements.

I. Produces food crops rich in lipids, vitamins and iron.
II. Uses biofertilisers which increase soil fertility.
III. There is more use of chemical fertilisers and pesticides.
IV. Raising unpolluted crops through the use of bacteria, fungi and cyanobacteria.

	I	II	III	IV		I	II	III	IV
(a)	T	T	F	F	(b)	F	T	F	T
(c)	T	F	T	F	(d)	T	F	F	F

Assertion and Reason

Direction (Q. Nos. 24-31) *In each of the following questions, a statement of Assertion (A) is given followed by corresponding statement of Reason (R). Of the statements, mark the correct answer as*

(a) Both A and R are true and R is the correct explanation of A
(b) Both A and R are true, but R is not the correct explanation of A
(c) A is true, but R is false
(d) A is false, but R is true
(e) Both A and R are false

24 **Assertion** (A) Yeasts such as *Saccharomyces cerevisiae* are used in baking industry.

Reason (R) Carbon dioxide produced during fermentation causes bread dough to rise by thermal expansion.

25 **Assertion** (A) The kneaded flour shows leavening, when yeast is added to it.

Reason (R) Enzymes secreted by yeast cause leavening.

26 **Assertion** (A) Extraction and purification of enzymes is laborious and expensive.

Reason (R) Protein engineering can be used to produce enzymes at large scale.

27 **Assertion** (A) Enzymes application in industry is enhanced by its immobilisation.

Reason (R) Immobilisation provides protection to enzymes without affecting their activity.

28 **Assertion** (A) Penicillin is obtained from *Penicillium griseofulvum.*

Reason (R) Ergot is obtained from *Penicillium notatum.*

29 **Assertion** (A) Invertase is manufactured from *Aspergillus oryzae.*

Reason (R) Amylase is produced by *Saccharomyces cerevisiae.*

30 **Assertion** (A) Champagne and wines are the products of fermentation.

Reason (R) Rum is an alcoholic distillate from the fermented juice of sugarcane.

31 **Assertion** (A) Alcohol contents of champagne wine is 12-16%.

Reason (R) Alcohol contents of rum is 60-70%.

(C) Medical Entrances' Gallery

(Collection of Questions Asked in NEET & in Various Medical Entrance Exams)

1 Cyclosporin-A used as immunosuppression agent is produced from **[NEET 2020]**

(a) *Monascus purpureus* (b) *Saccharomyces cerevisiae*
(c) *Penicillium notatum* (d) *Trichoderma polysporum*

2 Match the following columns and select the correct option from the codes given below.

	Column I		Column II
A.	Dragonflies	1.	Biocontrol agents of several plant pathogens
B.	*Bacillus thuringiensis*	2.	Get rid of aphids and mosquitoes
C.	*Glomus*	3.	Narrow spectrum insecticidal applications
D.	Baculoviruses	4.	Biocontrol agents of lepidopteran plant pests
		5	Absorb phosphorus from soil

[NEET 2020]

Codes

	A	B	C	D		A	B	C	D
(a)	3	5	4	1	(b)	2	1	3	4
(c)	2	3	4	5	(d)	2	4	5	3

3 Match the following organisms with the products they produce.

A.	*Lactobacillus*	1. Cheese
B.	*Saccharomyces cerevisiae*	2. Curd
C.	*Aspergillus niger*	3. Citric acid
D.	*Acetobacter aceti*	4. Bread
		5. Acetic acid

Codes **[NEET 2019]**

	A	B	C	D		A	B	C	D
(a)	2	4	3	5	(b)	3	4	5	1
(c)	2	1	3	5	(d)	2	4	5	3

4 Which of the following is a commercial blood cholesterol lowering agent? **[NEET 2019]**

(a) Statin (b) Streptokinase
(c) Lipases (d) Cyclosporin-A

5 Which one of the following equipment is essentially required for growing microbes on a large scale for industrial production of enzymes? **[NEET 2019]**

(a) Sludge digester
(b) Industrial oven
(c) Bioreactor
(d) BOD incubator

6 Match Column I (Antibiotic) with Column II (Source) and choose the correct option from the codes given below.

	Column I		Column II
A.	Fumagillin	1.	*Gliocladium virens*
B.	Bacitracin	2.	*Streptomyces griseus*
C.	Streptomycin	3.	*Bacillus polymyxa*
D.	Viridin	4.	*Aspergillus fumigatus*
E.	Polymyxin	5.	*Bacillus licheniformis*

Codes **[AIIMS 2019]**

	A	B	C	D	E
(a)	1	2	3	4	5
(b)	4	5	2	1	3
(c)	3	1	4	2	5
(d)	2	3	5	4	1

7 Select the correct group of biocontrol agents. **[NEET 2019]**

(a) *Trichoderma*, Baculovirus, *Bacillus thuringiensis*
(b) *Oscillatoria*, *Rhizobium*, *Trichoderma*
(c) *Nostoc*, *Azospirillum*, *Nucleopolyhedrovirus*
(d) *Bacillus thuringiensis*, tobacco mosaic virus, aphids

8 Which of the following can be used as a biocontrol agent in the treatment of plant disease? **[NEET 2019]**

(a) *Chlorella* (b) *Anabaena*
(c) *Lactobacillus* (d) *Trichoderma*

9 A biocontrol agent to be a part of an integrated pest management should be **[NEET 2019]**

(a) species-specific and symbiotic
(b) free-living and broad spectrum
(c) narrow spectrum and symbiotic
(d) species-specific and inactive on non-target organisms

10 Among the following pairs of microbes, which pair has both the microbes that can be used as biofertilisers? **[NEET 2019]**

(a) *Aspergillus* and *Rhizopus*
(b) *Rhizobium* and *Rhizopus*
(c) Cyanobacteria and *Rhizobium*
(d) *Aspergillus* and Cyanobacteria

11 Which of the following statements about methanogens is not correct? **[NEET 2019]**

(a) They can be used to produce biogas
(b) They are found in the rumen of cattle and their excreta
(c) They grow aerobically and breakdown cellulose rich food
(d) They produce methane gas

12 Conversion of milk to curd improves its nutritional value by increasing the amount of **[NEET 2018]**

(a) vitamin-B_{12} (b) vitamin-A
(c) vitamin-D (d) vitamin-E

13 *Azolla* is used as a biofertiliser because it **[AIIMS 2018]**

(a) has association of mycorrhiza
(b) multiplies at faster rate to produce massive biomass
(c) has association of nitrogen-fixing *Rhizobium*
(d) has association of nitrogen-fixing cyanobacteria

14 Roquefort cheese is ripened by using a **[JIPMER 2017]**

(a) type of yeast (b) fungus
(c) bacterium (d) cyanobacteria

15 Which of the following is incorrect matched in the given table? **[NEET-II 2017]**

	Microbes	Products	Applications
(a)	*Monascus purpureus*	Statins	Lowering of blood cholesterol
(b)	*Streptococcus*	Streptokinase	Removal of clot from blood vessel
(c)	*Clostridium butylicum*	Lipase	Removal of oil stains
(d)	*Trichoderma polysporum*	Cyclosporin-A	Immunosuppressive drug

16 Match Column I with Column II and select the correct option using the codes given below.

	Column I		Column II
A.	Citric acid	1.	*Trichoderma*
B.	Cyclosporin	2.	*Clostridium*
C.	Statins	3.	*Aspergillus*
D.	Butyric acid	4.	*Monascus*

Codes **[NEET 2017]**

	A	B	C	D
(a)	3	1	2	4
(b)	3	1	4	2
(c)	1	4	2	3
(d)	3	4	1	2

17 Which of the following is not used as a biopesticide? **[AIIMS 2017]**

(a) *Bacillus thuringiensis*
(b) *Xanthomonas campestris*
(c) Nuclear Polyhedrosis Virus (NPV)
(d) *Trichoderma harzianum*

18 Which of the following in sewage treatment removes suspended solids? **[NEET 2017]**
(a) Tertiary treatment
(b) Secondary treatment
(c) Primary treatment
(d) Sludge treatment

19 Biochemical Oxygen Demand (BOD) may not be a good index for pollution in water bodies receiving effluents from **[NEET-II 2016]**
(a) domestic sewage (b) dairy industry
(c) petroleum industry (d) sugar industry

20 The polluting strength of sewage is usually characterised by **[J&K CET 2015]**
(a) BOD (b) nitrogen content
(c) ozone content (d) eutrophication

21 Yeast is used in the production of **[J&K CET 2015]**
(a) bread and beer (b) cheese and butter
(c) citric acid and lactic acid (d) lipase and pectinase

22 The biological control of agricultural pests unlike chemical control is **[J&K CET 2015]**
(a) very expensive (b) polluting
(c) self-perpetuating (d) toxic

23 BOD refers to **[Karnataka CET 2015]**
(a) the oxygen required for bacteria to grow in 1 L of effluent
(b) the amount of oxygen consumed if all the organic matter in 1000 mL of water were oxidised by bacteria
(c) the amount of oxygen released if all the organic matter in 1000 mL of water were oxidised by bacteria
(d) the amount of oxygen released when all the organic matter was consumed by bacteria in 1 L of water

24 During sewage treatment, biogas produced includes **[Karnataka CET 2015; NEET 2013]**
(a) hydrogen sulphide, nitrogen, methane
(b) methane, oxygen, hydrogen sulphide
(c) methane, hydrogen sulphide, carbon dioxide
(d) hydrogen sulphide, methane, sulphur oxide

25 The term antibiotic was given by **[Chhattisgarh PMT 2015]**
(a) Funk (b) Mellanby
(c) Waksman (d) Pasteur

26 Which of the following are involved in and used for cheese manufacturing? **[Chhattisgarh PMT 2015]**
(a) Bacteria and fungi
(b) Bacteria and some algae
(c) Bacteria and mycoplasma
(d) Bacteria and cyanobacteria

27 High value of BOD (Biochemical Oxygen Demand) indicates that **[CBSE AIPMT 2015]**
(a) water is pure
(b) water is highly polluted
(c) water is less polluted
(d) consumption of organic matter in the water is higher by the microbes

28 Which one of following insecticides is of plant origin? **[WB JEE 2015]**
(a) Ecdysone (b) Rotenone (c) Parathion (d) Malathion

29 During wastewater treatment, trickling filter is used for **[WB JEE 2015]**
(a) primary treatment
(b) secondary aerobic treatment
(c) secondary anaerobic treatment
(d) tertiary treatment

30 Which one of the following organisms is not used as a biocontrol agent? **[WB JEE 2015]**
(a) *Bacillus sphaericus* (b) *Trichoderma viride*
(c) *Bacillus thuringiensis* (d) *Bacillus subtilis*

31 Match the Column I with Column II.

	Column I		Column II
A.	Statins	1.	Remove the clots in blood vessels
B.	Cyclosporin-A	2.	Competitive inhibitor of cholesterol synthesising enzyme
C.	Streptokinase	3.	Immunosuppresant
D.	Lipase	4.	Soap industry to remove oil strain

Codes **[EAMCET 2015]**

	A	B	C	D		A	B	C	D
(a)	2	3	1	4	(b)	4	2	3	1
(c)	3	2	4	1	(d)	4	1	3	2

32 Match the following Column I with Column II.

	Column I		Column II
A.	Fermenting malted cereals and fruit juices	1.	Clots in the blood vessels
B.	Production of large holes in Swiss cheese	2.	Digestion of sludge by bacteria and fungi resulting in emission of methane and other gases
C.	Myocardial infarction	3.	Production of ethanol
D.	Biogas	4.	Blood cholesterol lowering agent
		5.	Production of large amount of CO_2

Codes **[EAMCET 2015]**

	A	B	C	D		A	B	C	D
(a)	3	5	4	2	(b)	1	2	3	4
(c)	3	5	1	2	(d)	5	4	3	2

33 Which one of the following functions as symbiotic nitrogen-fixing plants? [JCECE 2012]
(a) *Azolla* (b) *Cycas*
(c) Moss (d) *Marchantia*

34 Which of the following can be controlled by using biopesticides? [JCECE 2012]
(a) Insects (b) Diseases
(c) Weeds (d) All of these

35 An organism used as a biofertiliser for raising soyabean crop production is [CBSE AIPMT 2011]
(a) *Azospirillum* (b) *Rhizobium*
(c) *Nostoc* (d) *Azotobacter*

36 Which one of the following is not a biofertiliser? [CBSE AIPMT 2011]
(a) *Rhizobium* (b) *Nostoc*
(c) Mycorrhiza (d) *Agrobacterium*

37 Ethanol is commercially produced through a particular species of [CBSE AIPMT 2011]
(a) *Clostridium* (b) *Trichoderma*
(c) *Aspergillus* (d) *Saccharomyces*

38 Some blue-green algae are used as biofertiliser as they [AIIMS 2010]
(a) fix nitrogen (b) are mucilaginous
(c) can grow everywhere (d) are deficient in nutrient

ANSWERS

Check Point 19.1

1. (b) 2. (b) 3. (b) 4. (a) 5. (b)

Check Point 19.2

1. (c) 2. (c) 3. (c) 4. (c) 5. (a) 6. (c)

Check Point 19.3

1. (a) 2. (b) 3. (c) 4. (a) 5. (c) 6. (a)

(A) Topical Exercise

1. (d) 2. (b) 3. (d) 4. (c) 5. (a) 6. (a) 7. (c) 8. (c) 9. (b) 10. (b)
11. (a) 12. (d) 13. (a) 14. (b) 15. (a) 16. (a) 17. (c) 18. (a) 19. (c) 20. (b)
21. (c) 22. (d) 23. (d) 24. (c) 25. (a) 26. (a) 27. (b) 28. (c) 29. (b) 30. (b)
31. (a) 32. (d) 33. (c) 34. (d) 35. (d) 36. (c) 37. (d) 38. (b) 39. (c) 40. (d)
41. (d) 42. (a) 43. (c) 44. (d) 45. (c) 46. (h) 47. (a) 48. (b) 49. (a) 50. (a)
51. (c) 52. (c) 53. (c) 54. (b) 55. (b) 56. (d) 57. (a) 58. (a) 59. (b) 60. (a)
61. (a) 62. (c) 63. (d) 64. (a) 65. (c) 66. (c) 67. (b) 68. (d) 69. (d) 70. (d)
71. (b)

(B) Cumulative Exercise

1. (d) 2. (b) 3. (c) 4. (c) 5. (a) 6. (b) 7. (d) 8. (b) 9. (a) 10. (c)
11. (c) 12. (a) 13. (b) 14. (b) 15. (c) 16. (d) 17. (c) 18. (d) 19. (c) 20. (c)
21. (b) 22. (a) 23. (b) 24. (a) 25. (a) 26. (b) 27. (a) 28. (e) 29. (e) 30. (b)
31. (b)

(C) Medical Entrances' Gallery

1. (d) 2. (d) 3. (a) 4. (a) 5. (c) 6. (b) 7. (a) 8. (d) 9. (d) 10. (c)
11. (c) 12. (a) 13. (d) 14. (b) 15. (c) 16. (b) 17. (b) 18. (c) 19. (c) 20. (a)
21. (a) 22. (c) 23. (b) 24. (c) 25. (c) 26. (a) 27. (b) 28. (b) 29. (b) 30. (d)
31. (a) 32. (c) 33. (a) 34. (d) 35. (b) 36. (d) 37. (d) 38. (a)

Explanations

(A) Topical Exercise

5 (*a*) Statement I is true, but II is false. Incorrect statement can be corrected as

Curd has more nutritional value than milk. The former contain more vitamin-B_{12} content than the latter.

18 (*a*) Statement in option (a) is correct, while other three are incorrect. These can be corrected as

Biogas is produced by the activity of anaerobic bacteria, e.g. *Methanobacterium*. Biogas is a mixture of gases like methane, CO_2, etc.

29 (*b*) Statement in option (b) is incorrect and can be corrected as

The floating cover keeps on rising as the gas is released in the tank.

31 (*a*) Option (a) is incorrectly matched pair and can be corrected as

Bioethanol is derived from starch and sugar crops through the amylase activity by *Bacillus licheniformis*.

Rest options are correctly matched pairs.

38 (*b*) Statement in option (b) is incorrect and can be corrected as

Kojic acid is produced as result of fermentation carried out by *Aspergillus oryzae*.

46 (*b*) Statement in option (b) is false and can be corrected as

Antibiotics are not capable of curing all diseases. These mainly help to treat bacterial infections but not viral infections.

67 (*b*) Option (b) is mismatched pair and can be corrected as

Mycar is a product obtained form the fungus, *Hirsutella thompsonii*. It controls citrus rust mite.

(B) Cumulative Exercise

1 (*d*) Statements I, III and IV are correct, while II is incorrect. Incorrect statement can be corrected as

Waksman is known for coining the term antibiotics.

7 (*d*) Diseases I, II and IV are correct as

These can be treated by antibiotics. Rest three are bacterial diseases. On the other hand, myocardial infarction is a heart disease that cannot be treated using antibiotics.

9 (*a*) Statements I, II and III are correct while IV and V are incorrect. Incorrect statement can be corrected as

The most abundant free-living nitrogen fixers in rhizosphere are *Azospirillum* and *Azotobacter*.

Azolla is a water fern which cannot fix nitrogen on its own. In non-leguminous plants, *Frankia* helps to fix nitrogen.

10 (*c*) Options (a) and (b) are correct, while (d) is incorrect. Incorrect option can be corrected as

Collego is obtained from fungus, *Aeschynomene virginica*.

Thus, option (c) is correct.

21 (*b*) Only pair III represents incorrectly matched pair and can be corrected as

Statins are derived from the yeast.

22 (*a*) Statements I and II are correct, while III is incorrect. Incorrect statement can be corrected as

Ashbya gossypii is used to obtain vitamin-B_2, i.e. riboflavin. Vitamin-B_{12} is obtained from bacteria called *Streptomyces olivaceus*.

23 (*b*) Statements II and IV are true, whereas I and III are false. Incorrect statements can be corrected as

Organic farming discourages the use of chemical fertilisers and pesticides. It has no role in increasing lipid, vitamin and iron content in crops.

24 (*a*) Both A and R are true and R is the correct explanation of A.

Baker's yeast (*Saccharomyces cerevisiae*) is added to flour during kneading. Yeast secretes enzymes like amylase (change some starch to maltose), maltase (maltose to glucose) and zymase (glucose to ethyl alcohol and CO_2). Leavened dough is baked and both alcohol and CO_2 evaporate due to which the bread becomes soft and porous.

25 (*a*) Both A and R are true and R is the correct explanation of A.

A small quantity of yeast is added to wheat flour and the same is kneaded. The kneaded flour is kept at a warm temperature for a few hours. It swells up. The phenomenon is called leavening. It is caused by the secretion of three types of enzymes by yeast. They are amylase, maltase and zymase.

26 (*b*) Both A and R are true, but R is not the correct explanation of A.

Although thousands of proteins have been characterised in prokaryotes and eukaryotes, only few became commercially important. This is due to the high cost of isolating and purifying enzymes in sufficient quantities. Through recombinant DNA technology, a protein can be obtained in abundant quantity. The objectives of protein engineering are to create superior enzymes to catalyse production of high value specific chemicals and to produce enzymes for large scale use.

27 (*a*) Both A and R are true and R is the correct explanation of A.

An immobilised enzyme is physically entrapped or covalently bonded by chemical means to an inert and usually insoluble matrix, where it can act upon its natural substrate. The matrix is usually a high molecular weight polymer such as polyacrylamide, cellulose, starch, glass, beads, etc. Because of its binding with a matrix, the immobilised enzyme has better stability in many cases. Efficiency of immobilised enzyme is better. The enzyme can be recovered at the end of the reaction and can be used repeatedly.

28 (*e*) Both A and R are false and can be corrected as

Penicillin is obtained from *Penicillium notatum* and *Penicillium chrysogenum*, whereas ergot is obtained from *Claviceps purpurea*.

29 (*e*) Both A and R are false and can be corrected as

Amylase is produced by *Aspergillus oryzae*, while invertase from *Saccharomyces cerevisiae*.

30 (*b*) Both A and R are true, but R is not the correct explanation of A.

Champagne and wines are the product of fermentation. It is bottled, before fermentation is complete. Rum is an alcoholic distillate from the fermented juice of sugarcane and sugarcane byproducts.

31 (*b*) Both A and R are true, but R is not the correct explanation of A.

About 12-16% of alcohol is found in champagne and wine, while the content of alcohol in rum is 60-70%.

(C) Medical Entrances' Gallery

1 (*d*) Bioactive molecule, cyclosporin-A is used as an immunosuppressive agent in organ transplant patients. It is produced by the fungus *Trichoderma polysporum.*

On the other hand, *Monascus purpureus* is a yeast which helps to produce statins (blood cholesterol lowering agent). *Saccharomyces cerevisiae* is a yeast which produces ethanol. *Penicillium notatum* is a yeast which produces penicillin (an antibiotics).

4 (*a*) Statins are commercial blood cholesterol lowering agent as they competitively inhibit the enzymes involved in cholesterol synthesis. They are obtained from a yeast, *Monascus purpureus.*

Other options can be explained as

- Streptokinase is a clot buster which is used to treat myocardial infarction.
- Lipases help to digest fat molecules, while cyclosporin-A is an immunosuppressant.

5 (*c*) Bioreactors are required for growing microbes on a large scale for the industrial production of enzymes.

These large vessels provide biologically active environment with appropriate conditions of pH, temperature, nutrients, aeration, etc.

On the other hand, sludge digesters are used to decompose organic solid waste. BOD incubators are used to maintain the temperature for test tissue culture growth, storage of bacterial cultures, etc. Industrial ovens are used for variety of processes like drying, curing, etc.

7 (*a*) The correct group of biocontrol agents is *Trichoderma*, Baculovirus and *Bacillus thuringiensis.* Baculoviruses are pathogens that attack insects and other arthropods. Most of Baculoviruses used as biocontrol agent belong to the genus *Nucleopolyhedrovirus.*

Trichoderma is extensively used against pathogenic fungi which causes soil borne diseases.

Bacillus thuringiensis secretes toxin crystals which kill the insect larvae.

On the other hand, *Rhizobium, Nostoc, Azospirillum* and *Oscillatoria* are used as biofertilisers. Tobacco mosaic virus is a pathogen and aphids are pests that harm crop plants.

8 (*d*) *Trichoderma* can be used as a biocontrol agent in the treatment of plant disease. It is a filamentous soil fungus having mycoparasitic activity. On the other hand, *Anabaena* helps in nitrogen-fixation, *Lactobacillus* helps in the production of curd from milk and *Chlorella* is a producer of single cell protein which acts as food supplement.

9 (*d*) A biocontrol agent to be a part of an Integrated Pest Management (IPM) programme should be species-specific and inactive or have no negative impacts on non-target organisms like plants, mammals, birds, fish and even on other non-target insects. It should kill only targeted insects/pests (organisms).

10 (*c*) Biofertilisers are organisms that enrich the nutrient quality of the soil. For example, cyanobacteria and *Rhizobium. Aspergillus* and *Rhizopus* are not used as biofertilisers.

11 (*c*) Statement in option (c) is not correct and can be corrected as

Certain bacteria which grow anaerobically on cellulosic material produce large amount of methane along with CO_2 and H_2. These bacteria are collectively called methanogens and one such example is *Methanobacterium.*

12 (*a*) Conversion of milk to curd improves its nutritional value by increasing the amount of vitamin-B_{12}.

Other options can be explained as

Vitamin-A is found in milk, carrot, tomato, etc., and it promotes good eyesight. Skin can synthesise vitamin-D in the presence of sunlight and it promotes bone growth. Vitamin-E acts as an antioxidant is found in wheat, green leafy vegetables, etc.

13 (*d*) *Azolla* is used as a biofertiliser because it has association of N_2-fixing cyanobacteria. The leaves of *Azolla* (fern) have as many as 80,000 blue-green algae belonging to *Anabaena azollae.* They have the capacity to fix atmospheric nitrogen and make it available to *Azolla. Azolla pinnata* is an excellent biofertiliser for rice fields. Farmers have reported 50% increase in yield of rice by using this biofertiliser.

14 (*b*) Roquefort cheese is ripened by fungus *Penicillium roqueforti*, which gives a particular flavour. It is a blue coloured cheese made from sheep's milk, which comes from the South of France.

15 (*c*) Option (c) is incorrectly matched and can be corrected as

Butyric acid is produced by fermentative activity of the bacteria called *Clostridium butylicum.* It does not produce lipase. Lipase is obtained from *Candida albicans.*

17 (*b*) The bacterium *Xanthomonas campestris* is not used as biopesticide. It is a causative agent of plant disease, i.e. black rot of cabbage.

18 (*c*) In sewage treatment, suspended solids are removed during primary treatment. It is also known as physical treatment. It consists of shredding, churning, screening and sedimentation. Sequential filtration removes floating and large suspended solids.

24 (*c*) During sewage treatment, biogas is produced. It is a mixture of gases such as methane, hydrogen sulphide and carbon dioxide.

33 (*a*) Biofertilisers are organisms, which bring about nutrient availability to crop plants by fixing the nitrogen. The main sources of biofertilisers are nitrogen-fixing bacteria, nitrogen-fixing cyanobacteria and mycorrhizal fungi, e.g. *Azotobacter, Azolla, Clostridium,* etc.

35 (*b*) *Rhizobium leguminosarum* is a symbiotic bacteria found in root nodules of legume. This bacterium has nitrogen *nif* gene and fixing N_2. Soyabean is a legume. Thus, *Rhizobium* is used as a biofertiliser for raising soyabean crop production.

36 (*d*) *Agrobacterium* is a Gram negative bacterium that causes tumours in plants. It is well-known for its ability to transfer DNA between itself and plants and for this reason it has become an important tool for genetic engineering.

A. tumefaciens causes crown gall disease in plants. It has Ti plasmid.

So, *Agrobacterium* is not a biofertiliser.

CHAPTER 20

Plant Breeding and Tissue Culture

Plants are the basic source of our food. Over 50% of the supply of food comes from the seven cereal grains including rice and wheat. But now, the world is facing a problem. Our food production is not in accordance with the increase in our population. Thus, in order to meet the food requirements of the growing population, we need to incorporate modern agricultural techniques like **plant breeding** and **tissue culture** to increase crop yield.

PLANT

It is the process of developing varieties of plants that are superior to the existing varieties in terms of their economic use. In this process, refined varieties of crops are developed by improving their genetic make up. Therefore, they become commercially successful and more desirable, both agronomically and economically.

The classical plant breeding involves crossing or hybridisation of pure lines, followed by artificial selection. However, due to advancements in genetics, molecular biology and tissue culture, the plant breeding activities are becoming much more advanced.

Objectives of plant breeding

Plant breeding is always carried out on the basis of certain objectives such as

- Development of high yielding varieties.
- Improvement of the quality, such as grain size, colour, shape, flavours and protein content, etc.
- Development of disease and insect resistant varieties.
- Change in duration in maturity of some crops. It permits crop rotations and often extends the crop area. For example, development of wheat varieties suitable for late planting has permitted rice-wheat rotation.
- Modification of agronomic characteristics, such as plant height, branching, tillering, erect or trailing habit, etc.
- Development of **photoinsensitive** and **thermoinsensitive** varieties.
- To improve synchronous maturity. It is highly desirable in crops where several picking is necessary, e.g. *Vigna radiata.*

Inside

- To develop non-shattering characteristics in crops, as shattering is a major problem in several commercial varieties.
- Development of varieties with determinate growth.
- To remove or produce dormancy, whatever is desirable to the particular crop plant.
- Development of varieties with moisture stress and salt tolerance for the rainfed areas and for saline soils.
- Elimination of toxic substances from the crops, so as to make them safe for consumption, e.g. β-N-Oxalylamine Alanine (β-N-OA), a neurotoxin from Khesari (*Lathyrus sativus*).
- To increase the responsiveness to fertilisers.

The understanding of various techniques involved in plant breeding contributed a lot to the establishment of green revolution.

Green revolution

- It is the rapid increase in agricultural production (especially wheat and rice) during 1960-1970s. It occurred as a result of the introduction of high yielding varieties, increased irrigation facilities, applications of fertilisers, weed pest and pathogen control, multiple cropping and better agricultural management.
- **Dr. NE Borlaug** is known as **Father of Green Revolution**. He was conferred Nobel Prize for peace in 1970. **Dr. MS Swaminathan** is known as **Father of Green Revolution** in India. He collaborated with Dr Borlaug and obtained semidwarf Mexican varieties of rice and wheat.
- After this, Indian scientists initiated the following five strategies for breeding a wide range of high yielding varieties possessing a broad spectrum of resistance to major biotic and abiotic stresses.
  (i) **Direct introduction** of promising Mexican wheats, which led to the release of **Lerma Roja 64A** and **Sonora 64**.
  (ii) **Selection** from the advanced generation material received from Mexico. This led to the release of **Kalyan Sona** and **Sonalika**.
  (iii) **Hybridisation** between Mexican strains and Indian varieties resulted in several high yielding and rust-resistant strains.
  (iv) **Mutation breeding** for changing the red grain colour of **Lerma Roja 64A** and **Sonora 64**. This, led to the release of **Pusa Lerma** and **Sharbati Sonora**.
  (v) **Crossing the semidwarf** *Triticum aestivum* with *Triticum durum* varieties. This permitted the release of **Malavika** (HD-452), which was the first dwarf high yielding durum wheat varieties.

High yielding varieties

The high yielding varieties produced during green revolution are described below

(i) Semidwarf wheat

- Dr. Borlaug and his associates developed semidwarf wheat varieties at **International Centre for Wheat and Maize Improvement** (ICWMI), Mexico.
- These wheat (*Triticum aestivum*) varieties are lodging resistant, fertiliser responsive, high yielding, photoinsensitive and generally resistant to rust and other major diseases of wheat.
- They used a Japanese variety, **Norin 10** (a high yielding semidwarf winter wheat variety) as a source of Norin 10 gene (dwarfing gene).

  An outline of the crosses done for the reproduction of semidwarf wheat varieties is given below

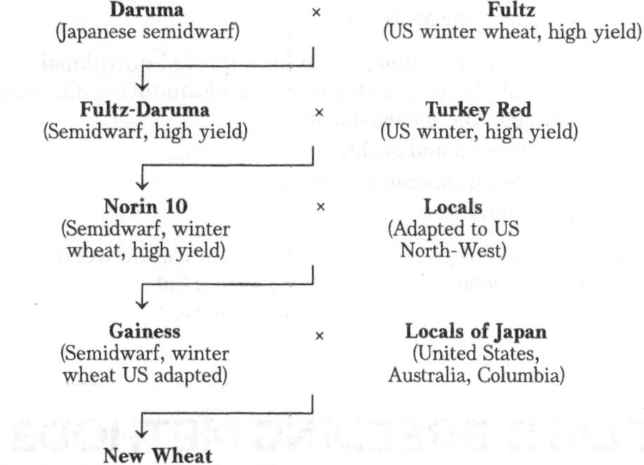

- **ICAR** (Indian Council of Agricultural Research) in 1963, introduced several dwarf varieties including **Sonalika** and **Kalyan Sona** in all wheat growing belts of India.
- Sonora-64 and Lerma Roja-64 were brought by India and modified though gamma mutation, so that these could become part of Indian, agriculture.

(ii) Semidwarf rice

- A dwarfing gene **'dee-geo-woo-gen of rice'** (*Oryza sativa*) was first noted in **Taiwan**. The scientists from Taichung and Phillipines used this gene and produced **Taichung Native-I** and **IR-8** respectively. It was produced at **International Rice Research Institute** (IRRI), Philippines.
- **TN-1** is the first semidwarf fertiliser responsive hybrid variety. It was developed at **Taichung District Agricultural Improvement Station** (TDAIS).
- **IR-8** variety earned the soubriquet **'miracle rice'**. It was short statured, sturdy stemmed, photoperiod insensitive,

high yielding and fertiliser responsive variety adapted to a wide range of environments.

- IR-8 was followed by a series of several IR varieties (i.e. IR-20, IR-24, IR-26, IR-54, IR-72, etc). **IR 36** is the most widely planted variety in history. It was developed by crossing 13 varieties of *Oryza nivara*.

  Later, better yielding semidwarf varieties **Jaya** and **Ratna** were developed in India.

(iii) Sugarcane

- *Saccharum barberi* (grown in North India) had poor sugar content and yield. However, *Saccharum officinarum* (did not grow well in North India) had higher sugar content and thicker stems.
- These two species were crossed together such that sugarcane varieties combined the desirable qualities of high sugar content, high yield, thick stems and ability to grow in the sugarcane area of North India.

(iv) Millets

- Hybrid jowar, maize and bajra have been developed in India.
- Hybrid variety has led to the development of several high yielding varieties resistant to water stress.

CHECK POINT 20.1

1. An objective of plant breeding is
(a) to produce low yielding crop
(b) to decrease responsiveness to fertilisers in crops
(c) to produce disease and insect resistant crops
(d) None of the above

2. Plant breeding is undertaken for improved nutritional quality of plants, with the objective of improving all, except.
(a) Protein content and quality
(b) Oil content and quality
(c) Increased cholesterol content
(d) Vitamin content

3. The period of green revolution in India was between
(a) 1990–2000 (b) 1930–1940
(c) 1960–1970 (d) 1950–1960

4. Norin 10 was produced by crossing between
(a) Daruma × Fultz
(b) Fultz-Daruma × Turkey Red
(c) Gainess × Locals of Japan
(d) Locals × Gainess

5. A dwarfing gene noted in Taiwan in rice variety, which led to production of IR-8 variety is
(a) dee-geo-woo-gen (b) TN-1
(c) Norin 10 (d) IR-24

6. IR-36 was developed through breeding of
(a) 6 rice varities of with *Oryza sativa*
(b) 13 rice varities with *Oryza nivara*
(c) *Oryza sativa* and *Oryza indica*
(d) *Oryza indica* only

PLANT BREEDING METHODS

The process of plant breeding is carried out in a controlled environment by undertaking following steps

1. Collection of variability

- All breeding programmes mainly depend on genetic variability. Collection of variability refers to collection of variable plants or their seeds.
- All these plants contain valuable alleles of genes. The entire collection of plants/seeds having all the diverse alleles for all genes in a given crop is called **'germplasm collection'**.

2. Evaluation and selection of parents

The whole germplasm is first evaluated for plants with desirable combination of characters. Then selection of parents is done by picking up the seeds of only those plants having the desired traits.

3. Crop improvement

The common methods of crop improvement are as follows

(i) Plant introduction

- It is the process of introducing a genotype or plant into a new environment from its native environment for the use of mankind.
- An introduced plant is called **exotic species** if it is brought from a foreign country or **indigenous species** if it is brought from same country.

  It may be classified into following two categories

  (a) **Primary introduction** The introduced variety is well-adapted to the new environment. Hence, it is directly released for commercial cultivation, e.g. Sonora 64, Lerma Roja, Taichung Native-1 (TN-1), TR-8, IR-28, IR-36, etc.

  (b) **Secondary introduction** The introduced variety is subjected to selection and hybridisation, e.g. Sonalika and Kalyan Sona wheat varieties.

Table 20.1 Some of the introduced plant varieties showing good performance in India

Crop	Variety	Introduced from
Wheat	(i) Relay (ii) Sonora 63 (iii) Sonora 64	Australia USA USA
Oat	Kent	Australia
Tomato	Sioux	USA
Onion	Texas	USA
Grape	Beauty seedless	USA
Rice	IR-8	Philippines
Maize	Dixie 11, 12	USA

(ii) Selection

- It is the oldest method of plant breeding and also the basis of all crop improvement programmes. It includes picking up of plants that possess some desirable characters.
  The selection may be natural. However, it takes a longer duration to bring about improvement. In contrast, artificial selection bring about improvement within few years.
  Various artificial selection methods applied in plants are as follows
  (a) **Mass selection** It is the simplest, easiest and the oldest method.
    - It is usually used to improve cross-pollinated crops.
    - The basis of mass selection is the presence of heterozygosity or variability.
    - In this process, a breeder selects a number of plants at the time of harvesting. This selection is based on the phenotypic characters such as, fruit size, number or size of seeds, etc.
    - In cross-pollinated crops, mass selection is usually practiced for population improvement purposes. In self-pollinated crops, it has only a limited use of maintaining purity of a variety.
    - Some important cotton varieties like Dharwar American, Dodahatti local, Cambodias, etc., are obtained from mass selection.
    - TMU-1, TMU-2, AK-10 and K-122, etc., are some groundnut varieties, which are the results of the mass selection.

  (b) **Pureline selection** The term 'pureline' was suggested by **Johannsen** (1903) for homozygous and self-pollinated plants.
    - In this selection, a large number of plants are selected from a self-pollinated crop and are harvested individually.
    - Individual plant progenies from them are evaluated and the best progeny is released as a pureline variety.
    - Pureline selection is the favourite method for improvement of local varieties having considerable genetic variability.

Table 20.2 Some improved varieties obtained from pureline selection

Crop	Varieties
Wheat	NP-4, NP-6, K-13, Kalyan Sona, Sonalika
Rice	Co-4, Co-10, Mu-3
Cotton	Co-2, RC-50, Gourani, Nandyal 14, Coconada 1
Tobacco	NP-28, T-59
Groundnut	TMV 3 Kt
Castor	HC-1, HC-6

  (c) **Progeny selection** It is mainly employed in cross-pollinated crops.
    - It is based on the principle of testing the progenies of selected plants.
    - In 1908, **Hopkins** developed an ear to row method of progeny selection. It is now a common method used to obtain maize.

  (d) **Clonal selection** A clone is a group of plants produced from a single plant through vegetative propagation.
    - Clonal selection is the selection of desirable clones from the mixed population of vegetatively propagated plants.
    - In these crops, the progenies derived from a plant resemble the parent plant in genetic constitution.
    - A generalised clonal selection involves the collection of possible clonal variability and critical evaluation of each member of a clone for better yield and quality following artificial inoculation of diseases and pests.
      The disease-free and high yielding clones may be selected, further evaluated and multiplied as a variety. It is the method mostly used in improving vegetatively propagated crops.

Table 20.3 The improved varieties developed by clonal selection

Crop	Varieties
Potato	Kufri Red, Kufri Safed
Mango	Mundapa, Padma, Neelam
Banana	Bombay Green, High Gate
Orange	Yuvraj, Blood Red

(iii) Hybridisation

- It is the method of producing new crop varieties, in which two or more plants of unlike genotype (genetically dissimilar) are crossed.
- It is practiced both in self-pollinated and cross-pollinated crops. In hybridisation, no new characters are formed, but new combinations are formed.
- The process of hybridisation involves
  - (a) **Combination breeding** The main aim of combination breeding is the transfer of one or more characters into a single variety from the other variety.
  - (b) **Transgressive breeding** It aims at improving yield or its contributing characters through transgressive segregation. This refers to the appearance of such plants in a F_2-generation that are superior to both parents for one or more characters.

Types of hybridisation

On the basis of taxonomic relationships of the parents involved in a cross, hybridisation may be of following types

(a) **Intravarietal hybridisation** It is a cross between two plants of the same variety having different genotypes. This is useful for the improvement of self-pollinated crops.

(b) **Intervarietal hybridisation** It is a cross between the plants of two different varieties of the same species. It is also known as **intraspecific hybridisation**. This process is employed in the improvement of both self-pollinated and cross-pollinated crops.

Table 20.4 Some varieties improved by intervarietal hybridisation

Wheat	NP-52 × NP-165 → NP-170
Paddy	TN-1 × TN-141 → Jaya
Cotton	Malvi 8 × Jarlia → Maljari Grade 1 × Co-2 → Laxmi
Tomato	Sioux × Meeruti → Pusa Rubi
Maize	Ganga hybrid, Ganga Safed, Ranjit hybrid, Histarch
Mango	Prabha Shankar

(c) **Interspecific hybridisation** The cross is made between plants of two different species of the same genus. Hence, it is also known as **intrageneric hybridisation.**

- These crosses are practiced to produce resistance for diseases, pests, drought, etc.
- By this method, the genes for resistance located in the wild species are brought into a single hybrid individual.
- Some varieties developed through interspecific hybridisation are as follows
  - **Cotton** *Gossypium hirsutum* × *Gossypium arboreum* → Deviraj
  - **Cotton** *Gossypium hirsutum* × *Gossypium herbaceum* → Devitej
  - **Tomato** *Lycopersicon esculentum* × *Lycopersicon pimpinellifolium* → Pusa red plum
  - **Wheat** *Triticum aestivum* × *T. durum* → PI 94587 (Resistant to hessian fly)

(d) **Intergeneric hybridisation** These crosses are made between the plants belonging to different genera of the same family.

- This is the most difficult method among all types of crosses.
- The hybrids produced by this method are both scientifically as well as agronomically significant.
- The useful varieties developed by this method are as follows
  - *Triticum aestivum* × *Secale cerale* → *Triticale*
  - Radish × cabbage → Rabbage
  - *Raphanus sativus* × *Brassica oleracea* → *Raphanobrassica*
  - Brinjal × Tomato → Bromato
  - Sugarcane × *Sorghum* → Sugarcane *Sorghum*
  - Potato × Tomato → Pomato

Triticale : The man-made cereal

It is the first man-made cereal. It is the result of artificial **allopolyploidy** between wheat (*Triticum*) and rye (*Secale*) species. Depending upon whether tetraploid ($2n = 4x = 28$) or hexaploid ($2n = 6x = 42$), wheat is utilised for the synthesis. *Triticale* may be hexaploid or octaploid. In each case, only diploid rye ($2n = 2x = 14$) is used.

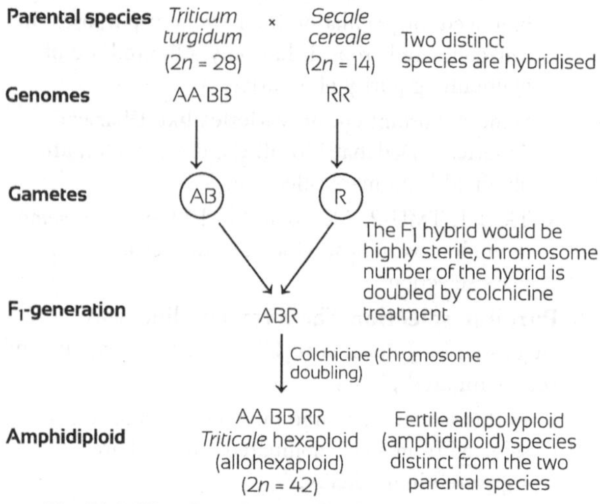

Fig. 20.1 Flowchart showing the development of Triticale

Steps of plant hybridisation

The following steps are involved in hybridisation

(a) **Selection of parents** This is based upon the objectives of the breeder. It is always better to select locally available plants as parents because they are already adapted to that climate.

(b) **Selfing of parents** In this step, parents are allowed to self-pollinate for several generations. The objective of selfing is to eliminate the undesirable genes.

(c) **Hybridisation** The selected plants marked as male and female are allowed to cross-breed. For effective cross-breeding, self-pollination is completely prevented.

This step is carried out by following manner

- **Emasculation** It is the process of removal of stamens of a flower, without affecting the female reproductive organs. Emasculation is usually done in bisexual flowers before the anthers mature and stigma has become receptive.
- It can be done by various methods, such as, hand emasculation, suction method, hot water emasculation, alcohol treatment, cold treatment and genetic emasculation. Among these methods, hand and suction method are mostly used.
- **Hand emasculation** is used for flowers with large anthers. In this method, the anthers are carefully removed with the help of fine-tip-forcep generally in the evening (between 4-6 pm).
- **Suction method** is used for small flowers. In this case, a thin rubber or glass tube is attached to a suction hose. It is used to suck the anthers from the flower.
- **Bagging** In this method, the emasculated flower or inflorescence is immediately bagged to avoid pollination by any foreign pollen. Emasculation bags made up of butter paper, fine cloth or polythene, etc., may be used depending upon the crop.
- **Tagging** In this process, the emasculated and bagged inflorescence or flowers are tagged and properly labelled.

  The labels contain following information

- Date of emasculation
- Date of pollination
- Name of female and male plants. The name of the female parent plant is written first and that of the male parent plant is written later.
- **Crossing** The properly labelled flowers are then allowed to cross-pollinate. The crossed flowers are then tagged again.

(d) **Harvesting F_1 seeds and raising F_1-generation** On maturity, the seeds developed after crossing, i.e. the F_1 seeds are harvested, dried and stored. The seeds from each cross should be kept separately. In the next season, these seeds are sown and F_1-plants are raised. Thus, F_1-plants are hybrids of parents with desirable characters.

Table 20.5 Some varieties developed by hybridisation

Crop	Varieties
Wheat	NP-165, NP-710
Rice	Padma, Jaya, Krishna, Sabarmati
Maize	Ganga, Ranjit, Decan, Histarch, Sweet Maize, Ganga Safed
Cotton	Vinar, Deiraj, Devitej, MCU, Lakshmi, Varlakshmi
Tomato	Pusa Red Plum, Pusa Ruby

Hybrid vigour or Heterosis

- The term 'heterosis' was first used by **Shull** in 1914. It was though, first studied by **Kolreuter** (1763) followed by **Darwin** (1876).
- **Heterosis** is the superiority of the hybrid over either of its parents in one or more traits. This is caused by hybridisation between unrelated strains.
- Hybrid vigour results in increased yield and growth. It may also increase resistance to various diseases.
- Heterosis is usually lost by inbreeding (self-fertilisation).
- It is generally expressed as an increase in size and yield, but it may be expressed in several ways. For example, earlier or later flowering and maturity, greater adaptability, faster growth rate, etc. It is observed both in cross and self-pollinated species.
- Following theories have been proposed to explain heterosis. These are as follows

  (a) **Dominance hypothesis** It states that heterosis is the result of masking of harmful effects of recessive alleles by their dominant alleles.

  (b) **Overdominance hypothesis** According to this, heterosis is the result of superiority of the heterozygote.
- It is generally believed that heterosis is the result of dominance and epistatic interactions.

Importance of heterosis

Heterosis is commercially exploited in the form of hybrid or synthetic varieties. It has been extensively used in many crop species, e.g. vegetables, fruits and in animals also.

Table 20.6 List of some examples of species in which heterosis is commercially exploited

Category	Example
Crop species	Asexually propagated species, cross-pollinated species, e.g. maize, jowar, bajra, sugarbeet, sunflower, forage grasses, forage legumes, cotton and some self-pollinated crops, e.g. rice.
Vegetable crops	Tomato, brinjal, onion, cucurbits and Brussel's sprouts.
Fruit trees	All fruit
Animals	Silkworm, poultry, cattle and swine

(iv) Polyploid breeding

- Presence of more than two sets of chromosomes in a plant is called **polyploidy**. This arises due to failure of mitosis in somatic cells where chromosomes duplicate in S-phase.
- When polyploids are exploited by plant breeders for crop improvement, it is known as **polyploid breeding.**
- It is performed by to achieve genetically stable plants with improved characteristics.
- Polypoids are produced by artificially inducing polyploidy.

Induction of polyploidy

Polyploidy can be induced by following methods

(a) **Physical agents,** such as heat or cold treatments, centrifugation and X-ray or γ-ray radiation. These may produce polyploids in low frequencies.
For example, heat treatment has been successfully used in barley (*Hordeum vulgare*), wheat (*Triticum aestivum*), rye (*Secale cereal*), etc.

(b) **By colchicine treatment,** which is the most effective and widely used for chromosome doubling. **Colchicine** is a poisonous chemical isolated from the seeds (0.2-0.8%) and bulbs (0.1-0.5%) of autumn crocus (*Colchicum autumnale*). It blocks spindle formation during cell division thus, inhibits the movement of sister chromatids to the opposite poles. The resulting restitution nucleus includes all the chromatids. As a result, the chromosome number of the cells is doubled.

(c) Various chemicals such as acenepthene, 8-hydroxyquinoline and nitrous oxide, etc., have polyploidisation effect. These chemicals are much less effective than colchicine and are not commonly used.

Achievements of polyploid breeding

The role of polyploidy in crop improvement is as follows

- Seedless watermelons ($3n$) and banana ($3n$) have been produced by polyploid breeding. They have been developed by to a cross between tetraploid female and diploid male.
- **TV-29**, a triploid variety of tea, has been produced by tea research association of India. It has large shoots and leaves and is tolerant to drought also.
- Pusa giant berseem ($4n$) is the polyploid variety that yields more fodder than diploid varieties.
- *Triticale* is a synthetic hexaploid.
- *Raphanobrassica* is a tetraploid man-made genus produced by colchicine treatment.
- The commercial bread wheat, *T. aestivum* is a hexaploid produced from a cross between *T. monococcum* ($2n = 14$) and *Aegilops speltoides* ($2n = 14$). The hybrid was a tetraploid, that was later crossed with *Aegilops squarrosa* ($2n = 14$). Their cross led to the formation of hexaploid bread wheat.

(v) Mutation breeding

- Mutation is a sudden heritable change in the characteristics of an organism. When mutations are artificially induced in a crop for crop improvement, it is known as mutation breeding.
- Mutations can be artificially induced by certain agents called **mutagens.** These mutagens are of two types
  (a) **Physical mutagens** They comprise mainly of radiations, e.g. X-rays, β-rays, γ-rays and UV-rays.
  (b) **Chemical mutagens** These include nitrous acid maleic hydrazide, hydrazine, Methyl Methane Sulphonate (MMS), Ethyl Methane Sulphonate (EMS), etc.

Achievements of mutation breeding

These are as follows

- Sharbati Sonora was produced from Sonora 64 by mutation breeding using γ-rays.
- Some new crop varieties developed by mutation breeding are **NP-386** (wheat), **Jagannath** (rice), **Aruna** (castor), **Mu-7** and **Indore 2** (cotton), **Pusa Lal Meeruti** (tomato), **Primex** (white mustard), etc.
- By mutation breeding, disease resistance has been induced in dwarf variety of paddy, i.e. IR-8.
- In total, about 200 mutant varieties have been released in India till now. The largest number of varieties that have been developed are rice (278), barley (229) and wheat (113).
- China has developed the largest number (281) of mutant varieties followed by India (200), Russia (82) and Japan (65).

Table 20.7 Some of the important mutant strains

Crop	Varieties
Wheat (*Triticum aestivum*)	Sharbati Sonora
Rice (*Oryza sativa*)	Jagannath, IIT-60, Padmini
Sugarcane (*Saccharum officinarum*)	Co-1852, 8153
Ground nut (*Arachis hypogea*)	TG-17, TG-19
Pea (*Pisum sativum*)	Hans
Pigeon pea (*Cajanus cajan*)	TV-1, TAT-70
Black gram (*Vigna mungo*)	TAU-1
Jute (*Corchorus olitorius*)	TKJ-40

4. Selection of superior recombinants

The progenies produced by the crop improvement method are selected on the basis of objective of plant breeding. Selected plants are self-pollinated for several generations to bring out a state of uniformity (homozygosity).

5. Commercialisation of new cultivars

The new cultivars are evaluated and tested for agronomic traits such as yield, quality, disease resistance, etc. **Indian Council of Agriculture Research** (ICAR) carries out all evaluations in India. After testing, the seeds of plants are certified by **National Seed Corporation** (NSC) and the new variety is released in the market.

CHECK POINT 20.2

1. In plant breeding, the entire collection of plants or seeds having all the diverse alleles far all genes in a given crop is known as
(a) gene pool (b) genome
(c) germplasm collection (d) None of these

2. Which of the following is a variety developed by primary introduction?
(a) IR 36 (b) TN 28
(c) PV 14 (d) HC 1

3. The variety of wheat improved by pureline selection is
(a) NP-6 (b) HC-1
(c) TMV-3 (d) HC-6

4. Emasculation of female plant having bisexual flowers is carried out in hybridisation programme with the help of forceps by removing
(a) style before dehiscence of anthers
(b) style after dehiscence of anthers
(c) anthers before their dehiscence
(d) anthers after their dehiscence

5. Hybrid vigour is mainly due to
(a) heterozygosity
(b) superiority of all the genes
(c) homozygosity of pure characters
(d) mixing up of cytoplasm of the male with that of the female exclusively

6. Polyploidy involves
(a) increase in chromosome number
(b) decrease in chromosome number
(c) increase in number of genome sets
(d) None of the above

PLANT BREEDING TO INCORPORATE DESIRED TRAITS

The main aim of plant breeding is to produce crops and seeds with traits like better yield, disease resistance, insect/pest resistance, improved nutritional quality, etc. The methods and advantages to these traits in plants are discussed below

Disease resistance

- A disease is a complex phenomenon that results in abnormal growth or dysfunction of a plant.
- The development of a disease in a plant depends on the interaction of various factors like host genotype, pathogen genotype and environment.
- The wide range of disease in plants are caused by fungi, bacteria, viruses and nematodes.
- Most of the diseases result into the reduction of crop yield. To overcome this situation, farmers use fungicides and bacteriocides. However, such chemicals have adverse effects on both environment and the human health.
- Hence, it is beneficial for farmers to opt for plant breeding methods for disease resistance.

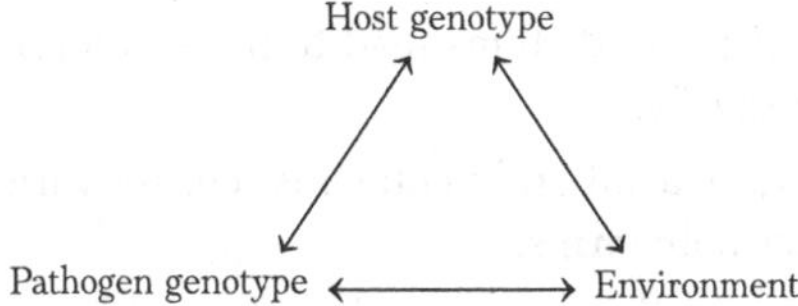

Fig. 20.2 Interaction of factors causing disease

- Resistance is the capacity of plants to resist, withstand, lessen and overcome the attack of pathogens. It denotes less disease development in a genotype than that in the susceptible variety.

- By developing disease resistance, food production can be increased. It will also reduce the application of fungicide and bacteriocides.
- Disease resistance can be developed by the use of conventional breeding, mutation breeding, etc.
- Some disease resistant crops developed by plant breeding are given in the table

Table 20.8 Some disease resistant crop varieties

Crop	Variety	Resistance to diseases
Wheat	Himgiri	Leaf and stripe rust, hill bunt
Brassica	Pusa Swarnim	White rust
Chilli	Pusa Sadabahar	Chilly mosaic virus, tobacco mosaic virus and leaf curl
Cauliflower	Pusa Shubhra, Pusa show ball K I	Black rot
Cowpea	Pusa Komal	Bacterial blight

Advantages of disease resistance breeding

- Disease resistance varieties provide the cheapest and hazard-free means of controlling disease.
- Once incorporated, resistant varieties go a long way in protecting crop loss due to diseases.
- Disease resistance is the only control measure against many diseases, where chemicals or other measures are not successful, e.g. wilts, wheat rusts and viral diseases, etc.

Insect/Pest resistant

- Another major cause for large scale destruction of crop plants is insect or pest infestation. Some plants are genetically resistant to insects/pests, while some are susceptible to certain insects.
- The inherited insect resistance in host crop plants may be due to morphological, biochemical or physiological characteristics as follows
  (i) Hairy leaves in several plants are associated with resistance to insect/pests. For example, resistance to jassids in cotton and cereal leaf beetle in wheat.
  (ii) In wheat, solid stems lead to non-preference by the stem sawfly.
  (iii) Smooth leaved and nectar less cotton varieties do not attract bollworms.
  (iv) High aspartic acid, low nitrogen and high sugar content in maize leads to resistance to maize stem borers.
- Breeding methods for insect/pest resistance involve the same steps as those for any other agronomic trait. The sources of resistant genes may be cultivated varieties and/or germplasm collections, etc.
- Some released insect/pest resistant crop varieties by hybridisation and selection are given below

Table 20.9 Insect/pests resistant crop varieties

Crop	Variety	Insect/Pests
Brassica (rapeseed mustard)	Pusa Gaurav	Aphids
Flat bean	Pusa Sem 2, Pusa Sem 3	Jassids, aphids and fruit borer
Okra (bhindi)	Pusa Sawani, Pusa A 4	Shoot and fruit borer

Improved nutritional quality

Crops are the chief source of carbohydrates, fats, proteins, vitamins and other various substances. Nutritional quality of a crop determines its effects on health of during being (human/animals).

The nutritional quality of a crop may be observed in terms of the following

- Protein content
- Protein quality
- Protein digestibility
- Oil content
- Oil quality (fatty acid consumption)
- Mineral content

Biofortification

Breeding methods developed to produce crops with high levels of vitamins, proteins and minerals, to improve public health are called biofortification.

Some of the varieties developed as a result of biofortification are as follows

- Maize hybrids having twice the amount of the amino acids, lysine and tryptophan, compared to existing varieties were developed. **Protina, Shakti** and **Ratna** are the three lysine rich maize hybrids developed in India.
- **Atlas 66**, a protein rich wheat variety has been used as a donor for the improvement of cultivated wheat.
- It has been possible to develop an iron fortified rice variety containing over five times as much iron as in commonly consumed varieties.
- The **Indian Agricultural Research Institute**, New Delhi has also released several vegetable crops that are rich in vitamins and minerals, e.g. **vitamin-A** enriched carrots, spinach, pumpkin, **vitamin-C** enriched bitter gourd, bathua, mustard, tomato; **iron** and **calcium** enriched spinach and bathua and **protein** enriched beans, lablab, French and garden peas.

Single Cell Protein (SCP)

- Conventional agricultural production of cereals, pulses, vegetables and fruits, etc., may not be able to meet the demand of food at the rate at which human and animal population is increasing.
- The shift from grain to meat diet also creates more demand for cereals as it takes 3-10 kg of grain to produce 1 kg of meat by animal farming.
- One of the alternate sources of proteins for animal and human nutrition is **Single Cell Protein** (SCP). For this, microbes are being grown on an industrial scale as a source of good protein.
- Microbes like *Spirulina* can be grown easily on materials like waste water from potato processing plants (containing starch), straw, molasses, animal manure and even sewage.
- It produces large quantities and can serve as food rich in protein, minerals, fats, carbohydrate and vitamins.
- Such utilisation also reduces environmental pollution. It has been estimated that in a day, 250 g of microorganisms like *Methylophilus methylotrophus,* can be expected to produce 25 tonnes of protein because of its high rate of biomass production and growth.

CHECK POINT 20.3

1. Which of the following is a bacterial blight resistant variety of cowpea?
(a) Pusa Shubra (b) Himgiri
(c) Pusa Komal (d) Pusa Swarnim

2. Hairy leaves in cotton provides resistance to
(a) cereal leaf bettle (b) ballworms
(c) jassids (d) sawfly

3. Biofertified maize hybrids are improved for
(a) protein content
(b) micronutrient and mineral content
(c) amino acid content
(d) All of the above

4. Himgiri variety of wheat, which was developed by hybridisation and selection is mainly resistant to
(a) white rust (b) bacterial blight
(c) chilly mosaic virus (d) leaf and stripe rust

5. A protein rich wheat variety is
(a) HN-10 (b) IR-8
(c) TN-1 (d) Atlas-66

6. Which of the following is source of single cell protein?
(a) *Bacillus thuringiensis*
(b) *Azospirillum*
(c) *Saccharomyces cerevisiae*
(d) *Methylophilus methylotrophus*

TISSUE CULTURE

- It is the *in-vitro* maintenance and growth of plant cells, tissues or organs on a suitable culture medium. This technique was developed as the conventional breeding methods that failed to keep pace with increasing demands of crop improvement.
- In tissue culture, a plant part is taken and grown under sterile conditions in special nutrient media. The plant part which is cultured is called **explant.** The technique of tissue culture is based on totipotency.

Totipotency

- The concept of totipotency is the basis of tissue culture.
- This was discovered by **Haberlandt** in (1902). Each living cell of a multicellular organisms is capable of independent development, when provided with suitable conditions.
- **Cellular totipotency** is the inherent capability of a somatic cell or explant to divide and differentiate into a complete organism.
- Vegetatively produced descendents of a somatic cell are collectively called **clone.**

Requirements of plant tissue culture

An experiment of plant tissue culture requires a well-equiped laboratory. Some other requirements of plant tissue culture are as follows

1. Explant

It is the tissue obtained from the plant for the purpose of tissue culture. The most commonly used explants are the meristematic ends of the plants. These include stem tip, auxillary bud tip and root tip. Meristematic tissues have high rate of cell division.
Before the procedure starts, explants are cleaned and surface sterilised with the help of disinfectants and detergents to remove germs.

2. Nutrient media

- The medium in which explants are cultured is known as **nutrient medium** or **culture medium** or simply **medium.**
- The culture media may be solid or liquid. The optimum pH of the media should be 5.7.
- The basic components of culture media are
  (i) **Inorganic nutrients** These include salts, that provides all essential macro and microelements.

(ii) **Organic nutrients** These are the sources of energy such as sucrose, glucose, fructose or carbohydrates, amino acids and vitamins, etc.

(iii) **Growth hormone** Auxin (2, 4-D) and cytokinins (benzyl mino purine) are commonly used in tissue culture experiments. A media without growth hormones is known as **base media.**

High auxins concentration induces root formation while high cytokinins promote shoots growth.

3. Sterilisation

- For plant tissue culture experiments, it is essential that the explants, culture vessel, media and instruments, etc., are free from microbes. For this purpose, explants are treated with specific antimicrobial chemicals. This procedure is called **surface sterilisation.**
- The vessels, media and instruments are suitably treated with steam, dry heat or alcohol or subjected to filtration. This makes them free from microbes. This is called **complete sterilisation.**

Types of tissue culture

The plant tissue cultures are often classified according to the type of *in vitro* growth, *viz,* callus and suspension culture or the explant used for culture initiation, e.g. embryo culture, anther culture, etc.

These cultures are described below

1. Callus and suspension culture

- In callus culture, cell division in the explant forms a callus. It is an amorphous mass of loosely arranged thin-walled parenchymatous cells. It develops from proliferating cells of the parent tissue.
- This is usually maintained in an agar medium. In case of suspension culture, explant is suspended in liquid medium. In both cases, callus differentiates into plantlets in different experimental conditions.
- Suspension cultures grow faster than callus cultures.
- In both types of tissue culture experiments, cell/ tissue dry water increases with the passage of time with the simultaneous decrease of nutrients.
- To prevent the damage of newly formed cells, part of the cultures are regularly transferred to new culture vessels containing fresh media. This process is called **subculturing.**

2. Meristem culture

- In this type of tissue culture experiments, meristematic tissues, i.e. shoot and root tips are used as the explants.
- By this method, virus-free clones of plants can be obtained because meristems are usually free of pathogens.

3. Embryo culture

- It involves the excision of young embryo from seeds and their cultivation. It is used in the rescue of aborted embryos, i.e. embryo rescue technique.
- This technique is applicable for the recovery of embryo of interspecific hybrids, e.g. hybrid between *Phaseolus vulgaris* (common bean) and *Phaseolus augustissimus* (wild bean).

4. Haploid culture

- This technique was developed by **Guha** and **Maheshwari** (1946) in *Datura innoxia.*
- In this technique, floral buds are opened to remove anthers. These anthers are then cultured for the production of haploid embryoids.
- The plants produced *via* haploid culture are sterile.
- This technique is also known as **androgenic culture** or **pollen grain culture**, e.g. winter wheat (jinghua-1) and rice (Guan-18).
- Gynogenic haploids are also obtained by using unfertilised ovules.

Uses of androgenic haploid

- It is useful in mutation breeding.
- Androgenic haploids are pure for its characters.
- Every gene can be express in the plant.

5. Somatic hybrid culture

- Somatic hybrids are formed through the fusion of protoplasts of two plants belonging to different varieties, species and even genera. The process through which somatic hybrids are formed is know as **somatic hybridisation.**
- In this culture, isolated protoplasts are selected by culturing them in such a medium where only somatic hybrid protoplast can grow.
- For instance somatic hybrids of *Petunia parodii* and *P. hybrid* can grow and regenerate on a specific medium containing actinomycin D.
- The fused protoplasts are either cultured in liquid or semi-liquid agar media plates. Other methods also used for culturing somatic hybrids, e.g. hanging drop, suspension culture, etc.
- The nutritional requirements of the protoplast culture are different from the nutritional requirements of tissue and cell culture.
- The process of somatic hybridisation is as follows

(i) **Isolation of protoplasts** It is readily achieved by treating cells/tissues with a suitable mixture of cell wall degrading enzymes. Usually pectinase and cellulase are used for the isolation of protoplasts.

(ii) **Fusion of protoplasts** of desired varieties/species. It is induced by **Polyethylene Glycol** (PEG) solution or by electrofusion technique. It can also be achieved using by sodium nitrate and calcium ions. After fusion, either synkaryon (single fused nucleus) or heterokaryon (having two unfused nuclei) are formed.

(iii) **Selection of hybrid cells** The somatic hybrids with desirable characters are selected. The hybrid protoplast is called **cybrid** or cytoplasmic hybrids.

(iv) **Culture of hybrid cells and regeneration of hybrid plants** When the protoplasts are cultured in a suitable medium, they generate cell walls and produce new plants. Thus, in this way somatic hybrid plants are produced.

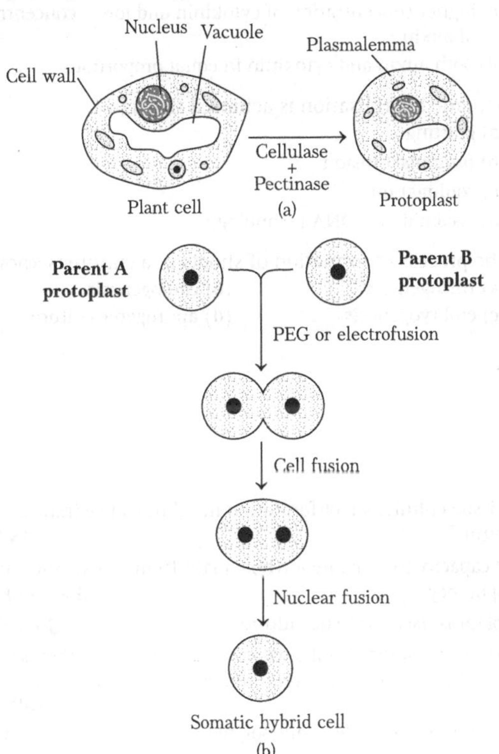

Fig. 20.3 (a) Isolation of protoplast, (b) Somatic hybridisation

- The first ever somatic hybrid was obtained by **Carlson** *et al* (1972). It was produced by fusing protoplasts of *Nicotiana glavca* and *N. langsdorfi.*
- The first intergeneric somatic hybrid, pomato was a result of fusion of tomato with potato.

Applications of somatic hybrids

- Somatic hybrids may be used for gene transfer, transfer of cytoplasm.
- They are used in the production of useful allopolyploids.
- Somatic hybrids, provide a distinct possibility of development of new crop plants.

Plant regeneration in tissue culture

Plant cells cultured *in vitro* can ultimately give rise to complete plants by the process of regeneration. Plantlets can be obtained from cultured cells by two different ways as follows

1. Organogenesis

- It involves the formation of plant organs, i.e. roots and shoots directly from cultured tissues. The process of formation of roots is known as **rhizogenesis**, while that of shoots is **caulogenesis.**
- Organogenesis is highly controlled by the relative concentrations of auxin and cyotokinin in medium.
- Generally, a high concentration of auxin promotes rhizogenesis. On the other hand, high concentration of cytokinin promotes caulogenesis.

2. Somatic embryogenesis

- A **Somatic Embryo** (SE) is an embryo derived from a somatic cell, other than zygote. SEs are obtained usually on culture of the somatic cells *in vitro* and this process is called **somatic embryogenesis.**
- It is induced by a relatively high concentration of auxin, like 2, 4-D.
- SEs are bipolar structures, i.e they have a radicle and a plumule. These young embryos develop into mature embryos either in the same medium or in another medium. Mature somatic embryos germinate to yield complete plantlets.

Establishment of plantlets in the field

- Plantlets are kept under reduced and high humidity conditions for a certain period of time. This process is known as **hardening.**
- It makes the plantlets capable of tolerating the relatively harsh environment outside the culture vessels. After the hardening, plantlets are established in the field.

Applications of plant tissue culture

Plant tissue culture has a number of commercial applications, which are as follows

- It can be used to produce a large number of plantlets vegetatively. This rapid vegetative multiplication of plants in artificial media under aseptic conditions from a small piece of plant is termed as **micropropagation.**
- It is widely used in forestry and floriculture. It can also be used to conserve rare or endangered plant species.
- A plant breeder may use tissue culture to screen cells rather than plants for advantageous characters, e.g. herbicide resistance/tolerance.

- Large scale growth of plant cells in liquid culture in bioreactors is used for the production of valuable compounds. For example, plant derived secondary metabolites and recombinant proteins are used as biopharmaceuticals.
- To cross distantly related species and then raising embryos by tissue culture which would otherwise normally die (embryo rescue).
- For the production of dihaploid plants from haploid cultures to achieve homozygous lines more rapidly in breeding programmes. It is achieved by the treatment with colchicine which causes the doubling of the chromosome number.
- Certain techniques such as meristem tip culture can be used to produce virus-free plants.

CHECK POINT 20.4

1. Tissue culture technique can produce infinite number of new plants from a small parental tissue. The economic importance of the technique is in raising
(a) genetically uniform population identical to the original parent
(b) homozygous diploid plants
(c) development of new species
(d) variants through picking up somaclonal variations

2. The nutrient medium without growth hormone is known as
(a) basal medium (b) incomplete media
(c) complete media (d) full media

3. The procedure of sterilisation of explant by antimicrobial chemicals is known as
(a) surface sterilisation (b) complete sterilisation
(c) explant heating (d) disinfection

4. In callus culture, roots can be induced by the supply of
(a) auxin and no cytokinin
(b) higher concentration of auxin and lower concentration of cytokinin
(c) higher concentration of cytokinin and lower concentration of auxin
(d) Both auxin and cytokinin in equal proportions

5. Somatic hybridisation is achieved through
(a) grafting
(b) protoplast fusion
(c) conjugation
(d) recombinant DNA technology

6. The process of formation of shoots in a culture is known as
(a) rhizogenesis (b) caulogenesis
(c) embryogenesis (d) androgenic culture

EXAM POINTS

- The purposeful manipulation of plant species is called plant breeding. **[UK PMT 2014]**
- A system of rotating crops with leguma or grass pasture to improve soil structure and fertility is called ley farming. **[NEET 2017]**
- Plant grown from hybrid protoplast are called somaclone. **[Kerala CEE 2014]**
- Parbhani Kranti, a variety of bhindi (ladyfinger) is resistant to yellow mosaic virus. **[JIPMER 2017, KCET 2014]**
- In mung bean, resistance to yellow mosaic virus and powdary mildew were brought by mutation breeding. **[NEET 2019]**
- Sonalika is an example of semi-dwarf variety of wheat. **[HP PMT 2012]**
- Breeding crops with higher level of nutrients is called biofortification. **[Kerala CEE 2014]**
- Atlas 66 has high protein content. It has been used as a donor for improving cultivated wheat. **[JIPMER 2019]**
- Virus-free plants can be formed by meristem culture. **[AIIMS 2019]**
- In plant breeding, the entire collection of plants/seeds having the diverse alleles of all genes in a particular organism is called germplasm. **[MHT CET 2012]**
- Sonalika and Kalyan Sona are high yield variety of wheat. **[CBSE AIPMT 2014]**
- In tissue culture, shoot formation in callus can be induced by kinetin. **[AMU 2015]**
- The capacity to generate a whole plant from an explant is called totipotency. **[Kerala CEE 2014]**
- Explant is used in tissue culture. **[JIPMER 2018]**
- Hormones, inorganic salts, vitamin, amino acid. carbon source like sucrose are the basic requirement of tissue culture. **[AIIMS 2019]**
- *Triticale* is an example of allopolyploidy. **[AMU 2015]**
- The common bread wheat has 42 chromosome. **[AMU 2015]**
- Genetically improved crop variety can be developed in laboratory by somatic hybridisation. **[WB JEE 2014]**
- In somatic hybrid, the plants grow from hybrid protoplasm. **[Kerala CEE 2014]**
- During somatic hybridisations in plant, the cell walls and the middle lamella are digested before fusion of the cell. **[KCET 2014]**
- Polyethylene glycol and sodium nitrate enhance or induce fusion of protoplasts. **[CBSE AIPMT 2015]**
- A technique of micropropagation is somatic embryogenesis. **[CBSE AIPMT 2015]**
- Micropropagation is producing large number of plants through tissue culture. **[Kerala CEE 2014]**
- *Cissus Querdranglelaris* plants are used to treat bone fractures. **[AIIMS 2018]**

Chapter Exercises

(A) Topical Exercise

Plant Breeding

1 In India earliest work in the field of plant breeding was initiated by

(a) Rao (b) Barber
(c) Borlaug (d) Vavilov

2 Consider the following statements.

I. Plant breeding has close relationship with genetics.
II. Modern plant breeding started in 1900.

Choose the correct option.

(a) Statement I is true, but II is false
(b) Statement I is false, but II is true
(c) Both statements I and II are true
(d) Both statements I and II are false

3 An important germplasm storing centre in India is

(a) CDRI (b) FRI
(c) ICRISAT (d) NEERI

4 Which one of the following is being tried in India as a biofuel substitute for fossil fuels?

(a) *Aegilops* (b) *Jatropha*
(c) *Azadirachta* (d) *Musa*

5 Match the following columns.

Column I	Column II
A. Venkatraman and Barber	1. Father of green revolution
B. Norman E Borlaug	2. Father of white revolution in India
C. MS Swaminathan	3. Father of green revolution in India
D. Verghese Kurien	4. Nobilisation of sugarcane

Codes

	A	B	C	D
(a)	4	1	3	2
(b)	1	4	3	2
(c)	2	1	3	4
(d)	4	1	2	3

6 The biggest constraint of plant breeding is **[NCERT Exemplar]**

(a) availability of desirable gene in the crop and its wild relatives
(b) infrastructure
(c) trained manpower
(d) transfer of genes from unrelated sources

7 If we were to list the traits or characters that the breeders have tried to incorporate into crop plants, the first will be

(a) resistance to pathogens
(b) increased tolerance to insect pests
(c) increased tolerance to salinity and drought
(d) crop yield and improved quality

8 Consider the following statements.

I. Pusa RH-10 is long and scented grained variety of rice.
II. Pusa Lerma and Sharbati Sonara are mutants of Indian varieties.

Choose the correct option.

(a) Statement I is true, but II is false
(b) Statement I is false, but II is true
(c) Both statements I and II are true
(d) Both statements I and II are false

9 Sonalika and Kalyan Sona are ...*A*... which are introduced in ...*B*... .

	A	B
(a)	High yielding	1967
(b)	High yielding	1963
(c)	High yielding and disease resistance	1967
(d)	High yielding and disease resistance	1963

10 The Mexican wheat variety Sonora-64 and Lerma Roja 64 were modified by gamma mutation for Indian agriculture and were named as ...*A*... and ...*B*..., respectively.

	A	B
(a)	Sharbati Sonora	Pusa Lerma
(b)	Jaya	Ratna
(c)	Pusa Komal	Pusa Sadabahar
(d)	Pusa Swarnim	Himgiri

11 Select the incorrect match.

	Variety	Resistance of diseases
(a)	Wheat (Himgiri)	1. Leaf and stripe rust hill bunt
(b)	*Brassica* (Pusa Swarnim)	2. Black rot
(c)	Cow pea (Pusa Komal)	3. Bacterial blight
(d)	Chilli (Pusa Sadabahar)	4. Chilli mosaic virus, TMV, leaf curl

12 Choose the composite varieties of maize, developed in India.

I. Protina II. Shakti
III. Ratna IV. Pusa 24

Codes
(a) I, II and III (b) I and II (c) Only IV (d) I and IV

13 Several South Indian states raise 2-3 crops of rice annually. The agronomic feature that makes this possible is because of **[NCERT Exemplar]**
(a) shorter rice plant
(b) better irrigation facilities
(c) early yielding rice variety
(d) disease resistant rice variety

14 The best way to increase the yield of wheat in India is
(a) to spread seeds of improved varieties
(b) to use tractors to till the soil
(c) to reduce the quantity of ration consumers
(d) to remove weeds from wheat fields

15 The quickest method of plant breeding is
(a) introduction
(b) selection
(c) hybridisation
(d) mutation breeding

16 Which of the following species has the chromosome complement similar to that of *Triticum aestivum*?
(a) *Zea mays* (b) *Secale cereale*
(c) *Gossypium* (d) *Aegilops*

17 In the hexaploid wheat, the haploid (n) and basic (x) numbers of chromosomes are
(a) $n = 7$ and $x = 21$
(b) $n = 21$ and $x = 21$
(c) $n = 21$ and $x = 14$
(d) $n = 21$ and $x = 7$

18 In bread, wheat chromosome number is
(a) 42 (6×7) (b) 14 (2×7)
(c) 24 (4×6) (d) 21 (7×3)

19 Which one of the following chemical induce polyploidy in plant cells?
(a) 2-4-dichlorophenoxy acetic acid
(b) rifampicin
(c) cytokinin
(d) colchicine

20 For the formation of diploid cells from haploid cells colchicine is used to
(a) stop the spindle fibres formation
(b) replicate DNA twice in one cell cycle
(c) stop the formation of centromere
(d) stop the mitotic division

21 Match the columns with respect to plant varieties developed by mutation breeding.

Column I	Column II
A. Cotton	1. Reimi and Jagannath
B. Rice	2. Erectiferum and Erectoids
C. Wheat	3. Indore-2
D. Barley	4. NP-836

Codes

	A	B	C	D		A	B	C	D
(a)	3	1	4	2	(b)	1	2	4	3
(c)	3	1	2	4	(d)	1	2	3	4

22 Consider the following statements.

I. Heterosis is hybrid vigour.
II. Hybrid vigour is due to homozygosity.

Choose the correct option.
(a) Statement I is true, but II is false
(b) Statement I is false, but II is true
(c) Both statements I and II are true
(d) Both statements I and II are false

23 Rice variety named ADT-37 is formed as a result of cross between
(a) *Oryza japonica* × *O. indices*
(b) *Oryza astevium* × *O. vulgare*
(c) *Oryza sativa* × *O. japonica*
(d) None of the above

24 Consider the following statements.

I. The term heterosis was first studied by Darwin.
II. Hybrid vigour is best maintained in crops by outbreeding.

Choose the correct option.
(a) Statement I is true, but II is false
(b) Statement I is false, but II is true
(c) Both statements I and II are true
(d) Both statements I and II are false

25 The reason why vegetatively reproducing crop plants are best suited for maintaining hybrid vigour is that
(a) these can be easily propagated
(b) once a desired hybrid has been produced there are few chances of losing it
(c) they have a longer lifespan
(d) they are more resistant to diseases

26 In high yielding 'hybrid crop varieties', to exploit hybrid vigour, the farmers need to purchase fresh hybrid seed every year, because
(a) they are not allowed to grow their own seed
(b) the hybrid vigour is lost due to inbreeding depression
(c) the government of India has accepted Dunkel's proposals
(d) it is cheaper to purchase fresh seed.

27 A cybrid is hybrid carrying
(a) genomes and cytoplast of two different plants
(b) cytoplasm of two different plants
(c) cytoplasm of two different plants, but genome of one plant
(d) genome of two different plants

28 Plant can be disease resistant by
(a) breeding with their wild relatives
(b) colchicine treatment
(c) hormone treatment
(d) heat treatment

29 Which one of the following pairs is incorrectly matched in respect to the 'crop varieties for disease resistance'?

	Crop variety	Resistant to
(a)	Pusa Sawani	Fruit borers
(b)	Pusa Sem 3	Jassids and aphids
(c)	Pusa Gaurav	Aphid
(d)	Pusa Sem 2	Shoot borers

30 Pusa Snowball K-1 and Pusa A-4 are resistant from
(a) white rust and jassids, respectively
(b) curl blight black rot and aphids, respectively
(c) black rot and shoot borer, respectively
(d) leaf curl and fruit borer, respectively

31 Find the incorrect match with respect to insect best resistance?

(a)	Pusa Gaurav variety of rapeseed (*Brassica*)	Resistant to aphids
(b)	Pusa Sem 2 variety of flat bean	Resistant to jassids aphids and fruit borer.
(c)	Pusa Sawani variety of okra	Resistant to shoot and fruit borer
(d)	Pusa A-4 variety of bhindi	Resistant to jassids and aphids

32 Consider the following statements.
I. The scientific process by which crop plant are enriched with certain desirable nutrient is called biofortification.
II. Atlas 66 is an example of biofortification.
Choose the correct option.
(a) Statement I is true, but II is false
(b) Statement I is false, but II is true
(c) Both statements I and II are true
(d) Both statements I and II are false

33 Atlas 66 is a variety of ...*A*... with high ...*B*... content.

	A	B
(a)	rice	protein
(b)	wheat	fatty acid
(c)	rice	fatty acid
(d)	wheat	protein

34 One of the alternate sources of proteins for animal and human nutrition is
(a) single cell protein
(b) non-vegetarian meal
(c) mushrooms
(d) pulses

35 Single Cell Protein (SCP) is
(a) protein obtained from a clone of cells
(b) protein obtained from unicellular organisms
(c) biomass got from microorganisms
(d) proteins obtained from biomass of microorganisms

36 SCP is commercially obtained at present from
(a) Yeast and *Fusarium* fungi
(b) *Morchella* and *Agaricus*
(c) *Methanomonas* and other bacteria
(d) All of the above

37 Capacity of a plant cell to give rise to whole plant body is known as
(a) reproduction (b) budding
(c) totipotency (d) regeneration

38 Consider the following statements.
I. *Spirulina* cannot grow on lava.
II. The most common source of SCP is yeast.
Choose the correct option.
(a) Statement I is true, but II is false
(b) Statement I is false, but II is true
(c) Both statements I and II are true
(d) Both statements I and II are false

39 Find out the incorrect statements.
(a) 250g of *Methylophilus methylotrophus* produce 25×10^3 kg of protein in a day
(b) The shift from meat to grain diets creates more demand for cereals
(c) 250 kg cow produce 200 g of protein per day
(d) *Spirulina* when grow on sewage also reduces environmental pollution besides producing large quantities of protein.

Tissue Culture

40 The ability of single cells to divide and produce all differentiated cells in the entity is called
(a) totipotency
(b) sterilisation
(c) pluripotency
(d) hybridisation

41 The first successful cellular totipotency was experimentally performed by
(a) Steward taking phloem cells of carrot root
(b) White taking tracheal cells
(c) Haberlandt taking cells or carrot root
(d) White taking xylem cells

42 In tissue culture medium, the embryoids formed from pollen grains is due to
(a) cellular totipotency (b) organogenesis
(c) double fertilisation (d) test tube culture

43 What is the basis of tissue culture technique that enables the cloning of plants?
(a) Plant cells have a rigid cell wall that increases their ability to divide
(b) Plants have no resistance to pathogens, so they need to be grow in sterile conditions
(c) Plant cells are pluripotent
(d) Plant cells are totipotent

44 In tissue culture why does culture medium contain sugar?
I. Green cells lost chloroplast.
II. Green cells require energy to divide.
III. Sugar maintains pH and does not allow cells to burst.
Choose the correct option.
(a) I and II (b) Only III
(c) I and III (d) I, II and III

45 The optimum pH the nutrient culture medium used in plant tissue culture is
(a) 5.7 (b) 3.8 (c) 7.5 (d) 8.5

46 Sterilisation of tissue culture medium is done by
(a) autoclaving of medium at 120°C for 15 minutes
(b) filtering the medium through fine sieve
(c) mixing the medium with antifungal agents
(d) keeping the medium at -20°C

47 In making a medium for culturing, agar is added because
(a) agar solidifies the medium
(b) agar is a good nutrient
(c) agar does not allow callus formation
(d) agar does not melt easily to 50°C

48 Consider the following statements.
I. The scientific process by which crop plants are enriched with certain desirable nutrients is called biofortification.
II. The term totipotency refers to the capacity of a cell to generate whole plant.
Choose the correct option.
(a) Statement I is true, but II is false
(b) Statement I is false, but II is true
(c) Both statements I and II are true
(d) Both statements I and II are false

49 Hardening in tissue culture is
(a) keeping at 30-50°C temperature for about 30 min
(b) acclimatisation of plants slowly before growing in the field
(c) plunging the vials into water at 37-40°C
(d) None of the above

50 Callus formation is promoted by
I. proper light and subculturing.
II. darkness and subculturing.
III. excess of NAA.
IV. absence of salts.
Choose the correct option.
(a) Only I (b) Only II
(c) I and III (d) II and III

51 In tobacco callus, which one shall induce shoot differentiation in combination of auxin and cytokinin?
(a) higher concentration of cytokinin and lower concentration of auxin
(b) lower concentration of cytokinin and higher concentration of auxin
(c) Only cytokinin and no auxin
(d) Only auxin and no cytokinin

52 It shows correct chronological order of the events occurring during callus culture.
(a) Callus → Cell division → Explant → Addition of cytokinin → Cell acquire meristematic property
(b) Explant → Callus → Cell division → Addition of cytokinin → Cells acquire meristematic property
(c) Explant → Cell division → Callus → Addition of cytokinin → Cells acquire meristematic property
(d) Callus → Explant → Cell division → Addition of cytokinin → Cells acquire meristematic property

53 Pollen grains of a plant ($2n = 28$) are cultured to get callus by tissue culture. What would be the number of chromosomes in the cells of callus?
(a) 56 (b) 28
(c) 21 (d) 14

54 Consider the following statements.
I. Callus is undifferentiated mass of cells.
II. In tissue culture, callus can be induced to form shoot or root by altering the ratio of auxin to cytokinin.
Choose the correct option.
(a) Statement I is true, but II is false
(b) Statement I is false, but II is true
(c) Both statements I and II are true
(d) Both statements I and II are false

55 The first successful experimental attempt of tissue culture was done by ...A... taking ...B... cells.

	A	B
(a)	Haberlandt	Xylem
(b)	Steward	Xylem
(c)	White	Tomato root
(d)	Haberlandt	Phloem

56 The growth regulators commonly used in plant tissue culture are
(a) 2, 4-D and BAP (b) AMO 16 and BAP
(c) 2, 4, 5-T and TIBS (d) TIBA and AMO 16

57 Haploid culture/Androgenic culture was first developed by
(a) Guha and Maheshwari in *Datura innoxia*
(b) Swaminathan in *Datura innoxia*
(c) Ramdeo Mishra in *Solanum*
(d) Venkatraman in *Saccharum*

58 Tissue culture technique can produce indefinite number of new plants from a small parental tissue. The economic importance of the technique is in raising
(a) variants through picking up somaclonal variations
(b) genetically uniform population of an elite species
(c) homozygous diploid plants
(d) development of new species

59 Which of the following is correct for nuclear status of the following during somatic hybridisation technique?
(a) Synkaryon = $4n$, Dikaryon = $2n + 2n$, Cybrid = $2n$
(b) Synkaryon = $2n$, Dikaryon = $n + n$, Cybrid = n
(c) Synkaryon = $2n + 2n$, Dikaryon = $n + n$, Cybrid = $2n$
(d) Synkaryon = $4n$, Dikaryon = $n + n$, Cybrid = $2n + 2n$

60 Sequentially arrange the steps of somatic hybridisation/protoplast fusion/parasexual hybridisation.
I. Chemofusion
II. Synkaryon formation
III. Treatment of plant cells by pectinases and cellulases
(a) I → II → III (b) II → I → III
(c) III → I → II (d) I → III → II

61 During somatic hybridisation in plants
(a) somaclones are produced in large numbers
(b) apical meristem are cultured to get virus free plants
(c) cell walls and middle lamella are digested before fusing the cells
(d) crop plants with higher levels of vitamins, protein and minerals are hybridised

62 In protoplast fusion/somatic hybridisation technique, two protoplasts are fused by
(a) electrofusion (b) PEG
(c) sendai virus (d) All of these

63 Micropropagation is a technique
(a) of somatic embryogenesis for production of true plants
(b) for production of haploid plants
(c) for production of somatic hybrids
(d) for production of somaclonal plants

64 Which one of the following statements regarding pomato is correct?
(a) It is a product of somatic hybridisation
(b) It is a product of gene manipulation
(c) Product of sexual hybridisation
(d) Product of cloning

(B) Cumulative Exercise

(Assorted Questions of the Chapter for Advanced Level Practice)

1 Among the following statements, which one represents top cross?
I. Inbreed variety cross.
II. Polycross.
III. Cross between an inbreed line and an open pollinated variety.
IV. Cross between a single cross and an inbreed line.
Choose the correct option.
(a) I, II and III (b) I and II
(c) II and IV (d) I and III

2 Read the given statements.
I. High aspartic acid, low nitrogen and sugar content in maize leads to resistance to maize stem borers.
II. Pusa Sadabahar is a food variety resistant to chilli mosaic virus.
III. Norman E Borlaug developed a semidwarf variety of wheat.
IV. Germplasm collection is the collection of all sexual genes of an individual.
Choose the incorrect statements.
(a) I and IV (b) II and III
(c) Only IV (d) II, III and IV

3 Which of the statements about breeding is wrong?
(a) By inbreeding purelines cannot be evolved
(b) Continued inbreeding especially close inbreeding reduce fertility and productivity
(c) Inbreeding exposes harmful recessive genes that are eliminated by selection
(d) A single outcross often helps to overcome inbreeding depression

4 Match the following columns.

Column I	Column II
A. Oldest cereal crop	1. Banana
B. Tallest cereal	2. Barley
C. Gossypol	3. Male antifertility chemical present in cotton and its oil
D. Oldest cultivated crop of the world	4. Maize

Codes

	A	B	C	D
(a)	2	1	4	3
(b)	2	4	3	1
(c)	1	3	4	2
(d)	3	1	2	4

5 Arrange the main steps of plant breeding sequentially.

I. Cross-hybridisation among the selected parents.
II. Evaluation and selection of parents.
III. Selection and testing of superior recombinants.
IV. Testing, release and commercialisation of new cultivars.
V. Collection of variability.

(a) II → V → I → IV → III
(b) V → II → III → I → IV
(c) V → II → I → III → IV
(d) II → I → V → III → IV

6 Which of the following is incorrectly matched.

(a) Explant – Excised plant part used for callus formation
(b) Cytokinins – Root initiation in callus
(c) Somatic embryo – Embryo produced from a vegetative cell
(d) Anther culture – Haploid plants

7 Match the following columns.

Column I	Column II
A. Guarana (*Paullinia cupana*)	1. A shrub or tree having tuberous roots for N_2-fixation
B. Paraguay tea	2. Colchicine
C. *Leucaena* plant	3. Beverage plant, rich in caffeine
D. Polyploidy	4. *Ilex paraguariensis*
E. Recalcitrant seeds	5. Seeds get killed on drying and freezing

Codes

	A	B	C	D	E
(a)	3	1	4	5	2
(b)	5	2	1	4	3
(c)	3	4	1	2	5
(d)	4	1	5	3	2

8 Read the following statements.

I. About 840 million people in the world suffer from hidden hunger.
II. About 3 billion people suffer from micronutrient protein and vitamin deficiencies.
III. About 25% population suffering from hunger and malnutrition.
IV. SCP is the one of the alternate source of proteins for animal and human nutrition.

Select the correct statements.

(a) I, II and III
(b) I, III and IV
(c) I, II and IV
(d) II, III and IV

9 Given below are a few statements regarding somatic hybridisation.

I. Protoplasts of different cells of the same plant are fused.
II. Protoplasts from cells of different species can be fused.
III. Treatment of cells with cellulase and pectinase is mandatory.
IV. The hybrid protoplast contains characters of only one parental protoplast.

Choose the correct statements.

(a) I and III (b) I and II (c) I and IV (d) II and III

10 Consider the following statements.

I. A line is a group of individuals related by decent and similar in genotype.
II. Pureline is a self-pollinated progeny of a homozygous plant.
III. The chances that hybrids combine the desirable characters is about 85%.
IV. The cross between Ranjit and Ganga varieties of maize is a type intravarietal hybridisation.
V. *Raphanobrassica* is an intergeneric hybrid.

Choose the correct option.

(a) I, II and V
(b) III and IV
(c) III, IV and V
(d) I and III

11 Consider the following statements, which of them are the advantages of tissue culture/micropropagation?

I. A large number of plants can be grown in short time.
II. Disease-free plants can be developed from diseased plants.
III. Seedless plants can be multiplied.
IV. Somatic hybrids can be raised by tissue culture, where sexual hybridisation is not possible.

Codes

(a) I, II and III
(b) II, III and IV
(c) I, II and IV
(d) I, II, III and IV

12 The first somatic hybrid by protoplast fusion technique was prepared by ...*A*... between ...*B*... and ...*C*...

	A	*B*	*C*
(a)	Carlson	*Nicotiana tabacum*	*Lycopersicum esculentum*
(b)	White	*Nicotiana glauca*	*Nicotiana langsdorfii*
(c)	Steward	*Nicotiana tabacum*	*Lycopersicum esculentum*
(d)	Carlson	*Nicotiana glauca*	*Nicotiana langsdorfii*

13 In the table given below, some of the crop plants, their diseases and the pathogens are given. Match the three columns and identify the correct choice.

Crop	Disease	Pathogen
A. Pigeon pea	I. Root knot	1. *Pseudomonas*
B. Brinjal	II. Ear cockle	2. *Fusarium*
C. Sugarcane	III. Wilt	3. *Anguinia*
D. Wheat	IV. Red stripe	4. *Meloidogyne*

(a) A-III-2, B-I-4, C-IV-1, D-II-3
(b) A-I-2, B-III-4, C-II-3, D-IV-3
(c) A-IV-3, B-I-2, C-III-1, D-II-3
(d) A-II-1, B-IV-3, C-I-2, D-III-4

14 Study the following columns.

Column I	Column II
A. Usage of bisexual flowers as female parents	1. Clonal selection
B. Incorporation of several desirable characters into a single variety	2. Pureline selection
C. Exploiting hybrid vigour for many generation	3. Emasculation
D. Improving local varieties of self-pollinated crops	4. Hybridisation
	5. Polyploidy breeding

Codes

	A	B	C	D
(a)	4	5	3	1
(b)	2	3	4	5
(c)	3	4	1	2
(d)	1	5	2	4

15 Find out the incorrect statements.

I. Monosomy and nullisomy are the two types of euploidy.
II. Polyploidy is more common in animals than in plants.
III. Polyploids occur due to the failure in complete separation of sets of chromosomes.
IV. $2n-1$ condition results in trisomy.

Codes
(a) I and III
(b) II and III
(c) I, II and IV
(d) II and IV

16 In virus-infected plants, the meristematic tissues in both apical and axillary buds are free of virus because
(a) the dividing cells are virus resistant
(b) meristems have antiviral compounds
(c) the cell division of meristems are faster than the rate of viral multiplication
(d) viruses cannot multiply within meristem cell(s)

17 Which one of following pairs is correctly matched?
(a) Inbreeding – Cross-pollination
(b) Hybrid vigour – Maintained due to inbreeding depression
(c) Male sterility – Self-pollination
(d) *Triticum boeticum* – First domesticated wheat

18 The following diagram refer to the process of somatic hybridisation. Select the right option in which *X*, *Y* and *Z* are correctly identified.

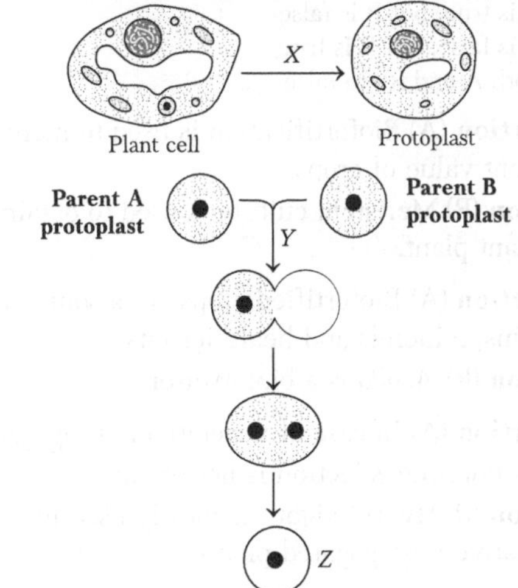

(a) *X*–Cellulase and pectinase, *Y*–Polyethylene glycol, *Z*–Zygotic cell
(b) *X*–Cellulase and pectinase, *Y*–Proteinase, *Z*–Somatic hybrid cell
(c) *X*–Proteinase, *Y*–Polyethylene glycol, *Z*–Somatic hybrid cell
(d) *X*–Cellulase and pectinase, *Y*-Polyethylene glycol, *Z*–Somatic hybrid cell

19 Match the following columns.

	Column I	Column II
A.	Emasculation	1. Mass production
B.	Micropropagation	2. Polyploidy
C.	Colchicine	3. Anther removal
D.	Mutation	4. X-rays

Codes

	A	B	C	D
(a)	2	3	1	4
(b)	4	2	3	1
(c)	1	2	4	3
(d)	3	1	2	4

20 Which one of the following is a case of wrong matching?
(a) Somatic hybridisation – Fusion of two diverse cells
(b) Vector DNA-Site for *t*RNA synthesis
(c) Micropropagation – *In vitro* production of plants in large numbers
(d) Callus – Unorganised mass of cells produced in tissue culture

Assertion and Reason

Direction (Q. Nos. 21-35) *In each of the following questions, a statement of Assertion (A) is given followed by the corresponding statement of Reason (R). Of the statements, mark the correct answer as*

(a) Both A and R are true and R is the correct explanation of A
(b) Both A and R are true, but R is not the correct explanation of A
(c) A is true, but R is false
(d) A is false, but R is true
(e) Both A and R are false

21 Assertion (A) Biofortification is used to increase nutrient value of crops.
Reason (R) Meristem culture is used to obtain virus resistant plant.

22 Assertion (A) Biofortified crops are a source of higher proteins, minerals and healthier fats.
Reason (R) *Azolla* is a biofertiliser.

23 Assertion (A) In case of vegetatively propagated crops, pureline selection is not required.
Reason (R) Hybrid vigour is mostly used in vegetatively propagated plants.

24 Assertion (A) Genetic variations provide raw material for selection.
Reason (R) Genetic variations are differences in genotypes of the individuals.

25 Assertion (A) Hybridisation is mating between two or more different lines.
Reason (R) Hybridisation is not a common method of creating genetic variation.

26 Assertion (A) Interspecific hybrids are important in breeding for diseases resistance.
Reason (R) All the sugarcane varieties being cultivated today are interspecific hybrids.

27 Assertion (A) HUW-486 wheat variety is self-pollinated.
Reason (R) Pollen from a flower, lands on the stigma of the same flower is known as self-pollination.

28 Assertion (A) Decrease in heterozygosity reduces the performance of cross-pollinated crops.
Reason (R) Decrease in heterozygosity enhances the performance of self-pollinated crops.

29 Assertion (A) Variation in pureline occurs due to the environment.
Reason (R) Purelines have identical genotype.

30 Assertion (A) Maize is completely dependent on human beings for their survival.
Reason (R) Maize cannot survive in wild.

31 Assertion (A) Mass selection is useful in self-pollinated plants.
Reason (R) Self-pollinated plants are homozygous which retain the selected traits in the progeny.

32 Assertion (A) Pureline selection is a modern day technique of plant selection.
Reason (R) Pureline selection involves obtaining good characters in homozygous state.

33 Assertion (A) Hybridisation is involved in the production of hybrid vigour or heterosis.
Reason (R) Hybrid is obtained by crossing the selected inbreed lines.

34 Assertion (A) The removal of male of a hermaphrodite flower is called emasculation.
Reason (R) Emasculation is easy in case of large-sized flowers.

35 Assertion (A) Hybrid vigour is superior over either of its parents.
Reason (R) Hybrid vigour is lost upon inbreeding.

(C) Medical Entrances' Gallery

(Collection of Questions Asked in NEET & in Various Medical Entrance Exams)

1 In mung bean, resistance to yellow mosaic virus and powdery mildew were brought about by **[NEET 2019]**
(a) mutation breeding (b) biofortification
(c) tissue culture (d) hybridisation and selection

2 Which one is correct about Atlas 66? **[JIPMER 2019]**
(a) It has high protein content
(b) It has been used as a donor for improving cultivated wheat
(c) Both (a) and (b)
(d) None of the above

3 Virus-free plants can be formed by **[AIIMS 2019]**
(a) meristem culture
(b) callus culture
(c) somatic cell culture
(d) protoplast fusion

4 What are the requirements in tissue culture?
(a) Hormones like auxin, cytokinin, agar-agar **[AIIMS 2019]**
(b) Inorganic salt, vitamin, amino acid only
(c) Carbon source like sucrose only
(d) All of the above

5 Consider the following four measures (I-IV) that could be taken to successfully grow chickpea in an area where bacterial blight is common. **[AIIMS 2018]**

I. Spray with Bordeaux mixture.
II. Control of the insect vector of the disease pathogen.
III. Use of disease-free seeds only.
IV. Use of varieties resistant to the disease.

Which of the above measures can control the diseases?

(a) I, II and IV (b) I, III and IV
(c) II, III and IV (d) I, II and III

6 Which of the following plants are used to treat bone fractures? **[AIIMS 2018]**

(a) *Digitalis purpurea*
(b) *Hevea brasiliensis*
(c) *Cissus quadrangularis*
(d) *Lawsonia inermis*

7 Which one is used in tissue culture? **[JIPMER 2018]**

(a) Explant (b) Somaclones
(c) Hybridisation (d) None of these

8 Parbhani Kranti, a variety of bhindi (ladyfinger) is resistant to **[JIPMER 2017, KCET 2014]**

(a) bacterial blight (b) yellow mosaic virus
(c) black rot (d) leaf curl

9 Identify the correct matches for crops and their improved varieties. **[AIIMS 2017]**

	Crops	Varieties	Disease
(a)	Wheat	Karan Rai	White rust
(b)	Cauliflower	Pusa Shubhra	Leaf and stripe rust
(c)	Cowpea	Pusa Komal	Hill bunt
(d)	Chilli	Pusa Sadabahar	Tobacco mosaic virus and leaf curl

10 A system of rotating crops with legume or grass pasture to improve soil structure and fertility is called **[NEET I 2017]**

(a) contour farming (b) strip farming
(c) shifting agriculture (d) ley farming

11 A technique of micropropagation is **[CBSE AIPMT 2017]**

(a) somatic hybridisation (b) somatic embryogenesis
(c) protoplast fusion (d) embryo rescue

12 Which of the following enhances or induces fusion of protoplasts? **[CBSE AIPMT 2017, 2015]**

(a) Sodium chloride and potassium chloride
(b) Polyethylene glycol and sodium nitrate
(c) IAA and kinetin
(d) IAA and gibberellins

13 A cell at telophase stage is observed by a student in a plant brought from the field. He tells his teacher that this cell is not like other cells at telophase stage. There is no formation of cell plate and thus the cell is containing more number of chromosomes as compared to other dividing cells. This would result in **[NEET-I 2016]**

(a) polyploidy (b) somaclonal variation
(c) polyteny (d) aneuploidy

14 In recent years some crops were improved by various methods for higher yield and better quality of food grains. Match the improved varieties with the related crop. **[EAMCET-I 2015, CBSE AIPMT 2011]**

	Column I		Column II
A.	Golden rice	1.	Cross breed hybrid
B.	IR-8 rice	2.	Somatic hybrid
C.	Himgiri wheat	3.	Semidwarf variety
D.	Pomato	4.	Genetically modified crop

Codes

	A	B	C	D		A	B	C	D
(a)	4	1	2	3	(b)	4	3	1	2
(c)	2	4	1	3	(d)	1	3	4	2

15 *Triticale* is an example of **[AMU 2015]**

(a) autopolyploidy (b) allopolyploidy
(c) aneuploidy (d) None of these

16 The common bread wheat has **[AMU 2015]**

(a) 14 chromosomes (b) 21 chromosomes
(c) 28 chromosomes (d) 42 chromosomes

17 In tissue culture, shoot formation in callus can be induced by **[AMU 2015]**

(a) IAA (b) ABA (c) GA_3 (d) kinetin

18 Sonalika and Kalyan Sona are high yielding varieties of **[CBSE AIPMT 2014]**

(a) sugarcane (b) rice
(c) wheat (d) maize

19 To obtain virus-free healthy plants from a diseased one by tissue culture technique, which part/parts of the diseased plant will be taken? **[CBSE AIPMT 2014]**

(a) Apical meristem only
(b) Palisade parenchyma
(c) Both apical and axillary meristems
(d) Epidermis only

20 In plant breeding, the entire collection of plants/seeds having the diverse alleles of all genes in a particular organism is called **[MHT CET 2014]**

(a) gene bank (b) *c*DNA library
(c) genomic library (d) germplasm

21 Match the following columns. **[Kerala CEE 2014]**

Column I	Column II
A. Totipotency	1. Breeding crops with higher levels of nutrients
B. Micropropagation	2. Plant grown from hybrid protoplast
C. Somaclone	3. Producing a large number of plants through tissue culture
D. Somatic hybrid	4. Capacity to generate a whole plant from an explant
E. Biofortification	5. Plants genetically identical to original plant

Codes

	A	B	C	D	E
(a)	4	3	5	2	1
(b)	1	5	2	4	3
(c)	3	2	5	4	1
(d)	4	5	1	2	3
(e)	4	5	2	1	3

22 Genetically improved crop varieties can be developed in laboratory by **[WB JEE 2014]**
(a) somatic hybridisation
(b) transgenic technology
(c) cell suspension culture
(d) somaclonal variation

23 The purposeful manipulation of plant species is called **[UK PMT 2014]**
(a) hybridisation
(b) germplasm collection
(c) plant breeding
(d) conventional plant breeding

24 Identify the correct pair of combinations. **[EAMCET 2014]**
I. Parbhani Kranti – Resistance to virus – Bhindi
II. Pusa Gaurav – Resistance to aphids – Mustard
III. Pusa Sadabahar – Resistance to fruit borer – Cowpea
IV. Pusa Shubhra –Resistance to white rust – Cauliflower

Codes
(a) II and III (b) II and IV (c) I and II (d) I and III

25 During somatic hybridisation in plants, **[KCET 2014]**
(a) somaclones are produced in large numbers
(b) the apical meristems are cultured to get virus-free plants
(c) the cell walls and the middle lamella are digested before fusing the cells
(d) crop plants with higher levels of vitamins, proteins and minerals are hybridised

26 In plant breeding programmes, the entire collection (of plants/seeds) having all the diverse alleles for all genes in a given crop is called **[NEET 2013]**
(a) cross-hybridisation among the selected parents
(b) evaluation and selection of parents
(c) germplasm collection
(d) selection of superior recombinants

27 An example for semidwarf variety of wheat is **[HP PMT 2012]**
(a) IR-8 (b) Sonalika (c) *Triticum* (d) *Saccharum*

28 Explant required for virus-free culture is **[HP PMT 2012]**
(a) root (b) shoot tip (c) leaf (d) leaf and root

ANSWERS

Check Point 20.1

1. (c)	2. (c)	3. (c)	4. (b)	5. (a)	6. (b)

Check Point 20.2

1. (c)	2. (a)	3. (a)	4. (c)	5. (a)	6. (c)

Check Point 20.3

1. (c)	2. (c)	3. (c)	4. (d)	5. (d)	6. (d)

Check Point 20.4

1. (a)	2. (a)	3. (a)	4. (b)	5. (b)	6. (b)

(A) Topical Exercise

1. (b)	2. (c)	3. (c)	4. (b)	5. (a)	6. (a)	7. (d)	8. (a)	9. (d)	10. (a)
11. (b)	12. (a)	13. (c)	14. (a)	15. (d)	16. (d)	17. (d)	18. (a)	19. (d)	20. (a)
21. (a)	22. (a)	23. (a)	24. (b)	25. (b)	26. (b)	27. (c)	28. (a)	29. (d)	30. (c)
31. (d)	32. (c)	33. (d)	34. (a)	35. (b)	36. (d)	37. (c)	38. (c)	39. (b)	40. (a)
41. (a)	42. (a)	43. (c)	44. (d)	45. (a)	46. (a)	47. (a)	48. (c)	49. (b)	50. (b)
51. (a)	52. (c)	53. (d)	54. (c)	55. (c)	56. (a)	57. (a)	58. (b)	59. (d)	60. (c)
61. (c)	62. (d)	63. (a)	64. (a)						

(B) **Cumulative Exercise**

1. (d)	2. (c)	3. (a)	4. (b)	5. (c)	6. (b)	7. (d)	8. (d)	9. (d)	10. (a)
11. (a)	12. (d)	13. (a)	14. (c)	15. (c)	16. (c)	17. (d)	18. (d)	19. (d)	20. (b)
21. (c)	22. (b)	23. (b)	24. (b)	25. (c)	26. (b)	27. (a)	28. (c)	29. (a)	30. (a)
31. (a)	32. (b)	33. (b)	34. (b)	35. (b)					

(C) **Medical Entrances' Gallery**

1. (a)	2. (c)	3. (a)	4. (d)	5. (b)	6. (c)	7. (a)	8. (b)	9. (d)	10. (d)
11. (b)	12. (b)	13. (a)	14. (b)	15. (b)	16. (d)	17. (d)	18. (c)	19. (c)	20. (d)
21. (a)	22. (a)	23. (c)	24. (c)	25. (c)	26. (c)	27. (b)	28. (b)		

Explanations

(A) Topical Exercise

8 (*a*) Statement I is true, but II is false and can be corrected as
Pusa Lerma and Sharbati Sonara are the mutants of Mexican varieties.

11 (*b*) Option (b) is incorrectly matched and can be corrected as
Brassica (Pusa Swarnim) is resistant to white rust. Cauliflower (Pusa Shubhra, Pusa show ball KI) is resistant to black rot.
Rest options are correctly matched.

22 (*a*) Statement I is true, but II is false. It can be corrected as
Hybrid virgour is a result of heterozygosity.

24 (*b*) Statement I is false, but II is true. Incorrect statement can be corrected as
The term 'heterosis' was first studied by George Shull in 1952.

29 (*d*) Option (d) is incorrect match and can be corrected as
Pusa Sem-2 and Pusa Sem 3 varieties resistance to Jassids, aphids and fruit borer.

31 (*d*) Pusa A-4 variety of okra (bhindi) is resistant to Jassids, aphids and shoot and root bores tolerant yellow vein mosaic virus. They are ideal for cultivation throughout the year except during low temperature.

32 (*c*) Both statements I and II are correct because
The scientific process by which crop plant are enriched with certain desirable nutrients is called biofortification. Through this process nutritional quality of food crops is improved by agronomic practices, conventional plant breeding or modern biotechnology.
Atlas 66 is an example of biofortification.

39 (*b*) Statement in option (b) is incorrect and can be corrected as
The shift from grain to meat diets has created more demands for cereals because to produce 1kg of meat, 3-10 kg of grains are spend on the cattle.
Rest statements are correct.

(B) Cumulative Exercise

2 (*c*) Statement IV is incorrect and can be corrected as
The entire collection of plant/seed having all the diverse alleles for all genes is called germplasm collection.

3 (*a*) Statement in option (a) is worng and can be corrected as
By inbreeding pureline can be envolved.
Rest statements are true.

6 (*b*) Option (b) is incorrectly matched pair and can be corrected as
Cytokinins play an important role in shoot initiation is callus.

20 (*b*) Matched pair in option (b) is wrong and can be corrected as
Vector DNA is a small piece of DNA that can stably maintained in an organism into which a foreign DNA fragment can be inserted. It is not a site for RNA synthesis. In eukaryotes *t*RNA synthesised in nucleus.

21 (*c*) A is true, but R is false because
Biofortification is used to increase nutrient value of crops, because it involves various methodologies to produce the hybrid crops with high levels of vitamins, proteins for improvement in public health, such as Atlas 66, which is a wheat variety with high protein content.
The meristem culture is used to obtain virus-free plants from a virus-infected parent plant.

22 (*b*) Both A and R are true, but R is not the correct explanation of A.
Biofortified crop is a source of higher proteins, minerals and healthier fats developed by new agronomic practices and biotechnological methods. *Azolla pinnata* is pteridophyte which is a biofertiliser used in rice fields.

23 (*b*) Both A and R are true, but R is not the correct explanation of A.
In case of vegetatively propagated crops pureline selection is not required. Pureline selection is useful only for sexually reproducing plants. Hybrid vigour is most profitably used in vegetatively propagated crops because they do not involve sexual reproduction.

24 (*b*) Both A and R are true, but R is not the correct explanation of A.
Creation of genetic variation and selection are the two critical steps in the plant breeding. Genetic variations are differences in genotypes of the individuals which arise due to genetic reasons. Genetic variation provides the raw material for selection and selection effects the desired improvement.

25 (*c*) A is true, but R is false. R can be corrected as Hybridisation is the most common method of creating genetic variation. Mating between two or more individuals/lines differing in genotypes is termed as hybridisation and the product of hybridisation is called as hybrid.

26 (*b*) Both A and R are true, but R is not the correct explanation of A.
Hybridisation between different related species is known as interspecific hybridisation. Interspecific hybrids are very important in plant breeding particularly in breeding for disease resistance. Some interspecific hybrids are being treated as varieties. All the sugarcane varieties being cultivated today are interspecific hybrids.

27 (*a*) Both A and R are true and R is the correct explanation of A. Self-pollination is a phenomenon, in which pollen from a flower lands on the stigma of the same flower, e.g. wheat varieties. In self-pollinated crops, the amount of cross-pollination is less than 5%. As a result of self-pollination, homozygosity is increased and purelines are developed.

28 (*c*) A is true, but R is false because
Populations of cross-pollinated crops are heterozygous for most of their genes. Any decrease in heterozygosity may reduce their performance. So, homozygous genotypes cannot be used as varieties in cross-pollinated crops. In case of self-pollinated species, the best homozygous genotype present in the population is selected.

29 (*a*) Both A and R are true and R is the correct explanation of A.
The self-pollinated progeny of a homozygous plant constitutes a pureline. All the plants have identical genotype, that is why variation present within a pureline is due to the environment which have no genetic basis.

30 (*a*) Both A and R are true and R is the correct explanation of A. Some species are currently known only in cultivation because domestication has deprived the plants from their natural defence system against predators. Many of them cannot survive in wild and depend entirely on human beings for their survival, e.g. maize.

31 (*a*) Both A and R are true and R is the correct explanation of A. Mass selection is the most ancient method of selection which involves the selection of seeds of a number of plants on the basis of phenotypic characters like seed size, fruit size, quality of fruit pollinated plants because they are usually homozygous and retain the selected traits in the progeny.

32 (*b*) Both A and R are true, but R is not the correct explanation of A.
Pureline selection involves obtaining good characters in homozygous state. Pureline selection or single plant selection is a modern day technique of plants selection. PV-18 wheat variety was obtained through pureline selection.

33 (*b*) Both A and R are true, but R is not the correct explanation of A.
Hybrid is the result of mating between two individuals or lines differing in genotypes. The main objectives of hybridisation are the development of hybrid vigour or heterosis and bringing together desirable characters of different races, varieties, etc., into hybrid.

34 (*b*) Both A and R are true, but R is not the correct explanation of A.
During hybridisation, removal of anthers from a bisexual flower to prevent the self-pollination is called emasculation. It is easy in case of large-sized flowers, while tedious, laborious and time consuming in case of small flowers.

35 (*b*) Both A and R are true, but R is not the correct explanation of A.
Hybrid vigour or heterosis is superior over either of its parents in one or more characters. Hybrid vigour is lost during inbreeding. It is lost in F_2-generation in self-pollinated plants, whereas in cross-pollinated plants, it slowly declines.

(C) Medical Entrances' Gallery

1 (*a*) In mung bean, resistance to yellow mosaic virus and powdery mildew were induced by mutation breeding.
Mutation breeding is the process of exposing the seeds to chemicals or radiation in order to generate mutants with desirable traits to be breed with other cultivars.

2 (*c*) Atlas 66 or soft wheat has been used since 1953 as a genetic source of higher protein in wheat. It has been used as a donor for improving cultivated wheat.

3 (*a*) Virus-free plants can be formed by meristem culture. The reason behind this is that virus cannot propagate in rapidly dividing cells, so the meristematic zone of plants always remains virus-free.
Protoplast fusion technique is used for making somatic hybrids.
Somatic cell culture technique is used to propagate plants from somatic cells using nutrient medium and combination of hormones. Callus is the undifferentiated mass of tissues. Growing callus from plant organs is callus culture.

4 (*d*) The requirements of tissue culture are hormones (auxin, cytokinin), agar-agar, inorganic salt, vitamins, amino acids, carbon source like sucrose, etc.
In plant tissue culture, the medium on which explants are cultured is known as nutrient or culture medium. It acts as a source of important nutrients which are required for proper development of explant.

5 (*b*) The measures given in statements I, III and IV are correct. Bacterial blight of chickpea is caused by the bacterium *Xanthomonas campestris*. The stem and leaves of the infected plant give a blighted or burnt up appearance.
Control measures include roguing, 3 years crop rotation, disease-free seeds, spray of copper fungicides (Bordeaux mixture) and antibiotics besides sowing disease resistant varieties.

6 (*c*) *Cissus quadrangularis* is an ancient medicinal plant of India. It has specific bone healing properties and helps in faster increase of the bone tensile strength. It acts as a glucocorticoid antagonist.

7 (*a*) Explant is used in plant tissue culture. It is an excised plant part which has the potential to give rise to a whole new plant. The plants obtained through this technique are morphologically and genetically similar to each other and to their parent plant.

8 (*b*) Parbhani Kranti (example of mutation breeding) is a variety of bhindi which has been made resistant to the yellow mosaic virus. Resistance to yellow mosaic virus in bhindi (*Abelmoschus esculentus*, i.e. okra) was transferred from a wild species to produce this new variety.

9 (*d*) Only option (d) is correct. Rest of the options are incorrect. The correct information regarding incorrect options are as follows

Himgiri is the variety of wheat developed by hybridisation and selection for disease resistance against leaf and stripe rust and hill bunt. Pusa Shubhra is a variety of cauliflower which is highly resistant to black rot and Pusa Komal is a variety of cowpea resistant to bacterial blight.

10 (*d*) Ley farming is a system of rotating crops with legumes or grass pasture in order to improve soil structure and fertility and also to disrupt pest and disease life cycles.

11 (*b*) Somatic embryogenesis is technique of micropropagation. It is the growing of plants from meristematic tissue or somatic cells of plants on suitable nutrient media, under controlled condition.

(i) **Organogenesis** is method of micropropagation that involves tissue regeneration of adventitious organs or axillary buds from explants.

(ii) **Somatic embryogenesis** is development of embryos without formation of zygote (i.e. development from somatic cells).

12 (*b*) **Polyethylene Glycol** (PEG) and **sodium nitrate** enhance fusion of protoplasts (protoplast fusion). Protoplast fusion is a physical phenomenon which occurs due to the fusion of protoplast (cell without cell wall) of two or more cells. It can be done either mechanically (spontaneous) or by inducing agents.

13 (*a*) Polyploid cells have a chromosome number that is more than double the haploid number, e.g. *Triticum aestivum* (wheat) is a hexaploid (6*n*).

15 (*b*) *Triticale* is a man-made allopolyploid cereal, which is of two types, allohaploid and allodiploid.

16 (*d*) The bread wheat genome is classified as a hexaploid genome. This means that it has 6 copies of each of its 7 chromosomes, the complete set numbering 42 chromosomes.

17 (*d*) Kinetin is a type of cytokinin, a class of plant hormone that promotes cell division. In tissue culture, kinetin helps to produce new leaves, chloroplast in leaves, lateral shoot growth and adventitious shoot formation.

18 (*c*) Sonalika and Kalyan Sona are wheat varieties that were introduced in India in 1963. These are high yielding drug resistant varieties.

19 (*c*) Both apical and axillary meristems are free of virus for healthy plant cultivation because of strong interferon activity in these region. These tissues form a protective impermeable covering around themselves, which is non-penetrable by any pathogen. Hence, these tissues are used in the production of disease-free plants by tissue culture.

22 (*a*) All three techniques given in the options, i.e. somatic hybridisation, transgenic technology and somaclonal variation are the methods which are used to produced genetically improved varieties in labs. Genetically improved varieties are those whose genome is altered artificially in laboratory by using different methods in order to favour the expression of desired physiological traits or for the production of desired biological products.

The cell suspension culture is used for the multiplication of cells by providing them culture or by suspending them in a suitable medium.

24 (*c*) Parbhani Kranti is a yellow vein mosaic virus resistant variety of bhindi released in 1985. Pusa Gaurav is a mustard variety resistant to aphids. Pusa Sadabahar is a variety of chilli. Pusa Shubhra is a resistant cauliflower variety to black rot and curd blight diseases.

25 (*c*) Somatic hybridisation is the technique used in laboratories in which protoplasts of two different plant species are fused together on a suitable nutrient medium to develop a hybrid known as somatic hybrid.

During this process, cell walls and middle lamella of the single cells are digested by the enzymes like pectinases and cellulases to expose the marked protoplasts.

After this, these isolated protoplasts are fused to obtain hybrid protoplast under sterile condition. This fusion is induced by Polyethylene Glycol (PEG).

CHAPTER 21

Biotechnology : Principles and Processes

The term **'Biotechnology'** is concerned with the use of biological agents or their components for generating useful products for mankind.

The term was first coined by **Karl Ereky** in 1917.

Biotechnology involves a group of techniques that share a common characteristic of working with living cells and their molecules. In recent years, biotechnology has become an important tool for the production of food crops, human health care, chemical industries, etc.

BIOTECHNOLOGY : THE DEFINITION

The European Federation of Biotechnology (EFB) in 1988 defined biotechnology as the integration of natural science and organisms, cells, parts thereof, and molecular analogues for products and services.

Traditional biotechnology

- Human beings have been using microorganisms for thousands of years to obtain products like curd, ghee, vinegar, alcoholic beverages, breads, etc., without knowing the microorganisms were involved in these processes.
- Microorganisms were first used to produce some organic compounds like citric acid following the first world war.
- Later on, microorganisms were employed to generate a variety of products, including antibiotics.
- *In vitro* culture techniques (tissue culture) of plant and animal cells are used to obtain various valuable products.
- Thus, the traditional biotechnology includes the processes that are based on the natural capabilities of microorganisms. But, the type of products obtained have remained same, as those from the natural strains/cell lines.
- The traditional biotechnology has established a huge and expanding world market.

Inside

- Various applications of traditional biotechnology are as follows
  - (i) **Fermentation to produce foods** It is the most ancient biotechnological discovery. It is used to produce products such as wine, beer, vinegar, bread, yoghurt, etc., using a range of microorganisms such as lactic acid bacteria, mold, etc. These processes are still in use today for the production of modern foods.
  - (ii) **Industrial fermentation** It involves the development of industrial processes for the manufacturing of chemicals such as **butanol**, **acetone** and **glycerol**.

    It is still in use for the production of enzymes, which are mainly used in pharmaceutical processes, environmental remediation and other industrial processes.
  - (iii) **Food preservation** The various preservation techniques like drying, salting and freezing are used to prevent the food from contamination. Thus, these processes aids in food preservation.
  - (iv) **Selective plant breeding** It is a part of early crop improvement technology. It includes the formation of new species.

Modern biotechnology

- It includes the combination of modern techniques that allows the isolation of desired genes from any organism and its transfer and expression into another organism.
- It is performed for the production of desired economic products.
- Now, the conventional industries, pharmaceutical industries, agro-industries, etc., are focusing their attention to produce modern biotechnology-based products.
- The two major features of technology which differentiates the modern biotechnology from the traditional biotechnology are as follows
  - The capability of science to change the genetic material for getting new products for specific requirements through **Recombinant DNA Technology** (RDT).
  - The ownership of technology and its socio-political impact.
- The method associated with modern biotechnology is genetic engineering, which includes recombinant DNA technology and gene cloning.
- These include isolating DNA fragments, joining them in new combinations and introducing the recombined DNA back into the new hosts as shown in the given figure below

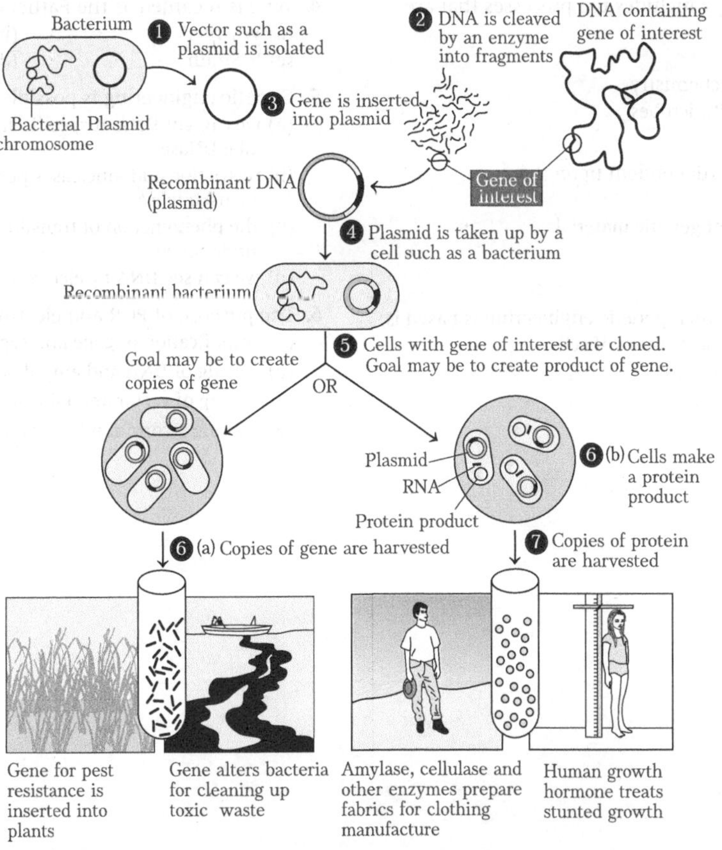

Fig. 21.1 Basic steps in biotechnology

Principles of biotechnology

Two main principles of biotechnology are given below

1. Maintenance of sterile ambience (chemical engineering)

- Microbial contamination free ambience (axenic culture) in biochemical engineering process enables the growth of desired cell in large quantities.
- It helps in the manufacture of desired products like vaccines, antibiotics, enzymes, etc.

2. Genetic engineering

- It is a process of manipulation of genetic material by humans *in vitro* for the benefit of mankind.
- One such technique used for performing genetic engineering is recombinant DNA technology.
- **Paul Berg** is regarded as the **Father of Genetic Engineering.**

Table 21.1 Some common techniques used in *r*DNA technology

Techniques	Purposes
*c*DNA	To make a DNA copy of *m*RNA. It is also called complementary DNA.
Restriction enzymes	To cut DNA at specific site, making small fragments.
DNA ligase	To join DNA fragments together.
Vectors	To carry DNA into cells and ensure replication.
Plasmids	Common kind of vector.
Gene transfer	To deliver a gene to a living cell.
Genetic markers	To identify cells that have been transformed.
Replica plating	To make exact copies of bacterial colonies on an agar plate.
PCR	To amplify very small samples of DNA.
DNA probes	To identify and label a piece of DNA containing a certain sequence.
Antisense genes	To stop the expression of a gene in a cell.
Electrophoresis	To separate fragments of DNA on gel.

CHECK POINT 21.1

1. Traditional biotechnology includes the processes that are based on
   (a) genetic engineering
   (b) modification of gene chemistry
   (c) natural capabilities of microbes
   (d) Both (a) and (b)
2. Modern biotechnology is dependent upon the
   (a) fermentation
   (b) change in chemistry of genetic material
   (c) plant breeding
   (d) Both (a) and(c)
3. Main phenomenon on which genetic engineering is based is,
   (a) alteration of genetic constitution of cells
   (b) insertion of plasmid in cells
   (c) alteration in cell organelles
   (d) joining of two cells
4. Who is regarded as the Father of Genetic Engineering?
   (a) W Arber (b) Paul Berg
   (c) H Smith (d) D Nathans
5. Genetic engineering is possible because.
   (a) we can cut DNA at specific sites by endouncleases like DNase
   (b) restriction endonucleases purified from bacteria can be used *in vitro*
   (c) the phenomenon of transduction in bacteria is well understood
   (d) we can see DNA by electron microscope
6. The purpose of PCR and electrophoresis is
   (a) amplification of gene and separation of DNA fragment
   (b) cutting of DNA and amplify of gene
   (c) cutting of vector and join DNA fragement
   (d) making a copy of *m*RNA and find a particular gene

RECOMBINANT DNA TECHNOLOGY

- It is the technique of combining genes from two different sources to create new gene combination.
- Recombinant DNA technology aims at isolating desired DNA sequences (genes) from different sources and then joining them to produce a recombinant DNA.
- It involves a complex procedure and a number of tools.

Tools of recombinant DNA technology

Various tools of *r*DNA technology are as follows

1. Enzymes

The enzymes mainly involved in *r*DNA are restriction enzymes, ligases and lyases, etc.
These are described below

I. Restriction enzymes

- The most important tool in genetic engineering is restriction enzymes or **restriction endonucleases** or **molecular scissors**.
- These enzymes have the ability to recognise and cut specific nucleotide sequences.
- Restriction enzymes belong to a larger class of enzymes called **nucleases**.
- These are of two types
  (i) **Exonucleases** remove nucleotides from the ends of the DNA.
  (ii) **Endonucleases** make cuts at a specific positions within the DNA.
- The credit for the discovery of first restriction enzymes were given to **Arber**, **Smith** and **Nathans** (1970).
- These enzymes destroy the DNA of invading foreign viruses in bacteria. However, bacterial DNA remains protected from these enzymes as it is methylated.
- The first discovered restriction enzyme was ***Hind* II**. It was isolated from *Haemophilus influenzae*. It always cuts DNA at the sequence given below

  5′ GT AC 3′
  3′ CA TG 5′.
- Due to this ability of cutting at specific sites, restriction enzymes are also called as **site specific nucleases**.

Naming of restriction enzymes

- The convention for naming these enzymes is that the first letter of the name denotes the genus.
- The second two letter denotes the species of prokaryotic cell from which they have been isolated, e.g.

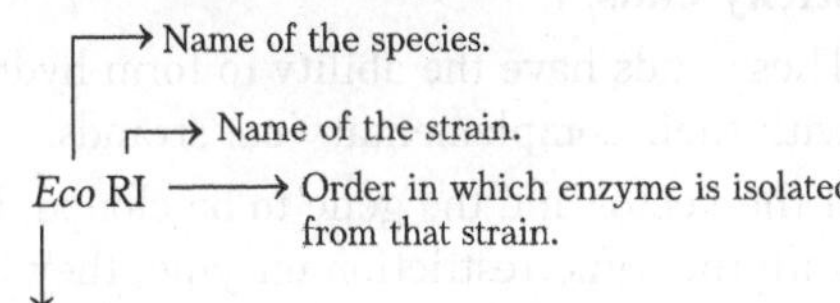

- Similarly in ***Bam* HI**, **'*B*'** is derived from *Bacillus*, **'*am*'** is derived from *amyloliquefaciens*, **'H'** is derived from name of strain and **I** indicates that this is the first enzyme isolated from this bacterium.

Recognition sites for restriction enzymes

- The recognition sites or target sites are those regions of DNA that are recognised by a particular enzyme.
- The sequences are usually 4-8 base pairs long and are palindromic in nature.
- A palindromic sequence is a nucleic acid sequence that is same when read in 5′-3′ direction on complementary strands, e.g.

  5′ – GAATTC – 3′
  3′ – CTTAAG – 5′

Different restriction enzymes produce different types of cuts on DNA.

Types of cuts made by restriction enzymes

The restriction enzymes cut the nucleotide sequence in DNA by cleavage in any of the following ways

(i) **Blunt end style** Restriction enzymes like *Alu* I, *Hae* III, *Hind* II, *Sma* I, etc., make cut across both the strands of DNA in the centre of recognised sequence. Thus, the DNA segments with blunt ends are produced. This type of cleavage helps to join two defined sequences.

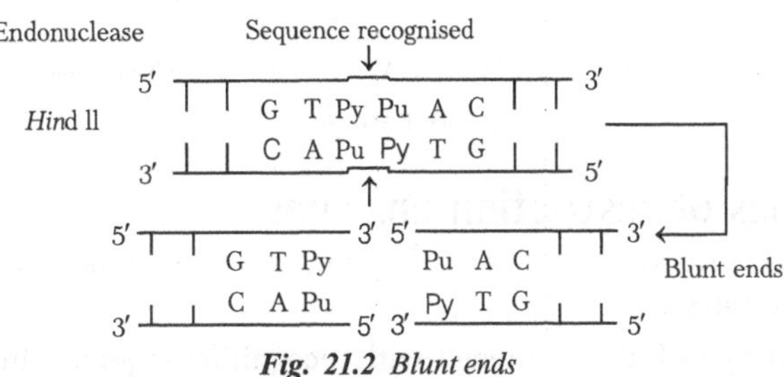

Fig. 21.2 Blunt ends

(ii) **Staggered cut or cohesive or sticky end style** In this type of cleavage, the cuts are made in two strands of DNA at two different sites, few nucleotides away from each other. As a result of this, two strands with protruding ends or overhanging stretches are produced. These strands are called **sticky ends**.

These ends have the ability to form hydrogen bonds with their complementary cut strands.

If the vector and the gene to be cloned, both are cut with the same restriction enzyme, they both will have complementary sticky ends, e.g. *Eco* RI, *Bgl* II, *Bam* HI, *Pst* I, etc., produce these type of ends.

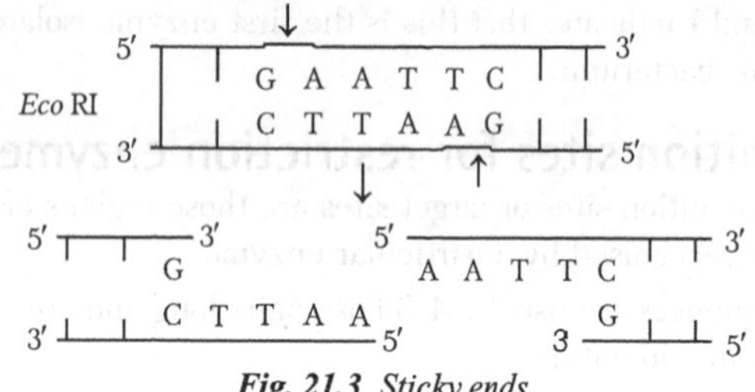

Fig. 21.3 Sticky ends

Table 21.2 Some restriction enzymes their sources and the target DNA sequences with cleavage sites

Enzymes	Organisms	Target DNA sequences (cleavage sites marked by arrow)	Ends produced
Eco RI	*Escherichia coli* Ry 13	5′–G↓ AATTC......3′ 3′ CTTAA↑ G......5′	Sticky ends
Hind II	*Haemophilus influenzae* Rd	5′....GTPy ↓Pu AC...3′ 3′....CAPu↑Py TG...5′	Blunt ends
Hae III	*Haemophilus aegypticus*	5′–GG↓ CC......3′ 3′ ...CC↑ GG......5′	Blunt ends
Hpa I	*Haemophilus parainfluenzae*	5′... GTT↓ AAC......3′ 3′ ...CAA↑ TTG......5′	Blunt ends
Sma I	*Serratia marcescens*	5′... CCC↓ GGG......3′ 3′ ...GGG↑ CCC......5′	Blunt ends
Sal I	*Streptomyces albus* G.	5′... G↓TCGAC......3′ 3′ ...CAGCT↑ G......5′	Sticky ends
Bgl I	*Bacillus globigii*	5′... A↓GATCT......3′ 3′ ...TCTAG↑ A......5′	Sticky ends

Types of restriction enzymes

The restriction enzymes can be categorised into following three categories.

(i) **Type I** These interact with recognition sequence in a double-stranded DNA and cleave only one strand of DNA at a random site. These enzymes require Mg^{2+} ions, ATP and S-adenosyl methionine cofactors for their functioning, e.g. *Eco* K, etc.

(ii) **Type II** These recognise specific DNA nucleotide sequences and cleave both the strands. Type II enzymes require only Mg^{2+} for their functioning. Only type II restriction endonucleases are used for restriction mapping and gene cloning in view of their cleavage action only at specific sites, e.g. *Eco* RI, *Hind* II.

(iii) **Type III** These are more or less similar to type II enzymes. These require ATP and S-adenosyl methionine along with Mg^{2+} for their functioning. These are intermediate between type I and type II, e.g. *Eco* P15.

In this chapter, we are specifically focusing on type II restriction enzymes.

End modification enzymes

These enzymes make changs at the ends of DNA molecules, e.g. some end modification enzymes are given below

(i) **Alkaline phosphatase** This enzyme removes phosphate groups from the 5′ end of DNA molecules. It prevents these molecules from being ligated to one another.

(ii) **T_4-polynucleotide kinase** It performs the reverse action to alkaline phosphatase and adds phosphate to 5′ ends of DNA.

II. DNA ligase (Molecular binders)

- These enzymes join two DNA strands together.
- These mediate the formation of phosphodiester bonds between adjacent 3′– OH and 5′-phosphate termini, hence join the nicks in double-stranded DNA.
- The sticky ends produced by restriction enzymes allow two complementary restriction fragments to anneal but only by weak hydrogen bonds. It can quite easily be broken by gentle heating.
- The backbone is still incomplete. DNA ligase completes the DNA backbone by forming covalent bonds. Restriction enzymes and DNA ligase can therefore, be used together to join the lengths of DNA from different sources.

Other enzymes used in *r*DNA technology

These include

(i) **Lyases** These are used to open the cells or dissolve the cell wall, e.g. lysozymes are used to digest the bacterial cell wall. Proteases, lipases, etc., also come in this category.

(ii) **Synthetases** They help in either *in vitro* synthesis of DNA or in the synthesis of complementary DNA (*c*DNA), e.g. DNA polymerases and reverse transcriptase.

2. Vectors (Vehicle DNA)

It is defined as a DNA molecule that can be used to carry a foreign DNA segment (gene) to be cloned. In actual sense, it is required for transferring and cloning the gene in a suitable host or bacterium.

- In *r*DNA technology, a foreign gene is inserted in the vector to form a **recombinant DNA** or a **recombinant vector.**
- The recombinant vector is also called as **hybrid vector** or **chimeric vector** (chimera = a mythological monster with lion's head, goat's body and serpent's tail).

Essential features of vectors

A good vector must have following characteristics

(i) **Origin of replication** (*ori*) This is the sequence from where the replication starts and any piece of DNA when linked to this sequence, can be made to replicate within the host cell.

- This sequence provides the ability to replicate autonomously, so as to generate its multiple copies within the host itself.
- Its representation in many copies in the cell provides more replicates of inserted DNA sequences. So, if one wants to recover many copies of target DNA, it should be cloned in a vector whose *ori* supports high copy number.

(ii) **Marker gene or Selectable markers** A vector should also have a selectable marker.

- It permits the selection of transformed host cells.
- The marker gene can easily distinguish the cell carrying vector (transformants) from those lacking vectors (non-transformants).
- It selectively permits the growth of transformants. Usually, the genes encoding resistance to antibiotics such as ampicillin, chloramphenicol, tetracycline or kanamycin, etc., are useful selectable markers for *E. coli.* Enzyme producing genes such as *lac* Z are also good markers.

(iii) **Recognition sites** A vector should have a unique restriction site that would allow only a particular enzyme to cut the vector only once. This site is recognised by the commonly used restriction enzymes.

When a vector possesses more than one recognition site in a small region of DNA, that region is called as **polylinker** or **Multiple Cloning Site** (MCS).

(iv) **Small size** Large vectors usually have a tendency to breakdown during purification. These cannot be easily manipulated. Thus, a vector should have a small size, i.e. generally < 10 kb.

(v) **High copy number** A vector should have a high copy number in order to provide more replicates of gene of interest.

Mostly, all these requirements are not found in naturally occurring vectors. Thus, these are engineered *in vitro* to obtain the features and finally to facilitate gene transfer.

Different types of vectors

The vectors commonly used in RDT are described below

(i) Plasmids

- These are most widely used vectors. Plasmids are extrachromosomal, self-replicating, double-stranded, closed and circular DNA molecules in the bacterial cells and few yeast cells.
- The size of plasmids ranges from 1×10^6 to 200×10^6 dalton.
- Plasmids can be of two types depending on their copy numbers
  - **Single copy plasmids** Low copy number, occur as one plasmid per cell.
  - **Multiple copy plasmids** High copy number, occur as 10-20 copies per cell.
- Plasmids can be cleaved at one site by **restriction endonucleases** to give a linear DNA molecule. A foreign DNA segment can then be inserted which lead to the formation of a bigger DNA molecule.

Artificial cloning vector based on plasmids

(a) **pBR322** It is one of the standard cloning vector which is widely used in recombinant DNA technology.

- In pBR322, **P** signifies **plasmid**, **B** indicates **Boliver** and **R** indicates **Rodriguez**. Boliver and Rodriguez were the scientists who developed pBR322 in 1977.
- It is 4.3 kb in size. 322 is a number given to distinguish this plasmid from others which were developed in the same laboratory.
- pBR322 has genes for resistance against **ampicillin** and **tetracycline**.
- They have restriction sites for enzymes like *Pvu* I, *Pst* I, *Sal* I, *Bam* HI.

(b) **pUC8** It is also a reconstructed **plasmid vector.** It was named after **University of California** (UC). It is 2.75 kb in size and has high copy number (500-700).

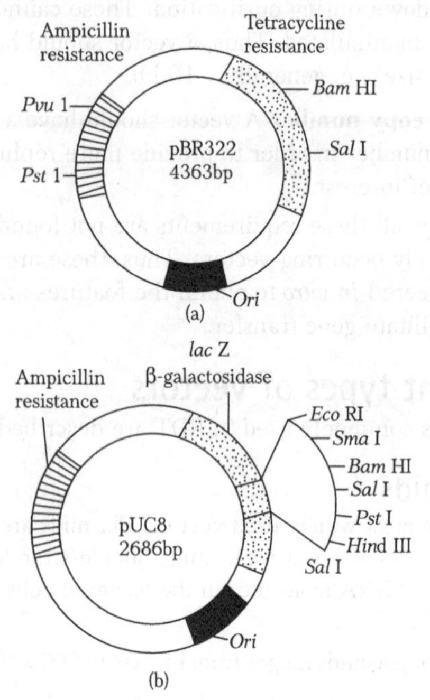

Fig 21.4 Different types of artificial cloning vectors : (a) pBR322, (b) pUC8 (one type of pUC vector)

(ii) Bacteriophage

- Plasmid vectors are normally used to clone DNA segments of small size, i.e. upto 10 kilo bases.
- When the size of gene of interest is more than 10 kb, bacteriophage vectors are used, e.g. M13, λ (lambda) phage, etc.
- From bacteriophage vectors, cloning of gene with size of 20-25 kilo bases is possible. These consist of linear double-stranded DNA molecules, which are engineered in the way that their lytic cycle is possible but lysogenic cycle is not possible.
- **Lambda (λ) phage** Its genome is a 50 kbp circular DNA. It follows either a lytic path or a lysogenic path. Lytic cycle may be switched to the lysogeny or *vice-versa.*
- In lambda phage, only about 60% genome is required for the lytic growth of phage. The central 40% can be replaced by the foreign DNA. The percentage of foreign DNA can be increased also. This is made possible by removing some of the non-essential parts of phage genome, but only upto certain limit.
- The lambda cloning vectors are of two types
  (a) The **insertion vector** accept inserts of only 12 kbp long at a single cloning site, e.g. λ gt10 and λ gt11 vectors.
  (b) The **replacement vector** accept inserts of 9-23 kbp long with the involvement of replacement of a non-essential part (stuffer) of genome, e.g. EMBL3 and EMBL4 vectors.

(iii) Cosmids (plasmid + lambda phage)

- These vectors can accommodate DNA segments of upto 45 kbp.
- These are actually plasmids to which *cos* sites of phage lambda are joined. These *cos* sites enable the DNA to be packed in the phage (λ) particle. So, we can say that the cosmids allow the packaging of DNA in phage, *in vitro.*
- Cosmids also perpetuate in bacteria. The advantage of cosmids for cloning is that their efficiency is high enough to produce a complete genome library of 10^6 - 10^7 clones from mere only 1 μg of insert DNA.
- The disadvantage is their inability to accept more than 40-50 kbp of DNA.

(iv) Phasmids/Phagemids (plasmid + filamentous phage)

- These are the vectors that contain plasmid with a fragment of filamentous phage DNA. Hence, it combines the features of both of them.
- Initially, the segments of foreign DNA cloned in these plasmids are multiplied normally. However, when these plasmid vectors are infected with a filamentous phage called **helper phage**, the phagemid genome behaves like a phage. As a result, the phagemid generates multiple copies of its one strand and the associated DNA inserted in it.
- The single-strand can be purified from these phage particles. These are used for sequencing, site-directed mutagenesis and the synthesis of strand specific probes.
- Phagemids have been developed by inserting intergenic regions of a variety of filamentous phages into plasmids.
- Phagemids have several advantages over other vectors like
  - They give high yield of foreign DNA just like plasmid vectors.
  - They can provide single-stranded DNA along with the double-stranded foreign DNA fragments.
  - Due to their small sizes, single-stranded DNA upto 10 kbp can be easily obtained from them.
- The examples of phagemids include M13, fd, f1, pUC118, pUC119, etc.

(v) Tumour inducing plasmids (Ti plasmids)

- These are found in *Agrobacterium tumefaciens,* which is the bacterium that infects dicot plants.
- Ti plasmid has tumour inducing properties, thus for genetic engineering, the modified *Agrobacterium* strains were developed (with deleted tumour forming genes) to infect the plant cell.
- The part of Ti plasmid which is transferred in the plant cell DNA is T-DNA. This T-DNA with desired DNA is spliced and inserted into the chromosome of the host plant where it produces copies of itself.

(vi) Yeast Artificial Chromosome (YAC)

- These vectors allow cloning of DNA that is about 500 kb in size, within yeast cells. They have heen exploited extensively in mapping the large genome, e.g. in the human genome project.
- These are based on chromosomes. They contain centromere, telomeric sequences, autonomously replicating sequences, recognition sites and selectable markers.

(vii) Bacterial Artificial Chromosome (BAC)

- It is a bacterial cloning vector based on F-factor of *E. coli.*
- These vectors can clone fragments of size 300-350 kb.
- They contain genes for the replication and maintenance of F-factor, selectable marker and cloning sites.

(viii) Jumping genes as vector

- These are units of DNA which can move from one DNA molecule to another, hence are called **mobile genes** or **jumping genes** or **transposons.**
- **Barbara MClintock** discovered transposons in maize.
- In *Drosophila,* **P element** (transposon) is used as vector. The P element is 2.9 kb in length and contains three genes that code for transposase enzyme. These enzymes carryout the transposition process.
- This vector carries two P elements. One of these contains the insertion site for the foreign DNA. Second P element of the vector carries out the transposition of foreign DNA.

3. Passenger DNA or Gene of Interest (GOI)

It is the DNA which is transferred from one organism into another by combining it with the vehicle DNA. Two types of DNA can be used as passenger DNA, i.e. **cDNA** and **synthetic DNA.**

Complementary DNA (cDNA)

- It is a DNA made from *m*RNA by using the enzyme **reverse transcriptase.** This enzyme acts by reversing transcription (i.e. it synthesises DNA from RNA template).
- The enzyme is produced naturally by a group of virus called the **retroviruses** (which include HIV) and it helps them to invade cells. Reverse transcriptase is obtained normally from the **Avian Myoblastosis Virus** (AMV).
- It is difficult to find gene of interest out of a complete genome.
- However, a given cell only expresses a few genes, so it only makes a few different kinds of *m*RNA molecule. Thus, it is easier to find specific *m*RNA.
- For example, the β-cells of the pancreas synthesise several *m*RNA molecules that code for insulin. This *m*RNA can be isolated and used to make *c*DNA of the insulin gene.

Synthetic DNA

- It is synthesised with the help of DNA polymerase on DNA template or from free deoxyribonucleotides without a template.
- The desired gene is synthesised using a computerised machine called **DNA synthesiser** or **DNA gene machine.**
- This machine can synthesise gene of more than 1000 nucleotides length according to a predetermined sequence.

4. DNA probes

- A probe is simply a short length of DNA (20-100 nucleotides long) with a label attached.
- These are used to identify and label DNA fragments that contain a specific sequence.
- Based on the type of label, DNA probe can be categorised into two types
  - (i) **A radioactively-labelled probe** It is synthesised using the radioactive isotope ^{32}P, H^3,N^{15}, etc. It can be visualised using photographic film (an autoradiograph).
  - (ii) **A fluorescently-labelled probe** It emits visible light when illuminated with invisible ultraviolet light. Probes can be made to fluoresce with different colours.
- Probes are always single-stranded and can be made of DNA or RNA.
- The universal DNA probe is made up of repeated GATA sequence.

- If a probe is added to a mixture of different pieces of DNA (e.g. restriction fragments), it anneals (base pair) with any lengths of DNA containing the complementary sequence. These fragments are then labelled and these stand out from the rest of the DNA.

Uses of probes

DNA probes have many uses in genetic engineering which are as follows

- Identify restriction fragments containing a particular gene out of the thousands of restriction fragments formed from a genomic library.
- Identify the short DNA sequences which are used in DNA fingerprinting.
- Identify genes from one species that are similar to those of another species. For example, a gene probe for a mouse gene would probably anneal with the same gene from a human. This has aided the identification of human genes.
- Identify genetic defects - DNA probes have been prepared that match the sequences of genes causing many human genetic diseases, such as muscular dystrophy and cystic fibrosis. Hundreds of these probes can be stuck to a glass slide in a grid pattern to form a DNA microarray (or DNA chip).

  A sample of human DNA is added to the array and any sequences that match any of the various probes stick to the array and gets labelled. Using these rapid testing, large number of genetic defects at a time can be detected.

5. **Genetic** (Selectable) **markers**

- These are the tools used to identify host cells that have successfully taken up a cloning vector.
- A common marker used is **R-plasmid**, i.e. resistance plasmid. It has a gene resistant to a certain antibiotics such as tetracycline, ampicillin, etc.
- Host cells that take up this marker and make the gene product are resistant to this antibiotic.
- So, if both transformed and non-transformed cells are grown in a medium containing tetracycline, only transformed cells would grow. This is because they possess the genetic marker conferring resistance to tetracycline.

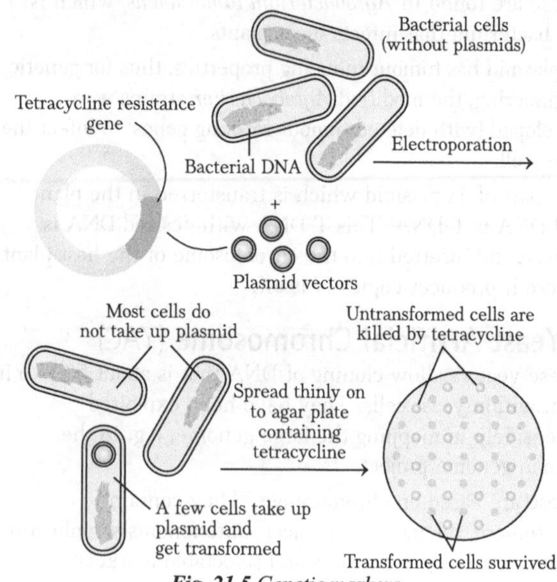

Fig. 21.5 Genetic markers

Other important tools

Some other important tools of *r*DNA technology are as follows

Shot gun

- This is used to find one particular gene in a whole genome. It is called so, because it starts by indiscriminately breaking up the genome like firing a shot gun at a soft target. Then, it sort through the debris for the particular gene.
- This tool also requires a DNA probe for recognising the required gene, which means atleast a short part of the gene sequence must be known.

Antisense genes

- These are used to turn off the expression of a gene in a cell.
- A copy of the gene to be switched off is inserted into the host genome in such a way that the complementary (antisense) strand is transcribed.
- The antisense *m*RNA anneal to the sense *m*RNA and form a double-stranded RNA.
- Ribosomes cannot bind to this, so the *m*RNA is not translated and the gene is effectively switched off.

CHECK POINT 21.2

1. Which of the following statements does not hold true for restriction enzyme?
   (a) It recognises a palindromic nucleotide sequence
   (b) It is an endonuclease
   (c) It is isolated from viruses
   (d) It produces the same kind of sticky ends in different DNA molecules
2. Which of the following palindromic sequence is recognised by *Eco* RI ?
   (a) 5′ G↓AATTC 3′ / 3′ CTTAA↑G 5′
   (b) 5′ CCC↓GGG 3′ / 3′ GGG↑CCC 5′
   (c) 5′ AG↓TACT 3′ / 3′ TCA↑TGA 5′
   (d) 5′ G↓GATTC 3′ / 3′ CCTAG↑G 5′
3. The role of DNA ligase in the construction of a recombinant DNA molecule is the
   (a) formation of phosphodiester bond between two DNA fragments
   (b) formation of covalent bonds between sticky ends of DNA fragments
   (c) formation of H-bonds between all purine and pyrimidine bases
   (d) None of the above
4. *E. coli* cloning vector pBR322 contains restriction sites in the region of amp^R, tet^R genes that codes for the
   (a) antibiotic resistance genes
   (b) foreign DNA
   (c) selection of recombinants from non-recombinants
   (d) proteins involved in the replication of the plasmid
5. Which of the following represents a cosmid?
   (a) Plasmids + filamentous phage
   (b) Ti-plasmid + phage
   (c) Plasmid + λ phage
   (d) None of the above
6. The major advantage of using artificial chromosome such as YAC and BAC for cloning genes is that
   (a) these can carry much larger DNA fragments than ordinary plasmids
   (b) these can express protein but plasmids cannot
   (c) Plasmids are unable to replicate in cells
   (d) they can produce only two copies

TECHNIQUES USED IN RECOMBINANT DNA TECHNOLOGY

*r*DNA technology involves a group of techniques. These techniques are utilised in different steps.
A general account of these techniques is given below

Gene synthesis

- It is possible to chemically synthesise a gene in the lab by laboriously joining nucleotides together in the correct order.
- Automated machines have made gene synthesis much easier, but only upto a limit of about 30 bp. Therefore, very few real genes could be made by this way.

Artificial synthesis of genes

The artificial synthesis of genes can be done *via* following two ways

(i) **Synthesis of gene by known DNA sequences** If the detailed structure of the gene is known then the gene can be synthesised with purely chemical approach.
It can be summarised in following two steps

- In this method, nucleotides assemble with short-stranded DNA fragments (10 to 100 nucleotides), which are called **oligonucleotides**.
- These oligonucleotides assemble into double-stranded clonable DNA enzymatically.

(ii) **Synthesis of gene by unknown DNA sequence or cDNA synthesis** If detailed structure of gene is not known, then the RNA directed DNA polymerase enzyme (reverse transcriptase) is used for *in vitro* synthesis.

Synthesis of complementary DNA is an essential technique in *r*DNA technology. It is described in the figure given below

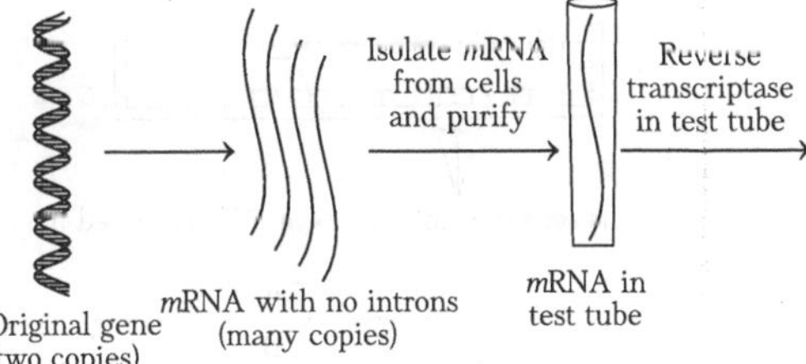

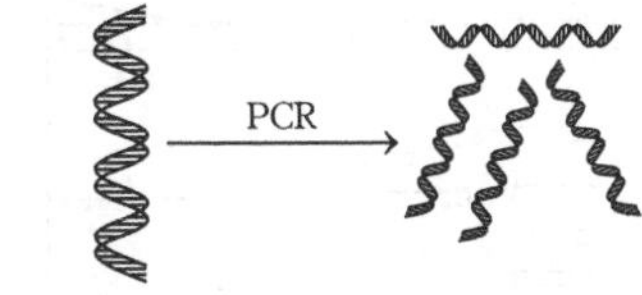

Fig. 21.6 cDNA formation

Electrophoresis

- It is a technique used to separate different pieces of DNA on the basis of their size, shape, surface area and molecular weight.
- Gel electrophoreis is used to separate fragments produced due to action of restriction enzymes.

- The DNA samples are placed into wells at one end of a thin slab of gel. It is made up of agarose or polyacrylamide and covered in a buffer solution.
- An electric current is passed through the gel. DNA has a negative charge due to the presence of negatively-charged phosphate group. Hence, in an electric field, DNA is attracted to the positive electrode, i.e. anode.
- The DNA molecules diffuse through the gel. The smaller fragments move faster than the larger ones. It is because the small size fragment experience lesser friction as compared to larger fragments.
- The DNA fragments on the gel cannot be seen, so they must be made visualised.
- There are two common methods to visualise DNA fragments
  (i) The gel can be stained with a chemical that specifically stains DNA, such as **Ethidium Bromide** (EtBr) or **Azure A**.
  EtBr is an intercalating dye, which gives colour in UV light. This method is simple, but not very sensitive.

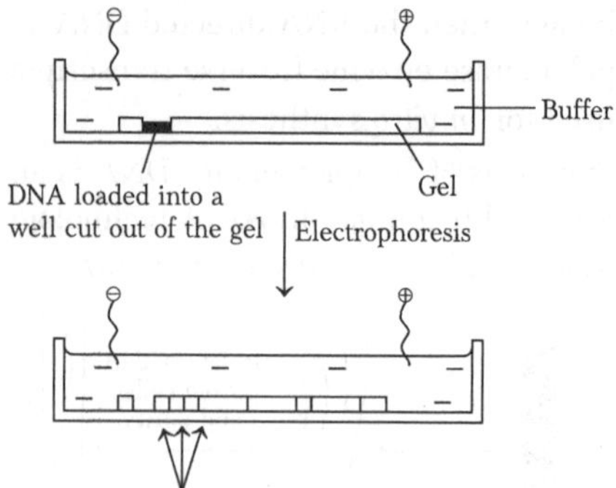

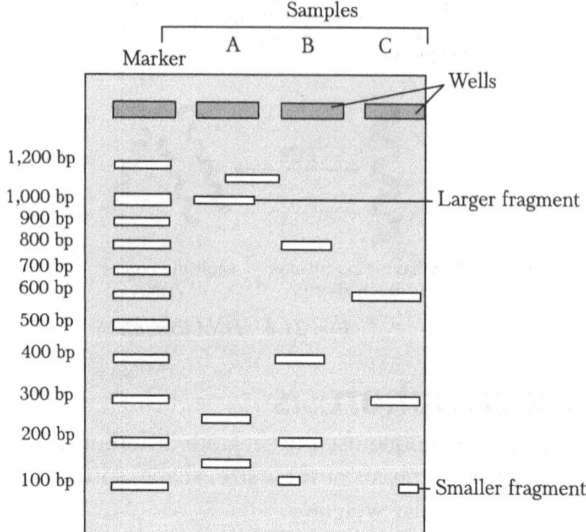

Gel after staining

***Fig 21.7** Electrophoresis*

  (ii) The DNA samples at the beginning can be radiolabelled with a radioactive isotope such as P^{32}. Photographic film is then placed on top of the finished gel in the dark. The DNA appears as dark bands on the film. This method is extremely sensitive.

Polymerase Chain Reaction (PCR)

- It is a technique to amplify specific DNA sequence, i.e. gene.
- PCR was developed by **Kary Mullis** in 1985. He got Nobel Prize for this discovery in 1993. PCR is best defined as the 'DNA replication *in vitro*'.

Principle of PCR

- PCR involves the heating of double-stranded DNA molecule at a high temperature.
- DNA strands get separated and single-stranded DNA molecules are formed.
- Then with the help of a DNA primer and DNA polymerase, the strands are copied again and again. This leads to the production of multiple copies of gene of interest.

Requirements of PCR

The basic requirements of PCR are as follows

(i) **DNA template** Segment of DNA or any desired DNA, which needs to be amplified serves as DNA template.

(ii) **Primers** These are short stretches of oligonucleotides. These are usually 10-18 nucleotides long. Usually two primers are utilised in PCR. These primers are oriented with their ends facing each other. This allows the synthesis of DNA towards one another.

(iii) **Enzyme** The enzyme used in PCR is derived from the thermophilic bacterium (*Thermus aquaticus*). This bacterium grows naturally in hot springs at a temperature of 300°C, due to its *Taq* polymerase enzyme. This enzyme does not get denatured at high temperatures.

The optimum temperature of *Taq* polymerase is about 72°C. Thus, when the mixture is heated to this temperature for a few minutes, the enzyme remains active and catalyses DNA synthesis.

Steps involved in PCR

The procedure of PCR involves three steps. These steps are as follows

(i) **Denaturation** It is the first step of PCR that involves separation of double-stranded DNA. The DNA is subjected to heating at 95 °C for two minutes. This leads to breakage of H-bonds between nucleotides and the formation of single-stranded DNA.

(ii) **Annealing** (hybridisation) It is the second step of PCR which involves annealing of primer to DNA strands. In this step, the DNA must be cooled to 50°C. At this temperature, the primers anneal to their complementary sequences on the separated DNA strands.

(iii) **Extension** This is the third step of PCR cycle. In this step, *Taq* polymerase enzyme extends the primers thus, completing the replication of the rest of the DNA.

Each original DNA strand replicates to form two new strands. The cycle is repeated and each time the number of DNA molecules get doubled. That is why, it is called a **chain reaction.**

Typically, PCR is run for 20-30 cycles. After the completion of PCR, several copies of gene of interest are generated. A diagrammatic representation of PCR is as follows

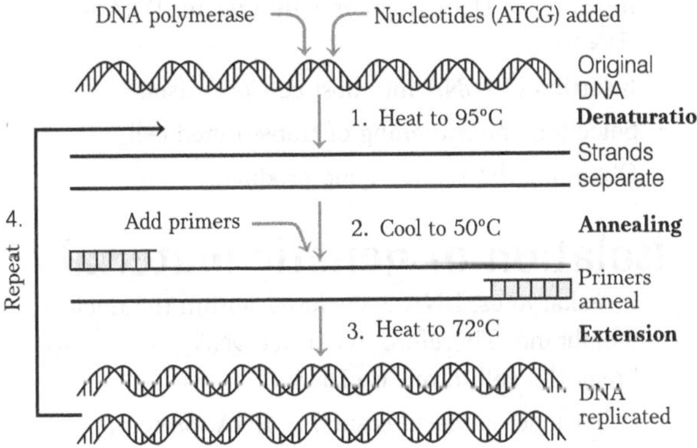

Fig. 21.8 PCR technique

Applications of PCR

Some of the applications of PCR are described below

(i) **Detection of pathogens** PCR detects infectious agents that are even very low in number.

(ii) **Diagnosis of specific mutations** PCR can be used to detect specific mutations causing a genetic diseases such as hepatitis, sickle-cell anaemia, etc.

(iii) **DNA fingerprinting** PCR is used to synthesise DNA for fingerprinting assays.

(iv) **Prenatal diagnosis** of genetic diseases can be done using PCR.

(v) **Palaeontology** PCR is used to copy DNA from mummified human bodies.

Southern blotting

This technique was invented by **Southern** in **1975.** It is used to detect the target DNA that have been transferred on to a blotting membrane with the help of a labelled probe.

Northern blotting

- This technique was developed by **James Alwin** and others in 1979. The Northern blotting is equivalent to Southern blotting. However, it is used to detect RNA.
- In this technique, *m*RNA separated by gel electrophoresis cannot bind to nitrocellulose membrane.
- Thus, RNA bands are blotted on to a DBM paper (Whatman's 540 paper). This paper is then hybridised to labelled probe and detected by autoradiography.

Western blotting

- It is developed by **Brunette** in 1979. This technique was developed by **W Neal.** It is used to detect proteins of a particular specificity.
- In this, proteins are electrophoresed in polyacrylamide gel and are then transferred on to a nitrocellulose membrane.
- These are later labelled with antibodies, lectins or some other compounds.

Replica plating technique

- It is a simple technique for making an exact copy of culture on an agar plate.
- In this technique, a pad of sterile cloth having same size as agar plate is pressed on the surface of agar plate with bacteria growing on it.
- Some cells from each colony stick to the cloth. The cloth is then pressed on to a new agar plate. Some cells get deposited and colonies grow in exactly the same positions on the new plate.
- This technique has a number of uses, but the most common use is to identify the transformed cells in *r*DNA technology.

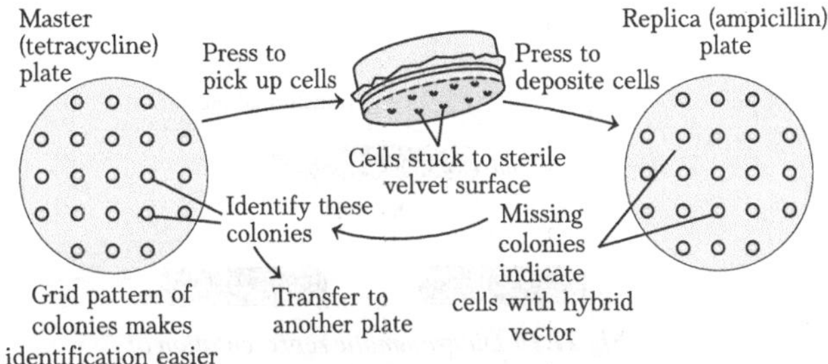

Fig. 21.9 Replica plate experiment

CHECK POINT 21.3

1. Synthesis of gene when DNA sequence is not known can be done *via*
   (a) combining nucleotides
   (b) *c*DNA synthesis
   (c) *t*RNA synthesis
   (d) All of the above

2. Gel electrophoresis is used for
   (a) cutting of DNA into fragments
   (b) separation of DNA fragments according to their size
   (c) construction of recombinant DNA by joining with cloning vectors
   (d) isolation of DNA molecule

3. Kary Mullis was awarded Nobel Prize in chemistry in 1993 for his work on
   (a) site directed mutagenesis (b) PCR
   (c) mobile genetic elements (d) antibody diversity

4. The polymerase chain reaction generates a fragment of distinct size even when an intact chromosome is used as template. What determines the boundaries of the amplified fragment?
   (a) The sites to which the primer anneal
   (b) The duration of the elongation step in each cycle
   (c) The temperature of the elongation step in each cycle
   (d) The concentration of one particular deoxynucleotide in the reaction

5. What is the first step in the Southern Blotting technique?
   (a) Denaturation of DNA on the gel for hybridisation with specific probe
   (b) Production of a group of genetically identical cells
   (c) Digestion of DNA by restriction enzyme
   (d) Denaturation of DNA from a nucleated cell such as the one from the scene of crime

6. Replica plating technique can be used for
   (a) identifying transformed cells
   (b) separation of DNA fragments
   (c) isolation of gene product
   (d) detetion of gene product

STEPS INVOLVED IN RECOMBINANT DNA TECHNOLOGY

Recombinant DNA technology is a complex process. Formation of a recombinant DNA occurs in a stepwise procedure.

The various steps involved in this process are as follows

- Isolation of genetic material (DNA).
- Cutting DNA at specific locations.
- Amplification/copying of gene of interest using PCR.
- Insertion of DNA fragments into vector DNA to form *r*DNA.
- Insertion of rDNA into host cell/organism.
- Selection and screening of transformed cell.
- Obtaining the foreign gene product.

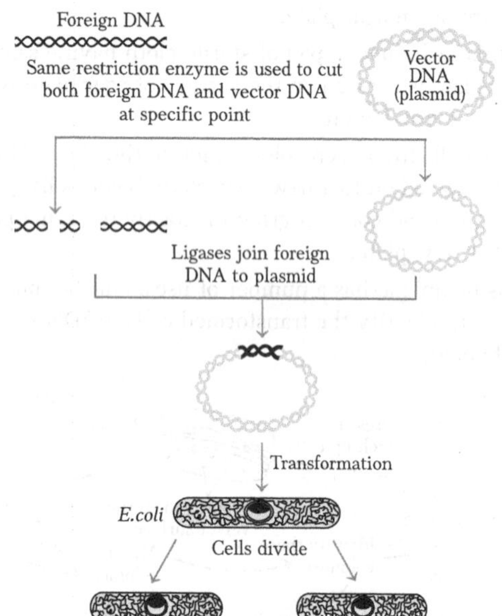

Fig 21.10 Diagrammatic representation of recombinant DNA technology

Isolation of genetic material

- In eukaryotes, DNA is enclosed within the nuclear membrane. Therefore to extract DNA, we have to break the cell to release DNA.
- Other macromolecules such as RNA, protein, polysaccharides and lipids are also released along with DNA. Extraction of DNA along with macromolecules is achieved by treating the cells with enzymes.
- Different enzymes are used for different type of cells, such as for breaking the cell membranes.

  For example

  (a) Lysozymes are used for bacterial cells

  (b) Cellulase are used for plant cells.

  (c) Chitinase are used for fungal cells.
- The purified DNA can be extracted from the crude product which is obtained after the cell lysis.
- The RNA and protein from the crude extract are removed by ribonucleases and proteases, respectively.
- The other molecules can be removed by appropriate treatment and purified DNA is ultimately precipitated

out after the addition of **chilled ethanol.** Purified DNA is seen as collection of fine thread in the suspension.

- In a process called **spooling,** DNA is removed from the suspension with the help of a glass rod. The rod is rotated over extracted DNA and it adheres to the glass rod.

Cutting of DNA at specific location

- The purified DNA fragments are treated with restriction enzymes at optimal conditions.
- A restriction enzyme function by inspecting the length of whole DNA sequence. Once it finds its recognition site, it binds to the DNA.
- After binding, it cuts each of the two strands at specific points in their sugar-phosphate backbone. As a result, desired fragments can be produced.
- The fragmented DNA are loaded on agarose gel for electrophoresis. It is employed to check the progression of restriction enzyme digestion. It also helps in the separation of DNA fragments.
- The separated DNA fragments are cut from the agarose gel and extracted from the gel piece. This step is known as **elution.** By elution, gene of interest can be isolated.

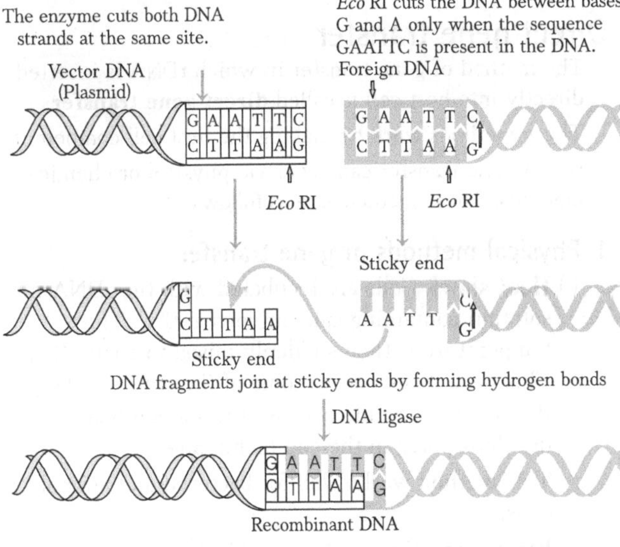

***Fig 21.11** Formation of recombinant DNA by different enzyme action*

Amplification of gene of Interest

- The gene of interest is amplified with the help of PCR.
- We have already studied the working of PCR, in techniques of recombinant DNA technology.

Insertion of gene of interest into vector

- The amplified gene of interest is joined with a cloning vector by using DNA ligase.
- The fragments produced by the action of restriction enzyme may have either blunt ends or sticky end. The ligation of blunt ends of gene and vector DNA is not an efficient process.
- In contrast, ligation of sticky ends is much more efficient. We often put sticky ends on to a blunt end molecule. This can be achieved by homopolymer tailing method. It was first used by **Jackson *et. al.*** in 1972.
- The insertion of gene of interest into the vector is based on the ability of enzyme, terminal transferase. It adds sequences of same nucleotides (homopolymers) to 3′ end of DNA.
- For example, polymer G is added to the 3′ end of foreign DNA molecule. Similarly, complementary homopolymer-C is added to the cloning vector. Thus, complementary homopolymer 3′ tails are generated.
- These tails help in joining of Gene Of Interest (GOI) with cloning vector thus, resulting in the formation of recombinant DNA. After the ligation of GOI with cloning vector, this cloning vector is called as *r*DNA.

Insertion of *r*DNA into host cell

- Recombinant DNA, i.e. vectors containing the gene of interest must be inserted into living cells for their replication.
- The insertion of *r*DNA into the cell is most commonly called as **gene transfer.**
- The cells receiving the recombinant DNA are called **host cells.** Once these cells have successfully incorporated the *r*DNA, they are said to be transformed.

Gene transfer

It may take place in two ways, which are as follows

Indirect gene transfer

When the rDNA is inserted into host cell by the use of a vector, the method of gene transfer is called **indirect gene transfer.** It can occur through following means

(i) **Plant tumours** This method has been used successfully to transform plant cells. This method uses tumour causing microbe, e.g. *Agrobacterium tumefaciens.*

The recombinant DNA (Ti plasmid + Gene of interest) enter the cells when bacterium infects the plant.

The figure given below describes the steps involved in *Agrobacterium* mediated gene transfer.

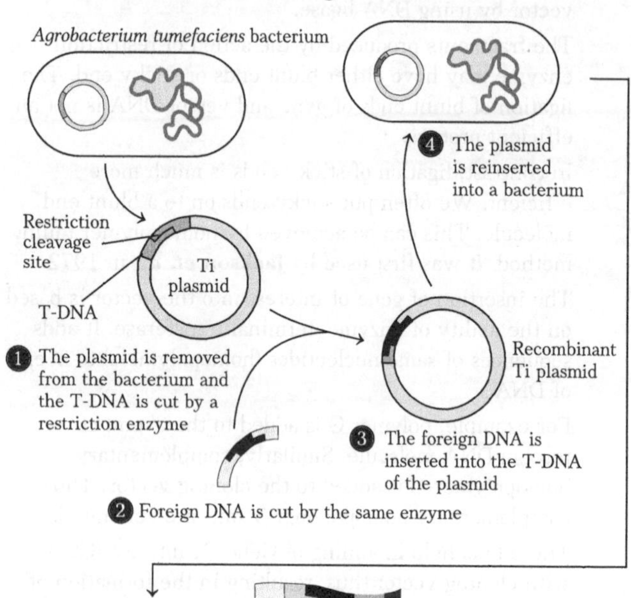

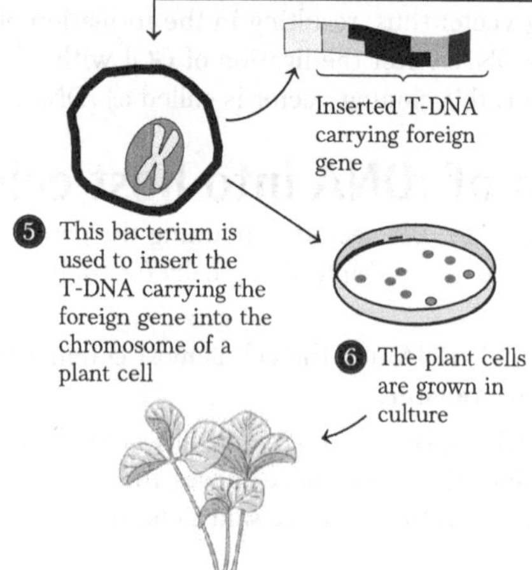

Fig. 21.12 Introduction of DNA segment to plant cell through Ti plasmid

(ii) **Viruses** In this method, DNA is first transferred into a virus. The virus infects a cell and transfers the recombinant DNA along with its own genetic material. Thus, they have been utilised for developing a successful method of gene delivery. The virus is genetically engineered to make it safe, so that it cannot reproduce itself or make toxins.

Three commonly used viruses are as follows

(a) **Bacteriophages** (phages) These viruses infect bacteria. They are a very effective way of delivering large genes into bacterial cells in culture (as discussed earlier in this chapter).

(b) **Adenoviruses** These are human viruses that cause respiratory diseases including common cold. Their genetic material is double-stranded DNA. They are ideal for delivering genes into living patients in gene therapy. Their DNA is not incorporated into the host's chromosomes, so it is not replicated, but their genes are expressed.

Adenovirus is genetically altered, so that its coat proteins are not synthesised. Therefore, new virus particles cannot be assembled and the host cell is not killed.

(c) **Retroviruses** They are enclosed in a lipid membrane. Their genetic material is the double-stranded RNA. On infection, this RNA is copied to DNA and the DNA is incorporated into the host's chromosome. This means that the foreign genes are replicated into every daughter cell.

Direct gene transfer

- The method of gene transfer in which rDNA is inserted directly into host cell is called **direct gene transfer.**
- These methods work by making the host cell competent.
- Direct gene transfer can occur *via* physical or chemical methods. These methods are as follows

1. Physical methods of gene transfer

(i) **Heat shock** Cells are incubated with the rDNA in a solution containing calcium ions at 0°C. The temperature is then suddenly raised to about 40°C. This heat shock causes some of the cells to take up the rDNA. It occurs because the sudden heat develops pores in the cell membrane.

This method works well for bacterial and animal cells.

(ii) **Electroporation** Cells are subjected to a high voltage pulse, which temporarily disrupts the membrane. The rDNA enters to enter the cell. This is the most efficient method of delivering genes to bacterial cells.

(iii) **Gene gun or Biolistics** This technique fires microscopic gold particles coated with the foreign DNA at the cells using a compressed air gun (burst of helium). It is designed to overcome the problem of the strong cell wall in plant tissue as gold particles can penetrate the cell wall.

(iv) **Microinjection** A cell is held on a glass pipette under a microscope. The foreign DNA is injected directly into the nucleus using an incredibly fine micropipette. This pipette can puncture the plasma membrane. This method is used when very few cells are available.

(v) **Liposomes** Vectors can be encased in liposomes, which are small membrane vesicles. The liposomes fuse with the cell membrane (sometimes the nuclear membrane too) thus, delivering the DNA into the cell. This works for many types of cells, but it is particularly useful for delivering genes to cells *in vivo* (such as in gene therapy).

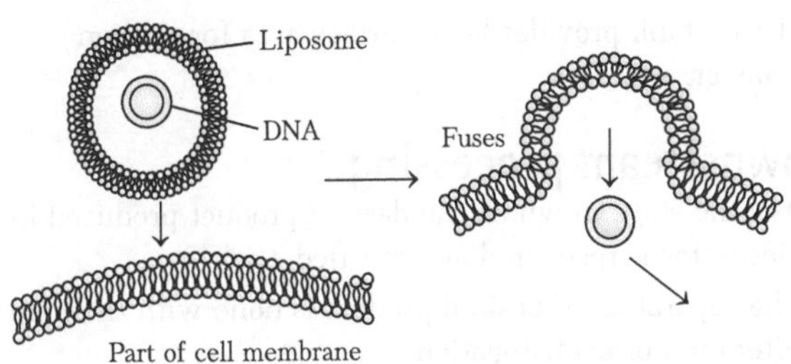

Fig. 21.13 Liposomes

2. Chemical methods of direct gene transfer

(i) **Poly-Ethylene Glycol** (PEG) **mediated transfer** The first integration of Ti plasmid DNA into plant protoplast was reported in *Petunia* and tobacco in the presence of PEG. The 40% solution of PEG creates small pores in plasma membrane, which helps in the integration of rDNA.

(ii) **Calcium-phosphate coprecipitation** In this method, the DNA $CaPO_4$ complex is added to the dividing cells to transfer rDNA.

Selection and screening of transformed cells

The selection of transformed cells from the non-transformed cells (cells without rDNA) can be achieved by selectable markers (already discussed). After the selection of transformed cells, these cells are screened for recombinant cells (cells with rDNA) and non-recombinant cells (cells without rDNA).

This can be done by following methods

(i) Immunological method

- It was developed by **Broom** and **Gilbert** (1978).
- In this method, first the transformed cells are plated on agar in petridish.
- Each of these develops into an isolated independent colonies. This is followed by replica plating, then application of unlabelled immunoglobin and finally labelled immunoglobin.
- At the end, the clones are detected by Western blotting method.

(ii) The nucleic acid hybridisation

- It is also called **colony hybridisation method**.
- This method was developed by **Grunstein** and **Hogness** in 1975.
- In this method, the recombinant DNA is detected by molecular probes, i.e. either radioactive DNA or RNA probes.

(iii) Blue white screening or Insertional inactivation

- In this methodology, the recombinants are differentiated from non-recombinants on the basis of their ability to produce colour in the presence of a chromogenic substrate.
- The rDNA is inserted within the coding sequence of an enzyme, β-galactosidase. This enzyme is encoded by ***lac*-Z gene.**
- As a result, the enzyme gets inactivated. The presence of a chromogenic substrate gives blue coloured colonies if the plasmid in the bacteria, does not have an insert (non-recombinants).
- The presence of inserts results in the inactivation of enzyme β-galactosidase, due to which colourless colonies are produced (recombinants).

Obtaining the foreign gene product

- To obtain the foreign gene product, the transformed host cells are cultured in nutrient medium at large scale.
- This can be done with the help of bioreactors.
- It is a chamber in which transformed cells or microorganisms are cultured in a liquid or solid medium.

- In bioreactors, raw materials are biologically converted into specific product like enzymes, etc.
- It provides optimal conditions, i.e. temperature, pH, substrate, etc., for achieving the desired product. Bioreactors are mostly utilised when 100-1000 L of culture need to be processed.

Design of a bioreactor

- The most commonly used bioreactors are **stirred tank bioreactors.** It is of mainly two types, i.e. **simple stirred-tank** and **sparged stirred-tank.**
- Simple stirred-tank is cylindrical or may have a curved base to facilitate the mixing of reactor contents.
- A stirrer is present that allows mixing and oxygen availibility to all the cells present in a bioreactor.

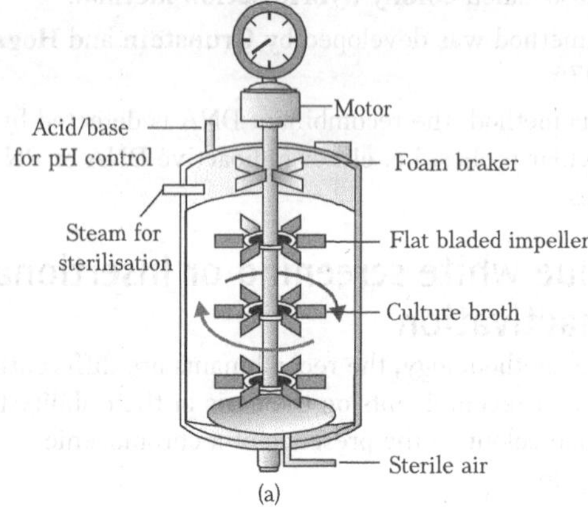

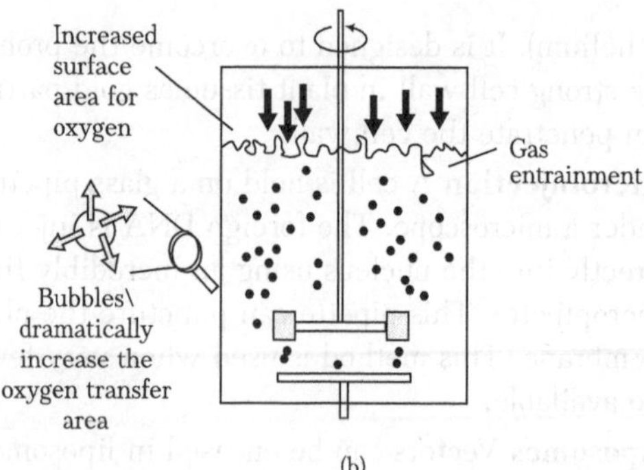

Fig 21.14 (a) A stirred-tank bioreactor, (b) Sparged stirred-tank bioreactor

- A bioreactor has an agitator system, oxygen delivery system, a foam control system, pH control system, temperature control system and a sampling port that periodically withdraw culture.
- Stirred-tank provides large surface area for oxygen transfer.

Downstream processing

- It is the stage in which the desired product produced in bioreactor is recovered and purified.
- The separation of desired product is done with the help of filteration or centrifugation.
- A number of biochemical techniques are also available for this purpose. These include drying, chromatography, solvent extraction, distillation, etc.

CHECK POINT 21.4

1. Which of the following enzyme is used for the isolation of genetic material from fungal cells?
(a) Lysozyme (b) Cellulase (c) Chitinase (d) Ligase

2. Significance of heat shock method in bacterial transformation is to facilitate
(a) binding of DNA to the cell wall
(b) uptake of DNA through membrane transport proteins
(c) uptake of DNA through transient pores in the bacterial cell wall
(d) expression of antibiotic resistance gene

3. In immunological method, which technique is used to detect clones at the end?
(a) Western blotting
(b) Insertional inactivation
(c) Replica plating
(d) None of the above

4. In blue-white screening, the recombinants can be identified as
(a) colourless colonies
(b) blue coloured colonies
(c) red coloured colonies
(d) None of the above

5. In blue-white screening, ... is used in medium.
(a) chromogenic substrate
(b) ampicillin
(c) tetracycline
(d) All of the above

6. Stirred tank bioreactors have been designed for the
(a) purification of the product
(b) addition of preservatives to the product
(c) availability of oxygen throughout the bioreactor
(d) ensuring anaerobic conditions in the culture vessel

OTHER ADVANCED TECHNOLOGIES ASSOCIATED WITH GENETIC ENGINEERING

There are number of advanced technologies or techniques and tools associated with genetic engineering. Some of them are as follows

Genomic library

A genomic library or gene bank is the collection of entire genome of an organism either in the form of plasmid clones or phage lysates with recombinant DNA inserts.

Construction of genomic library

A genomic library is generally constructed by applying the shotgun sequencing, which involves following three steps

- The entire genome is randomly broken into fragments of clonable size with the help of restriction endonucleases.
- These fragments are then joined to suitable cloning vectors *in vitro*.
- The recombinant DNA molecules thus produced are introduced into prokaryotic cells, inside which these rDNA molecules replicate to form the clones. Hence, gene bank or gene library is constructed.

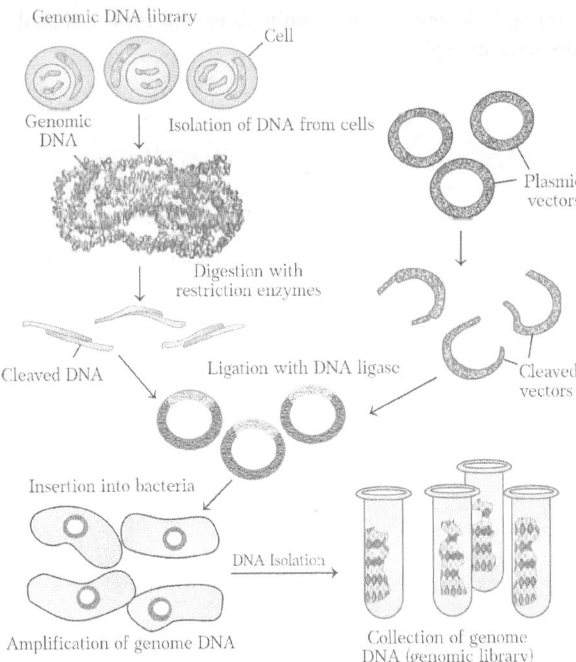

Fig. 21.15 Construction of gene library

Application of genomic library

Genomic libraries are essential for maintaining and retrieving the DNA clones.

Note *Genomic library contains complete genome, i.e. coding and non-coding DNA, whereas cDNA library consists of only coding DNA sequences.*

Biochip

- It is also called as **gene microarray**. It is a discrete collection of gene fragments on a stamp-sized chip.
- It is made up of thin wafers of silicon glass. This chip can be used to screen the presence of a particular gene variant.
- These chips allow rapid screening of gene profiles.
- **Biochips** are most commonly used for identifying precise forms of cancer. For example, leukemia from different patients can be distinguished.

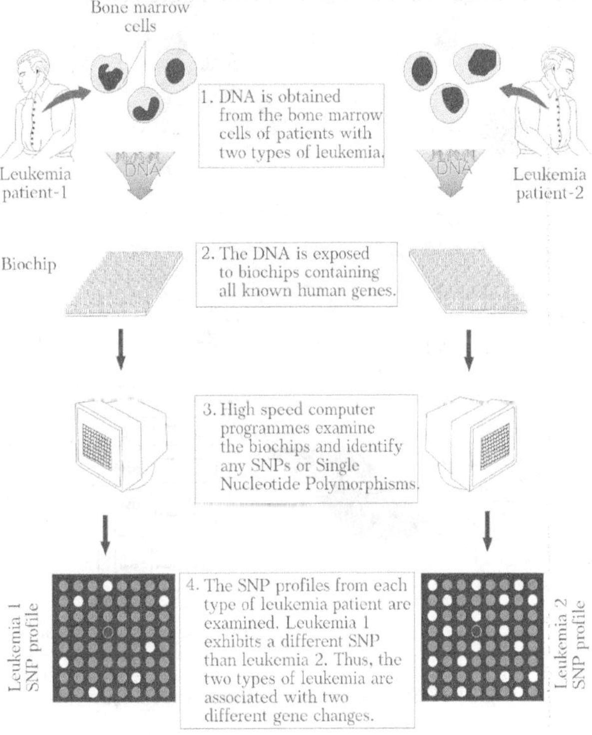

Fig. 21.16 Biochips can help in identifying precise forms of cancer

DNA fingerprinting

- DNA fingerprinting or DNA typing or genetic fingerprinting or DNA profiling is a technique to identify a person on the basis of person's DNA specificity. This technique was developed by **Alec Jeffreys** in 1984.

- The technique is based upon the fact that the DNA constitution of an individual carries some specific sequences of nucleotides.
- These sequences do not carry any information for protein synthesis.
- These specific sequences are repeated many times and found at many places within the genome.
- The loci at which these sequences are present are known as the **Variable Number Tandem Repeats** (VNTRs) or **minisatellites**. These sequences are 10 to 100 nucleotides long with repetition of certain combination within them.
- These sequences are variable in their number from person to person.
- VNTRs, thus are used as genetic markers, which individuals inherit from their parents.
- VNTRs are similar in monozygotic twins only. The process of DNA fingerprinting is given in the figure below

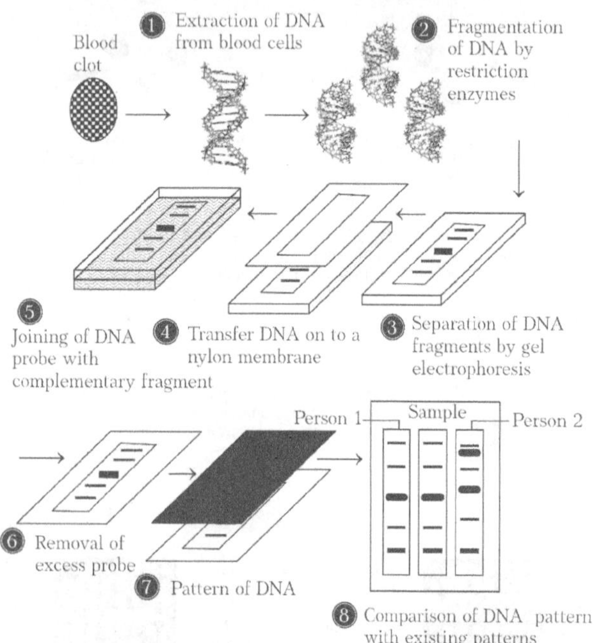

Fig 21.17 Steps in DNA fingerprinting technique

Applications of DNA fingerprinting

- DNA fingerprinting is highly reliable method for identification of individuals involved in rape, murder and other crimes, using samples like blood (erythrocytes), hair, etc.
- It is a sure method in solving paternity and maternity disputes.
- It is useful in guiding breeding programmes for endangered animals.
- It can help in identifying the individuals and races with specific genes carrying inherited diseases, susceptibility to various (parasitic) diseases as well as resistance to them.
- This method provides information about human lineage and relationship with great apes.
- It is being used to study relationships amongst various groups of people for knowing historical migrations and invasions.

Note *Forensic scientists have recently developed a different set of similar markers that are analysed by the PCR, rather than RFLP analysis. These markers are called **Short Tandem Repeats (STRs)** or **microsatellites**. In these markers, the segment is similar to the VNTRs, but the repeated portion is shorter (2-9 base pairs long) than VNTRs.*

Cloning

- It is the production of organisms, which are genetically identical to their parents.
- These identical structures are called **clones.** These can be defined as exact carbon copies of a single parent.
- The idea of cloning was first suggested by **Hans Spemann** in 1938. He is considered as the **Father of Modern Embryology**.
- Spemann proposed what he called a Fantastical experiment, i.e. to remove the nucleus from an egg then putting nucleus from another cell into that egg.
- Cloning is absent in higher animals except for occasional monozygotic split ups.

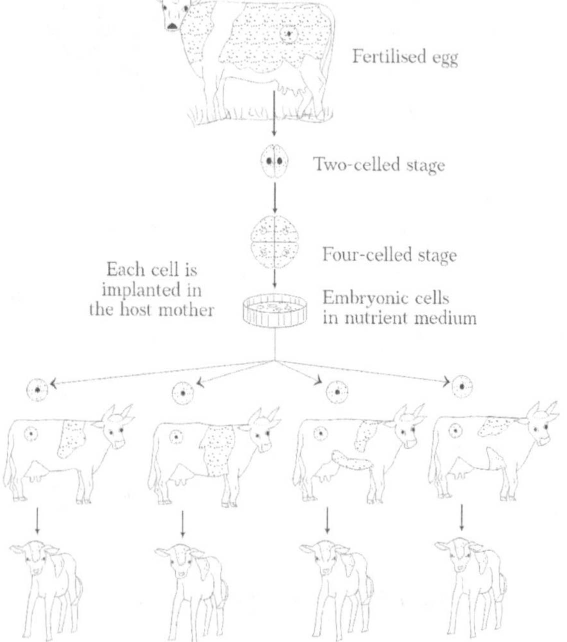

***Fig. 21.18** Clonal calves*

Types of cloning

It is of three types as follows

(i) **Gene cloning** is the formation of multiple copies of the same gene, which is achieved by DNA technology.

(ii) **Cell cloning** is the formation of multiple copies of the same cell. Cells of a clone are identical genetically, morphologically and physiologically.

(iii) **Organismal cloning** is the formation of one or more genetically identical individuals from a single parent. The lamb **Dolly** is the first successful clone derived from differentiated animal cell (**Wilmut** and **Campbell** in 1997). Similarly, **Noori** (Pashmina goat) was cloned by the scientists of **University of Agricultural Science and Technology, Kashmir**.

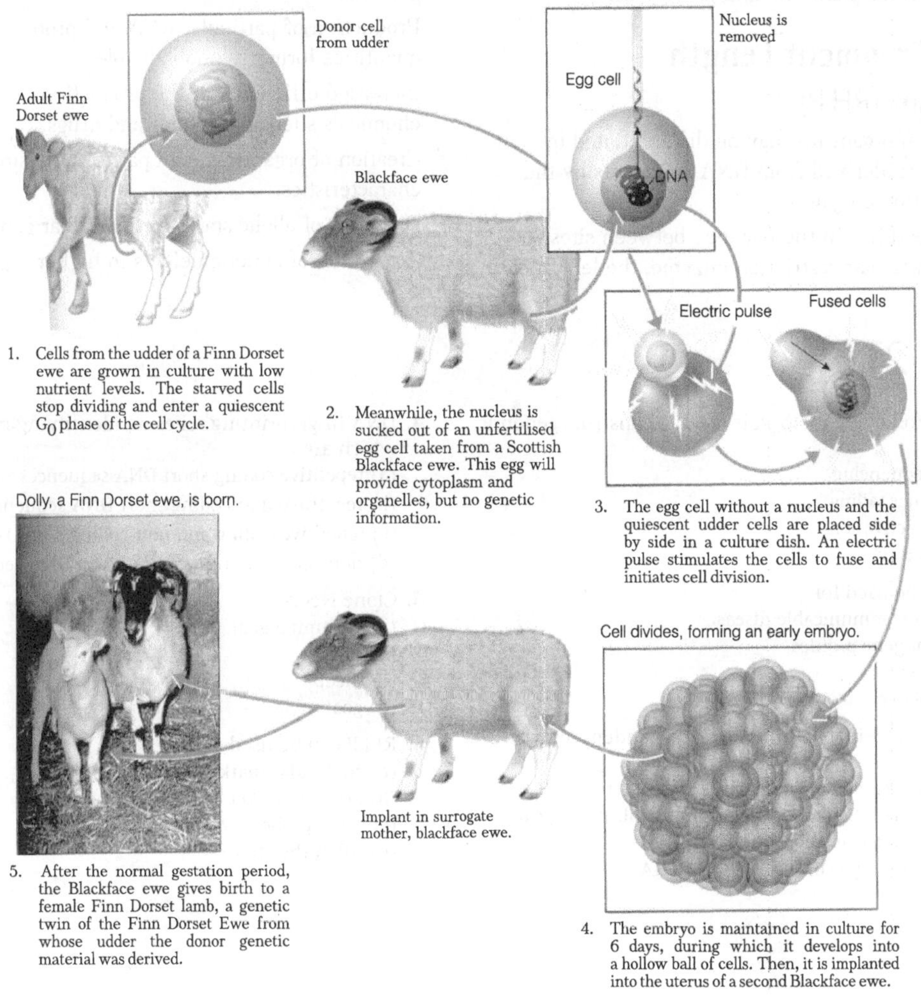

Fig. 21.19 Formation of Dolly (Wilmut's experiment)

Random Amplification of Polymorphic DNA (RAPD)

- It is a type of PCR in which the DNA segments to be amplified are random.
- RAPD does not require any specific knowledge of DNA sequence of target organism.
- In RAPD, several random short primers (8-12 nucleotides) and a large template of DNA are used.
- This technique is widely used to characterise and trace the phylogeny of diverse plant and animal species.

Restriction Fragment Length Polymorphism (RFLP)

- In this technique, organisms may be differentiated by analysis of pattern derived from DNA fragments by the action of restriction enzymes.
- If two organisms differ in the distance between sites of cleavage of a particular restriction enzyme, the length of the fragments produced will differ when the DNA is digested with a restriction enzyme.
- The similarity of patterns generated can be used to differentiate species from one another.
- RFLPs are used as molecular markers.

Current research areas of biotechnology

Current interest in genetic engineering centres are as follows

- Isolation of a particular gene, part of gene or region of the genome.
- Production of particular RNA and protein molecules in quantities formerly unobtainable.
- Increased efficiency in the production of biological chemicals such as enzymes and drugs.
- Creation of organisms with particular desired characteristics.
- Diagnosis of allelic status for molecular genetic diseases.
- Correction of genetic defects in higher organisms.

CHECK POINT 21.5

1. Which of the following method is used to construct genomic library?
(a) Shot gun sequencing
(b) Homopolymer tailing
(c) Insertion inactivation
(d) Both (b) and (c)

2. A biochip can be used for
(a) detection of communicable diseases
(b) screening of gene profiles
(c) Palaeontology
(d) All of the above

3. Which of the following statements about tandem repetitive DNA are correct?
(a) Tandem means two repeats next to each other
(b) It is usually classified according to the number of repeats
(c) STRs are the same as microsatellite DNA
(d) VNTRs are not a type of minisatellite DNA

4. DNA fingerprinting relies on identifying minisatellite which are
(a) repetitive coding short DNA sequences
(b) repetitive non-coding short DNA sequences
(c) repetitive coding and non-coding short DNA sequences
(d) non-repetitive non-coding short DNA sequences

5. Clone Noori is a
(a) Pashmina goat
(b) calf
(c) sheep
(d) goat

6. RFLP can be used as
(a) molecular marker
(b) protein marker
(c) DNA probe
(d) All of the above

EXAM POINTS

- *Hind* II is a restriction endonuclease. **[NEET 2016]**
- *Eco* RV restriction enzyme produces blunt ends. **[NEET 2016]**
- The enzyme catalysing the removal of nucleotides from ends of DNA is exonuclease. **[NEET Odisha 2019]**
- Restriction endonucleases are synthesised by bacteria as part of their defence mechanism. **[AMU 2015]**
- Restriction nuclease enzyme binds DNA at specific sites and cuts only one of the two stands. **[NEET 2019]**
- Restriction endonucleases are the enzymes that break phosphodiester bond between specific nucleotides of DNA. **[Chhattisgarh PMT 2015]**
- First discovered restriction endonuclease that always cut DNA molecule at a particular part by recognising a specific sequence of six base pair is *Hind* II. **[NEET 2020]**
- The specific palindromic sequence which is recognised by *Eco* RI is

  $5'-\text{GAATTC}-3'$
  $3'-\text{CTTAAG}-5'$ **[NEET 2020]**
- Retrovirus is commonly used as a vector for introducing a DNA fragment in human lymphocytes. **[NEET 2019]**
- The sequence that contols the copy number of the linked DNA in the vector is termed *ori* site. **[NEET 2020]**
- In recombinant DNA technology, antibiotics are used as selectable markers. **[NEET 2020]**
- A selectable marker is used in eliminating the non transformants, so that the transformants can be regenerated. **[NEET 2019]**
- The two antibiotic resistance genes on vector pBR322 are ampicillin and tetracycline. **[NEET 2019]**
- In Ti plasmid, virulent gene is removed. **[AIIMS 2019]**
- A foreign DNA and plasmid cut by the same restriction endonuclease can be joined to form a recombinant plasmid using ligase. **[NEET 2016]**
- DNA precipitation out of mixture of biomolecules can be achieved by the treatment with chilled ethanol. **[NEET 2019]**
- In gel electrophoresis, separated DNA fragments can be visualised with the help of ethidium bromide in UV radiation. **[NEET 2020]**
- In a mixture, DNA fragments are separated by electrophoresis. **[NEET 2020, 2013]**
- The criterion for DNA fragments movement on agarose gel during gel electrophoresis is that smaller the fragment size, the further it moves. **[NEET 2017]**
- The *Taq* polymerase enzyme is obtained from *Thermus aquaticus*. **[NEET 2019]**
- The Polymerase Chain Reaction (PCR) is a technique that is used for *in vitro* replication of specific DNA sequences using thermostable DNA polymerase. **[Kerala CEE 2014]**
- The correct order of steps in Polymerase Chain Reaction (PCR) is denaturation, annealing and extension. **[NEET 2018]**
- Gene transfer is achieved by biolistics. **[JIPMER 2018]**
- In annealing, primers anneal to the DNA template. **[JIPMER 2019]**
- If a recombinant DNA bearing gene for ampicillin resistance is transferred into *E. coli* cells and the host cells are spread on agar plates containing ampicillin, then transformed recipient cells will grow and untransformed recipient cells will die. **[NEET 2018]**
- Chimeric DNA is recombinant DNA. **[AIIMS 2019]**
- Gene library or DNA library has collection of *c*DNA only. **[AIIMS 2019]**
- Spooling is the collection of isolated DNA . **[NEET 2020]**
- Stirred-tank bioreactors have been designed for availability of oxygen throughout the process. **[NEET 2016]**
- Alec Jeffreys developed the DNA fingerprinting technique. The probe he used was VNTR. **[Rajasthan PMT 2011, Kerala CEE 2011]**

Chapter Exercises

(A) Topical Exercise

Biotechnology and Its Principles

1 The technique of using living organism or enzymes from organisms to produce products and processes useful to humans is called
(a) biopiracy
(b) biotechnology
(c) bioprospecting
(d) biomagnification

2 The core technique(s) that enabled the birth of modern biotechnology is/are
(a) genetic engineering
(b) maintenance of sterile ambience (chemical engineering)
(c) Both (a) and (b)
(d) None of the above

3 Yeast has become important in genetic engineering because it
(a) has plasmids that can be genetically engineered
(b) allows the study of eukaryotic gene regulation and expression
(c) grows readily and rapidly in the laboratory
(d) All of the above

4 Consider the following statements.
I. Term which can be used as synonym of genetic engineering in many cases is known as recombinant DNA technology.
II. A gene carried by recombinant DNA is cloned when its host bacterium divides by binary fission.
Choose the correct option.
(a) Statement I is true, but II is false
(b) Statement I is false, but II is true
(c) Both statements I and II are true
(d) Both statements I and II are false

Tools of Recombinant DNA Technology

5 The word 'restriction' in restriction enzyme refers to
(a) cutting of DNA at specific position only
(b) cleaving of phosphodiester linkage
(c) prevention of the multiplication of bacteriophage in bacteria
(d) All of the above

6 The role of restriction enzymes in DNA technology is to
(a) provide a vector for the transfer of recombinant DNA
(b) produce *c*DNA from *m*RNA
(c) produce a cut (usually staggered) at specific recognition sequences on DNA
(d) reseal 'sticky ends' after base-pairing of complementary bases

7 A piece of DNA, cut by restriction enzyme, forms bonds with other DNA molecules which have
(a) methyl groups attached to them
(b) unpaired bases
(c) plasmid components
(d) been fragmented by the same restriction enzyme

8 A restriction enzyme breaks between the
(a) base pairs of a DNA molecule
(b) base pairs of a DNA-RNA hybrid molecule
(c) sugar and phosphate components of a nucleic acid molecule
(d) exons and introns of a DNA molecule

9 Consider the following statements.
I. Exonucleases are restriction enzymes, which cut DNA internally.
II. Exonuclease can destroy both DNA and RNA.
Choose the correct option.
(a) Statement I is true, but II is false
(b) Statement I is false, but II is true
(c) Both statements I and II are true
(d) Both statements I and II are false

10 GAATTC is the recognition site for the restriction endonuclease
(a) *Eco* RI (b) *Hind* II (c) *Eco* RII (d) *Bam* HI

11 When a typical restriction enzyme cuts a DNA molecule, the cuts are uneven, so that the DNA fragments have single-stranded ends. These ends are useful in recombinant DNA work because
(a) they serve as starting points for DNA replication
(b) only single-stranded DNA segments can code for proteins
(c) they enable researchers to use the fragments as molecular probes
(d) the fragments will bind to other fragments with complementary ends

12 In restriction enzymes like *Eco* RI, the Roman numbers following the names indicate the
(a) order in which the enzyme were dicovered from that strain of bacteria
(b) order in which the enzyme were isolated from that strain of bacteria
(c) genus of the prokaryotic cell or bacteria
(d) strain of the bacteria

13 Match the following columns.

	Column I (Vectors)		Column II (Derivative microorganisms)
A.	*Eco* RI	1.	*E. coli* R 245
B.	*Hind* III	2.	*Bacillus amyloliquefaciens*
C.	*Bam* HI	3.	*Haemophilus aegyptus*
D.	*Eco* RII	4.	*Escherichia coli* RY13

Codes

	A	B	C	D		A	B	C	D
(a)	1	2	3	4	(b)	3	2	1	4
(c)	4	3	2	1	(d)	4	2	3	1

14 Which of the following produces blunt ends?
(a) *Hind* III and *Sma* I
(b) *Hae* III and *Sma* I
(c) *Eco* RI and *Eco* RII
(d) *Hind* II and *Hind* III

15 Consider the following statements
I. Type-1 restriction enzymes cleave only one strand of DNA.
II. Type-II restriction enzyme requires Mg^{2+} ion and S-adenosylmethionine for their functioning.
Choose the correct option.
(a) Statement I is true, but II is false
(b) Statement I is false, but II is true
(c) Both statements I and II are true
(d) Both statements I and II are false

16 Type-II restriction enzymes are preferred over type-I in cleaving DNA strand because they
(a) cleave DNA very fast
(b) do not require additional energy for cleavage
(c) cleave DNA at specific site
(d) Both (a) and (c)

17 Stickiness of the ends of the DNA facilitates the
(a) action of DNA ligase and these ends joined together laterally
(b) action of DNA ligase and these ends joined together end-to-end
(c) action of *Taq* polymerase
(d) action of restriction enzyme

18 The role of DNA ligase in the construction of a recombinant DNA molecule is
(a) formation of phosphodiester bond between two DNA fragments
(b) formation of hydrogen bonds between sticky ends of DNA fragments
(c) ligation of all purine and pyrimidine bases
(d) All of the above

19 The linking of antibiotic resistance gene with the plasmid vector become possible with
(a) DNA ligase
(b) endonucleases
(c) DNA polymerase
(d) exonucleases

20 Which of the following features are required to facilitate cloning into a vector?
I. Origin of replication (*ori*)
II. Selectable marker
III. Cloning site
(a) I and II
(b) II and III
(c) I and III
(d) I, II and III

21 Construction of recombinant DNA involves
(a) cleaving and rejoining of DNA segments with endonuclease
(b) cleaving DNA segments with endonuclease and rejoining with ligase
(c) cleaving and rejoining DNA segments with ligase
(d) cleaving DNA segments with ligase and rejoining with endonuclease

22 Consider the following statements.
I. A plasmid can replicate independently.
II. DNA of plasmid is double-stranded and circular.
Choose the correct option.
(a) Statement I is true, but II is false
(b) Statement I is false, but II is true
(c) Both statements I and II are true
(d) Both statements I and II are false

23 The most important feature in a plasmid to be used as a vector is
(a) origin of replication (*ori*)
(b) presence of a selectable marker
(c) presence of sites for restriction endonuclease
(d) All of the above

24 Plasmids are suitable vectors for gene cloning because these
(a) are small circular DNA molecules, which can integrate with host chromosomal DNA
(b) are small circular DNA molecules with their own replication origin site
(c) can shuttle between prokaryotic and eukaryotic cells
(d) often carry antibiotic resistance genes

25 To prevent recirculation of vector DNA and to increase the frequency of production of recombinant DNA technology
(a) reverse transcriptases are used
(b) alkaline phosphatases are used
(c) acid phosphatases are used
(d) All of the above

26 *Ori* sequence in plasmid refers to sequence
(a) for antibody resistance
(b) from which replication will start in plasmid
(c) for restriction site
(d) Both (a) and (c)

27 Consider the following statements.

I. Large amount of recombinant protein can be produced by gene cloning.

II. pBR322 vector was constructed by using DNA derived from naturally occurring plasmids of *E.coli.*

Choose the correct option.

(a) Statement I is true, but II is false
(b) Statement I is false, but II is true
(c) Both statements I and II are true
(d) Both statements I and II are false

28 What is the disadvantage of using pBR322 as cloning vector?

(a) Reasonably high copy number is produced
(b) Size is 4.3 kb
(c) Both (a) and (b)
(d) Selection of recombinants due to inactivation of antibiotics require simultaneous plating on two plates having different antibiotics

29 In recombinant DNA technology, a plasmid vector must be cleaved by

(a) four separate enzymes
(b) modified DNA ligase
(c) a heated alkaline solution
(d) the same restriction enzyme that cleaves the donor gene

30 Using recombinant DNA technology, genes from a donor cell can be implanted into a bacterium for DNA replication and protein synthesis. The kinds of cells that can be used as gene donors in this technology are

(a) bacteria only
(b) either yeast or bacteria only
(c) eukaryotic cells only
(d) any kind of cell

31 Consider the following statements.

I. Plasmids that carry genes to provide resistance to antibiotics are called R-plasmid.

II. *c*DNA-*m*RNA hybrids are made by using reverse transcriptase.

Choose the correct option.

(a) Statement I is true, but II is false
(b) Statement I is false, but II is true
(c) Both statements I and II are true
(d) Both statements I and II are false

32 Which of the following is not true for recognition sequences?

(a) Modification by methylation of bases within them prevents restriction of bacterial DNA
(b) They are usually symmetrical sequences of four to eight nucleotides
(c) They signal the attachment of RNA polymerase
(d) Each recognition sequence is cut by a specific restriction enzyme

33 The presence of more than one recognition site, for commonly used restriction enzymes, within the cloning vector will

(a) generate several fragments
(b) complicate the gene cloning
(c) Both (a) and (b)
(d) Not allow gene cloning

34 Which of the following statements incorrectly explains the part of the normal process during the cloning of recombinant DNA in bacteria?

(a) Restriction enzymes are used to cut DNA fragments from cellular and plasmid DNA
(b) A copy of the required gene is inserted into a bacterial plasmid by using DNA ligase
(c) The Southern blotting technique is used to separate the recombinant DNA plasmids
(d) The bacterium is transformed by the recombinant DNA plasmids

35 Match the following columns.

Column I	Column II
A. Bacterial enzymes used to cut DNA at defined sequences	1. Recognition sequences
B. Sequences cut by restriction enzymes	2. Plasmids
C. Ends left on DNA segments cut by DNA restriction enzymes	3. Sticky ends
D. Circular pieces of DNA found in bacteria	4. Restriction enzymes

Codes

	A	B	C	D
(a)	1	4	3	2
(b)	4	1	3	2
(c)	1	4	2	3
(d)	4	3	2	1

36 Consider the following statements.

I. Cosmid is fragment of DNA inserted in bacteria for forming copies.

II. These are unable to accept more than 40-50 kbp of DNA.

Choose the correct option.

(a) Statement I is true, but II is false
(b) Statement I is false, but II is true
(c) Both statements I and II are true
(d) Both statements I and II are false

37 The first restriction endonuclease, to be discovered was

(a) *Hind* III
(b) *Hae* II
(c) *Hind* II
(d) *Hae* III

38 In the year 1963, the two enzymes responsible for restricting the growth of bacteriophage in *E. coli* were isolated. They were ...*A*... and ...*B*... .

	A	*B*
(a)	ligase	restriction endonuclease
(b)	helicase	restriction endonuclease
(c)	methylase	restriction endonuclease
(d)	DNA polymerase	restriction endonuclease

39 YAC contains which of the following elements?

(a) Centromeres only
(b) Telomeres only
(c) Centromeres, telomeres and *ori*-site
(d) Telomeres and centromeres

40 For transformation with recombinant DNA, the bacterial cells must first made competent which means

(a) should increase their metabolic reactions
(b) should decreae their metabolic reactions
(c) increaese efficiency with which DNA enters the bacterium
(d) ability to divide fast

41 Which of the following are considered as useful selectable markers for *E. coli.*

I. Ampicillin resistane gene
II. Chloramphenicol resistance gene
III. Tetracycline resistance gene
IV. Kanamycin resistance gene

Codes

(a) Only I (b) I and II
(c) I, II and III (d) I, II, III and IV

42 Consider the following statements for selectable marker.

I. It helps to select the host cells which contain the vector and eliminate the non-transformants.
II. Genes encoding resistance to antibiotics like ampicillin, chloramphenicol, tetracycline or kanamycin are useful selectable markers for *E.coli.*

Which of the statements given above are correct?

(a) Only I (b) Only II
(c) I and II (d) None of these

Techniques Used in RDT

43 Consider the following statements.

I. Gel electrophoresis is used for construction of recombinant DNA by joining with cloning vectors.
II. During gel electrophoresis for separation of DNA fragment, smallest fragment will move to the farthest point towards anode.

Choose the correct option.

(a) Statement I is true, but II is false
(b) Statement I is false, but II is true
(c) Both statements I and II are true
(d) Both statements I and II are false

44 After electrophoresis, the separated DNA fragment can be visualised in ethidium bromide gel exposed to UV light. These DNA fragments appear as what coloured bands?

(a) Orange (b) Blue
(c) Silver (d) Green

45 Which of the given statements is correct in the context of observing DNA separated by agarose gel electrophoresis?

(a) DNA can be seen in visible light
(b) DNA can be seen without staining in visible light
(c) Ethidium bromide stained DNA can be seen orange in visible light
(d) Ethidium bromide stained DNA can be seen under exposure to UV light

46 Which of the following has popularised the PCR (Polymerase Chain Reaction)?

(a) Easy availability of DNA template
(b) Availability of synthetic primers
(c) Availability of cheap deoxyribonucleotides
(d) Availability of 'thermostable' DNA polymerase

47 The copies of a DNA molecule in a test tube are produced by

(a) Polymerase Chain Reaction (PCR)
(b) Molecular Chain Reaction (MCR)
(c) Ephemeral Chain Reaction (ECR)
(d) All of the above

48 Which of the following steps are catalysed by *Taq* polymerase in a PCR reaction?

(a) Denaturation of template DNA
(b) Annealing of primers to template DNA
(c) Extension of primer end on the template DNA
(d) All of the above

49 Select the correct statement(s).

(a) If any protein encoding gene is expressed in a homologous host, it is called a recombinant protein
(b) In PCR, the multiple copies of gene of interest is synthesised *in vitro* using one set of primers
(c) A thermostable enzyme (*Taq* polymerase) is obtained from cyanobacterium, *Thermus aquaticus*
(d) None of the above

50 In PCR, short primers are added to single-stranded DNA molecules in a test tube and the appropriate enzymes are included to make a copy of the DNA. Which of the following primers is needed for copying the single-stranded DNA sequence 5′ TACGGTAGGTC ?

(a) 5′ ATGCC
(b) 5′ GACCT
(c) 5′ TACGG
(d) 5′ GGCAT

51 Match the following columns.

Column I	Column II
A. PCR	1. Join or hybridise
B. Denaturation of DNA	2. Polymerisation
C. Annealing	3. *Thermus aquaticus*
D. Extension	4. Kary Mullis

Codes

	A	B	C	D
(a)	4	3	2	1
(b)	1	2	3	4
(c)	3	1	2	4
(d)	4	3	1	2

52 The procedure, in which DNA fragments are separated by gel electrophoresis and then transferred on to a filter for radioactive probing is known as

(a) gene mapping
(b) gene cloning
(c) polymerase chain reaction
(d) Southern blotting technique

53 Choose the incorrect match.

(a) Northern blotting - W Neal
(b) PCR - Kary Mullis
(c) Southern blotting - EM Southern
(d) Father of Genetic Engineering-Paul Berg

54 Choose the incorrect match.

(a) Western blotting — Protein
(b) Northern blotting — RNA
(c) Southern blotting — DNA
(d) DNA fingerprinting — Protein

55 Choose the incorrect statement.

(a) Transformation is a procedure through which a place of DNA is introduced in a host bacterium
(b) Normally the genes encoding resistance to antibotics like ampicillin, chloramphenicol, tetracycline, kanamycin, etc., are considered useful selectable markers for *E. coli*
(c) The normal *E. coli* cells carry genes resistant against ampicillin, chloramphenicol, tetracycline and kanamycin
(d) In order to link the alien DNA the vector needs to have very few, preferably single, recognition site for the commonly used restriction enzymes

56 Find out the incorrect statement.

(a) If any protein encoding gene is expressed in a heterologous host, is called a recombinant protein
(b) In PCR, primers with exposed 3′-OH group is used
(c) The natural habitat of *Thermus aquaticus* is the Hot Spring Ecosystem of Yellow Stone National Park
(d) Cells of continuous culture system are maintained in stationary phase

57 Significance of the 'heat shock' in bacterial transformation is to facilitate

(a) expression of the antibiotic resistance gene in the vector
(b) ligation of DNA to the cell membrane
(c) uptake the DNA to the cell membrane
(d) uptake of DNA through pores in the bacterial cell wall

58 Consider the following statements.

I. The almost pure DNA which gets precipitated by chilled ethanol is removed from solution by spooling.
II. During heat shock to the bacterium, the templates used for giving thermal shock is 42°C.

Choose the correct option.

(a) Statement I is true, but II is false
(b) Statement I is false, but II is true
(c) Both statements I and II are true
(d) Both statements I and II are false

59 Which of the following statements is/are correct about heat shock?

(a) Given at 42°C
(b) A step of the process that enables linking of alien DNA to the plasmid
(c) A step of the process that enables introduction of alien DNA into the host cells
(d) Both (a) and (c)

60 Match the following columns with respect to insertion of recombinant DNA into host cell.

Column I	Column II
A. Transformation	1. Animal cell
B. Biolistics/Gene gun	2. Plant cell
C. Microinjection	3. Bacterial cell

Codes

	A	B	C		A	B	C
(a)	1	2	3	(b)	3	2	1
(c)	3	1	2	(d)	2	1	3

61 Alternate selectable markers have ability to differentiate recombinants from non-recombinants due to the

(a) inactivation of the recombinants DNA
(b) inactivation of the enzyme β-galactosidase
(c) insertional inactivation
(d) Both (b) and (c)

62 Due to difficulty in inactivation of antibiotics, alternate selectable markers developed to differentiate recombinants from non-recombinants on the basis of ability to

(a) produce bright orange colour in the presence of a chromogenic substrate
(b) produce colour in the presence of a chromogenic substrate
(c) produce blue colour colonies due to insertional inactivation
(d) All are correct

63 Identify the correct match for the given apparatus.

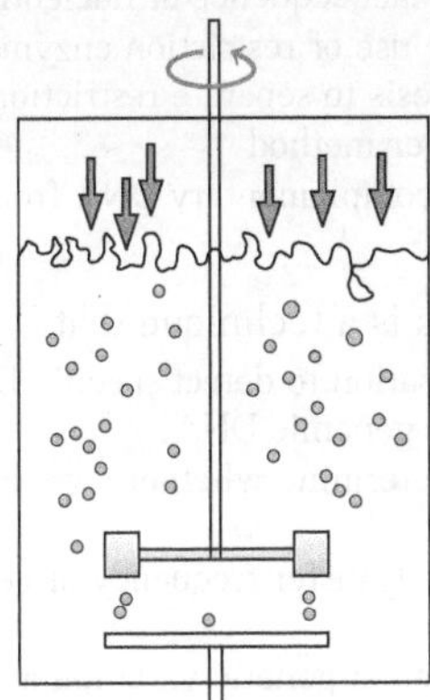

Apparatus	Functions
(a) Gene gun	Vectorless direct gene transfer
(b) Column chromatograph	Separation of chlorophyll pigments
(c) Sparged tank bioreactor	Carryout fermentation process
(d) Respirometer	Finding out rate of respiration

64 Which of the following is true for downstream processing?

(a) The product is formulated with suitable preservatives
(b) The formulations undergo clinical trial in case of drugs
(c) Strict quality control testing for each product is done
(d) All of the above

65 Which of the following should be chosen for best yield if one were to produce a recombinant protein in large amounts?

(a) Laboratory flask of largest capacity
(b) A stirred-tank bioreactor without inlets and outlets
(c) A continuous culture system
(d) Any of the above

66 Consider the following statements.

I. Bioreactor provides optimum temperature, pH, salt, vitamins and oxygen.
II. Sparged stirred tank bioreactor is a stirred type reactor in which air bubbled.

Choose the correct option.

(a) Statement I is true, but II is false
(b) Statement I is false, but II is true
(c) Both statements I and II are true
(d) Both statements I and II are false

67 Consider the following statements.

I. The downstream processing and quality control testing vary from product to product.
II. In bioreactors raw materials are biologically connected into specific products.

Choose the correct option.

(a) Statement I is true, but II is false
(b) Statement I is false, but II is true
(c) Both statements I and II are true
(d) Both statements I and II are false

68 The device in which substances are treated to stimulate biochemical transformation by living cells is

(a) PCR (b) electrophoresis device
(c) bioreactor (d) biochips

69 Recombinant DNA is forced to enter the host cells by incubating the cells with *r*DNA first

(a) on ice followed by heat shock and then again on ice
(b) at low temperature followed by heat ahock and then on ice
(c) in ethidium bromide followed by calcium salts
(d) into chilled ethanol followed by ice and then into CsCl

70 A bacterial cell was transformed with a recombinant DNA that was generated using a human gene. However, the transformed cells did not produce the desired protein. Reasons could be

(a) human gene may have intron which bacteria cannot process
(b) amino acid codons for humans and bacteria are different
(c) human protein is formed, but degraded by bacteria
(d) All of the above

71 Forensic scientists have to work often with extremely small samples of DNA obtained from the hair or other sources of suspected criminals. However, it is possible to produce DNA 'fingerprint' from these small samples by using

(a) gene gun
(b) gene cloning
(c) polymerase chain reaction
(d) genetically engineered microorganisms

72 What is genomic library?

(a) A collection of recombinant molecule with insects that contain all the genes of organism
(b) A collection of recombinant molecule that contains all of an organism genome
(c) A collection of recombinant molecule that expresses all of the genes of an organism
(d) A collection of recombinant molecule that have been sequenced

73 Complementary DNA does not create a complete gene library because

(a) it has eliminated introns from the genes
(b) cell produces *m*RNA for only small portion of its genes
(c) the shotgun approach produces more restriction fragments
(d) *c*DNA can easily integrated into plasmids or phage genomes

74 In order to express human gene in a bacterium, *c*DNA must be made because bacteria
(a) splice RNA
(b) destroy human DNA
(c) cannot remove introns
(d) have reverse transcriptase

75 Which of the following is not a difference between genomic library and *c*DNA library?
(a) The presence or absence of introns in cloned genes
(b) The presence or absence of promoless in cloned gene
(c) The presence or absence of a prokaryotic origin of replication on the vector
(d) The presence or absence of DNA from intergenic regions

76 Gene for cloning may be chemically synthesised
(a) when the exact sequence of nucleotides is known
(b) through the use of restriction enzymes and gel electrophoresis to separate restriction fragments
(c) by the Sanger method
(d) by making complementary DNA from genes without introns

77 RFLP analysis is a technique that
(a) use hybridisation to detect specific DNA restriction fragment in genomic DNA
(b) is used to determine whether a gene is transcribed in specific cell
(c) measure the transfer frequency of gene during conjugation
(d) is used to detect genetic variation at the protein

(B) Cumulative Exercise

(Assorted Questions of the Chapter for Advanced Level Practice)

1 Among the following, select the tools of recombinant DNA technology.
I. Restriction enzymes
II. Polymerase enzymes
III. Ligases
IV. Vectors
V. Host organisms

Codes
(a) I, II III, IV and V
(b) I, III, IVand V
(c) I, II, III and IV
(d) I, II, III and V

2 Which of the following steps are involved in recombinant DNA technology?
I. The cells having desired DNA molecule are separated and cultured to increase their number.
II. A suitable vector and donor DNA both are treated with similar restriction endonucleases.
III. Self ligation is increased with alkaline phosphatase.
IV. The host cell cannot be a bacterium.

Codes
(a) I and IV (b) I and II
(c) II and III (d) None of these

3 Read the following statements.
I. Primers used in PCR are small chemically synthesised oligosaccharides.
II. *E. coli* is closely related to *Salmonella.*
III. There are 3 basic steps in genetically modifying an organism.
IV. The techniques of the genetic engineering over come the limitation of traditional hybridisation procedures.

In these statements, how many are correct?
(a) 4 (b) 3 (c) 1 (d) 2

4 A plasmid has two antibiotic-resistance genes, one for ampicillin and one for tetracycline. It is treated with a restriction enzyme that cuts in the middle of the ampicillin gene. DNA fragments containing a haemoglobin gene were cut with the same enzyme. The plasmids and fragments are mixed, treated with ligase and used to transform bacterial cells. Clones that have taken up the recombinant DNA are the ones that
(a) are blue and can grow on plates with both antibiotics
(b) can grow on plates with ampicillin, but not with tetracycline
(c) can grow on plates with tetracycline, but not with ampicillin
(d) cannot grow with any antibiotics

5 Palaeonotologists unearthed a human skull during excavation. A small fragment of the scalp tissue was still attached to it. Only little DNA could be extracted from it. If the genes of the ancient man need to be analysed, the best way of getting sufficient amount of DNA from this extract is
(a) hybridising the DNA with a DNA probe
(b) subjecting the DNA to polymerase chain reaction
(c) subjection the DNA to gel electrophoresis
(d) treating the DNA with restriction endonucleases

6 Following enzymes/techniques are used in the process of recombinant DNA technology .

I. *Eco* RI to cut the isolated genome.
II. DNA ligase.
III. Protease and ribonuclease for removal of proteins and RNA from DNA.
IV. Production of recombinant hosts.
V. Lysozyme for isolation of the genetic material (DNA).
VI. Gel electrophoresis for separation and isolation of DNA fragments.

Mark the correct sequence of their use.

(a) III, V, II, VI, I, IV (b) V, III, I, II, VI, IV
(c) V, III, I, VI, II, IV (d) I,V, III, II, IV, VI

7 Match the following columns.

Column I	Column II
A. A molecule used to carry foreign genes into bacteria	1. Restriction enzymes
B. A rapid way to amplify DNA in the laboratory	2. Recombinant DNA
C. A way to separate DNA fragments based on their size	3. PCR
D. Molecular scissors	4. Vector
E. A gene sequence from more than one origin	5. Gel electrophoresis

Codes

	A	B	C	D	E
(a)	4	3	5	1	2
(b)	2	4	3	1	5
(c)	5	4	3	2	1
(d)	1	5	4	2	3

8 There are three basic steps in genetically modifying an organism. Arrange these steps in correct sequence.

I. Introduction of the identified DNA into the host.
II. Maintenance of introduced DNA in the host and transfer of the DNA to its progeny.
III. Identification of DNA with desirable genes.

Codes

(a) I $\rightarrow$ II $\rightarrow$ III (b) II $\rightarrow$ III $\rightarrow$ I
(c) III $\rightarrow$ II $\rightarrow$ I (d) III $\rightarrow$ I $\rightarrow$ II

9 Read the following statements and find out the incorrect statements with reference to agarose gel electrophoresis.

I. Now-a-days the most commonly use matrix is agarose which is a synthetic polymer extracted from seaweeds.
II. Larger the fragment size, the farther it moves.
III. We cannot see prue DNA in UV light without staining .
IV. DNA fragments separate (resolve) according to their size through sieving effect provided by the agarose gel.

Codes

(a) I, II and III (b) II, III and IV
(c) III and IV (d) I and II

10 This segment of DNA has restriction site-I and II, which create restriction fragments a, b and c. Which of the following gel(s) produced by electrophoresis would represent the separation and identification of these fragments?

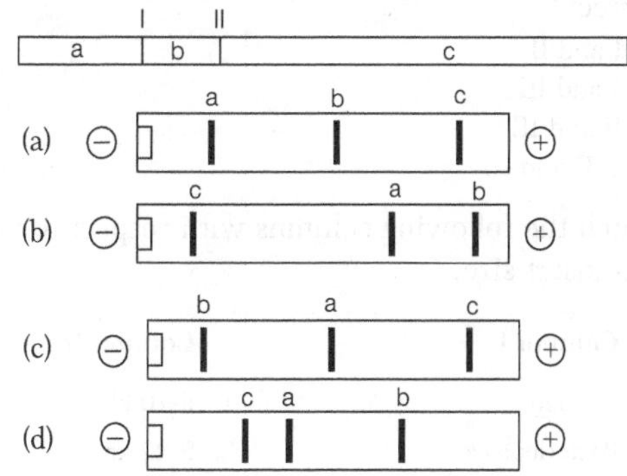

11 Identify the correct statements.

I. The first recombinant DNA was constructed by using a piece of DNA from plasmid carrying antibiotic- resistance gene in the bacterium *Salmonella typhimurium* and linked it to the plasmid of *E. coli*.
II. When cut by the same restriction enzyme, the resultant DNA fragments have the same kind of sticky ends and these can be joined together using DNA ligases.
III. The presence of more than one recognition site within the vector will generate several fragments, which will complicate the gene cloning.

Codes

(a) I, II and III (b) I and II (c) Only I (d) II and III

12 This figure shows the restriction site of *Eco* RI.

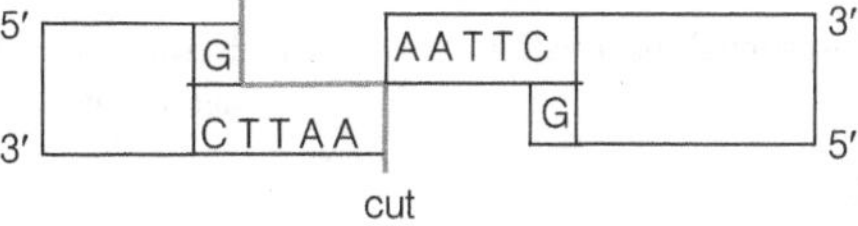

This restriction enzyme recognition site is palindromic and has specified base pairs. This means that the recognition site has

(a) base sequences identical to one another
(b) base sequences that consist of only four bases
(c) the base sequence in one DNA strand reading from one end the same as the sequence in the complementary strand reading from the opposite end
(d) base sequences with attached probe

13 Consider the following statements.

I. Recombinant DNA technology popularly known as genetic engineering is a stream of biotechnology which deals with the manipulation of genetic material by man *in vitro*.

II. pBR322 is the first artificial cloning vector developed in 1977 by Boliver and Rodriguez from *E. coli* plasmid.

III. Restriction enzymes belong to a class of enzymes called nucleases.

Which of the following statements given above are correct?

(a) I and II
(b) I and III
(c) II and III
(d) I, II and III

14 Match the following columns with respect to vectors and insert size.

Column I	Column II
A. Plasmid	1. 6-10 kb
B. Bacteriophage	2. 9-22 kb
C. Cosmid	3. 33-47 kb
D. BAC	4. 75-350 kb
E. YAC	5. 100-1000 kb

Codes

	A	B	C	D	E
(a)	2	4	5	1	3
(b)	1	5	2	4	3
(c)	5	4	3	2	1
(d)	1	2	3	4	5

15 Match the following columns.

Column I	Column II
A. Elution	1. Gene gun
B. Competence	2. Ca^{2+}
C. Biolistics	3. β-galactosidase gene
D. Insertional inactivation	4. Extraction of DNA from agarose gel

Codes

	A	B	C	D
(a)	1	2	4	3
(b)	3	4	1	2
(c)	1	2	3	4
(d)	4	2	1	3

16 In the year ...*A*.., the two enzymes responsible for ...*B*... the growth of bacteriophage in *E. coli* were isolated. One of these added ...*C*... group to DNA , while other ...*D*... DNA. The later was called ...*E*... .

	A	*B*	*C*	*D*	*E*
(a)	1967	promoting	ethyl	join	DNA ligase
(b)	1963	restricting	methyl	join	DNA ligase
(c)	1972	restricting	methyl	act	restriction endonuclease
(d)	1963	restricting	methyl	cut	restriction endonuclease

17 Which of the following creates problem getting prokaryotic cells to express eukaryotic genes?

(a) The signals that control gene expression are different and prokaryotic promoter regions must be added to the vector
(b) The genetic code differs between the two because prokaryotes substitute the base uracil for thymine
(c) Prokaryotic cells cannot transcribe exons because their genes do not have them
(d) The ribosomes of prokaryotes are not large enough to handle long eukaryotic genes

18 Recognise the figure and find out the correct matching.

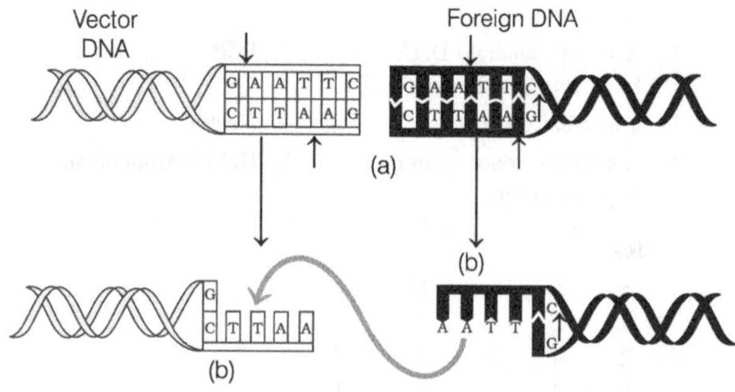

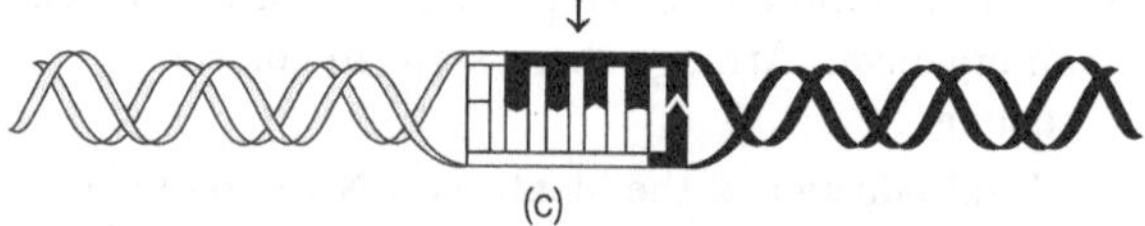

(a) *A-Hind* II, *B*-Blunt end, *C*-Non-recombinant DNA
(b) *A-Bam* HI, *B*-Sticky end, *C*-Recombinant DNA
(c) *A-Eco* RI, *B*-Sticky end, *C*-Non-recombinant DNA
(d) *A-Eco* RI, *B*-Sticky end, *C*-Recombinant DNA

19 Which of the following statements are incorrect?

I. Term PCR is used for organisms, which carry foreign genes.

II. SCID includes genetic disorders only.

III. Cloning is the production of GMOs, e.g. *Flavr Savr* tomato.

IV. The bacteria use restriction endonucleases to destroy the DNA of invading foreign viruses.

Codes

(a) Only I
(b) Only II
(c) II and IV
(d) I, II and III

20 Simplified steps of recombinant DNA preparation is shown below. Identify I, II, III and IV.

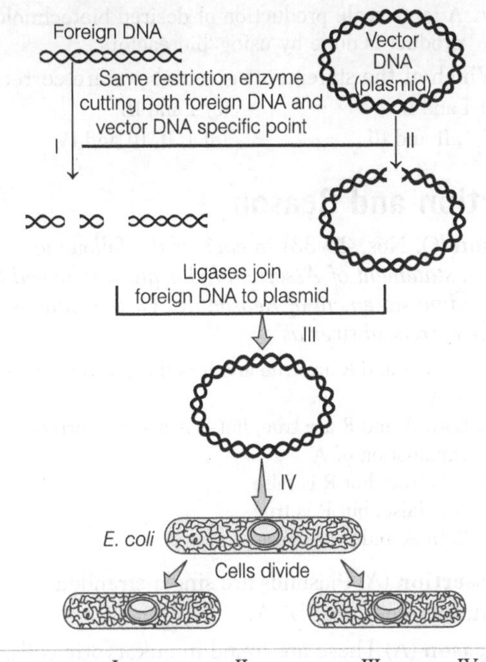

	I	II	III	IV
(a)	Exonuclease	Endonuclease	Ligase	Competence
(b)	Restriction endonuclease	Restriction endonuclease same as I	Ligase	Transformation
(c)	Restriction endonuclease	Exonuclease	Ligase	Competence
(d)	Exonuclease	Restriction endonuclease	Ligase	Transformation

21 Consider the following statements.

I. Ability to replicate autonomously.
II. Single sites for a large number of restriction enzymes.
III. Easy transformation to the host cells.
IV. High molecular weight for enhanced stability.

Choose the statements that are requirements of a vector.

(a) I and II
(b) II and IV
(c) I, II and III
(d) I, II, III and IV

22 The EFB has given a definition of biotechnology that encompasses both traditional view and modern molecular biotechnology. The definition given by EFB is as follows.

(a) The use of bioresources by multinational companies and other organisation without proper authorisation from the countries and people concerned without compensatory payment
(b) The integration of natural sciene and organisms, cells, parts thereof and molecular analogues for products and services
(c) Industrial scale production of biopharmaceuticals and biologicals using genetically modified microbes, fungi, plants and animals
(d) Techniques to alter the chemistry of genetic material (DNA and RNA) to introduce these into host organisms and thus change the phenotype of the host organism

23 Which of the following is correct for DNA fingerprinting?

I. It is used to identify a person on the basis of person DNA specificity.
II. It is based upon the fact that DNA constitution of an individual carries some specific sequences of nucleotides.
III. It is used to produce transgenic organisms.
IV. It starts with one gene sized piece of RNA.

Codes

(a) Only I
(b) Only II
(c) I and II
(d) I, II and III

24 Match the following columns.

Column I	Column II
A. Stanley Cohen and Herbert Boyer	1. Father of Genetic Engineering
B. Arber, Smith and Nathan	2. Isolated the antibiotic resistant genes from a plasmid
C. Paul Berg	3. Developed PCR
D. Kary Mullis	4. Nobel Prize winner for the discovery of restriction endonucleases

Codes

	A	B	C	D		A	B	C	D
(a)	1	2	4	3	(b)	2	4	3	1
(c)	2	4	1	3	(d)	3	2	1	4

25 Consider the following statements.

I. Recombinant DNA technology is used to improve crop plants by increasing their productivity by making them more nutritious and by developing disease resistance.
II. *Bt* cotton is resistant to bollworm infestation.
III. *Bacillus thuringiensis* forms Cry protein during any phase of their growth.
IV. *Bacillus thuringiensis* is not harmed by self Cry protein because of its occurrence as protoxin (inactive).
V. Protoxin Cry protein is changed into active Cry protein in the stomach of insects due to alkaline pH in stomach.

(a) All statements are correct
(b) Statements I and IV are correct
(c) Only statement III is incorrect
(d) All statements are inocrrect

26 Match the following columns.

Column I	Column II
A. Bacterial viruses	1. Transformation
B. Process by which bacteria take up pieces of DNA from the environment	2. Cloning vector
C. *Hind* II	3. *Haemophilus influenzae*
D. Vehicle that moves DNA from one organism to another	4. Bacteriophages

Codes

	A	B	C	D
(a)	2	3	4	1
(b)	1	3	4	2
(c)	4	1	3	2
(d)	1	4	3	2

27 Simple stirred-tank bioreactor is given below. Identify the parts labelled as *A*, *B*, *C*, *D* and *E*.

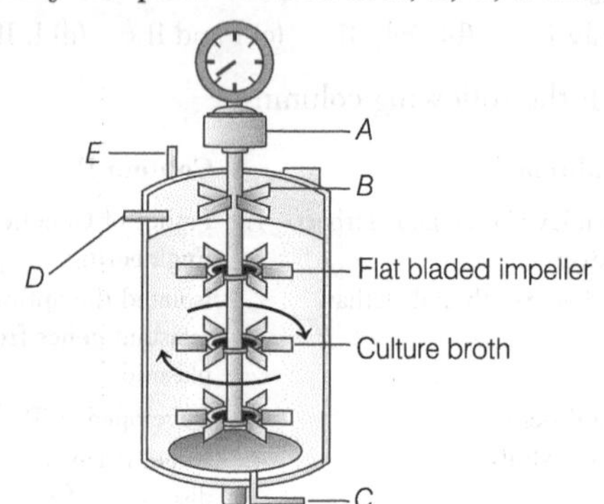

	A	B	C	D	E
(a)	Motor	Foam breaker	Sterile air	Steam for sterilisation	Acid/Base for pH control
(b)	Foam breaker	Sterile air	Steam for sterilisation	Acid/Base for pH control	Motor
(c)	Acid/Base for pH control	Motor	Foam breaker	Sterile air	Steam for sterilisation
(d)	Sterile air	Steam for sterilisation	Foam breaker	Motor	Acid/Base for pH control

28 Consider the following statements.

I. Bioreactors are vessels of large volumes in which raw materials are biologically converted into specific products.

II. One of the most commonly used bioreactor is of stirring type.

III. Shake flasks are used for growing and mixing the desired materials on a small scale in the laboratory.

IV. A large scale production of desired biotechnological product is done by using 'bioreactors'.

Which of the statements given above are correct?

(a) I and II (b) I and III
(c) I, II and III (d) I, II, III and IV

Assertion and Reason

Direction (Q. Nos. 29-33) *In each of the following questions, statement of Assertion (A) is given followed by corresponding statement of Reason (R). Of the statements, mark the correct answer as*

(a) Both A and R are true and R is the correct explanation of A
(b) Both A and R are true, but R is not the correct explanation of A
(c) A is true, but R is false
(d) A is false, but R is true
(e) Both A and R are false

29 **Assertion** (A) Plasmids are single-stranded extrachromosomal DNA.

Reason (A) These are found in eukaryotic cells.

30 **Assertion** (A) Recombinant DNA can be chimeric DNA.

Reason (R) The chimeric DNA is the recombinant DNA, which is formed of two or more sources.

31 **Assertion** (A) DNA fingerprinting is very useful in forensic science.

Reason (R) It is the method, in which individual pattern of DNA fragments is determined through the number and position of specific repeated sequences.

32 **Assertion** (A) Vector is very useful in recombinant DNA technology.

Reason (R) It is a tool that carries a foreign DNA molecule to the living cell.

33 **Assertion** (A) A genetic probe is helpful in the detection of specific DNA sequence.

Reason (R) Genetic probe is a radiolabelled *c*DNA, which has complementary base sequence, to DNA fragment which is to be detected.

(C) Medical Entrances' Gallery

(Collection of Questions Asked in NEET & Various Medical Entrance Exams)

1 In gel electrophoresis, separated DNA fragments can be visualised with the help of [NEET 2020]

(a) ethidium bromide in UV radiation
(b) acetocarmine in UV radiation
(c) ethidium bromide in infrared radiation
(d) acetocarmine in bright blue light

2 The sequence that controls the copy number of the linked DNA in the vector is termed [NEET 2020]

(a) *ori* site (b) palindromic sequence
(c) recognition site (d) selectable marker

3 The specific palindromic sequence which is recognised by *Eco* RI is [NEET 2020]

(a) 5′ - G G A A C C - 3′
3′ - C C T T G G - 5′
(b) 5′ - C T T A A G - 3′
3′ -G A A T T C - 5′
(c) 5′ - G G A T C C - 3′
3′ - C C T A G G - 5′
(d) 5′ - G A A T T C - 3′
3′ - C T T A A G - 5′

4 Identify the wrong statement with regard to restriction enzymes. [NEET 2020]

(a) They cut the strand of DNA at palindromic site
(b) They are useful in genetic engineering
(c) Sticky ends can be joined by using DNA ligases
(d) Each restriction enzyme functions by inspecting the length of a DNA sequence

5 Match the following columns of organisms with their uses in biotechnology.

Column I	Column II
A. *Bacillus thuringiensis*	1. Cloning vector
B. *Thermus aquaticus*	2. Construction of first *r*DNA molecule
C. *Agrobacterium tumefaciens*	3. DNA polymerase
D. *Salmonella typhimurium*	4. Cry protiens

Codes [NEET 2020]

	A	B	C	D		A	B	C	D
(a)	4	3	1	2	(b)	3	2	4	1
(c)	3	4	1	2	(d)	2	4	3	1

6 Choose the correct pair from the following.

(a) Polymerases — Break the DNA into fragments
(b) Nucleases — Separate the two strands of DNA
(c) Exonucleases — Make cuts at specific positions within DNA
(d) Ligases — Join the two DNA molecules

7 First discovered restriction endonuclease that always cuts DNA molecule at a particular point by recognising a specific sequence of six base pairs is [NEET 2020]

(a) *Eco* RI
(b) Adenosine deaminase
(c) Thermostable DNA polymerase
(d) *Hind* II

8 In recombinant DNA technology, antibiotics are used [NEET 2020]

(a) to keep medium bacteria-free
(b) to detect alien DNA
(c) to impart disease-resistance to the host plant
(d) as selectable marker

9 In a mixture, DNA fragments are separated by [NEET 2020]

(a) bioprocess engineering
(b) restriction digestion
(c) electrophoresis
(d) polymerase chain reaction

10 Select the correct statement from the following. [NEET 2020]

(a) Gel electrophoresis is used for amplification of DNA segment
(b) The polymerase enzyme joins the gene of interest and the vector DNA
(c) Restriction enzyme digestions are performed by incubating purified DNA molecules with the restriction enzymes of optimum conditions
(d) PCR is used for isolation and separation of gene of interest

11 Match the following columns in techniques or instruments with their uses.

Column I	Column II
A. Bioreactor	1. Separation of DNA fragments
B. Electrophoresis	2. Production of large quantities of products
C. PCR	3. Detection of pathogen, based on antigen-antibody reaction
D. ELISA	4. Amplification of nucleic acids

Codes [NEET 2020]

	A	B	C	D		A	B	C	D
(a)	3	2	4	1	(b)	2	1	4	3
(c)	4	3	2	1	(d)	2	1	3	4

12 Spooling is [NEET 2020]

(a) amplification of DNA
(b) cutting of separated DNA band from the agarose gel
(c) transfer of separated DNA fragments to synthetic membranes
(d) collection of isolated DNA

13 Following statements describe the characteristics of the enzyme restriction endonuclease. Identify the incorrect statement. [NEET 2019]

(a) The enzyme binds DNA at specific sites and cuts only one of the two strands
(b) The enzyme cuts the sugar-phosphate backbone at specific sites on each strand
(c) The enzyme recognises a specific palindromic nucleotide sequence in the DNA
(d) The enzyme cuts DNA molecule at identified position within the DNA

14 Match the following columns in enzymes with their functions.

	Column I	Column II
A.	Restriction endonuclease	1. Joins the DNA fragments
B.	Restriction exonuclease	2. Extends primers on genomic DNA template
C.	DNA ligase	3. Cuts DNA at specific position
D.	*Taq* polymerase	4. Removes nucleotides from the ends of DNA

Codes [NEET 2019]

	A	B	C	D		A	B	C	D
(a)	3	1	4	2	(b)	3	4	1	2
(c)	4	3	1	2	(d)	2	4	1	3

15 The two antibiotic resistance genes on vector pBR322 are for [NEET 2019]

(a) ampicillin and tetracycline
(b) ampicillin and chloramphenicol
(c) chloramphenicol and tetracycline
(d) tetracycline and kanamycin

16 A selectable marker is used to [NEET 2019, Karnataka CET 2015]

(a) help in eliminating the non-transformants, so that the transformants can be regenerated
(b) identify the gene for a desired trait in an alien organism
(c) select a suitable vector for transformation in a specific crop
(d) mark a gene on a chromosome for isolation using restriction enzyme

17 An enzyme catalysing the removal of nucleotides from ends of DNA is [NEET 2019]

(a) DNA ligase (b) endonuclease
(c) exonuclease (d) protease

18 Chimeric DNA is [AIIMS 2019]

(a) gene clone (b) recombinant DNA
(c) transposon (d) vector shuttle

19 In Ti plasmid, which of the following is removed? [AIIMS 2019]

(a) Auxin gene (b) Virulent gene
(c) Cytokinin gene (d) Auxin and cytokinin gene

20 Gene library or DNA library has collection of [AIIMS 2019]

(a) DNA and RNA
(b) Any one type of gene of organism
(c) cDNA only
(d) All possible genes of all organisms

21 Match the following columns in enzymes with their functions.

Column I	Column II
A. KC Mehta	1. Fluid mosaic model
B. P Maheshwari	2. First recombinant plasmid
C. Cohen and Boyer	3. Haploid culture
D. Singer and Nicolson	4. Rust disease

Codes [AIIMS 2019]

	A	B	C	D		A	B	C	D
(a)	1	3	2	4	(b)	4	3	2	1
(c)	1	2	3	4	(d)	2	3	4	1

22 Which is also called molecular glue? [JIPMER 2019]

(a) DNA gyrase (b) DNA helicase
(c) DNA ligase (d) DNA polymerase

23 DNA precipitation out of a mixture of biomolecules can be achieved by treatment with [NEET 2019]

(a) chilled ethanol (b) methanol at room temperature
(c) chilled chloroform (d) isopropanol

24 Given below are four statements pertaining to separation of DNA fragments using gel electrophoresis. Identify the incorrect statements.

I. DNA is negatively charged molecule and so it is loaded on gel towards the anode terminal.
II. DNA fragments travel along the surface of the gel whose concentration does not affect movement of DNA.
III. Smaller the size of DNA fragment larger is the distance it travels through it.
IV. Pure DNA can be visualised directly by exposing UV-radiation.

Select the correct option from the following. [NEET 2019, 17]

(a) I, III and IV (b) I, II and III
(c) II, III and IV (d) I, II and IV

25 Match the following columns.

Column I (Substrates)	Column II (Enzymes)
A. Ribonucleotide	1. Chitinase
B. Chitin	2. Cellulase
C. Cellulose	3. Ribonuclease

Codes [AIIMS 2019]

	A	B	C		A	B	C
(a)	1	2	3	(b)	3	1	2
(c)	3	2	1	(d)	2	1	3

26 In annealing, [JIPMER 2019]
(a) primers anneal to the DNA template
(b) *Taq* polymerase adds nucleotides to the annealed primer
(c) two strands of the DNA separate
(d) temperature is 92°C

27 Which of the following is commonly used as a vector for introducing a DNA fragment in human lymphocytes? [NEET 2018]
(a) λ-phage (b) Ti plasmid
(c) Retrovirus (d) pBR322

28 If a recombinant DNA bearing gene for ampicillin resistance is transferred into *E. coli* cells and the host cells are spread on agar plates containing ampicillin, then [AIIMS 2018]
(a) both transformed and untransformed recipient cells will die
(b) both transformed and untransformed recipient cells will grow
(c) transformed recipient cells will grow and untransformed recipient cells will die
(d) transformed recipient cells will die and untransformed recipient cells will grow

29 Gene transfer is present in [JIPMER 2018]
(a) biolistics (b) hybridisation
(c) tissue culture (d) vegetative propagation

30 The correct order of steps in Polymerase Chain Reaction (PCR) is [NEET 2018, EAMCET 2015]
(a) denaturation, extension, annealing
(b) annealing, extension, denaturation
(c) extension, denaturation, annealing
(d) denaturation, annealing, extension

31 **Assertion** (A) *Agrobacterium tumefaciens* is a popular genetic engineer because this bacterium is associated with the roots of all cereal and pulse crops.

Reason (R) A gene incorporated in the bacterial chromosomal genome gets automatically suppressed into the crop with which the bacteria is associated. [CBSE AIPMT 2015, AIIMS 2017]
(a) Both A and R are true and R is the correct explanation of A
(b) Both A and R are true, but R is not the correct explanation of A
(c) A is true, but R is false
(d) Both A and R are false

32 Stirred-tank bioreactors have been designed for [NEET-II 2016]
(a) purification of product
(b) addition of preservatives to the product
(c) availability of oxygen throughout the process
(d) ensuring anaerobic conditions in the culture vessel

33 A foreign DNA and plasmid cut by the same restriction endonuclease can be joined to form a recombinant plasmid using [NEET-II 2016]
(a) *Eco* RI (b) *Taq* polymerase
(c) polymerase III (d) ligase

34 Which of the following is not a component of downstream processing? [NEET-II 2016]
(a) Separation (b) Purification
(c) Preservation (d) Expression

35 Which of the following restriction enzymes produces blunt ends? [NEET-II 2016]
(a) *Sal* I (b) *Eco* RV
(c) *Xho* (d) *Hind* III

36 **Assertion** (A) Restriction endonucleases recognise short palindromic sequence and cut at specific sites.

Reason (R) When a restriction endonuclease acts on palindrome, it cleaves both the strand of DNA molecule. [Gujarat CET 2015]
(a) Both A and R are true and R is the correct explanation of A
(b) Both A and R are true, but R is not the correct explanation of A
(c) A is true, but R is false
(d) Both A and R are false

37 DNA polymerase is isolated from bacteria [Gujarat CET 2015]
(a) *E. coli*
(b) *B. thuringiensis*
(c) *Thermus aquaticus*
(d) *Agrobacterium*

38 Restriction endonucleases are [AMU 2015, J&K CET 2015]
(a) used for *in vitro* DNA synthesis
(b) synthesised by bacteria as part of their defence mechanism
(c) present in mammalian cells for degradation of DNA when the cells dies
(d) used in genetic engineering for ligating two DNA molecules

39 Consider the following statements with respect to DNA fragmentation.

Statement (A) Gel electrophoresis and elution are two important processes.

Statement (B) After staining with ethidium bromide, it has to be exposed to UV light. [Karnataka CET 2015]
(a) Only A is correct
(b) Both A and B are correct
(c) Only B is correct
(d) A is correct but B is incorrect

40 Which vector can clone a small fragment of DNA? **[Karnataka CET 2015, CBSE AIPMT 2014]**
(a) Plasmid
(b) Bacterial artificial chromosome
(c) Cosmid
(d) Yeast artificial chromosome

41 In insertional inactivation of β-galactosidase gene, the bacteria in white colonies have **[EAMCET 2015]**
(a) non-recombinant plasmid (b) recombinant plasmid
(c) no plasmid (d) linear foreign DNA

42 The recognition sequence of restriction enzyme 'A' is GGCC and that of 'B' is GAATTC. Which statement among the following is true regarding the probable frequency of cutting sides in a genome. **[EAMCET 2015]**
(a) Both 'A' and 'B' cut equally frequently
(b) 'A' cuts once every 676 nucleotides and 'B' 1024 nucleotides
(c) 'A' cuts once every 256 nucleotides and 'B' 4096 nucleotides
(d) 'A' cuts once every 256 nucleotides and 'B' 1024 nucleotides

43 The cloning vector M13 has genetic material **[MHT CET 2015]**
(a) *ss*RNA (b) *ds*RNA (c) *ss*DNA (d) *ds*DNA

44 Restriction endonucleases are the enzymes that **[Chhattisgarh PMT 2015]**
(a) restrict the action of other enzymes
(b) break phosphodiester bond between specific nucleotides of DNA
(c) break nucleus into pieces
(d) break H-bond between two strands of DNA

45 The DNA molecule to which the gene of interest is integrated for cloning is called **[CBSE AIPMT 2015]**
(a) transformer (b) vector (c) template (d) carrier

46 An analysis of chromosomal DNA using the Southern hybridisation technique does not use **[CBSE AIPMT 2014]**
(a) electrophoresis (b) blotting
(c) autoradiography (d) PCR

47 Commonly used vectors for human genome sequencing are **[CBSE AIPMT 2014]**
(a) T-DNA (b) BAC and YAC
(c) Expression vectors (d) T/A cloning vectors

48 The first recombinant DNA was constructed by linking an antibiotic resistant gene with the native plasmid of **[Kerala CEE 2014]**
(a) *Escherichia coli* (b) *Salmonella typhimurium*
(c) *Clostridium butylicum* (d) *Acetobacter aceti*
(e) *Bacillus thuringiensis*

49 The Polymerase Chain Reaction (PCR) is technique that is used for **[Kerala CEE 2014]**
(a) *in vivo* replication of specific DNA sequence using thermostable DNA polymerase
(b) *in vitro* synthesis of *m*RNA
(c) *in vitro* replication of specific DNA sequence using thermostable DNA polymerase
(d) *in vivo* synthesis of *m*RNA
(e) separation of DNA fragments according to their size

50 Bioreactors are useful in **[Kerala CEE 2014]**
(a) separation and purification of a product
(b) processing of large volumes of culture
(c) microinjection
(d) isolation of genetic material
(e) amplification of genes

51 During gene cloning, the enzyme used to join the insert DNA with the plasmid vector is **[WB JEE 2014]**
(a) DNA ligase
(b) restriction endonuclease
(c) alkaline phosphatase
(d) exonuclease

52 During gene cloning, which is called as 'gene taxi'? **[UK PMT 2014]**
(a) Vaccine
(b) Plasmid
(c) Bacterium
(d) Protozoa

53 Some foreign DNA fragments are attached to *Cla* I site of pBR322. This recombinant vector is used to transit *Escherichia coli* host cells. The cells subjected to transformation are plated on two different media, one containing ampicillin and the other containing tetracycline. The transformed cells containing the recombinant vector **[EAMCET 2014]**
(a) will grow on both tetracycline containing and ampicillin containing media
(b) will not grow on either tetracycline containing or ampicillin containing media
(c) will grow on tetracycline, but not on ampicillin containing medium
(d) will grow on ampicillin, but not on tetracycline containing medium

54 Minisatellites or VNTRs are used in **[EAMCET 2014]**
(a) DNA fingerprinting
(b) Polymerase Chain Reaction (PCR)
(c) gene therapy
(d) gene mapping

55 *Eco* RI is **[KCET 2014]**
(a) a restriction enzyme
(b) a plasmid
(c) used to join two DNA fragments
(d) the abbreviation for bacterium, *Escherichia coli*

56 Which of the following option is correct for recombinant DNA technology? **[Gujarat CET 2014]**

(a) Endonuclease enzyme removes nucleotides from the ends of DNA
(b) Exonuclease enzyme removes nucleotides from site within DNA
(c) Endonuclease enzyme cuts long polandric DNA strand
(d) Exonuclease enzyme removes nucleotides from ends of DNA

57 The colonies of recombinant bacteria appear white in contrast to blue colonies of non-recombinant bacteria because of **[NEET 2013]**

(a) insertional inactivation of α-galactosidase in non-recombinant bacteria
(b) insertional inactivation of β-galactosidase in recombinant bacteria
(c) inactivation of glycosidase enzyme in bacteria
(d) non-recombinant bacteria containing β-galactosidase

58 DNA fragments generated by the restriction endonucleases in a chemical reaction can be separated by **[NEET 2013]**

(a) polymerase chain reaction
(b) electrophoresis
(c) restriction mapping
(d) centrifugation

59 The figure below is the diagrammatic representation of the *E. coli* vector pBR322. Which one of the given options correctly identifies its certain components ?

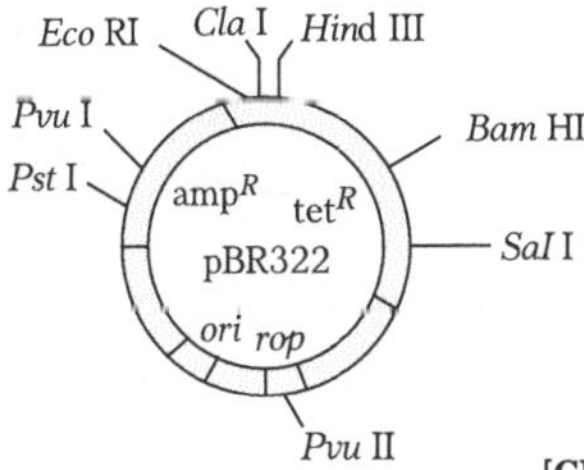

[CBSE AIPMT 2012]

(a) *ori* — original restriction enzyme
(b) *rop* — reduced osmotic pressure
(c) *Hind* III, *Eco* RI — selectable markers
(d) amp^R, tet^R — antibiotic resistance genes

60 For transformation, microparticles coated with DNA to be bombarded with gene gun are made up of **[CBSE AIPMT 2012]**

(a) silver or platinum
(b) platinum or zinc
(c) silicon or platinum
(d) gold or tungsten

61 PCR and Restriction Fragment Length Polymorphism are the methods for **[CBSE AIPMT 2012]**

(a) study of enzymes (b) genetic transformation
(c) DNA sequencing (d) genetic fingerprinting

62 A single-strand of nucleic acid tagged with a radioactive molecule is called **[CBSE AIPMT 2012, Rajasthan PMT 2011]**

(a) vector (b) selectable marker
(c) plasmid (d) probe

63 Which one is a true statement regrading DNA polymerase used in PCR? **[CBSE AIPMT 2012]**

(a) It is used to ligate introduction DNA in recipient cells
(b) It serves as a selectable marker
(c) It is isolated from a virus
(d) It remains active at high temperature

64 When bacterial chromosome is attached to plasmid, this is called **[BHU 2012]**

(a) episome (b) chromosome
(c) genome (d) None of these

65 Cohen and Boyer isolated an antibiotic resistance gene, by cutting out a piece of DNA from a plasmid which was responsible for conferring antibiotic resistance, in the year **[AMU 2012]**

(a) 1962 (b) 1965
(c) 1972 (d) 1982

66 Restriction enzyme *Eco* RI cuts the DNA between bases G and A only when the sequence in DNA is **[AMU 2012]**

(a) GATATC (b) GAATTC
(c) GATTCC (d) GAACTT

67 A mixture containing DNA fragments a, b, c and d, with molecular weights of a + b = c, a > b and d > c, was subject to agarose gel electrophoresis. The positions of these fragments from cathode to anode sides of the gel would be **[AIIMS 2012]**

(a) b, a, c, d (b) a, b, c, d
(c) c, b, a, d (d) b, a, d, c

68 Cloning is a process where **[AFMC 2012]**

(a) gene is cloned in an animal
(b) fragments of DNA are transferred from one organism to another, usually carried on a DNA vector
(c) fragments of DNA cloned in the same organism using carrier
(d) DNA is cloned in plants

69 Enzyme that cleaves nucleic acids within the polynucleotide chain is known as **[AFMC 2012]**

(a) endonuclease (b) exonuclease
(c) arylsulfatase (d) phosphotriesterase

70 The restriction enzyme(s) used in recombinant DNA technology making staggered cuts in DNA leaving sticky ends is/are **[AMU 2012]**

(a) *Eco* RI (b) *Hind* III
(c) *Bam* HI (d) All of these

71 A clone is a [BCECE 2012]
(a) heterozygote obtained asexually
(b) homozygote obtained asexually
(c) heterozygote produced by sexual methods
(d) homozygote produced by sexual reproduction

72 There is a restriction endonuclease called *Eco* RI. What does '*co*' part in it stand for? [CBSE AIPMT 2011]
(a) Coelom (b) Coenzyme (c) *coli* (d) Colon

73 Alec Jeffreys developed the DNA fingerprinting technique. The probe he used was [Kerala CEE 2011, RPMT 2011]
(a) ribozyme (b) sex chromosomes
(c) SNP (d) VNTR
(e) *r*DNA

74 Which of the following statements is not true for a clone? [UP CPMT 2011]
(a) Clones are descended from a single parent
(b) Identical twins are not clones
(c) Clone is a result of sexual reproduction
(d) Both (a) and (c)

75 Which one of the following techniques has helped to solve many mysteries involving murders, robberies and rapes? [UP CPMT 2011]
(a) Gene splicing
(b) Computer technology
(c) DNA fingerprinting
(d) Gene cloning

76 A kind of biotechnology involving manipulation of DNA is [Rajasthan PMT 2011]
(a) DNA replication (b) genetic engineering
(c) denaturation (c) renaturation

77 A suitable vector for gene cloning in higher organisms is [Rajasthan PMT 2011]
(a) adenovirus (b) retrovirus
(c) *Salmonella typhimurium* (d) *Neurospora crassa*

78 Which of the following radioisotope is not suitable for DNA labelling based studies? [J&K CET 2011]
(a) H^3 (b) P^{32}
(c) N^{15} (d) S^{35}

ANSWERS

Check Point 21.1

1. (c)	2. (b)	3. (a)	4. (b)	5. (b)	6. (a)

Check Point 21.2

1. (c)	2. (a)	3. (a)	4. (a)	5. (c)	6. (a)

Check Point 21.3

1. (b)	2. (b)	3. (b)	4. (a)	5. (c)	6. (a)

Check Point 21.4

1. (c)	2. (c)	3. (a)	4. (a)	5. (a)	6. (c)

Check Point 21.5

1. (a)	2. (b)	3. (c)	4. (b)	5. (a)	6. (a)

(A) Topical Exercise

1. (b)	2. (c)	3. (d)	4. (c)	5. (a)	6. (c)	7. (d)	8. (c)	9. (b)	10. (a)
11. (d)	12. (b)	13. (c)	14. (b)	15. (a)	16. (d)	17. (b)	18. (a)	19. (a)	20. (d)
21. (b)	22. (c)	23. (d)	24. (b)	25. (b)	26. (b)	27. (c)	28. (d)	29. (d)	30. (d)
31. (c)	32. (c)	33. (c)	34. (c)	35. (b)	36. (c)	37. (c)	38. (c)	39. (c)	40. (c)
41. (d)	42. (c)	43. (b)	44. (a)	45. (d)	46. (d)	47. (a)	48. (c)	49. (d)	50. (a)
51. (d)	52. (d)	53. (a)	54. (d)	55. (c)	56. (d)	57. (d)	58. (c)	59. (d)	60. (a)
61. (d)	62. (b)	63. (c)	64. (d)	65. (c)	66. (c)	67. (c)	68. (c)	69. (a)	70. (a)
71. (c)	72. (b)	73. (b)	74. (c)	75. (c)	76. (a)	77. (a)			

(B) Cumulative Exercise

1. (a)	2. (b)	3. (b)	4. (c)	5. (c)	6. (c)	7. (a)	8. (d)	9. (d)	10. (b)
11. (a)	12. (c)	13. (d)	14. (d)	15. (d)	16. (d)	17. (a)	18. (d)	19. (d)	20. (b)
21. (c)	22. (b)	23. (c)	24. (c)	25. (c)	26. (c)	27. (a)	28. (d)	29. (e)	30. (a)
31. (b)	32. (a)	33. (a)							

(C) Medical Entrances' Gallery

1. (a)	2. (a)	3. (d)	4. (c)	5. (a)	6. (d)	7. (d)	8. (d)	9. (c)	10. (c)
11. (b)	12. (d)	13. (a)	14. (b)	15. (a)	16. (a)	17. (c)	18. (b)	19. (b)	20. (c)
21. (b)	22. (c)	23. (a)	24. (d)	25. (b)	26. (a)	27. (c)	28. (c)	29. (a)	30. (d)
31. (d)	32. (c)	33. (d)	34. (d)	35. (b)	36. (b)	37. (c)	38. (b)	39. (b)	40. (a)
41. (b)	42. (d)	43. (c)	44. (b)	45. (b)	46. (d)	47. (b)	48. (b)	49. (c)	50. (b)
51. (a)	52. (b)	53. (d)	54. (a)	55. (a)	56. (d)	57. (b)	58. (b)	59. (d)	60. (d)
61. (d)	62. (d)	63. (d)	64. (a)	65. (c)	66. (b)	67. (a)	68. (a)	69. (a)	70. (d)
71. (b)	72. (c)	73. (d)	74. (c)	75. (c)	76. (b)	77. (b)	78. (d)		

Explanations

(A) Topical Exercise

5 (*a*) The term restriction in the restriction enzyme refers to the function of these enzymes in restricting the propagation of foreign DNA of bacteriophage in host bacterium, i.e. cutting of DNA at specific position only.

9 (*b*) Statement I is false, but II is true. Incorrect statement can be corrected as

Endonucleases are restriction enzymes, which cut the DNA internally.

15 (*a*) Statement I is true, but II is false. Incorrect statement can be corrected as

Type III restriction enzyme requires Mg^{2+} ion and S-adenosylmethionine for their functioning.

29 (*d*) Plasmid vector is cleaved by the same restriction enzyme that cleaves donor DNA leading to the creation of sticky ends.

34 (*c*) Statement in option (c) incorrectly explains the part of the normal process during the cloning of recombinant DNA in becteria and can be corrected as

Southern blotting is not used for sparation of recombinant DNA plasmids. Southern technique is used to confirm the presence of specific DNA in sample.

49 (*d*) All statements are incorrect and can be corrected as

- If any protein encoding gene is expressed in a heterologous host, it is called a recombinant protein.
- In PCR, the multiple copies of gene of interest is synthesised *in vitro* using two sets of primers.
- A thermostable enzyme (*Taq* polymerase) is obtained from bacterium, *Thermus aquaticus.*

Thus, option (d) is correct.

53 (*a*) Option (a) is incorrect matched can be corrected as

- Northern blotting -James Alwin.
- Western blotting technique was developed by W Neal.

Rest options are correct match.

54 (*d*) Option (d) is incorrect matched pair and can be corrected as

DNA fingerprinting or DNA profiling is a technique to identify a person on the basis of person's DNA specificity.

Rest options are correct matched pairs.

55 (*c*) The incorrect statement is option (c) and can be corrected as

The normal *E. coli* cell does not carry genes resistant against ampicillin, chloramphenicol, tetracycline and kanamycin.

56 (*d*) The incorrect statement is option (d) and can be corrected as

Cells of continuous culture system are maintained in log phase because in continuous culture system product is forming continuously and cells will grow exponentially in log phase.

61 (*d*) Alternate selectable markers have ability to differentiate recombinants from non-recombinants due to the inactivation of the enzyme β-galactosidase or insertional inactivation.

Thus, option (d) is correct.

(B) Cumulative Exercise

2 (*b*) Statements I and II are involved in recombinant DNA technology while III and IV are not involved.

Incorrect statements can be corrected as

- Self ligation is prevented with alkaline phoshatase.
- Bacterium can be the host cell for recombinant DNA technology.

3 (*b*) Only three statements II, III and IV are correct, while I is incorrect. Incorrect statement can be corrected as

Primers used in PCR are small chemically synthesised oligonucleotides.

4 (*c*) Due to insertion of haemoglobin gene, the bacterium losses its property of resistance against ampicillin, therefore it will not grow with ampicillin but can grow with tetracycline. Hence, option (c) is correct.

9 (*d*) Statements I and II are incorrect about agarose gel electrophoresis and can be corrected as

- Agarose is the most common matrix used in gel electrophoresis, it is a natural polymer which is extracted from seaweed.
- The smaller fragment size, the farther it moves.

Rest statements are correct about agarose gelelectrophoresis.

10 (*b*) DNA is negatively charged and it moves from negative to positive electrode in gel electrophoresis. Smaller fragments move fast and more distance towards positive electrode. Fragment (b) is smaller and move, more distance towards positive electrode.

25 (*c*) Only statement III is incorrect and can be corrected as *Bacillus thuringinesis* synthesis crystal (cry) and cytolytic (cyt) toxin during the stationary growth phase.
Rest statements are correct.

29 (*e*) Both A and R are false and can be carrected as Plasmids are extrachromosomal self-replicating, double-stranded, small circular DNA usually found in bacterial cell in addition to main genetic material.

30 (*a*) Both A and R are true and R is the correct explanation of A.

The DNA, which is formed of two or more sources are called chimeric DNA. The recombinant DNA can also be called as chimeric DNA.

31 (*b*) Both A and R are true, but R is not the correct explanation of A.
DNA fingerprinting or DNA typing is a technique to identify a person, on the basis of person's DNA specificity. The technique is based upon the fact that the DNA constitution of an individual carries some specific sequences of nucleotides, which do not carry any information for protein synthesis.
These specific sequences are repeated many times and found at many places within the genome. These loci are known as the Variable Number Tandem Repeats (VNTRs) or minisatellites, which are very specific in nature and with variability in their number from person to person.

32 (*a*) Both A and R are true and R is the correct explanation of A.
A vector is defined as the DNA molecule capable of self-replication and used as the carrier of DNA segment to be cloned. In practice, it is required for transferring and cloning the gene in a suitable host or bacterium.

The gene is inserted in the vector forming recombinant DNA or recombinant vector. The recombinant vector is also called the hybrid vector or chimeric vector. The vectors can be cloning vectors or expression vectors.

33 (*a*) Both A and R are true and R is the correct explanation of A.
Probes are small nucleotide sequences used to detect the presence of complementary sequences in nucleic acid samples.
This is achieved by permitting the probes to base pair with the sample nucleic acids and then identifying the samples that show base pairing with probes, i.e. hybridisation.
The probes can either be labelled with (i) radioactive isotopes, e.g. P^{32} or (ii) with non-radioactive labels, e.g. biotin, digoxigenin, etc.

(C) Medical Entrances' Gallery

1 (*a*) In gel electrophoresis, separated DNA fragments can be visualised with the help of ethidium bromide in UV radiation because DNA fragments cannot be seen in visible light without staining. So, they are stained with ethidium bromide and made observable through UV radiation as bright orange coloured bands.

2 (*a*) The sequence that controls the copy number of linked DNA in the vector is called *ori* site. Origin of replication is a sequence from where replication starts and any foreign DNA is linked to this region. *Ori* site is also responsible for controlling copy number of linked DNA.
Therefore, if any person wants to produce many copies of the target DNA he/she should clone in a vector whose *ori* site supports high copy number.

3 (*d*) The correct option is (d) because the specific palindromic sequence which is recognised by *Eco* RI is

5′ - G A A T T C - 3′
3′ - C T T A A G - 5′

A palindromic sequence is a sequence made up of nucleic acids within the double helix of DNA or RNA that is the same when read from 5′ to 3′ on one strand and 3′ to 5′ on the other complementary strand.

4 (*c*) Statement in option (c) is incorrect and can be corrected as Restriction endonucleases make cut at specific position within the DNA known as palindromic site. They function by inspecting the length of DNA sequence. They are used in genetic engineering to form recombinant molecules of DNA. DNA ligases join the DNA fragments.

Rest statements are correct with regard to restriction enzymes.

6 (*d*) The correct pair is option (d). Rest options are incorrect pair and can be corrected as

- The main function of DNA polymerase is to synthesise DNA from deoxyribonucleotides, the building blocks of DNA.
- Nuclease hydrolyse the phosphodiester bond of DNA and RNA.
- Exonucleases are a broad class of enzymes that cleave off nucleotides one at a time from the 3′ or 5′ ends of DNA and RNA chains.

7 (*d*) *Hind* II was the first discovered endonuclease. It was isolated by Smith Wilcox and Kelley in 1968 from *Haemophilus influenzae* bacterium. It always cuts bacterium. DNA at particular point by recognising a specific sequence of six base pairs. It is known as the recognition sequence for *Hind* II and reads as

5′-GTC GAC-3′
3′-CAG CTG-5′.

8 (*d*) In recombinant DNA technology, antibiotics are used as selectable markers, which help in identifying and eliminating non-transformants and selectively permitting the growth of the transformants. Normally, the genes encoding resistance to antibiotics such as chloramphenicol, ampicillin, tetracycline or kanamycin, etc., are considered useful selectable markers for *E. coli.*

9 (*c*) Electrophoresis is a technique used for the separation of substances of different ionic properties. It is used in RDT to separate the DNA fragments that are being cut by restriction endonuclease. In this technique, DNA fragments are loaded on agarose gel and then electric field is applied. Due to being negatively charged, DNA fragments move toward anodes (+ charge).

The smaller fragments move farther away as compared to larger fragments and thus, these get separated.

10 (*c*) Statement in option (c) is correct.
Restriction enzyme digestions are performed by incubating purified DNA molecule with the restriction enzymes of optimum conditions.
Other statements are incorrect and can be corrected as
- Gel electrophoresis is used for separation and isolation of DNA fragments.
- The polymerase enzyme uses DNA template to catalyse polymerisation of deoxynucleotides.
- PCR is Polymerase Chain Reaction, it is used for amplification of a DNA segment.

12 (*d*) Spooling is the method of collection of isolated DNA in the form of fine threads in the suspension. This is done to isolate DNA from the cell during the process of recombinant DNA technology.

13 (*a*) The statement about restriction enzymes that the enzyme binds DNA at specific sites and cuts only one of the two strands is incorrect. It can be corrected as
These enzymes cut both the strands of DNA helix at specific sites in their sugar phosphate backbone. The sequences being recognised by restriction enzymes are called palindromic sequences which have same reading frame in both $5' \rightarrow 3'$ and $3' \rightarrow 5'$ directions.
Rest of the statements are correct.

15 (*a*) The two antibiotic resistance genes on *E.coli* cloning vector pBR322 are for ampicillin and tetracycline. Cloning vectors are DNA molecules that carry a foreign DNA segment and replicate inside host cell. Plasmid in *E.coli* is a cloning vector.

16 (*a*) To facilitate cloning into a vector, the vector requires a selectable marker, which helps in identifying and eliminating non-transformants and selectively permitting the growth of the transformants.

17 (*c*) An enzyme catalysing the removal of nucleotides from ends of DNA is exonuclease.
On the other hand, endonuclease made cuts at specific positions within the DNA. DNA ligase joins DNA fragments. Proteases are protein-degrading enzymes.

18 (*b*) A chimeric DNA is a recombinant DNA generated by joining sequences derived from different species. Other options are explained as
- Gene clone is an exact copy (clone) of a particular gene or DNA sequence produced by genetic engineering techniques.
- Transposons or jumping genes are DNA sequences produced by genetic engineering techniques.
- Vector shuttle is a vector with ability to propagate in two different host species, e.g. pJDB219.

19 (*b*) In Ti plasmid, virulent gene is removed to get modified strain of *Agrobacterium.* Thus, tumour forming virulent genes are replaced with desired genes and this way it acts as a vector to carry desired gene to a new organism when it gets expressed to produce the product.
On the other hand, auxin gene, cytokinin genes are not present in *Agrobacterium.* These are present in green plants.

20 (*c*) Gene library or DNA library has collection of *c*DNA only. It is a cloned/copy DNA of cells/tissues, organs of an organism in a preserved form for future use. DNA and RNA are nucleic acid and constitute genetic materials of an organisms.
Option (b) and (d) are incorrect with reference to gene library.

22 (*c*) Enzyme DNA ligase is also called as molecular glue as it works to repair broken DNA by joining two nucleotides in a DNA strand. It is commonly used in genetic engineering to do the reverse of restriction enzyme, i.e. join together complementary restriction fragments.
Other options are explaind as
- DNA gyrase is an enzyme of class topoisomerase that relieves torque or strain in DNA during DNA replication.
- DNA helicase unwinds the double helix to make site of DNA synthesis.
- DNA polymerase catalyses the formation of new DNA on template strand.

23 (*a*) Chilled ethanol is used to precipitate DNA out of a mixture of biomolecules.
Low temperature protects the DNA by slowing down the activity of enzymes that could break it apart and ethanol helps in the quick precipitation of DNA.

24 (*d*) Statements I, II and IV are incorrect and can be corrected as
- DNA fragments are negatively charged molecules they can be separated by forcing them to move toward the anode under an electric field through a medium/matrix. The concentration of gel does affect the resolution of DNA separation.
- The separated DNA fragments can be visualised only after staining the DNA with a compound known as ethidium bromide followed by exposure to UV radiation.

Rest statement III is correct.
The DNA fragments separate (resolve) according to their size through sieving effect provided by the agarose gel. Hence, the smaller the fragment size, the farther it moves.

26 (*a*) In annealing, primers anneal to the DNA template to provide a site for intiation of polymerisation by enzyme, *Taq* polymerase. Before this, denaturation of DNA takes place in which two strands of DNA separate from each other at high temperature of 92-95° C.

27 (*c*) Usually a retrovirus is used as a vector for introducing a DNA fragment in human cells like lymphocytes. They are used as vector in gene, therapy to introduce the desired gene, so as to replace the functioning of a defective gene.
On the other hand, λ-phage allows cloning of DNA fragments upto 23 Kb lengths. Ti plasmid is usually used for DNA transfer in plants. pBR322 is an artificial cloning vector, usually used for bacteria.

28 (*c*) Transformation is a procedure through which a piece of DNA is introduced in a host bacterium. DNA bearing ampicillin resistance gene (transformed recipient cells) when introduced into the plate containing ampicillin will grow, while DNA without the ampicillin resistance gene (untransformed recipient cells) will die.
The genes encoding resistance to antibiotics such as ampicillin, chloramphenicol, tetracycline or kanamycin, etc., are considered useful selectable markers for *E.coli.* The normal *E. coli* does not carry resistance against any of these antibiotics.

29 (*a*) Gene transfer is present in biolistics. This technique involves firing of microscopic gold particles coated with the foreign DNA at the cells using a compressed air gun.

It is designed to overcome the problem of strong cell wall in plant tissues. These particles can penetrate the cell wall, the cell and the nuclear membrane to deliver the DNA to the nucleus.

30 (*d*) The Polymerase Chain Reaction (PCR) was developed by Kary Mullis in 1983.

It involves three basic steps in the order as denaturation, where strand separation takes. In place, annealing, primers are annealed to DNA strands and during extension, nucleotides are added by *Taq* polymerase to extend the primers. During PCR, amplification of desired gene/DNA is done.

31 (*d*) Both A and R are false and can be corrected as *Agrobacterium* tumefaciens infects certain plants, in which Ti plasmid causes the formation of tumour like growth, called crown gall. *Agrobacterium* does not infect grasses, i.e. cereals. It is a pathogen of dicots.

32 (*c*) A stirred-tank bioreactor is usually cylindrical, possessing a stirrer which facilitates mixing of the reactor contents and oxygen availability through out the bioreactor. The bioreactor has an agitator system, an oxygen delivery system, foam control, pH and temperature control systems.

Thus, option (c) is correct.

33 (*d*) DNA ligases (genetic gum) are used in recombinant DNA technology to join two individual fragments of double-stranded DNA by forming phosphodiester bonds between them to produce a recombinant DNA (plasmid).

34 (*d*) Option (d) is not a component of downstream processing.

Downstream processing is the process of separation and purification of products synthesised in bioreactors. After the completion of biosynthetic stage, the product has to be subjected through a series of processes before it is ready for marketing as a finished product.

Whereas the processes separation and purification, collectively referred to as downstream processing. The product is then formulated with suitable preservatives.

35 (*b*) *Eco* RV is a type II restriction endonuclease isolated from strains of *E.coli*. It creates blunt ends. The enzyme recognises the palindromic 6-base DNA sequence and makes a cut at vertical line. The blunt ends are formed as

↓

5′ -GATATC-3′

3′ -CTATAG-5′

↑ Coverage site

↓ *Eco* RV

5′–GAT] [ATC – 3′

3′– CTA] [TAG – 5′

Blunt ends

36 (*b*) Both A and R are true, but R is not the correct explanation of A.

The restriction endonucleases cut the DNA sequences at a specific site and produce DNA strands with the sticky ends. It cuts both the strands of DNA at the palindrome sites.

38 (*b*) Restriction endonucleases are synthesised by bacteria as part of their defence mechanism. It is an exnzyme that cuts DNA at or near specific recognition nucleotide sequences known as restriction sites. These enzymes are found in bacteria to provide a defence mechanism against viruses by cleaning the toxic viral DNA

39 (*b*) Both statements A and B are correct.

Agarose gel electrophoresis plays a critical role in analysing DNA in laboratory experiments. It is a method of separating biological molecules using an electrical current.

Ethidium bromide is a molecule commonly used to visualise DNA in agarose gel electrophoresis experiments. If both binds to DNA and fluorescence under the proper conditions. Ethidium bromide is known as an intercalating agent.

40 (*a*) Plasmid is a small fragment of DNA (about 10 Kbp size) that is physically separate from and can replicate freely of chromosomal DNA within a cell. It can clone small DNA fragments.

Cosmid	–	45 Kbp
BAC	–	300-350 Kbp
YAC	–	1 Mbp/1000-2500 Kbp

42 (*d*) There are four nucleotides, i.e. A, T, G and C. In case of A enzyme, it is four nucleotides sequence cutter. Therefore, the probable frequency of fragments produced by A is $4^4 = 256$ nucleotides. Similarly, with B enzyme, the number of fragments produced by it is $4^6 = 1024$ nucleotides.

Thus, A cut (s) at every 256 nucleotides and B produces cut at 1024 nucleotides in sequence.

46 (*d*) Southern hybridisation is a technique used in molecular biology for detection of a specific DNA sequence in DNA samples. Except PCR, we use all three methods such as electrophoresis, blotting and autoradiography.

PCR is a method used for the amplification of DNA sample. *In vitro* clonal propagation is characterised by PCR and RAPD.

47 (*b*) Commonly used vectors for human genome sequencing are BAC and YAC. BAC is a DNA construct, based on a functional fertility plasmid (F-plasmid) used for transforming and cloning in bacteria (*E. coli*) and YAC are genetically engineered chromosomes derived from the DNA of the yeast, *Saccharomyces cerevisiae* which is then ligated into a bacterial plasma.

48 (*b*) The construction of first recombinant DNA emerged from the linking of gene encoding antibiotic resistance gene with a native plasmid of *Salmonella typhimurium.*

It was accomplished by Stanley Cohen and Herbert Boyer in 1972. They isolated the antibiotic resistance gene by cutting out a piece of DNA. This cutting of DNA at specific locations is carried out by molecular scissors also known as restriction enzymes.

49 (*c*) Polymerase Chain Reaction (PCR) is a technique which was developed by Kary Mullis in 1985. It is used for *in vitro* replication of specific DNA sequence using thermostable DNA polymerase.

50 (*b*) Bioreactors are the large volume vessels in which raw materials are biologically converted into specific products, individual enzymes, etc., using microbial, plant, animal or human cells. It provides the optimal conditions for achieving the desired product by providing optimum growth conditions like pH, temperature, substrate, salt, vitamins and oxygen.

51 (*a*) In molecular biology, DNA ligase is a special type of enzyme that is used to seal the double-stranded breaks, i.e. breaks in both complementary strands of DNA or is used to join insert DNA with the plasmid vector.

52 (*b*) Plasmids are considered as vectors. The vectors are DNA molecules that can carry a foreign DNA segment and replicate inside the host cell. That is why during gene cloning plasmid is called as gene taxi.

53 (*d*) The transformed cells will grow on ampicillin but not on tetracycline. This is because the foreign DNA fragment is attached to *Cla* I site, which is present in the region of tet^R gene. Thus, it causes disintegration of tet^R gene.

54 (*a*) Minisatellites or Variable Number of Tandem Repeats (VNTRs) are used in DNA fingerprinting technique. In VNTR, satellite DNA as probe is used that shows very high degree of polymorphism. The technique used Southern blot hybridisation using radiolabelled VNTR as a probe.

55 (*a*) Restriction enzymes are also known as molecular scissors, which are used for cutting DNA at specific locations. *Eco* Rl, is a restriction enzyme isolated from the strain *Eco* RY13.

56 (*d*) The most correct and appropriate option is that exonuclease enzyme removes nucleotides from the terminal ends of DNA and cut a short palindromic DNA strand. Endonuclease removes nucleotides from specific positions within the DNA.

57 (*b*) The colonies of recombinant bacteria appear white in contrast to blue colonies of non-recombinant bacteria due to inactivation of beta-galactosidase enzyme in recombinant bacteria.

58 (*b*) Electrophoresis is used to separate different pieces of DNA on the basis of their size, shape, surface area and molecular weight. Restriction fragments can easily be separated using this technique.

59 (*d*) Option (d) is correct

amp^R and tet^R are the antibiotic resistant genes. Other options are incorrect and can be corrected as

ori represents the site of origin of replication, *rop* represents the proteins that take part in the replication of plasmid. *Hind* III, *Eco* RI are the recognition sites of restriction endonucleases.

60 (*d*) Biolistics or gene gun is a direct or vectorless way used to introduce alien DNA into host cells. In this method of gene transfer, high velocity microparticles of gold or tungsten, coated with DNA are bombarded on the plant cells.

61 (*d*) Polymerase Chain Reaction (PCR) and Restriction Fragment Length Polymorphism (RELP) are used in genetic fingerprinting. RELP identifies the length polymorphism of genes among individuals and PCR is used to amplify that particular DNA fragment (gene).

63 (*d*) Statements in option (d) is true.

PCR is used to amplify a DNA segment or to synthesise *in vitro* the multiple copies of gene (DNA) of interest, using two sets of primers and the enzyme DNA polymerase. This enzyme is isolated from a bacterium, *Thermus aquaticus* and it remains active during the high temperature, but high temperature induces denaturation of double-stranded DNA.

67 (*a*) The positions of these DNA fragments on the electrophoresis gel depends upon relative molecular weight. The fragment with lowest molecular weight will appear farther from the wall and fragment with higher molecular weight will appear near the wall. So, on the basis of information given, molecular weight of d is maximum and molecular weight of b is minimum. So, the order of fragments will be b, a, c, d.

71 (*b*) Clone is a homozygote obtained asexually or it is a group of individuals or cells derived from single parent or cell through asexual reproduction. All the cells in a clone have the same genetic material and are exact copies of the original.

72 (*c*) Restriction endonuclease recognises a particular palindromic sequence and degrades the same. It was so, called because it restricted the growth of bacteriophage in the bacterium (e.g. *E. coli*).

The convention for naming these enzymes is the first letter (*E*) of the name comes from the bacterial genus; the second two letters *co* come from the species and the fourth letter from strain, e.g. *Eco* RI comes from *Escherichia coli* RY13. Roman numbers following the names indicate the order in which the enzymes were isolated.

74 (*c*) Statement in option (c) is not true and can be corrected as

A clone consists of asexual progeny of a single individual or cell. The process of producing a clone is called cloning. All the individuals of a clone have the same genotype, which is also identical with that of the individual from which the clone was derived.

Rest statements are true for a clone.

76 (*b*) In genetic engineering, *r*DNA technology is applied to several biotechnological processes for obtaining particular biochemical improvement of genetic makeup of an organism and fighting genetic defects.

77 (*b*) Vector is a DNA molecule that has the ability to replicate autonomously in an appropriate host cell and into which the DNA fragment to be cloned is integrated for cloning. In higher organism, retrovirus vectors are used, while Baculovirus vectors are used for production of transgenic proteins in silkworm.

78 (*d*) S^{35} radioisotope is not suitable for DNA labelling based studies as DNA does not contain sulphur. S^{35} radioisotope is suitable for protein labelling based studies because protein contains sulphur.

CHAPTER 22

Biotechnology and Its Applications

Biotechnology essentially deals with industrial scale production of biopharmaceuticals and other biological materials using genetically modified microorganisms, fungi, plants and animals. It has tremendous applications in healthcare (medical), crop production, agriculture, non-food uses of crops, other useful products (e.g. biodegradable plastics, vegetable oil, biofuels) and in environmental issues.

Types of biotechnology based on application

Based on its applications, biotechnology is classified as red, white, green, grey and blue biotechnology.

(i) **Red biotechnology** is applied to medical processes. It includes designing of organisms to produce antibiotics and the bio-engineering to cure genetic disease through genomic manipulation.

(ii) **White biotechnology** is applied to industrial processes.

(iii) **Green biotechnology** is applied to agricultural processes. An example of green biotechnology is the designing of transgenic plants that can grow under specific environmental conditions or in the presence of certain agricultural chemicals.

(iv) **Grey biotechnology** include all those applications of biotechnology that are directly related to the environment.

(v) **Blue biotechnology** is based on the exploitation of sea resources to create products and applications of industrial interest.

Other applications of biotechnology include direct use of organisms for the manufacturing of products such as beer and milk products. Similarly, naturally occurring bacteria can be used in mining industry for bioleaching. Biotechnology is also used to recycle and treat waste products, clean up sites contaminated by industrial activities (bioremediation) and to produce biological weapons, etc.

Inside

Based on these informations, it can be concluded that biotechnology has given several useful products to humans by using microbes, plants, animals and their metabolic machinery.

Three critical research areas of biotechnology are

- Providing the best catalyst in the form of improved organism (a microbe or pure enzyme).
- Creating a novel conditions through engineering for a catalyst to perform its action.
- Downstream processing methods to purify the organic compound/protein.

Therefore, biotechnology proves its immense applications at every step of human progress. In this chapter, we will discuss the updated information of various applications of biotechnology.

BIOTECHNOLOGY IN CROP IMPROVEMENT

There are broadly three benefits of biotechnology in relation to agriculture and crop improvement programmes. The first benefit is the reduction of the duration of breeding programmes, which is done by using the method of tissue culture. The second benefit is the development of new hybridisation methods. The third and most promising benefit is obtained through the use of recombinant DNA techniques. This technique has been exploited to form transgenic crops or GM crops.

Transgenic crops or GM crops

It is a crop which contains and expresses a transgene, i.e. a gene transferred into an organism by genetic engineering. A popular term for the transgenic crop is Genetically Modified or GM crops. The technique of GM crops has two unique advantages

(i) Any gene from any organism or a chemically synthesised gene, can be used for transfer.

(ii) Change in genotype can be precisely controlled because only the transgene is added into the crop genome.

When a gene is introduced into the genome of an organisms, it can achieve one of the following

(i) **Produces a protein of interest** It may produce a protein that is the product in which we are interested, e.g. hirudin protein found in leech prevents blood clotting.

The gene encoding hirudin was chemically synthesised. This gene was then transferred into *Brassica napus,* where hirudin accumulates in seeds. Thus, hirudin obtained from seed is purified and used as medicine. In such cases, the transgene product itself is the product of interest.

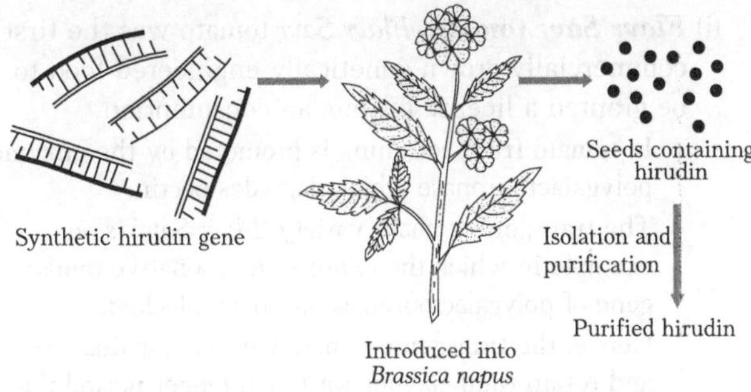

Fig. 22.1 A simplified representation of the production of hirudin from transgenic Brassica napus seeds

(ii) **Produces a desired phenotype** It produces a protein responsible for the desired phenotype.

- For example, a soil bacterium, *Bacillus thuringiensis* produces a Crystal (Cry) protein that is toxic to the larvae of certain insects.
- There are several different types of Cry proteins and each Cry protein is toxic to different group of insects. The gene encoding Cry protein (*cry* gene) has been isolated and transferred into several crops.
- The crop expressing a *cry* gene is usually resistant to the group of insects for which the concerned Cry protein is toxic. In such cases, the transgene product directly produces the phenotype of interest.
- *cry* gene have been transferred into corn. It enables the corn to produce its own pesticides against insects, such as the European corn borer.
- It is interesting to note that the symbols for a gene and for its product are similar. However, gene symbol has small letters and is invariably in italics, e.g. *cry,* whereas, the first letter of the protein symbol is always capital and is always written in roman letters, e.g. Cry.
- The *cry* gene are of different types, e.g. the proteins encoded by the genes *cry* IAc and *cry* IIAb control the cotton bollworms and that of *cry* IAb controls corn borer.

(iii) **Modifies an existing biosynthetic pathway** It modifies an existing biosynthetic pathway, so that a new end product is obtained. Transgenic rice and transgenic potato produce higher content of vitamin-A and protein, respectively.

(iv) **Masks expression of a native gene** It prevents the expression of an existing native gene, e.g. *Flavr Savr* tomato.

Examples of GM crops

Some examples of genetically modified crops are as follows

(i) ***Flavr Savr* tomato** *Flavr Savr* tomato was the first commercially grown genetically engineered food to be granted a license for human consumption.

- In tomato fruit, softening is promoted by the enzyme polygalactouronase which degrades pectin.
- The transgenic tomato variety '*Flavr Savr*' is an example in which the expression of a native tomato gene of polygalactouronase has been blocked.
- Hence, the transgenic tomato variety remains fresh and retain their flavour for much longer period than that of the fruits of normal tomato varieties. In addition, these fruits have a superior taste and increased amount of total soluble solids.
- It was produced by the Californian Company **'Calgene'** and submitted to the US Food and Drug Administration (FDA) in 1992.
- On May 17, 1994, the FDA competed its evaluation of the *Flavr Savr* tomato and the use of APH (3')II.
- They concluded that the tomato is as safe as tomatoes breed by conventional means. Also, the use of aminoglycoside 3'-phosphotransferase (APH) II is safe for use as a processing aid in the development of new varieties of tomato, oilseed rape and cotton.
- It was first sold in 1994 and was only available for a few years before production ceased in 1997. Calgene made history, but mounting costs prevented the company from becoming profitable and it was eventually acquired by Monsanto Company.

Contribution of different fields of biology in the production of *Flavr Savr*

Biotechnology

- In tomato, enzyme Polygalactouronase (PG) is responsible for softening of fruits by degrading pectin of cell wall.
- The expression of polygalactouronase has been reduced in *Flavr Savr*, which lead to improvement in flavour, longer shelf-life (2 weeks) and total soluble solids.

Genetics

- *Flavr Savr* is the result of antisense RNA technology.
- Antisense construct of the gene encoding polygalactouronase show drastically reduced expression of PG in transgenic tomato and slower fruit softening.
- The antisense construct of ACC synthase gene was transferred in tomato, which reduced ethylene production to < 1% of the normal.

Physiology

- The antisense RNA technology has been used to suppress ethylene biosynthesis.
- The fruits remain green and hard on the plants, so that they accumulate more sugar and organic acids that make the fruit sweeter and tasty.
- The new variety called 'Endless summer' remain fresh for about four weeks.

(ii) ***Bt* cotton** It is made by using a bacterium called as, *Bacillus thuringiensis* (*Bt*).

- This bacterium produces a protein that kills certain insects such as *Lepidopterans* (moths and butterflies), *Coleopterans* (beetles) and *Dipterans* (flies, mosquitoes), etc.
- *B. thuringiensis* forms protein crystals (Cry) during a particular phase of their growth. These crystals contain a toxic insecticidal protien.
- *Bt* toxin does not kill the *Bacillus* because it exists as inactive protoxins in the body of *Bacillus*. Once an insect ingest the inactive toxin, it gets exposed to the alkaline pH of the gut, which solubilises the crystals and converts it into active form.
- The activated toxin binds to the surface of midgut epithelial cells and create pores. It causes cell swelling and lysis and eventually death of the insect.
- Specific *Bt* toxin genes were isolated from *Bacillus thuringiensis* and incorporated into several crop plants like cotton, tomato, rice, soybean, etc.

(iii) **Golden rice** It is a variety of *Oryza sativa* produced through the genetic engineering to biosynthesise β-carotene, a precursor of vitamin-A.

Golden rice differs from its parental strain in having three β-carotene biosynthesis genes. Golden rice was created by transforming rice with only two β-carotene biosynthesis genes

(a) ***psy*** (Phytoene synthase) from daffodil *(Narcissus pseudonarcissus).*

(b) ***crtl*** (Phytoene desaturase) from the soil bacterium *Erwinia uredovora.*

The third gene *lcy* (lycopene cyclase) is already produced in wild type of rice endosperm.

RNA interference in pest-resistant plants (antisense RNA)

- A nematode, *Meloidogyne incognita* infects the roots of tobacco plants and causes great reduction in yield.
- RNA interference (RNAi) had been adopted to prevent this infestation. All eukaryotic organisms use RNAi as a method of cellular defence. This method involves silencing of a specific *m*RNA due to a complementary *ds*RNA molecule that binds to and prevents translation of the *m*RNA (silencing).
- The source of this complementary RNA could be either an infection (by viruses having RNA genomes) or transposons (mobile genetic elements) that replicate *via* an RNA intermediate.
- Using *Agrobacterium* vectors, nematode specific genes were injected into the host plant. The introduced gene produced both sense and antisense RNA in the host cells.
- These two RNAs formed a *ds*RNA that initiated RNAi and thus, silenced the specific *m*RNA of the nematode.
- The result was that the parasite could not survive in a transgenic host expressing specific interfering RNA. In this way, the transgenic plant became resistant to parasite.

Advantages of GM crops

These are as follows

(i) **Nutrition** Researchers have created food crops which gives better nutrition variety of rice, i.e. 'Golden rice' has higher content of β-carotene (vitamin-A), *Flavr Savr* tomato has better nutrient quality, delayed ripening and long shelf life. Potato varieties have high starch content.

(ii) **Cold tolerance** These plants are able to tolerate cold climate.

(iii) **Drought tolerance and salinity tolerance** These plants can withstand long periods of drought or high salt content in soil.

(iv) **Herbicide tolerance** Herbicides (weed killers) do not harm the GM crops, e.g. *Bt* cotton, soybean and maize.

(v) **Disease resistance** Plant biologists are working to create plants which are resistant to viruses, bacteria and fungi.

(vi) **Pest resistance** Growing GM crops can help to eliminate the use of chemical pesticides.

Criticism against GM crops

There are following criticism against GM crops

(i) **Unintended harm to other organisms** Recently, a laboratory study was published in the reputed science magazine 'Nature'.

- It highlighted that the pollens from *Bt* corn caused high mortality rates in monarch butterfly caterpillars.
- Monarch caterpillars consume milkweed plants, not the corn, but fear is that if pollens from *Bt* corn are blown by the wind onto milkweed plants in the neighbouring fields, the caterpillars could eat the pollen and perish.

(ii) **Gene transfer to non-target species** Another concern is that the crop plants engineered for herbicide tolerance and weeds would cross-breed.

- It may result in the transfer of the herbicide resistance genes from the crops into the weeds. These 'superweeds' would then be herbicide tolerant as well.
- Other introduced genes may cross over into non-modified crops and then planted next to the GM crops.

(iii) **Reduced effectiveness of pesticides**

- We all know that some populations of mosquitoes developed resistance to the pesticide DDT.
- Similarly, insects may also become resistant to *Bt* or other crops that have been genetically modified to produce their own pesticides.

Table 22.1 Some other genetically modified crops and their modifications

Crops	Modification
Insect-resistant crops	• Genes for various powerful protein toxins have been transferred from the bacterium, *Bacillus thuringiensis* to crop plants including maize, rice and potatoes. • These *Bt* toxins are thousands of times more powerful than chemical insecticides. • Since they are built into the crops, insecticide spraying (which is non-specific and damages the environment) is not required.
Virus-resistant crops	• Gene for virus coat protein has been cloned and inserted into tobacco, potato and tomato plants. • The coat protein seems to 'immunise' the plants, which are much more resistant to viral attack.
Herbicide-resistant crops	• The gene for resistance to the non-volatile herbicide basta has been transferred from *Streptomyces* bacteria to tomato, potato, corn and wheat plants, making them resistant to basta. • Crop fields can safely be sprayed with this herbicide which would kill all weeds, but the crops will not be affected. • Using more agrochemicals, crops like soybean, maize have been modified to provide herbicide tolerance to plants.
Pest-resistant legumes	• The gene for an enzyme synthesises a chemical toxic to weevils (small bettals with an elongated snout). It has been transferred from *Bacillus* bacteria to the *Rhizobium* bacteria that live in the root nodules of legume plants. These root nodules are now resistant from the attack by weevils. Thus, these crops helps to eliminate the use of chemical pesticide.
Nitrogen-fixing crops	• This is a huge project, which aims to transfer about 15 or more genes required for nitrogen-fixation (*nif* genes) from the nitrogen-fixing bacteria, *Rhizobium* into cereals and other crop plants. • These crops would then be able to fix their own atmospheric nitrogen and would not need any fertiliser. However, the process is extremely complex and the project is nowhere near success.
Crop improvement	• Proteins in some crop plants, including wheat, are often deficient in essential amino acids (which is why vegetarians have to watch their diet so carefully). • Therefore, the protein genes are being altered to improve their composition for human consumption.

Genetically modified food

The food prepared from the products of genetically modified (transgenic) crops is called as genetically modified food or **GM food.** The GM food differs from the food prepared from the products of conventionally developed varieties mainly in the following aspects

(i) It contains the protein produced by the transgene. For example, Cry protein in case of insect-resistant varieties.

(ii) It contains the enzymes produced by the antibiotic resistance gene that was used during gene transfer by genetic engineering.

(iii) It contains the antibiotic resistance gene itself.

Disadvantages of GM food

The global community is now-a-days facing challenges associated with public perception of transgenic crops. It has been argued that the above features of GM foods could lead to the following problems when they are consumed.

(i) The transgene products may cause toxicity and/or produce allergies. There is a fear of transferring allergens (usually glycoprotein) from GM food to human and animals, e.g. peanuts and other nuts.

(ii) The enzyme produced by the antibiotic resistance gene could cause allergies because it is a foreign protein.

(iii) The bacteria present in the alimentary canal of the humans could take up the antibiotic resistance gene, which is present in the GM food. These bacteria would then become resistant to the concerned antibiotic. Thus, these bacteria could become difficult to manage.

(iv) Bringing GM food to market is a lengthy and expensive process and of course agribiotech companies wish to ensure a profitable return on their investment.

The scientists involved in the production of transgenic crops are addressing to these concerns. Therefore, efforts are being made to use other genes in place of antibiotic resistance genes.

The toxic and allergic actions of the transgene product can be adequately examined by detailed assays using suitable animal models.

CHECK POINT 22.1

1. Which of the following enzymes was transferred into golden rice from *Narcissus pseudonarcissus*?

(a) Polygalacturonase (b) Acetyltransferase
(c) Phytoene synthase (d) Carotene desaturase

2. A gene encoding Cry protein (*cry* gene) has been isolated and transferred into several crops. Which of the following result can be observed?

(a) Produce its own gene
(b) Offspring will carry the recessive gene
(c) Produce the phenotype of interest
(d) Reduce efficiency of pesticides

3. '*nif*' gene for nitrogen-fixation in cereal crops like wheat, jowar, etc., is introduced by cloning.

(a) *Rhizobium melilioti* (b) *Bacillus thuringiensis*
(c) *Rhizobium stolonifer* (d) *Agrobacterium tumefaciens*

4. The toxin protein produced by *B. thuringiensis* act in alkaline medium and binds with the epithelial cell of

(a) foregut (b) hindgut
(c) midgut (d) foregut and midgut

5. *Bt* toxin gene is isolated from *Bacillus thuringiensis* and incorporated into crop plants making them insecticidal. The choice of genes depend upon

(a) crop plant only
(b) targeted pest only
(c) neither type of crop nor targeted pest
(d) Both (a) and (b)

BIOTECHNOLOGY IN MEDICINE

Biotechnology has very few successful commercial applications in the field of medicine. Although, these are increasing each year.
The applications so far can be considered in the following groups

Medicinal gene products

- The biggest and the most successful kind of genetic engineering is the production of gene products of medical interest.
- The following table shows some of the examples of genetically engineered products that are already available.

Table 22.2 Some medicinal gene products, their uses and host organisms involved

Products	Uses	Host organisms
Insulin	Human hormone used to treat diabetes.	Bacteria/Yeast
hGH	Human growth hormone, used to treat dwarfism.	Bacteria
BSHT	Bovine growth hormone, used to increase milk yield of cows.	Bacteria
Factor-VIII	Human blood clotting factor, used to treat haemophilics.	Bacteria
Penicillin	Antibiotic used to kill bacteria.	Fungi/Bacteria
Vaccines	Hepatitis-B antigen for vaccination.	Yeast
α-glucosidase	Enzyme used to treat Pompe's disease.	Rabbit
DNase	Enzyme used to treat cystic fibrosis	Bacteria

- The gene products are mostly proteins and produced directly when a gene is expressed. However, they can also be non-protein products produced by genetically engineered enzymes.
- The basic principle here is to transfer a gene (often human) to another organism (usually a microbe). As a result of this, gene product is formed quickly, cheaply and ethically.
- It is also possible to make 'designer proteins' by altering gene sequences. Such products are useful research tool, but have no commercial applications yet.
- The most common group of host organisms used to make gene products are the bacteria. It is because they can be grown quickly and the product can be purified from their cells easily.
- Recently animals and even plants have been used to make gene products as bacteria cannot always make human proteins. It is more appropriate to extract the product from their cells. In animals, the product must be secreted in milk or urine, while in plants, the product must be secreted from their roots.

Examples of genetically engineered products

Some examples of genetically engineered products are given below

(i) Human insulin

- Insulin is a small protein hormone, produced by the pancreas. It regulates the blood sugar concentration.
- In diabetes mellitus, the pancreas cells do not produce enough insulin. The disease can be successfully treated by injection of insulin extracted from the pancreas of slaughtered cows and pigs.
- Insulin from these species has a slightly different amino acid sequence from human insulin and thus, this may lead to immune reaction and side effects.

History of insulin production

- The human insulin gene was isolated, cloned and sequenced in 1970s. Therefore, it became possible to insert this gene into bacteria to produce human insulin in large amounts.
- In humans, pancreatic cells first make proinsulin, which then undergoes post-translational modification to make the final, functional insulin.
- Proinsulin contains an extra stretch called the C-peptide. The C peptide is not present in the mature insulin and is removed during the maturation into insulin.

Humulin production

- Bacterial cells cannot perform post-translational modification.
  Eventually, a synthetic *c*DNA gene was made and inserted into the bacterium *E. coli.*
- Proinsulin was made in bacteria and post-translational conversion to insulin was carried out chemically.
- This technique was developed by Eli Lily and Company in 1982 and the product, '**humulin**' became the first genetically engineered product approved for medical use.
- In 1990s, the procedure was improved by using the yeast, *Saccharomyces cerevisiae* instead of *E. coli.*
- Yeast, a eukaryote, is capable of post-translational modification. This simplifies the production of human insulin.
- Another company has developed a method of converting pig insulin into human insulin by chemically changing few amino acids.

This turned to be cheaper than the genetic engineering methods.

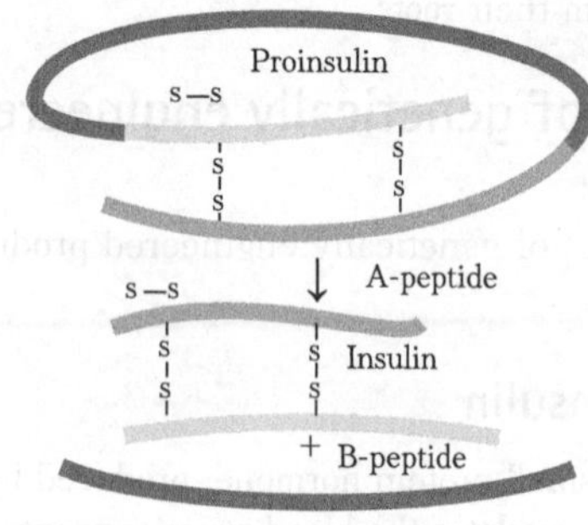

Fig. 22.2 Maturation of proinsulin into insulin (simplified)

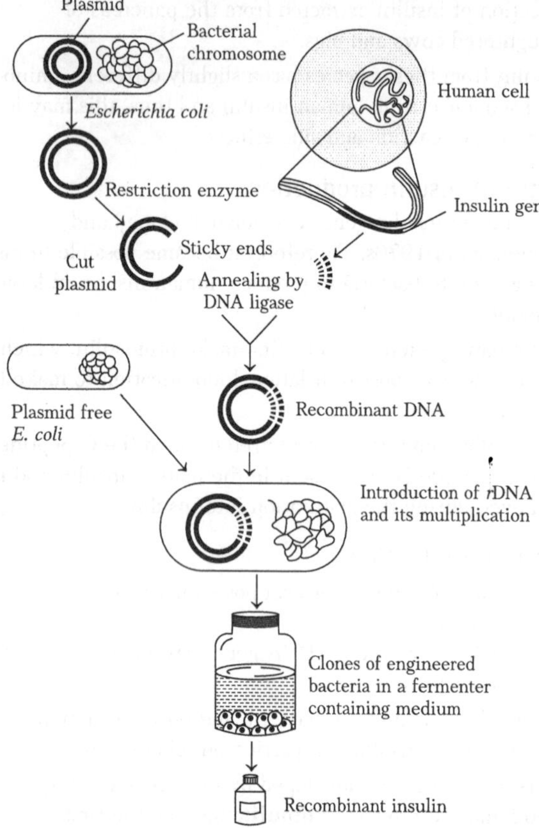

Fig. 22.3 Steps involved in gene transfer for the production of human insulin

(ii) human Growth Hormone (hGH)

- This is a protein hormone secreted by the pituitary gland. It can stimulate tissue growth.
- Low production of hGH in childhood results in pituitary dwarfism. This can be treated with hGH extracted from dead humans.
- This treatment may cause some side effects such as, Creutzfeldt Jacob Disease (CJD). Hence, this treatment was withdrawn.
- The hGH was cloned and an artificial *c*DNA gene was inserted into *E. coli*. A single sequence was added into it. It not only caused the gene to be translated but, also caused the protein to be secreted from the cell.
- This genetically engineered hGH was produced by Genetech that could successfully restore normal height in children with hGH deficiency.

(iii) α-1 Antitrypsin (AAT)

- It is a human protein made in the liver and found in the blood. It is an inhibitor of protease enzymes like trypsin and elastase.
- There is a rare mutation of the AAT gene (a single base substitution) that causes AAT to be inactive, so the protease enzymes become uninhibited.
- The most noticeable effect of this is in the lungs. In lungs, elastase digests the elastic tissue of the alveoli. This leads to the lung disease called **emphysema**.
- It can be treated by inhaling an aerosol spray containing AAT. This reaches the alveoli and inhibits the elastase activity.
- AAT for this treatment can be extracted from blood donations, but only in very small amounts. Therefore, to make AAT extract in sufficient amounts, AAT genes can be expressed in some animals, e.g. sheeps.
- Genes for AAT cannot be expressed in bacteria. It is because AAT is a glycoprotein that needs to have sugars added by post-translational modification. Such kinds of modifications can only be carried out by animals.
- In this method, AAT gene was coupled to a promoter for milk protein β-lactoglobulin. This promoter is only activated in mammary gland cells. Thus, AAT is produced in mammary glands and secreted by means of milk. The firstever sheep to produce milk with AAT was named **Tracy**.

Stem cell technology

- Since, the isolation of embryonic stem cells in 1998, laboratories all over the world have been exploring the possibility of using stem cells to restore damaged or lost tissue.
- A sperm fertilises an egg to create a single cell destined to become a child. As development commences, the cell begins to divide and produce a small ball of a few dozen cells.
- At this point each of these cells, called embryonic stem cells, are identical. Each one of them is capable of developing into a healthy individual.
- These cells can develop into any tissue. Hence, they can be used to restore damaged heart or spine tissue.
- In stem cell technology, embryonic stem cells are isolated from inner cell mass of **blastocyst**. These are preserved and used later for the treatment of abnormal conditions.

- Heart muscle cells have been grown from mouse embryonic stem cells and successfully integrated with the heart tissue of a living mouse. This suggests that the damaged heart muscle of heart attack victims might also be repairable with stem cells.
- Similarly, injured spinal cord can also be repaired. Stem cells can also be used in leukemia, alzheimer's disease, Parkinson's diseases, huntington's disease, burns, etc.
- These very promising experiments are being pursued aggressively. They are however, quite controversial, as embryonic stem cells are typically isolated from the tissue of discarded or aborted embryos which raises serious ethical issues.

Gene therapy

Gene therapy means altering the genotype of a tissue or even a whole human. The idea of gene therapy is to genetically alter human genome sequence in order to treat a disease.

This is perhaps the most significant and most controversial kind of genetic engineering. This could represent the first opportunity to cure incurable diseases. This technique is quite different from using genetically engineered microbes to produce a drug, vaccine or hormone to treat a disease by conventional means.

Somatic cell therapy

It means genetically altering somatic cells, e.g. bone marrow cells, pancreas cells, etc. This therapy may treat or cure the disease, but any genetic changes will not be passed on to offspring. Hence, it is important to appreciate the difference between somatic cell therapy and germ line therapy.

Germ line therapy

It means genetically altering germ line cells, i.e. sperm cells, sperm precursor cell, ova, ova precursor cells, zygotes or early embryos, etc.

Alterations to any of these cells affect every cell in the resulting offsprings and in all the descendants.

Examples of gene therapy

Few examples of diseases which are curable (temporarily) through gene therapy are listed below

Severe Combined Immunodeficiency Disease (SCID)

- This is a rare genetic disease that affects the immune system. It is also known as **baby in a bubble syndrome**.
- It is caused by a mutation in the gene for the enzyme **Adenosine Deaminase** (ADA).
- Without ADA white blood cells cannot be made, so patients do not have an effective immune system. The affected individuals would quickly contract a fatal infection unless they spend their lives in sterile isolation.
- This disease can be treated by either bone marrow transplantation or by enzyme replacement therapy. However, both of these are not completely curative.
- The treatment of Adenosine Deaminase (ADA) deficiency was the first clinical gene therapy given in 1990 to a 4 year old girl.

Mechanism of SCID treatment

- In this method, lymphocytes from the blood of the patient are grown in a culture outside the body.
- A functional *c*DNA of ADA is then introduced into these lymphocytes, and then subsequently returned to the patient. These genetically engineered lymphocytes have to be periodically infused in the patient.
- Gene therapy has also been attempted on few children in USA and UK by surgically removing their bone marrow cells. These are then transferred with a genetically engineered virus containing the ADA gene. These cells are later transferred to the patient.
- The hope is that these transformed cells would multiply in the bone marrow and make white blood cells. The trials are still underway, so the success is unknown. However, if the gene isolated from bone marrow cells producing ADA is introduced into cells at early embryonic stages, it could be a permanent cure.

Cystic Fibrosis (CF)

- It is the most common genetic disease. It is caused by a mutation in the gene for protein called **CFTR** (Cystic Fibrosis Transmembrane Regulator).
- Common mutation causes a deletion of three bases, thus removing one amino acid out of 1480 amino acids in the protein.
- CFTR is a chloride ion channel protein found in the cell membrane of epithelial (lining) tissue cells. The mutation stops this protein working. Therefore, chloride ions cannot cross the cell membrane.

Etiology

- Chloride ions inside the cells causes sodium ions to enter into the cell to balance the charge.
- The increased concentration of both these ions inside the epithelial cells decreases the osmotic potential.
- Water is therefore, retained inside the cells. Hence, the mucus secreted by these cells is drier and more sticky than normal.

- This sticky mucus blocks the tubes into which it is secreted, such as the small intestine, pancreatic duct, bile duct, sperm duct, bronchioles and alveoli, etc.
- In this disease, breathlessness, lung infections such as bronchitis and pneumonia, poor digestion, absorption and infertility may be seen.

Treatment

- This disease can be treated with the help of antibiotics and DNase enzyme which loosen the mucus. Regular physiotherapy is also performed during treatment. These are very complicated methods. Thus, gene therapy can be employed to treat cystic fibrosis.
- The gene for CFTR was identified in 1989 and a *c*DNA clone was made soon after.
- The idea was to deliver the copies of this gene to the epithelial cells of the lung, where they could be incorporated into the nuclear DNA to make functional CFTR chloride channels. If about 10% of the cells could be corrected, this would cure the disease.
- Two methods of delivery of gene are being tried, liposomes and adenoviruses. Both of these are delivered with an aerosol inhaler, like those used by asthmatics. Clinical trials are currently underway, but till now, no therapy has been shown to be successful.

Future of gene therapy

Gene therapy should not be limited to treating genetic diseases, but could also help in treating infections and environmental diseases. Despite being highly effective, gene therapy is illegal in most of countries. It may be because of the following reasons

- Gene therapy can be potentially dangerous because its long term effects are unknown.
- It is unethical as it could lead to eugenics.
- Gene therapy is considered immoral as it involves altering and destroying human embryos.

It is currently illegal in most of the countries and the current research is focusing on somatic cell therapy only.

Development of new phenotypes

New phenotypes are being developed continuously by adding new genes or by manipulating the existing genes. Phenotypes of various plants and animals have been continuously modified for the welfare of humans. New phenotypes are developed by transgenic animals, plants and microorganisms.

Transgenic animals

- These are animals which carry foreign genes. In them, the desired gene is introduced, using the recombinant DNA technology.
- The potential of the technology has also made it possible to employ it in cattle, swine, sheep and goat as processing units.
- These animals are then used to manufacture proteins or can be used as organ donors, e.g. tissue plasminogen activator in milk (goat) and blood clotting factor-VIII (sheep from progeny of ewe).
- The possible benefits and reasons of producing transgenic animals are as follows

(i) **Study of physiology and development** Transgenic animals can be specifically used to study the biological effects of certain products on the normal physiology and development.

(ii) **Study of diseases** Transgenic animals can be designed to understand the contribution of genes in the development of diseases. These animals serve as models to study human diseases, e.g. transgenic models for cancer, cystic fibrosis, rheumatoid arthritis and alzheimer's disease.

(iii) **Vaccine safety** Transgenic animals that are sensitive to vaccines can be developed. These animals can be used for testing the safety of vaccines, e.g. transgenicmice is used to test the safety of polio vaccine.

(iv) **Chemical safety testing** In order to test the safety against a chemical, transgenic animals can be produced. These animals are highly sensitive to certain chemicals.

Transgenic microorganisms

Various microorganisms, particularly bacteria have been modified through genetic engineering to meet specific needs in various fields such as agriculture, medicine, environment protection, etc. A few examples are given below

1. **Degradation of oil spills** Plasmids of four different strains of *Pseudomonas putida* have genes to degrade the toluene , camphor, octane and xylene. A 'superbug' strain was developed that contained all these four sets of genes. This superbug has been used in controlling water pollution due to oils spills.
2. **Crop improvement** The N_2-fixing ability of bacteria can be increased by increasing the expression of *nif* gene.
3. **Medicine** Various bacteria including *E. coli* has been successfully transformed to produce human growth hormone, blood clotting factors, etc.

(v) **Biological products** Production of medicine containing a biological product is an expensive task. By the introduction of gene encoding the particular biological product, transgenic animal can be produced.

This animal then produce the required protein that can further be utilised to make medicines, e.g. α-1-antitrypsin was introduced in sheep.

A few examples of certain transgenic animals are given in the table below

Table 22.3 Gene inserted in transgenic animals and their benefits

Transgenic animals	Gene inserted	Effects of inserted gene	Benefits
Sheep	Anti-haemophilic factor-IX.	Secretes human clotting factor-IX in their milk.	Administered to haemophilic patients.
	Amino acid cysteine.	Cysteine is important component of keratin protein in wool.	High yield of wool.
	Growth hormone.	More growth is observed in animal.	More mutton production.
	Human γ-1 antitrypsin.	Produce milk with AAT-1.	Treatment of patient suffering from emphysema and cystic fibrosis.
	Lactoferrin coding gene.	Kill ticks by digesting their exoskeleton.	Sheep resistant to tick parasites thus, disease resistant sheep are produced.
Goat	Blood clot dissolving gene, i.e. TPA gene.	Produce milk with high TPA concentration.	Easy extraction of TPA resulting a cost effective treatment of patients suffering from coronary thrombosis.
	Anti-thrombin gene	Produce milk with high antithrombin concentration.	Improved milk yield.
Bull	Lactoferrin coding gene.	Resistance to infection that cause udder disease mastitis.	The new progeny produced was not suffering from mastitis.
Cows	DNA coding lactoferrin.	Milk with high lactoferrin concentration.	To cure patients suffering from cystic fibrosis, thus providing immunity to such patients.
	Bovine somatotropin gene.		High milk production.
Pigs	bovine Growth Hormone (bGH) gene.	Pigs grows faster than normal, with reduced subcutaneous fats.	Production of leaner pork with lower fat content.
Fish	human Growth Hormone (hGH) gene.	Fish with twice growth.	Increased meat production.

Vaccines production

- Vaccination (administration of vaccine) was discovered by **Edward Jenner** (1708). The technique of attenuating or weakening of pathogen was discovered by **Louis Pasteur** (1879, against cholera).
- Vaccines are suspensions or killed or modified pathogenic microorganisms. When injected into an animal, these produce immunity against a particular disease.
- Biotechnology has proved successful in the development of recombinant vaccines, also known as **second generation vaccines** and even **third generation vaccines**. Hepatitis-B vaccine is the second generation vaccine.
- The vaccines produced using genetic engineering can usually be made faster than those manufactured by traditional methods.

Note *The method of manufacturing drugs in transgenic animals is called **molecular farming** or **molecular pharming**.*

Monoclonal antibodies

- In 1984, **Caeser Milstein** (of England) and **George Kohler** (of Switzerland) were awarded Nobel Prize for engineering 'monoclonal antibodies'.
- These are made outside the body by the fusion of B-cells and myeloma cells (cancerous cells). These hybrid cells are known as **hybridomas**.
- To produce monoclonal antibodies, B-cells are removed from the spleen of an animal that has been challanged with the relevant antigen.
- These B-cells are then fused with myeloma tumour cells that can grow indefinitely in cultures (myeloma is a B-cell cancer). This fusion is performed by making the cell membranes more permeable.
- The fused hybrid cells, being cancerous multiply rapidly. As a result, large amounts of the desired antibodies are produced.
- These are selected and subsequently cloned by limiting dilution. Supplemental media (HAT) containing interleukin-6 are essential for this step.
- Monoclonal antibodies are thus, true magic bullets that strike specific molecules and leave the rest of the body unharmed.
- Monoclonal antibodies have been used in genetic engineering for identifying and measuring levels of gene product. These bodies are also used in pregnancy testing, diagnosis of disease, treatment of disease, preventing rejection of transplants and tissue typing for transplants.

CHECK POINT 22.2

1. The lactalbumins of 'Rosie' (transgenic cow) contains which peptide chain?
(a) Delta (b) Beta (c) Gamma (d) Alpha

2. A bacterial product used to treat cystic fibrosis is
(a) penicillin
(b) DNase
(c) factor VIII
(d) BSHT

3. An example of somatic cell therapy is the treatment of
(a) Parkinson's disease
(b) Huntington's disease
(c) SCID
(d) None of the above

4. Genentech has successfully produced
(a) human growth hormone (b) humulin
(c) *c*DNA of ADA (d) All of these

5. The maximum application of animal cell culture technology today is in the production of
(a) vaccine (b) edible protein
(c) insulin (d) interferon

6. Monoclonal antibodies are produced from hybrid cells called hybridomas. The cells employed to obtain these hybridoma cell are
(a) B-lymphocytes and myeloma cells
(b) lymphoma cells and bone marrow cells
(c) T-lymphocytes and myeloma cells
(d) B-lymphocytes and carcinoma cells

ETHICAL ISSUES IN BIOTECHNOLOGY

With the development of GMO's (Genetically Modified Organisms), a continuous challenge is also growing against them. The people all over the world feels that use of GMO's is unethical and such manipulations of living being should not continue without regulations. Thus, several societies have started objecting to genetic modifications, and regulatory measures has been established to take care of morality on such issues and biological importance of these studies.

Biopatent

A patent is the right granted by the government to an inventor which prevent others to make commercial use of one's invention. Different countries have different patent laws, which are changed with the advent of time.

A patent is granted for

- An invention (including a product).
- An improvement in an earlier invention.
- The process of generating a product.
- A concept or a design.

The patents granted for biological entities and products derived from them are called as biopatents.

Primarily, industrialised countries like USA, Japan and members of European Union, award the biopatents. Biopatents are awarded for the achievements in the following areas of biotechnology

- Strains of microorganisms
- Cell lines
- Genetically modified strains of plants and animals
- DNA sequences
- The proteins encoded by DNA sequences
- Various biotechnological procedures
- Production processes
- Products
- Product applications

There is a great opposition from various social groups to biopatents. The nature of these objectives is mainly ethical and political. The arguments in favour of biopatents are primarily of increased economic growth.

Several biotechnology patents are very broad in their coverage, e.g. one patent covers 'all the transgenic plants of *Brassica* family'.

Some cases of patenting

Patents on natural product inventions are subjected to attack, unless all public knowledge about the species in question and its uses are fully disclosed. For example,

(i) **In turmeric** in 1995, the USA lab granted a patent to the Medical Centre, University of Missisippi (USA) for the use of turmeric (haldi) powder as a wound healing agent. Council of Scientific and Industrial Research (CSIR), New Delhi (India) objected this patent and the patent was cancelled in 1998. The new evidence established that the use of turmeric to promote wound healing had been known for generations in India.

(ii) **In neem oil** in 1997, the EPO (European Patent Organisation) had given a favourable interim judgement on the challenge of an European Patent on the fungicidal effect of neem oil owned by W Grace and coworkers. The challenge to neem patent was done by Dr. Vandana Shiva, Magda Aevoet (President of the green group of The European Parliament) and the other NGOs of neem campaign. This patent was also revoked in 2004 on the basis of evidence that such aided properties of neem had already been reported in Indian literature.

(iii) **In ayahuasca**, the 1986 patent claimed an ostensibly new, distinct variety of *Banisteriopsis caapi*, known in the Amazon as **ayahuasca**. However, new evidences establish that the claimed plant is actually the wild uncultivated variety and is neither new nor distinctive.

(iv) **In basmati**, the US government has patented the Indian 'basmati' rice as 'Rice tech'. The Government of India challenged on April 28, 2001. Consequently, USPTO (United States Patent and Trademark Office) served a notice to M/S Rice Tech. Inc., for the amendments in claims restricting to only three strains developed by it.

(v) **In superbug** Dr. Anand Mohan Chakrabarty, an India born American scientist created a superbug by using a bacterium, *Pseudomonas.* It eats upon oils. This superbug could not be patented because the US laws before 1980 did not allow the patent of liveforms. Later on, the patent laws were amended.

In 1988 in US, a patent was issued to genetically engineered mouse **'oncomouse'**, which contains human cancer gene and is again a liveform. Then, he filed a case in the US Supreme Court and won it. In 1990, the US government allowed him to treat oil spills by using *Pseudomonas* based superbug.

Significance of biopatents

- Biopatent system permits private, monopoly rights over cells, genes, animals and plants. It means that people will not share vital research informations because they are afraid that it will be patented by someone else. The people would not research in such areas, which are dominated by patents.
- It will lead to research programmes dominated by potentiability and profitability rather than need.
- It provides the patent holder monopoly control over resources for food and medicine.
- The important advantage of biopatents is that they are a direct incentive for genetic engineering.
- The strong arguments in favour of biopatents are primarily increased economic growth.

Biopiracy

It can be defined as an illegal use of biological materials. Some organisations and multinational companies exploit and/or patent biological resources (bioresources) of other nations without proper authorisation from the countries concerned. This is called as biopiracy.

Various institutions and companies of industrialised nations are collecting and exploiting the bioresources in several ways, such as

- Useful genes are isolated from the bioresources and patented. These genes are then used to generate commercial products.
- The bioresources are being analysed for the identification of valuable biomolecules. The biomolecules are then patented and used for commercial modes.
- The traditional knowledge related to bioresources is utilised to achieve the above objectives. In some cases, this knowledge itself may be the subject of a patent.

Examples of biopiracy

India is rich in traditions, communal knowledge and expertise in natural medicines, spices, food preparations, biological pesticides and diverse agriculture. That is why, it is under surge from biopirates. Some examples of biopiracy are given below

(i) Through patenting without consent, foreign companies have acquired at least 22 plants for their beneficial derivatives. The patents have been taken out on plants such as basmati rice (*Oryza sativa*), black pepper (*Piper nigrum*), pomegranate (*Punica granatum*), Indian mustard (*Brassica campestris*), turmeric (*Curcuma longa*) and neem (*Azadirachta indica*). US, Japanese and German companies are the principal patenting pirates.

(ii) Nestle India has lined up a processing patent on cooked cereals, parboiled rice and vegetarian pulao, at the Indian Patent Office, even though Indians have been making parboiled rice, often as a staple diet for centuries.

(iii) Brazzein is a protein, which is produced by a West African plant, *Pentadiplandra brazzeana* and is approximately 2000 times as sweet as sugar. It is used as a low calorie sweetener. Local people have been using the super-sweet berries of the plant for centuries. But the protein was patented by USA. The gene encoding brazzein was isolated, sequenced and patented by USA as well.

It is proposed to transfer the brazzein gene into maize and express it in maize kernels. Such kernels will then be used for the extraction of brazzein.

This development could have serious implications for the countries who export large quantities of sugar.

Biowar

The war, which is fought with the help of biological organism using them as weapons against humans, their crops and animals is called as biowar or **biological war**. In biowar, viruses, bacteria and some other harmful organisms are used and are called as **Bioweapons** (BW).

Some historical biowars

1. **Pre-modern era**
   - In 5th century BC, Greco-Romans contaminated water resources with animal carcasses.
   - In 400 BC, Scythian archers 'weaponised' biological agents by dipping arrowheads in faeces and cadavers.
   - In 190 BC, Harmibal launched pottery with poisonous snakes onto enemy ships.
   - During 14th century, Mongols catapulated plague infected cadavers into Ukrainian city of Koffa.
   - In 1763, British officers gave blankets infected with smallpox to native Americans during French and Indian war.
   - In 1860s, US civil war confederate surgeon imported clothes infected with yellow fever.
2. **During 20th century**
   - In World War-I, Germany used *Bacillus anthracis* (anthrax) and *Bacillus mallei* (glanders) to infect livestock and animal feed exported to allies.
   - In 1932-1945, Japan conducted research on *Bacillus anthracis, Shigella* sp., *Vibrio cholerae*, etc.
   - In 1942, Britain developed strategic amounts of anthrax.
   - In 1940s, Nazi prisoners infected with *Rickettsia* sp., hepatitis-A, *Plasmodia* sp., and treated with investigational vaccines and some drugs.
   - During 1940s, Nazi secret agent Reinhardt Heydrich assassinated with botulinum toxin.
3. **US Biological Weapons Programme**
   - In 1942, approximately 5000 bombs filled with *Bacillus anthracis* were produced.
   - In 1950s, programmes expanded during Korean war.
   - In 1955, human experiments with *F. tularensis* and *C. burnetti.*
   - During 1949-1968, simulant organisms released off coast of San Francisco and in New York City subway.
   - In 1969, US terminated offensive biological weapons programmes.
   - In 1972, biological weapons convention and treaty.

Biological weapon

Bioweapons can cause the following diseases

- Smallpox
- Anthrax
- Q-fever (fever, chills, fatigue, etc.)
- Plague
- Tularemia (it can occur in humans in two forms–typhoidal and ulceroglandular)
- Botulinum toxin (skeletal muscle paralysis)
- Viral encephalitis
- Viral haemorrhagic fevers

Characteristics of bioweapons

Few characteristics that make bioweapons attractive to countries and terrorists are mentioned below

- Bioweapons are low cost weapons.
- They cause more casualities than conventional or chemical weapons.
- Bioweapons are invisible, odourless and tasteless once released.

Defence against bioweapons

These are as follows

- Protective shelter
- Proper vaccination
- Effective detection systems
- Respirator or gas mask
- Decontamination
- Antibiotics

Bioethics

It is the branch of ethics, philosophy and social commentary that deals with the biological sciences and their potential impact on society.

Major bioethical concerns

The major bioethical concerns pertaining to genetic modification of organisms are as follows

- Use of animals in biotechnology causes immense sufferings and pain to them.
- Introduction of a transgene from one species into another species goes against the integrity of species.
- Transfer of human genes into animals and plants weakens the concept of humanity.
- Biotechnology is discourteous to living beings and only makes use of them for the advantage of human beings.
- Biotechnology may pose unforeseen risks to the environment, including risk to the biodiversity.

Thus, we can say that genetic modification of organisms can have unpredictable results when such organisms are introduced into ecosystem.

Therefore, the government of India has setup **GEAC**, i.e. genetic engineering approval committee. The organisation make decisions regarding validity of GM research and their safety issues.

CHECK POINT 22.3

1. For which of the following biopatents are not awarded?
   (a) The protein encoded by DNA sequences
   (b) Production processes
   (c) Invention that are well-known
   (d) Product applications

2. Illegal and unlawful development of biomaterials without payment to concerned authorities or organisation is called
   (a) bioethics (b) biopatent
   (c) biowar (d) biopiracy

3. US government has patented the Indian 'Basmati' rice as 'Rice tech' which of the following sence notice to Rice tech?
   (a) CSIR (b) USPTO
   (c) EPO (d) ICAR

4. A genetically engineered microorganism used successfully in the bioremediation of oil spills is a species of
   (a) *Xanthomonas*
   (b) *Bacillus*
   (c) *Pseudomonas*
   (d) *Neisseria*

5. The microorganism which causes respiratory disorder in worker in wool industries is used as bioweapon to infect livestock and animal feed during World War-I is
   (a) *Bacillus anthracis*
   (b) *Neisseria gonorrhoeae*
   (c) *Mycobacterium tuberculosis*
   (d) *Streptococcus pyogenes*

EXAM POINTS

- In *Bt* cotton, the specific *Bt* toxin gene was isolated from *Bacillus thuringiensis*. **[NEET 2020]**
- Alkaline pH of gut triggers activation of protoxin to act on *Bacillus thuringiensis* in bollworm. **[NEET 2019, CBSE AIPMT 2015]**
- The Golden rice is enriched with vitamin-A, with a gene from daffodil. The grain appears yellow due to high β-carotene in it. Golden rice is neither drought tolerant, nor pest resistant. **[NEET 2019]**
- The root of the tobacco plant is infected by *Meloidogyne incognita*. **[NEET-I 2016]**
- In all eukaryotic organisms, RNAi is used as cellular defence. **[NEET 2020]**
- RNA interference is used to develop a pest-resistant plant against infestation by nematode. **[NEET 2020]**
- In RNAi, genes are silenced using *ds*RNA. **[NEET 2019]**
- Silencing of a gene/specific *m*RNA translation could be achieved through the use of both RNA and antisense RNA. **[KCET 2018]**
- In humans, insulin is synthesised as a proinsulin, the proinsulin has an extra peptide called C-peptide. **[NEET 2020]**
- The two polypeptides of human insulin are linked together by disulphide bridges. **[Gujarat CET 2016, NEET-I 2020, 16]**
- Genetically engineered insulin is produced in *E. coli*. **[NEET 2020]**
- Gene therapy was given in 1990 to a 4-years-old girl with Adenosine Deaminase (ADA) deficiency. **[NEET 2020, 16]**
- An example of gene therapy is production of injectable hepatitis-B vaccine. **[NEET 2017]**
- PCR is now routinely used to detect HIV in suspected AIDS patients. **[NEET 2020]**
- The laws and rules to prevent unauthorised exploitation of bioresources are termed as bioethics. **[NEET 2020]**
- The exploitation of bioresources of a nation by multinational companies without authorisation from the concerned country is referred as biopiracy. **[NEET 2019, 18]**

Chapter Exercises

(A) Topical Exercise

Biotechnological Applications in Agriculture

1 Red biotechnology is applied to
(a) agricultural processes (b) medical processes
(c) Both (a) and (b) (d) industrial processes

2 Production of value added products like nutrition supplements, pharmaceuticals, fuels, etc., using transgenic crop is called
(a) genetic farming (b) molecular farming
(c) biotech farming (d) All of these

3 Which of the following depicts white biotechnology?
(a) Agricultural processes (b) Industrial processes
(c) Medical processes (d) All of these

4 Hirudin gene was first transferred into .... with the help of recombinant DNA technology.
(a) *Oryza sativa* (b) *Brassica napus*
(c) Wheat (d) Maize

5 Which of the following is an insecticidal protein produced by *Bacillus thuringiensis?*
(a) Rop (b) Hir
(c) Cry (d) Both (a) and (c)

6 Which *Bt* crop is recently recommended for cultivation in India?
(a) Cotton (b) Wheat (c) Soyabean (d) Rice

7 Which of the following statements is incorrect?
(a) *Bt* toxin gene has been cloned from the bacteria
(b) Genetic engineering works only on animals and has not yet been sucessfully used on plants
(c) Strains of *Bacillus thuringiensis* are used in producing bioinsecticidal plant
(d) Both (b) and (c)

8 Choose the incorrect match.
(a) *Bt* tobacco - *Escherichia coli*
(b) Lepidopterans - Tobacco budworm
(c) *Bt* cotton - High yield and pest resistant
(d) Golden rice - Vitamin-A

9 In Golden rice, phytoene synthase was transferred from
(a) *Erwinia* (b) *Narcissus*
(c) *Oryza sativa* (d) Both (a) and (c)

10 Which one of the following bacteria is to be used extensively in genetic engineering work in plants?
(a) *Clostridium septicum* (b) *Xanthomonas citri*
(c) *Bacillus coagulens* (d) *Agrobacterium tumefaciens*

11 Genetically modified tobacco plant with *Bt* gene is resistant to
(a) bollworms (b) hornworms
(c) hookworms (d) roundworms

12 Which of the following is a variety genetically engineered for masking the expression of native gene?
(a) *Bt* cotton (b) *Flavr Savr* tomato
(c) Golden rice (d) Both (a) and (c)

13 Which of the following plants have been genetically engineered to provide herbicide tolerance?
(a) Soyabean (b) Maize
(c) Apple (d) Both (a) and (b)

14 The slow ripening transgenic tomato was developed in USA by using
(a) antisense RNA technology
(b) ribozyme technology
(c) cosuppression approach
(d) transgene silencing approach

15 An artificial seed is raised from
(a) meristem (b) root tip
(c) somatic embryo (d) immature seed

16 Which of the following statements is correct about SCID?
(a) It is caused by a mutation in Adenosine Deaminase (ADA) gene
(b) WBCs are not formed in SCID
(c) A functional DNA of ADA introduced into lymphocytes to cure SCID
(d) All of the above

17 Which of the following is correct?
(a) The proteins encoded by the genes *cry* IAc and *cry* IIAb control cotton bollworms
(b) Protein encoded by *cry* IAb controls corn borer
(c) Proteins encoded by *cry* IAc and *cry* IAb control flies
(d) Both (a) and (b)

18 Source of genes for high vitamin content in Golden rice is
(a) daffodils (b) *Erwinia*
(c) Both (a) and (b) (d) None of these

19 A transgenic plant is one in which
(a) a gene from another plant is introduced
(b) a gene from an animal is introduced
(c) a gene from a microorganism is introduced
(d) All of the above

Biotechnological Applications in Animal

20 Pathophysiology is the [NCERT Exemplar]
(a) study of physiology of pathogen
(b) study of normal physiology of host
(c) study of altered physiology of host
(d) None of the above

21 C-peptide of human insulin is [NCERT Exemplar]
(a) a part of mature insulin molecule
(b) responsible for formation of disulphide bridges
(c) removed during maturation of proinsulin to insulin
(d) responsible for its biological activity

22 Which of the following is a second generation vaccine?
(a) DPT (b) Cholera
(c) Hepatitis-B (d) None of these

23 Why is insulin not administered orally to diabetic patient?
(a) Insulin is bitter in taste
(b) Insulin is a peptide
(c) Insulin will lead to sudden decrease in blood sugar if given orally
(d) Insulin leads to peptic ulcer if given orally

24 Which of the following statements is false?
(a) Insulin was originally extracted from pancreas of slaughtered pigs and cattle
(b) Animal insulin is difficult to obtain
(c) Animal insulin is identical to human insulin
(d) Non-human insulin caused some patients to develop allergy

25 The company which developed human insulin is
(a) Eli Lilly (b) Calgene
(c) Caltech (d) Genentech

26 In which year, the first genetically engineered product was approved for medical use?
(a) 1972 (b) 1982
(c) 1992 (d) 1973

27 hGH extracted from dead human may result into genetic disease known as
(a) Severe combined immuno deficiency disease
(b) Pituitary dwarfism
(c) Creutzfeldt Jakob
(d) Cystic fibrosis

28 Transgenic animal has
(a) Foreign DNA in all its cells
(b) Foreign RNA in all its cells
(c) Foreign DNA in some of the cell
(d) Both (b) and (c)

29 α-1 antitrypsin is
(a) an antacid (b) an enzyme
(c) used to treat arthritis (d) used to treat emphysema

30 Human gene therapy requires
(a) gene isolation
(b) introduction of DNA into target cells
(c) inclusion of a promoter sequence
(d) All of the above

31 Hybridomas are employed for
(a) production of antibiotics
(b) treatment of cancer
(c) synthesis of monoclonal antibodies
(d) alcohol fermentation

32 Myeloma cells are used in hybridoma technology because
(a) they cannot grow in tissue culture
(b) they can grow infinitely
(c) they are non-cancerous cells
(d) they are easily available

33 Monoclonal antibodies are
(a) single parent type that attack many antigens
(b) single parent type and attack specific antigen
(c) various parent types and attack many antigens
(d) various parent types and attack single antigen

34 Which gene was introduced in the first transgenic cow?
(a) Human α-lactalbumin (b) α-1-antitrypsin
(c) β-1-antitrypsin (d) *cry* IAc

35 The ions which cannot cross the cell membrane due to cystic fibrosis are
(a) Cl^- ions (b) Na^{2+} ions
(c) H^+ ions (d) Mg^{2+} ions

36 Nexia biotechnologies spliced spider genes into the cells of lactating
(a) cow (b) sheep
(c) goat (d) buffalo

37 Resistance to antibiotics is a genetic trait that spreads naturally from one type of bacterium to
(a) almost any other type of bacterium
(b) another bacterium of the same strain
(c) eukaryotic cells of all types
(d) any other cell containing copy DNA

38 Silencing of a gene could be achieved through the use of
(a) short interfering RNA (b) antisense RNA
(c) Both (a) and (b) (d) None of these

Ethical Issues

39 A patent is granted for
I. An invention
II. Strains of microorganisms
III. Process of generating a product
IV. An improvement in an earlier invention
Codes
(a) I, II and III (b) II, III and IV
(c) I, III and IV (d) I, II, III and IV

40 Biopatents are usually awarded for the discovery of
(a) new cell lines
(b) new DNA sequences
(c) GM strains
(d) All of the above

41 Biopiracy is
(a) the use of biological patent
(b) thefts of plants and animals
(c) the use of bioresources of a country without proper authorisation
(d) stealing of biological resources

42 Which Indian plants have either been patented or attempts have been made to patent them by Western nations for their use?
(a) Basmati rice (b) Turmeric
(c) Neem (d) All of these

43 Which one is known as 'Superbug'?
(a) *Pseudomonas putida*
(b) *E. coli*
(c) *Aspergillus niger*
(d) *Acetobacter aceti*

44 The superbug can be used to control ....
(a) oil spills
(b) water pollution
(c) eutrophication
(d) air pollution

45 Brazzein is produced by
(a) *Pentadiplandra brazzeana*
(b) *Curcuma longa*
(c) *Azadirachta indica*
(d) None of the above

46 In which year, a USA lab granted a patent to the medical centre, University of Missisippi for the use of turmeric?
(a) 1959 (b) 1995
(c) 1986 (d) 1997

47 Biosensors are
(a) enzymes used in industries
(b) analytic devices used to monitor the product of biological process
(c) used to detect abnormal toxins in body
(d) Both (b) and (c)

48 Biological weapons convention and treaty given in
(a) 1972 (b) 1942
(c) 1932 (d) 1955

49 Which of these can be a defence against bioweapon?
(a) Protective shelter (b) Immunisation
(c) Gas mask (d) All of these

50 Which of the following diseases are caused by bioweapon agents?
I. Smallpox II. Anthrax
III. Tularemia IV. Cancer
Codes
(a) Only I (b) Only II
(c) II and IV (d) I, II and III

51 A branch of ethics, philosophy and social commentary that deals with the biological sciences and their impact on society is known as
(a) bioethics (b) biopatent
(c) biopiracy (d) biowar

52 Rules of conduct that may be used to regulate our activities in relation to the biological world is called
(a) Bioethics (b) Biowar
(c) Biopiracy (d) Biopatent

53 GEAC stands for **[NCERT Exemplar]**
(a) Genome Engineering Action Committee
(b) Ground Environment Action Committee
(c) Genetic Engineering Approval Committee
(d) Genetic and Environment Approval Committee

54 Select the correct statement(s).
virus or bacteria
(a) In biowar, virus or bacteria can be used as bioweapons
(b) Botulinum toxin can be a potent bioweapon
(c) Tularemia, *Bacillus anthracis*, *Vibrio* are used in biowar
(d) All the above statements are correct

(B) Cumulative Exercise

(Assorted Questions of the Chapter for Advanced Level Practice)

1 Find out the pairs, which are correctly matched?

I. Cyanobacteria – Biopesticides
II. Mycorrhiza – Solubilisation of phosphate
III. *Bacillus thuringiensis* – Cry protein
IV. Single cell protein – *Rhizobium*

Codes

(a) I and II (b) II and III
(c) III and IV (d) I, II and III

2 Match the following columns.

	Column I		Column II
A	Gene therapy	1.	Effort to fix functional gene
B.	Humulin	2.	A single-stranded DNA or RNA tagged with a radioactive molecule
C.	Probe	3.	Diagnostic test
D.	ELISA	4.	Diabetes

Codes

	A	B	C	D		A	B	C	D
(a)	1	4	2	3	(b)	4	2	3	1
(c)	2	3	1	4	(d)	3	1	4	2

3. Consider the following statements.

I. In ADA deficiency, bone marrow treatment does not help in curing the disease.
II. The human Growth Hormone (hGH) was produced by genetically engineered methods by Calgene.
III. The N_2 fixing ability of bacteria can be increased by expression of *nif* gene.
IV Tracy was the first goat that produced milk with AAT.

Choose the option with containing correct statement(s).

(a) I, II and III (b) I and IV
(c) Only III (d) II, III and IV

4 When DNA is transcribed into *m*RNA, usually the *m*RNA remains single-stranded but in some cases, an RNA can be made that is complementary to the *m*RNA. This is called .... and its main function is to ....

(a) antisense RNA, block gene expression
(b) antisense RNA, amplify *m*RNA
(c) antisense RNA, enhance translation
(d) reverse transcription, enhance translation

5 The bacterium, *Pseudomonas* is useful because of its ability to

(a) transfer gene from one plant to another
(b) decompose a variety of organic compounds
(c) fix atmospheric nitrogen in the soil
(d) produce a wide variety of antibiotics

6 Match the following columns.

Column I	Column II
A. Virus resistance	1. 2, 4-D
B. Somatic hybridisation	2. Coat protein gene
C. Callus culture	3. PEG
D. Vinegar	4. *cry* gene
E. Insect resistance	5. Fermentation

Codes

	A	B	C	D	E
(a)	3	2	1	4	5
(b)	5	4	2	3	1
(c)	2	3	1	5	4
(d)	1	2	3	4	5

7 Consider the following statements.

I. In CFTR treatment, *c*DNA is introduced in epithelial cells of lungs.
II. HAT medium is used for the production of monoclonal antibodies.
III. In monoclonal antibodies production, hybridomas are hybrid cells of myeloma and B-cells.
IV. CFTR is a chloride ion channel protein in epithelial and endothelial cells.
V. CFTR is caused by addition of three bases in gene.

Choose the correct option.

(a) I, II and III
(b) II, III and IV
(c) I, III, IV and V
(d) I, II, III, IV and V

8 Match the following columns.

Column I	Column II
A. *Bacillus thuringiensis*	1. Production of chitinases
B. *Rhizobium meliloti*	2. Scavenging of oil spills
C. *Escherichia coli*	3. Incorporation of '*nif*' gene
D. *Pseudomonas putida*	4. Production of *Bt* toxin
E. *Trichoderma*	5. Production of human insulin

Codes

	A	B	C	D	E
(a)	2	4	1	5	3
(b)	2	4	5	1	3
(c)	4	3	5	2	1
(d)	4	2	5	3	1

9 Frequent coughing or wheezing that produce mucus, shortness of breath, tightness in chest are some symptoms of emphysema. Which of the following transgenic human protein product has been used to treat it?

I. α-1-antitrypsin
II. α-1-globulin
III. Cry IAb protein
IV. Cry II Ac protein

Codes
(a) I and III
(b) II and IV
(c) I and II
(d) Only II

10 Consider the following statements.

I. Milstein and Kohler discovered hybridoma technology.
II. Creutzfeldt Jakob Disease (CJD) occurs due to side effect of insulin.
III. Factor VIII is a blood clotting factor and is used to treat haemophilia.
IV. The promoter of β lactoglobulin can be activated in mammary gland cells.
V. *Brassica campestris*, *Punica granatum* and *Curcuma longa* had been patented by US companies.

Choose the correct option.
(a) I, II, III, IV
(b) III, IV, V
(c) II, III, IV, V
(d) I, III, IV, V

11 Kohler and Milstein developed biotechnology for the production of
(a) myelomas
(b) steroid conversion
(c) monoclonal antibodies
(d) immobilised enzymes

Assertion and Reason

Direction (Q. Nos. 12-17) *In each of the following questions, a statement of Assertion (A) is followed by corresponding statement of Reason (R). Of the statements mark the correct answer as*

(a) Both A and R are true and R is the correct explanation of A
(b) Both A and R are true, but R is not the correct explanation of A
(c) A is true, but R is false
(d) A is false, but R is true
(e) Both A and R are false

12 **Assertion** (A) Transgenic plant production is an application of plant tissue culture.

Reason (R) An organism that contains and expresses a transgene is called transgenic organism.

13 **Assertion** (A) Hirudin is a protein that stimulates blood clotting.

Reason (R) The gene encoding hirudin is transferred into *Brassica napus*, where hirudin is accumulated in seeds.

14 **Assertion** (A) A crop expressing a *cry* gene is usually resistant to a group of insects.

Reason (R) Cry protein produced from *Bacillus thuringiensis* is toxic to larvae of certain insects.

15 **Assertion** (A) *Flavr Savr*, a transgenic tomato remains fresh and retains their flavour for a long time.

Reason (R) Production of polygalacturonase enzyme, which degrades pectin, was blocked in *Flavr Savr.*

16 **Assertion** (A) Ti-plasmid obtained from *Agrobacterium tumefaciens* is effectively used as a vector for gene transfer in plant cells.

Reason (R) The part of Ti-plasmid transferred into the DNA of plant cells is called as T-DNA.

17 **Assertion** (A) Transgenic mouse is termed as 'supermouse' because it is twice as big in size than the normal mouse.

Reason (R) In 'supermouse', the gene for human growth factor has been introduced and expressed.

(C) Medical Entrances' Gallery

(Collection of Questions Asked in NEET & in Various Medical Entrance Exams)

1 RNA interference is used for which of the following purposes in the field of biotechnology? **[NEET 2020]**

(a) to develop a plant tolerant to abiotic stresses
(b) to develop a pest resistant plant against infestation by nematode
(c) to enhance the mineral usage by the plant
(d) to reduce post harvest losses

2 The laws and rules to prevent unauthorised exploitation of bioresources are termed as **[NEET 2020]**

(a) biopatenting
(b) bioethics
(c) bioengineering
(d) biopiracy

3 Match the following columns and select the correct option.

	Column I		Column II
A.	*Bt* cotton	1.	Gene therapy
B.	Adenosine deaminase deficiency	2.	Cellular defence
C.	RNAi	3.	Detection of HIV infection
D.	PCR	4.	*Bacillus thuringiensis*

Codes **[NEET 2020]**

	A	B	C	D
(a)	3	2	1	4
(b)	2	3	4	1
(c)	1	2	3	4
(d)	4	1	2	3

4 Which of the following statements is not correct? **[NEET 2020]**

(a) The proinsulin has an extra peptide called C-peptide
(b) The functional insulin has A and B chains linked together by hydrogen bonds
(c) Genetically engineered insulin is produced in *E. coli*
(d) In man, insulin is synthesised as a proinsulin

5 What triggers activation of protoxin to act of *Bacillus thuringiensis* in bollworm? **[NEET 2019, CBSE AIPMT 2015]**

(a) Moist surface of midgut
(b) Alkaline pH of gut
(c) Acidic pH of stomach
(d) Body temperature

6 In RNAi, genes are silenced using **[NEET 2019]**

(a) *ss*DNA
(b) *ds*DNA
(c) *ds*RNA
(d) *ss*RNA

7 Which of the following is true for Golden rice? **[NEET 2019]**

(a) It is pest resistant, with a gene from *Bacillus thuringiensis*
(b) It is drought tolerant, developed using *Agrobacterium* vector
(c) It has yellow grains, because of a gene introduced from a primitive variety of rice
(d) It is vitamin-A enriched, with a gene from daffodil

8 Exploitation of bioresources of a nation by multinational companies without authorisation from the concerned country is referred to as **[NEET 2019, 18]**

(a) bioweapon (b) biopiracy
(c) bioethics (d) biowar

9 Silencing of a gene/specific *m*RNA translation could be achieved through the use of **[KCET 2018]**

(a) RNA only
(b) Antisense RNA only
(c) Both RNA and antisense RNA
(d) None of the above

10 Choose the correct option for the toxic protein produced by *B. thuringiensis.* **[Gujarat CET 2017]**

(a) It acts in acidic medium and binds to epithelial cells of foregut
(b) It acts in neutral medium and binds to epithelial cells of hindgut
(c) It acts in alkaline medium and binds to epithelial cells of foregut
(d) It acts in alkaline medium and binds to epithelial cells of midgut

11 An example of gene therapy is **[NEET 2017]**

(a) Production of injectable hepatitis-B vaccine
(b) Production of vaccines in food crops like potatoes, which can be eaten
(c) Introduction of gene for adenosine deaminase persons suffering from Severe Combined Immuno Deficiency (SCID)
(d) Production of test tube babies by artificial insemination and implantation of fertilised eggs

12 Which part of the tobacco plant is infected by *Meloidogyne incognita*? **[NEET-I 2016]**

(a) Flower (b) Leaf (c) Stem (d) Root

13 Which kind of therapy was given in 1990 to a 4-years-old girl with Adenosine Deaminase (ADA) deficiency? **[NEET 2016]**

(a) Gene therapy (b) Chemotherapy
(b) Immunotherapy (d) Radiation therapy

14 The two polypeptides of human insulin are linked together by **[NEET-I 2016]**

(a) phosphodiester bonds
(b) covalent bonds
(c) disulphide bridges
(d) hydrogen bonds

15 What is indicated by *A* in the figure?

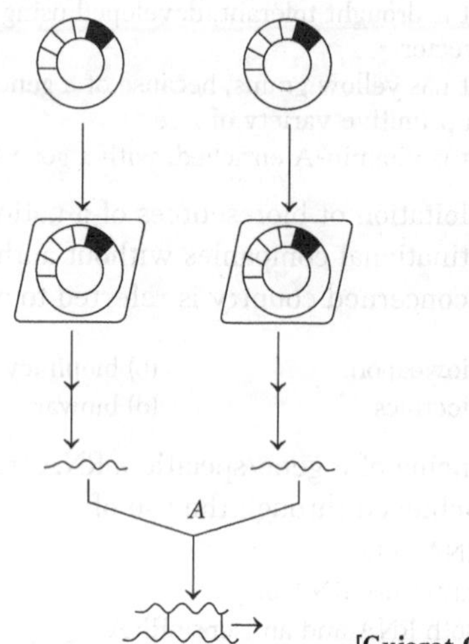

[Gujarat CET 2016]

(a) Peptide bond (b) Disulphide bond
(c) Glycosidic bond (d) Hydrophobic bond

16 Match the following columns.

Column I	Column II
A Golden rice	1. Cross breed hybrid
B. IR-8 rice	2. Somatic hybrid
C. Himgiri	3. Semi-dwarf variety
D. Pomato	4. Genetically modified crop

Codes **[EAMCET 2015]**

	A	B	C	D
(a)	4	1	2	3
(b)	4	3	1	2
(c)	2	4	1	3
(d)	1	3	4	2

17 Hepatitis-B vaccine is **[UK PMT 2015]**

(a) combined vaccine
(b) recombinant antigen vaccine
(c) polysaccharide vaccine
(d) DNA vaccine

18 Human insulin is being commercially produced from transgenic species of **[UK PMT 2015]**

(a) *E. coli*
(b) *Brassica napus*
(c) *Bacillus thuringiensis*
(d) *Agrobacterium*

19 One of the advantages of developing transgenic mice is that it is very useful **[COMEDK 2015]**

(a) to study vaccine safety
(b) in producing new varieties of mice
(c) in developing a show piece example
(d) in gene targeting

20 Clot formation can be prevented by treatment with ..... in gene therapy. **[MHT CET 2015]**

(a) DNase (b) Recombinant vaccine
(c) TPA (d) TGF-B

21 Transgenic animals are generally produced for all of the following needs except **[MHT CET 2015]**

(a) testing of chemical safety
(b) testing of vaccine safety
(c) stimulation of pathogenicity
(d) production of pharmacologically important proteins

22 In which field, application of biotechnology occurs? **[Gujarat CET 2015]**

(a) Bio-medicine (b) Agriculture
(c) Environment field (d) All of these

23 What is true about *Bt* toxin? **[CBSE AIPMT 2009]**

(a) The inactive protoxin gets converted into active form due to alkaline pH of the insect gut
(b) *Bt* protein exists as an active toxin in the *Bacillus*
(c) The activated toxin enters the ovaries of the pest to sterilise it and thus prevent its multiplication
(d) The concerned *Bacillus* has antitoxins

24 A desirable change in genotype of an organism is obtained by **[MHT CET 2015]**

(a) DNA replication (b) protein synthesis
(c) *r*DNA technology (d) *m*RNA formation

25 More than 95% of transgenic animals are **[MHT CET 2015]**

(a) rabbits (b) mice (c) fish (d) cows

26 Select the wrong statement. **[Kerala CEE 2015]**

(a) Human insulin is being commercially produced from a transgenic species of *Escherichia coli*
(b) Genetically modified *Bacillus thuringiensis* is used as biopesticide on commercial scale
(c) Human protein, α-1 antitrypsin, is used to treat emphysema
(d) *Bt* toxin gene *cry* IAc controls corn borer
(e) First transgenic cow, Rosie produced α-lactalbumin enriched milk

27 What is the advantage of clinical use of humulin over use of conventional ox or pig insulin? **[COMEDK 2015]**

(a) It does not cause immunological problems
(b) It is cheaper for the patient
(c) It is produced by *E. coli* in our intestine
(d) There is no advantage

28 Which one is wrong in relation to transgenic *Bt* cotton plant? **[WB JEE 2015]**

(a) Crop yield loss due to attack by *Bacillus thuringiensis* bacterium is reduced
(b) Crop yield loss due to attack by lepidopteran insect pest is reduced
(c) Use of chemical insecticides in the cotton field is minimised
(d) Better quality cotton is produced

29 Antibodies produced by a group of identical B-cells against a single epitope of an antigen is called **[UK PMT 2015]**

(a) polyclonal antibodies
(b) monoclonal antibodies
(c) antihapten antibodies
(d) somaclonal antibodies

30 Gene therapy has been successful in curing genetic diseases in laboratory animals through **[UK PMT 2015]**

(a) exposure to X-ray to rectify the defective gene
(b) replacing the defective gene with a functional gene
(c) oral delivery of genes
(d) use of therapeutic medicines to rectify the defective genes

31 The first human hormone produced by recombinant DNA technology is **[CBSE AIPMT 2014]**

(a) insulin (b) oestrogen
(c) thyroxine (d) progesterone

32 *In vitro* clonal propagation in plants is characterised by **[CBSE AIPMT 2014]**

(a) PCR and RAPD
(b) Northern blotting
(c) electrophoresis and HPLC
(d) microscopy

33 The inactive protoxin is activated in the gut of the insect by **[MHT CET 2014]**

(a) acidic pH (b) alkaline pH
(c) low temperature (d) high temperature

34 In India, research in genetic modification of organisms and safety issues are controlled by **[MHT CET 2014]**

(a) DBT (b) IARI
(c) CSIR (d) GEAC

35 Which is correct regarding genetically engineered insulin using *E. coli* ? **[MHT CET 2014]**

(a) Difficult to purify
(b) Obtained in large unlimited quantities
(c) Possibility of transmission of animal diseases
(d) Insulin obtained varies in chemical structure

36 Ernst Chain and Howard Florey's contribution was **[Kerala CEE 2014]**

(a) discovery of streptokinase
(b) establishing the potential of penicillin as an effective antibiotic
(c) discovery of the DNA sequences
(d) isolating the bacterial plasmid
(e) production of genetically engineered insulin

37 Insect pest resistant *Bt* cotton plant was developed using **[B JEE 2014]**

(a) somaclonal variation (b) micropropagation
(c) somatic hybridisation (d) transgenic technology

38 The strategy used to prevent the nematode infection in the roots of tobacco plants is called **[J&K CET 2014]**

(a) use of agrochemicals (b) *Bt* toxin gene
(c) gene mutation (d) RNA interference

39 Name the nematode which infects the roots of tobacco plants **[UK PMT 2014]**

(a) *Bacillus thuringiensis* (b) *cry* IAc
(c) *Meloidogyne incognita* (d) None of these

40 A transgenic food crop which may help in solving the problem of night blindness in developing countries is **[UK PMT 2014]**

(a) *Bt* soyabean (b) Golden rice
(c) *Flavr Savr* tomatoes (d) Starlink maize

41 Match the following columns. **[EAMCET 2014]**

Column I	Column II
A RNAi	1. Cotton bollworms
B. ELISA	2. Early detection of HIV
C. PCR	3. *Meloidogyne* resistance
D. *cry* IAb	4. Antigen-antibody
	5. Corn borer

Codes

	A	B	C	D		A	B	C	D
(a)	3	4	2	5	(b)	4	3	1	5
(c)	2	3	5	4	(d)	5	1	3	2

42 RNA interference which is employed in making tobacco plant resistant to *Meloidogyne incognita* is essentially involved in preventing the process of **[Karnataka CET 2014]**

(a) translation of *m*RNA
(b) transcription
(c) replication of DNA
(d) splicing of *hn*RNA

43 ADA deficiency results in **[Karnataka CET 2014]**

(a) increased risk of infertility
(b) inability of the immune system to function normally
(c) chromosomal disorders
(d) decrease in the yield of crop plants

44 Select the correct option for the given statements I, II and III.

I. A transgenic cow, Rosie produced human protein-enriched milk, which was nutritionally more balanced product for human babies than natural cow milk.

II. Milk produced by transgenic cow, Rosie contains 2.4 gm protein/L.

III. In the above mentioned milk in II statement, alpha-lactalbumin is present. **[Gujarat CET 2014]**

Codes

(a) Statements I, II and III are true and statement III does not give correct explanation of I
(b) Statements I, II and III are true and statement III gives correct explanation for I
(c) Statements I and II are true, statement III is false
(d) Statements I and II are false, statement III is true

45 Which of the following *Bt* crops is being grown in India by the farmers? **[NEET 2013]**

(a) Soyabean (b) Maize
(c) Cotton (d) Brinjal

46 Which of the following represents the action of insulin? **[NEET 2013]**

(a) Increases blood glucose levels by stimulating glucagon production
(b) Decreases blood glucose levels by forming glycogen
(c) Increases blood glucose level by promoting cellular uptake of glucose
(d) Increases blood glucose levels by hydrolysis of glycogen

47 Which one of the following vectors is used to replace the defective gene in gene therapy? **[NEET 2013]**

(a) Adenovirus (b) Cosmid
(c) Ri-plasmid (d) Ti-plasmid

48 *Bt* cotton is resistant to **[Manipal 2013]**

(a) Insects (b) Herbicides
(c) Salt resistant (d) Drought resistant

49 Which one of the following bacterium is used for the production of transgenic plants? **[WB JEE 2013]**

(a) *Escherichia coli* (b) *Pseudomonas*
(c) *Staphylococcus aureus* (d) *Agrobacterium tumefaciens*

50 *Bt* brinjal is an example of transgenic crops. In this, *Bt* refers to **[KCET 2013]**

(a) *Bacillus tuberculosis* (b) Biotechnology
(c) β-carotene (d) *Bacillus thuringiensis*

51 Choose the correct option for the toxic protein produced by *B. thuringiensis*, it acts in **[Gujarat CET 2013]**

(a) neutral medium and binds to epithelial cells of hindgut
(b) acidic medium and binds to epithelial cells of foregut
(c) alkaline medium and binds to epithelial cells of foregut
(d) alkaline medium and binds to epithelial cells of midgut

52 Cells obtained from cancerous tumours are known as **[MP PMT 2012]**

(a) hybridomas (b) myelomas
(c) lymphocyte (d) monoclonal cells

53 Consumption of which of the following foods can prevent the kind of blindness associated with vitamin-A deficiency? **[CBSE PMT (Pre) 2012]**

(a) *Bt* soyabean (b) Golden rice
(c) *Flavr Savr* tomatoes (d) Starlink maize

54 The first clinical gene therapy was given for treating **[CBSE AIPMT 2012]**

(a) diabetes mellitus
(b) chicken pox
(c) rheumatoid arthritis
(d) adenosine deaminase deficiency

55 Tobacco plants resistant to a nematode have been developed by the introduction of DNA that produced (in the host cells). **[CBSE AIPMT 2012]**

(a) Both sense and antisense RNA
(b) A particular hormone
(c) An antifeedant
(d) A toxin protein

56 '*cry*' gene is obtained from **[MHT CET 2014, COMEDK 2014, KCET 2012]**

(a) *Agrobacterium tumefaciens* (b) *Bacillus thuringiensis*
(c) *Rhizobium leguminosarum* (d) *Rhizobium phaseoli*

57 α-1 antitrypsin (AAT) protein is used to treat which disease? **[AFMC 2012]**

(a) Dwarfism (b) CJD
(c) Both (a) and (b) (d) Emphysema

58 Basic principle of developing transgenic plant and animals is to introduce the gene of interest into the nucleus of **[WB JEE 2012]**

(a) somatic cell (b) vegetative cell
(c) germ cell (d) body cell

59 In transgenic, expression of transgene in target tissue is determined by **[Manipal 2012]**

(a) enhancer (b) transgene
(c) promoter (d) reporter gene

60 Which transgenic animal has been given human genes for organ transplantation into human without risk of rejection? **[MP PMT 2011]**

(a) Cow (b) Sheep (c) Goat (d) Pig

61 Maturation of genetically engineered proinsulin into insulin takes place after **[MP PMT 2011]**

(a) Joining of C-peptide
(b) Removal of C-peptide
(c) Removal of disulphide bridge
(d) All of the above

62 GM brinjal in India has been developed for resistance against **[Rajasthan PMT 2011]**
(a) virus
(b) bacteria
(c) fungi
(d) insects

63 The protein products of the following *Bt* toxin genes *cry* I Ac and *cry* II Ab are responsible for controlling **[DUMET 2011]**
(a) bollworm
(b) roundworm
(c) moth
(d) fruitfly

64 Some of the characteristics of *Bt* cotton are **[CBSE AIPMT 2011]**
(a) long fibre and resistance of aphids
(b) medium yield, long fibre and resistance to beetle pests
(c) high yield and production of toxic protein crystals which kill dipteran pests
(d) high yield and resistance to bollworms

65 *cry* II Ab and *cry* I Ab produced toxins that control **[Kerala CEE 2011]**
(a) cotton bollworms and corn borer, respectively
(b) corn borer and cotton bollworms, respectively
(c) tobacco budworms and nematodes, respectively
(d) nematodes and tobacco budworms, respectively
(e) corn borer and tobacco budworms, respectively

66 The bacterium *Bacillus thuringiensis* is widely used in contemporary biology as a/an **[CBSE AIPMT 2011]**
(a) indicator of water pollution
(b) insecticide
(c) agent for production of dairy products
(d) source of industrial enzyme

67 What is true about *Bt* toxin? **[CBSE AIPMT 2011]**
(a) The inactive protoxin gets converted into active form in the insect gut
(b) *Bt* protein exists as active toxin in the *Bacillus*
(c) The activated toxin enters the ovaries of the pest to sterilise it and thus, prevents its multiplication
(d) The concerned *Bacillus* has antitoxins

68 Product of biotechnology is **[BHU 2011]**
(a) transgenic crops (GM crops)
(b) humulin
(c) biofertiliser
(d) All of the above

69 Main objective of production/use of herbicide resistant GM crops is to **[CBSE AIPMT 2011]**
(a) eliminate weeds from the field without the use of the manual labour
(b) eliminate weeds from the field without the use of herbicides
(c) encourage eco-friendly herbicides
(d) reduce herbicide accumulation in food articles for health safety

70 Cultivation of *Bt* cotton has been much in the news. The prefix *Bt* means **[AIIMS 2011]**
(a) barium-treated cotton seeds
(b) bigger thread variety of cotton with better tensile strength
(c) produced by biotechnology using restriction enzymes and ligases
(d) carrying an endotoxin gene from *Bacillus thuringiensis*

ANSWERS

Check Point 22.1

1. (c)	2. (c)	3. (a)	4. (c)	5. (d)

Check Point 22.2

1. (d)	2. (b)	3. (c)	4. (a)	5. (a)	6. (a)

Check Point 22.3

1. (c)	2. (d)	3. (b)	4. (c)	5. (a)

(A) Topical Exercise

1. (b)	2. (b)	3. (b)	4. (b)	5. (c)	6. (a)	7. (b)	8. (a)	9. (b)	10. (d)
11. (a)	12. (b)	13. (d)	14. (a)	15. (c)	16. (d)	17. (d)	18. (c)	19. (d)	20. (c)
21. (c)	22. (c)	23. (b)	24. (c)	25. (a)	26. (a)	27. (c)	28. (a)	29. (d)	30. (d)
31. (c)	32. (b)	33. (b)	34. (a)	35. (a)	36. (c)	37. (b)	38. (c)	39. (c)	40. (d)
41. (c)	42. (d)	43. (a)	44. (a)	45. (a)	46. (b)	47. (d)	48. (a)	49. (b)	50. (d)
51. (a)	52. (a)	53. (c)	54. (d)						

(B) Cumulative Exercise

1. (d)	2. (a)	3. (c)	4. (a)	5. (b)	6. (c)	7. (a)	8. (c)	9. (c)	10. (d)
11. (c)	12. (b)	13. (d)	14. (a)	15. (a)	16. (b)	17. (a)			

(C) Medical Entrances' Gallery

1. (b)	2. (b)	3. (d)	4. (b)	5. (b)	6. (c)	7. (d)	8. (b)	9. (c)	10. (d)
11. (a)	12. (d)	13. (a)	14. (c)	15. (b)	16. (b)	17. (b)	18. (a)	19. (a)	20. (c)
21. (c)	22. (d)	23. (a)	24. (c)	25. (b)	26. (e)	27. (a)	28. (d)	29. (a)	30. (b)
31. (a)	32. (a)	33. (b)	34. (d)	35. (b)	36. (b)	37. (d)	38. (d)	39. (c)	40. (b)
41. (a)	42. (a)	43. (b)	44. (b)	45. (c)	46. (b)	47. (a)	48. (a)	49. (d)	50. (d)
51. (d)	52. (b)	53. (b)	54. (d)	55. (a)	56. (b)	57. (d)	58. (c)	59. (c)	60. (d)
61. (b)	62. (d)	63. (a)	64. (d)	65. (a)	66. (b)	67. (a)	68. (d)	69. (d)	70. (d)

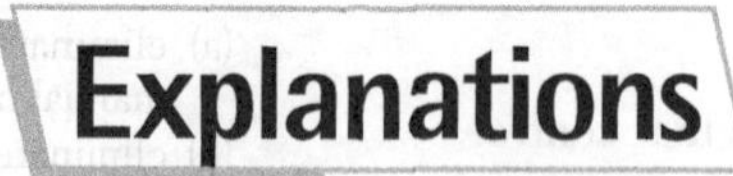

Explanations

(A) Topical Exercise

7 (*b*) Statement in option (b) is incorrect and can be corrected as

Genetic engineering can be used to produce plants having desired traits like higher nutritional value, disease resistance, etc.

8 (*a*) Option (a) represents incorrect match and can be corrected as

Bt tobacco is genetically engineered crop which is obtained by a gene from *Bacillus thuringiensis* (*Bt*) bacteria.

24 (*c*) Statement in option (c) is false and can be corrected as

Animal insulin differs from human insulin in one or a few amino acids. Due to this, it elicit allergic responses in some people.

(B) Cumulative Exercise

3 (*c*) Only statement III is correct. Rest other statements are incorrect and can be corrected as

- In ADA deficiency, both bone marrow transplantation and enzyme replacement therapy helps in treating the disease.
- The human growth hormone was engineered genetically by the company Genentech.
- Tracy was the first sheep that produced milk with AAT.

11 (*c*) Kohler and Milstein developed biotechnology for the production of monoclonal antibodies. Monoclonal antibodies are produced by a single clone of cells and consists of identical antibodies. They are produced *via* hybridoma technology.

12 (*b*) Both A and R are true, but R is not the correct explanation of A.

Plant tissue culture has various applications in different fields of biology. An example of this is the production of transgenic plants and animals. Transgenic organisms contain genes, which are transferred through genetic engineering. These genes are known as transgenes.

13 (*d*) A is false, but R is true because

Hirudin is a protein which prevents blood clotting. The genes responsible for the production of this blood preventing protein have been chemically synthesised and then transferred into *Brassica napus* (Brassicaceae). In the seeds of this plant, hirudin protein accumulates.

14 (*a*) Both A and R are true and R is the correct explanation of A.

Bacillus thuringiensis (*Bt*), a soil bacterium produces a Cry protein (crystal protein). This protein is toxic to larvae of certain insects. There are several kinds of Cry proteins. Each Cry protein is toxic to a different group of insects. The gene encoding Cry protein that is *cry* gene has been isolated and transferred into several crops.

A crop expressing a *cry* gene is usually resistant to the groups of insects.

15 (*a*) Both A and R are true and R is the correct explanation of A.

'*Flavr Savr*' is a transgenic tomato variety. Fruits of this variety remain fresh and retain their flavour much longer than normal fruits. It happens in the blockage of the production of pectin degrading enzyme, polygalacturonase.

16 (*b*) Both A and R are true, but R is not the correct explanation of A.

Agrobacterium tumefaciens, a pathogen of several dicot plants can transfer a piece of DNA called (T-DNA) to transform normal plant cell into a tumour cell. Ti-plasmid of *Agrobacterium tumefaciens* and Ri plasmid of *A. rhizogens* are best known plant cloning vectors. *Agrobacterium* is natural genetic engineer of plants.

17 (*a*) Both A and R are true and R is the correct explanation of A.

Palmiter and Brinster (1981) developed the first transgenic animal 'supermouse'. It has human growth hormone gene. It has been introduced and expressed. Size of supermouse is big in size than the normal mouse.

(C) Medical Entrances' Gallery

1 (*b*) RNA interference is used to develop a pest resistant plant against infestation by nematode. RNA interference takes place in all eukaryotic organisms as a method of cellular defence. This method involves silencing of a specific *m*RNA due to a complementary *ds*RNA molecule that binds to and prevents translation of the *m*RNA (silencing).

2 (*b*) Bioethics are sets of laws and rules to prevent unauthorised exploitation of bioresources. Other options are explained as

Biopiracy is the use of bioresources by multinational companies and other organisations without proper authorisation from the countries and people concerned without compensatory payment.

Biopatenting is patent granted on biological products, organisms processes or bioresources.

Bioengineering is the application of the life sciences, physical sciences, mathematics and engineering principles to define and solve problems in biology, medicine, healthcare and other fields.

4 (*b*) Statement in option (b) is not correct and can be corrected as

Insulin is composed of two peptide chains referred to as the A chain and B chain. A and B chains are linked together by two disulphide bonds and an additional disulphide is formed within the A chain. Insulin molecules have a tendency to form dimers in solution due to hydrogen-bonding between the C-terminal of B-chain.

5 (*b*) Alkaline pH of the insect gut triggers activation of protoxin to active *Bt* toxin of *Bacillus thuringiensis* in bollworm. The inactive protoxins contain toxic insecticidal protein crystals. When the alkaline pH of insect gut solubilises the crystals, the activated toxin binds to the epithelial cells of the midgut and creates pores. It causes the cell to swell and burst, eventually leads to the death of the insect.

6 (*c*) In RNAi, the genes are silenced using *ds*RNA. RNA interference (RNAi) takes place in all eukaryotic organisms as a method of cellular defence. This method involves silencing of a specific *m*RNA due to a complementary *ds*RNA molecule that binds to and prevents translation of the *m*RNA (silencing).

7 (*d*) Statement in option (d) is true.

Golden rice is genetically engineered variety of rice to biosynthesise β-carotene which is a precursor of vitamin-A. It contains *psy* gene (phytoene synthease) which is derived from daffodil.

Other statements are incorrect for Golden rice and can be corrected as

- Golden rice is neither drought tolerant nor pest resistant.
- The grains of Golden rice appear yellow due to high level of β-carotene in it.

8 (*b*) Exploitation of bioresources of a nation by multinational companies without authorisation from concerned country is referred to as biopiracy. For example, a patent granted in USA covers the entire basmati rice germplasm of our country.

10 (*d*) Toxin produced by *Bacillus thuringiensis* acts in alkaline medium and binds to epithelial cells of midgut and causes pores that leads to death of the insects.

Thus, option (d) is correct.

17 (*b*) Hepatitis-B vaccine is a second generation vaccine. It is a recombinant antigen vaccine.

19 (*a*) Transgenic mice is very useful in the studies of polio vaccine safety.

31 (*a*) Insulin is a peptide hormone, which controls the level of blood sugar. It is formed by joining of two polypeptide chains by disulphide bonds. In 1983, Eli Lilly Co., launched the first genetically engineered human insulin by the name humulin.

32 (*a*) *In vitro* clonal propagation in plants is characterised by PCR and RAPD.

RAPD stands for Random Amplified Polymorphic DNA. It is a type of PCR reaction, but the segments of DNA that are amplified are random. Often, PCR is used to amplify a known DNA sequence.

33 (*b*) *Bacillus thuringiensis* forms a protein crystal (Cry) during a particular phase of their growth. These crystals contain a toxic insecticidal protein.

Bt toxin protein exists as an inactive protoxins, but once it is ingested by the insect, the inactive toxin gets converted to the active form due to the alkaline pH of the gut, which helps in the solubilisation of these crystals.

The activated toxin then binds to the surface of midgut epithelial cells, creating pores that causes cell swelling and lysis. It leads to the death of the insects.

34 (*d*) The genetic modification of organisms can have unpredictable results due to introduction of such organisms into the ecosystem. Public is very concerned that certain companies are being granted patents for the products and technologies that make use of the genetic materials, plants and other biological resources that have long been developed by the farmers and indigenous people of a specific region/country.

In order to control these issues, Indian Government has set an organisation Genetic Engineering Approval Committee (GEAC) which controls all research in genetic modifications of organisms and other safety issues.

35 (*b*) The only correct option about genetically engineered insulin using *E. coli* is that it can be obtained in huge amounts and unlimited quantities. The other options given are not appropriate for insulin and can be corrected as

It is not difficult to purify. It does not allow transmission of animal diseases and insulin obtained does not vary in chemical structure.

36 (*b*) The first antibiotic was discovered by Alexander Fleming, while working on *Staphylococci* bacteria. The potential use of *Penicillium* as an effective antibiotic was established by Ernst Chain and Howard Florey. They were awarded Nobel Prize in 1945 for this work. *Penicillium* was extensively used in treating wounded American soldiers in World War-II.

37 (*d*) *Bt* cotton is a genetically modified variety of cotton producing an insecticide. It was produced by Monsanto by inserting *cry* gene coding for *Bt* toxin into cotton plant genome by using transgenic technology, causing cotton to produce this natural insecticide in its tissues.

This gene was obtained from *Bacillus thuringiensis*, while other techniques mentioned in the options such as somaclonal variation, somatic hybridisation and micropropagation are the methods that rely on tissue culture techniques of producing plants by using different plant parts. They do not involve the gene transfer.

38 (*d*) Nematode is a group of organisms which parasitise a large number of plants and animals including human beings. One of the most common nematodes (*Meloidogyne incognita*) infects the roots of tobacco plants and causes a great loss by causing reduction in yield. This infestation was prevented by using a novel strategy which was based on the process of RNA interference (RNAi).

39 (*c*) *Meloidogyne incognita* infects the roots of tobacco plant and causes great reduction in yield. RNAi is the strategy adopted to prevent this infection.

40 (*b*) Golden rice is a transgenic variety of rice (*Oryza sativa*) which contains good quantities of β-carotene (provitamin-A inactive state of vitamin-A). β-carotene is further converted into vitamin-A. Deficiency of vitamin-A causes night blindness and skin disorder. Thus, Golden rice may help in solving the problem of night blindness in developing countries.

42 (*a*) A nematode, *Meloidogyne incognita* infects the roots of tobacco plant and causes a great reduction in the yield. RNAi takes place in all eukaryotic organisms as a method of cellular defence. This method involves silencing of specific *m*RNA due to a complementary *ds*RNA molecule that binds to and prevent translation of *m*RNA.

43 (*b*) Adenosine deaminase deficiency is an autosomal recessive metabolic disorder which results in immunodeficiency. It is caused due to deficiency of enzyme adenosine deaminase. The defective gene leads to the accumulation of deoxyadenosine triphosphate which further blocks several metabolic pathways, i.e. inability of the immune system to function normally.

44 (*b*) Statements I, II, III are true and statement III gives correct explanation for I.

α-lactalbumin is one of the major proteins in milk (approx 1.5 gm/L). It is considered to be highly nutritious and this is the protein which is not only involved in the synthesis of lactose but it is also responsible for the milk production. The fact that the milk is nutrionally enriched (statement I) can be attributed to the increased production of α-lactalbumin (statement III).

47 (*a*) Adenovirus is non-enveloped *ds*DNA virus which causes respiratory diseases. It is used to transfer a gene of interest in animal cells. So, adenovirus is used to replace the defective gene in gene therapy.

48 (*a*) *Bt* cotton is produced by the insertion of insect resistance genes from bacterium *Bacillus thuringiensis* to cotton plant. This gene produces an insect resistant protein toxin crystals, called parasporal body (delta endotoxin) that can act as a microbial insecticide for specific insect groups.

49 (*d*) Plant cells do not have endogenous plasmids. The plasmid vectors used for plant cell transformation are mostly based on *Agrobacterium tumefaciens* Ti-plasmid. These are plant pathogenic Gram positive soil bacteria which cause crown gall disease of dicot plants.

50 (*d*) *Bt* brinjal is genetically modified insect resistance brinjal. It has gene for insect resistance from *Bacillus thuringiensis.*

52 (*b*) Cells obtained from cancerous tumour are known as myelomas. The myelomas are of the plasma cells cancer which is mature form of lymphocyte that produces β-lymphocyte.

53 (*b*) Golden rice is vitamin-A rich variety developed by *r*DNA technology and used in the treatment of vitamin-A deficiency.

55 (*a*) RNA interference technique, sense and antisense RNA fused to form *ds*RNA that silent the expression of *m*RNA of nematode.

So, tobacco plants resistant to a nematode have been developed by the introduction of DNA that produced both sense and antisense RNA.

56 (*b*) *Bacillus thuringiensis* is the bacterium which produces *Bt* toxin. The gene encoding *Bt* toxin, i.e. *cry* gene is widely cloned and expressed in plants to provide resistance to insects without the need of insecticides. This bacterium produces a protein that kills certain insects such as Lepidopterans, Coleopterans and Dipterans.

59 (*c*) In transgenics, expression of transgene in target tissue is determined by same tissue specific promoter. A promoter is the main regulatory portion of a gene. The simplest analogy is that a promoter is a switch that turns a gene 'on' or 'off'. It is the portion of the gene where cellular machinery binds before transcribing the DNA blueprint into a useful RNA.

61 (*b*) Insulin is synthesised as a prohormone. It contains an extra stretch called the C-peptide. The C-peptide is not present in mature insulin and is removed during maturation into insulin. So, maturation of genetically engineered proinsulin into insulin takes place after.

63 (*a*) The *cry* gene of *Bacillus thuringiensis* produces a protein which forms crystalline inclusions in the bacteria. These crystal proteins are responsible for the insecticidal activities of bacterial strain. *cry* I Ac and *cry* II Ab genes are responsible for controlling cotton bollworms.

64 (*d*) Characteristics of *Bt* cotton are high yield and resistance to bollworms. The *Bt* toxin is coded by a gene named, *cry* II Ab and *cry* IAc that control the cotton bollworms.

65 (*a*) *Bt* toxin is coded by a gene named *cry*. These are of many forms, e.g. the proteins encoded by the genes *cry* I Ac and *cry* II Ab control the cotton bollworms, *cry* I Ab controls corn borer, etc.

67 (*a*) *Bacillus thuringiensis* toxin is an inactive protoxin, which gets converted into active form in the insect gut. It works as an insecticide.

68 (*d*) Biotechnology is helpful in producing transgenic crops or Genetically Modified (GM) crops, transgenic animals, biofertilisers, antibodies, hormones like humulin (genetically engineered human insulin), antibodies and various other useful products.

Thus, option (d) is correct.

69 (*d*) Main objective of production/use of herbicide resistant genetically modified crops is to reduce herbicide accumulation in food articles for health safety. These plants have been developed in such a way that they continue to produce normal crop yield, while remaining unaffected by activity of herbicides.

CHAPTER 23

Organisms and Populations

Ecology (Gk. *Oikos*-home, *logos*-study) is the branch of biology that deals with the interrelationship amongst organisms and their interaction with the environment. In simple words, it is the study of organisms in their habitat. The essence of ecological understanding is to know about the mutual interactions of organisms as well as their correlation with the physical environment as a group.

Hence, it behaves like an organised population, community, ecosystem or even as the whole biosphere. The term **ecology** was first coined by **Ernst Haeckel** in 1869. However, its first authentic use was made by **Reiter** in 1885. This chapter describes various ecological aspects, mainly emphasising more on its organismic and population levels.

Branches of ecology

Ecology has been divided into several branches. The main branches are given below

1. **Autecology** It is concerned with the study of an individual organism (an individual species). The term was coined by Schroeter and Kirchner (1896).
2. **Synecology** It deals with the study of a group of organisms, which are associated together as a unit. The synecology is further subdivided into the population ecology, community ecology and ecosystem ecology. This term was also coined by **Schroeter** and **Kirchner** (1896).
3. **Demecology** It is the ecology of a population.
4. **System ecology** It deals with the interpretation of ecological concepts and processes in terms of mathematical models and formulae.
5. **Genecology** It deals with the genetic composition and changes in relation to the origin of ecads, ecotypes, new species, etc.
6. **Population ecology** It is the study of growth, trophic structure, metabolism and regulation of a population.
7. **Community ecology** It is the study of different populations present in same habitat and environmental conditions.
8. **Taxonomic ecology** It deals with the study of different taxonomic group such as plant, insects, human, etc.

Inside

9. **Applied ecology** It deals with the study of applications of ecological concepts to human needs including wildlife management, biological control and forestry.
10. **Habitat ecology** It deals with the study of plants and animals inhabiting different habitats.

Terms used in ecology

Various terms used in ecology are explained below

1. **Population** It is a group of individual organisms of the same species in a given area.
2. **Community** It is a group of populations of different species in a given area.
3. **Environment** It is the complex sum of many factors therefore, it is also referred as the environmental complex.
4. **Habitat** It is a place, where an organism lives. It represents a particular set of environmental conditions that are suitable for the survival of its inhabitants.
5. **Adaptation** It is a specialised feature of an organism that allows it to exist under the conditions of its habitat.
6. **Ecads** (of a plant species) It is a population of individuals, which although belong to the same genetic stock (i.e. are genetically similar), but differ in vegetative characters such as size, shape, number of leaves and stems, etc.
7. **Ecotype** It is a population of individuals of a species, which are genetically different.
8. **Ecospecies** One or more ecotype in a single coenospecies (a collection of related species which are able to hybridise).
9. **Ecotone** It is a transition zone present between two different types of communities. The species found in this region are called **edge species** and the effect that these species have on each other is called **edge effect**.
10. **Biological spectrum** It is the percentage distribution of species among the various life forms of a particular flora.
11. **Biological clock** An internal mechanism in organism that controls the periodicity of various functions or activities.
12. **Ecological succession** It is a natural process by which different groups or communities colonise the same area over a period of time in a definite sequence.
13. **Climax community** During succession, the final terminal community that can maintain itself more or less indefinitely in an equilibrium with the prevailing environment is known as climax community. The stage is called as **climax stage**.
14. **Biome** A complex of several types of communities maintained under more or less similar climatic conditions is known as biome.
15. **Ecosystem** An ecosystem is a whole biotic community in a given area including its abiotic environment.
16. **Biosphere** The planet earth along with its atmosphere (air, land and water) that sustain life is called biosphere.
17. **Standing state** The amount of inorganic substances such as P, S, N, C, H, etc., present at a given time in the environment of an ecosystem is called standing state or **standing quality**.
18. **Standing crop** The amount of living material (organic material) present in a population at any time is called standing crop.
19. **Biomass** It is the standing crop expressed in terms of weight of the living matter present in particular habitat.
20. **Ecological pyramid** It is the graphic representation of the structure and function of successive trophic levels of an ecosystem. It is represented in terms of number, biomass or energy content.
21. **Food chain** The transfer of food energy from the source in plants through a series of organisms with repeated eating and being eaten is called food chain in an ecosystem.
22. **Food web** It is an interlinked pattern of a number of food chains that form a web-like arrangement in an ecosystem.
23. **Productivity** The rate of production, i.e. amount of organic matter accumulated in the living component of an ecosystem in a unit time is referred to as the productivity of an ecosystem.
24. **Biogeochemical cycle** More or less circular pathways, through which the chemical elements including all the essential elements of the protoplasm circulate in the biosphere from the environment to organisms and back to the environment are known as biogeochemical cycles.
25. **Ecological niche** It includes the physical space occupied by an organism, its functional role in the community and the conditions of its existence.

26. **Ecological equivalents** These are the organisms, which occupy the same or similar ecological niches in different geographical regions.
27. **Conservation** The planning and management of resources, so as to secure their wide use and continuity of supply, while maintaining and enhancing their quality, value and diversity.
28. **Pollution** It is an undesirable change in the physical, chemical or biological characteristics of air, land and water that may harmfully affect on human life directly or indirectly.

Table 23.1 Alternate terms used by some scientists for ecology

Terms	Scientists
Oecology	Ernst Haeckel
Biocoenosis	Karl Mobius
Hexicology	St. George and Jackson Mivart
Ethology	St. Hilaire
Bioecology	Shelford and Clements

ENVIRONMENT

The word 'environment' means everything that is around us. It may be defined as 'the whole complex of climatic, edaphic, physiographic and biotic factors that act upon an organism or an ecological community and ultimately determine its form and survival.

Components of environment

The surface of the earth consists of three elements, i.e. land, sea and air. On the basis of these elements, the environment is divided into

(i) **Lithosphere** It represents land.

(ii) **Pedosphere** It is composed of disintegrating compounds of rock and stone-forming soil.

(iii) **Hydrosphere** It represents water.

(iv) **Atmosphere** It is a layer of air around the earth.

These components of environment are interdependent on and interact with each another.

Atmosphere

It is an insulating blanket of air around the earth. It shields the earth from the lethal concentration of ultraviolet radiations. The atmosphere selectively filters the sun's rays, so that only two small segments of the electromagnetic spectrum penetrate the earth's surface in appreciable amounts. The atmosphere is divided into troposphere, stratosphere, mesosphere and ionosphere. These are as follows

(i) **Troposphere** First 20 km of earth's atmosphere is called troposphere. The rate of temperature drop is about 6.4°C per 1000 metre. This is called the **normal environmental lapse rate**. Cloud formation, lightning, thundering and thunderstorm takes place in troposphere. More than 90% of atmospheric gases are found in troposphere.

(ii) **Stratosphere** About 30 km zone over troposphere is called stratosphere. At about 25 km in stratosphere lies an ozonosphere that lacks dust and water vapours. This zone absorbs most of the UV radiations due to the presence of ozone in this part.

(iii) **Mesosphere** The mesosphere is found up to 30 km above the stratosphere. In this zone, temperature decreases around – 80°C.

(iv) **Ionosphere** It is the uppermost zone of the atmosphere. In this zone, all the gases are in their ionised form.

Table 23.2 Major regions of the atmosphere

Regions	Altitude ranges (km)	Temperature ranges (°C)	Significant chemical species
Troposphere	0-8 to 18	15°C to – 56 °C	N_2, O_2, CO_2, H_2O
Stratosphere	8 to 18.50	– 56°C to 2 °C	O_3
Mesosphere	50 to 85	– 2°C to – 92 °C	O_2^+, NO^+
Ionosphere	85 to 500	– 92°C to 1200 °C	O_2^+, O^+, NO^+

Climate

- The conditions of the atmosphere at any place at a specific time, with respect to various elements (temperature, sunshine, wind, clouds, fog, etc.) is known as **weather**.
- The long-term weather conditions and factors peculiar to a given environmental area due to its geographical distribution is called climate.
- It is chiefly determined by meteorological influences such as relative humidity of air, temperature, wind pressure and evaporation rate.
- The scientific study of climate is called **climatology**.
- Four climatic and vegetation zones have been recognised on the basis of mean temperature along the latitude.

Table 23.3 Different zones of climate and their characteristics

Zones	Latitudes	Mean annual temperatures	Winters	Vegetations
Tropical	0 to 20	Above 24°C	No winter	Tropical forest
Subtropical	20 to 40	17 to 24°C	Mild winter	Subtropical deciduous forests
Temperate	40 to 60	7 to 17°C	Winter with snow	Coniferous forest
Arctic and Antarctic	60 to 80	Below 7°C	Winter with heavy snow	Arctic vegetation

Microclimate (Microenvironment)

- It can be defined as local variation of a climate that occurs in an area of limited size. Microclimate is the effective climate upon which life of an organism depends.
- An interesting example of microclimate is the desert animal's burrows, in which the physical conditions are very much different from those of the region as a whole.
- When kangaroo rat (*Dipodomys*) retreats within its burrow, it breathes air that is two to five times more humid than that of outside. If this animal remains out of its burrow continuously, the rate of evaporation from its lung exceeds the rate at which it obtains water. It results into death of kangaroo.

Biomes

A large regional unit characterised by a major vegetation type and associated fauna found in a specific climatic zone is referred to as a biome. Rainfall, temperature range, nature of soil, barriers, latitude and altitude determine the nature and extent of different biomes present on the earth.

Causes of biome formation

- These biomes are formed as the solar radiations from the sun falls vertically in tropical areas, but obliquely in temperate and polar areas.
- The rotation of earth and tilt of its axis causes the seasonal changes.
- Variation in temperature together with annual variation in precipitation results into the formation of major biomes.
- The various types of biomes found all over the world are summarised in the table given below

Table 23.4 Different types of biomes of the world

Biome names	Life forms	Climates	Location	Temperature	Rainfall	Remarks
Tundra	Permafrost (subsoil remains frozen). Trees absent. Lichens, grasses, sedges and mosses present. Birches and willows.	Polar continental has the driest climate, cold conditions and low humidity.	Found in Arctic region, North America, Europe and Asia.	Freezing (< 0°C)	Little precipitation < 25 cm annually.	Covers 1/5th of earth's land surface. Absent in Southern hemisphere.
Temperate deciduous forest (broad leaf forest)	Trees like maple beachoaks grow well. Leaf fall occurs in the autumn, fauna includes deer, racoon, beaver, etc.	Temperate maritime (coastal) has the wet conditions needed for tree growth.	Found in the mid-latitudes, along the coasts. These are found in American, European and Asian coastlines.	Warm and moist (22-32°C)	Moderate precipitation 75-150 cm/yr.	Warm summers and plentiful rains promote the growth of forest.
Temperate grassland	It is a fragile ecosystem that naturally sustains a variety of grasses and plants with broad leaves. Large herbivores are sustained, including horses and bison.	Further inlands from maritime another climate is found– Temperate continental. Here, freezing winters and hot summers are typical, whilst rainfall is low.	Found in the mid latitudes, in the continental interiors. This natural biome type is called Steppes - Russia Prairies - North America Pampas - South America Veldts - South Africa Tussock - New Zealand Dawns - Australia	Warm (20-30°C)	Seasonal droughts common. Medium amounts of moisture rainfall 25-75 cm/yr.	Highly productive, but their overgrazing leads to desertification. Found at midway of equator and poles.

Biome names	Life forms	Climates	Location	Temperature	Rainfall	Remarks
Deserts	Specialised plants exist in the desert, which cope up with the extreme absence of water, e.g. desert cactus. Animal forms like gila monster larkin and rattle snake are found. Vegetation sparse. Ephermerals and short lived annuals herbs. Succulent xerophytes. Deep rooted shrubs and small trees, e.g. *Prosophis, Salvadora, Tamarix.*	Arid climate	The desert belt is found at around 20-30 degrees North or South of the equator, e.g. Africa (Sahara), Asia (Gobi).	Hot (> 30°C) in day Cold (< 0°C) at night	Low precipitation, Less than 30 cm/yr.	They cover 30% of the earth land.
Savanna	This biome is grassland with tall scattered trees. Large mammals, e.g. lions, cheetah, giraffe, etc., are present.	Tropical seasonal climate with a long dry season, preventing the development of rainforest.	Tropical regions, between the desert and rainforest. Sometimes further South, e.g. Serongeti (Africa).	(26-50°C) Hot dry	Low annual rainfall 90-150 cm/yr.	Plants have horizontal root system by which they obtain water during rainy season. Grasses have vertical leaves that expose their less surface area to hot sun.
Tropical rainforest	A tall, thick canopy at around 40 cm, with emergent trees up to 80 cm. Animals abundant.	Tropical equatorial. The best rainforest grows where it rains everyday.	At the equator and up to around 10 degrees North or South, e.g. South America, Africa, Asia.	Hot (20-30°C) Normally warm and constant.	Very high precipitation, more than 250 cm/yr.	Richest ecosystem on the earth. Soil is nutrient limited and acidic in nature.

Table 23.5 Differences between tropical rainforests and temperate rainforests

	Tropical rainforests	Temperate rainforests
Temperature	Warm	Cool
Number of tree species	Many (hundreds)	Few (10-20)
Types of leaves	Broad	Needle-shaped
Age of trees	50-100 yrs	500-1000 yrs
Epiphytes	Different kinds including orchids and bromeliads	Mostly mosses and ferns
Decomposition rate	Rapid	Slow

Habitat and microhabitat

- The natural home of an organism including its total environment is called its **habitat**. It is an area where all the needs of its inhabitants are fulfilled.
- Earth has four major habitats including marine, freshwater, terrestrial and estuarine habitats.
- Each of these habitats is characterised by their own physical conditions or limiting factors, such as salinity, temperature, etc. It influences the presence and survival of organisms in their habitat and their distribution.
- Organisms are usually adapted to the physical conditions of the habitat.
- **Microhabitat** is a small part of the habitat with its own characteristic and environmental features, e.g. forest floors, tree canopies, edges of a pond, etc. It is a smaller habitat within a habitat.

Niche/Ecological niche

It refers to the functional role of species in its habitat rather more precisely in its microhabitat.

The term 'niche' was first used by **J Grinnel** (1971) to explain microhabitats. But niche differs from habitat, as habitat is the address of the organism whereas niche is its profession (role).

There are three aspects for the existence of ecological niche. These are as follows

(i) **Spatial or Habitat niche** It is concerned with the physical space occupied by an organism. For example, seven species of millipedes of a maple-oak forest belong to the same trophic level, i.e. decomposers, but each species is found in a different layer of the forest floor. This is because each species of millipede predominates in its own specific different microhabitat.

(ii) **Trophic niche** It is concerned with the trophic position of an organism. For example, various species of birds in Galapagos islands in South America. Each bird has different beak inspite of the fact that they live in the same general habitat. This is because they differ in their trophic positions. As some feeds on fruit and buds whereas rest are insect eaters. Out of the insect eater birds, different species feed on insects of different size.

(iii) **Multifactor or Hypervolume niche** In this concept, a niche is considered as an abstract multidimensional space or hypervolume, which is amenable to the measurement and mathematical manipulation (**Hutchinson**; 1958).

Diagrammatic representation of hypervolume niche

- Ecological niche involves competition among different populations. Any population can only survive and reproduce within certain environmental limits.
- If temperature and humidity, two abiotic factors are considered as niche dimensions, a two dimensional graph could be obtained.
- If a third factor, like size of food eaten, is added, the graph can be represented three dimensionally. The resulting rectangular box is the **niche space** in which the population can revive and reproduce.

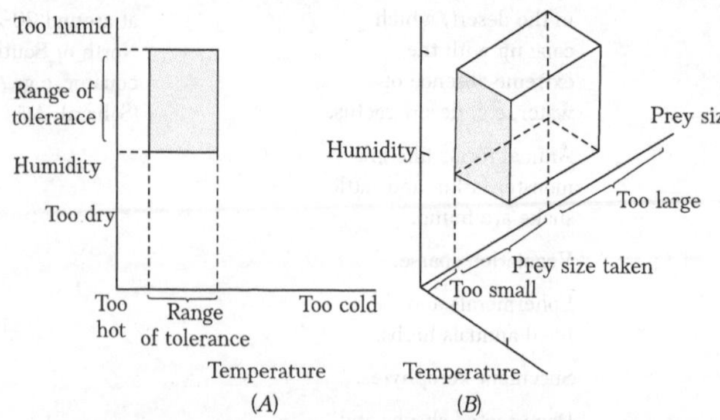

Fig 23.1 Diagrammatic sketch to show hypervolume niche. A. In two dimensions (For example, temperature and humidity), B. In three dimensions (For example, prey size added).

- The fundamental niche of a species is the hypervolume that a population can fill in the absence of competitors.
- Closely related species of competitors would have similar requirements. Therefore, they can fully or partially overlap each other. In that case, the niche occupied by a species is termed as **realised niche**.

Niche theory

- It states that no two organisms can occupy the same niche for an indefinite period of time. Also, that the niche of an organism is defined by its need and tolerance.
- The modern niche concept developed independently by **Pitel Ka** (1941), **Mac Fadyen** (1957) and **Hutchinson** (1957), describe the niche as a quality of the environment rather than a quality of a species.

Table 23.6 Differences between habitat and niche

Habitat	Niche
The place or set of environmental conditions in which a particular organism lives.	It is a functional description of the role, a species play in a community.
It is the address of an organism.	It is the profession of an organism.
It can have number of niches.	It does not have any components.
It can have or support a number of species.	It comprises of only one species.
A variety of environmental variables are present in a habitat.	Every niche has its own specific environment.

CHECK POINT 23.1

1. One biome is characterised by precipitation of less than 25 cm per year, temperatures fluctuate widely during the day and plants living here have adaptations such as poisons and thorns. This is a
   (a) temperate grassland (b) taiga
   (c) tropical rainforest (d) desert
2. Which of the following is not a characteristic of the tropical rainforest biome?
   (a) About 200 cm of precipitation
   (b) Canopy of fall evergreen trees
   (c) Climbing lianas
   (d) Permafrost
3. The assemblage of all the populations of different species that function as an integrated unit through co-evolved metabolic transformation in a specific area is called
   (a) biome (b) biotic community
   (c) population (d) ecosystem
4. Two plants can be conclusively said to belong to the same microspecies if they
   (a) can reproduce freely with each other and form seed
   (b) have more than 90% similar gene
   (c) look similar and possess identical secondary metabolites
   (d) have same number of chromosomes
5. Which of the following is correct for ecological niche?
   (a) It is the surface area of the ocean
   (b) It is an ecologcially adapted zone
   (c) It is the physical position and functional role of a species within the community
   (d) It is formed in all plant and animals living at the bottom of lake

ECOLOGICAL FACTORS

These are constituents of the environment which directly or indirectly influence the form and functioning of organisms in a specific way.

Ecological factors may be either living or biotic (e.g. plants, animals, microbes, etc.) or non-living or abiotic (environmental).

Abiotic factors
(Environmental factors)

- These are non-living factors, substances and conditions of the environment. These may influence the physiology, survival, function, behaviour and reproduction of organisms.
- Abiotic factors are subdivided into climatic factors, topographic factors and edaphic factors.
- Climatic factors are light, temperature, water and wind.
- Edaphic factors are related to soil.
- Topographic factors involves the physical geography of earth that include altitude, slope, etc.

The major abiotic factors are described below

Temperature

- It is the most ecologically relevant environmental factor. It is the degree of hotness or coldness of a substance.
- Latitude, altitude, topography, vegetation and slope are some aspects, which influence the temperature.
- Temperature may affect the climatic conditions, growth responses of plants and activities of organisms.
- Temperature on land varies seasonally. It decreases progressively from the equator towards the poles and from plains towards the mountain tops.
- It ranges from subzero levels in polar areas and high altitudes to more than 50°C in tropical deserts in summers.
  (i) **Periodic activity** (in animals) Every animal is active at a particular period of day and night. It may be diurnal (active during day), nocturnal (active during night), auroral (active at dawn), vesperal (active during evening) and crepuscular (active in twilight).
  (ii) **Thermoperiodicity** Thermoperiodism in plants is the response of living organisms to regular changes of temperature. It is of two types
    (a) **Diurnal thermoperiodicity** It is the response of organism to daily changes in temperature. Generally, day time temperature is higher, while night time temperature is lower.
    (b) **Seasonal thermoperiodicity** It is the response of organism to seasonal changes in temperature. Along with photoperiodicity, it also controls the phenology of plants.
- Types of organisms based on their zone of occurrence in relation to temperature are as follows
  (i) **Megatherms** Organisms that are adapted to high temperature throughout the year. These are found in tropical zone.
  (ii) **Mesotherms** Organisms that are adapted to mild winters and high summer temperature. These are found in subtropical zone.
  (iii) **Microtherms** Organisms that are adapted to low winter temperature and moderate summer temperature and are found in temperate areas.
  (iv) **Hekistotherms** Organisms that are adapted to a brief summer period and long snowy winter period and are found in Arctic or Alpine zone.

- Types of organisms based on the tolerance of temperature are as follows
  (i) **Stenothermals** The organisms that can tolerate only a narrow range of variation in temperature. These organisms live in areas where the temperature remains nearly uniform throughout the year, e.g. amphibians, lizards, etc.
  (ii) **Eurythermals** The organisms that can tolerate a wide range of temperature variations, e.g. most mammals, birds, etc.
- Types of organisms on the basis of regulation of their body temperature are as follows
  (i) **Cold-blooded** or **Poikilothermic** (ectothermic) **animals** The organisms that can adjust their body temperature with the temperature of the environment, e.g. all non-vertebrates, fish, amphibian and reptiles.
  (ii) **Warm-blooded** or **Homeothermic** (endothermic) **animals** The organisms which keep their body temperature constant despite changes in their external environmental temperature, e.g. birds and mammals, etc.

- **Gloger's rule** In warm blooded animals, pigmentation is little in colder areas. Yellow brown to red in arid climate and black in humid hot areas.
- **Bergmann's rule** Warm blooded animals of colder areas are of larger size as compared to those of warmer areas.
- **Allen's rule** Extremities of mammals (ears, snout, tail, legs) of colder areas are shorter than those of warmer regions.
- **Jordan's rule** Fish of colder waters tend to have more vertebrae.

Thermal stratification of water body

The occurrence of different temperatures in different horizontal layers in a forest or in a deep water body is called thermal stratification. A water body has three thermal strata (layers). These are as follows

(i) **Epilimnion** is upper stratum of water` with highest concentration of dissolved oxygen. The temperature gradient is less than 1°C per metre of depth. This region is exposed to maximum sunlight.

(ii) **Metalimnion** is a transitional stratum of marked thermal change between the hypolimnion and epilimnion. The middle part of metalimnion is called **thermocline.**

It is the area of maximum temperature change. The temperature gradient is more than 1°C per metre of depth.

(iii) **Hypolimnion** is lower stratum of water. It is characterised by a temperature gradient of less than 1°C per metre. Temperature fluctuation is less in this layer.

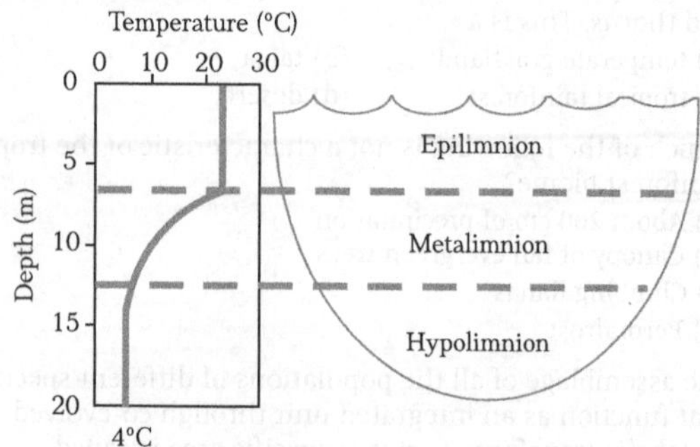

Fig 23.2 Representing the thermal zonation of water body

Note *The **epilimnion** is affected by surface mixing. The mixing between the hypolimnion and epilimnion is inhibited by a sharp temperature and density difference at the thermocline.*

Water

- It is the essence of all living processes. It is the most abundant and versatile chemical of life.
- Water forms most of our flesh and blood. A cell's protoplasm also consists about 75-80% water.
- The ocean occupies 70% of the earth's surface. It contains around 97% of all the water on the earth. But not all this water is consumable by all organisms. This water contains dissolved salt in it.
- Water present on land is called **freshwater** with less than 0.5% of salt content. This water is mostly consumed by the organisms.
- Sea water contains salt content of more than 3.5%.
- The salt concentration is less than 5% in inland water, 30-35% in sea water and more than 100% in some hypersaline lagoons. Nearly pure water occurs in the form of vapour in the atmosphere.
- In fact, life on the earth originated in water and is unsustainable without water.
- Types of organisms based on tolerance to salinity are as follows
  (i) **Stenohaline organisms** These organisms can tolerate a narrow range of salinity, e.g. freshwater fishes.
  (ii) **Euryhaline organisms** These organisms can tolerate a wide range of salinity, e.g. salmons, eels, etc.
- The productivity and distribution of plants is also dependent on water. For aquatic organisms, the quality (chemical composition, pH) of water is very important.

- Animals found in coastal water are called **neritic** and those found in open water are termed as **pelagic**.
- These organisms include **plankton** (suspended deep inside the water), **neuston** (inhabiting surface layer of water) and **nekton** (actively swimming aquatic organisms).
- Organism found at the bottom of water bodies are called **benthos**.

- On the basis of water availability, plants are grouped into three communities namely hydrophytes, xerophytes and mesophytes (which are discussed later in this chapter).

Light

- It is the radiant energy emitted by the sun. But only 48% of it reaches the earth. It has a wavelength of 300-2600 nm.
- Solar radiation with a wavelength over 760 nm is invisible to the eye and is called **infra-red**.
- The visible part of electromagnetic spectrum ranges from 390-740 nm. It is the most important factor for living organisms.
- Radiations below the visible light are **ultraviolet** (UV) **radiations.**

Useful and harmful effects of light

- The light which is effective in photosynthesis is called **Photosynthetically Active Radiation** (PAR). Its wavelength ranges from 400-700 nm. This band provides the radiant energy for the photosynthesis and thus, supports all autotrophic organisms.
- The light of wavelength below 400 nm is ultraviolet light. It is of three types, UV-A (320-400 nm), UV-B (290-320 nm) and UV-C (< 290 nm). UV-C is the most damaging radiation followed by UV-B and UV-A.
- The amount of these radiations entering into earth is chiefly regulated by ozone layer. It virtually eliminates UV-C and greatly reduces the amount of UV-B reaching the surface of planet.
- On the basis of requirement of light intensity, plants may be of two types, i.e. heliophytes and sciophytes (which are discussed later in the chapter).

Light zones in aquatic habitat

There are four major light zones of lake ecosystem as described below

(i) **Littoral zone** It adjoins the shore and extends down to a point called the light compensation level. It is the depth at which the rate of photosynthesis becomes equal the rate of respiration. In this zone, rooted plants and phytoplanktons are found.

(ii) **Limnetic zone** It includes all the water beyond the littoral zone and light compensation level.

- The limnetic zone derives its oxygen content from the photosynthetic activity of phytoplanktons.
- It is the home of plankton and nekton.
- This zone has two parts, upper euphotic zone and lower disphotic zone.
- **Euphotic zone** receives light more than compensation point.
- **Disphotic zone** receives light at or below the compensation point for photosynthesis. Here, producers can survive, but cannot flourish.

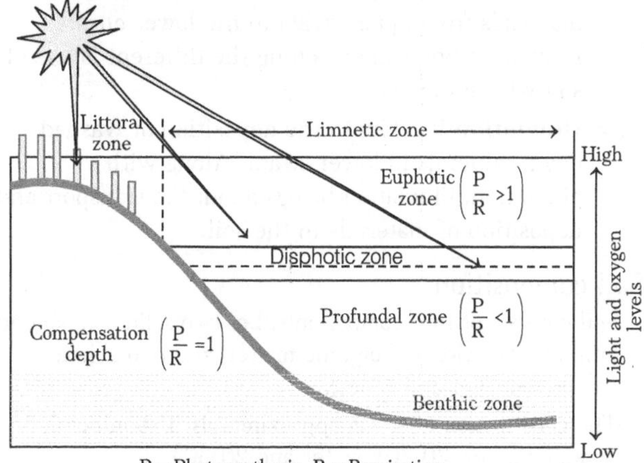

Fig 23.3 Light zones in lake ecosystem

- **Compensation depth** The point in a light gradient at which plants can balance between food production and its use, is called compensation depth, P/R = 1.

(iii) **Profundal** (dark) **zone** The light intensity in this zone is very low for photosynthesis, so only respiration occurs at the bottom zone. Producers do not occur in this part, instead only consumers are found.

(iv) **Benthic zone** It is the lowest zone that usually remains in perpetual darkness.

Soil

It is the weathered top surface of earth's crust. Various mineral, organic matter and microorganisms constitute the soil.

Soil formation or Pedogenesis

The process of soil formation is called as pedogenesis. It is divided into four stages, which are as follows

(i) **Weathering** It is the breaking of rocks into fine powder. It is of three types

(a) **Physical weathering** It is caused by water, wind, gravity, glacier, etc.

(b) **Chemical weathering** Various chemical reaction such as oxidation, reduction, hydrolysis, carbonation, etc., cause breakage of rocks.

(c) **Biological weathering** It is caused by living organisms, e.g. lichens, mosses and other organisms.

(ii) **Humification** It is a biological phenomenon. In this process, living organisms such as lichens, bacteria, fungi, etc., degrade organic matter into humus. This humus contains many useful nutrients for healthy soil. It is a colloidal substance that increases the soil's cation exchange capacity.
It helps in the formation of soil crumbs, has high water holding capacity, etc.

(iii) **Eluviation** It is a process of washing down of materials from upper strata to the lower ones. Eluviation helps in enriching the different layers of soil with minerals.

(iv) **Illuviation** It refers to the deposition of washed down minerals in lower strata. Along with eluviation, illuviation brings about the transport and deposition of materials in the soil.

Soil composition

- Soil consists of four components, i.e. two solid components (mineral particles and organic matter) and two abiotic components (air and water).
- The constitution of soil is approximately 45% mineral, 5% organic matter, 20-30% water and 20-30% air.
- The composition of the soil can fluctuate on a daily basis, depending on numerous factors such as water supply, cultivation practices or soil type.

(i) **Soil minerals** There are various types of minerals found in soil. These minerals vary greatly in size and chemical composition.

The contents of soil play a vital role in soil fertility. Based on the size of soil particle and type of minerals, soil can be of four types as given in the table below.

Table 23.7 Soil particles size according to International Code of Nomenclature

Soil	Size of particles (mm)
Clay (fined grained natural rock)	0.002 or less
Silt (very fine quartz grains)	0.002 to 0.02
Fine sand (SiO_2)	0.02 to 0.2
Coarse sand (quartz and SiO_2)	0.2 or more than 2

(ii) **Organic matter** It stores nutrient in the soil. More fertile soil contains high amount of organic matter. It includes all organic substances within the soil. It acts as a binding agents for mineral particles.

(iii) **Soil water** It provides a pool of dissolved nutrients that are readily available for plant uptake.

- The water in soil may be present in three forms, i.e. gravitational water, capillary water and hygroscopic water.
- The free water that moves through the soil due to the gravity is the **gravitational water.**
- **Capillary water** remains in the soil after the water drains. It can be easily utilised by the plants.
- **Hygroscopic water** forms very thin films around soil particles and it is not available to the plant. This water is held so tightly with the soil particle that it cannot be taken up by roots.

(iv) **Soil air** There are air spaces in between soil particles. These spaces are occupied by various liquids and gases that make the atmosphere of soil. Oxygen concentration is less in soil, whereas carbon dioxide concentration is high. Anaerobic soils such as waterlogged soils are highly deficient in oxygen.

Soil texture

It refers to the physical structure of soil. It directly influences soil-water relationship, aeration and root penetration. Based on soil texture, three types of soil are recognised.

(i) **Sandy soils** contain more sand than clay. They are nutrient deficient due to high porosity.

(ii) **Clayey soils** possess more clay than sands. They contain inorganic nutrients. It has the lowest porosity.

(iii) **Loamy soils** have nearly proportionate mixture of clay and sand. They have good mineral nutrition, aeration and hydration. Therefore, loam soils are best for plant growth.

Soil profile

The various processes of soil development result in the differentiation of soil into a series of horizontal zones. These zones differ from each other in morphology, chemical composition and biological activity. These are called as **soil horizons**. The arrangement of horizons in a soil is termed as soil profile.

The various horizons of the soil are discussed below

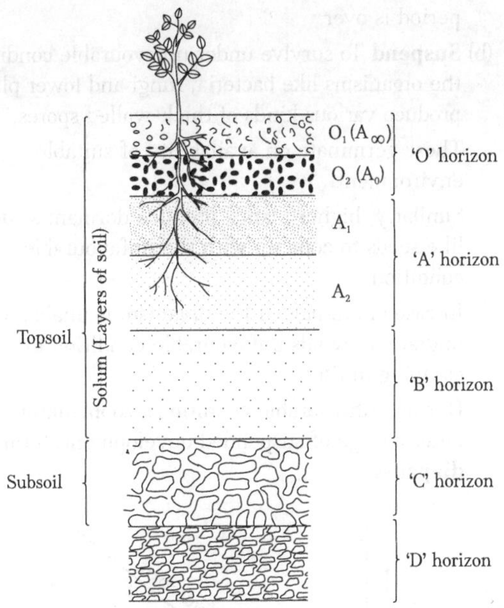

Fig 23.4 Hypothetical diagram of the soil profile to show principal horizons

(i) **O-horizon** It is the organic layer mainly composed of fresh or partially decomposed organic matter.

It is divided into following two sub-layers

(a) **O_1 (A_∞) region** It is the uppermost layer consisting of freshly fallen dead organic matter. It has undercomposed organic debris.

(b) **O_2 (A_0) region** It is present just below the O_1 region. In this region, decomposition takes place. Bacteria, fungi, Actinomycetes are frequently found in this region. The upper layer contains detritus in initial stages of decomposition, in which materials can be recognised. The lower layers contain fairly decomposed matter, the duff.

(ii) **A-horizon** It is the uppermost horizon of the soil, also called as **topsoil**.

This horizon is divided into following two sub-layers

(a) **A_1 region** This region is dark and rich in organic matter. The amorphous, finely divided organic matter here becomes mixed with the mineral matter, which is now known as **humus.**

(b) **A_2 region** This region is of light colour with little amount of organic matter. This region is found chiefly in areas with heavy rainfall. The mineral elements and organic chemicals are rapidly lost downwards in this region, making it light coloured. This region is also known as **podsolic** or **eluviation zone** or **zone of leaching**.

(iii) **B-horizon** It is also called as **subsoil**. This horizon receives various materials leached from the top soil. It is thus, the area of deposit of materials or **illuviation**. This horizon is poor in aeration and biological activity. It is rich in plant nutrients including humus. Illuviation also causes formation of compact and hard sublayers. It is differentiated into following three subhorizons

(a) **B_1 subhorizon** It is a dark-coloured, humified and somewhat compact subhorizon. It receives deposits of organic matter or humus from the above.

(b) **B_2 subhorizon** It contains deposits of inorganic nutrients, clay and heavy metals.

(c) **B_3 subhorizon** It contains small rock fragments stained with materials leaching from the above.

(iv) **C-horizon** It contains irregular rock fragments. The horizon is saturated with moisture and represents the water table.

(v) **D-Horizon** It represents the unbroken and unweathered parent bed rock.

Reponses to abiotic factors

An organism may evolve various mechanisms to maintain its internal environment at homeostasis. This property permits all biochemical reactions and physiological functions to proceed with the maximal efficiency. It also enhances the overall fitness of the species. Homeostasis may be maintained naturally or artificially. Various organisms may cope up with the stressful conditions by opting any of the following methods

(i) **Regulate** Some organisms are able to maintain a constant body temperature and osmotic concentration despite change in the external environment.

- All birds and mammals and a very few lower vertebrate and invertebrate species are capable of such regulation by physiological adjustment through thermoregulation and osmoregulation.
- Most of the mammals regulate their body temperature to about 37°C. However at many places, the external temperature rises to 45°C or sometimes may fall to zero or even below that. To these environmental fluctuations, the body may respond by sweating (at higher temperature) and shivering (at lower temperature).
- Most reptiles regulate their body temperature by staying in burrows during summer and by basking in the sun during winters. However, plants do not have such mechanisms to maintain an internal temperature.

(ii) **Conform** A majority of organisms cannot maintain a constant internal environment, i.e. their osmotic concentration and their body temperature changes with their environment (ectotherms). Such organisms are conformers.

- The efficiency of conformers is reduced under stressful conditions.
- Conformers had not evolved mechanisms like regulators because thermoregulation and osmoregulation mechanisms are energetically expensive for many small-sized organisms.
- The small-sized animals have large surface area relative to their volume, they tend to loose body heat very fast when its cold outside. Therefore, they have to spend more energy to generate body heat through metabolism. This is the main reason why, small-sized animals are rarely found in polar regions.
- Some organisms have evolved only a limited ability to alter their body temperature in accordance with the environment in which they live in. They are known as **partial** or **limited conformers.**
- If stressful external conditions are localised or remain only for short duration then these organisms have two other alternatives, i.e. migrate or suspend as described further

(a) **Migrate** The organisms can move away temporarily from the stressful habitat to a more favourable one. They return back when the unfavourable (stressful) period is over.

(b) **Suspend** To survive under unfavourable condition, the organisms like bacteria, fungi and lower plants produce various kinds of thick-walled spores.

- These germinate on availability of suitable environment.
- Similarly, higher plants, produce dormant structures like seeds to cope up with the unfavourable condition.
- In case of animals, if the organism is unable to migrate, it avoids unfavourable condition by escaping in time.
- During unfavourable conditions, zooplanktons may enter a stage of suspended development, termed as **diapause.**

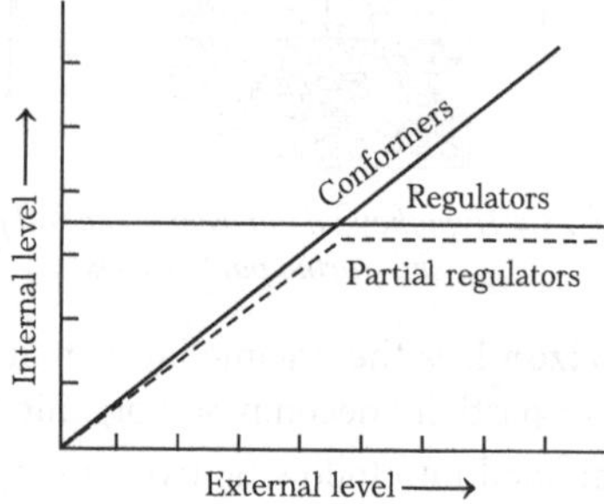

Fig 23.5 Diagrammatic representation of organismic response

CHECK POINT 23.2

1. A fertile agricultural soil appears deep coloured at the surface as compared to soil one metre down. The reason for colour of top soil is
(a) more moisture
(b) rich in organic matter
(c) rich in iron, calcium and magnesium
(d) recent formation

2. The maximum amount of water retained per unit dry weight of soil after the stoppage of gravitational flow is called
(a) gravitational water
(b) field capacity
(c) water logging
(d) Permanent Wilting Percentage (PWP)

3. Choose the incorrect match.
(a) Glacial — Transported by glaciers
(b) Aeolian — Transported by running water
(c) Colluvial — Transported by gravity
(d) Both (b) and (c)

4. An organism found in tropical zone which is adapted to high temperature throughout the year falls under which of the following group?
(a) Hekistotherms (b) Microtherms
(c) Megatherms (d) Mesotherms

5. Temperature is considered as the most ecological relevent environmental factor because it affects
(a) physiology (b) morphology
(c) geographical distribution (d) All of these

6. Organisms which are able to maintain homeostasis by physiological and behavioural changes are
(a) conformers (b) eurythermals
(c) regulators (d) stenothermals

7. The percentage of soil volume occupied by pore space is called porosity of soil. It is minimum in which of the following?
(a) Sandy soil (b) Clay soil
(c) Loam soil (d) Silt

ECOLOGICAL ADAPTATIONS

These are the specialised features of an organism that enhance its capacity to withstand a particular ecological condition.

Adaptations may be morphological, physiological, behavioural or the combination of all. These develop through the natural selection of suitable variations appearing in living beings through mutations and recombinations.

The ultimate aim of adaptation is to make the individual fit to obtain food and space for its survival, opportunities, for its reproduction and rearing of young ones.

Types of ecological adaptations

These are of two types

(i) **Genotypic adaptations** These adaptations are the genetic variations that allow a subpopulation to adapt itself to a particular habitat and environmental condition.

(ii) **Phenotypic adaptations** These are the favourable changes in the morphology and physiology, which develop in response to changes in environmental conditions. They disappear when the environmental conditions become normal. The ability of genetically similar populations to undergo phenotypic changes in response to variation in environment is called **phenotypic plasticity**.

Strategic adaptations in plants

Various types of plants possess special traits that help them to tolerate a wide range of light regimes, dry conditions, high temperature, water saturated condition as well as saline environments, etc.

Plant adaptation to light regime

According to the ability of plants to tolerate the light intensity, the plants are classified into various strata. This phenomenon is known as **stratification**.

On the basis of stratifications, plants are of two types

(i) Plants growing in bright light are called **sun plant** or **heliophytes**.

- These plants have short and thick internodes, small and thick leaves. They also possess thick cuticle and epidermal cells. Sunken stomata are found in these plants.
- The leaves are pale green with shining surface or hairy growth.
- Palisade parenchyma is well-developed. Cells are smaller. Intercellular spaces are small.
- Root system is extensive. There is good amount of flowering and fruiting.

(ii) Plants growing in a partial shade or low light intensity are called **shade plants** or **sciophyte**.

- These are slender plants with soft stems and long internodes. These leaves are thin and large-sized. They are bright green in colour.
- Leaf cells are large, cuticle is thin, stomata are in level with the surface. They are present in both the surfaces.
- Palisade parenchyma is less developed.
- The vegetative growth is more as compared to flowering and fruiting.

Plant adaptations to aquatic environment

The plants growing in aquatic habitat are known as **aquatic plants** or **hydrophytes**. The hydrophytes are grouped into five categories as follows

(i) **Submerged hydrophytes** These plants grow entirely under water. They are initially anchored, but later on they become suspended, e.g. *Hydrilla*, *Potamogeton* and *Vallisneria*, etc.

(ii) **Suspended hydrophytes** These are non-rooted submerged hydrophytes, which remain suspended in water.

These are never found in contact with the bottom. e.g. *Utricularia* and *Ceratophyllum*.

(iii) **Free-floating hydrophytes** These plants do not have any connection with the bottom and float freely over the surface of water, e.g. *Trappa*, *Wolffia* (plant devoid of leaf), *Pistia*, *Azolla* and *Salvinia*, etc.

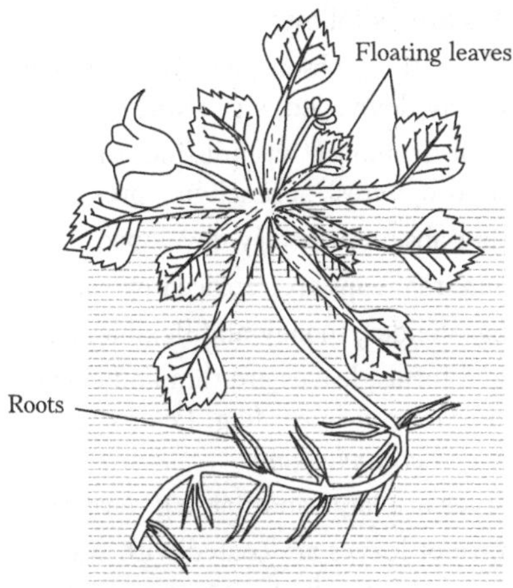

Fig. 23.6 Free-floating hydrophytes Trappa

(iv) **Rooted hydrophytes with floating leaves** These hydrophytes grow in shallow water. They are anchored to the bottom.
The mature leaves may come out of water as in case of *Nelumbo* (lotus). Heterophylly occurs in some plants, where submerged leaves occur along with the floating leaves, e.g. *Potamogeton notaus* and *Nymphoides.*

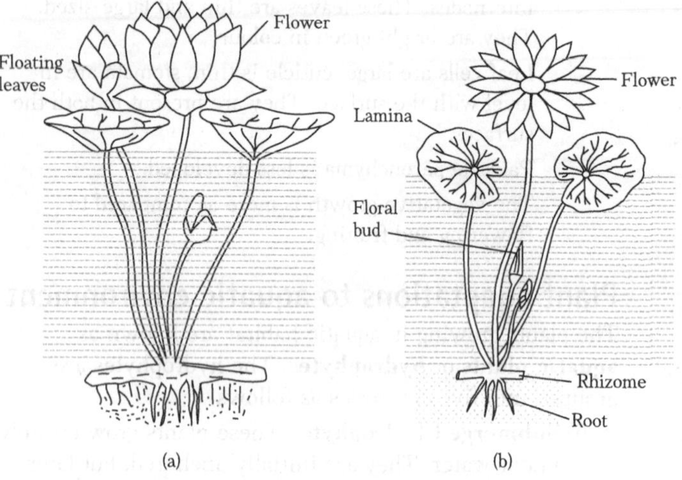

Fig 23.7 Free-floating hydrophytes: (a) Nelumbium, (b) Nymphaea

(v) **Emergent hydrophytes** (Amphibious plants) These plants grow in shallow water with their shoots extending above the surface of water. These are also known as **helophytes.** The plant shows both hydrophytic and mesophytic characteristics, e.g. *Typha, Sagittaria, Ranunculus aquatilis, Phragmites, Limnophylla* and *Heterophylla.*

Adaptations in hydrophytes

Some common morphological adaptations seen in different types of hydrophytes are as follows

- Roots may be entirely absent, e.g. *Wolffia, Salvinia.* Roots are poorly developed, e.g. *Hydrilla.*
- Roots are well-developed with distinct root caps, e.g. *Ranunculus* (emergent hydrophytes), aerenchyma present.
- Root hairs are absent or poorly developed.
- In *Eichhornia,* root caps are replaced by root pockets.
- Stem is long, slender, spongy and flexible, e.g. *Hydrilla.*
- In submerged forms, leaves are thin and ribbon-shaped (e.g. *Vallisneria*) or long or linear (e.g. *Potamogeton*) and finely dissected (e.g. *Ceratophyllum*).
- Floating leaves are large and flat, e.g. *Nymphaea* and *Nelumbo.*
- Upper surface of leaves are coated with wax.
- *Ranunculus* and *Sagittaria* show heterophylly.

Plant adaptations to moist habitat-Mesophytes

Mesophytes grow in moist habitats and need well-aerated soils.

- Root system is well-developed. They are branched with root caps and root hairs.
- Stems are aerial and freely branched.
- Leaves are large, broad and thin.
- Cuticle in all aerial parts is moderately developed.
- Vascular and mechanical tissues fairly developed and well-differentiated.

Plant adaptations to water scarcity and heat-Xerophytes

Xerophytes are adapted to dry regions and have high rate of transpiration than absorption of water.

These are mainly of three types as discussed below

(i) **Ephemerals** or **Drought escapers** These plants live for a brief period of 4-6 weeks during the rain. The rest of the year is passed in the form of seeds, e.g. *Euphorbia* species, *Argemone, Mexicana, Solanum, Xanthocarpum,* etc.

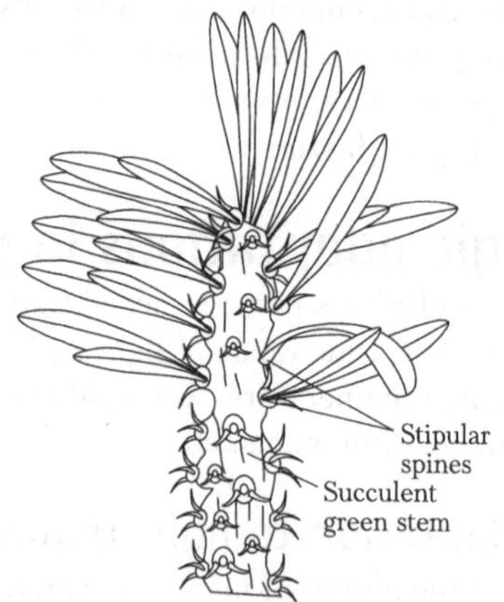

Fig 23.8 Shoots of E. royleana

(ii) **Succulent** or **Drought resistant** These plants suffer from dryness in external environment only.

- Their succulent, fleshy organs serve as water storage organs, which accumulate large amount of water. The plants store water and mucilage in their succulent organs.
- Depending upon the organs where succulence occurs, the succulents show chylophylly (fleshy leaves, e.g. *Aloe*), chylorhizy (fleshy

roots, e.g. *Asparagus*), chylocauly (fleshy stems, e.g. *Opuntia*).

- The stems are green, photosynthetic and have thick cuticle. They are called **phylloclades** (stems of indefinite growth) and **cladodes** (1-2 internodes long stems).
- The leaves are reduced to spines.
- Stomata are sunken and open during night only.
- Succulents are adapted to perform CO_2 fixation by **Crassulacean Acid Metabolism** (CAM).

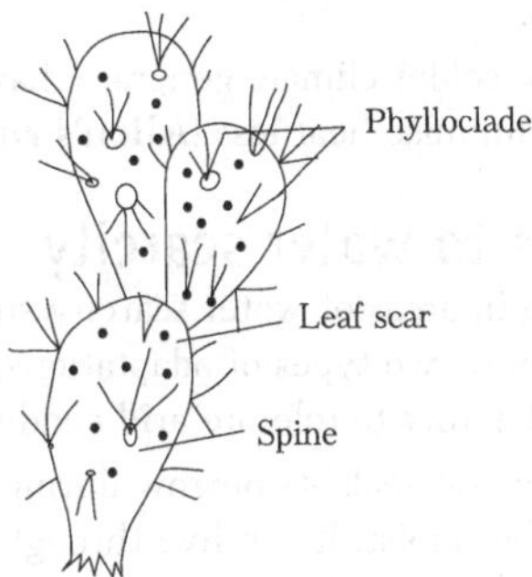

Fig 23.9 Shoot of Opuntia showing phylloclades

(iii) **Non-succulents** or **Drought endurers** These plants suffer from dryness both in their internal as well as external environments. Root system is very extensive, e.g. *Prosopis, Calotropis.* Rolling and folding of leaves occur, e.g. *Tamarix, Prosopis.*

Adaptations in xerophytes

The common adaptations seen in xerophytes are as follows

- Roots are very extensive, long, tap roots, with branching spread over wide areas.
- Root hairs and root caps are very well-developed.
- Stems are stunted, woody, dry, hard and covered with thick bark.
- In *Opuntia*, stem becomes green and fleshy (phylloclade).
- On stems and leaves, there are generally hairs and waxy coatings.
- Leaves are reduced, sometimes modified into spines.
- Leaf surfaces are generally shiny and glazed to reflect light and heat.
- In *Ammophila, Poa* and *Agropyron*, leaves become folded and rolled to reduce transpiration.
- In *Euphorbia, Acacia* and *Capparis*, stipules become modified into spines.
- Stomata are of sunken type.
- Oil and resins are often present.
- Non-succulent plants such as *Prosopis, Calotropis,* etc., contain prolines and chaperones (heat-shock proteins).

Plant adaptations to saline habitat-Halophytes

Halophytes are plants of saline habitats. They grow in saline soils, i.e. soil rich in NaCl, $MgCl_2$ and $MgSO_4$. They usually have a high osmotic pressure. These plants have the ability to tolerate high concentration of salts. They are also able to obtain their water supply from their rooting medium.

Adaptations in halophytes are as follows

- Plants of saline soil show characteristics similar to xerophytes. They may have succulence in leaves, stems or both.
- The succulent parts have large size cells which store water and mucilage. Though, it is a means of storing and retaining water, succulence also helps in diluting salts.
- Many halophytes may secrete salts through chalk or salt glands, e.g. *Atriplex, Spartina. Tamarix* also excretes salts, but directly through epidermis.
- Thick cuticle, sunken stomata, anthocyanin and tannins occur to reduce insolation and prevent desiccation, e.g. *Suaeda, Salsola, Salicornia, Tamarix, Atriplex* and *Spartina.*
- The plants growing near sea shore shows xerophytic characters as the concentration of salt is too high for such plants to absorb sufficient water from the soil.

Plants adaptations to marshy areas-Mangrove

Mangroves are the marshy areas found in tropical deltas and saline ponds near sea shore. These areas face the challenges of excess salt and water. The plants growing in these areas usually face difficulty in respiration and seed germination (salty areas).

Adaptations in mangroves are as follows

- A few of them secrete salts from roots and leaf surfaces (e.g. *Avicennia*).
- Their cuticle is thick.
- Some leaves have corky cells.
- Stomata are sunken.
- Anthocyanins, tannins and oils occur to reduce insolation.

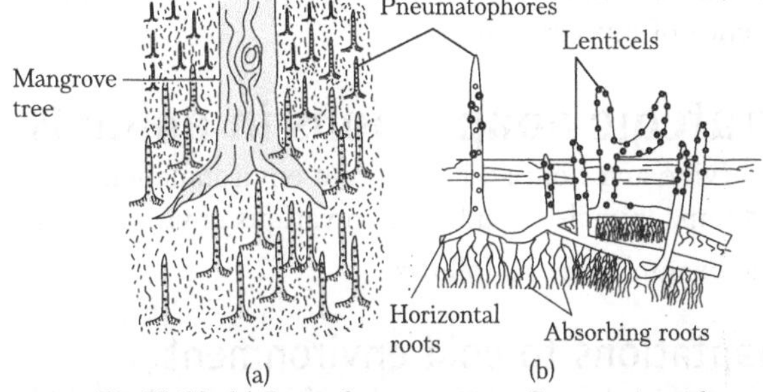

Fig 23.10 (a) Base of mangrove tree Sonneratia with pneumatophores coming out of mud, (b) Pneumatophores present in horizontal roots

- Proline and sorbitol are organic solutes often found in these plants for osmoregulation.
- A number of these plants possess negatively geotropic vertical roots called **pneumatophores**. These are connected with internal aerenchymatous tissue.
- Supporting roots such as horizontal roots, knee roots, buttress roots, stilt roots, prop roots, etc., are also present in them.
- Lenticels occur for gaseous exchange.
- These plants also exhibit **vivipary**. In this mechanism, a seedling grows sufficiently before it falls into the saline marsh. Only the radicle part passes into mud or water, while the plumule part remains above the surface of water, e.g. *Rhizophora*, *Aegiceras* and *Ceriops*.

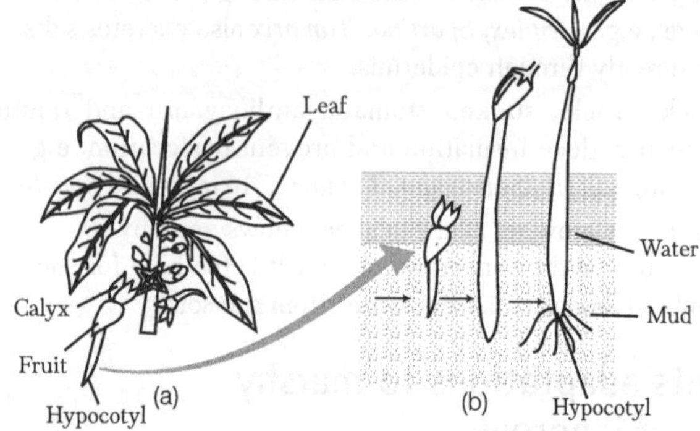

Fig 23.11 Vivipary in Rhizophora : (a) Shoot with fruits having viviparous seeds, (b) Seedling established in mud

Note *A green alga, Dunaliella found in hypersaline lakes, possess a lot of glycerol in its cells for osmoregulation.*

Plant adaptations to oligotrophic soils

Oligotropic soils are poor in nutrients. One such type of soil, which supports dense vegetation is found in tropical rainforests. Here, the top soil is shallow, while subsoil has dense clay mixed with iron-aluminium compounds. Despite growing in oligotrophic soil, nutrient accumulation is high in vegetation.

More than 84% of nutrients undergo biogeochemical circulation. A major adaptation of tropical plants is the presence of mycorrhizae.

Strategic adaptations in animals

To survive and flourish in different environmental condition, animals are adapted to various environments.

Some examples are as follows

Adaptations to cold environment

- Some animals protect themselves from excessive cold by developing cold hardiness. It is the ability of animals to resist injury during exposure to low temperature. These animals do not undergo hibernation and do not migrate, e.g. barnacles and molluscs of intertidal zone of cold areas, several insects and spiders.
- These animals are adapted to colder environment by developing extra solutes in the body fluids and special ice nucleating proteins in the extracellular spaces.
- The extra solutes which prevent freezing are glycerol and antifreeze proteins.
- Ice fish (*Chaenocephalus*) or Antarctic fish (*Trematomus*) remains active even in extremely cold sea water due to this hardiness.
- Mammals from colder climate generally have shorter ears and limbs to minimise heat loss (**Allen's rule**).

Adaptations to water scarcity

- Animals living in areas of water scarcity such as arid or desert areas show two types of adaptations, i.e. reducing water loss and ability to tolerate arid conditions.
- Kangaroo desert rat seals its burrow during daytime to keep its chamber moist. It can live throughout year without drinking water. Loss of water is minimised by producing nearly solid urine and faeces.
- Camel has a number of adaptations to desert conditions, i.e. economical in water consumption, minimising surface exposure, tolerance to variations of temperature. The animal produces dry faeces and urine. When water is available, the camel can rehydrate itself quickly. It is estimated that camel stores about 80 L of water in its hump.

Adaptations to environmental stress

During unfavourable conditions, animals change their physiology. These are of three types as follows

(i) **Hibernation and aestivation** Hibernation or winter sleep and aestivation or summer sleep are quite common in ectothermal (cold-blooded) animals.

- These, also occur in those warm-blooded or endothermal animals, which do not migrate from area of intense cold or heat.
- Frog, an ectothermal animal shows both hibernation and aestivation.
- Northern ground squirrels are endothermal mammals and they undergo hibernation during winter in comparatively warm places.
- During hibernation, their body temperature drops but remains above the outside atmosphere.
- Breathing and heartbeat become slow to reduce consumption of stored food.
- Endothermal ground squirrels of South-Western deserts undergo aestivation and lie in torpid or lifeless state inside the burrows during hot dry periods. Hibernation is a periodic event.

(ii) **Acclimatisation** It is the development of a favourable morphological and physiological response to a change in the environment. Change occurs due to change in season or due to some other reasons.
- People living in plains if move to high altitude places, experience nausea, fatigue and heart palpitation condition called **altitude sickness.** This occurs due to low atmospheric pressure of high altitude, as the body does not get enough oxygen. However, gradually the body stop feeling all these symptoms as it is acclimatised to new conditions.
- If the change in an environmental factor is beyond the tolerance range of an organism, the later can migrate, come to the resting stage, get acclimatised or die.

(iii) **Migration** It is the movement of an animal to other places for food, climate and other reasons.
It is of four types

(a) **Diurnal migrations** These are correlated with circardian rhythms of animals. For example, the movement of planktons towards the surface of aquatic bodies during night and descend to depth during day.

(b) **Metamorphic migrations** These are the movement of organism from one habitat to other in different stage of animal's life cycle. Salmon fishes living in pacific ocean ascend freshwater stream once in life for spawning. After laying eggs, breeders die and offspring return back to the ocean to develop for period of years before they again repeat the event.

(c) **Periodic migrations** These migrations are commonly found in locusts. When their population exceeds beyond the feeding capacity of place of living then they migrate to different directions in search of food.

(d) **Annual migrations** They are correlated with the circardian rhythm of organism and can involve the change of latitude, altitude or may be local.

Adaptations for protection from predators

Animal possesses different morphological behaviour to protect itself from the predators.

These adaptations are as follows

Camouflage

- It is the ability of an organism to blend with the surroundings or background.
- It is the most common type of adaptation by animals to remain unnoticed for protection or aggression, e.g. many insects, reptiles and mammals.
- It is difficult to distinguish leaf like grasshopper (*Arantia rectifolia*) or praying mantis (*Mantis religiosa*) from the surrounding foliage.
- Stick insect, leaf insect and dead leaf butterfly (*Phyllocrania paradoxa*) cannot be noticed unless and until they show movement.
- Camouflage is protective to animals, which are preyed upon by others. It is advantageous in predation for predators like praying mantis as they remain unnoticed till the prey comes within their striking range.

Mimicry

- It is the resemblance of one species with another in order to obtain advantage, especially, against predation.
- The species, which is imitated is called **model,** while the species, which imitates is known as **mimic** or **mimictic.** Model is either ferocious or distasteful to predator.
- Mimicry is of two types
  (i) **Batesian mimicry** In this mimicry, the mimic is defenceless. Due to its resemblance to a dangerous or unpalatable model, the predator usually does not prey upon it, e.g. viceroy butterfly mimics unpalatable toxic monarch butterfly.
  (ii) **Mullerian mimicry** In this mimicry, there is resemblance to two animals species, especially insects, both unpalatable/ferocious, to their mutual benefit, e.g. monarch butterfly and queen butterfly.

Warning colouration

Dart frogs (*Phyllobates bicolor, Dendrobates pumilio*) found in tropical rainforests of South America are highly poisonous as well as brightly coloured to be easily noticed. Predators usually avoid them.

- **Cope's law** states that there is a tendency of an organism to increase in size during the long course of evolution.
- **Bergman's law** states that the warm blooded animals become larger in the Northern and colder parts of their range.
- **Gause's law** (Gause, 1934) **Competitive exclusion principle** (Hardin, 1960) states that the two species having the same ecological requirements cannot continue to occupy the same habitat indefinitely.
- **Gloger's rule** states that among warm-blooded animals those living in warm and moist climate develop more melanin (pigment) whereas those living in dry hot climates have more yellow and red pigment.
- **Jordan's rule** states that temperature influences the morphology of certain fishes. It was supported by the fact that the number of vertebrae fishes inhabiting water of low temperature tend to have more vertebrae than those of warm water.

CHECK POINT 23.3

1. The plants growing near sea shore will usually have xerophytic characters, like thick leaves because
   (a) there is plenty of water in the soil
   (b) the concentration of salts is too high for the plants to absorb sufficient water from the soil
   (c) light available to the plants is not sufficient
   (d) the soil is muddy
2. The leaves of desert plants are not torn away by high wind velocity because of
   (a) spines
   (b) bending of leaves towards opposite side
   (c) sclerenchymatous tissue that provides extra mechanical support
   (d) tearing of corners, while the middle remains saved
3. A leaf showing a greatly thickened palisade layer, thickened cuticle and stomata located in pits came from a plant that probably lived in
   (a) tropical forest
   (b) lake
   (c) desert
   (d) mountain top
4. Many freshwater organisms cannot live for long in sea water because the surrounding water will be ...... to body cells and .... may occur.
   (a) hypertonic, exosmosis (b) hypertonic, endosmosis
   (c) hypotonic, exosmosis (d) hypotonic, endosmosis
5. Through which one of the following ways, our body at higher altitudes compensate low oxygen availability?
   (a) By increasing RBC production
   (b) By decreasing breathing rate
   (c) By decreasing the binding affinity of haemoglobin
   (d) by increasing the synthesis of ATP
6. Small animals are not found in polar region as they loss their body heat very fast as compare to big animals what can be the reason?
   (a) Intake of energy by small animals in the form of food is very less
   (b) Surface area of small animals is less than the big animals
   (c) Metabolic rate of small animals is very low as compared to big animals
   (d) Surface area of small animals is larger relative to their volume

POPULATION

The term 'population' can be defined as an assemblage of organisms of the same species living in a particular area at a given time. For example, the lion population of the Gir forest or the peacock population of India, etc.

The population may be subdivided into **demes** or local populations, which are a group of interbreeding organisms. It is the smallest collective unit of a plant or animal population. Metapopulation consists of whole set of local populations which are connected by dispersing individuals.

Table 23.8 Differences between community and population

Community	Population
It is a grouping of individuals of different species found in an area.	It is a grouping of individuals of a single species found in an area.
Interbreeding is absent amongst different members of a community.	Individuals interbreed freely.
Different members of a community are morphologically and behaviourly dissimilar.	Morphologically and behaviourly similar individuals are found in a population.
It is a large unit of organisation.	It is a small unit of organisation.
In a biotic community, there is often a relationship of eating and being eaten.	There is no relationship of eating and being eaten.

Population characteristics

A population has certain attributes that an individual organism does not possess.

Some important characteristics of a population are discussed below

Dispersion

- It indicates how the individuals of a population are distributed in space and time.
- There are three possible ways in which the individuals in a population may be spaced relative to one another. It may be **uniform, random** or **clumped.**
- Invertebrates form populations that contain uniformly spaced individuals. In uniform dispersion, individuals are more or less spaced at equal distance from one another.
- Random spacing occurs particularly among the plants, in which position of one individual is unrelated to the position of its neighbour.
- In clumped dispersion, individuals aggregated into patches interspersed with no or few individuals. Such aggregation may result from social aggregations such as family.
- Besides such clumping for reproductive purposes, animals aggregate in swarms, herbs, flocks or colonies for greater facility of feeding and protection.

- Each species has an optimum clumping value and overcrowding. Beyond this stage, it tends to act as a limiting factor in population regulation (**Allen's principle**).

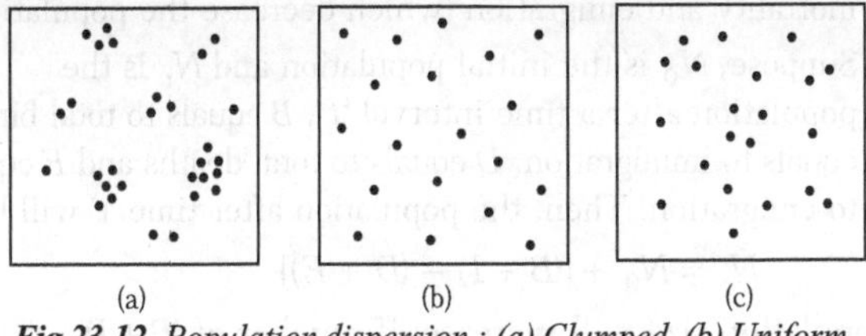

Fig 23.12 Population dispersion : (a) Clumped, (b) Uniform, (c) Random

Population density (*N*)

Density of a population is the number of individuals per unit area or volume. The complete count of individuals in an area is called **census**.

- Density is represented as $D = \frac{N}{S}$,

  Where, N = Total number of individual, S = Space/Area.
- In some cases, it is difficult or meaningless to determine number of individual. For example, in an area if there are 150 *Parthenium* plants, but only a single huge banyan tree with large canopy. Therefore, the percentage cover or biomass is a more meaningful measure of population size.
- Sometimes for certain ecological investigation, there is no need to know the absolute population densities as relative density serves the purpose equally well. For instance, the number of fish caught per trap is a good measure of its population density in lake and the population size is calculated indirectly without actually counting their number.
- Tiger census in our country's National Park and Reserves is often based on pug marks and faecal pellets.
- The density of a population can be studied in several ways. These are as follows
  (i) **Average or Regional density** It is the abundance of a population in a given geographical region.
  (ii) **Economic or Niche density** It refers to the abundance of a population within its niche.
  (iii) **Crude density** It is the density per unit of total space.
  (iv) **Ecological density** It is the density per unit of habitat space (i.e. available area or volume that can actually be colonised by the population).

Natality (birth rate)

- It is the rate of production of new individuals per unit of population per unit time.
- The maximum natality or birth rate achieved under ideal conditions is called **biotic potential**.
- Natality is expressed as

  $\Delta N_n / \Delta t$ = The absolute natality rate

  $\Delta N_n / N\Delta t$ = The specific natality rate (i.e. natality rate per unit of population)

  Where, N = Initial number of organisms

  n = New individuals in the population

  t = Time

Mortality (death rate)

It is the rate of loss of individuals per unit time due to death. It is of two types

(i) **Specific mortality** is the minimum death rate that occurs under ideal conditions due to natural process of senescence.

(ii) **Realised mortality** is the actual rate of death occurring in a unit population due to different environmental changes, competition, disease, predation, etc.

It is seen that maximum mortality occurs in egg, larva, seedling and in old age.

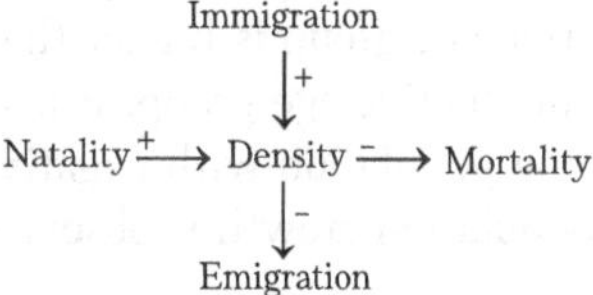

Population dispersal

It is the inward or outward movement of the individuals from the population for preventing overcrowding, obtaining food, avoiding predators and adverse conditions, etc. It also affects the size of a population. Population dispersal may occur in two ways

(i) **Emigration** is permanent outward movement of individuals from a given population to elsewhere. It decreases the size of a population.

(ii) **Immigration** is permanent inward movement of individual of the same species from outside into a habitat from elsewhere. It increases the size of population.

Age distribution

The distribution of individuals of different age groups in a population is known as age distribution. There are three major ecological ages (age groups) in any population (proposed by **AS Bodenheimer**; 1985), which are as follows

(i) Pre-reproductive (ii) Reproductive
(iii) Post-reproductive

The relative duration of these age groups in proportion to the lifespan varies greatly with different organisms.

Age pyramid

A graphic representation of proportion of different age group of a population is called age pyramid. The shape of the pyramids reflect the growth status of the population. The age pyramid can be of following types

(i) **Triangular age pyramid** In this, number of pre-reproductive individual is very large, number of reproductive individuals is moderate, while post-reproductive individuals are fewer. This type of age pyramid shows that population is growing. The rate of growth depends upon the size of pre-reproductive population. This type of population growth is observed in developing countries like India, Brazil, etc.

(ii) **Bell-shaped age pyramid** In this, the number of pre-reproductive and reproductive individual is almost equal. Post-reproductive individuals are comparatively fewer. The rate of growth becomes slow and stable. This type of population growth is observed in countries like USA, Denmark, etc.

(iii) **Urn-shaped pyramid** The proportion of reproductive age group is higher than the individuals in pre-reproductive age group. It is declining or diminishing population with negative growth. This type of population growth is observed in countries like Japan.

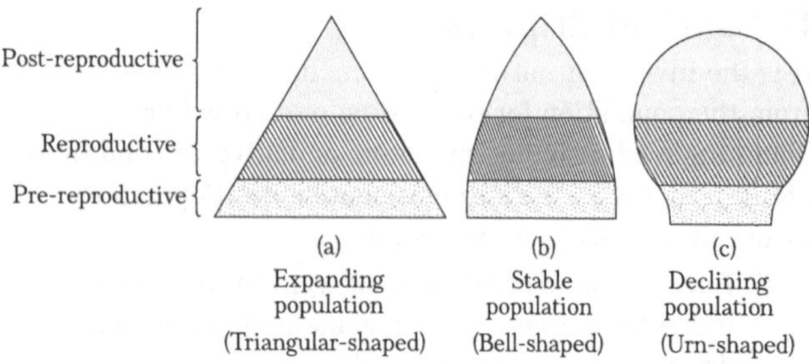

Fig 23.13 Age pyramid in different types of population

Population growth

- It is the number of individuals added per unit population per unit time due to higher birth rate and immigration over the rate of death and emigration.
- The percentage ratio of natality to mortality is called **vital index** ($N/M \times 100$).
- The density of a population in a given habitat during a given period changes by four basic processes, i.e. natality and immigration (which increase the population) and mortality and emigration (which decrease the population).
- Suppose, N_0 is the initial population and N_t is the population after a time interval 't', B equals to total births, I equals to immigration, D equals to total deaths and E equals to emigration. Then, the population after time 't' will be

$$N_t = N_0 + [(B + I) - (D + E)]$$

Population size will increase, if number of $(B + I) >$ number of $(D + E)$

Population size will reduce, if number of $(B + I) <$ number of $(D + E)$

Note
- ***Fecundity*** *is the reproductive output, usually of an individual or number of offsprings produced or capacity of reproduction.*
- ***Total Fertility Rate*** *(TFR) is the total number of offsprings produced per female during her lifetime. TFR should be 2-2.5 for a stable population.*
- ***Survival rate*** *is expressed by survival ship curve (i.e. curve, which plots the number of surviving individuals at a particular age).*

Population growth curves

They represent specific pattern of population growth. There are two basic patterns of population growth, which may be represented as follows

(i) S-shaped growth curve or Sigmoid growth curve

It is also known as **logistic growth** or **Verhulst-Pearl logistic growth.** This kind of graph represents the population growing in a habitat with limited resources.

This type of growth pattern have five phases namely

(a) **Lag phase** In this phase, an organism adapt itself to the new environment.

(b) **Positive acceleration phase** Increase in population starts. It occurs at slow rate in the beginning.

(c) **Exponential** or **Lag phase** Increase in the population become rapid and soon attains its full potential rate due to constant requirement (with respect to availability of food and other requirements).

(d) **Negative acceleration phase** The growth rate finally slows down as the environmental resistance increases due to increase in competition for food, space and mortality, etc.

(e) **Stationary phase** The population become stabilised. A stable population is said to be in equilibrium or at saturation level.

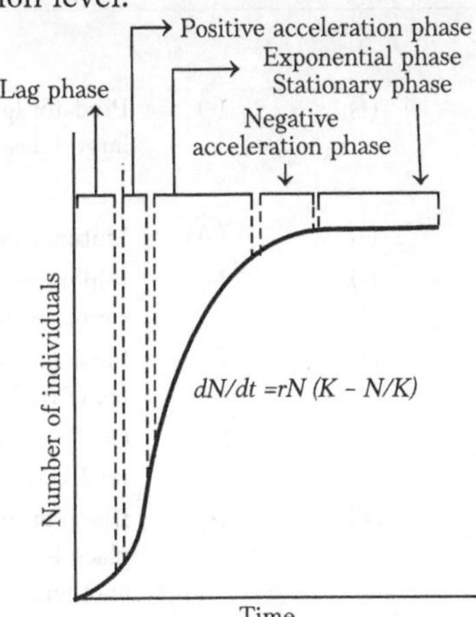

Fig 23.14 Sigmoid growth curve

- In this growth curve, the population size increases, but the population growth rate declines as it approaches carrying capacity (K).
- It is the maximum number of individuals in a population that can be supported sustainably by a given environment.
- Beyond the carrying capacity, the size of the population begins to decrease due to lower natality and higher mortality.
- Sigmoid growth is thus, density dependent and can be expressed by the following equation

$$\frac{dN}{dt} = rN\frac{(K-N)}{K} = rN\left(1-\frac{N}{K}\right)$$

Where, N = Population size

t = Time

K = Carrying capacity

$\frac{dN}{dt}$ = Rate of change in population size

$\frac{K-N}{K}$ = Environmental resistance

r = Natality - Mortality

r = Intrinsic rate of natural increase or biotic potential

When, N = K, the growth rate becomes zero and population reaches to equilibrium. Such type of growth pattern is common in bacteria, yeast and humans.

(ii) J-shaped growth curve or Exponential growth curve

This kind of graph represents the growth of a population in a habitat with unlimited resources.

This type of growth pattern has only two phases namely

(a) **Lag phase** In this phase, there is no significant increase in population for sometime as the organism become adapted to their environment.

(b) **Exponential phase** On becoming adapted to environment, organism starts reproducing rapidly. Finally, when the supply of resources exhausts, this leads to mass starvation and finally leads to death. e.g. lemmings of tundra, some insects, algal blooms, annual plants, etc.

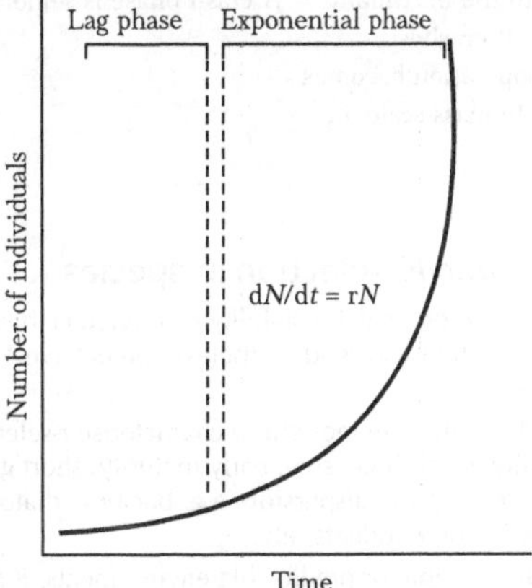

Fig 23.15 Population growth curve when resources are not limiting the growth

- This growth can be expressed by the following equation

$$\frac{dN}{dt} = rN$$

Where, N = Population size

t = Time

r = Intrinsic rate of natural increase

- The value of r is maximum when resources are unlimited.
- The integral form of the exponential growth would be

$$N_t = N_0 e^{rt}$$

Where, N_0 = Population density at time (zero)

N_t = Population density at time t

e = The base of natural logarithms

r = Intrinsic rate of natural increase

Since, resources for growth of most organisms are finite and become limiting sooner or later, the logistic growth model is considered a more realistic model.

Table 23.9 Differences between J-shaped and S-shaped growth curve

J-shaped growth curve	S-shaped growth curve
It occurs when the resources are abundant.	It occurs when the resources are limited.
Population passes well beyond the carrying capacity of the ecosystem.	Population seldom grow beyond the carrying capacity of ecosystem.
An inflection in phase of diminishing growth is not reached.	Prior to reaching the equilibrium phase, population growth shows a phase of declining growth.

J-shaped growth curve	S-shaped growth curve
Minor fluctuations are not observed.	After reaching maximum size, population shows minor fluctuation.
Exponential phase is prolonged.	Exponential phase for shorter duration.
After growing to the maximum population size, it crashes suddenly and population becomes very small due to mass scale death.	A crash phase is seldom reached.

r-selection and *K*-selection in species

(i) ***r*-selection** Environmental instability or unpredictability favours quick reproduction and renders useless competitive adaptations.

- Among the traits that are thought to characterise *r*-selection are high fecundity, small body size, early maturity, short generation time and wide offspring dispersion, e.g. bacteria, diatoms, insects, weeds, some rodents, etc.

(ii) ***K*-selection** In stable or predictable environments, *K*-selection predominates as the ability to compete successfully for limited resources is crucial. The population of *K*-selected organisms typically are very constant and close to maximum that the environment can bear.

- These species have large body size, long life expectancy and the production of fewer offspring and extensive parental care, e.g. elephants, humans, whales, etc.

Population interactions

Members of different populations often interact with each other as well as with their environment. These interactions between the two or several species are based on some factors like

(i) Nature of food and mode of obtaining it.

(ii) Habitat

There are mainly three types of interactions seen among a biological community.

(i) **Negative interaction** (antagonistic) where members of one population may kill members of the other population, compete for food and shelter, etc.

(ii) **Positive interaction** (beneficial) where populations help one another, the interaction being either one way or reciprocal.

(iii) **Neutral interaction** in which neither species is harmed nor benefitted. Relationship between the organisms of two species is known as **interspecific relationship**. It could be negative, positive and neutral interaction.

Table 23.10 Nature of population interactions

Interactions	Effects on species A	Effects on species B	Natures of interaction
With negative effect			
Predation	(+)	(–)	Predator (generally larger) destroys the prey.
Competition			
(a) Direct	(–)	(–)	Mutual inhibition
(b) Indirect	(–)	(–)	Inhibition due to short supply of resources.
Parasitism	(+)	(–)	Parasite (usually smaller) benefitted, host harmed.
Amensalism	(–)	Nil	One inhibited, other unaffected.
Antibiosis	Nil	(–)	Death of organism takes place by the product of another.
With positive effect			
Commensalism	(+)	Nil	Commensal benefitted, other unaffected.
Protocooperation	(+)	(+)	Beneficial to both, not obligatory.
Mutualism	(+)	(+)	Beneficial to both, obligatory.

I. Neutralism

It is an interaction in which a species is not affected by the presence of other species in its environment. This lack of interaction is known as neutralism, e.g. shrew, rabbit and rats inhabit the grassland but none takes the other's food. Shrew feeds on insects, rat feeds on seeds and fruits and rabbits eat grasses.

II. Negative interaction

It is a harmful interaction between two different species, in which at least one of the species is harmed. The antagonistic relationship between organisms is shown by competition, predation, parasitism and antibiosis.
These are described below

Competition

It is interaction between two or more organisms for obtaining the same resources such as food, shelter, etc. It can lead to death for some competitors. It occurs due to fighting or being deprived of food or space.

Competition is of two types

(i) **Intraspecific competition** It occurs between the members of the same population. It is more acute because all organisms of same species. They have similar requirements of food, space, light, mate, etc.

(ii) **Interspecific competition** It occurs between the members of different species. The competition is likely to have two outcomes. These are as follows

(a) **Competitive exclusion** According to Gause's competitive exclusion principle, two closely related species competing for same resources cannot co-exist indefinitely and the competitively inferior species will be eliminated eventually.

e.g. two species of beetles (*Tribolium castaneum* and *T. confusum*) feed on stored flour, one species would survive and other would die.

(b) **Co-existence** Species facing competition might evolve a mechanism to live in the same niche by changing the feeding time or foraging pattern. This is called **resource partitioning**.

Predation

It is an interaction between members of two sepcies in which members of one species capture, kill and eat up members of other species. Former are called **predators,** while later are called **preys.**

Predators are mostly carnivorous animals that eat up other animals. Some plants also act as predators. Typical examples of predator plants are insectivorous plants like sundew (*Drosera*), aquatic bladderwort (*Utricularia*) and pitcher plant (*Nepenthes*).

- **Cannibalism** is a special form of predation in which the predator and the prey belongs to the same species. Thus, in predation, one organism kills another for food.

Importance of predation

- The predator keeps the population of the prey under check, so that an equilibrium is maintained.
- Biological control of weeds and pests, e.g. *Opuntia* turned out to be serious weed in Australia. A herbivore, i.e. *Cactobastis* was introduced to control it.
- Predators also help in maintaining species diversity in a community.
- Predators help in the growth of vegetation all over the globe by restricting the population of herbivore.

Parasitism

It is an interaction between two individuals, wherein the parasite gets the benefit at the expense of the host.

The parasites are divided into different categories

(i) **Ectoparasites** These parasites live on the surface of host, e.g. human body lice *(Pediculus humanus),* human flea (*Pulex irritans*), rat flea (*Xenopsylla cheopsis*), etc.

(ii) **Endoparasites** These parasites live in the digestive tract, body cavities, various organs or blood or other internal tissues of the host, e.g. *Plasmodium malariae, Trypanosoma gambiense, Taenia solium, Fasciola hepatica,* etc.

Table 23.11 Differences between ectoparasites and endoparasites

Ectoparasites	Endoparasites
These are found on the surface of the host.	They are found inside the body of the host.
They can be temporary, intermittent or permanent.	These are always permanent.
These can be holo or hemiparasite.	These are holoparasites.
Aerobic respiration.	Often anaerobic respiration.

(iii) **Facultative parasites** These are the parasites, which can live entirely as saprophytes but become parasites under certain conditions, e.g. oyster, prawn and peacrab.

(iv) **Obligate parasites** These are parasites which live only as parasite, e.g. *Plasmodium* species causing malaria.

(v) **Holoparasites** These parasites are completely dependent on the host for all their requirements, e.g. *Rafflesia, Cuscuta,* etc.

(vi) **Hemiparasites** These parasites receive a part of nourishment from the host, e.g. *Loranthus* (parasitic plant), etc.

(vii) **Hyperparasite** These parasites live on another parasite, e.g. *Cicinnobolus cesatii* (fungus), found on powdery mildew fungi.

(viii) **Brood parasitism** It is a kind of parasitism found in a parasitic bird, which lays its eggs in the nest of its host bird and let the host incubate them. During the course of evolution, the eggs of parasitic birds evolve to resemble the host eggs in size and colour to reduce the chances of host bird detecting the foreign eggs and ejecting them from nest. e.g. cuckoo lays its egg in crow's nest.

Table 23.12 Differences between predator and parasite

Predator	Parasite
It feeds on another organism called prey.	It feeds on another organism called host.
Predator is stronger than the prey.	Parasite is smaller and weaker than the host.
Predator kills the prey.	Parasite does not kill the host immediately, but the host can die due to exploitation.
It feeds on killed prey.	It feeds on living host.
Predator comes in contact with prey for catching and eating.	Temporary or permanent contact with the host.

Co-evolution of parasites

Many parasites have evolved to be host specific in such a way that both host and parasite tend to coevolve, i.e. if the host evolves special mechanism for rejecting or resisting the parasite, the parasite also has to evolve the mechanism to counteract and neutralise them.

- In accordance with their lifestyle, parasites have evolved special adaptations such as
  (a) Loss of unnecessary sense organs.
  (b) Presence of adhesive organs or suckers to cling on to host.
  (c) Loss of digestive system, e.g. *Taenia.*
  (d) High reproductive capacity.

Amensalism

It is an interaction between two living individuals of different species, in which an organism does not allow other organism to grow or live near it. This inhibition is achieved through the secretion of chemicals called **allochemies**, e.g.

(i) *Penicillium* does not allow the growth of *Staphylococcus* bacterium.
(ii) *Convolvulus arvensis* inhibits the germination and growth of wheat.
(iii) Roots of black walnut (*Juglans nigra*) produce a chemical named **juglans.** It is toxic to apple, tomato and alflfa.
(iv) *Tagetes* (marigold) secretes chemicals toxic to soil nematodes.

Antibiosis

It is a type of negative interaction in which complete or partial inhibition or death of one organism takes place by the products of another organism. Here, none of them derive any benefit from each other.
For example, antibiotics derived from fungi are antagonistic to microbes.

III. Positive interaction

It means 'living together'. It is a beneficial coaction between two or more different species, in which one or both the species are benefitted and neither species is harmed. It includes commensalism, protocooperation and mutualism.

These are as follows

Commensalism

It is an association or relationship between two different organisms in which one is always benefitted, while the other is neither benefitted nor harmed. All commensalistic unions are facultative. For example,

(i) **Sucker fish** (*Echenesis*) attaches itself to the under surface of shark with the help of its dorsal fin, which is modified into holdfast. Sucker fish gets a free ride and remains of food which a shark eats.
The shark neither benefits nor suffers in any respect.

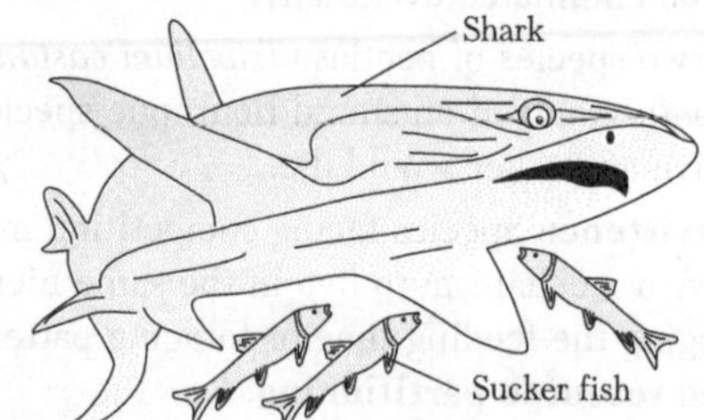

Fig 23.16 Commensalism between sucker fish and shark

(ii) An orchid growing as epiphyte on mango tree.
(iii) Barnacles growing on the back of whale.
(iv) Clown fish that lives among sea anemone gets protection from predators, which stay away from the stinging tentacles of sea anemone.
(v) The most extraordinary example of a commensal living within its host is that of a small tropical fish, *Fierasfer.* It finds shelter in the cloaca of sea cucumbers. The fish comes out for food and returns to the cloacal cavity on its own will.

Protocooperation

It is the interaction between two living organisms of different species, in which both are mutually benefitted but they can also live without each other. e.g.

(i) Association of hermit crab and a coelenterate (sea anemone). The sea anemone (*Adamsia palliata*) grows on the back of the hermit crab (*Eupagurus prideauxi*). It protects the crab with the help of its nematocysts and in turn, obtains shelter from the crab.
(ii) Red billed ox pecker sits on the back of rhinoceros and feed on the ticks.

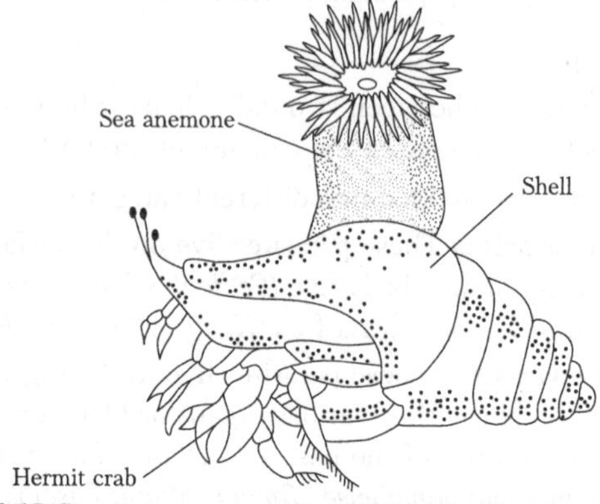

Fig 23.17 Sea anemone on snail's shell inhabited by a hermit crab

Mutualism

It is a relationship between two or more individuals of different species in which all are benefitted by one another.

(i) **Lichen** It is a mutualistic association between some species of algae and fungi. The main body of the lichen is formed of fungus. The fungus (myobiont) provides fixation, water, minerals and shelter to the algae. The algae (phycobiont) in turn, manufactures food not only for itself but also for the fungus. This interaction or relationship allows the lichens to grow in highly hostile environment.

(ii) **Mutualism** between the plants and bacteria. It is an interaction between the roots of certain leguminous plants and the **nitrogen-fixing bacteria** (e.g. *Rhizobium radicicola*). The plant provides shelter to the bacteria and bacteria fix the N_2 for the plants.

(iii) **Mycorrhiza** (Gr. *myo*-fungus; *rhiza*—root) It is a mutualistic association of a fungus with the roots of higher plants. The root provides food and shelter to the fungus.

The fungus helps the plants in solubilisation and absorption of mineral, water and protection against pathogenic fungi. It is mainly found in vascular plants. These plants grow mainly in oligotrophic soil, i.e. soil poor in nutrients.

They are of two types

(a) **Ectomycorrhiza** They form a thick sheath of fungal mycelium around the roots. Mantle is present outside and intercellular hyphae is present in the cortex of root, which penetrates between the cortical cells. The cortical cells themselves are not penetrated by the fungal hyphae.

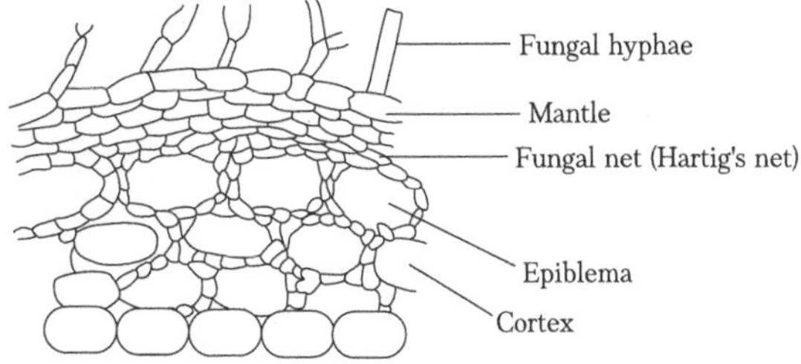

***Fig 23.18** Ectomorphic mycorrhiza : Part of a section showing mantle and Hartig's net*

Cortical cells are surrounded by a network of hyphae called **Hartig's net.** They occur in several trees, shrubs of temperate areas and some tropical species as well, e.g. pine, oak, *Eucalyptus.*

Ectomycorrhiza is found in about 80% of all the vascular plants. These mycorrhiza are most widely distributed through plant kingdom geographically. It is a type of endoinfection formed by the member of Zygomycota or order—Glomales.

(b) **Endomycorrhiza** In this association, the penetrating hyphae forms a haustorial branches (arbus cules) and vesicles. Therefore, the fungus is also called **Vesicular Arbuscular Mycorrhizae** (VAM). Intercellular hyphae and external hyphae are present, but are fewer in number.

Animal-plant mutualism

Plants need help of animals for pollinating their flowers and dispersing their seeds, e.g.

(i) Female wasp uses the fig fruits as a site of oviposition (egg lying) and developing seeds for nourishing its larvae. The wasp in turn, pollinates the fig inflorescence.

(ii) In orchids, it employs sexual deceit to get pollination done by a species of bee. One petal of its flower bears an uncanny resemblance to the female bee.

The male bee is attracted to what it perceives as a female, pseudocopulates with the flower and in that process, pollination is done.

Table 23.13 Differences between mutualism and commensalism

Mutualism	Commensalism
It is an association between two organisms, in which both are benefitted.	It is an association between two organisms, in which one is benefitted. The second is neither benefitted nor harmed.
Contact between the two organisms is obligatory.	All commensalism unions are facultative.

Symbiosis and mutualism

The term '**symbiosis**' and '**mutualism**' are sometimes confused with each other. Symbiosis is only a **beneficial interaction** between the organisms, which in real sense means **living together**.

In broad sense, it includes all such interactions, which are possible between any two or more organisms or their population living together and sharing same habitat. **Mutualism** is one such category under symbiosis.

CHECK POINT 23.4

1. When the carrying capacity is equal to the population size, the net rate of increase in the population equals to
   (a) the carrying capacity
   (b) less than zero
   (c) the intrinsic rate of growth
   (d) zero

2. Under which of the following circumstances, would interspecific competition be most obvious?
   (a) In the presence of a keystone species
   (b) When organisms have quite different ecological niches
   (c) Among species, whose trophic levels are different
   (d) When a non-native organism is introduced to a community

3. The flower fly resembles a honeybee, but the flower fly has no stings. This is an example of
   (a) Batesian mimicry
   (b) Mullerian mimicry
   (c) Cryptic colouration
   (d) Interspecific competition

4. Competition for food, light and space is most severe between two
   (a) distantly related species growing in different habitat
   (b) distantly related species growing in the same habitat
   (c) closely related species growing in different habitat
   (d) closely related species growing in the same area

5. Two species competing for the same resource can avoid competition by choosing different habits. This phenomenon is called ...... and was supported by ....
   (a) competitive exclusion, Cause
   (b) competitive exclusion, MacArthur
   (c) resource partitioning, Gause
   (d) resource partitioning, MacArthur

6. The interdependent evolution of flowerig plants and pollination insects together is known as
   (a) mutualism
   (b) co-evolution
   (c) commensalism
   (d) co-operations

7. A bird introduced from another country became a serious pest due to
   (a) better adaptation to new area
   (b) more sexual reproduction
   (c) better nesting habitats
   (d) absence of natural competition

8. Scavenging is
   (a) an interaction between two living individuals of different species, in which one organism does not allow other organism to grow or live near it
   (b) a relationship between two living individuals of different species, in which one is benefitted, while the other is neither harmed nor benefitted except to a negligible extent
   (c) a rivalry between two or more organisms for obtaining the same resources
   (d) feeding on flesh of an animal, which had died naturally or has been killed by another animal

EXAM POINTS

- The basic unit of study in ecology is organism. **[DUMET 2011]**
- Plant species having a wide range of genetic distribution evolve into local population is known as ecotype. **[J&K CET 2015]**
- Adaptations in an organism are meant for optimum lifespan. **[AMU 2015]**
- Major ecological community of plants and animals extending over large natural area is known as biome. **[J&K CET 2016]**
- Mean annual precipitation in tropical forest is 150-400 cm, coniferous forest is 50-250 cm, grassland is 50-100 cm and desert is 0-50 cm. **[AIIMS 2016]**
- 45-66° is the range of latitudes for temperate region. **[Gujarat CET 2014]**
- The term 'Niche' was first used by Grinnel. **[UP CPMT 2011]**
- The niche of a population is defined as place where it lives. **[JCECE 2012]**
- Some organisms are tolerant to a narrow range of salinity and are termed as stenohaline. **[AMU 2012]**
- Edaphic factors are related to soil texture. **[EAMCET 2015]**
- Water holding capacity of sandy soil as compared to clayey soil is less. **[UK PMT 2015]**
- Majority of animals and nearly all plants cannot maintain a constant internal environment. **[Kerala CEE 2014]**
- All birds and mammals are capable of thermoregulation. **[Kerala CEE 2014]**
- Roots play insignificant role in absorption of water in *Pistia*. **[CBSE AIPMT 2015]**
- Plants growing on sandy soil are psammophyte. **[CPMT 2015]**
- Marine fishes have aglomerular kidneys. Aglomerular kidneys increase the loss of water through urine. **[EAMCET 2015]**
- The resting state of reptiles in winter is hibernation. **[WB JEE 2015]**
- Hibernating animals have tissues containing mitochondria with a membrane protein that accelerates electron transport while blocking synthesis of ATP. The consequence of this is that energy of respiration is converted into heat. **[CBSE AIPMT 2015]**
- The characters such as pointed elongated snout, strong and stout forelimbs, well-developed claws are observed in fossorial adaptation. **[MHT CET 2015]**
- Shivering is a kind of exercise which produces heat and raises body temperature. **[Kerala CEE 2014]**
- Diapause is a stage of suspended development seen in zooplankton. **[Kerala CEE 2014]**
- Most animals that live in deep oceanic waters are detritivores. **[CBSE AIPMT 2015]**
- Allen's rule stated that animals with shorter limbs and ears minimize heat loss. **[Karnataka CET 2016]**
- The age pyramid with broad base indicates high percentage of young individuals. **[DUMET 2011]**
- In growing population of a country, pre-reproductive individuals are more than the reproductive individuals. **[NEET 2018]**
- Triangular pyramid shows growing or expanding population. Bell-shaped pyramid shows stable population and spindle-shaped shows declined population. **[AIIMS 2019]**
- Natality (birth rate), mortality (death rate) and sex ratio are attributes of a population whereas species interaction is not. **[NEET 2020]**
- Natality refers to the number of birth during a given period of time. **[NEET 2018]**
- The impact of immigration on population is positive as the population density increases. **[NEET 2020]**
- Exponential growth in plants can be expressed as $W_1 = W_0 ert$.
- Asymptote is a logistic growth curve. It is obtained when $K=N$. **[NEET 2017]**
- The carring capacity of enviornment for a given population can be represented by $\frac{dN}{dt} = rN\left(1 - \frac{N}{K}\right)$ **[AMU 2012]**
- r -selected are the species having the ability to produce large number of progenies with small size. **[NEET-II 2016]**
- A population growing in a habitat with limited resources shows four phases of growth are as follows
  Lag phase – Acceleration – Deceleration – Asymptote. **[AFMC 2012]**
- The growth of a population without limit at its maximal rate and also that, rates of immigration and emigration are equal, than it is called biotic potential. **[EAMCET 2012]**
- Maximum survival and reproductive capacity shown by a population under optimal environmental conditions is called biotic potential. **[J&K CET 2011]**
- In competition, species fight over same resources, e.g. sheep and cow for grass. **[NEET 2019]**
- Relation between herbivores and plants is prey and predator type where herbivores are predator and plants are prey. **[NEET 2017]**
- Carnivores animals, lions and leopards occupy the same niche, but lions predate mostly larger animals. This mechanism of competition is referred as resource partitioning. **[NEET 2019]**
- Gause's principle of competitive exclusion states that no true species can occupy the same niche indefinitely for the same limiting resources. **[NEET-II 2016]**
- Predation and parasitism are the two ways of exploitation. **[Gujarat CET 2011]**
- Parasitism represented by +, – as in this, one species is benefitted and the other is harmed. **[NEET-II 2016]**
- In commensalism, neither the species is harmed nor benefitted, e.g. orchid and tree cattle egret and grazing cattle, sea anemone and clown fish. **[NEET 2020, 19, JIPMER 2019]**
- A sedentary sea anemone gets attached to the shell lining of hermit crab. The association is called commensalism. **[NEET 2013]**
- Small fish get stuck near the bottom of a shark and derives its nutrition from it. This kind of association is called as commensalism. **[BCECE 2012]**
- An interaction favourable to both population, but no obligatory to either is protocoperation. **[UP CPMT 2011]**
- Amensalism is an interaction between different species in which one species is harmed and the other is neither benefitted nor harmed. **[NEET 2018]**
- In mutualism, both species are benefitted, e.g. mycorrhiza. **[NEET 2020, 2017]**
- Allelopathy is a phenomenon associated with plants in which one species suffer and other remains unaffected. **[AIIMS 2017]**
- The association of mycorrhiza is relationship of fungi and higher plants. **[BCECE 2012]**
- The coralloid root of *Cycas* has *Anabaena* (BGA), this type of association is called symbiotic. **[UP CPMT 2012]**

Chapter Exercises

(A) Topical Exercise

Branches and Terms of Ecology, Environment

1 The study of interaction between the living organism and their environment is called

(a) Phytogeography (b) Ecology
(c) Ecosystem (d) Phytosociology

2 The study of inter-relationship between the species/individual and its environment in all stages of its life cycle

(a) synecology (b) forest ecology
(c) autecology (d) ecology

3 The study of inter-relationship between an entire community and its environment is

(a) autecology (b) resource ecology
(c) species ecology (d) synecology

4 A boundary between two plant communities of major rank is called

(a) ecotone (b) niche (c) ecotypes (d) ecade

5 Species found exclusively in ecotone are called

(a) morphospecies (b) edges species
(c) allopatric species (d) sympatric species

6 The phenomenon of having higher number of species in ecotone is called

(a) edge effect (b) abundance
(c) frequency (d) dominance effect

7 Find the incorrect matched pair.

(a) Ecology – Haeckel
(b) Niche – Grinnell
(c) Bioecology – Shelford and Clements
(d) None of the above

8 Consider the following statements.

I. Mean annual temperature of tropical zone is more than 24°C.

II. Climate zone between 20-40°C is in temperate and sub-Arctic.

Choose the correct option.

(a) Statement I is true, but II is false
(b) Statement I is false, but II is true
(c) Both statements I and II are true
(d) Both statements I and II are false

9 Choose the correct statement.

(a) A local variation of climate is called microclimate
(b) Winters are absent in tropical climatic zone
(c) The factor related to structure of earth surface is edaphic
(d) All of the above

10 Consider the following statements.

I. Cow in India and kangaroo in Australia (both herbivores) are ecological equivalents.

II. The organisms having similar niche in different geographical regions are known as ecological equivalents.

Choose the correct option.

(a) Statement I is true, but II is false
(b) Statement I is false, but II is true
(c) Both statements I and II are true
(d) Both statements I and II are false

11 Choose the incorrect statement.

(a) Biome characterised by a layer of permanently frozen forest is cold deserts
(b) Biome having the highest species diversity is tropical rainforest
(c) The typical biome of an area having 25-75 cm of rainfall is grassland
(d) Two species cannot live in the same niche due to Allen's law

12 Niche of an organism denotes

(a) habitat
(b) microhabitat
(c) habitat as well as inter-relations
(d) habitat as well as climate

13 What will happen to a well growing herbaceous plant in the forest if it is transplanted outside the forest in a park?

(a) It will grow normally
(b) It will grow well because it is planted in the same locality
(c) It may not survive because of change in its microclimate
(d) It grows very well because the plant gets more sunlight

14 Choose the incorrectly matched pair.

(a) Productivity - Amount of organic matter accumulated in living being
(b) Biomass -Standing mass in terms of weight of living matter
(c) Hypervolume niche-Explained by Hutchinson
(d) None of the above

15 Formation of tropical forests needs mean annual temperature and mean annual precipitation of
(a) 18-25°C and 150-400 cm
(b) 5-15°C and 50-100 cm
(c) 30-50°C and 100-150 cm
(d) 5-15°C and 100-200 cm

Ecological Factors

16 The most important factor for living organisms is
(a) water (b) temperature
(c) light (d) All of these

17 Warm, oxygen-rich, upper layer of water in a lake or water body is called
(a) thermocline (b) epilimnion
(c) hypolimnion (d) All of these

18 Aquatic animals which can tolerate only a narrow range of salinity are said to be
(a) euryhaline (b) stenohaline
(c) poikilotherms (d) catadromus

19 In which zone of the lake ecosystem, the production is greater than respiration?
(a) Littoral zone (b) Profundal zone
(c) Limnetic zone (d) Both (a) and (b)

20 Shallow lakes with abundant organic matter are
(a) saprotrophic (b) oligotrophic
(c) eutrophic (d) heterotrophic

21 In an aqueous environment, microscopic animals and plants are collectively known as
(a) plankton (b) herbivore
(c) commensals (d) flora and fauna

22 Abyssal zone in ocean has
(a) no sunlight, but contains consumers and decomposers
(b) no sunlight, but contains producers
(c) no sunlight, but contains living beings
(d) sunlight as well as producers

23 Edaphology is connected with
(a) plant and biosphere
(b) soil and living microorganisms
(c) animals and ecosystem
(d) soil and biosphere

24 An area of soil thoroughly wetted and allowed to drain till percolation stops will have a water content called
(a) capillary water
(b) storage water
(c) field capacity
(d) gravitational water

25 The amount of water a soil can hold against the pull of gravity is called
(a) field capacity
(b) gravitational water
(c) storage water
(d) hygroscopic water

26 Water held tightly by soil particles as a thin film over their surface is
(a) hygroscopic water (b) capillary water
(c) chemical water (d) gravitational water

27 Top soil is darker and
(a) contains more sodium and magnesium
(b) is drier than subsoil
(c) contains more organic matter
(d) is better than subsoil

28. A_0 layer of the soil is made up of
(a) decaying litter
(b) rocky matter
(c) soil mixed with organic matter
(d) soil rich in inorganic matter

29 Soil particles arranged in a series of increasing size is
(a) silt → sand → clay (b) sand → silt → clay
(c) clay → sand → silt (d) clay → silt → sand

30 Choose the correct statement.
(a) River water deposits alluvial soil
(b) Least porous soil is clayey soil
(c) Soil water available to roots is capillary water
(d) All of the above

31 What is the best pH of soil for cultivation?
(a) 3.4-5.4 (b) 4.5-5.5 (c) 5.5-6.5 (d) 6.5-7.5

32 Insectivorous plants are adapted to soils
(a) rich in water
(b) deficient in water
(c) deficient in nitrogenous compounds
(d) deficient in trace elements

33 Animals of coastal water are called
(a) pelagic (b) neritic
(c) benthos (d) stenothermals

34 Consider the following statements.
I. Deposition of washed minerals in lower strata is illuviation.
II. Sandy soil is deficient in nutrients.
Choose the correct option.
(a) Statement I is true, but II is false
(b) Statement I is false, but II is true
(c) Both statements I and II are true
(d) Both statements I and II are false

Ecological Adaptations

35 Heliophytes are plants grawing in
(a) low light intensity
(b) partial shade intensity
(c) bright light intensity
(d) Both (a) and (b)

36 Consider the following statements.
I. Stem of submerged hydrophytes is soft and weak because of the absence of xylem.
II. *Typha* is a emergent hydrophytes.
Choose the correct option.
(a) Statement I is true, but II is false
(b) Statement I is false, but II is true
(c) Both statements I and II are true
(d) Both statements I and II are false

37 A plant devoid of roots is
(a) *Wolffia/Ceratophyllum*
(b) *Vallisneria*
(c) *Hydrilla*
(d) *Azolla*

38 Consider the following statements.
I. Aquatic plants generally have a well-developed vascular system.
II. The floating leaves of an aquatic plant have stomata on the upper surfaces.
Choose the correct option.
(a) Statement I is true, but II is false
(b) Statement I is false, but II is true
(c) Both statements I and II are true
(d) Both statements I and II are false

39 Choose the incorrect match pair.
(a) *Eichhornia crassipes* – Mesophyte
(b) *Rhizophora* – Vivipary
(c) *Sagittaria* – Amphibious plant
(d) None of the above

40 Stomata are sunken types in
(a) mesophytes (b) xerophytes
(c) hygrophytes (d) hydrophytes

41 Which one is an exclusive xerophytic adaptation?
(a) Absence of stomata (b) Long tap root system
(c) Stipular leaves (d) Presence of spines

42 The type of plants having adaptations to check transpiration is
(a) xerophytes (b) lithophytes
(c) halophytes (d) epiphytes

43 Ephemerals are a type of xerophytes, which are
(a) drought-escaping (b) drought-resisting
(c) drought-enduring (d) None of these

44 Thick cuticle occurs on the leaves of plants belonging to
(a) cool habitats (b) warm habitats
(c) dry habitats (d) wet habitats

45 Succulents occur in
(a) deserts
(b) tundra
(c) temperate deciduous forests
(d) tropical rainforests

46 Plants of salty sea shore wet lands are
(a) heliophytes (b) hydrophytes
(c) halophytes (d) saprophytes

47 Viviparity and pneumatophores are the features of
(a) hydrophytes (b) halophytes
(c) mesophytes (d) xerophytes

48 Deserts can be converted into grass land by
(a) tropical trees (b) psammophytes
(c) halophytes (d) xylophytes

49 Mangrove of marshy sundarbans is characterised by
(a) pneumatophores (b) prop roots
(c) vivipary (d) All of these

50 Which of the following forest plants controls the light conditions at the ground?
(a) Lianas and climbers (b) Shrubs
(c) Tall trees (d) Herbs

51 Dormancy in animals through a hot season is called
(a) hibernation (b) aestivation
(c) diapause (d) None of these

52 A terrestrial mammal who seldom drink water is
(a) hippopotamus (b) rhinoceros
(c) kangaroo rat (d) camel

53 Cryptic appearance/camouflage is found in
(a) praying mantis
(b) leaf insect
(c) stick insect/dead leaf butterfly
(d) All of the above

Population, its Characteristics and Interaction

54 Population natality is
(a) realised natality (b) biotic potential
(c) vital index (d) carrying capacity

55 Which one of the following is a qualitative character?
(a) Dispersion (b) Life forms
(c) Growth forms (d) Diversity

56 Which of the following would necessarily decrease the density of a population in a given habitat?
(a) Natality > mortality
(b) Immigration > emigration
(c) Mortality and emigration
(d) Natality and immigration

57 The age structure of a population is its
(a) relative number of individuals at each age
(b) number of newborns each year
(c) number of young reaching puberty each year
(d) relative number of deaths at each age

58 The representation of age pyramid for human population given here, shows

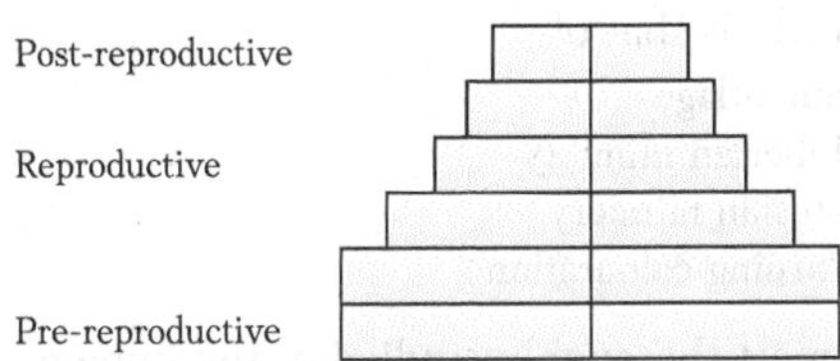

(a) declining population (b) stable population
(c) increasing population (d) fluctuating population

59 The formula, $dN/dt = g$ represents
(a) environmental resistance
(b) vital index
(c) carrying capacity
(d) exponential growth

60 The equation, $\frac{(K-N)}{K}$ represents
(a) carrying capacity
(b) environmental resistance
(c) vital index
(d) crash phase

61 The graph shows two types of population growth curve *A* is exponential and *B* is logistic.

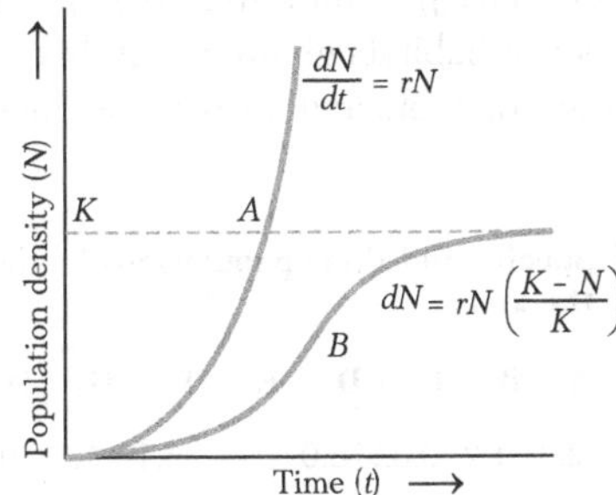

Which one of the following growth model considered as more realistic one?
(a) Exponential growth curve
(b) Logistic growth curve
(c) Z-shaped growth curve
(d) All of the above

62 Choose the correct statement.
(a) Population connected by dispersing individuals is called metapopulation
(b) In ecology, *N/S* represents population density
(c) dN/dt represents change in population size
(d) All statements are correct

63 Consider the following statements.
I. Minor fluctuations are not observed in J.shaped growth curve.
II. Environmental instability favours quick reproduction in *r*-selected population.
Choose the correct option.
(a) Statement I is true, but II is false
(b) Statement I is false, but II is true
(c) Both statements I and II are true
(d) Both statements I and II are false

64 If a population of 50 *Paramecium* present in a pool increases to 150 after an hour, what would be the growth rate of population?
(a) 50 per hour (b) 200 per hour
(c) 5 per hour (d) 100 per hour

65 Two opposite forces operate in growth and development of every population. One of them has ability to reproduce at a given time rate. The opposite force is
(a) morbidity (b) fecundity
(c) biotic potential (d) environmental resistance

66 At the equilibrium stage of sigmoid curve, population size
(a) shows minor fluctuation (b) shows slow growth
(c) remains static (d) declines very slowly

67 Exponential growth in human population is done in
(a) lag phase (b) log phase
(c) plateau stage (d) first stage

68 When birth rate equals death rate, it is called
(a) plateau stage (b) exponential growth stage
(c) early growth stage (d) acceleration stage

69 At asymptome stage, the population is
(a) stabilised (b) increasing
(c) decreasing (d) changing

70 All the listed organisms would exhibit *K*-selection except.
(a) elephant (b) bacteria
(c) whale (d) human

71 Dominant species represent most abundant
(a) species having major effect on physical environment
(b) shrubs that appears for the first time
(c) trees
(d) herbs that binds the soil

72 The association of mycorrhiza with angiospermic root is referred as

(a) amensalism (b) mutualism
(c) parasitism (d) commensalism

73 Mutualism and protocooperation are

(a) positive interactions (b) negative interactions
(c) neutral (d) Both (a) and (b)

74 Choose the correct statements.

(a) Species interaction with negative influence on both is called competition
(b) The non-obligatory mutually beneficial relationship is represented by protocooperation
(c) The relationship between epiphytes and tree is commensalism
(d) All of the above

75 When an animal group is centred around a dominant female, it is called

(a) patriarchy (b) matriarchy
(c) monarchy (d) polyarchy

76 The relationship between the two organisms or species in which both the partners derive benefit from each other is known as

(a) parasitism (b) symbiosis
(c) commensalism (d) None of these

77 Symbiosis may be defined as a relationship, in which

(a) Both the partners derive benefit from each other
(b) Both the partners are harmed
(c) Only one partner derives the benefit
(d) None of the partner derives the benefit

78 The relationship between species and another within a community that has evolved through interaction is based upon

(a) requirement and mode of obtaining food only
(b) requirement and mode of obtaining shelter only
(c) on the habits of the species only
(d) All of the above

79 Relation between viceroy butterfly and monarch butterfly is that of

(a) Camouflage
(b) Mullerian mimicry
(c) Batesian mimicry
(d) Warning colouration

80 The most thoroughly studied of the known bacteria-plant interactions is the

(a) cyanobacterial symbiosis with some aquatic ferns
(b) gall formation on certain angiosperms by *Agrobacterium*
(c) nodulation of *Sesbania* stems by nitrogen-fixing bacteria
(d) plant growth stimulation by phosphate solublising bacteria

(B) Cumulative Exercise

(Assorted Questions of the Chapter for Advanced Level Practice)

1 Match the following columns.

Column I	Column II
A. Competition	1. Favourable relationship between two species, but not obligatory
B. Antagonism	2. Relationship between two organisms in which both are benefitted
C. Mutualism	3. Harmful co-action between two species
D. Protocooperation	4. Rivalry between two or more organisms for same resource

Codes

	A	B	C	D		A	B	C	D
(a)	1	2	3	4	(b)	4	3	2	1
(c)	4	2	1	3	(d)	1	2	4	3

2 The following diagrams show possible ways of population dispersion.

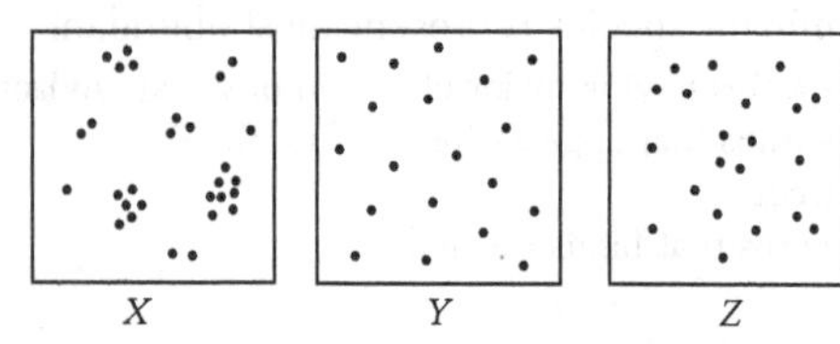

Which one of the following is the most common pattern of dispersion in a human population?

(a) *X* (b) *Y*
(c) *Z* (d) *X* and *Y*

3 The table below gives the populations (in thousands) of ten species (A-J) in four areas (I-IV) consisting of the number of habitats given within brackets against each. Study the table and answer the question, which follows.

Area and number of habitats	Species and their populations (in thousands) in the areas									
	A	B	C	D	E	F	G	H	I	J
I (11)	2.3	1.2	0.52	6.0	–	3.1	1.1	9.0	–	10.3
II (11)	10.2	–	0.62	–	1.5	3.0	–	8.2	1.1	11.2
III (13)	11.3	0.9	0.48	2.4	1.4	4.2	0.8	8.4	2.2	4.1
IV (12)	3.2	10.2	11.1	4.8	0.4	3.3	0.8	7.3	11.3	2.1

Which area out of I to IV shows maximum species diversity?

(a) II (b) III
(c) IV (d) I

4 Match the following columns.

Column I		Column II
A. Plants growing in water	1.	Mesophytes
B. Plants growing in arid region	2.	Xerophytes
C. Plants growing in wet region	3.	Hydrophytes
D. Plants growing on land	4.	Halophytes

Codes

	A	B	C	D
(a)	3	2	4	1
(b)	1	2	3	4
(c)	4	3	1	2
(d)	1	2	3	4

5 The figure given below is a diagrammatic representation of response of organisms to abiotic factors. What do *A*, *B* and *C* represent, respectively?

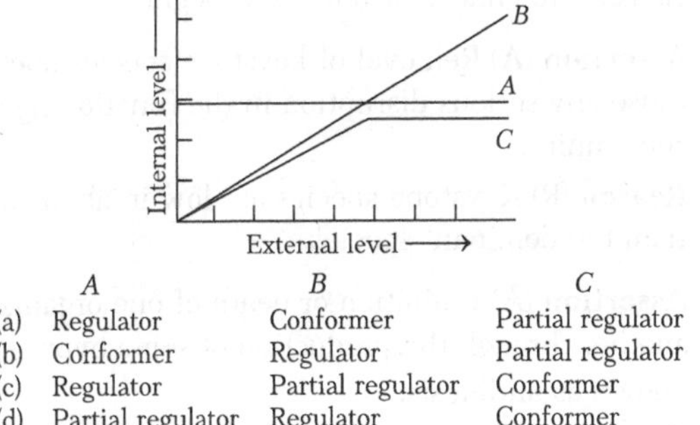

	A	*B*	*C*
(a)	Regulator	Conformer	Partial regulator
(b)	Conformer	Regulator	Partial regulator
(c)	Regulator	Partial regulator	Conformer
(d)	Partial regulator	Regulator	Conformer

6 Which of the following statements are correct?

I. Mortality is the rate of loss of individuals per unit time due to death.

II. Population dispersion affects the size of population.

III. Age distribution influences both natality and mortality of the population.

IV. Realised natality is the actual death rate found under existing conditions.

Codes

(a) I and IV (b) II and IV
(c) I and II (d) I, II and III

7 In lake ecosystems, in

I. littoral zone, the rate of photosynthesis equals the rate of respiration.

II. profundal zone, only respiration occurs.

III. limnetic zone, production is lower than respiration.

IV. profundal zone, production is greater than respiration.

Choose the option containing correct statement(s).

(a) Only I (b) III and IV (c) I and III (d) I and II

8 A country with a high rate of population growth took measures to reduce it. The figure below shows age sex pyramids of populations. Where '*A*' and '*B*' are twenty years apart. Select the correct interpretation about them.

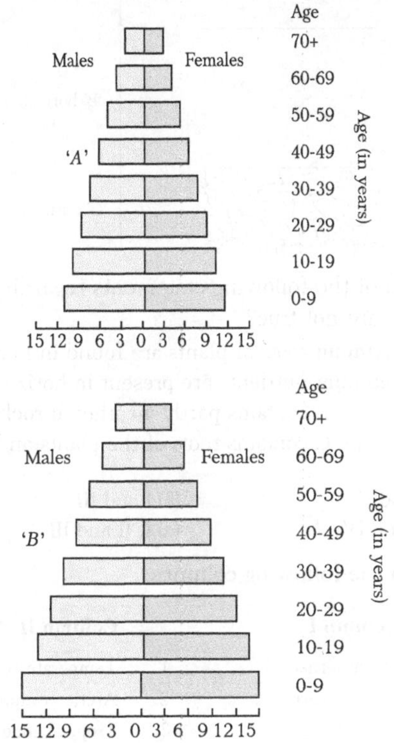

Interpretations

(a) '*A*' is more recent and shows slight reduction in the growth rate

(b) '*B*' is earlier pyramid and shows stabilised growth rate

(c) '*B*' is more recent showing that population is very young

(d) '*A*' is the earlier pyramid and no change has occurred in the growth rate

9 Which of the following statement(s) is/are correct?

I. Population is a group of individual organisms of the same species in a given area.

II. An ecotype is a population of individuals of a species, which are genetically different.

III. Environment is influnced by many biotic and abiotic factors.

IV. Ecade is a place, where an organism lives.

Choose the correct option from the codes given below.

(a) Only III
(b) I and III
(c) I and II
(d) I, II and III

10 Given figure represents the soil profile, showing different layers/horizons of soil.

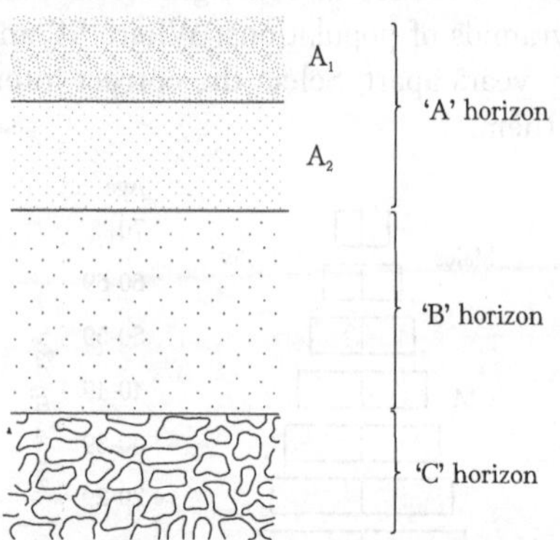

Which of the following statements regarding the soil profile are not true?

I. Maximum roots of plants are found in horizon A.
II. Maximum nutrients are present in horizon B.
III. Horizon B contains partly weathered rocks.
IV. Horizon C contains roots of the plants and minerals.

Codes

(a) I and II (b) I and III
(c) II and IV (d) I, II and III

11 Match the following columns.

	Column I		Column II
A.	Megatherms	1.	Temperate zone
B.	Mesotherms	2.	Arctic or alpine zone
C.	Microtherms	3.	Tropical zone
D.	Heikstotherms	4.	Subtropical zone

Codes

	A	B	C	D		A	B	C	D
(a)	1	2	3	4	(b)	4	3	2	1
(c)	1	2	4	3	(d)	3	4	1	2

Assertion and Reason

Direction (Q. Nos. 12-23) *In each of the following questions, a statement of Assertion (A) is given followed by corresponding statement of Reason (R). Of the statements, mark the correct answer as*

(a) Both A and R are true and R is the correct explanation of A
(b) Both A and R are true, but R is not the correct explanation of A
(c) A is true, but R is false
(d) A is false, but R is true
(e) Both A and R are false

12 **Assertion** (A) Genecology is the study of genetic composition and changes in relation to the origin of ecads, ecotypes, new species, etc.

Reason (R) Autecology deals with the study of a group of organisms.

13 **Assertion** (A) Leaf butterfly and stick insect show mimicry to dodge their enemies.

Reason (R) Mimicry is a method to acquire body colour blending with the surroundings.

14 **Assertion** (A) Animals adopt different strategies to survive in hostile environment.

Reason (R) Praying mantis is green in colour, which merges with plant foliage.

15 **Assertion** (A) Xeromorphic characters are inherited.

Reason (R) Plants obtain xeromorphic characters from xeric conditions.

16 **Assertion** (A) Drought escaping plants survive in the form of seeds and fruits.

Reason (R) Drought evader plants do not have the capacity to endure or tolerate drought.

17 **Assertion** (A) Removal of keystone species does not cause any serious disruption in the functioning of the community.

Reason (R) Keystone species are low in abundance than the dominant species.

18 **Assertion** (A) Inhibition or death of one organism by another through the production of some byproducts is known as antibiosis.

Reason (R) Antibiosis is a type of negative interaction.

19 **Assertion** (A) Commensalism is a type of positive interaction.

Reason (R) In commensalism, one organism is benefitted, while other is harmed.

20 **Assertion** (A) Mycorrhiza is an mutualistic inter-relationship.

Reason (R) Mycorrhiza is an association between fungi and roots of higher plants.

21 **Assertion** (A) Individual of a species makes a community.

Reason (R) Groups of different species of individuals make a population.

22 **Assertion** (A) Epiphytes are attached on the other plants.

Reason (R) They obtain their nutrition from host plants.

23 **Assertion** (A) Symbiosis is a kind of positive interaction.

Reason (R) It is a one-sided relationship.

(C) Medical Entrances' Gallery

(Collection of Questions Asked in NEET & in Various Medical Entrance Exams)

1 Which of the following is not an attribute of a population? **[NEET 2020]**

(a) Natality (b) Mortality
(c) Species interaction (d) Sex ratio

2 Match the items in Column I with those in Column II.

Column I	Column II
A. Herbivores-Plants	1. Commensalism
B. Mycorrhiza-Plants	2. Mutualism
C. Sheep-Cattle	3. Predation
D. Orchid-Tree	4. Competition

Codes **[NEET 2020]**

	A	B	C	D		A	B	C	D
(a)	4	2	1	3	(b)	3	2	4	1
(c)	2	1	3	4	(d)	1	3	4	2

3 The impact of immigration on population density is **[NEET 2020]**

(a) negative (b) positive
(c) Both (a) and (b) (d) neutralised by natality

4 Match Column I with Column II.

Column I	Column II
A. Saprophyte	1. Symbiotic association of fungi with plant roots
B. Parasite	2. Decomposition of dead organic materials
C. Lichens	3. Living on living plants or animals
D. Mycorrhiza	4. Symbiotic association of algae and fungi

[NEET 2019]

Codes

	A	B	C	D		A	B	C	D
(a)	3	2	1	4	(b)	2	1	3	4
(c)	2	3	4	1	(d)	1	2	3	4

5 Carnivorous animals like lions and leopards, occupy the same niche but lions predate mostly larger animals and leopards take smaller ones. This mechanism of competition is referred to as **[NEET 2019]**

(a) character displacement
(b) altruism
(c) resource partitioning
(d) competitive exclusion

6 Between which among the following, the relationship is not an example of commensalism? **[NEET 2019]**

(a) Orchid and the tree on which it grows
(b) Cattle egret and grazing cattle
(c) Sea anemone and clown fish
(d) Female wasp and fig species

7

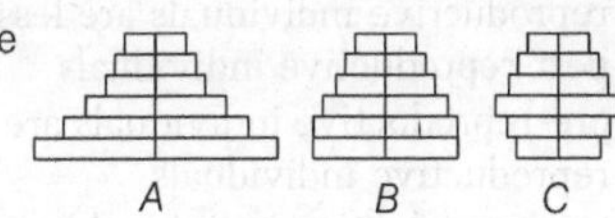

Select the correct option with respect to age pyramids. **[AIIMS 2019]**

(a) *A*-Expanding, *B*-Stable, *C*-Declining
(b) *A*-Stable, *B*-Expanding, *C*-Declining
(c) *A*-Stable, *B*-Declining, *C*-Expanding
(d) *A*-Declining, *B*-Stable, *C*-Expanding

8 **Assertion** (A) In commensalism, one organism is benefitted and other is unaffected.

Reason (R) Cattle egret bird and cattle is an example of commensalism. **[AIIMS 2019]**

(a) Both A and R are true and R is the correct explanation of A
(b) Both A and R are true, but R is not the correct explanation of A
(c) A is true, but R is false
(d) Both A and R are false

9 An interaction in which one organism is benefitted and other is unaffected. **[JIPMER 2019]**

(a) Predation (b) Commensalism
(c) Mutualism (d) Parasitism

10 Match Column I with Column II and choose the correct option from the codes given below.

Column I	Column II
A. Pacific salmon fish	1. Verhulst-Pearl logistic growth
B. $Nt = N_0 e^{rt}$	2. Breeds only once in lifetime
C. Oyster	3. Exponential growth
D. $dN/dt = rN\left(\frac{K-N}{K}\right)$	4. A large number of small-sized offspring

Codes **[Karala CEE 2018]**

	A	B	C	D		A	B	C	D
(a)	4	3	1	2	(b)	3	4	1	2
(c)	3	1	4	2	(d)	2	3	4	1
(e)	2	4	3	1					

11 Natality refers to **[NEET 2018]**

(a) number of individuals leaving the habitat
(b) birth rate
(c) death rate
(d) number of individuals entering a habitat

12 Which one of the following population interactions is widely used in medical science for the production of antibiotics? **[NEET 2018]**

(a) Parasitism (b) Mutualism
(c) Commensalism (d) Amensalism

13 In a growing population of a country, **[NEET 2018]**
(a) reproductive and pre-reproductive individuals are equal in number
(b) reproductive individuals are less than the post-reproductive individuals
(c) pre-reproductive individuals are more than the reproductive individuals
(d) pre-reproductive individuals are less than the reproductive individuals

14 From the graph of population growth, select the correct option having correct value of '*r*' and bar graph. **[AIIMS 2018, Gujarat CET 2011]**

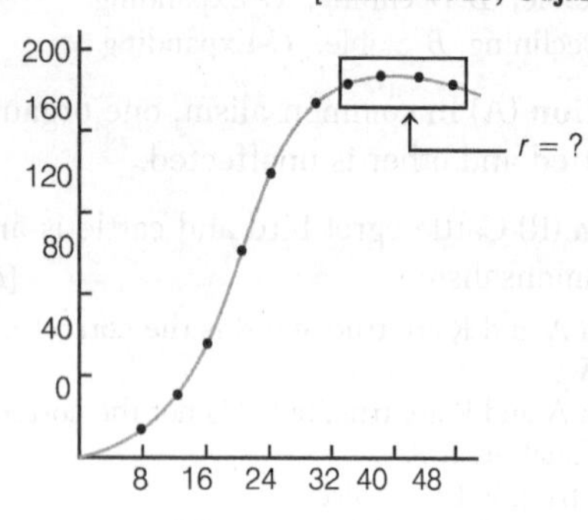

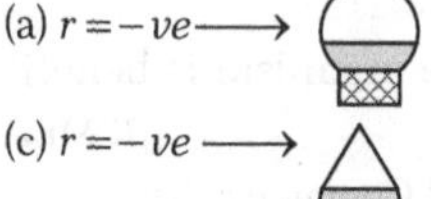

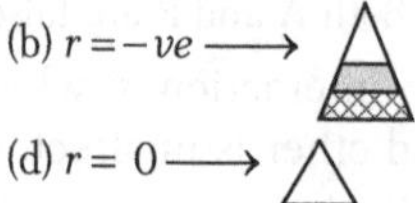

15 What is true about the isolated small tribal populations? **[AIIMS 2018]**
(a) Wrestlers who develop strong body muscles in their lifetime pass this character on their progeny
(b) There is no change in population size as they have a large gene pool
(c) There is a decline in population as boys marry girls only from their own tribe
(d) Hereditary diseases like colour blindness do not spread in the isolated population

16 Asymptote in a logistic growth curve. It is obtained, when **[NEET 2017]**
(a) the value of '*r*' approaches zero
(b) $K = N$
(c) $K > N$
(d) $K < N$

17 Mycorrhizae are the example of **[NEET 2017]**
(a) fungistasis
(b) amensalism
(c) antibiosis
(d) mutualism

18 **Assertion** (A) Allelopathy is a form of amensalism that occurs in plants.
Reason (R) It is the symbiotic association of the roots of higher plant and fungi. **[AIIMS 2017]**
(a) Both A and R are true and R is the correct explanation of A
(b) Both A and R are true, but R is not the correct explanation of A
(c) A is true, but R is false
(d) A is false, but R is true

19 Major ecological community of plants and animals extending over large natural areas is known as **[J&K CET 2016]**
(a) bioregion
(b) biosphere
(c) biota
(d) biome

20 Match mean annual precipitation in Column I with the biome in Column II and choose the correct option from the codes given below.

Column I	Column II
A 0-50 cm	1. Tropical forest
B 50-100 cm	2. Coniferous forest
C 150-400 cm	3. Grassland
D 50-250 cm	4. Desert

Codes

	A	B	C	D
(a)	4	3	1	2
(b)	3	1	2	4
(c)	3	4	1	2
(d)	2	4	1	3

21 Which of the following is correct for *r*-selected species? **[NEET-II 2016]**
(a) Large number of progeny with small size
(b) Large number of progeny with large size
(c) Small number of progeny with small size
(d) Small number of progeny with large size

22 If '+' sign is assigned to beneficial interaction, '–' sign to deterimental and '0' sign to neutral represented by '+' '–' refers to **[NEET-II 2016]**
(a) mutualism
(b) amensalism
(c) commensalism
(d) parasitism

23 The principle of competitive exclusion was stated by **[NEET-II 2016]**
(a) C Darwin
(b) GF Gause
(c) MacArthur
(d) Verhulst and Pearl

24 Gause's principle of competitive exclusion states that **[NEET-I 2016]**
(a) competition for the same resources excludes species having different food preferences
(b) no two species can occupy the same niche indefinitely for the same limiting resources
(c) larger organisms exclude smaller ones through competition
(d) more abundant species will exclude the less abundant species through competition

25 When does the growth rate of a population following the logistic model equal zero? The logistic model is given as $dN/dt = rN(1-N/K)$ [NEET-I 2016]

(a) when N nears the carrying capacity of the habitat
(b) when N/K equals zero
(c) when death rate is greater than birth rate
(d) when N/K is exactly one

26 Match the following columns.

	Column I		Column II
A.	Sea gulls	1.	Chloride secreting glands
B.	Kangaroo rat	2.	Water cells in rumen
C.	Turtle	3.	Salt secreting glands
D.	Salmon	4.	Oxidation of fats to generate water
		5.	Anadromous migration

Codes [EAMCET 2016]

	A	B	C	D
(a)	2	4	3	1
(b)	3	2	1	5
(c)	2	3	4	1
(d)	3	4	1	5

27 The following graph depicts change in two populations (*A* and *B*) of herbivores in grassy field. A possible reason for these changes is that

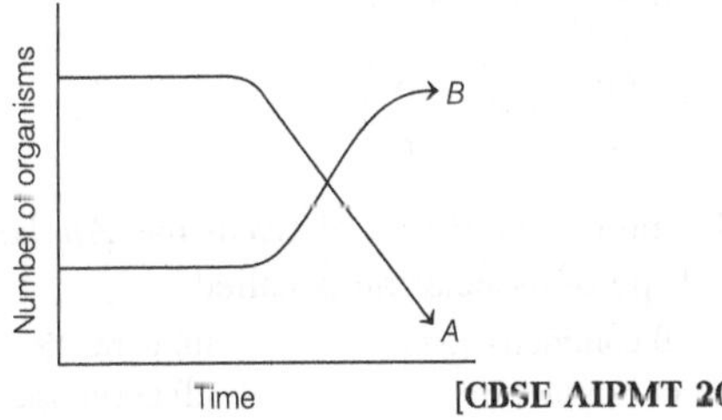

[CBSE AIPMT 2016]

(a) Both plant populations in this habitat decreased
(b) population *B* competed more successfully for food than population *A*
(c) population *A* produced more offspring than population *B*
(d) population *A* consumed the members of population *B*

28 Which one refers to Allen's rule? [Karnataka CET 2016]

(a) If stressful conditions are localised or remain only for a short duration an organism either migrates or suspends itself
(b) Mammals from colder climates have shorter ears and limbs to minimise heat loss
(c) An organism can move from a stressful habitat to a more hospitable area and return when the stressful period is over
(d) Low atmospheric pressure in higher altitudes results in altitude sickness

29 The resting state of reptiles in winter is [WB JEE 2015]

(a) hibernation
(b) aestivation
(c) diapause
(d) moulting

30 The characters such as pointed elongated snout, strong and stout forelimbs, well-developed claws are observed in .... adaptation. [MHT CET 2015]

(a) arboreal (b) aerial
(c) cursorial (d) fossorial

31 Plant species having a wide range of genetic distribution evolve into local population known as [J&K CET 2015]

(a) ecotype (b) population
(c) ecosystem (d) biome

32 Water holding capacity of sandy soil as compared to clayey soil is [Uttarakhand PMT 2015]

(a) more (b) less
(c) equal (d) None of these

33 Plants growing on sandy soil are [Uttarakhand PMT 2015; CPMT 2013]

(a) lithophytes (b) psammophyte
(c) hydrophytes (d) xerophytes

34 Identify the correct pair of combinations.

I. *Vallisneria* – Long stalked female flowers – Hydrophily
II. *Tribulus* – Annual – Root succulent
III. *Hydrilla* – Submerged rooted hydrophyte Aerenchyma
IV. *Casuarina* – Perennial – Phylloclades

Codes [EAMCET 2015]

(a) III and IV (b) II and IIII
(c) I and IV (d) I and III

35 **Assertion** (A) Marine fishes have aglomerular kidneys.
Reason (R) Aglomerular kidneys increase the loss of water through urine. [EAMCET 2015]

(a) Both A and R are true and R is the correct explanation of A
(b) Both A and R are true, but R is not the correct explanation of A
(c) A is false, but R is true
(d) A is true, but R is false

36 Edaphic factors are related to [EAMCET 2015]

(a) humidity
(b) soil texture
(c) rainfall
(d) wind velocity

37 Adaptations in an organism are meant for **[AMU 2015]**
(a) optimum primary production
(b) optimum lifespan
(c) optimum mobility
(d) optimum survival and reproduction

38 Roots play insignificant role in absorption of water in **[CBSE AIPMT 2015]**
(a) sunflower (b) *Pistia*
(c) pea (d) wheat

39 Most animals that live in deep oceanic waters are **[CBSE AIPMT 2015]**
(a) primary consumers
(b) secondary consumers
(c) tertiary consumers
(d) detritivores

40 Hibernating animals have tissues containing mitochondria with a membrane protein that accelerates electron transport while blocking synthesis of ATP. What is the consequence of the this? **[CBSE AIPMT 2015]**
(a) The energy of respiration is converted into heat
(b) Pyruvate is converted to lactic acid by anaerobic fermentation
(c) Energy is saved because glycolysis and citric acid cycle are shut down
(d) Hibernating animals can synthesise fat instead of wasting energy on respiration

41 Which statements regarding response of organisms to abiotic factors is false? **[Kerala CEE 2014]**
(a) All birds and mammals are capable of thermoregulation
(b) Majority of animals and nearly and nearly all plants cannot maintain a constant internal environment
(c) Shivering is a kind of exercise which produces heat and raises body temperature
(d) Very small animals are commonly found in polar regions as they have to spend less energy to generate heat
(e) Diapause is a stage of suspended development seen in zooplankton

42 Which of the following is correct range of latitudes for temperate region? **[Gujarat CET 2014, 2011]**
(a) 45-66° (b) 0-20°
(c) 20-40° (d) 60-80°

43 A biologist studied the population of rats in a barn. He found that the average natality was 250, average mortality 240, immigration 20 and emigration 30. The net increase in population is **[NEET 2013]**
(a) 15 (b) 05
(c) zero (d) 10

44 A sedentary sea anemone gets attached to the shell lining of hermit crab. The association is **[NEET 2013]**
(a) symbiosis (b) commensalism
(c) amensalism (d) ectoparasitism

45 A population growing in a habitat with limited resources shows four phases of growth in the following sequence. **[AFMC 2012]**
(a) Acceleration-Deceleration-Lag phase-Asymptote
(b) Asymptote-Acceleration-Deceleration-Lag phase
(c) Lag phase-Acceleration-Deceleration-Asymptote
(d) Acceleration-Lag phase-Deceleration-Asymptote

46 Some organisms are tolerant to a narrow range of salinity and are termed as **[AMU 2012]**
(a) euryhaline (b) stenohaline
(c) narrowhaline (d) saline

47 The carring capacity of environment for a given population can be represented by the following equation **[AMU 2012]**
(a) $dN = rN - \frac{N}{K}$
(b) $\frac{dN}{dt} = rN - \frac{N}{K}$
(c) $\frac{dN}{dt} = rN - \frac{1}{K}$
(d) $\frac{dN}{dt} = rN\left(1 - \frac{N}{K}\right)$

48 The coralloid root of *Cycas* has *Anabaena* (BGA), this type of association is called **[UP CPMT 2012]**
(a) commensalism (b) parasitic
(c) symbiotic (d) antibiosis

49 The niche of a population is defined as **[JCECE 2012]**
(a) set of condition that interacts
(b) place where it lives
(c) set of conditions and resources
(d) geographical area that it covers

50 The association mycorrhiza is **[BCECE 2012]**
(a) relationship of algae and fungi
(b) relationship of fungi and higher plants
(c) relationship of algae and higher plants
(d) None of the above

51 Small fish get stuck near the bottom of a shark and derives its nutrition from it. This kind of association is called as **[BCECE 2012]**
(a) antibiosis (b) commensalism
(c) predation (d) parasitism

52 Sigmoid growth curve is represented by **[AFMC 2012]**
(a) $dN/dt = rN$
(b) $dN/dt = r\,N(1 - N/K)$
(c) $Nt = No + B + I - D - E$
(d) $dN/dt = 1 - N/K$

53 The growth of a population without limit at its maximal rate and also that, rates of immigration and emigration are equal, then it is called **[EAMCET 2012]**
(a) carrying capacity (b) biotic potential
(c) positive growth (d) negative growth

54 What type of human population is represented by the following age pyramid? **[CBSE AIPMT 2011]**

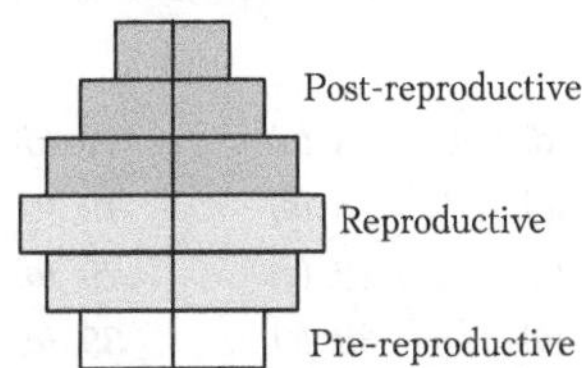

(a) Stable population (b) Declining population
(c) Expanding population (d) Vanishing population

55 The basic unit of study in ecology is **[DUMET 2011]**
(a) population (b) organism
(c) community (d) species

56 The age of pyramid with broad base indicates
(a) high percentage of young individuals **[DUMET 2011]**
(b) low percentage of young individuals
(c) high percentage of old individuals
(d) low percentage of old individuals

57 Maximum survival and reproductive capacity shown by a population under optimal environmental conditions is called **[J&K CET 2011]**
(a) carrying capacity (b) natality
(c) biotic potential (d) vitality

58 There are two optional ways of exploitation. One way is parasitism. Which is the other one? **[Gujarat CET 2011]**
(a) Antibiosis (b) Competition
(c) Predation (d) Commensalism

59 The term 'Niche' was first used by **[UP CPMT 2011]**
(a) Clements (b) Grinnel
(c) Warming (d) Odum

60 An interaction favourable to both population, but no obligatory to either is **[UP CPMT 2011]**
(a) protocooperation
(b) mutualism
(c) commensalism
(d) parasitism

61 Match the following columns.

Column I (Population interaction)	**Column II** (Examples)
A. Mutualism	1. Ticks on dogs
B. Commensalism	2. *Balanus* and *Chathamalus*
C. Parasitism	3. Sparrow and any seed
D. Competition	4. Epiphyte on a mango branch
E. Predation	5. Orchid, *Ophrys* and bee

Codes **[Kerala CEE 2011]**

	A	B	C	D	E
(a)	1	5	4	3	2
(b)	2	1	5	4	3
(c)	3	2	1	5	4
(d)	4	3	2	1	5
(e)	5	4	1	2	3

62 Exponential growth in plants can be expressed as **[Kerala CEE 2011]**
(a) $L_t = L_0 + rt$ (b) $L_e = L_t rt$
(c) $W_1 = W_0 e^{rt}$ (d) $W_1 = W_0 e\ rt$
(e) $W_1 = W_0 + e^{rt}$

63 In a population, unrestricted reproductive capacity is called **[WB JEE 2011]**
(a) biotic potential
(b) fertility rate
(c) carrying capacity
(d) birth rate

ANSWERS

Check Point 23.1

1. (d)	2. (d)	3. (b)	4. (a)	5. (c)

Check Point 23.2

1. (b)	2. (c)	3. (b)	4. (c)	5. (d)	6. (c)	7. (b)

Check Point 23.3

1. (b)	2. (c)	3. (c)	4. (a)	5. (a)	6. (d)

Check Point 23.4

1. (d)	2. (d)	3. (c)	4. (d)	5. (d)	6. (b)	7. (d)	8. (d)

(A) Topical Exercise

1. (b)	2. (c)	3. (d)	4. (a)	5. (b)	6. (a)	7. (d)	8. (a)	9. (d)	10. (c)
11. (d)	12. (c)	13. (c)	14. (d)	15. (a)	16. (d)	17. (b)	18. (b)	19. (c)	20. (b)
21. (a)	22. (a)	23. (b)	24. (c)	25. (a)	26. (a)	27. (c)	28. (a)	29. (d)	30. (d)
31. (c)	32. (c)	33. (b)	34. (c)	35. (c)	36. (b)	37. (a)	38. (c)	39. (a)	40. (b)
41. (d)	42. (a)	43. (a)	44. (c)	45. (a)	46. (c)	47. (b)	48. (b)	49. (d)	50. (c)
51. (b)	52. (c)	53. (d)	54. (b)	55. (d)	56. (c)	57. (a)	58. (a)	59. (d)	60. (b)
61. (b)	62. (d)	63. (c)	64. (d)	65. (d)	66. (a)	67. (b)	68. (a)	69. (a)	70. (b)
71. (a)	72. (b)	73. (a)	74. (d)	75. (b)	76. (b)	77. (a)	78. (d)	79. (c)	80. (b)

(B) Cumulative Exercise

1. (b)	2. (a)	3. (c)	4. (a)	5. (a)	6. (d)	7. (d)	8. (a)	9. (d)	10. (c)
11. (d)	12. (c)	13. (e)	14. (b)	15. (c)	16. (a)	17. (d)	18. (a)	19. (c)	20. (b)
21. (e)	22. (c)	23. (c)							

(C) Medical Entrances' Gallery

1. (c)	2. (b)	3. (b)	4. (c)	5. (c)	6. (d)	7. (a)	8. (b)	9. (b)	10. (d)
11. (b)	12. (d)	13. (c)	14. (d)	15. (c)	16. (b)	17. (d)	18. (c)	19. (d)	20. (a)
21. (a)	22. (d)	23. (b)	24. (b)	25. (d)	26. (d)	27. (b)	28. (b)	29. (a)	30. (d)
31. (a)	32. (b)	33. (b)	34. (b)	35. (d)	36. (b)	37. (b)	38. (b)	39. (d)	40. (a)
41. (d)	42. (a)	43. (c)	44. (b)	45. (c)	46. (b)	47. (d)	48. (c)	49. (b)	50. (b)
51. (b)	52. (b)	53. (b)	54. (b)	55. (b)	56. (a)	57. (c)	58. (c)	59. (b)	60. (a)
61. (e)	62. (c)	63. (a)							

Explanations

(A) Topical Exercise

8 (*a*) Statement I is true, but II is false and it can be corrected as

Climatic zone between 20-40°C is only temperate not sub-Arctic.

11 (*d*) Statement in option (d) is incorrect. It can be corrected as

Two species cannot live in the same niche due to Gause's competitive exclusion hypothesis.

36 (*b*) Statement I is false, but II is true. Statement I can be corrected as

Stem of submerged hydrophytes have xylem.

(B) Cumulative Exercise

6 (*d*) Statements I, II and III are correct, while IV is incorrect. Incorrect statement can be corrected as

Realised natality is the actual birth rate found under existing conditions.

7 (*d*) Statements I and II are correct. Other statements are incorrect and can be corrected as

In limnetic zone, production is higher than respiration.

In profundal zone, production is lower than respiration.

8 (*a*) Pyramid *B* has greater member of young individuals that represents earlier population. Pyramid *A* has slight reduction as shown by narrow base. It represents newer stable population.

9 (*d*) Statements I, II and III are correct while IV is incorrect. Incorrect statement can be corrected as

Niche is a place, where an organism lives. Whereas ecads is a population of individual which are genetically similar but differ in negative characters, such as size, shape, etc.

12 (*c*) A is true, but R is false because

Genecology is the study of genetic composition and changes in relation to the origin of ecads, ecotypes, new species, etc. Synecology deals with the study of a group of organisms.

13 (*e*) Both A and R are false and can be corrected as

Mimicry is the resemblance of one organism to another for the purpose of protection from predators, e.g. Viceroy butterfly mimics the unpalatable toxic monarch butterfly. Stick insect and leaf butterfly show camouflage.

14 (*b*) Both A and R are true, but R is not the correct explanation of A.

Adaptation is an important feature of animals in which they adopt different strategies to survive in the hostile environment. The stick insect or praying mantis having green body colour exhibits close resemblance with twigs and foliages. It is an adaptation known as camouflage.

15 (*c*) A is true, but R is false.

Xeromorphic characters are genetically fixed characters, which are inherited from one xerophytic plant to their offsprings. These characters will appear in xerophytes irrespective of conditions where they are growing in desert or in humid regions.

For example, halophytic mangroves although grow in moist conditions, but always develop xeromorphic characters.

16 (*a*) Both A and R are true and R is the correct explanation of A.

Drought escapers or ephemerals are short-lived xerophytes, which do not have the capacity to tolerate drought. During critical dry periods, they survive in the form of fruits and seeds, which have hard, resistant seed coats and pericarp, respectively. During favourable conditions, which are of very short duration, these seeds germinate into new plants, which complete their life cycle within few weeks.

17 (*d*) A is false, but R is true because

Dominant species are one or few species in a community, which influence the other species in terms of numbers, production of biomass and distribution of animals, while keystone species are present in low abundance and influence other community.

These species play an important role in checking the relative abundance of other species. So, the removal of keystone species causes serious disruption in the functioning of the community.

18 (*a*) Both A and R are true and R is the correct explanation of A.

In a negative interaction, one organism or both the organisms (associating) are harmed in any way during their life period. Antibiosis is a type of negative interaction, in which complete or partial inhibition or death of one organism has taken place by the products of another organism. Here, none of them derive any benefit, e.g. antibiotics derived from fungi are antagonistic to microbes.

19 (*c*) A is true, but R is false because

Positive interactions are those, in which organisms help one another and either one or both the species (associating) are benefitted. Commensalism is a type of positive interaction in which one organism is benefitted and other is neither benefitted nor harmed.

20 (*b*) Both A and R are true, but R is not the correct explanation of A.

Mutualism is a type of positive interaction in which the organisms forming an association are benefitted. For example, mycorrhiza is an association of fungi and roots of higher plants. In this association, fungi helps in the absorption of water and mineral for plant. In exchange, fungi obtain prepared food material from plant.

21 (*e*) Both A and R are false and can be corrected as

Individuals of same species make up a population of organisms, while a community is a group of populations of different species living together in a particular area at a particular time.

22 (*c*) A is true, but R is false. R can be corrected as

Epiphytes grow on the branches of other plants for support and not for nourishment.

23 (*c*) A is true, but R is false because

Symbiosis is a positive interaction in which both organisms are benefitted.

(C) Medical Entrances' Gallery

1 (*c*) Species interaction is not an attribute of a population. Rest natality (birth rate), mortality (death rate) and sex ratio are population attributes.

3 (*b*) Population density is the member of individuals present per unit area or volume at a given time. It is calculated by the formula $D = N/S$, where D = Density, N Total number of individuals and S Number of units of space. Since, immigration increases the number of individuals in an area, population density increases. Thus, immigration has positive impact on population density.

5 (*c*) Carnivorous animals, lions and leopards occupy the same niche, but lions predate mostly larger animals and leopard takes smaller ones. This is called resource partitioning. It is a mechanism in which there is the division of limited resources by species to avoid competition in an ecological niche and by this way, they find ways to coexist with one another.

That is why, lions predate mostly larger animals and leopards eat smaller ones.

6 (*d*) Among the given examples, relationship between female wasp and fig species does not show commensalism. In the commensalism, one species derives the benefit and other neither harmed nor benefitted.

Wasp and fig tree show mutualism. Here, fig flower is pollinated by wasp and the female wasp uses the fig fruit for oviposition. By this way, both the organisms are benefitted. Other options show examples of commensalism.

8 (*b*) Both A and R are true, but R is not the correct explanation of A.

In commensalism type of community interaction, one organism is benefitted and other is neither benefitted nor harmed, such as in the case of cattle egret bird and the cattle. The egrets are benefitted by obtaining insects as food, which gets exposed due to the grazing action of cattle, but the cattle remains unaffected, i.e. it is neither benefitted from the presence of egret nor harmed.

9 (*b*) Commensalism is a type of interaction where one organism is benefitted and other remains unaffected. In predation, one organism feeds (benefitted) on another organism (harmed). In parasitism, one organism (parasite) gets the benefit at the expense of the host.

Mutualism is a type of positive interaction in which both the individuals are benefitted by one another.

11 (*b*) Natality is equal to birth rate. It refers to the number of births during a given period in the population that are added to the initial density.

Other options are explained as

Death rate or mortality refers to the number of deaths in the population during a given period.

Immigration is the number of individuals of the same species that have come into the habitat. Emigration is the number of individuals of the population who left the habitat.

12 (*d*) Amensalism is widely used in medical science for the production of antibiotics. It is an interaction between different species in which one species is harmed and the other is neither benefitted nor harmed.

It involves the secretion of chemicals called allochemics by one microbial group to harm other microbes, e.g. *Penicillium* fungus secretes chemicals (penicillin) to inhibit the growth of *Staphylococcus* bacteria.

On the other hand, no such chemicals are secreted in parasitism, mutualism and commensalism.

13 (*c*) In a growing population, younger population (or pre-reproductive individuals) are more than that of reproductive individuals. Such population is represented by a expanding (triangular-shaped) age pyramid.

Whereas, the equal number of reproductive and pre-reproductive individuals represents a stable population and the age pyramid is bell-shaped.

Less number of pre-reproductive individuals than reproductive individuals represents declining population and age pyramid appears urn-shaped.

14 (*d*) The correct value of r in the graph is $r = 0$ and the bar graph is a bell-shaped polygon, indicates a moderate proportion of young to old. As the rate of growth becomes slow and stable, the pre-reproductive and reproductive age group become more or less equal in size and post-reproductive group remains the smallest.

15 (*c*) Statement in option (c) is true about the isolated small tribal populations.

Rest of the statements are incorrect and can be corrected as

- Characters developed during lifetime do not pass on from parents to progeny.
- People of small tribal population have a small gene pool.
- Hereditary diseases like colour blindness spread in such isolated populations.

16 (*b*) When $K = N$ in a logistic growth curve, it is asymptote.

It means a population growing in a habitat with limited resources shows initially a lag phase, followed by phase of acceleration and deceleration and finally an asymptote, i.e. when the population density (N) reaches the carrying capacity (K)

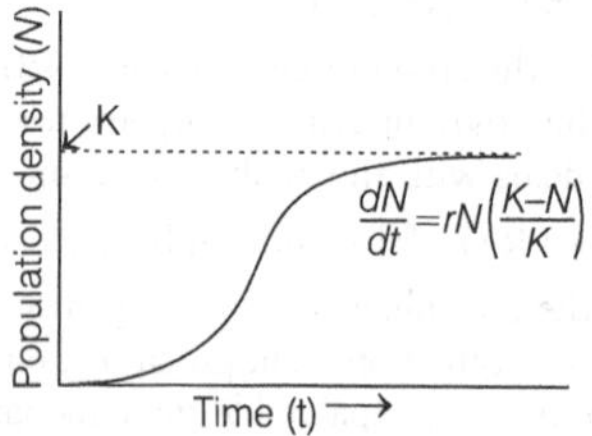

Population growth curve is logistic, when resources are limiting the growth, here K is carrying capacity and N is population density.

17 (*d*) Mutualism is an association of two species in which both species are benefitted.

Mycorrhiza is a mutualistic relationship between fungal hyphae and roots of higher plants. The fungus helps in mineral nutrition absorption for the plants with which they are associated and in turn, obtained food and shelter from plants.

18 (*c*) A is true, but R is false because

Allelopathy is a phenomenon associated with plants, in which one plant produces a substance or chemical which inhibits the growth of other plant species, while in amensalism also, one species suffers and other remains unaffected. Mycorrhiza is a symbiotic association of roots of higher plant and fungi.

19 (*d*) Biome is a major ecological community which consists of a major vegetation type (plants) and associated fauna (animals) in a particular climatic zone. Tropical rainforest, deciduous forest, sea coast, deserts, etc., are the major biomes in India.

21. (*a*) *r*-selected are the species having the ability to produce large number of progenies (offsprings) with small size. The population growth of these species is a function of biotic potential.
Hence, option (a) is correct.

22. (*d*) Parasitism is a relationship between two living organisms of different species in which one organism, i.e. parasite obtains its food directly from the host.
In this relationship, the parasite is benefitted positive (+) and the host is harmed negative (-), so this type of population interaction is represented by '+' '–'.

25. (*d*) In logisitic growth model population, growth equation is described as

$$\frac{dN}{dt} = rN\left(\frac{K-N}{K}\right)$$

Where, N = Population density at time t
r = Intrinsic rate of natural increase
K = Carrying capacity

when, $\frac{N}{K} = 1$ then $\frac{K-N}{K} = 0$

Therefore, $\frac{dN}{dt} = 0$

Thus, option (d) is correct

27 (*b*) Individuals of population *B* is increased because they have adapted better to their environment and competed more successfully for food than population *A*.

42 (*a*) The correct range of latitudes for temperate region extends between 45-66° in Northern and 45-66° in Southern hemisphere (temperate zone). This zone lies between the Arctic circle and the tropic of Cancer and between Antarctic circle and the tropic of Capricorn.

43 (*c*) Net increase in population : (Natality + Immigration) – (Mortality + Emigration)
(250 + 20) – (240 + 30)
270 - 270 = 0

48 (*c*) In symbiosis, both the organisms in association are benefitted and this association is obligatory. The blue-green alga, *Anabaena* reside in coralloid roots of *Cycas* for nitrogen fixation.

50 (*b*) Mycorrhiza is the symbiotic association between fungus and roots of higher plants. The mycorrhizal roots are usually covered with fungal woolly outgrowth. Fungus growth does not cause any harm to the plant. Along with water, phosphorus and nitrogen are also absorbed.

51 (*b*) In commensalism, association between the members of different species is made in the way that nor one is benefitted and neither is harmed. For example, small fish (sucker fish) gets stuck near the bottom of a shark with the help of its holdfast (modified dorsal fin) and is dispersed to distant areas. It also gets protection due to association with shark and derives its nutrition also. However, the shark does not get any benefit or harm from the sucker fish.

54 (*b*) For human population, the age pyramids show age distribution of males and females in a combined diagram. The shape of the age pyramids reflects the growth status of the population. In a declining population, the shape of pyramid is urn-shaped.

57 (*c*) Chapman (1928) proposed the term 'biotic potential' to define maximum reproductive power. An inherent power of a population or organism to survive or increase in number under optimal environmental conditions is called biotic potential.

58 (*c*) In exploitation, one species harms the other by making its direct or indirect use for support, shelter or food. In contrast to parasite, which derives nourishment from its host without killing, a predator is free-living which catches and kills another species for food.

60 (*a*) Protocooperation is the interaction between two living organisms of different species in which both are mutually benefitted, but they can live without each other.

62 (*c*) The exponential growth can be expressed as

$$W_1 = W_0\, e^{rt}$$

where, W_1 = Final size (weight, height, number, etc.)
W_0 = Initial size at the beginning of the period
r = Growth rate
t = Time of growth
e = Base of natural logarithms.

Here, r is the relative growth rate and is also the measure of ability of the plant to produce plant material, referred to as efficiency index. Hence, the final size of W_1 depends on the initial size W_0

CHAPTER 24

Ecosystem

Living organisms continuously interact among themselves and also with their environment to maintain a balance in nature. This forms a broad self sustaining functional unit of the living world called **ecosystem**. It may be as small as drop of water or as large as an ocean. Within an ecosystem, there is a flow of energy from sunlight, through food chain, food web, ecological pyramids and nutrient cycles.

ECOSYSTEM

The term 'Ecosystem' was proposed by **Tansley** in 1935. He defined it as the system that is formed by the integration of biotic community and its physical environment.

Odum defined it as any unit that includes all the organisms in a given area, interacting with the physical environment, so that a flow of energy leads to clearly defined trophic structure, biotic diversity and material cycles within the system.

Types of ecosystem

We can classify the ecosystem in the following ways

1. **Natural ecosystems** These ecosystems are capable of operating and maintaining themselves without any major interference by human. These are further divided as
   (i) **Terrestrial ecosystems** Forest, grassland, desert, etc.
   (ii) **Aquatic ecosystems** Freshwater ecosystems (pond, lake, river) and marine ecosystems (ocean, sea or estuary).
2. **Artificial ecosystems** These are maintained and manipulated by human for different purposes. Artificial or man-made ecosystem have little diversity (generally monocultures), little recycling of minerals and no self-regulatory mechanism, e.g. croplands, artificial lakes and reservoirs, townships and cities, etc.

Note
- *Nano-ecosystem is very small-sized ecosystems, e.g. aquarium, kitchen garden.*
- *Microecosystem is a small ecosystem, e.g. pond.*
- *Mesoecosystem is a moderate size ecosystem, e.g. forest.*

These ecosystems can be well-understood only after studying the components of ecosystem in detail.

Inside

COMPONENTS OF ECOSYSTEM

According to Odum, an ecosystem has two major components, i.e. abiotic and biotic components.

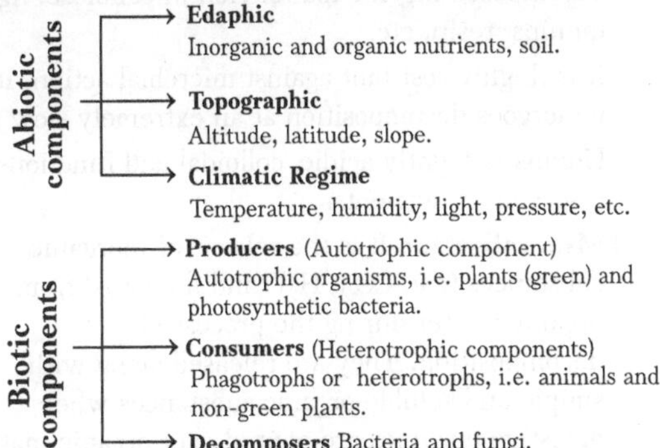

Fig. 24.1 Components of an ecosystem

Abiotic components

The abiotic components or the non-living components which consist of two things, the materials and energy. The materials are like water, minerals, atmospheric gases, salts, etc. They also include some organic matter, such as the amino acids and other products of decay of living things. These all abiotic components are already discussed in Chapter No. 23.

Biotic components

They constitute all the living member of an ecosystem. On the basis of their role in the ecosystem, biotic components are divided into following categories

1. Autotrophic component (Autotrophic-self-nourishing)

- These are the living organism who fix light energy to manufacture their own food from simple inorganic substances. Thus, they are called **autotrophs**.
- These are producers, i.e. green plants, as they convert solar radiations into chemical energy. These producers are largely photosynthetic plants.
- Their kind varies with the kind of ecosystem.
  - For example, in a dense forest, the trees are the most important producers. In lakes and ponds, the producers are rooted or large floating plants and microscopic plants (phytoplankton).
  - In the ocean, the rooted and floating algae are the producers.

> **Lifeform**
>
> It is the vegetative appearance of the plants, which is based on their size, shape branching and longevity, etc. **Raunkiaer** (1903) proposed the lifeform system for the description of vegetation. He categorised the various lifeforms into five types as follows
>
> 1. **Phanerophytes** These are generally trees. Majority of them occur in tropics having moist and warm climate. Perennating buds are present much above the ground level and they are least protected.
> 2. **Chamaephytes** These plants occur in cold regions at high altitudes and latitudes. Buds are situated close to the ground surface or upto a maximum height of 25 cm.
> 3. **Hemicryptophytes** This group of species is predominantly present in cold climatic regions. The perennating buds are present just under the surface of soil. The aerial parts of the plant die back with the onset of winter, e.g. rosette plants.
> 4. **Cryptophytes** Perennating buds are completely hidden in the ground. These plants are adapted to survive in regions having long dry periods. These are of three types, i.e. hydrophytes, geophytes and halophytes.
> 5. **Therophytes** This group includes such annual summer plant, which survive under unfavourable seasons in the form of seeds.

2. Consumers (Heterotrophic component)

These organisms ingest other organisms and therefore, called **heterotrophs**. They derive their food directly or indirectly from the producers or the green plants.

These can be divided into following categories

(i) **Primary consumers** These animals directly feed on producer. They are called **herbivore**. These are also known as key industry animals.The primary consumers vary with the kind of ecosystem, i.e. grasshopper, cow and deer in terrestrial ecosystem; molluscs, tadpole and mosquito larvae in aquatic ecosystem.

(ii) **Secondary consumers** These animals feed on herbivores, e.g. toad, spiders, lizards, centipedes and insectivorous birds in terrestrial ecosystem; *Hydra*, frog and some fishes in aquatic ecosystem.

(iii) **Tertiary consumers** These animals feed upon secondary consumers, e.g. large fishes (aquatic ecosystem), snakes (terrestrial ecosystem), etc.

(iv) **Top carnivores** These animals are not killed or eaten by other animals, e.g. lion, vulture, falcon, etc.

3. Decomposers

- These organisms are saprophytic, i.e. feeds upon dead bodies of animals and plants and organic wastes of living organisms.
- They secrete digestive enzyme to digest the organic matter externally.

- Since, they release minerals trapped in organic waste, they are also known as **mineralisers**. They bring about cyclic exchange of materials between biotic community and the environment.
- They also reduce organic remains, so they are also called as **reducers**, e.g. fungi, bacteria, moulds, etc.

Decomposition

- It is the physical and chemical breakdown of complex organic remains with the help of decomposers.
- The process of decomposition completely takes place outside the body of decomposers.
- They release enzyme from their body on dead remains and decompose it into simple inorganic substances and then absorb it. So, they are also called **osmotrophs** (absorptive).

Decomposition process

There are three important steps in the process of decomposition. These are as follows

(i) **Fragmentation of detritus** Small invertebrate animals called **detritivores**, e.g. earthworms and termites feed on detritus. They bring about its fragmentation.
   - A part of detritus eaten by detritivores comes out in highly pulverised state in their faeces.
   - Due to fragmentation during eating and pulverisation in digestive tracts, detritus is changed into fine particles which have a large surface area.

(ii) **Leaching** Part of soluble substances present in the fragmented and decomposing detritus (e.g. sugars, inorganic nutrients) get leached to deeper layers of soil by percolating water.

(iii) **Catabolism** It is carried out by saprotrophic bacteria and fungi.
   - They secrete digestive enzymes over the fragmented detritus.
   - The enzymes change insoluble complex organic compounds into soluble simple organic compounds. Inorganic substances are also released in this process.
   - A part of broken down food is taken by decomposers are immobilised. The phenomenon of incorporation of nutrient in living microbes is called **nutrient immobilisation**.
   - After death of microbes, the immobilised nutrient become available again for solubilisation.
   - Immobilisation protects the nutrient from being washed out and lost from ecosystem.
   - The rate of catabolic action or breakdown of different complex substances is different. This differential decomposition produces two substances, **humus** by humification and **inorganic nutrients** by **mineralisation** within the soil.

(a) **Humification** It is the process of partial decomposition of detritus to form humus.
   - **Humus** is dark coloured, amorphous, partially decomposed organic matter rich in cellulose, lignin, tannins, resin, etc.
   - It is highly resistant against microbial action. It undergoes decomposition at an extremely slow rate.
   - Humus is slightly acidic, colloidal and functions as reservoir of nutrients.

(b) **Mineralisation** It is the release of inorganic substances (e.g. CO_2, H_2O and minerals) from organic matter during the process of decomposition. They are released along with simple and soluble organic substances when digestive enzymes are poured over organic matter by saprotrophic microbes.

Factors affecting decomposition

The rate of decomposition of detritus is controlled by a number of factors. These are as follows

(i) **Chemical nature of detritus** Decomposition of detritus is slow if it contains lignin, chitin, tannins (phenolics) and cellulose. The process occurs rapidly if detritus contains more of nitrogenous compounds (like proteins, nucleic acids) and carbohydrates.

(ii) **Soil pH** Detritivores are rarely found in acidic soils. Thus, microbial activity is also low and rate of decomposition of organic matter is also slow in acidic soil. Partially decomposed organic matter piles up over such soils.

   Detritivores are abundant in neutral and slightly alkaline or slightly acidic soils.

(iii) **Temperature** Decomposers are active at more than 25°C of temperature. In humid tropical regions, complete decomposition of detritus occurs in about 3-4 months. However under low temperature conditions (>10°C), the rate of decomposition is very slow even if the moisture and aeration are optimum.

(iv) **Moisture** An optimum moisture level helps in faster decomposition of detritus. Reduction in moisture or excessive moisture, both cases reduces the rate of decomposition.

(v) **Aeration** It is required for the activity of decomposers and detritivores. The reduced aeration would slowdown the process of decomposition because it is oxygen requiring process.

Some natural ecosystems and their components

Some of the natural ecosystem and their important distinguished features are summarised in the table given below

Table 24.1 Comparative summary of marine, grassland, forest and desert ecosystems

Components	Marine ecosystem	Grassland ecosystem	Forest ecosystem	Desert ecosystem
Abiotic components	Temperature zones, air, O_2, minerals, salts, etc.	CO_2, H_2O, nitrate, phosphate and sulphates, roughly 19% of the earth's crust.	Soil, temperature, light, minerals, air.	Rainfall less than 25 cm, extreme of temperature and cold.
Biotic components	Phytoplanktons, diatoms and dinoflagellates	Grasses	Mainly trees teak, sal	Shrubs, bushes, some grasses and very few trees.
Producers	Microscopic algae. Members of Phaeophyta and Rhodophyta	*Digitaria, Dactyloctenium, Setaria* and also few shrubs.	*Quercus* in temperate forest *Pinus, Abies, Cedrus, Juniperus* and *Rhododendron.*	Cycads, cacti, palm, coconut, etc.
Macroconsumers				
Primary	Crustaceans, molluscs and fishes	Deer, sheep, cow, buffaloes, rabbit and mouse. Also some insects, termites and millipedes.	Leafhoppers, flies, beetle, bugs, spider, deer, mouse and moles.	Insects, some reptiles and camel.
Secondary	Carnivorous fishes	Fox, jackal, snake, frogs, lizards and birds.	Lizard, fox, snake and birds.	Snake, lizards.
Tertiary	Herring, shark and mackeral carnivore fishes like cod, haddock, halibut, etc.	Hawk and vulture.	Lion, tiger, wild cats, etc.	Vultures
Microconsumers				
Decomposers	Chiefly bacteria and fungi	*Mucor, Aspergillus, Penicillium, Fusarium, Cladosporium* and *Rhizopus*	Mostly fungi, *Aspergillus, Polyporus, Fusarium,* bacteria *Bacillus, Clostridium* and *Streptomyces.*	Fungi and bacteria, which are thermophilic.

Food chain

- The transfer of food energy from the producers through a series of organisms from herbivores to carnivores and to decomposers with repeated eating and being eaten is called food chain. It can be traced in any ecosystem.
- A simple food chain consists of three steps as follows

Producers ⟶ Herbivores ⟶ Carnivores

- For example, in a pond ecosystem, the food chain consists of phytoplanktons, herbivorous zooplanktons, small carnivorous fish, large carnivorous fish and finally, the decomposers.
- In a grassland ecosystem, the food chain consists of grasses, grasshoppers, frogs, snakes, vultures and decomposers.
- Each level or step in a food chain where transfer of energy takes place is called **trophic level**. It is a functional level. A single species may occupy more than one trophic level. In terrestrial ecosystem, generally 5 trophic levels are present. In aquatic ecosystem, trophic level can be upto 7.
- The various trophic levels in an ecosystem are as follows

(i) Producers ⟶ Green plants ⟶ I Trophic level
(ii) Primary consumers ⟶ Herbivores ⟶ II Trophic level
(iii) Secondary consumers ⟶ Carnivores and insectivores ⟶ III Trophic level
(iv) Tertiary consumers ⟶ Higher carnivores, insect, hyperparasites ⟶ IV Trophic level

- Thus in any ecosystem, the food chain extends from producers to primary consumers (herbivores) then to secondary consumers (small carnivores), tertiary consumers (large carnivores) and finally to the decomposers.

Table 24.2 Food chains and trophic levels in some ecosystems

Types	Producers	Primary consumers	Secondary consumers	Tertiary consumers	Quaternary consumers
Trophic level	**Ist trophic level**	**IInd trophic level**	**IIIrd trophic level**	**IVth trophic level**	**Vth trophic level**
Aquatic	Phytoplankton	Zooplankton	Fish (perch)	Fish (bass)	Man
Aquatic	Phytoplankton	Fish (minnow)	Frog	Raccoon	—
Terrestrial	Grass	Grasshopper	Frog	Snake	Hawk
Terrestrial	Dead leaves	Fungi	Squirrel	Hawk	—
Terrestrial	Leaves, twigs and bark	Rabbit	Lion	—	—

Types of food chain

Food chain system can be divided into three basic categories

(i) **Predator food chain or Grazing food chain** starts from a plant at the base and goes from the smaller to larger animals.

(ii) **Parasitic food chain or Auxiliary food chain** goes from the larger to smaller organisms.

(iii) **Saprophytic food chain or Detritus food chain** moves from dead matter to microorganisms.

Note *In nature, basically two types of food chains are recognised, i.e. grazing food chain and detritus food chain.*

Grazing food chain

It starts from green plants and ends at carnivores. In between, there are various herbivores. It is major conduit of energy flow in aquatic and terrestrial ecosystem. It binds up inorganic nutrients.

Thus, the gross production of a plant may meet by following three end results

- It may be oxidised during respiration.
- It may die and decay.
- It may be eaten and stored as carbohydrates, fats, proteins and transformed into relatively simpler substances. Energy to perform the secondary transformations is provided by respiration.

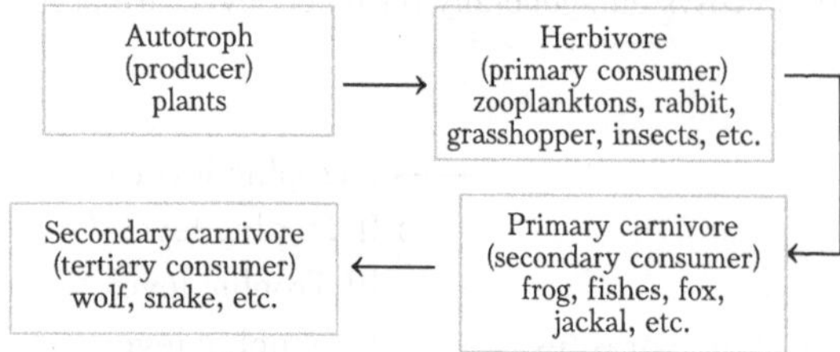

Detritus food chain

- It begins from dead organic matter or detritus. The microbes degrade dead organic matter. These microbes are also known as **saprotrophs** or **decomposers**.
- This food chain helps in releasing inorganic nutrients to the cycling pool.
- A good example of detritus food chain was given by **Heald** and **Odum**. The chain is based on mangrove (*Rhizophora mangle*) leaves, which fall into shallow estuarine waters of South Florida. Leaf fragments acted upon by saprotrophs and colonised by algae. These are eaten and re-eaten by a group of small detritus consumers, which in turn, provide the main food for game fish (small carnivore) and fish eating birds (top carnivores).

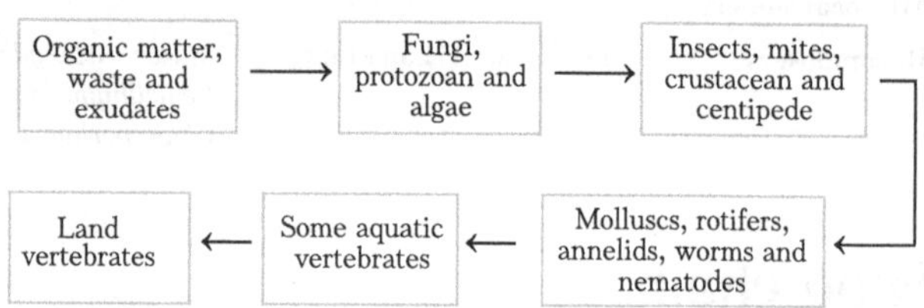

Food web

- In an ecosystem, various food chains are linked together and intersect with each other to form a complex network called **food web.**
- In nature, the same organisms may operate at more than one trophic level, i.e. it may derive its food from more than one source.
- Even the same organism may be eaten by several organisms of a higher trophic level or an organism may feed upon several different organisms of a lower trophic level.
- The complexity of food web can vary greatly and we can express this complexity by a measure called the **connectance of the food web.**

$$\text{Connectance} = \frac{\text{Actual number of interspecific interactions}}{\text{Potential number of interspecific interactions}}$$

- Food chains, in general tend to be short and rarely exceedes four links. No matter how productive an ecosystem, the number of links remain essentially the same. An ecosystem does not support longer food chains.

- As the number of species in the food web increases, the connectance decreases.

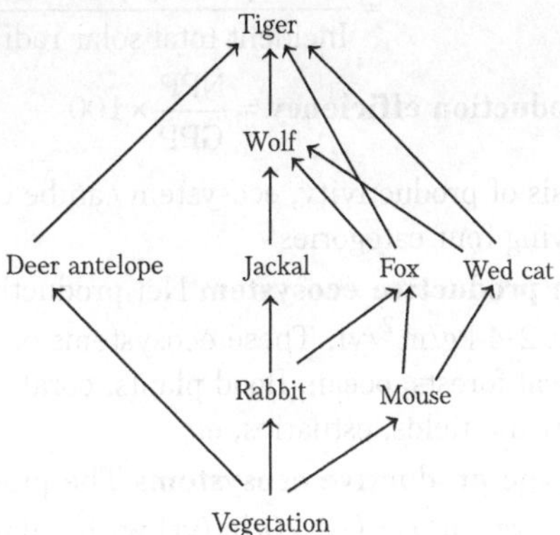

Fig. 24.2 Terrestrial food web

Table 24.3 Differences between food chain and food web

Food chain	Food web
It is a straight single pathway through which food energy travels in an ecosystem.	It consists of a number of interconnected food chains through which food energy passes in the ecosystem.
Members of higher trophic level feed upon a single type of organisms of lower trophic level.	Members of higher trophic level can feed as a number of alternative organisms of the lower trophic level.
Presence of separate or isolated food chains adds to the instability of the ecosystem.	Presence of food webs increases the stability of the ecosystem.
It does not add to the adaptability and competitiveness of the organisms.	Food webs increase adaptability and competitiveness of the organisms.

CHECK POINT 24.1

1. Global ecosystem is too much big and difficult to be studied at one time. It is convenient to divide it into
(a) natural and man-made ecosystem
(b) biotic and abiotic ecosystem
(c) terrestrial and aquatic ecosystem
(d) Both (b) and (c)

2. Physical structure, the characteristic for each type of ecosystem is formed due to the
(a) interaction of biotic and abiotic components
(b) stratification
(c) vertical distribution of different species
(d) Both (b) and (c)

3. Which of the following pairs is not correct?
(a) Ecosystem – Functional unit of nature
(b) Global ecosystem – Entire biosphere
(c) Aquatic ecosystem – Wetland
(d) Natural ecosystem – Crop field

4. In plants found in cold regions, the perennating buds which are present close to the ground are called
(a) chamaephytes
(b) phanerophytes
(c) cryptophytes
(d) hemicryptophytes

5. Which consumer directly feed upon producer?
(a) Primary
(b) Secondary
(c) Tertiary
(d) Top carnivores

6. Which of the following is an enzymatic process?
(a) Fragmentation
(b) Leaching
(c) Catabolism
(d) All of the above

FUNCTIONS OF ECOSYSTEM

- In all ecosystems, there is a self-regulatory mechanism of checks and balances. This is called **homeostasis.**
- For example, in a balanced ecosystem, the amount of O_2 and CO_2 is usually maintained at certain levels so that neither of the two become limiting or in excess.
- However, a fluctuation in the density of animal and plant population tends to disturb this balance. But it is interesting to note that within a certain limit, the ecosystem itself regulates the fluctuations.
- If the system is unable to regulate the fluctuations, the balance naturally gets disturbed and a new structural and functional balance tends to develop.
- An ecosystem is self-sufficient and self-regulating. A number of delicately balanced and controlled processes occur in every ecosystem.
- Identification and enumeration of plant and animal species of an ecosystem gives its species composition.
- Vertical distribution of different species occupying different levels is called **stratification.** For example, tree occupy top vertical strata or layer of a forest, the shrubs the second and herbs and grasses the bottom layers.
- Plants use biogenetic nutrients from the soil. Their availability largely depends upon the decomposition and mineralisation of organic detritus.
- Animals found in an ecosystem are balanced by the number of herbivores and the degree of herbivory.
- The important functional aspects of ecosystems are
  1. Productivity
  2. Energy flow
  3. Nutrient cycle

1. Productivity and its measurement

The rate of biomass production, i.e. the amount of organic matter accumulated per unit area in unit time is called productivity. Production ecology is the branch of ecology that deals with the rate of production of organic matter in different components of an ecosystem.

It is of following two types

(i) **Primary Productivity** (PP) It is defined as the rate at which radiant energy of the sun is stored by the photosynthetic and chemosynthetic activities of producers.

It is further of following two types

(a) **Gross Primary Productivity** (GPP) It is the rate of production or synthesis of organic matter by producers during photosynthesis in a given unit area. GPP depends on the chlorophyll content. The rate of gross primary productivity is estimated in terms of chlorophyll content as chlorophyll/gm dry weight/unit area.

(b) **Net Primary Productivity** (NPP) It is the total amount of GPP minus energy lost by plant during respiration. Thus, NPP is equal to the rate of organic matter stored by photosynthesis minus the rate of respiration and other losses.

$$\text{NPP} = \text{GPP} - R$$

Hence, NPP is the available biomass for the consumption of heterotrophs, i.e. both herbivores and decomposers.

(ii) **Secondary Productivity** (SP) It is the rate of energy storage at consumer's level, i.e. herbivores, carnivores and decomposers. Consumers tend to utilise already produced food materials during their respiration.

(iii) **Net Productivity** (NP) It is the rate of storage of organic matter not used by the heterotrophs or consumers. It is equal to NPP minus consumption by the heterotrophs during the unit period in a season or year.

Measurement of productivity

Productivity of an ecosystem can be measured by following ways

- **Ecological efficiency** is the percentage of energy converted into biomass by a higher trophic level over the energy of food resources available at the lower trophic level.

$$\text{Ecological efficiency} = \frac{\text{Energy converted into biomass at trophic level}}{\text{Energy present in biomass at lower trophic level}} \times 100$$

- **Photosynthetic efficiency**

$$= \frac{\text{Gross primary productivity}}{\text{Incident total solar radiation}} \times 100$$

- **Net production efficiency** $= \frac{\text{NPP}}{\text{GPP}} \times 100$

On the basis of productivity, ecosystem can be classified into following four categories

(i) **High productive ecosystem** Net productivity is about 2-4 kg/m^2/yr. These ecosystems occur in tropical forests, ocean, flood plants, coral reefs, sugarcane fields, estuaries, etc.

(ii) **Average productive ecosystems** The productivity is 1-2 kg /m^2/yr (10-20/ha/yr) with a daily output of 3-5 g/m^2, e.g. common agricultural crops and temperate forests.

(iii) **Less productivity ecosystem** The annual productivity is 200-1000 g/m^2 (2-10/ha) with a daily increment of 0.5 - 3.0 g/m^2, e.g. grassland ecosystems and savanna.

(iv) **Low productivity ecosystems** The net productivity is less than 200 g/m^2/yr. It is as low as 0.03 t/ha/yr in certain deserts, e.g. deep sea and arid lands.

2. Energetics of ecosystem or Energy flow

- Energy flow is a sequential process of the movement of energy in an ecosystem through a series of organisms. It is always unidirectional.
- The source of energy in an ecosystem is solar energy. Approximately 50% of the solar energy incident on the earth is Photosynthetically Active Radiation (PAR).
- Incident radiation of plants is about 1×10^6 kJ/m^2/yr. Of this, as much as 95-99% is immediately lost from the plants by reflection, radiation or heat of evaporation.
- The remaining 1-5% of incoming radiation is absorbed by the chlorophyll and used in the production of organic molecules.

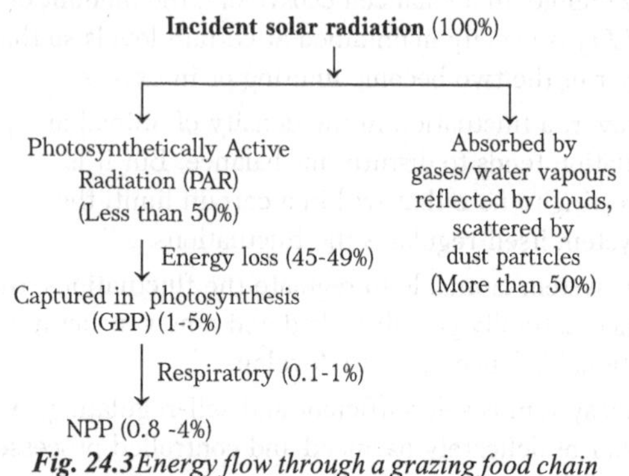

Fig. 24.3 Energy flow through a grazing food chain

Transfer of energy through trophic levels

- A part of energy captured by producers (GPP) is used for the maintenance and as food for herbivores. The remaining net productivity is either used by consumers or passes into detritus chain.
- When an organism dies, it is converted to detritus that serves as an energy source for decomposers.
- Organism at each trophic level depends on lower trophic level for their energy requirements.
- Each trophic level contains certain mass of living matter at a particular time called as **standing crop**.

Ten per cent (10%) law of energy transfer

- The number of trophic levels in the food chain is restricted as the transfer of energy follows 10% law.
- This law was given by **Lindeman** (1942). It states that only 10% of the energy is transferred to each upper trophic level from the lower trophic level.
- When the plants are eaten by herbivore, about 10% of energy in the food is fixed into animal flesh while 90% is consumed in ingestion, respiration, etc.

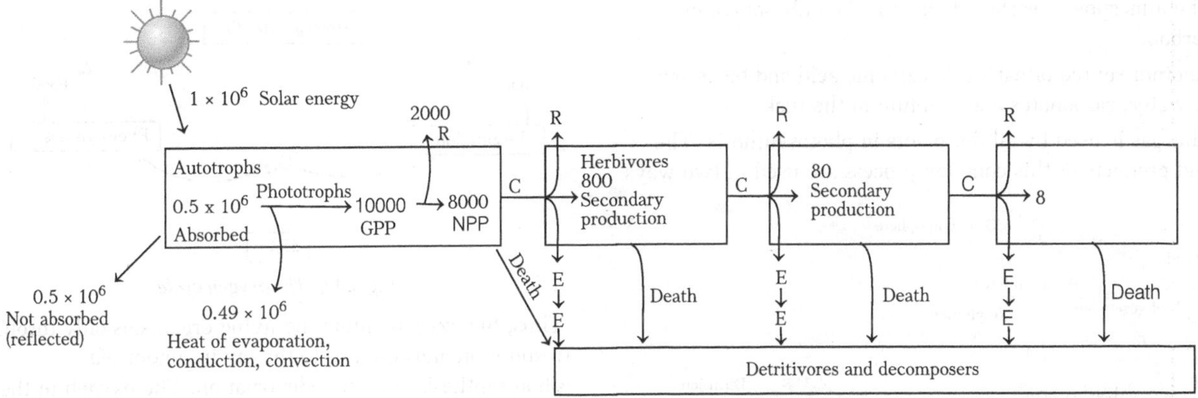

Fig. 24.4 Energy flow through a grazing food chain

3. Nutrient cycling

- An ecosystem has a limited supply of biogenetic nutrients in its abiotic environment.
- From producers, the nutrients in the form of organic matter pass to the higher trophic level.
- They are released back to abiotic environment by decomposers as these act on organic wastes and dead bodies of organisms.
- In this way, the same nutrients repeatedly move through living and non-living components of the ecosystem.
- The essential elements required by organisms for their body building and metabolism are known as **biogenetic nutrient** or **biogeochemicals**. These are provided by earth and return to earth again after their death and decay.
- The amount of biogenetic nutrients present at any time in the ecosystem is called **standing state**. The whole living matter is made up of nutrients, either as structural components, biochemicals as enzymes.
- The two stores of nutrients in the ecosystem are as follows
  - (i) **Reservoir pool** It is the reservoir of biogenetic nutrients from which they are slowly transferred to cycling pool, e.g. phosphates in rocks.
  - (ii) **Cycling pool** In this pool, biogenetic nutrients are emptied and filled repeatedly by the exchange between biotic and abiotic components of biosphere.

Types of nutrient cycle

The biogeochemical cycles are classified into two main types

(i) **Gaseous cycles** In these cycles, the main reservoirs of chemicals are the atmosphere and the ocean. Exchange of nutrients occur in gaseous or vapour form, e.g. carbon cycle, nitrogen cycle, oxygen cycle, etc.

(ii) **Sedimentary cycles** The biogenetic material is basically non-gaseous. In these cycles, the main reservoirs are soil and rocks, e.g. sulphur cycle, phosphorus cycle, etc.

Components of nutrient cycles

Nutrient cycles have three main components as follows

(i) **Input** An ecosystem receives an input of nutrients from the external sources, which it stores to utilise in biological processes. These nutrients are of four types, i.e. wet deposition, dry deposition, biological nitrogen-fixation and weathering of rocks.

(ii) **Output** Loss of nutrients from an ecosystem due to run-off water and soil erosion, etc.

(iii) **Internal nutrients cycling** Nutrients present in the soil are absorbed by plants. These are made available to soil in the form of detritus. The nutrients are released from the detritus through the activity of decomposers. In mature ecosystems, the amount of nutrients uptake is equal to the amount of recycled nutrients.

Carbon cycle

- The atmospheric carbon dioxide is the only source of carbon.
- Another source of carbon is carbonic acid and bicarbonate in water, carbonates and graphite in the rocks.
- This gas is used by all the plants in photosynthesis. The end products of this complex process are used in two ways

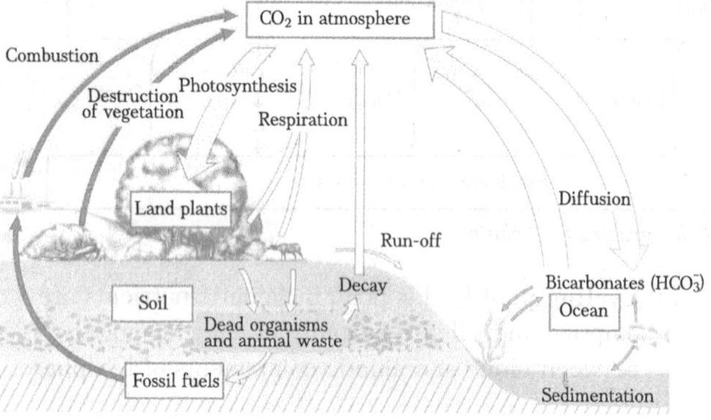

Fig. 24.5 The carbon cycle

- One product is used in the construction of living matter. Another product of the organic substance is used as fuel in respiration by both plants and animals. This process releases CO_2 as a byproduct.
- The carbon and oxygen supplied by CO_2 remain in living matter till death. Decaying of detritus returns CO_2 to the atmosphere and this completes one possible carbon cycle.
- This CO_2 may now be used in photosynthesis again, or it may return to the environment thus, completing the second possible carbon cycle.
- The CO_2 content of the atmosphere is replenished not only through biological oxidation (respiration), but also through non-living combustion, i.e. forest fires and burning of industrial fuels which release CO_2 into the air. Occasionally, volcanic eruptions also add CO_2 to the atmosphere.

Oxygen cycle

- The cycling of O_2 between biotic and abiotic system is called oxygen cycle.
- The atmospheric O_2 enters the living organism by respiration. During this process, CO_2 and H_2O are formed.
$$C_6H_{12}O_6 + 6O_2 \longrightarrow 6CO_2 + 6H_2O + \text{Energy}$$
- Oxygen returns to air either by photosynthesis or photodissociation.
- In photodissociation, water vapour is dissociated to release H_2 and O_2 in the presence of light.
- This free oxygen may again be used in respiration or it may be returned to the environment as molecular atmospheric oxygen, hence completing the cycle.

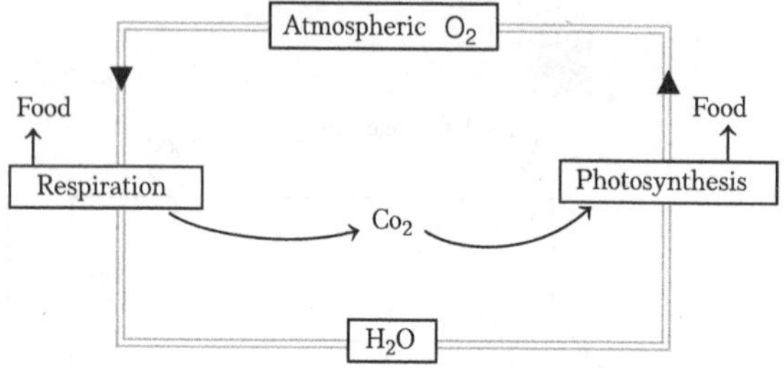

Fig. 24.6 The oxygen cycle

- Thus, the oxygen enters the living organisms only through respiration and re-enter to the environment *via* photosynthesis and photodissociation. The oxygen in the atmosphere is the source of ozone (O_3).
- The most important factors affecting the oxygen cycle and the oxygen budget of the earth is the man himself. In addition to inhaling oxygen and exhaling CO_2, man decreases the oxygen level and increases the CO_2 level by burning of fossil fuels.

Phosphorus cycle

- This cycle lacks an atmospheric component. The basic source and the great reservoir of phosphorus are the rocks or other deposits. These have been formed in the past geological ages.
- They gradually erod and release phosphates to the ecosystems. But, most of the phosphate escapes into the sea which deposits into shallow sediments and deep sediments.
- For the nutrition, plants absorb water dissolved inorganic phosphates from the soil, Phosphates absorbed from the soil in the form of $H_2PO_4^-$.
- They convert these into organic phosphates. The latter is transferred to consumers and decomposers.
- Phosphate is returned to soil as organic residuces *via* dead plant and animals. They are converted to humus.

- The floating algae or phytoplanktons rapidly absorb soluble inorganic phosphates and convert them into **organophosphates.**
- Algae provide food for zooplanktons, which in turn are consumed by other animals. All plants and animals eventually die and in due time, their organic remains or debris decay through the action of microorganisms. Thus, the phosphates are released into the water for recycling.
- The fish and marine birds are also important in phosphorus cycle. The bird guano's excreta also contains a large amount of phosphate.

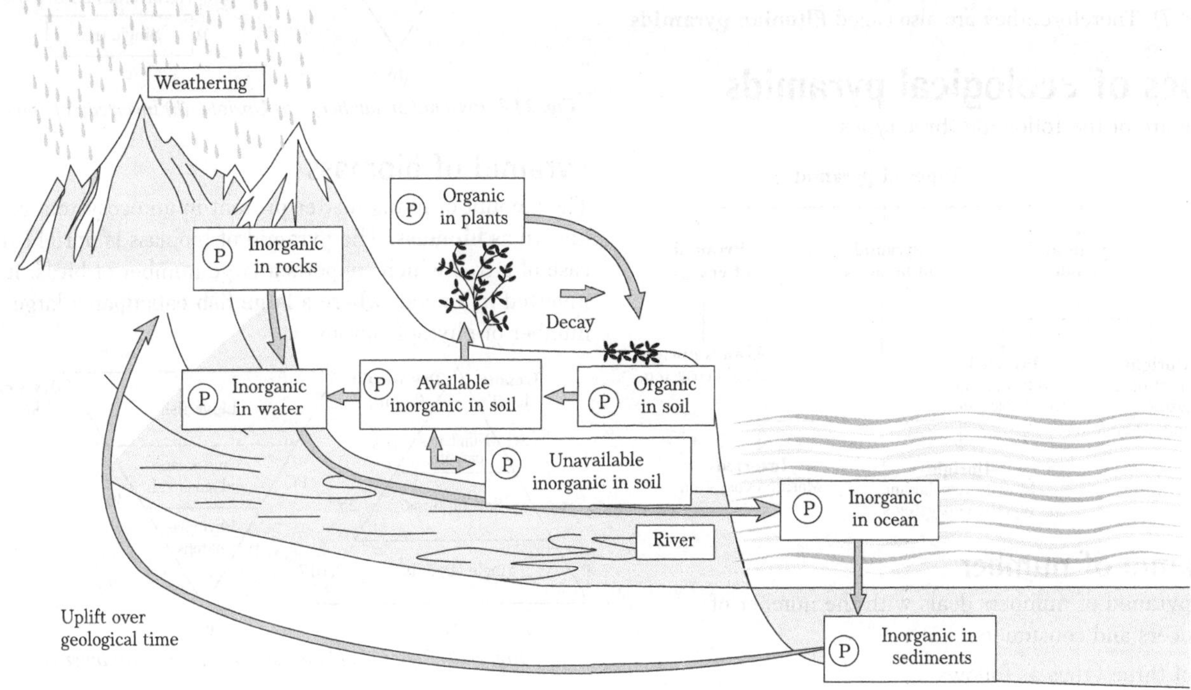

Fig. 24.7 Phosphorus cycle

CHECK POINT 24.2

1. Transfer of energy from one trophic level to other trophic level is according to the second law of thermodynamics. The efficiency of energy transfer from herbivorous to carnivorous is
(a) 20% (b) 30% (c) 90% (d) 10%

2. The rate of formation of new organic matter by rabbit in a grassland is called
(a) net productivity
(b) secondary productivity
(c) net primary productivity
(d) gross primary productivity

3. Study of biogeochemical cycle is called biogeochemistry. It involves
(a) cycling of energy
(b) cycling of gases
(c) cycling of nutrients
(d) cycling of water

4. The amount of nutrients, such as carbon, nitrogen, phosphorus, calcium, etc., present in the soil at any given time is referred as
(a) standing state (b) standing crop
(c) biogeochemical cycling (d) trophic level

5. All these processes contribute to the CO_2 pool in atmosphere except
(a) Respiration by producers
(b) Photosynthesis by producer
(c) Respiration by consumer
(d) Decomposition by decomposers

6. Which of the following is not one of the thus aspects studied in biogeochemical cycling?
(a) The rate of movement between reservoir
(b) Interaction between different biogeochemical cycles
(c) Creation of their own biogeochemical cycle by new species
(d) The nature and size of natural reservior

ECOLOGICAL PYRAMIDS

- There is some sort of relationship between the numbers, biomass and energy contents of the producers and consumers of different orders in any ecosystem. These relationships when represented in diagrammatic ways, are called ecological pyramids.
- The concept of pyramid was proposed by **Charles Elton** (1927). Therefore, they are also called **Eltonian pyramids.**

Types of ecological pyramids

These are of the following three types

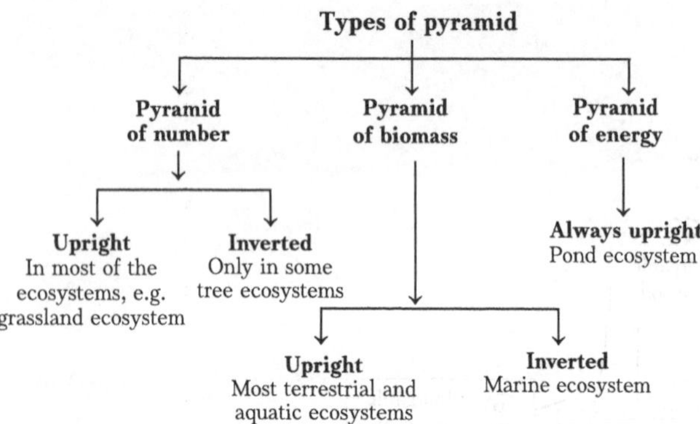

Pyramid of number

The pyramid of numbers deals with the number of producers and consumers.

It is of three types as follows

(i) **Upright pyramids** These are found in most ecosystem, e.g. grasslands, pond, etc. In a grassland, the number of producers are more than the number of top carnivores.

(ii) **Inverted pyramid** In a tree ecosystem, a large-sized tree (producer) may provide food to several birds. The number of ectoparasite dependent on birds are more than number of birds, e.g. parasitic food chain. Thus, the shape of pyramid may be inverted.

(iii) **Spindle pyramid** A tree supports a number of birds. These birds are eaten by one or two hawks of the area.

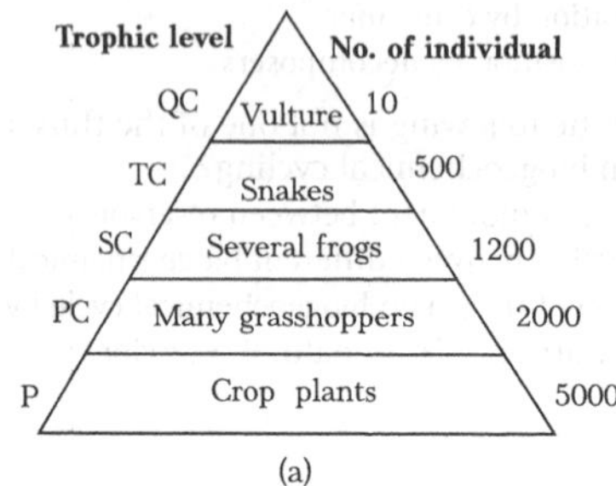

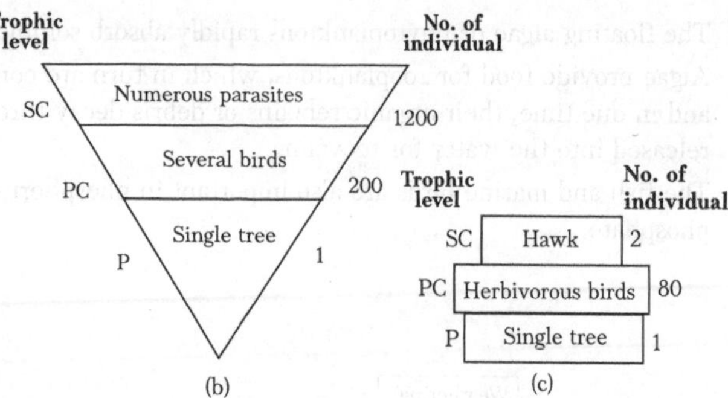

Fig. 24.8 Pyramid of numbers: (a) Upright, (b) Inverted, (c) Spindle

Pyramid of biomass

The amount of living matter present in an ecosystem is known as **biomass.** The pyramid of biomass is upright in case of a tree which supports a large number of birds. It is inverted in a pond, where a large fish eats upon a large number of phytoplanktons.

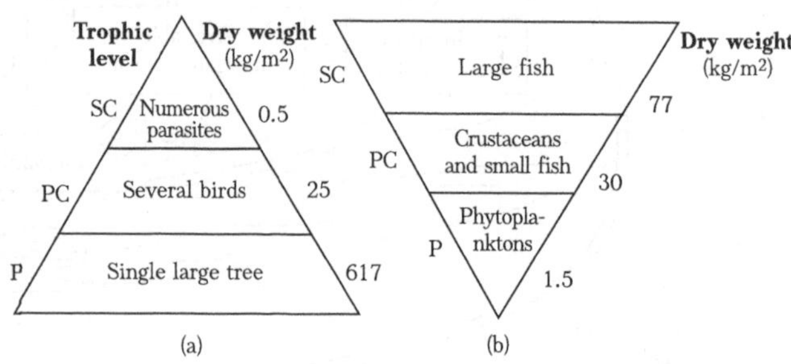

Fig. 24.9 Pyramid of biomass: (a) Upright, (b) Inverted

Pyramid of energy

It represents the total amount of energy utilised by organisms of different trophic level in unit area over a period of time. The pyramid of energy is always upright. The producers always have more energy than other trophic level. The energy continuously decreases as it passes from one trophic level to another trophic level. Some energy is lost in respiration, growth or reproduction and some in the form of heat.

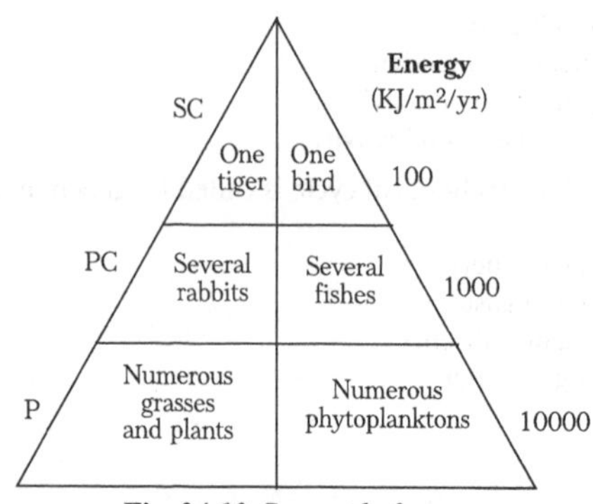

Fig. 24.10 Pyramid of energy

ECOLOGICAL SUCCESSION

- An ecosystem development and stabilisation can be best understood through ecological succession.
- It is a sequence of seres from barren land to the climax community.
- In ecological terms, the developmental stages of a biological community are known as **seral stages** and the final stage is called the **climax community**.
- The initial community of the area, which is replaced in time by a sequence of succeeding communities, is called **pioneer stage** or **pioneer community**.
- The entire series of communities that is a characteristic of given site is called a **sere**.

Table 24.4 Differences between pioneer community and climax community

Pioneer community	Climax community
It is the first biotic community, which develops in bare area.	It is the final biotic community that develops in an area.
Diversity little	Diversity more
Pioneer community is established over a previously bare area.	Climax community occurs over an area previously occupied by several communities.
Pioneer community consists of a fewer small-sized organisms.	Climax community consists of numerous, large and small-sized organisms.
The area is hostile for pioneer community.	The area is favourable for the climax community.
Lifespan is short.	Lifespan is long.
Growth is fast.	Growth is slow.
It is soon replaced by the next seral community.	Climax community is stable. It is not replaced by any other community.

Causes of succession

The important causes of ecological succession are as follows

(i) **Initial or Initiating causes of succession** These include climatic as well as biotic causes. The climatic causes include factors such as erosion and deposits, wind, fire, etc. These causes destroy the existing populations in an area.

(ii) **Ecesis causes** These are the processes such as migration, aggregation, etc.

(iii) **Stabilising causes** The climatic conditions of an area determine the type of the climax community.

While the process of succession in the tropics is similar to that in temperate regions, the plant populations are quite different. This is due to different climate conditions.

Changes during biotic succession

The following changes may occur due to biotic succession

- Small short-lived plants to large long-lived plants.
- Unstable biotic community to stable biotic community.
- Little diversity to high diversity.
- Greater niche specialisation.
- Increase in biomass.
- Increase in soil differentiation.
- Increase in humus content of the soil.
- Aquatic or dry conditions to mesic conditions.
- Simple food chains to complex food webs.

Types of ecological succession

The various types of succession have been grouped in different ways on the basis of different aspects.

1. On the basis of occurrence of succession on bare area, these are as follows

   (i) **Primary succession** According to **Clarke** (1954), ecological succession that begins on a bare area, where no life has existed, or where the previous flora and fauna have been completely destroyed, is known as primary succession.

   Soil is absent at the beginning of succession. Pioneer community comes from the outside to new area, e.g. newly exposed sea, igneous rocks, etc.

   (ii) **Secondary succession** It occurs in an area, which has been renewed recently. Soil is already present, pioneer community develops partly from the previous occupants and partly from the migrants. It takes less time for completion, e.g. forest fire, flood plain, etc.

2. On the basis of successive changes occur *via* autonomous or any external factor, these are as follows

   (i) **Autogenic succession** The succession resulting from the changes brought about by the organisms themselves is called autogenic succession.

   An abandoned agricultural field changing into mature forest over long span of time is an example of autogenic succession.

   (ii) **Allogenic succession** When replacement of the existing community is caused by any other external condition, it is called allogenic succession.

3. On the basis of successive changes in nutritional and energy contents, these are as follows

   (i) **Autotrophic succession** It is characterised by early and continued dominance by autotrophic organisms.

(ii) **Heterotrophic succession** This succession is characterised by early dominance of heterotrophs, e.g. bacteria, fungi, etc.
- It occurs in the special and rare case, where the environment is predominantly organic. For example, in a stream heavily polluted with sewage.
- The organisms in heterotrophic succession use the energy of the dead organic matter.
- In this type of succession, energy is maximum at the beginning and gradually declines as succession proceeds until additional organic matter is added from the outside.

General process of succession

The whole process of a primary autotrophic succession is actually completed through a number of sequential steps, which follow one another. These steps in sequence are as follows

(i) **Nudation** This is the development of a bare area without any form of life. The area may develop due to several causes, such as land slides, erosion, deposition or other catastrophic agency. The cause of nudation may be topographic, climatic or biotic.

(ii) **Invasion** This is the successful establishment of a species in a bare area. The species actually reaches the new site from any other area.

The process of invasion is completed in three steps
- **Migration** The seed, spores and propagules reach the bare area through water or air medium.
- **Ecesis** After reaching to new area, the process of successful establishment, i.e. the germination of seed or propagules of the species is known as ecesis. Only few species are capable to establish under harsh conditions.
- **Aggregation** After ecesis, as a result of reproduction, the individuals of the species increase in number. They also come close to each other.

(iii) **Competition and co-action** It usually occurs after aggregation of a large number of individuals of the species at the limited place. Inter as well as intraspecific competition develops due to limited space and nutrition. Individuals of a species affect each other's life in various ways and this is called co-action.

(iv) **Reaction** It is the modification of environment. Due to this, environment is modified and becomes unsuitable for the existing community, which sooner or later is replaced by another community. The whole sequence of community that replaces the another community is called **seres**.

(v) **Stabilisation** (climax) It is the process, when the final terminal community becomes more or less stabilised for a longer period of time. It can maintain itself in equilibrium with the climate of the area. The final community cannot be replaced and is known as **climax community**. This stage is known as **climax stage**.

Sometimes due to changes in local conditions, the process of succession becomes deflected in a different direction than that presumed under climatic condition of the area. Thus, the climax communities are likely to be different from the presumed climatic climax community. This type of succession is called **deflected succession**.

Examples of biological succession

Xerosere and hydrosere are two main biological successions. They are discussed as follows

1. Xerosere/Lithosere

The sequence of successional stages that occur on bare rocks is called lithosere. The bare rock is deficient in water, thus lithosere is also called xerosere.

It originates on bare rock surfaces, where the original substratum is deficient of water and lacks any organic matter. The various stages of a xerosere are as follows

(i) **Crustose lichen stage** The pioneers community of this stage are crustose lichens of species- *Rhizocarpon, Rinodina* and *Lecanora.*
- Lichens can tolerate desiccation, heating during summer noon or excessive cooling during winter nights.
- They produce some acids (e.g. lichen acid and carbonic acid), which bring about weathering of rocks.
- The dead organic matter of lichens become mixed with the small particles of rocks. However, this process is very slow.
- The crustose lichens are then replaced by foliose type of lichens.

(ii) **Foliose lichen stage** The individuals of this stage includes species of *Parmelia, Dermatocarpon,* etc., which have large leaf-like thalli. These lichens increase shading of the rock and hence, cause deep depressions. They accumulate more soil particles as well as organic matter.

(iii) **Moss stage** The soil condition then favours the growth of some mosses, e.g. *Polytrichum* and *Grimmia.*
- Mosses are of larger size, have gregarious habit and their rhizoids penetrate deeper in the rocks.

- It accumulates more soil and organic matter. The substratum remains moist for longer periods. Therefore, it invites more moisture loving mosses (e.g. *Hypnum, Bryum,* etc.)

(iv) **Annual grass stage** Mosses mat becomes sufficiently moist during the rainy season. This facilitates germination of seeds of annual grasses and other hardy herbs, e.g. *Aristida, Poa, Eleusine,* etc. Their roots penetrate deeper into the rock and cause its further fragmentation.

(v) **Perennial grass stage** Annual grasses are replaced by perennial grasses due to increased moisture and soil in the rock crevices, e.g. *Cymbopogon* and *Heteropogon.*

(vi) **Shrub stage** Due to much accumulation of soil, the habitat becomes suitable for shrubs, e.g. *Rhus, Phytocarpus, Zizyphus,* etc. Their roots reach greater depth thus, causing further cracks in the rocky substratum. The shrubs shade the area, make it more moist and invite hardy trees.

(vii) **Forest stage** Some xerophytic trees invade the area. Slowly environment becomes more moist and shadier, so that plants of climax community spread in the area. Types of climax community depends upon the climate. Therefore, it is also called **climatic climax community.**

Table 24.5 Pioneer, seral and climax communities of xerosere

Pioneer community	Seral community				Climax community
Crustose lichens stage	**Foliose lichen stage**	**Moss stage**	**Herb stage**	**Shrub stage**	**Forest stage**
Rhizocarpon	*Parmelia, Dermatocarpon*	*Polytrichum*	*Rhus*	*Rhus*	Mesophytic trees
Rinodina		*Tortula*	*Pestuca*	*Phyto-carpus*	
Lecanora		*Grimnia*			

2. Hydrosere

In this succession, a pond and its community are converted into a land community.

Various stages of hydrosere are as follows

(i) **Plankton stage** It is the pioneer stage of hydrosere. Different spores reach the water body through wind or animals.

- The first organisms appear minute autotrophs called phytoplanktons, e.g. diatoms, green flagellates, single-celled colonial or filamentous green algae.
- They multiply rapidly and soon a balance is created by the appearance of zooplankton which feed on phytoplankton.
- Death and decomposition of planktons produce organic matter.
- The latter get mixed up with clay and silt at the bottom to form soft mud. These processes are favourable for the growth of next seral stage.

(ii) **Submerged stage** The bottom, lined by soft mud is favourable for the growth of submerged plants like *Hydrilla, Potamogeton, Vallisneria, Utricularia,* etc. They are rooted in the mud and form dense growth. As a result, sand, silt and humus get deposited around the plants.
This enriches the newly built up bottom and makes it favourable for the growth of next stage.

(iii) **Floating stage** Floating leaves anchored plants (e.g. *Nymphaea, Nelumbo*) appear where water is shallow. The plants make the water rich in mineral and organic matter. It becomes suitable for the growth of free-floating plants like *Wolffia, Azolla,* etc. They cover the surface of water quickly.

(iv) **Reed swamp stage** Amphibious plants grow where the water body becomes shallow (0.3-1.0 m), e.g. *Sagittaria, Typha,* etc. The plants of swamp stage transpire huge quantities of water. They also produce abundant organic matter. Their tangled growth accumulates silt.

(v) **Sedge or Marsh meadow stage** The shores built up by reed swamp stage are invaded by *Carex* (sedge), *Juncus,* grasses like *Themeda* and *Dichanthium* and herbs like *Caltha, Polygonum,* etc. They form mat-like vegetation towards the centre of the pond with the help of their much branched rhizomatous system. These plants transpire rapidly and add abundant humus. Therefore, soil is buildup to invite the next stage.

(vi) **Woodland stage** The periphery of previous stage is invaded by some rhizome bearing shrubs.

- These can tolerate bright sunlight as well as waterlogged conditions, e.g. bogwood, *Cephalanthus* (button brush).
- The shrubs shade away the plants of sedge meadow stage. They invite invasion of trees which are capable of bearing sunlight and waterlogging. For example, *Populus* (cotton wood), *Alnus* (alder), etc.
- The plants of woodland stage lower the water table by their transpiration. They also built up more soil.

Climax forest

- New trees invade the area. They have shade loving seedlings. These trees grow to greater heights. The trees and shrubs of woodland stage disappear.
- The climax forest depends upon the climate, i.e. rainforest in moist tropical area and mixed coniferous in temperate area.
- A mixed temperate forest includes broad leaved tree like oak.

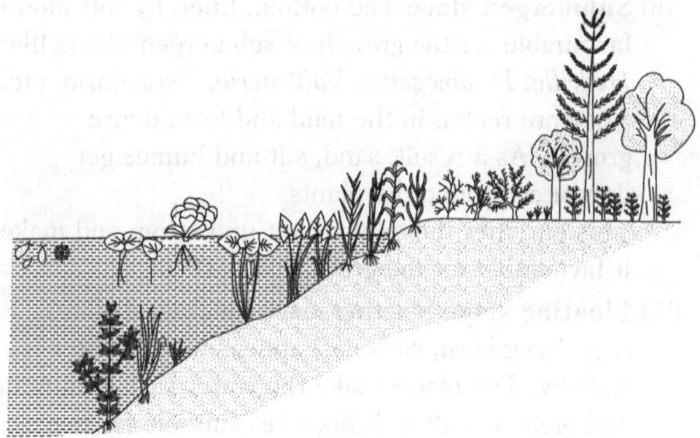

Fig. 24.11 Ecological succession from a pond to the climax forest

ECOSYSTEM SERVICES

- Healthy ecosystems are the base for a wide range of economic, environmental, aesthetic goods and services.
- The products of ecosystem processes are named as ecological or ecosystem services.
- **Millenium ecosystem assessment** is an international synthesis of over 1000 of the world's leading biologist that analyses the state of the earth's ecosystem.
- It divides ecosystem services into four types as follows
  - (i) **Supporting services** These include services such as nutrient recycling, primary production and soil formation.
  - (ii) **Provisioning services** These include products obtained from ecosystems.
  - (iii) **Regulating services** These include benefits from the regulation of ecosystem processes.
  - (iv) **Cultural services** These include non-material benefits people obtain from ecosystem through spiritual enrichment, cognitive development, reflection and aesthetic experiences.
- These services maintain biodiversity and the production of ecosystem goods, such as seafood, forage, timber, biomass fuels, natural fibres and many pharmaceuticals, industrial products and their precursors.
- **Robert Constanza** and his colleagues have put an average price tag of US $ 33 trillion a years on these fundamental services, i.e. nearly twice the value of a global GNP- US $18 trillion.
- The cost is distributed in following way.

  The soil formation accounts for about 50% and contributions of other services like recreation and nutrient cycling are less than 10% each. The cost of climate regulation and habitat for wildlife are about 6% each.

CHECK POINT 24.3

1. Which of the following is not the limitations of ecological pyramids?
   (a) Pyramids accommodate a food web
   (b) Saprophytes are not given any place in ecological pyramid
   (c) Pyramid does not take into account the same species belonging to two or more trophic levels
   (d) Pyramid assumes a simple food chain, something that almost never exist in natures
2. 'Pyramid of biomass is more real than the pyramid of number'. Which of the following correctly justify the statement?
   (a) The pyramid of number does not take into consideration the size of the individual
   (b) Maximum biomass occurs in top carnivores
   (c) It can be inverted in terrestrial ecosystem and upright in aquatic ecosystem
   (d) Both (a) and (c)
3. Which of the following is the last stabilising community of plant succession?
   (a) Seral community
   (b) Pioneer community
   (c) Ecosere
   (d) Climax community
4. ...... is the series of natural changes in the dominance of a community developing on a previously baren/virgin area.
   (a) Primary autotrophic succession
   (b) Primary heterotrophic succession
   (c) Secondary autotrophic succession
   (d) Secondary heterotrophic succession
5. Correct sequence of plants in a hydrosere is
   (a) *Pistia* → *Volvox* → *Scirpus* → *Hydrilla* → Oak → *Lantana*
   (b) Oak → *Lantana* → *Volvox* → *Hydrilla* → *Pistia* → *Scirpus*
   (c) Oak → *Lantana* → *Scirpus* → *Pistia* → *Hydrilla* → *Volvox*
   (d) *Volvox* → *Hydrilla* → *Pistia* → *Scirpus* → *Lantana* → Oak

EXAM POINTS

- The term ecosystem was coined by AG Tansley. **[NEET-I 2016]**
- Fragmentation is the breakdown of detritus into small particles by detritivores. **[KCET 2015, NEET 2013]**
- Steps of decomposition process are fragmentation, leaching, catabolism, humification and mineralisation. **[AMU 2012]**
- The rate of decomposition is fast when the environment is favourable for aerobic microbes and detritus is rich in sugar. But if the detritus is rich in lignin and chitin, decomposition rate slows down. **[NEET 2020]**
- The primary producers of the deep sea hydrothermal vent ecosystem are Archaebacteria. They have chemosynthetic mode of nutrition hence, also called chemosynthetic bacteria. **[NEET-II 2016]**
- Stratification is the vertical distribution of different species occupying different levels in a biotic community. It is not a functional unit of ecosystem. **[CBSE AIPMT 2015, 12]**
- The presence of plants arranged into well-defined vertical layers depending on their height can best seen in tropical rainforest. **[NEET 2017]**
- Most animals are tree dwellers in tropical rainforests. **[CBSE AIPMT 2015]**
- Primary productivity depends on plant species inhabiting a particular area. **[Kerala CEE 2014]**
- The rate at which organic matter is produced during photosynthesis is known as gross primary productivity. **[CBSE AIPMT 2015]**
- Gross Primary Productivity (GPP) is always more than Net Primary Productivity (NPP) because $NPP = GPP - R$ **[NEET 2020, 2017]**
- 1.9 g organic matter is produced by 1g CO_2. **[EAMCET 2016]**
- The biomass energy available for consumption by herbivores is called net primary productivity. **[BHU 2012]**
- Secondary productivity is the rate of formation of new organic matter by consumer. **[NEET 2013]**
- Least genetic diversity is the characteristic feature of cropland ecosystem. **[NEET-I 2016]**
- In ecosystem, energy flow is unidirectional. **[J&K CET 2015, AFMC 2009]**
- Standing crop is the mass of living material at trophic level at a specific time. **[CBSE AIPMT 2015]**
- The energy content decreases from the first (produce) to fourth (consumer) level because at each level, 90% energy is lost and 10% is passed to next level. **[NEET 2020]**
- Availability of nutrients limits the number of trophic levels in a stable ecosystem. **[AIIMS 2013]**
- Autotrophs are the primary trophic level and have the greatest amount of energy. **[BCECE 2012]**
- In an ecosystem, there are different trophic levels based on eating habits. The producers are eatten by primary consumer, primary consumers are eatten by secondary and so on. Hence, in grassland ecosystem, following food chain is seen. **[NEET 2020]**

  Grass (Producer) → Rabit (Primary consumer) → Crow (Secondary consumer) → Vulture (Tertiary consumer)

- Earth's crust is the reservoir for sedimentary type or biogeochemical cycle. **[CBSE AIPMT 2015]**
- There is no respiratory release of phosphorus into atmosphere as phosphorus is an inorganic nutrient, which does not take part in respiration. **[NEET 2020]**
- The pyramid of energy is always upright, pyramid of biomass is upright in forest while inverted in sea. The pyramid of number is upright for grassland, lake and ponds. **[NEET 2019, 18, CBSE AIPMT 2012, 11]**
- Forest ecosystem has the maximum biomass. **[NEET 2017]**
- Lichens are pioneer species in xerarch succession and phytoplanktons are pioneer species in hydrarch succession. **[KCET 2015, NEET 2016]**
- During ecological succession, gradual and predictable change in species composition occurs in a given area. **[AMU 2015]**
- Secondary succession takes place on degraded forest. It is the process of regrowth of an ecosystem which undergoes destructive events. The rate of succession is faster, e.g. Abandoned grass. **[CBSE AIPMT 2016, 15, 11, EAMCET 2016]**
- Sequence of hydroseric succession is Phytoplanktons → Rooted submerged plants → Reed swamp → Sedge meadow **[Gujarat CET 2015]**
- Limnetic zone is the area in lake where phytoplanktons grow in abundance **[J&K CET 2015]**
- According to Robert Constanza, 50% of the total cost for ecosystem services goes to nutrient cycling. **[KCET 2015, Kerala CEE 2014]**

Chapter Exercises

(A) Topical Exercise

Ecosystem and its Components

1 Biological community and components of the physical environment with which the community interacts is known as

(a) atmosphere (b) ecosystem
(c) biosphere (d) hydrosphere

2 Agroecosystem is unstable because of

(a) lack of variety
(b) lack of biological control
(c) being man-made
(d) Both (a) and (b)

3 Aquatic ecosystem consists of

(a) biotic factor
(b) biotic and abiotic factors
(c) consumers only
(d) producers only

4 Aquatic ecosystems cover approximately how much of the earth's surface?

(a) 20% (b) 40% (c) 75% (d) 90%

5 Biotic components include

(a) producers
(b) consumers
(c) producers and consumers
(d) producers, consumers and decomposers

6 The organisms which physically and chemically break the complex organic remains are known as

(a) scavangers (b) decomposers
(c) parasites (d) saprophytes

7 Decomposers like fungi and bacteria are

I. Autotrophs
II. Heterotrophs
III. Chemoautotrophs

Codes

(a) I and III (b) I and III
(c) II and III (d) I and II

8 Excessive moisture inhibit the process of decomposition due to

(a) anaerobiosis (b) aerobiosis
(c) photooxidation (d) photophosphorylation

9 The organic substances which decompose slowly are

(a) chitin (b) lignin
(c) cellulose (d) All of these

10 Which one of the following components of ecosystem comes from outside?

(a) Oxygen (b) Temperature
(c) Insects (d) Energy

11 If phytoplanktons are destroyed in the sea,

(a) it will affect food chain
(b) no effect
(c) algae will get more space
(d) primary consumer will grow more

12 Which of the following is not a producer? **[NCERT Exemplar]**

(a) *Spirogyra* (b) *Agaricus*
(c) *Volvox* (d) *Nostoc*

13 The species which occupy the initial stages of an ecosystem are named as

(a) climax species (b) pioneer species
(c) divergent species (d) All of these

14 Stratification occurs in

(a) Tropical rainforests (b) Deciduous forest
(c) Desert (d) Both (a) and (b)

15 How much of the chemical energy within the producer tissues becomes chemical energy within the herbivore tissue?

(a) 1% (b) 10%
(c) 30% (d) 50%

16 Primary consumers and secondary consumers belong to which trophic level, respectively?

	Primary consumers	Secondary consumers
(a)	Trophic level - II	Trophic level - III
(b)	Trophic level - I	Trophic level - II
(c)	Trophic level - II	Trophic level - I
(d)	Trophic level - III	Trophic level - II

17 Consider the following statements.

I. The most productive area of the ocean is near the shore.
II. Decomposition takes place on upper layer of soil at maximum rate.

Choose the correct option.

(a) Statement I is true, but II is false
(b) Statement I is false, but II is true
(c) Both statements I and II are true
(d) Both statements I and II are false

18 Most animals that live in deep oceanic waters are

(a) producers (b) primary consumers
(c) secondary consumers (d) detritivores

19 The type of food chain in which decomposed organic matter is converted into energy rich compound is called

(a) detritus food chain (b) grazing food chain
(c) cybernetics (d) None of these

20 The process of release of inorganic substances both non-mineral and minerals from organic matter is known as

(a) mineralisation (b) humification
(c) photophosphorylation (d) pollination

21 In terrestrial ecosystem, maximum energy is present in

(a) T_3 (b) T_2
(c) T_1 (d) T_4

22 A sequence of species through, which the organic molecule in a community pass is called

(a) pyramid of energy (b) food chain
(c) food web (d) nutrient cycle

23 The region of sea having maximum productivity is

(a) coastal
(b) continental shelf water level
(c) deep sea
(d) bery deep sea

24 Importance of ecosystem maintenance lies in

(a) cycling of materials (b) flow of energy
(c) food chain (d) Both (a) and (b)

25 Consider the following statements.

I. Detritus food chain in comparison to grazing food chain is generally longer.
II. In the food chain, the saprophytic organisms are decomposers.

Choose the correct option.

(a) Statement I is true, but II is false
(b) Statement I is false, but II is true
(c) Both statements I and II are true
(d) Both statements I and II are false

26 Frog $\xrightarrow{\text{Eats}}$ Grasshopper $\xrightarrow{\text{Eats}}$ Green plant. Frog is a

(a) Primary producer (b) Herbivore
(c) Primary carnivore (d) Top consumer

27 At each trophic level of a food chain, the energy which is not used or passed along is given off as

(a) matter (b) free energy
(c) heat (d) water

28 Rate of storage of organic matter by heterotrophs is termed as

(a) Net productivity
(b) Net primary productivity
(c) Gross primary productivity
(d) Secondary productivity

29 Arrange the following in correct order.

I. Annual grass stage.
II. Foliose lichen stage.
III. Moss stage.
IV. Forest stage.

Codes

(a) II, III, IV and I (b) II, III, I and IV
(c) III, I, II and IV (d) I, IV, II and III

30 Most food chains are composed of

(a) 1 or 2 species (b) 3 to 4 species
(c) 90 or 10 species (d) more than 16 species

31 Which of the following type of ecosystem is expected in an area where evaporation exceeds precipitation, and mean annual rainfall is below 100 mm?

(a) Grassland (b) Shrubby forest
(c) Desert (d) Mangrove

Functions of Ecosystem

32 Which one of the following best describes the base of a pyramid of net production?

(a) Its size depends on the energy available from detritivores
(b) It contains the energy left after the producers have died
(c) It represents the energy available to the secondary consumers
(d) It contains the energy captured by photosynthesis

33 Which of the following is most responsible for increasing atmospheric CO_2 levels and upsetting the balance of the carbon cycle?

(a) Photosynthesis
(b) Activities of decomposers
(c) Aerobic respiration by plants and animals
(d) Combustion of fossil fuels

34 The rate at which light energy is converted to the chemical energy of organic molecules is the ecosystem's

(a) Net primary productivity
(b) Gross primary productivity
(c) Net secondary productivity
(d) Gross secondary productivity

35 The word 'standing state' in ecosystem refers to

(a) living components (b) non-living components
(c) producers (d) Both (a) and (b)

36 The rate at which new tissues are formed in producers in the ecosystem.

(a) Net primary productivity
(b) Gross primary productivity
(c) Net secondary productivity
(d) Gross secondary productivity

37 How do iron levels affect phytoplankton populations in a marine ecosystem?
(a) Without iron, eukaryotic phytoplankton population fall because they cannot convert atmospheric N_2 to nitrogenous minerals
(b) In the presence of too much iron, eukaryotic phytoplankton populations fall because they cannot convert atmospheric N_2 to the nitrogenous minerals
(c) Iron stimulates the growth of cyanobacteria, which converts atmospheric N_2 to nitrogenous minerals; stimulating the growth of phytoplankton
(d) Iron halts the growth of cyanobacteria, which convert atmospheric N_2 to nitrogenous minerals. Therefore, phytoplankton populations are limited

38 The reservoir for the gaseous type of biogeochemical cycle exists in **[NCERT Exemplar]**
(a) stratosphere (b) atmosphere
(c) ionosphere (d) lithosphere

39 Which is the most direct way that the carbon present in starch stored in cereal grains can return to the atmosphere as carbon dioxide?
(a) Grains are destroyed by fire during storage
(b) Grains are eaten by birds
(c) Grains are made into bread and eaten by humans
(d) Grains are stored in damp conditions goes mouldy and decay

40 Which is incorrectly matched?
(a) *Rhizobium* – Free-living nitrogen fixer
(b) Humus –Biotic component
(c) Phosphorus – Sedimentary
(d) *Shorea robusta* – Sal tree

41 The largest reservoir of phosphorus in the biosphere is the
(a) atmosphere (b) ocean
(c) organisms (d) rock

42 In an ecosystem, the population of
(a) primary producer is larger than primary consumers
(b) secondary consumer is largest
(c) primary consumers are more than primary producers
(d) primary consumers are least dependent upon primary producers

43 Organisms, which can convert ammonium or nitrates into amino acids are
(a) scavenger (b) producers
(c) primary consumers (d) primary detritivores

44 Phosphorus cycles in the form of
(a) HPO_3^- (b) P_2 (a gas) (c) PO_4^{2-} (d) $AlPO_4$

45 Which of the following atoms most often limits the primary productivity of an ecosystem?
(a) Carbon (b) Nitrogen
(c) Sulphur (d) Phosphorus

46 Biogeochemical cycles are also known as
(a) sedimentary cycling (b) gaseous cycle
(c) material cycling (d) cycles of water

47 Nitrogen is a critical element of the ecosystem because it is
(a) essential element (b) abundant in atmosphere
(c) labile (d) fixed by microbes

48 The phosphorus cycle is entirely
(a) within aquatic systems
(b) within terrestrial ecosystem
(c) sedimentary
(d) gaseous

49 Which of the following aquatic ecosystems has very little primary productivity?
(a) River (b) Estuary (c) Lake (d) Marsh

50 Most primary productivity in the surface waters of lakes and oceans is by
(a) floating plants (b) red and brown algae
(c) zooplankton (d) phytoplankton

51 If the carbon atoms fixed by producers already have passed through three species, the trophic level of the last species would be
(a) scavenger (b) tertiary producer
(c) tertiary consumer (d) secondary consumer

52 The energy utilised by the living world is primarily
(a) heat (b) electricity (c) sunlight (d) kinetic

53 Approximately how much of the solar energy that falls on the leaves of a plant is converted to chemical energy by photosynthesis?
(a) Less than 1% (b) 2-10% (c) 30% (d) 50%

54 Which one is sedimentary cycle?
(a) Oxygen cycle (b) Nitrogen cycle
(c) Hydrogen cycle (d) None of these

55 Which of them can be put in the category of primary consumers?
(a) Eagle and tigers (b) Fishes and whales
(c) Snakes and frogs (d) Insects and cattles

Ecological Pyramids

56 An ecological pyramid of biomass is a representation of the ecosystem's
(a) energy flow through each trophic level
(b) dry mass at each trophic level
(c) populations in each food web
(d) biological material in relation to abiotic material

57 Climax community is in a state of
(a) non-equilibrium (b) equilibrium
(c) disorder (d) constant change

58 Creating force of any ecosystem is
(a) organic fuels, carbohydrates (b) biomass
(c) solar energy (d) producers

59 The biomass of each succeeding trophic level is
(a) more than the one preceding
(b) less than the one preceding
(c) constantly fixed
(d) equal to next trophic level

60 Which of the following least affects succession in a community?
(a) Population growth rates
(b) The niches occupied by different species
(c) Evolutionary relationships between organisms
(d) Competition between organisms

61 The Millennium Ecosystem Assessment distinguished ecosystem services into classes
(a) two (b) three (c) four (d) None of these

62 In parasitic food chain, the pyramid of number is
(a) linear (b) upright
(c) inverted (d) inverted upright

63 Consider the following statements.
I. Succession occurs in an area, which has been bare from the beginning is known as primary succession.
II. An abandoned agriculture field changing into mature forest over long span of time is an example of autogenic succession.
Choose the correct option.
(a) Statement I is true, but II is false
(b) Statement I is false, but II is true
(c) Both statements I and II are true
(d) Both statements I and II are false

64 Choose the incorrect matched pair.
(a) Sere stage – Floating stage
(b) Woodland stage – *Rhus*
(c) Submerged stage – *Hydrilla*
(d) Plankton stage – Hydrosere

65 Which of the following acid is secreted by lichens or rocks?
(a) Carbonic acid (b) Hydrocarbonic acid
(c) HCl (d) H_2SO_4

66 During the process of ecological succession, the changes that take place in communities are
(a) orderly and sequential
(b) random
(c) very quick
(d) not influenced by the physical environment

67 The process of transformation of a set of natural soil, plants, air, water and animals into things that we value is known as
(a) Ecological services (b) Ecological products
(c) Ecological benefits (d) Ecological conserves

68 A lake community suddenly suffers from algal blooms. Using the strategy of biomanipulation, an ecologist may propose
(a) add fish that feed on algae
(b) adding mineral nutrients to the water
(c) adding fish that eats zooplankton
(d) removing fish that eats zooplankton

69 Which of the following is an ecosystem service provided by a natural ecosystem? **[NCERT Exemplar]**
(a) Cycling of nutrients
(b) Prevention of soil erosion
(c) Pollutant absorption and reduction of the threat of global warming
(d) All of the above

70 Choose the correct statements for pyramids.
I. Energy pyramid is always upright.
II. For forest, the pyramid of biomass is inverted.
III. For grassland, the pyramid of number is upright.
Codes
(a) I and II (b) II and III (c) I and III (d) I, II and III

71 Which of the following statements is incorrect regarding ecological pyramids?
(a) The pyramid of energy is inverted in ocean ecosystem
(b) The pyramid of biomass is inverted in aquatic ecosystem
(c) The pyramid of numbers is upright in grassland ecosystem
(d) The pyramid of biomass is upright in grassland ecosystem

72 The sequence of communities of primary succession in water is
(a) Phytoplankton, sedges, free-floating hydrophytes, rooted hydrophytes, grasses and trees
(b) Phytoplankton, free-floating hydrophytes, rooted hydrophytes, sedges, grasses and trees
(c) Free-floating hydrophytes, sedges, phytoplankton, rooted hydrophytes, grasses and trees
(d) Phytoplankton, rooted submerged hydrophytes, floating hydrophytes, reed swamp, sedges, meadow and trees

73 Which one of the following regarding ecological pyramid is not correct?
(a) In most ecosystems, the pyramid of number and biomass are inverted
(b) In tree-dominated ecosystem, the pyramid of number is inverted
(c) The pyramid of energy expresses mainly the rate of food production
(d) In deep water ecosystem, the pyramid of biomass is upright

74 Select the correct statement about hydrosere.
(a) Decomposers are not found in a hydrosere
(b) *Hydrilla* and *Utricularia* are floating stage organism
(c) Woodland stage is formed by *Populus* and *Alder* trees
(d) *Nelumbo* is species of submerged stage

(B) Cumulative Exercise

(Assorted Questions of the Chapter for Advanced Level Practice)

1 Oxidation of ammonia by nitrifying bacteria produces
(a) Only nitrate ion
(b) Only nitrite ion
(c) Nitrite ion and nitric oxide
(d) Both nitrites and nitrate ions

2 Match the following columns.

Column I	Column II
A. Xerosere	1. Ecological succession on aquatic habitat
B. Lithosere	2. Ecological succession on sandy soil
C. Psammosere	3. Ecological succession on dry habitat
D. Hydrosere	4. Ecological succession on rocks

Codes

	A	B	C	D
(a)	3	4	2	1
(b)	3	2	1	4
(c)	1	2	4	3
(d)	4	2	3	1

3 Consider the following statements.
I. Plant absorbed phosphates in the form of $H_2PO_4^-$.
II. Reservoir of phosphorus is atmosphere.
III. Most of the phosphates deposited in deep ocean as sediments.
IV. Plant absorbed organic phosphates.
Choose the option containing incorrect statements.
(a) II and IV (b) II and III
(c) I and IV (d) I and III

4 Productivity is the rate of production of biomass expressed in terms of
I. $(kcal^{-1}m^{-3})yr^{-1}$ II. $g^{-2}yr^{-1}$
III. $g^{-1}yr^{-1}$ IV. $(kcal^{-1}m^{-2})yr^{-1}$
Codes
(a) I and II (b) Only III
(c) II and IV (d) I and IV

5 Consider the following statements concerning food chains.
I. Removal of 80% tigers from an area resulted in greatly increased growth of vegetation.
II. Removal of most of the carnivores resulted in an increased population of deers.
III. The length of food chains is generally limited to 3-4 trophic levels due to energy loss.
IV. The length of food chains may vary from 2-8 trophic levels.
Which two of the given statements are correct?
(a) II and III (b) III and IV
(c) I and IV (d) I and II

6 Match the following columns.

Column I	Column II
A. Ammonification	1. Conversion of atmospheric nitrogen (N_2) into ammonia (NH_3)
B. Denitrification	2. Conversion of organic nitrogen (e.g. in amino acids) into ammonia
C. Nitrification	3. Conversion of nitrite (NO_2^{2-}) or nitrate (NO_3^-) into atmospheric nitrogen
D. Nitrogen-fixation	4. Conversion of ammonium (NH_4^+) into nitrite and nitrate

Codes

	A	B	C	D
(a)	3	2	1	4
(b)	1	2	3	4
(c)	2	3	4	1
(d)	4	3	2	1

7 Consider the given statements and identify which of the following statements is correct?
I. Quantity of biomass in a trophic level at a particular period is called as standing crop.
II. The energy content in a trophic level is determined by considering individuals of a species in that trophic level.
III. The succession that occurs in newly cooled lava is called primary succession.
IV. Rate of succession is faster in secondary succession.
Codes
(a) II and III (b) I and IV (c) Only II (d) Only IV

8 Study the four statements (I-IV) given below and select the two correct ones out of them.
I. A lion eating deer and a sparrow feeding on grain are eologically similar in being consumers.
II. Predator starfish *Pisaster* helps in maintaining species diversity of some invertebrates.
III. Predators ultimately leads to the extinction of prey species.
IV. Production of chemicals such as nicotine, strychnine by the plants are metabolic disorders.
The two correct statements are
(a) II and IV (b) III and IV
(c) I and III (d) I and II

9 Humans interfere with the natural phosphorus cycle by
I. utilisation of water.
II. adding phosphatic fertilisers to agricultural soils.
III. dumping sewage into lakes and rivers.
IV. temporary or permanent loss of hearing.

Choose the correct option.
(a) I, III and IV
(b) II and III
(c) I, II and IV
(d) I, II, III and IV

10 Match the following columns.

Column I	Column II
A. Producers	1. Trophic level-II
B. Primary consumers	2. Trophic level-III
C. Secondary consumers	3. Trophic level-I
D. Tertiary consumers	4. Trophic level-IV

Codes

	A	B	C	D		A	B	C	D
(a)	1	2	3	4	(b)	3	1	2	4
(c)	3	1	4	2	(d)	4	2	3	1

11 Dried plant parts such as leaves, bark, flowers, etc., and dead remains of animals including faecal matter drop over the soil, constitute the
I. below ground detritus
II. above ground detritus
III. detritus
IV. litter fall

Codes
(a) I and III (b) I and II (c) II and IV (d) I and IV

12 Select the formula for ecological efficiency.

(a) $\frac{\text{Gross primary productivity}}{\text{Incident total solar radiation}} \times 100$

(b) $\frac{\text{Food energy assimilated}}{\text{Food energy ingested}} \times 100$

(c) $\frac{\text{Net primary productivity}}{\text{Gross primary productivity}} \times 100$

(d) $\frac{\text{Energy converted in biomass production at a trophic level}}{\text{Energy present in biomass production at previous trophic level}} \times 100$

13 The diagram shows parts of the carbon cycle.

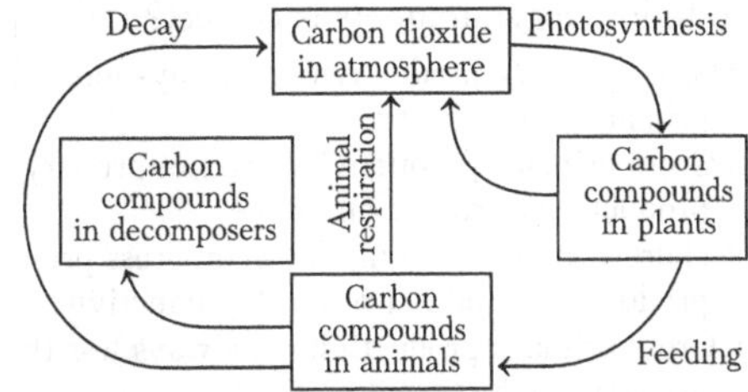

Which process converts most carbon from one form to the another?
(a) Animal respiration (b) Decay
(c) Feeding (d) Photosynthesis

14 The diagram shows losses from a rat to the environment.

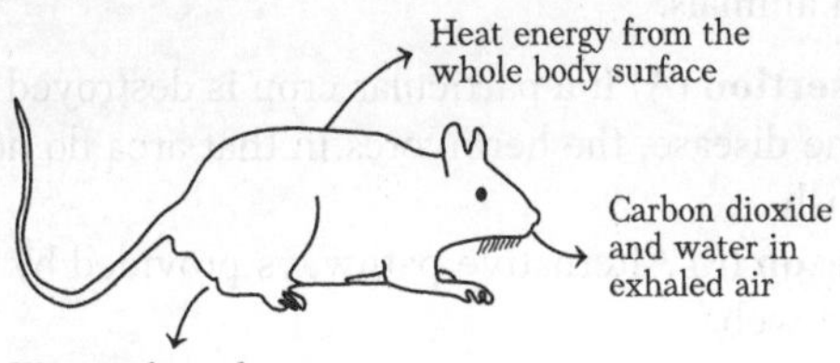

Which of the following will not be returned to the ecosystem and recycled?
(a) Carbon dioxide
(b) Heat energy
(c) Salts
(d) Urea

15 Consider the following statements.
I. The bare area supporting the growth of lichens is known as primary succession.
II. In secondary succession, the land is occupied with some kinds of propagules.
III. In heterotrophic succession, the energy is minimum in the beginning and gradually increases with time.
IV. An abandoned grassland changing into mature forest over long span of time is an example of allogenic succession.

Select the option containing correct statements.
(a) I, II and III (b) II, III and IV
(c) I and II only (d) I and III only

Assertion and Reason

Direction (Q. Nos. 16-27) *In each of the following questions, a statement of Assertion (A) is given followed by corresponding statement of Reason (R). Of the statements, mark the correct answer as*
(a) Both A and R are true and R is the correct explanation of A
(b) Both A and R are true, but R is not the correct explanation of A
(c) A is true, but R is false
(d) A is false, but R is true
(e) Both A and R are false

16 **Assertion** (A) An ecosystem is an interaction between biotic and abiotic components.
Reason (R) AG Tansley coined the term 'ecosystem'.

17 **Assertion** (A) Autotrophs are included in biotic components of an ecosystem.
Reason (R) Man can prepare food for their own.

18 **Assertion** (A) Consumers are heterotrophs.
Reason (R) They use a very little part of living plants and animals.

19 **Assertion** (A) Bacteria and fungi are microconsumers.
Reason (R) They use a very little part of living plants and animals.

20 **Assertion** (A) If a particular crop is destroyed due to some disease, the herbivores in that area do not perish.
Reason (R) Alternative pathways provided by the food web.

21 **Assertion** (A) The pyramid of number of pond ecosystem is upright.
Reason (R) Phytoplanktons are maximum and secondary consumers are least in number.

22 **Assertion** (A) The pyramid of energy is always upright.
Reason (R) Number of autotrophs in the pyramid of energy are maximum.

23 **Assertion** (A) The rate of decomposition of detritus is reduced in the regions of high altitude.
Reason (R) It happens due to immobilisation of nutrients.

24 **Assertion** (A) Nutrient cycle means cycling of glucose or reserved food material within the plant body.
Reason (R) Transfer of biogenetic nutrients between living and non-living components is called biogeochemical cycle.

25 **Assertion** (A) Reserve pool of nutrient cycle becomes emptied and filled repeatedly.
Reason (R) Filling and empting of reserved pool is due to exchange between living and non-living components of biosphere.

26 **Assertion** (A) The source of ozone is O_2.
Reason (R) Ozone protects us from harmful ultraviolet rays.

27 **Assertion** (A) Although atmosphere contains about 78% of N_2, but plants directly cannot use it.
Reason (R) Plant cells contain cell wall.

(C) Medical Entrances' Gallery

(Collection of Questions Asked in NEET & in Various Medical Entrance Exams)

1 Which of the following statements is incorrect? [NEET 2020]
(a) Biomass decreases from first to fourth trophic level
(b) Energy content gradually increases from first to fourth trophic level
(c) Number of individuals decreases from first trophic level to fourth trophic level
(d) Energy content gradually decreases from first to fourth trophic level

2 Which of the following statements is incorrect regarding the phosphorus cycle? [NEET 2020]
(a) Phosphates are the major form of phosphorus reservoir
(b) Phosphorus solubilising bacteria facilitate the release of phosphorus from organic remains
(c) There is appreciable respiratory release of phosphorus into atmosphere
(d) It is sedimentary cycle

3 The rate of decomposition is faster in the ecosystem due to following factors except [NEET 2020]
(a) detritus is rich in sugars
(b) warm and moist environment
(c) presence of aerobic soil microbes
(d) detritus is rich in lignin and chitin

4 Match the trophic levels with their correct species examples in grassland ecosystem.

Column I		Column II	
A.	Fourth trophic level	1.	Crow
B.	Second trophic level	2.	Vulture
C.	First trophic level	3.	Rabbit
D.	Third trophic level	4.	Grass

Codes [NEET 2020]

	A	B	C	D		A	B	C	D
(a)	3	2	1	4	(b)	4	3	2	1
(c)	1	2	3	4	(d)	2	3	4	1

5 In relation to gross primary productivity and net primary productivity of an ecosystem. Which one of the following statements is correct? [NEET 2020]
(a) Gross primary productivity is always more than net primary productivity
(b) Gross primary productivity and net primary productivity are one and same
(c) There is no relationship between gross primary productivity and net primary productivity
(d) Gross primary productivity is always less than net primary productivity

6 Which of the following ecological pyramids is generally inverted? **[NEET 2019]**
(a) Pyramid of energy
(b) Pyramid of biomass in a forest
(c) Pyramid of biomass in a sea
(d) Pyramid of numbers in grassland

7 What type of ecological pyramid would be obtained with the following data?
Secondary consumer : 120 g, Primary consumer : 60 g, Primary producer : 10 g **[NEET 2018]**
(a) Upright pyramid of numbers
(b) Pyramid of energy
(c) Inverted pyramid of biomass
(d) Upright pyramid of biomass

8 Select the incorrect match. **[AIIMS 2018]**
I. Sedimentary nutrient cycle- Nitrogen cycle
II. Pioneer species - Lichens
III. Secondary succession - Burned forests
IV. Pyramid of biomass in sea - Upright
Codes
(a) I and IV (b) I and III
(c) II and III (d) II and IV

9 Which ecosystem has the maximum biomass? **[NEET 2017]**
(a) Forest ecosystem (b) Grassland ecosystem
(c) Pond ecosystem (d) Lake ecosystem

10 **Assertion** (A) Gross primary productivity is always more than net primary productivity.
Reason (R) Consumers exhibit secondary productivity in an ecosystem. **[AIIMS 2017]**
(a) Both A and R are true and R is the correct explanation of A
(b) Both A and R are true, but R is not the correct explanation of A
(c) A is true, but R is false
(d) Both A and R are false

11 The presence of plants arranged into well-defined vertical layers depending on their height can be best seen in **[NEET 2017]**
(a) Tropical savannah (b) Tropical rainforest
(c) Grassland (d) Temperate forest

12 Which one of the following is a characteristic feature of cropland ecosystem? **[NEET-I 2016]**
(a) Least genetic diversity
(b) The absence of weeds
(c) Ecological succession
(d) The absence of soil organisms

13 The term ecosystem was coined by **[NEET-I 2016]**
(a) AG Tansley (b) E Haeckel
(c) E Warming (d) EP Odum

14 Which of the following would appear as the pioneer organisms on bare rocks? **[NEET-I 2016]**
(a) Liverworts (b) Mosses
(c) Green algae (d) Lichens

15 The primary producers of the deep sea hydrothermal vent ecosystem are **[NEET-II 2016]**
(a) green algae (b) chemosynthetic bacteria
(c) blue-green algae (d) coral reefs

16 Match the following columns.

Column I	Column II
A. Phytoplanktons	1. Pioneers of succession
B. Lichens	2. Grow in shady places
C. Sciophytes	3. Abandoned grasslands
D. Secondary succession	4. Lungs of the world

Codes **[EAMCET 2016]**

	A	B	C	D
(a)	4	1	2	3
(b)	2	3	4	1
(c)	4	1	3	2
(d)	2	1	4	3

17 The amount of carbon dioxide required for the production of 3 g of dry organic matter is **[EAMCET 2016]**
(a) 1.63 g (b) 4.89 g
(c) 180 g (d) 234 g

18 Secondary succession takes place on/in **[CBSE AIPMT 2016, 2015]**
(a) bare rock (b) degraded forest
(c) newly created pond (d) newly cooled lava

19 The breakdown of detritus into small particles by detritivores is called **[Karnataka CET 2015]**
(a) leaching (b) humification
(c) fragmentation (d) catabolism

20 The pioneer species in xerarch and hydrarch succession are respectively **[Karnataka CET 2015]**
(a) lichens and phytoplanktons
(b) lichens and sedges
(c) phytoplanktons and lichens
(d) lichens and rooted hydrophytes

21 Which of the following is a correct trend of succession in hydroseric succession? **[Gujarat CET 2015]**
(a) Rooted submerged → Phytoplankton → Reed swamp → Sedge meadow
(b) Phytoplankton → Reed swamp → Rooted submerged → Sedge meadow
(c) Phytoplankton → Sedge medow → Reed swamp → Root submerged
(d) Phytoplankton → Rooted submerged → Reed swamp → Sedge meadow

22 Vertical distribution of different species occupying different levels in a biotic community is known as **[CBSE AIPMT 2015]**
(a) divergence (b) stratification
(c) zonation (d) pyramid

23 The mass of living material at a trophic level at a particular time is called **[CBSE AIPMT 2015]**
(a) Gross pimary productivity
(b) Standing state
(c) Net primary productivity
(d) Standing crop

24 In an ecosystem, the rate of production of organic matter during photosynthesis is termed as **[CBSE AIPMT 2015, MHT CET 2014]**
(a) Net primary productivity
(b) Gross primary productivity
(c) Secondary productivity
(d) Net productivity

25 During ecological succession, **[AMU 2015]**
(a) The gradual and predictable change in species composition occurs in a given area
(b) The establishment of a new biotic community is very fast in its primary phase
(c) The numbers and types of animals remain constant
(d) The changes lead to a community that is in near equilibrium with the environment and is called pioneer community

26 In a lake, phytoplanktons grow in abundance in **[J&K CET 2015]**
(a) Littoral zone (b) Limnetic zone
(c) Profundal zone (d) Benthic zone

27 Energy flow in ecosystem is **[J&K CET 2015, AFMC 2009]**
(a) bidirectional (b) multidirectional
(c) unidirectional (d) All of these

28 Match the following columns.

Column I	Column II
A. Producer	1. Herbivores
B. Primary consumer	2. Green plants
C. Secondary consumer	3. Saprotrophs
D. Decomposer	4. Carnivores

Codes **[WB JEE 2015]**

	A	B	C	D
(a)	1	2	3	4
(b)	2	1	4	3
(c)	2	4	3	1
(d)	3	2	1	4

29 The overlapping zone in between two ecosystems is known as **[WB JEE 2015]**
(a) ecozone (b) biotope
(c) ecotone (d) buffer zone

30 The animal species controlling the ecosystem functioning is known as **[WB JEE 2015**
(a) edge species
(b) pioneer species
(c) keystone species
(d) umbrella species

31 Most animals are tree dwellers in a **[CBSE AIPMT 2015]**
(a) Coniferous forest
(b) Thorn woodland
(c) Temperate deciduous forest
(d) Tropical rainforest

32 For the sedimentary type of biogeochemical cycles, the reservoir is **[CBSE AIPMT 2015]**
(a) atmosphere (b) water
(c) earth's crust (d) living organisms

33 According to Robert Constanza, 50% of the total cost for ecosystem services goes to **[Karnataka CET 2015, Kerala CEE 2014]**
(a) nutrient cycling (b) recreation
(c) soil formation (d) climate regulation
(e) None of these

34 If 30 J of energy is trapped at producer level, then how much energy will be available to peacock as food in the following chain?
Plant → Mice → Snake → Peacock
[Karnataka CET 2015, CBSE AIPMT 2014]
(a) 0.3 J (b) 0.03 J (c) 0.0003 J (d) 0.003 J

35 Identify the incorrect statement from the following. **[Karnataka CET 2014]**
(a) Pyramid of energy is mostly upright, but sometimes it may be inverted
(b) Pyramid of number and biomass may be either upright or inverted
(c) Pyramid of biomass in sea is generally inverted as the biomass of fish far exceeds that of phytoplanktons
(d) Food chains are generally short few trophic levels as only 10% of the energy is transferred to each trophic level from the lower trophic level

36 Match the following columns.

Column I	Column II
A. Earthworm	1. Detritivore
B. Succession	2. Pioneer species
C. Ecosystem service	3. Natality
D. Population growth	4. Pollination

Codes **[CBSE AIPMT 2014]**

	A	B	C	D
(a)	1	2	3	4
(b)	4	1	3	2
(c)	3	2	4	1
(d)	1	2	4	3

37 Given below is a simplified model of phosphorus cycling in a terrestrial ecosystem with four blanks (*A-D*). Identify the blanks. **[CBSE AIPMT 2014]**

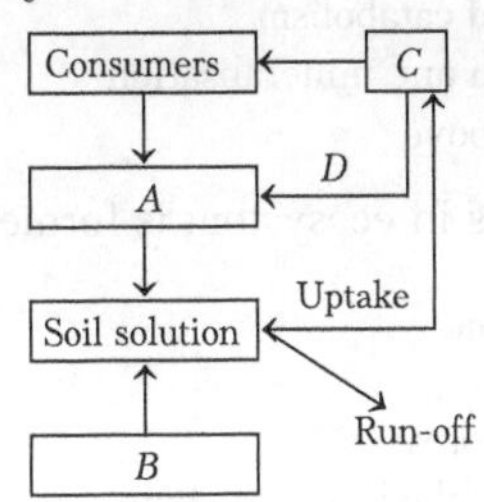

	A	*B*	*C*	*D*
(a)	Rock minerals	Detritus	Litter fall	Producers
(b)	Litter fall	Producers	Rock minerals	Detritus
(c)	Detritus	Rock minerals	Producer	Litter fall
(d)	Producers	Litter fall	Rock minerals	Detritus

38 Which of the following statements about productivity is correct? **[Kerala CEE 2014]**

(a) Primary productivity of all ecosystems is a constant
(b) The annual net primary productivity of the whole of the biosphere is 17 billion tons (dry weight) of organic matter
(c) Net primary productivity is the amount of biomass available for consumption by carnivores
(d) Secondary productivity is defined as the rate of formation of new organic matter by decomposers
(e) Primary productivity depends on the plant species inhabiting a particular area

39 Which of the following statements regarding energy flow are false?

I. The detritus food chain begins with dead organic matter.
II. In aquatic ecosystem, detritus food chain is the major conduit for energy flow.
III. In terrestrial ecosystem, there is a larger fraction of energy flows through grazing food chain.
IV. Producers belong to the first trophic level of the food chain.

Codes **[Kerala CEE 2014]**

(a) II and III (b) I and III
(c) I and IV (d) I and II
(e) I, II and III

40 Lindeman for the first time gave energy transfer law, which states that **[J&K CET 2014]**

(a) only 20% of the energy is transferred to each trophic level
(b) only 10% of the energy is transferred to each trophic level
(c) only 30% of the energy is transferred to each trophic level
(d) only 50% of the energy is transferred to each trophic level

41 Which one of the following process during decomposition is correctly described ? **[NEET 2013]**

(a) Fragmentation – Carried out by organisms such as earthworm
(b) Humification – Leads to the accumulation of a dark coloured sustance humus, which resistant to microbial action at a very fast rate
(c) Catabolism – Last step in the decomposition under fully anaerobic condition
(d) Leaching – Water soluble inorganic nutrients rise to the top layers of soil

42 In a stable ecosystem, which of the following limits the number of trophic levels? **[AIIMS 2013]**

(a) Biomass
(b) The number of nutrients
(c) Availability of nutrients
(d) Presence of contaminants that increase in concentration along the food chain

43 Energy and nutrients enter a community by **[Odisha JEE 2013]**

(a) sun (b) producers
(c) microbes (d) biogeochemical cycle

44 Natural reservoir of phosphorus is **[NEET 2013]**

(a) animal bones (b) rock
(c) fossils (d) sea water

45 Secondary productivity is the rate of formation of new organic matter by **[NEET 2013]**

(a) parasite (b) consumer
(c) decomposer (d) producer

46 Which one of the following organism form the decomposers? **[Manipal 2013; 2008]**

(a) *Pteris* (b) bacteria
(c) saprophytic fungi (d) Both (b) and (c)

47 Trophic level of food chain having greatest amount of energy, is **[BCECE 2012]**

(a) carnivores (b) herbivores
(c) autotrophs (d) omnivores

48 The upright pyramid of number is absent in **[CBSE AIPMT 2012]**

(a) pond (b) forest (c) lake (d) grassland

49 Maximum contribution of O_2 in the environment comes from **[BHU 2012]**

(a) ocean (b) forest (c) grassland (d) None of these

50 The biomass energy available for consumption by herbivores is called **[BHU 2012]**

(a) secondary productivity
(b) net primary productivity
(c) standing crop
(d) gross primary productivity

51 In an ecosystem at a particular time, standing crop includes [Manipal 2012]
(a) total living material
(b) total detritus
(c) Both (a) and (b)
(d) total nutrients present in crop

52 In a pyramid of biomass, if the total dry weight ($kg m^{-2}$) of primary producers is about 809. It will decrease at tertiary consumer level upto [Manipal 2012]
(a) 37 $kg m^{-2}$ (b) 11 $kg m^{-2}$ (c) 5 $kg m^{-2}$ (d) 1.5 $kg m^{-2}$

53 Given below is an imaginary pyramid of numbers. What could be one of the possibilities about certain organisms at some of the different levels?

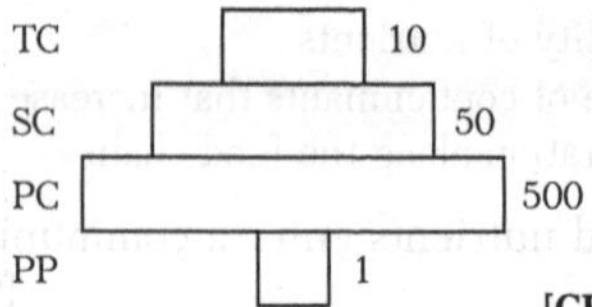

[CBSE AIPMT 2012]
(a) Level PC is insects and level SC is small insectivorous birds
(b) Level PP is phytoplanktons in sea and whale on top level TC
(c) Level one PP is pipal trees and the level SC is sheep
(d) Level PC is rats and level SC is cats

54 Which one of the following is not a functional unit of an ecosystem? [CBSE AIPMT 2012]
(a) Energy flow (b) Decomposition
(c) Productivity (d) Stratification

55 Identify the likely organisms I, II, III and IV in the food web shown below. [CBSE AIPMT 2012]

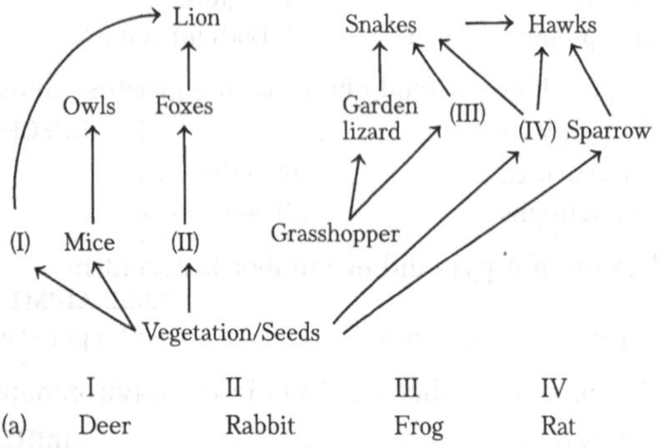

	I	II	III	IV
(a)	Deer	Rabbit	Frog	Rat
(b)	Dog	Squirrel	Bat	Deer
(c)	Rat	Dog	Tortoise	Crow
(d)	Squirrel	Cat	Rat	Pigeon

56 The important steps in the process of decomposition are [AMU 2012]
(a) fragmentation and mineralisation
(b) leaching and catabolism
(c) humification and mineralisation
(d) All of the above

57 Trophic levels in ecosystem is formed by [WB JEE 2012]
(a) Only bacteria
(b) Only plants
(c) Only herbivores
(d) Organisms linked in food chain

58 Which one of the following statements is correct for secondary succession? [CBSE AIPMT 2011]
(a) It occurs on a deforested site
(b) It follows primary succession
(c) It is similar to primary succession except that it has a relatively fast pace
(d) It begins on a bare rock

59 Which one of the following statements for pyramid of energy is incorrect, whereas the remaining three are correct? [CBSE AIPMT 2011]
(a) It shows energy content of different trophic level of organisms
(b) It is inverted in shape
(c) It is upright in shape
(d) Its base is broad

60 Select the matched ones.

I. Sedimentary nutrient	–	Nitrogen cycle
II. Pioneer species	–	Lichens
III. Secondary succession	–	Burned forests
IV. Pyramid of biomass in sea	–	Upright

Codes [Kerala CEE 2011]
(a) I, II and IV
(b) I and III
(c) II and III
(d) II and IV
(e) I, II and III

61 Which of the following statements regarding food chain is false? [Kerala CEE 2011]
(a) In an aquatic ecosystem, grazing food chain is the major conduit for energy flow
(b) In terrestrial ecosystems, a large fraction of energy flows through detritus food chain
(c) The detritus food chain begins with dead organic matter
(d) Primary consumers belong to the first trophic level
(e) Animals like cockroaches and crows are omnivores

ANSWERS

Check Point 24.1

1. (b) *2. (a)* *3. (d)* *4. (a)* *5. (a)* *6. (c)*

Check Point 24.2

1. (d) *2. (b)* *3. (c)* *4. (a)* *5. (b)* *6. (c)*

Check Point 24.3

1. (a) *2. (c)* *3. (d)* *4. (b)* *5. (d)*

(A) Topical Exercise

1. (b)	2. (d)	3. (b)	4. (c)	5. (d)	6. (b)	7. (c)	8. (a)	9. (d)	10. (d)
11. (a)	12. (b)	13. (b)	14. (b)	15. (b)	16. (a)	17. (c)	18. (d)	19. (a)	20. (a)
21. (c)	22. (c)	23. (b)	24. (d)	25. (b)	26. (c)	27. (c)	28. (d)	29. (b)	30. (b)
31. (c)	32. (d)	33. (d)	34. (b)	35. (b)	36. (a)	37. (c)	38. (b)	39. (a)	40. (a)
41. (d)	42. (a)	43. (b)	44. (c)	45. (a)	46. (c)	47. (a)	48. (c)	49. (a)	50. (d)
51. (c)	52. (c)	53. (b)	54. (d)	55. (d)	56. (b)	57. (b)	58. (c)	59. (a)	60. (c)
61. (c)	62. (c)	63. (c)	64. (b)	65. (a)	66. (a)	67. (a)	68. (a)	69. (d)	70. (c)
71. (a)	72. (d)	73. (a)	74. (c)						

(B) Cumulative Exercise

1. (d)	2. (a)	3. (a)	4. (c)	5. (a)	6. (c)	7. (d)	8. (a)	9. (b)	10. (b)
11. (c)	12. (d)	13. (d)	14. (b)	15. (c)	16. (b)	17. (c)	18. (c)	19. (b)	20. (a)
21. (a)	22. (c)	23. (a)	24. (d)	25. (d)	26. (b)	27. (b)			

(C) Medical Entrances' Gallery

1. (b)	2. (c)	3. (d)	4. (d)	5. (a)	6. (c)	7. (c)	8. (a)	9. (a)	10. (b)
11. (b)	12. (a)	13. (a)	14. (d)	15. (b)	16. (a)	17. (a)	18. (b)	19. (c)	20. (a)
21. (d)	22. (b)	23. (d)	24. (b)	25. (a)	26. (b)	27. (c)	28. (b)	29. (c)	30. (c)
31. (d)	32. (c)	33. (a)	34. (b)	35. (a)	36. (d)	37. (c)	38. (e)	39. (a)	40. (b)
41. (a)	42. (c)	43. (b)	44. (b)	45. (b)	46. (d)	47. (c)	48. (b)	49. (b)	50. (b)
51. (d)	52. (d)	53. (a)	54. (d)	55. (a)	56. (d)	57. (d)	58. (a)	59. (b)	60. (c)
61. (d)									

Explanations

(A) Topical Exercise

7 (*c*) Heterotrophs are defined as organisms that feed on other organisms for food (nutrition) and energy. Fungi and some bacteria are heterotrophic.

Chemoautotrophs are defined as organisms that will obtain or synthesise food (nutrition) by utilising chemical energy obtained from organic compounds oxidation. Bacteria are chemoautotrophic.

8 (*a*) Sustenance of life in the absence of oxygen is known as anaerobiosis.

Decomposition is a highly oxygen requiring process. Decomposition rate is maintained and regulated with the help of climatic factors like temperature and soil moisture and by chemical composition of detritus.

Therefore, warm and moist surrounding environment will elevate decomposition whereas low temperature and anaerobiosis (because of excessive moisture) will halt decomposition.

13 (*b*) The species that will occupy new habitats generated due to disturbance are called pioneer species. Other options are explained as

Plant species that can grow and germinate in limited amount of resources are known as climax species.

Closely related species that diverged into two or more groups due to evolution are called divergent speices.

25 (*b*) Statement I is false, but II is true. Incorrect statement can be corrected as

Detritus food chain is usually shorter than grazing food chain as it starts with dead organic materials. The dead organic substances are decomposed by microorganisms.

40 (*a*) Option (a) is incorrectly matched and can be corrected as *Rhizobium* is Gram negative soil bacterium. It is found in symbiotic association with the root nodules of the leguminous plants.

Rest options are correctly matched.

70 (*c*) Statements I and III are correct, but I is incorrect and can be corrected as

The pyramid of biomass for terrestrial ecosystem (grassland, forests), the biomass usually decreases at each trophic level from plant to top carnivores. Therefore, the pyramid of biomass is upright in terrestrial ecosystem.

71 (*a*) Statement in option (a) is incorrect and can be corrected as

The pyramid of energy is always upright in any ecosystem.

Rest statements are correct.

73 (*a*) Statement in option (a) is not correct and it can be corrected as

In most ecosystems, the pyramid of numbers and biomass are upright. Producers are more in number and biomass than the herbivores and herbivores are more in number and biomass than the carnivores.

Rest statements are correct.

74 (*c*) Statement in option (c) is correct. *Populus* and *Alder* are woodland stage species. Rest other statements are incorrect and can be corrected as

- In hydrosere, decomposers are found. They produce organic matter of planktons and other organisms by decomposition.
- *Hydrilla* and *Utricularia* are submerged stage plant.
- *Nelumbo* and *Nymphaea* are floating stage plant.

(B) Cumulative Exercise

3 (*a*) Statements II and IV are incorrect and can be corrected as

- The reservoir of phosphorus are rocks and other deposits. Most of the phosphate deposited in deep sea, ocean as sediments.
- Plants absorbe inorganic phosphates.

16 (*b*) Both A and R are true, but R is not the correct explanation of A.

AG Tansley coined the term ecosystem. It is an integrated system resulting from the interaction of living and non-living factors of the environment. In other words, the ecosystem is inter-relationship between biotic (living) and abiotic (non-living) components of the environment.

17 (*c*) A is true, but R is false because

Biotic components include the living elements of the ecosystem. It includes both autotrophic and heterotrophic animals. Autotrophs include the green plants, photosynthetic bacteria and cyanobacteria. These are capable of manufacturing their organic food from simple inorganic substances. Man is a consumer, because he cannot synthesise his own food. He obtains it from plants and animals.

18 (*c*) A is true, but R is false. R can be corrected as

Heterotrophic animals are unable to manufacture food for their own because, they do not have chlorophyll. These include those organisms, which consume either readymade organic food or decompose the complex organic compounds. These are also called consumers.

19 (*b*) Both A and R are true, but R is not the correct explanation of A.

Microconsumers are microscopic organisms such as bacteria and fungi. These microorganisms breakdown the complex organic compounds of dead bodies of both plants and animals and absorb some of the decomposed products, while releasing most of the inorganic compounds into the environment. From there, these are used by the plants. These are biotic components of an ecosystem.

20 (*a*) Both A and R are true and R is the correct explanation of A.

If a particular crop is destroyed due to some disease, the herbivores in that area do not perish, because the food web provides alternative pathways. Herbivores can graze on other type of crop or herbs.

21 (*a*) Both A and R are true and R is the correct explanation of A.

The pyramid of number of pond ecosystem is upright, because base of this pyramid is occupied by the maximum number of phytoplanktons (autotrophs) and number of individuals gradually decreases towards primary and secondary consumer, respectively.

22 (*c*) A is true, but R is false because

Pyramid of energy is a graphical representation of amount of energy trapped per unit time and area in different levels of a food chain.

Pyramid of energy is always upright because the flow of energy is unidirectional. All of the energy stored by the autotrophs in the form of food is available to the herbivores as food. Herbivores can store only 10% of this energy in their biomass and remaining 90% is used by them in metabolic activities. In the same way, only 10% of energy of lower trophic level can be captured by the organisms of next higher trophic level. Thus, this pyramid depends upon energy and not the number of individuals in a trophic level.

23 (*a*) Both A and R are true and R is the correct explanation of A.

Breakdown of complex organic matters into simple inorganic raw materials such as carbon dioxide, water and various nutrients by the activity of microorganisms, is known as decomposition. The chemical quality of detritus or climatic factors regulates the rate of decomposition of dead animals and plant parts (detritus).

At high altitude, the temperature becomes very low ($< 10°C$). It greatly reduces the activity of microbes. Nutrients immobilisation means tiding up of nutrients material with the biomass of microbes. This immobilisation prevents the nutrients from being washed out from the ecosystem.

24 (*d*) A is false, but R is true. A can be corrected as

Recycling of biogenetic nutrients through abiotic and biotic components of an ecosystem is called biogeochemical cycle or nutrient cycle.

25 (*d*) A is false, but R is true. A can be corrected as Reserve pool of biogeochemical cycle is the reservoir of biogenetic nutrients.

26 (*b*) Both A and R are true, but R is not the correct explanation of A.

Ozone formation takes place by O_2 in the influence of sunlight. Ozone absorbs harmful ultraviolet rays coming from sun. Thus, the ozone protects us from UV rays, which otherwise cause serious skin problems. Such as skin cancer.

27 (*b*) Both A and R are true, but R is not the correct explanation of A.

Although, atmosphere contains about 78% of N_2, but plants cannot use it directly due to the absence of enzymes, which directly metabolise this crude N_2. The characteristic feature of plant cells is the presence of cell wall.

(C) Medical Entrances' Gallery

1 (*b*) Statement in option (b) is incorrect and can be corrected as The energy content decreases from the first (producer) to fourth (consumer) level. At each level, about 90% of energy is lost and only 10% is passed to next level.

Rest statements are correct.

2 (*c*) Statement in option (c) is incorrect and can be corrected as Phosphorus cycle is a sedimentary cycle, i.e. main reservoirs are soil and rocks. It is mainly found as phosphates in rocks. During this cycle, phosphorus solublising bacteria like *Pseudomonas*, *Acetobacter*, etc., help to release phosphorus from organic remains. A large amount of phosphate is lost in sea by sedimentation. There is no respiratory release of phosphorus into atmosphere because phosphorus is an inorganic nutrient that does not take part in respiration.

Rest statements are correct.

3 (*d*) The rate of decomposition is faster in the ecosystem if detritus is rich in nitrogen and water soluble substances like sugars. Warm and moist environment also favour decomposition. Similarly high temperature and presence of aerobic soil microbes also helps in decomposition. When detritus is rich in lignin and chitin decomposition rate gets slower. Thus, option (d) is correct.

4 (*d*) A–2, B–3, C–4, D–1

The correct match is option (d) as

Grassland ecosystem is a terrestrial ecosystem. Which includes various trophic levels. In grassland ecosystem, grass is the producer (Ist trophic level). Rabbit is the primary consumer (IInd trophic level). Crow is secondary consumer (IIIrd trophic level). Vulture is tertiary consumer (IVth trophic level). The primary consumers eat the producers. Secondary consumers eat the primary consumers and so on.

Grass $\rightarrow$ Rabbit $\rightarrow$ Crow $\rightarrow$ Vulture

5 (*a*) Statement in option (a) is correct.

Gross primary productivity of an ecosystem is the rate of production of organic matter during photosynthesis. Net primary productivity is Gross primary productivity minus energy lost by plant during respiration. Hence, gross primary productivity is always more than NPP.

Rest statements are incorrect.

6 (*c*) Pyramid of biomass in sea is generally inverted. Biomass is the amount of living matter present in an ecosystem. In a sea, the biomass of phytoplanktons is usually lesser than that of zooplanktons, while the biomass of carnivores is greater than small carnivores and zooplanktons. On the other hand, pyramid of energy is always upright. Pyramid of biomass in forest and pyramid of numbers in grasslands is also upright. Thus, option (c) is correct.

7 (*c*) An inverted pyramid of biomass will be obtained from the given data because the biomass is continuously decreasing from secondary consumer (120 g) to primary consumer (60 g) to primary producer (10 g). Therefore, upright pyramid of biomass cannot be obtained. The data is given in the form of biomass, therefore pyramid of number and energy cannot be obtained.

8 (*a*) I and IV are incorrectly matched and can be corrected as Nitrogen cycle is an example of gaseous cycle where the gaseous materials are involved in circulation between biotic and abiotic components of biosphere. The reservoir pool is atmosphere.

On the other hand, in sedimentary cycle, the reservoir pool is lithosphere and the circulating material is non-gaseous, e.g. phosphorus, sulphur, etc. The pyramid of biomass in aquatic environment, e.g. sea is inverted.

Rest others are correctly matched.

9 (*a*) Biomass refers to the amount of living organic matter. Forest ecosystem have the maximum biomass, because it includes organisms of all trophic levels as compared to pond, lake or grassland ecosystem. In forest ecosystems, productivity is also high that contributes to maximum biomass.

10 (*b*) Both A and R are true, but R is not the correct explanation of A.

Net primary productivity is equal to gross primary productivity, minus loss due to respiration and other reasons. So, gross primary productivity is always more than net primary productivity. Secondary productivity is defined as the rate of formation of new organic matter by consumers.

11 (*b*) Tropical rainforests show stratification. It can be defined as the grouping of plants into 5-7 well-defined layers depending upon their height. These layers are called strata or storeys. These storeys consist of very tall emergent trees, tall trees, small trees, a shrub layer and mosses, herbs and grass.

15 (*b*) The primary producers of the deep sea hydrothermal vent ecosystem are Archaebacteria. These have chemosynthetic mode of nutrition. Thus, option (b), i.e. chemosynthetic bacteria is correct.

17 (*a*) Since 1.9 g organic matter is produced by 1 g CO_2.

That is why, 1 gm organic matter $= \frac{1}{1.9}$

3 g organic matter $= \frac{1}{1.9} \times 3 = 1.63\text{ g}$

18 (*b*) Secondary succession takes place on degraded forest. It is the process of regrowth of an ecosystem which undergoes a destructive event such as fire, avalanche, agricultural clearing, deforestation or disease. The rate of succession and establishment of communities is faster as compared to growth in primary succession.

19 (*c*) The breakdown of detritus into small particles by detritivores is fragmentation. In biology, detritus is dead particulate of organic material. It typically includes the bodies or fragments of dead organisms as well as faecal material.

20 (*a*) Xerarch succession takes place in dry areas where lichens are the pioneer species. They secrete acids that dissolve rocks by weathering and help in soil formation.

Hydrarch succession takes place in wet areas and pioneer species in the area is phytoplanktons, which are replaced by free-floating angiosperms in next stage.

21 (*d*) Hydroseric succession starts in the water bodies, which are newly formed. The sequence would be

Phytoplankton → Rooted submerged plants → Reed swamp → Sedge meadow.

Thus, option (d) is correct.

22 (*b*) Stratification is the vertical distribution of different species occupying different levels in a biotic community. It is the formation of vertical layers where vegetation is dense, e.g. 5-7 strata (layer) in tropical rainforests with emergent tall trees, canopy trees, shrub layer below tree layer, bottom layer of herbs and grass at ground level. Whereas zonation is the horizontal categorisation of biomass into zones based on their distribution or arrangement in habitat as determined by environmental factors, e.g. altitude, latitude, temperature, biotic factors, etc.

23 (*d*) The total dried biomass of living organisms present at a trophic level at a particular time is known as standing crop. Standing state is the amount of inorganic nutrients present at any time in the soil or water of ecosystem. The gross primary productivity is the total organic matter synthesised by producers during photosynthesis per unit time and area. Net primary productivity is total amount of GPP minus energy lost by plant during respiration.

29 (*c*) The overlapping zone or transition zone between two different ecosystems is called ecotone.

Other options are explained as

Ecozones are a method of dividing up the earth's surface. Each ecozone is a large area that contains a number of habitats, linked by the evolutionary history of the organisms within them. Biotope is an area` of uniform environmental conditions providing a living place for a specific assemblage of plant and animals.

A buffer zone is generally an area that lies between two or more other areas (often but not necessarily countries). It is often created to enhance the protection of areas under management for their biodiversity importance.

30 (*c*) The animal species controlling the ecosystem functioning is known as keystone species. These are the species that has a disproportionately large effect on its environment relative to its abundance. Such species will play critical role in maintaining the structure of an ecological community, affecting many other organisms in ecosystem and helping to determine the types and number of various other species in the community.

31 (*d*) Tropical rainforest biome is in equatorial or sub-equatorial regions with abundant rainfall and warmth.

The vegetation is stratified, i.e. each stratum has different flora contributing to the diversity because of this, most animals in this biome are tree dwellers.

32 (*c*) The main reservoir pool for sedimentary cycle is earth's crust (lithosphere). Atmosphere does not play any significant role. The materials involved in circulation between biotic and abiotic components of biosphere are non-gaseous, e.g. phosphorus, calcium, etc.

34 (*b*) According to 10% law energy flow by Raymond Lindeman (1942), the total amount of energy that can be transferred to the next trophic level is only 10%. Hence, peacock will receive 0.03 J of energy as top consumer. Energy received by the organisms at different trophic level can be seen as follows

Plant $\rightarrow$ 30 J

Mice $\rightarrow 30 \times 10\% = 3\text{J}$

Snake $\rightarrow 3 \times 10\% = 0.3\text{J}$

Peacock $\rightarrow 0.3 \times 10\% = 0.03\text{J}$

36 (*d*) A–1, B–2, C–4, D–3

Option (d) shows the correct match.

Detritivores are organisms that break the detritus into small particles, e.g. earthworm. The species that invade a bare area in succession is called pioneer species.

Ecosystem services are the products of ecosystem process, e.g. pollination.

Natality is the term used for population growth or birth rate in population ecology.

43 (*b*) Energy and minerals enter a community through producers. It manufactures organic food from simple inorganic substances by fixing energy which is then passed to the heterotrophic components (consumers).

44 (*b*) The natural reservoir of phosphorus is rock, which contains phosphorus in the form of phosphates. Sea water, animal bones and fossils are reservoir of carbon.

47 (*c*) In an ecosystem, all energy is provided by the sun. Autotrophs (plants) use 1-3% of sun light and store it in the form of food to the herbivores. So, the greatest amount of energy is present in autotrophs.

48 (*b*) Pyramid of number represents the number of individuals per unit area at various trophic levels. It is always upright in grassland, pond and lake ecosystems. But in forest or single tree ecosystem, it is spindle-shaped and if parasitic food chain is considered, then it will be an inverted pyramid.

So, the upright pyramid of number is absent in forest ecosystem.

49 (*b*) The forests play important role in recycling of oxygen as plants/trees evolve oxygen as byproduct of photosynthesis.

50 (*b*) The rate of storage of organic matter in plant tissues in excess of respiratory utilisation is available to herbivores as food. It is called net primary productivity.

52 (*d*) Nearly 90% of energy (dry weight) is lost when it moves from one trophic level to the next trophic level.

Producer $\rightarrow 1^\circ$ consumer $\rightarrow 2^\circ$ consumer $\rightarrow 3^\circ$ consumer

$809 \rightarrow 80.9 \rightarrow 8.09 \rightarrow 0.809$

So, about 1.5 k gm^{-2} remains at tertiary consumer in food chain.

53 (*a*) The given figure shows spindle-shaped pyramid of number in single tree ecosystem. Here, a single large-sized tree provides food to a large number of herbivores which support a few carnivores and the later are eaten by small number of top carnivores. So, here PP is used for producer, i.e. single tree, PC is Primary Consumers, i.e. large number of insects, SC is Secondary Consumers, i.e. small insectivorous birds and TC is Top Consumers, which may be eagles or falcon, etc.

54 (*d*) Vertical distribution of different species occupying different levels is called stratification. It represents the structural (not a functional) unit of an ecosystem. For example, trees occupy top vertical strata or layer of a forest, shrubs, the second and herbs and grasses occupy the bottom layers.

55 (*a*) Producers utilise the radiant energy of sun which is transformed to chemical form during photosynthesis. Thus, green plants occupy the first trophic level. The herbivores constitute the secondary trophic level and the carnivores the third trophic level. Deer is herbivores, rabbit and rat are also herbivores, but frog eats the grasshoppers.

56 (*d*) A number of processes are involved in decomposition. They are grouped into three catagories, i.e. fragmentation of detritus, catabolism and leaching. Decomposition leads to the formation of two products humus and inorganic nutrients (minerals). Processes involved in their formation are called humification and mineralisation, respectively.

58 (*a*) Statement in option (a) is correct.

Secondary succession or subsere is ecological succession that takes place in a recently denuded area which still contains a lot of organic debris, remains and propagules of previous living organisms. It is more common and caused by baring of an area due to forest fires, deforestation, excessive over grazing, landslides, earthquakes, repeated floods, etc. Only 50-100 yrs are required for establishment of a grassland over a recently denuded area. Formation of forest requires 100-200 yrs.

59 (*b*) Statement in option (b) is incorrect for pyramid of energy and can be corrected as

Pyramid of energy is graphic representation of energy per unit area sequencewise in various rising trophic levels with producers at the base and top carnivores at the apex. Pyramid of energy is upright in all cases.

60 (*c*) The successive development of different biotic communities at the same site till a climax community develops there, is called ecological succession (Hult; 1885). The species that invade a bare area are called pioneer species. In primary succession on rocks (xerarch succession), these are usually lichens which are able to secrete acids (lichenic acid) to dissolve rock, helping in weathering and soil formation. These later pave way to some very small plants like bryophytes (e.g. mosses), which are able to take hold in the small amount of soil.

61 (*d*) Statement in option (d) is false and can be corrected as

All animals depend on plants directly or indirectly for their food needs. They are hence, called consumers and also heterotrophs. If they feed on the producer, the plants (belonging to the first trophic level), they are called primary consumers. Obviously the primary consumers will be herbivores. Some common herbivores are insects, birds and mammals in terrestrial ecosystem and molluscs in aquatic system. Thus, primary consumers belong to the second trophic level.

Rest statements are true regarding food chain.

CHAPTER 25

Biodiversity and Its Conservation

The most striking feature of the earth is its varied lifeforms that constitute its diversity. The biological diversity has long been a source of wonderment and scientific curiosity, but now it is increasingly a source of concern. Human domination of earth's ecosystem is markedly reducing the diversity of various species in different habitats. Thus, many species are accelerating towards extinction. Loss of biodiversity reduces gene pool of species, number of interaction in the biota and ability of species to adapt themselves to change in the environment.

BIODIVERSITY

It is the degree of variation of life. It can either be genetic variation, species variation or ecosystem variation in an area of biome. It includes difference in genes among individual of same species, their variety and richness. The term biodiversity was coined by **Rosen** in 1985, but later popularised by **Edward Wilson**. The integration of several sciences such as ecology and genetics to sustain biological diversity at all its levels is called **conservation biology**.

Degree of biodiversity on earth

- According to the IUCN (2004), the total number of plants and animal species described so far is slightly more than 1.5 million. However, we have no clear idea of species that are yet to be discovered and described. Some extremes estimate range from 20-50 million.
- **Mayer** placed the global species diversity at about 7 million. He estimated that more than 1,00,000 plant species and 3,00,000 animal species are yet to be discovered.
- Approximately 15,000 new species are discovered every year.
- According to a latest study (2012), the total number of terrestrial species is estimated to be around 8.7 million and in ocean, around 2.2 million.
- The study also estimates that more than 70% of all the species recorded are animals and plants (including algae, fungi, bryophytes, gymnosperms and angiosperms).
- Insects are the most species rich taxonomic group amongst animals. It makes up more than 70% of the total animal groups. These are the most successful animals of nature due to its protective exoskeleton.
- The number of fungi species in the world is more than the combined total of the species of fishes, amphibians, reptiles and mammals.

Inside

India as megadiversity region

- India's special geographical position is responsible for its rich and vast biodiversitiy. It is located between three distinctive centres of biological evolution and radiation of species.
- It is one of the 12 megabiodiversity countries of the world. The Deccan Peninsula is the largest biogeographical region. In addition, the Western Ghats and the North-East are the most biodiversity rich regions in India.

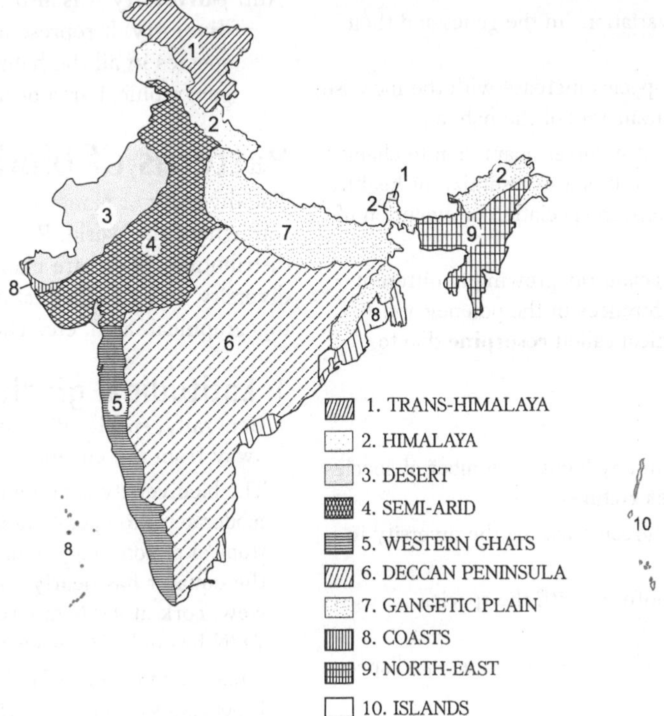

Fig 25.1 Biogeographical regions of India

- Approximately 18% of plants in India are endemic.
- In addition, about 62% amphibians and 50% lizard species are also endemic to India.
- The traditional cultivars include 30,000-50,000 varieties of rice and number of cereals.
- India has 27 indigenous breeds of cattle, 40 breeds of sheep, 22 breeds of goats and 8 breeds of buffaloes.

Table 25.1 Approximate number of species described from India

Numbers of species of plants and bacteria		Numbers of species of animals	
Groups	**Numbers of species**	**Group**	**Numbers of species**
Angiosperms	17,500	Mammalia	390
Gymnosperms	64	Aves	1232
Pteridophytes	1100	Reptilia	456
Bryophytes	2850	Amphibia	209
Lichens	2000	Pisces	2546
Fungi	14,500	Protochordata	119
Algae	6500	Invertebrates	8329
Bacteria	850	Arthropoda	68,389
		Mollusca	5070
		Protozoa	2577

Hierarchical levels of biodiversity

There are three interrelated hierarchical levels as given below

1. Genetic diversity

- It is the diversity in the number and types of genes as well as chromosomes present in different species.
- Further more, it is also the variations in the genes and their alleles in the same species.
- Variations in the genes of a species increase with the increase in size and environmental parameters of the habitat.
- Genetic diversity is useful as it involves adaptation to changes in the environmental condition. It is also essential for healthy breeding. Further more, it helps in speciation or evolution of new species.
- Medicinal plants, *Rauwolfia vomitaria*, growing in different Himalayan region, shows differences in the potency and concentration of active chemical called **reserpine** due to genetic diversity.

2. Species diversity

- It indicates species richness in any habitat. Number of species per unit area is called **species richness**.
- Greater the species richness, greater will be the diversity in the region.
- However, it should not be confused with the species abundance.
- Species diversity is the product of species richness and species evenness.
- Species evenness is the proportionate number of individuals of different species.
- India is among the world's 12 nations that are exceptionally rich in species diversity.
- Also, Western Ghats have a greater amphibian species diversity than the Eastern Ghats.

3. Ecosystem diversity

- It is the variety of ecosystem which indicates diversity in the number of niches, trophic levels, food webs, nutrient cycles and ecological processes sustaining energy flow.
- India with its deserts, rainforests, mangroves, coral reefs, wetlands, estuaries and alpine meadows has a great ecosystem diversity.
- Diversity at the level of community and ecosystem has three perspectives, i.e. α, β and γ-diversity (Whittaker; 1965).
  (i) α**-diversity** (within community diversity) It is also called **local diversity**. It is a diversity within a community.
  (ii) β**-diversity** (between community diversity) It is a diversity between two communities. It appears in a range of communities due to replacement of species with the change in community/habitat. This is due to the presence of different environmental conditions.
  (iii) γ**-diversity** It is also called the **regional diversity**. It represents the total richness of species in all the habitats found within a region, geographical area or landscape.

Patterns of biodiversity

The diversity of plants and animals is not uniform throughout the world. Rather, it shows uneven distribution. There are many different patterns of diversity in latitudinal, altitudinal, geographical and topographical area, etc. These are given below

1. Latitudinal gradient

- Generally, species diversity decreases as we move away from the equator towards the poles.
- The biodiversity is minimum in the Arctic region, moderate in temperate area and the maximum in tropical regions, e.g. Columbia, which is located near the equator has nearly 1400 species of birds, while New York at 41°N has 105 species and Greenland at 71°N has only 56 species.
- India has much of its land area in the tropical latitudes, It possesses as more than 1200 species of birds.
- The tropical Amazonian rainforest in South America has the greatest biodiversity on the earth.
- A tropical forest in equator has upto ten times as many species of vascular plants as in equal area of temperate forest in Midwest of USA.

Why biodiversity is rich in tropics?

Biodiversity is very rich in tropics due to the following reasons

- Tropics have a more stable climate than the temperate zones.
- **Tropical communities** are older than temperate ones and therefore, there has been more time for them to evolve. This could have allowed them for greater degree of specialisation and local adaptations to occur.
- **Warm temperatures** and **high humidity** in most tropical areas provide favourable conditions for many species that are unable to survive in temperate areas.
- **Tropical areas** receive more solar energy over the year. Therefore, the tropical communities are more productive or have greater resource base that can support a wider range of species.

2. Altitudinal gradient

A decrease in species diversity at high mountains is due to drop in temperature and greater seasonal variation.

Species-area relationship

- Alexander von Humboldt observed that within a region, species richness increases with increasing explored area, but upto a certain limit.
- In fact, the relation between species richness and area, for a wide variety of taxa (angiosperms, birds, bats, freshwater fishes) turn out to be a rectangular hyperbola as shown in the following graph

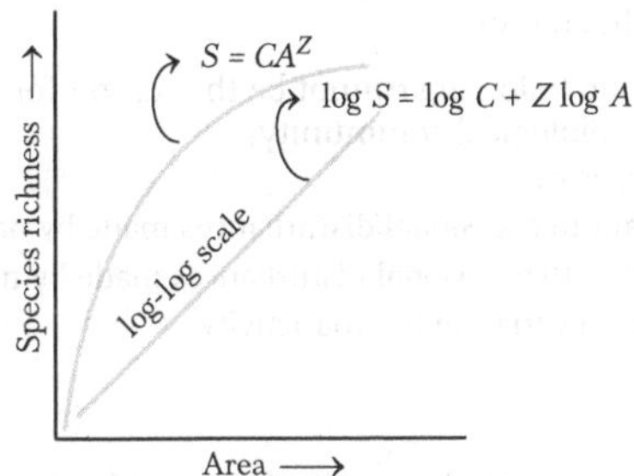

Fig. 25.2 Graph showing species area relationship.

- On a logarithmic scale, the relationship is a straight line or linear and is described by the following equation

$$\log S = \log C + Z \log A$$

where, S = Species richness

A = Area

Z = Slope of the line (regression coefficient)

C = Y-intercept

- Slope of regression (Z) of species-area relationship indicates that species richness decreases with the decrease in area. The value of Z lies in the range of 0.1-0.2 irrespective of the taxonomic group or the region, e.g. plant in Britain, birds in California. But, if we analyse the species-area relationships among very large areas like entire continents, we will find the slope of the line to be much steep (Z values in the range of 0.6-1.2).
- Diversity decreases form lower to higher altitudes on a mountain, i.e. it is maximum at the base.
- Condition favouring growth does not induce biodiversity or speciation. It is called as the **paradox of enrichment**.

Importance of biodiversity

It is very difficult to make people understand that every organism, big or small is important for the ecosystem. Rich diversity is essential not only for ecosystem, but also for the survival of human race.

The importances of biodiversity are given below

1. Stability

- Communities with more species tend to be more stable than those with less species.
- Here, stability means that the biological communities should be able to resist occasional disturbance.
- Also, it must be resistant to invasions by alien species. It should not show too much variations in productivity from year to year.
- David Tilman's long term ecosystem experiments using outdoor plots confirmed that these attributes are linked to the species richness in a community.
- He found that plots with more species show less year to year variation in total biomass. Also, increased diversity contributes to higher productivity.

2. Productivity

Ecosystem with higher biodiversity (e.g. tropical forests) are more productive than ecosystem with lower biodiversity (e.g. temperate forest).

3. Ecosystem health

- Biodiversity is essential for the maintenance and health of the ecosystem through the occurrence of various checks, controls, negative and positive feedbacks, critical link and keystone species.
- **Paul Ehlrich** had proposed a rivet popper hypothesis for the effect of decrease in biodiversity on the ecosystem. As per this hypothesis, an aeroplane (like an ecosystem) has thousand of rivets (species).
- Removal of rivets by passengers may not affect flight safety in the beginning, but the plane will become dangerously weak over a period of time.
- Similarly, removal of species from an ecosystem can adversely affect the balance of the ecosystem.

CHECK POINT 25.1

1. Biodiversity of a geographical region represents
   (a) endangered species found in the region
   (b) the diversity in the organisms living in the region
   (c) genetic diversity present in the dominant species of the region
   (d) species endemic to the region
2. Complete the analogy.
   Intraspecific diversity : Genetic diversity : : Interspecific diversity : ....
   (a) Ecosystem diversity
   (b) Species diversity
   (c) Ecological diversity
   (d) Allelic diversity
3. The state of Gujarat has river, desert, forest and lake ecosystem thus, exhibiting a variety of habitat, then which measure donates total diversity in such case?
   (a) Alpha (b) Beta
   (c) Gamma (d) Delta
4. Different arrangements of places are given in increasing order, on the basis of biodivesity of species birds. Choose the correct sequence.
   (a) Columbia → New York → Greenland → India
   (b) Greenland → New York → India → Columbia
   (c) New York → India → Columbia → Greenland
   (d) India → Columbia → Greenland → New York
5. If 'Z' value is found to be 1.15, which of the following species richness is studied?
   (a) Plants in Britain
   (b) Birds in California
   (c) Frugivores birds of tropical forest of different continent
   (d) Both (b) and (c)
6. Which of the following cannot be the reason for the stability of biological community?
   (a) More species
   (b) Resistant to occasional disturbances made by nature
   (c) Surrender to occasional disturbances made by nature
   (d) Not much variation in productivity

LOSS OF BIODIVERSITY

The loss of biological diversity is a global crisis. The tropical forests are disappearing at an alarming rate. This is one of the most urgent global environmental issues.

Tropical forests are estimated to contain 50-90% of the world's total biodiversity.

In general, loss of biodiversity in a region may lead to

- Decline in plant production.
- Lowered resistance to environmental perturbations such as drought, flood, etc.
- Increased variability in certain ecosystem processes, such as plant productivity, water use and pest and disease cycles.

Causes of biodiversity loss

The loss of biodiversity mainly occurs due to extinction of species. The accelerated rates of species extinctions that the world is facing now are largely due to human activities. The four major causes of biodiversity losses are habitat loss and fragmentation, overexploitation, alien-species invasion and coextinction. These are termed as **'Evil Quartet'**.

These can be explained as follows

Habitat loss and fragmentation

- This is the most important cause of driving animals and plants to extinction.
- The most dramatic example of habitat loss comes from the tropical rainforests.
- Once covering more than 14% of the earth's land surface, these rainforests now cover only upto 6% of the land area.
- By the time, you finish reading this chapter, 1000 more hectares of rainforest would have been lost.
- The Amazon rainforest is so huge that it is called as the **'Lungs of the Planet'**. It harbours millions of species. It is being cut and cleared for cultivating soyabeans or for the conversion to grasslands for raising beef cattle.
- The loss of these forests ultimately leads to the loss or extinction of the species.

Overexploitation

- Humans always depend on nature for food and shelter, but when 'need' turns to 'greed', it leads to overexploitation of the natural resources.
- Many species have become extinct in the last 500 years, e.g. dodo, passenger pigeon, subspecies of tiger (Bali, Javan and Caspian), Tasmanian wolf, Steller's sea cow were extinct due to overexploitation by humans.
- Presently, many marine fish population around the world are overharvested, which is endangering the continued existence of some commercially important species.

Alien-species invasion

When alien-species (non-native) are introduced unintentionally or deliberately for a specific purpose, some of them turn invasive and cause decline or extinction of indigenous species.

Some examples of alien species invasion are given below

- The Nile perch introduced into Lake Victoria in East Africa eventually caused the extinction of an ecologically unique assemblage of more than 200 species of cichlid fish in the lake.
- Water hyacinth was introduced in Indian water to reduce pollution. However, now it is resulting in death of several aquatic plants and animals.
- *Lantana* is a struggling shrub of tropical America which got introduced in the India accidentally. Now, it has replaced many species in the forests of UP and MP.
- *Eupatorium odoratum* has reduced the population of *Tectona grandis.*
- *Parthenium* has pushed out several herbs and shrubs from open places in the plains.
- African catfish, *Clarias gariepinus* became threat to native catfishes.

Extinction

- The major threat to biodiversity is extinction of species.
- Extinction is the total elimination or dying out of species from the earth.
- The colonisation of tropical Pacific Islands by humans caused the extinction of more than 2000 species of native birds.
- Careful analysis of records shows that the extinctions across taxa are not random; some groups like amphibians appear to be more vulnerable to extinction.
- More than 15,500 species worldwide are facing the threat of extinction. Presently, 12% of all bird species, 23% of all mammal species, 32% of all amphibian species and 31% of all gymnosperm species in the world face the threat of extinction.
- A species becomes prone to extinction due to drastic environmental changes and population characteristics.

Susceptibility to extinction

Some population traits, which make a species susceptible to extinction are given below

- Large body size, e.g. elephant, rhinoceros and lion.
- Small population size.
- Low reproductive potential, e.g. blue whale, giant panda.
- Higher states of trophic level, e.g. Bengal tiger, bald, eagle.
- Fixed migratory route and habitat, e.g. blue whale, whooping crane.
- Narrow range distribution or small geographical range, e.g. Woodland Caribou.
- Island species.
- Lack of genetic variability.
- Inability to switch over to alternate foods.

Types of extinction

There are generally three types of extinction

(i) **Natural extinction** It is a slow process of replacement of existing species with the better adapted species.

- This may be due to alternate evolution, changes in environmental condition, predators and diseases.
- Extinction vertex is a combination of genetic and demographic factors.

(ii) **Mass extinction** It occurs due to catastrophes, which had struck on the earth several times.

- A mass extinction occurred about 225 million years ago in Permian period when 90% of shallow marine invertebrates disappeared.
- Another mass extinction occurred between Cretaceous and Tertiary period over 60 million years ago when dinosaurs and a number of other organisms disappeared. It is also called **K-T** (Cretaceous-Tertiary) **boundary**.
- K-T boundary extinctions are connected with deposits of iridium, which is otherwise rare on the earth.

(iii) **Anthropogenic extinction** It is extinction of organisms by human activities like hunting, overexploitation and habitat destruction, e.g. dodo (*Raphus cucullatus*), Tasmanian wolf, etc. Anthropogenic extinction is causing a sixth extinction of species. It is 100-1000 times more faster than the rate of natural extinctions.

Coextinction

- In natural habitat, sometimes extinction of one species also results in extinction of the plant and animal species associated with it. It is an obligatory way of extinction.
- When a host fish species becomes extinct, its unique assemblage of parasites also meets the same fate.
- Another example is the case of a coevolved plant-pollinator mutualism where extinction of one invariably leads to the extinction of the other.

IUCN and red list categories

IUCN is International Union of Conservation of Nature and Natural Resources which is now called **World Conservation Union** (WCU). Its headquarters is at Morges, Switzerland. It maintains a Red Data Book or Red List which is a catalogue of taxa facing risk of extinction. Red Data Book was initiated in 1963. The purpose of preparation of red list is to

- Provide awareness to the degree of threat to biodiversity.
- Provide global index about already declined of biodiversity.
- Provide identification and documentation of species at high risk of extinction.
- Preparing conservation priorities and help in conservation plan.
- Provide information about international agreements like conservation on biological diversity and CITES (Convention on International Trade in Endangered Species of Wild Fauna and Flora).
- Red list has categories of species, which are as follows
  - (i) **Extinct** A taxon is extinct when there is no reasonable doubt that its last individual has died, e.g. dodo.
  - (ii) **Extinct in the Wild** (EW) A number of domesticated animals and plants have become extinct in the wild. A taxon is extinct in the wild when it is known only to survive in cultivation.
  - (iii) **Critically endangered** (CR) A taxon is critically endangered when it is facing an extremely high risk of extinction in the wild in immediate future. In IUCN list, 925 animals and 1014 plants are caritically endangered.
  - (iv) **Endangered** (EN) A taxon is endangered when it is not critically endangered, but facing a very high risk of extinction in the wild in near future.
  - (v) **Vulnerable** (VU) A taxon is vulnerable when it is not critically endangered or endangered, but it is facing a high risk of extinction in the wild in the medium term future.
  - (vi) **Threatened species** is the one which is liable to become extinct if not allowed to realise its full biotic potential by providing protection from the exotic species.
  - (vii) **Low Risk** (LR) A taxon is at low risk when evaluated, it does not qualify for any of the categories like critically endangered, endangered or vulnerable.
  - (viii) **Data Deficient** (DD) A taxon is data deficient when there is inadequate information to make a direct or indirect assessment of its risk of extinction based on its distribution or population status.
  - (ix) **Not Evaluated** (NE) A taxon is under the category of not evaluated, when it has not yet been assessed against above criteria.
- On 29th January in 2010, the IUCN Red List of threatened species identified 842 (746 Animalia, 96 Plantae) extinct species, subspecies and varieties, stocks and sub-populations.
- The Red List of 2012 was released on 19th July 2012, at Rio Earth Summit. Nearly 2000 species were added to the list with four species to the extinct list and two to the rediscovered list.
- The IUCN assessed a total of 63837 species which revealed 19,817 are threatened with extinction, 3947 described as critically endangered and 5766 as endangered, while more than 10,000 species are listed as vulnerable.
- About 41% of amphibian species, 33% of reef-building corals, 30% of conifers, 25% of mammals and 13% of birds are threatened.
- The IUCN Red List has listed 132 species of plants and animals from India as 'critically endangered'.

Table 25.2 Examples of threatened species

Categories	Plants	Animals
Critically endangered	*Berberis nilghiriensis*	*Sus salvanius* (Pigmy hog)
Endangered	*Bentinckia nicobarica* (Indian aconite), Blue vanda (orchid), *Podophyllum* (medicinal plant), *Nepenthes* (pitcher plant), *Rauwolfia serpentina, Santalum album* (sandal wood), *Cycas beddomei*	Asiatic lion, Giant panda, one horn rhinoceros, Kashmiri stag (Hangul), red panda (*Ailurus*), Indian elephant, Blue whale, Lion tailed macaque, Musk deer, Tiger, Indian wild ass, Great Indian bustard, Siberian crane.
Vulnerable	*Cupressus cashmeriana*	*Antilope cervicapra* (blackbuck), *Dyscophus antongilii*

Note

- *Clouded Leopard (Neofelis nebulosa), Hawaiian Monk seal (Monochus schavinslandii and great Indian bustard (Ardeotis nigriceps) are rare species.*
- *The 3-banded armadillo of Brazil, short eared rabbit of Sumatra and Mexican Prairie dog are indeterminate species.*
- *Snow Leopard (Leo uncia) was listed as indeterminate in 1968 and endangered in 1970.*

CHECK POINT 25.2

1. Which of the alien-species were introduced in India now have become a threat?
   (a) *Ficus religiosa, Lantana camara*
   (b) *Lantana camara ,Eichhornia crassipes*
   (c) Nile perch, *Ficus religiosa*
   (d) *Prosopis cineraria,* Nile perch

2. 'Extinction of wasp population will also lead to extinction of fig species'. This statement indicates towards which of the following cause of biodiversity loss?
   (a) Overexploitation (b) Coextinction
   (c) Alien-species invasion (d) Habitat loss

3. If any extinction of a mutualistic pollinator takes place, what would be its effect on the plants where it pollinates?
   (a) Decreased pollination
   (b) No effect because substitute pollinator is available
   (c) The plant would not be pollinated
   (d) Both (b) and (c)

4. The given characteristics are related to susceptibility of extinction of species except one
   (a) small population size
   (b) fixed habitat and migratory bird
   (c) high reproductive rate
   (d) large body size

5. A designation applied to species that possess a very high risk of extinction as a result of rapid population decline of 50-70% our three generations.
   (a) LC (b) VU
   (c) EN (d) NT

6. Species which occurs in small populations and are restricted to only certain geographical area are placed in which category?
   (a) Endangered species
   (b) Rare species
   (c) Vulnerable species
   (d) Threatened species

CONSERVATION OF BIODIVERSITY

It is protection, uplift and scientific management of biodiversity to maintain it at its optimum level and derive sustainable benefits for the present as well as future generation. In 2002, India passed its conservation act.

Note *A keystone species is a species that has a very large effect on the community through both direct and indirect pathways. Protection of keystone species is a priority for conservation efforts, because if a keystone species is lost from an area, numerous other species might be lost as well.*

Reasons to conserve biodiversity

There are many reasons as to why we should conserve biodiversity.

It can be grouped into the following three categories

(i) **Narrowly utilitarian** (Direct or economic uses)
Humans derive countless direct economic benefits from nature such as food, firewood, fibre, construction materials, industrial products and products of medicinal importances (further details given in chapter 24 ecosystem).

(ii) **Broadly utilitarian** (Ecosystem services)
Biodiversity a plays an important role in many ecosystems of the earth. For example, Amazon forest produces 20% of the total oxygen in the earth's atmosphere through photosynthesis. Bees, bumblebees, birds and bats play a very important role in pollination.

(iii) **Ethical** We must realise that every species has its own value, even if it may not be of current economic value to us. From ethical point of view, we have a moral duty to care about every existing form of life, so that we can pass on our biological legacy in good order to our future generations.

Strategies of conservation

Some main strategies of conservation are as follows

- All the threatened species should be protected. Priority should be given to ones belonging to the monotypic genera, endangered over vulnerable, vulnerable over rare and rare over other species.
- All the possible varieties (old or new) of food, forage and timber, medicinal plants, livestock, aquaculture animals, microbes should be conserved.
- Wild relatives of economically important organisms should be identified and conserved in protected areas.
- Critical habitats for feeding/breeding/resting/nursing of each species should be identified and safeguarded.
- Resting/feeding places of migratory/wide ranging animals should be protected. Their exploitation should be regulated.
- National Wildlife Protection Law should be enacted in India (1972), wildlife protection strategies (1983) and protection programmes should be integrated with the international programmes.
- Unique ecosystems can be preserved on priority basis.
- The reproductive capacity of the exploited species and productivity of the ecosystem should be determined.

- International trade in wildlife should be highly regulated.
- Development of reserves or protected areas should be initiated.
- Introduction of new species should be in strict control of regulatory laws.
- Pollution reduction and public awareness should be promoted.

Biodiversity can be conserved *via* two main strategies. These are as follows

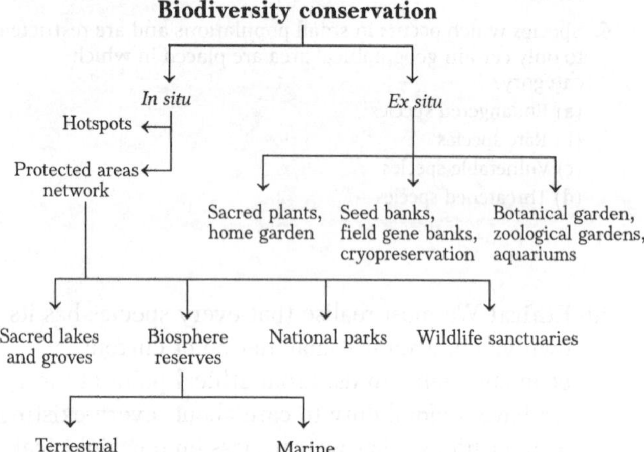

In situ conservation

- It is the conservation of living resources within their natural ecosystems.
- The *in situ* approach is preferable for both flora and fauna.
- Much of the diversity can be conserved in the natural habitat.
- Biodiversity at all its levels can be conserved *in situ* by comprehensive system of protected areas such as the national parks, sanctuaries, natural reserves, natural monuments, cultural landscapes, biosphere reserves and wetlands, etc.
- These areas vary considerably in size, design, purpose and effectiveness of management. They serve as a repositories for much of the world's biological diversity.
- *In situ* conservation is of two types

1. Hotspots

- The concept of hotspot was given by **Norman Myers** in 1988.
- Hotspots are areas that are extremely rich in species diversity, have high endemism and are under constant threat.
- Out of the 34 hotspots (cover less than 2% of earth land area) of the world, three are found in India and they extend into neighbouring countries too. The Western Ghats/Sri Lanka, Himalayas and Indo-Burma region are also known as **cradle of speciation.**
- These areas are particularly rich in floral wealth and endemism. These are also home to many reptiles, amphibians, swallow-tailed butterflies and some mammals.
- The key criteria for determining a hotspot are
  (i) Number of endemic species, i.e. the species, which are not found anywhere else.
  (ii) Degree of threat, which is measured in terms of habitat loss.
- Tropical forests appear in 15 hotspots, Mediterranean type zones in 5 whereas 9 hotspots are mainly made up of islands and 16 hotspots are in the tropics. About 20% of the human population lives in the hotspot regions.

Hotspots in India

The three hotspots in India are as follows

(i) **Indo-Burma** It extends from Bhutan to Myanmar, covering most of the North-Eastern India.

(ii) **Himalaya** It is one of the richest hotspot of biodiversity.

(iii) **Western Ghat** It lies parallel to the Western coast of Indian Peninsula. It extends almost 1600 km in Maharashtra, Karnataka, Tamil Nadu and Kerala. The Agasthyamalai hills, the Silent valley and the new Amambalam reserve, are the main centres of biological diversity.

Hotspots in world

Out of 34 hotspots of world, fifteen are as follows

- Caribbean
- Brazil's Atlantic forests
- Choco/Darien/Western Ecuador
- Brazil's Cerrado
- Central Chile
- Madagascar
- West African forests
- Mediterranean Basin
- Caucasus
- Wallacea
- Philippines
- South-Central China
- South-West Australia
- New Caledonia
- New Zealand

Ramsar sites

- Wetlands are called **Ramsar sites** because the 1st international convention on their conservation was held in Ramsar in Iran in 1971.
- In India, recently much attention has been towards *in situ* conservation of wetlands. These are an integral part of the watersheds and generally lie at the interface between the land and water.
- Wetlands are classified according to their location, water chemistry, dominant vegetation and human intervention.
- They occupy about 60% of total land of the world. They are very rich in biodiversity and are highly productive.

2. Protected areas

These are the part of land and sea, especially dedicated to protection and maintenance of biological diversity along with its natural and associated cultural resources. India has the largest network of protected areas in the world. These are managed through legal or other effective means.

These include the following

(i) Sacred groves and lakes

- These are the forest patches around places of worship which are held in high extreme by tribal communities. These are also known as **Island of Pristine forests.**
- These are found in several parts of India, e.g. Khasi and Jaintia Hills in Meghalaya. Aravalli Hills of Rajasthan, Western Ghat regions of Karnataka, Maharashtra and Sarguja and Chanda and Bastar area of Madhya Pradesh.
- In Meghalaya, the sacred groves are the last refuges for a large number of rare and threatened plants.
- Sacred lakes are Pushkar Lake in Rajasthan and Khecheopalri Lake in Sikkim.
- Sacred plants are *Ocimum sanctum, Ficus religiosa* and *Elaeocarpus floribundus* (Rudraksha), etc.

(ii) National parks

- These are areas maintained by government and are reserved for betterment of wildlife, cultivation, grazing, forestry and habitat manipulation.
- Cultivations are not allowed in these area.
- The earliest national parks, the Yellow stone National park in USA and the Royal Park near Sydney, Australia were famous for their scenic beauty and recreational values.
- A few national park of India have been declared as world heritage sites, i.e. Kaziranga, Keoladeo and Manas. India's first National Park (IUCN Category-II Protected area) was Hailey National Park, now known as Jim Corbett National Park, established in 1935.
- Anshi National Park is famous for Bengal tigers, black panther and Indian elephant.
- South Button Island National Park is famous for *Dugong*, dolphin, water monitor lizard and blue whale.
- Balpakram National Park is famous for wild water buffalo, red panda, elephant and eight cat species including tiger and marbled cat.
- Mount Harriet National Park is an important bird area attributed by Bird Life International.
- New species of frog, *Rana charlesdarwini* is also found in this park.
- As on April 2012, there are 102 national parks. Some of the national parks in India are listed below

Table 25.3 Some national parks in India

Names	States	Important animals
Bandhavgarh National Park (Highest tiger population)	Madhya Pradesh	Tiger
Bandipur National Park	Karnataka	Tiger
Bannerghatta National Park	Karnataka	Elephants, Tiger
Buxa Tiger Reserve	West Bengal	Tiger
Corbett National Park	Uttarakhand	Tiger
Dachigam National Park (Famous for Kashmir stags)	Jammu and Kashmir	Kashmir stags
Dudhwa National Park	Uttar Pradesh	Tigers, Swamp deers (Barasingha)
Gir National Park (Famous for Asiatic lion)	Gujarat	Asiatic lion
Gulf of Kutch Marine National Park	Gujarat	Wild ass
Indravati National Park	Chhattisgarh	Tiger
Kanha National Park	Madhya Pradesh	Tiger
Kaziranga National Park (Famous for Indian rhinoceros)	Assam	One-horned rhinoceros, Elephant
Kanchenjunga National Park	Sikkim	Snow leopard
Manas National Park	Assam	Elephant
Nanda Devi National Park	Uttarakhand	Snow leopard and Himalayan musk deer, Bharal or blue sheep
Panna National Park	Madhya Pradesh	Tiger
Rajaji National Park	Uttarakhand	Tiger
Simlipal National Park	Odisha	
Sundarbans National Park	West Bangal	Royal Bengal Tiger

Note ***National Forest Policy*** *was enunciated in 1988. According to it, the forest cover for the hills is about 67%, while the total forest area in India is about 19%.*

(iii) Wildlife sanctuaries of India

- India has over 448 wildlife sanctuaries (IUCN category-IV protected area). Among these, the 28 tiger reserves are concerned under Project Tiger and are of special significance in the conservation of the tigers.
- Some wildlife sanctuaries are specifically named as Bird sanctuary, e.g. Keoladeo National Park before it attained national park status.
- Many national parks were initially wildlife sanctuaries.
- The basic difference between wildlife sanctuaries and national park is that in wildlife sanctuaries, protection is given only to animal life while in national parks, both flora and fauna are protected.

Table 25.4 Some important sanctuaries in India

Name and location	Key vertebrate species being protected
Chilka Lake (Odisha)	Flamingos, sandpipers, ducks, water fowls, cranes, golden plovers and ospreys.
Keoladeo (Ghana) Bird Sanctuary (Rajasthan)	**Migratory birds** Siberian crane, spoonbill, herons, egrets and variety of other local birds.
	Mammals Blue bull, wild bear, blackbuck and spotted deer.
	Reptiles Python.
Mudumalai Wildlife Sanctuary, Nilgiri (Tamil Nadu)	**Mammals** Flying squirrel, porcupine, elephant, sambhar, cheetal, barking deer, mouse, deer, four-horned antelope, giant squirrel, wild dog, cat and civet.
	Reptiles Rat snake, python, flying lizard and monitor lizard.
Manas Wildlife Sanctuary, Kamrup (Assam)	Tiger, wild boar, sambhar, golden langoor, one-horned rhinoceros, panther, swamp deer, wild dog and wild buffalo.
Periyar Sanctuary (Kerala)	**Mammals** Elephants, leopard, black langoor, sambhar, gaur, bison. **Birds** Egret and hornbills.
Sultanpur Lake Bird Sanctuary (Uttar Pradesh)	**Birds** Cranes, duck, green pigeon, drake and spotbill.
	Reptiles Python and crocodile.
Gahirmatha Marine Sanctuary (Odisha)	Olive ridley turtles

(iv) Biosphere reserves

- These are a special category protected areas of land and/or coastal environments, wherein people are an integral component of the system.
- These are the representative examples of natural biomes and contain unique biological communities within.
- Biosphere reserves represent a specified area alloted for particular activity. These consist of
  (a) **Core zone** No human activity is allowed in this zone.
  (b) **Buffer zone** Limited activity is permitted.
  (c) **Transition zone** Several human activities are allowed.

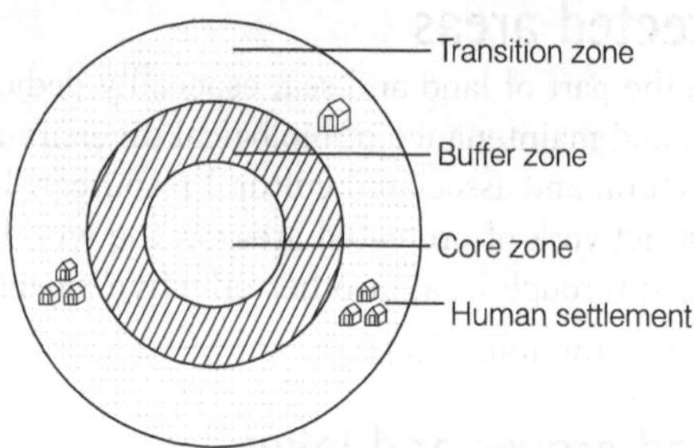

Fig 25.3 Different zones in a biosphere reserve

- Biosphere reserves were initiated in 1975 under **MAB** (Man and Biosphere) programme of UNESCO.
- The Indian government has established 14 biosphere reserves.
- In India, 18 biosphere reserves have been setup so far. Four of them are recognised as world heritage sites, e.g. Nanda Devi, Sunderbans, Nilgiri and Gulf of Mannar.
- The other important biosphere reserves of India include
  - Manas Biosphere Reserve (Assam)
  - Agasthyamalai Biosphere Reserve (Kerala-TN)
  - Dehang-Debang Biosphere Reserve (Arunachal Pradesh)
  - Simlipal Biosphere Reserve (Odisha)
  - Pachmarhi Biosphere Reserve (MP)
  - Great Nicobar Biosphere Reserve (Andaman Nicobar)
  - Nokrek Biosphere Reserve (Meghalaya)
  - Khangchendzonga Biosphere Reserve (Sikkim)
  - Dibru-Saikhowa Biosphere Reserve (Assam)
  - Achaanak maar-Amarkantak Biosphere Reserve (Chhattisgarh)

Wildlife conservation projects in India

- The **Project Tiger** was started in April 1973 to check the depletion of population of tiger (*Panthera tigris*). Initially, it was undertaken in 17 national parks. Recently, the project has been extended to six more national parks (a total of 23).
- **Lion Project** (*Panthera leo persica*) was started in 1972. It was initiated in **Gir National Park**, Junagarh (Gujarat).
- **Snow Leopard Project** (*Panthera uncia*) is in action throughout Himalayas, e.g. Kanchenjunga National Park (Gangtok).
- **Musk Deer Project** (*Moschus moschiferus*) is functioning in Kedarnath sanctuary (Uttarakhand), Manali sanctuary and Shikari Devi Sanctuary (Himachal Pradesh).
- **Hangul Project** was started in 1970 at Dachigam Sanctuary, Kashmir to protect Kashmir stag (*Cervus elephus hanglu*).
- **Rhino Conservation Project** was started in 1987 at Dudhwa National Park (Lakhimpur Kheri, Uttar Pradesh) to introduce Rhino under this project.
- **Crocodile Breeding Project** intially started in Odisha to save crocodile in 1975, it has three species of crocodile in India, (i) salt water (*Crocodylus porosus*), (ii) freshwater muggar (*C. palustris*), (iii) Gharial (*Gavialis gangeticus*).
- **Great Indian Bustard Project** is being run at Desert National Park (Rajasthan) and Great Indian Bustard Sanctuary (Maharashtra).
- **Lion Tailed Macaque Project** began at Silent Valley Park in Kerala.

Table 25.5 Differences between national park, wildlife sanctuary and biosphere reserve

National parks	Sanctuaries	Biosphere reserves
Attention is not given on biotic community as a whole. For example, conservation being connected to habitat for particular wild animal species such as lion, tiger, rhino, etc.	Attention is not given on biotic community, i.e. conservation is species oriented.	Attention is focused on biotic community as a whole, i.e. conservation is ecosystem oriented.
The size ranges from 0·04-3162 sq km. The usual size being between 100-500 sq km and between 500-1000 sq km.	The size ranges from 0·61-7818 sq km, usual size being between 100 and 500 sq km and between 500 and 1000 sq km.	The size is well over 5670 sq km.
Boundaries are circumscribed by state legislation.	Limits are not circumscribed.	Boundaries are circumscribed by the state legislation.
There occurs no biotic interference except in buffer zone.	There occurs limited biotic interference.	There occurs no biotic interference except in buffer zone.
Tourism is permissible, but often discouraged.	Tourism is permissible.	Tourism is not permissible.
Research and scientific management are lacking.	Research and scientific management are lacking.	Research and scientific management are carried out.
Proper attention is not given to gene pool conservation of economic species, particularly of plants.	Proper attention is not given to gene pool conservation of economic species, particularly of plants.	Attention is given to the conservation of plants as well as animal species.

Ex situ conservation

It means conservation of flora and fauna outside the habitats, e.g. zoos, botanical gardens, culture collections, etc. These can also be covered in the form of gene pools, gamete storage and germplasm banks for seeds, pollen, semen, ova and cell, etc.,

1. Zoos

Many zoos have various rare species of wild animals. Many of these animals have evidenced success in captive breeding of animals.

2. Botanical garden

- It plays an important role in the conservation of plant species. There are several instances when plants believed to be extinct, were found living only in a botanical garden.
- *Sophora toromiro* is the famous example. Record of threatened plants in cultivation have been kept in Green Books.
- The Indian Green Book prepared by Botanical Survey of India (BSI), has 100 such species which are rare, endangered or endemic, but all are growing in a living state in various botanical gardens.

3. Seed bank

- It is a fairly good way of conserving diversity. Seeds are stored under 'minimal life'.
- These are kept for many years with a minimum loss of viability. Such type of conservation is practiced in cold storage in seed banks.
- The recalcitrant seeds, i.e. those, which cannot be stored at low moisture content are stored for shorter duration.
- Efforts to develop improved method for storing recalcitrant seeds involves a three fold strategy; **dry storage**, **cryogenic storage** and **storage of fully hydrated seeds**.
- A seed bank has been setup at the **National Bureau of Plant Genetic Resource** (NBPGR, New Delhi) for the conservation of recalcitrant seeds.

- A plant biodiversity garden has also been established at NBPGR on 7th August in 2000.

4. Pollen storage

- It has considerable importance in the conservation of genetic diversity. However, the life of pollen is much shorter than the seed.
- A maximum of three years of life has been reported in some species.

5. Cryopreservation

- Preservation of tissue culture, explants, embryos, animal cells/tissues, gametes, etc., can be indefinitely stored at −196° C in liquid nitrogen.
- This method is useful in maintaining a large number of genotypes in small areas.

Conventions on biodiversity

Biodiversity knows no political boundaries and its conservation is therefore, a collective responsibility of all nations. These are as follows

(i) **Earth Summit** at Rio-de-Janeiro (1992), Brazil, promoted convention on biological diversity which is signed by 152 nations. India became a part to this convention on biological diversity in May (1994).

The various commitments are listed below

- Adoption of ways and means to conserve biodiversity.
- Managing biodiversity for sustainable use.
- Ensuring equitable sharing of benefits from the biological diversity including utilisation of genetic resources.

(ii) **Agenda 21**, a product of Earth Summit, is a blue print for encouraging sustainable development of biodiversity.

(iii) **Green peace** is a non-governmental organisation. It provides international support for conservation.

Some important abbreviations

- NEERI – National Environmental Engineering Research Institute
- UNEP — United Nations Environment Programme
- CAZRI — Central Arid Zone Research Institute
- MAB — Man and Biosphere
- CITES — Convention on International Trade in Endangered Species of Wild Fauna and Flora
- IPCC — Intergovernmental Panel on Climate Change
- UNCBD — United Nations Convention on Biological Diversity
- EPA — Environmental Protection Agency
- IUCN — International Union for Conservation of Nature and Natural Resource

CHECK POINT 25.3

1. Keystone species deserve protection because these
   (a) are capable of serving in harsh environment conditions
   (b) indicate presence of certain minerals in the soil
   (c) play an important role in supporting other species
   (d) have become rare due to overexploitation
2. The integral part of water shed which lie between land and water rich in biodiversity are
   (a) hotspot
   (b) biosphere
   (c) Ramsar sites
   (d) Both (b) and (c)
3. Sacred groves in India are related with
   (a) aesthetic pleasure
   (b) the place where threatened species are projected
   (c) the place where only artificial plant breeding is allowed
   (d) forest patches around the place of worship
4. Which of the following is true for National Parks?
   (a) Tourism is allowed in buffer zone
   (b) No human activity is allowed
   (c) Hunting allowed in core zone
   (d) Cattle grazing is allowed in buffer zone
5. Bioresources are different from national parks as
   (a) humans are integral part of biosphere reserve
   (b) plants and animals are protected in biosphere reserve
   (c) humans are not integral part of biosphere
   (d) Both (a) and (b)
6. Which is correct about white tiger?
   (a) White tiger is reccessive mutant
   (b) It is a part of subspecies of Indian tiger
   (c) It is a type of albino
   (d) It is a transgenic animals

EXAM POINTS

- According to Robert May, the global species diversity is about 7 million. **[NEET 2020]**
- The Amazon rainforest in South America has the greatest biodiversity on the earth. **[NEET 2020]**
- Fungi represent maximum number of species among global biodiversity. **[NEET 2013, 12]**
- India has only 204% of world's land area, its share of the global species diversity is 801%. **[AMU 2012]**
- The National aquatic animal of India is river dolphin. **[NEET 2016]**
- Western ghats have a very higher degree of species richness and endemism. **[CBSE AIPMT 2012]**
- Depletion in genetic diversity of crop plants is mainly due to introduction of better varieties with high yield, disease resistance, etc. **[KCET 2014]**
- The term alpha diversity refers to species diversity **[WB JEE 2013]**
- Beta (β) diversity refers to diversity between communities. **[WB JEE 2015]**
- Most of the tree dwellers are found in tropical rainforest. **[Kerala CEE 2013]**
- Biodiversity increases with higher altitudes to lowers altitudes. **[KCET 2014]**
- According to Alexander von Humboldt, species richness increases with increase area but only up to limit. **[NEET 2020, 17]**
- Endemic species are those species which are not found anywhere else. **[NEET 2019, 15]**
- Species diversity increases as we move away from the equator towards the pole. **[AIIMS 2014]**
- *Clarias gariepinus* were introduced in India which become threat for the native fishes. Similarly, *Lantana* and *Eichhornia* are invasive weeds in India. **[NEET-I 2016, AIIMS 2019]**
- *Parthenium hysterophorus* is an alien-species which is introduced for some economic uses but now it is a threat to indigenous species. **[NEET-I 2016]**
- The important cause of animals and plants being driven to extinction is due to habitat loss and fragmentation. **[NEET 2016]**
- Breeding ground for migratory Flamingo is area between khadir and Pachham island in great Rann of kachchh (kutch). **[Gujarat CET 2014]**
- When browsing goats were introduced into Galapagos island, Abangdon tortoise become extinct. **[EAMCET 2016]**
- Red list contains data or information on threatened species. **[NEET-II 2016]**
- In IUCN Red list, 2004 documents, the extinction of 784 species, it includes 338 vertebrates, 359 invertebrates and 87 plants. **[J&K CET 2014]**
- A species facing extremely high risk of extinction in the immediate future is called critically endangered. **[NEET 2014]**
- IUCN stand for International Union for Conservation of Nature and Natural Resources. **[JIPMER 2017]**
- The organisation which publishes the Red list of species is IUCN. **[NEET 2014]**
- *In situ* conservation includes biosphere reserve, national parks, wildlife sanctuaries and sacred lakes and groves. **[NEET 2020, 18, 19]**
- The concept of hotspot was first introduced by Norman Myers. **[WB JEE 2014]**
- The 34 biodiversity hotspot in the world have been identified till date by Norman Myers. **[NEET-II 2016]**
- The objective of 'Ramsar convention' was wetland conservation. **[WB JEE 2014]**
- Sacred groves are specially useful in conserving rare and threatened species. **[CBSE AIPMT 2012]**
- An area is declared as hotspot when it has 1500 more endemic species and 75% of its original habitat is lost. **[WB JEE 2015]**
- Management of national parks is controlled by central government. **[WB JEE 2014]**
- Dachigam National Park in Jammu and Kashmir is the home to the famous musk deer. **[NEET-II 2016]**
- Kanha National Park is located in Madhya Pradesh and is famous for tiger. **[AMU 2012, Odisa JEE 2011]**
- The single-horned rhinoceros is protected at Kaziranga National Park. **[BHU 2012, Chandigarh CET 2012]**
- Biodiversity hotspots are the biogeographic regions which are both, biologically rich reserviors and deeply threatened by habitat loss and other human activity destruction. **[KCET 2014]**
- Biosphere reserve programme was started in India in 1986. **[Manipal 2013]**
- In bioreserve, which are legally protected and where no human activity is allowed is called core zone. **[NEET 2017]**
- In buffer zone, limited activity is permitted. **[NEET 2017]**
- *Ex situ* conservation includes botanical gardens, wildlife safari parks, seed banks, cryopreservation, gene bank. **[EAMCET 2016, NEET 2020]**
- Gene bank is a type of *ex situ* conservation which involves the maintenance of stock of viable seeds, living growing plants tissue culture. **[AIIMS 2017]**
- Widlife Protection Act, India was implemented in the year 1972. **[WB JEE 2015]**
- The Earth summit held in Rio de Janeiro in 1992 was called for conservation of biodiversity and sustainable utilisation of its benefits. **[NEET 2019]**
- The government of India in 1980s had introduced a concept to work closely with local communities for protecting and managing forests. The concept is joint Forest Management. **[AIIMS 2013]**
- The full form of MAB is Man And Biosphere programme. **[WB JEE 2015]**

Chapter Exercises

(A) Topical Exercise

Biodiversity

1 The term biodiversity was given by
(a) WG Rosen (b) John Roy
(c) William Hornaday (d) Myers

2 Biological Diversity Day is celebrated on
(a) 3rd June (b) 22nd May
(c) 13th April (d) 4th December

3 The integration of several sciences such as ecology and genetics to sustain biological diversity at all levels is known as
(a) conservation biology (b) restoration ecology
(c) ecology (d) bioremediation

4 The number of known species of organisms on this earth is about
(a) 5.0 million (b) 3.2 million
(c) 10.9 million (d) 13.2 million

5 Among the ecosystem mentioned below,where can one find maximum biodiversity?
(a) Mangroves (b) Desert
(c) Coral reefs (d) Alpine meadows

6 The diversity of the habitat over the total geographical area is called
(a) alpha diversity (b) gamma diversity
(c) beta diversity (d) delta diversity

7 Discovery of new species has recently picked up due to project
(a) species 2000
(b) global diversity and information facility
(c) agenda 21
(d) Both (a) and (b)

8 Match the following columns.

	Column I		Column II
A.	Rivet popper hypothesis	1.	Paul Ehrlich
B.	Communities with more species	2.	Edward Wilson
C.	Communities with less species	3.	Less stable
D.	Term biodiversity	4.	More stable

Codes

	A	B	C	D		A	B	C	D
(a)	2	4	3	1	(b)	1	4	3	2
(c)	1	3	4	2	(d)	1	4	2	3

9 When a graph is plotted to describe a relationship between species richness and its area for a variety of taxa the relationship appears as
(a) a rectangular hyperbola
(b) a sigmoid
(c) a straight line
(d) None of the above

10 Rate of replacement of species along the gradient of habitats/communities is called
(a) α-diversity (b) β-diversity
(c) γ-diversity (d) ω-diversity

11 Which of the following is classified as β-diversity?
(a) Habitat diversity (b) Ecosystem diversity
(c) Resource diversity (d) Species diversity

12 The three levels of biodiversity are
(a) genetic, species, biome
(b) molecular, species, biome
(c) genetic, population, ecosystem
(d) genetic, species, ecosystem

13 Genetic diversity is related to the
(a) types of species within a community
(b) types of community in an area
(c) gene based diversity
(d) diversity and evolution of species with a genus

14 A species spread over a large tract with varied environmental condition, will have
(a) higher genetic diversity (b) uniform gene pool
(c) little genetic diversity (d) None of these

15 At which height in Himalayan region of our country are Taiga forests located?
(a) At the height of 1000-1500 m
(b) At the height of 2000-3000 m
(c) At the height of 500-1000 m
(d) At the height of 1000-1200 m

16 Consider the following statements.
I. Total number of all species of organism in a given region is known as the region of biota.
II. Tropical rainforest of South Africa possesses the greatest biodiversity on the earth.

Choose the correct option.
(a) Statement I is true, but II is false
(b) Statement I is false, but II is true
(c) Both statements I and II are true
(d) Both statements I and II are false

Loss of Biodiversity

17 The major causes of biodiversity reduction are termed as
(a) quartet (b) devil quartet
(c) biodiversity loss (d) evil quartet

18 Which of the following factors does not play a role in increased biodiversity?
(a) Complex population interactions
(b) Introduced species
(c) A higher degree of habitat heterogeneity
(d) Narrower niches

19 Which example below is not a threat to biodiversity?
(a) Habitat destruction (b) Bioremediation
(c) Introduced species (d) Overexploitation

20 Which of the following forests is known as the 'lungs of the earth'?
(a) Taiga forest (b) Tundra forest
(c) Amazon rainforest (d) Rainforests of North-East India

21 Troublesome weed of agricultural fields is
(a) *Chenopodium album* (b) *Parthenium hysterophorus*
(c) *Cyperus rotundus* (d) *Lantana camara*

22 *Parthenium hysterophorus* is a native of South America, but it grows luxuriantly in most of the area of India. In India, it is considered as
(a) introduced species (b) native species
(c) exotic species (d) endemic species

23 Species which are susceptible to extinction have
(a) large body size (b) low reproductive potential
(c) lack of genetic variability (d) All of these

24 Species which became extinct due to low reproductive rate
(a) eagle (b) whooping crane
(c) giant panda (d) elephant

25 Dinosaurs disappeared from earth due to
(a) natural extinction (b) mass extinction
(c) anthropogenic extinction (d) artificial extinction

26 Susceptibility to extinction is due to
(a) large body size (b) small population
(c) high trophic level (d) All of these

27 Red Data Book is maintained by
(a) CITES (b) WCU (c) CBD (d) IUPAC

28 According to Red list released in 2012, how many species are added to the extinct list?
(a) 4 (b) 3 (c) 5 (d) 10

29 Species very near to extinction, if conservation measures are not promptly taken is
(a) threatened species (b) rare species
(c) endangered species (d) vulnerable species

30 The organisation, which protects the trade in endangered species at international level is
(a) IBWL (b) CITES (c) WHO (d) WWJ

31 The cause of extinction of blue whale is
(a) small population size and low reproductive rate
(b) crushing of bones under body weight
(c) incapability to breath
(d) cracking of skin

32 Dodo of Mauritius became extinct due to
(a) overexploitation (b) habitat destruction
(c) global warming (d) Both (a) and (b)

33 Those species, whose population have been seriously depleted and whose ultimate security is not assured, are known as
(a) threatened species (b) endangered species
(c) vulnerable species (d) rare species

34 What is the symbol of 'Bombay National History' is
(a) hornbill (b) spoonbill
(c) egret (d) sunbird

35 Recently extinct bird is
(a) Carolina parakeet (b) Peacock
(c) Kirtland's warbler (d) Reed bunting

36 The only ape found in India is
(a) gorilla (b) chimpanzee
(c) hoolock gibbon (d) leaf monkey

37 Bald eagle has been at high risk of extinction due to its
(a) large size
(b) low reproduction potential
(c) high trophic level
(d) change in migrating route

38 Choose the incorrect match.
(a) Vulnerable species – *Antilope cervicapra*
(b) Endangered species – *Vanilla pilifera*
(c) Extinct species – Great Indian Bustard
(d) All of the above

39 Introduction of Nile Perch in Lake Victoria of South Africa resulted in
(a) excessive growth of water weeds
(b) elimination of water weeds
(c) elimination of many species of cichlid fish
(d) excessive growth of cichlid fish

40 Match the following columns.

Column I	Column II
A. Low risk plant species in India	1. 167
B. Threatened species in 2012 Red list	2. 109
C. Low risk animal species in India	3. 73
D. Cultivated species originated in India	4. 19817

Codes

	A	B	C	D
(a)	2	4	3	1
(b)	3	4	2	1
(c)	4	2	3	1
(d)	3	2	1	4

41 Which one of the following is not observed in biodiversity hotspots?
(a) Endemism
(b) Accelerated habitat loss
(c) Lesser interspecific competition
(d) Species richness

Conservation of Biodiversity

42 Which of the following comes under the broad utilitarian category?
(a) Pollination (b) Food
(c) Fibre (d) Industrial product

43 National 'Wildlife Protection Act' was passed in
(a) 1962 (b) 1972
(c) 1982 (d) 1987

44 Conservation and maintenance of wildlife within the natural ecosystem is
(a) *in situ* conservation (b) *ex situ* conservation
(c) botanical gardens (d) All of these

45 In which zone, limited human activity is permitted?
(a) Core zone
(b) Buffer zone
(c) Manipulation zone
(d) Restoration zone

46 The biosphere which is recognised as world heritage sites is
(a) Manas Biosphere Reserve
(b) Nanda Devi
(c) Nokrek Biosphere Reserve
(d) Dibru-Saikhowa Biosphere Reserve

47 Choose the correct pair.
(a) Rajaji National park – Uttarakhand
(b) Periyar sanctuary – Andhra Pradesh
(c) Dudhwa National Park – Madhya Pradesh
(d) All of the above

48 Arboretum is
(a) a forest patch
(b) a piece of social forestry
(c) botanical garden with trees and shrubs
(d) botanical garden with cacti and herbs

49 Rare endangered and endemic taxa can be found intact and flourishing in
(a) sacred groves (b) buffer zone
(c) tropical forests (d) temperate forests

50 Buffer zone of biosphere reserve is where
(a) no human activity is allowed
(b) human activity is limited
(c) free human activity
(d) wild animals are absent

51 The sanctuary, which has maximum number of rare animals is
(a) Manas National Park (b) Kaziranga National Park
(c) Dudhwa National Park (d) Corbett National Park

52 Silent valley of Kerala is preserved because
(a) it contains very rare species of plants and animals
(b) the soil is rich in minerals
(c) the areas of land were used extensively for agricultural purposes
(d) it has pine trees

53 The key criteria for determining a hotspot are
(a) biological augmentation
(b) disruption of interaction networks
(c) number of endemic species and degree of threat
(d) habitat destruction

54 Identify the odd combination of the habitat and the particular animal concerned.
(a) Dachigam National Park – Snow leopard
(b) Sundarbans – Bengal tiger
(c) Periyar – Elephant
(d) Rann of Kutch – Wild ass

55 Match the following columns.

Column I	Column II
A. Number of ecological hotspot in world	1. 37,000
B. Number of botanical garden and arboretum in world	2. 34
C. Number of zoological parks in world	3. 1500
D. Number of area protected in world	4. 800

Codes

	A	B	C	D		A	B	C	D
(a)	3	4	2	1	(b)	3	2	4	1
(c)	2	3	4	1	(d)	4	3	2	1

56 Choose the correct match pair.
(a) World summit on sustainable development – 4th April, 2002
(b) Convention of biodiversity – 29th December, 1993
(c) Plant biodiversity garden established in NBPGR – 6th August, 2000
(d) Earth summit at Rio de Janeiro – 4th September, 1996

57 Choose the incorrect match pair.
(a) Kanha National Park – Madhya Pradesh
(b) Dudhwa National Park – Gujarat
(c) Nanda Devi – Uttarakhand
(d) All of the above

58 Project musk deer was launched in 1974 in
(a) Dudhwa National Park – Uttar Pradesh
(b) Jim Corbett National Park – Uttarakhand
(c) Kedarnath Sanctuary – Uttar Pradesh
(d) Dachigam National Park – Jammu and Kashmir

59 The first white tiger safari in the world is in
(a) Nagarjun Sagar – Andhra Pradesh
(b) Kalakad Mundanthurai – Tamil Nadu
(c) Periyar – Kerala
(d) Nandan Kanan Zoo Park – Odisha

60 The only surviving habitat of the Asiatic lion is
(a) Gir Forest – Gujarat
(b) Jim Corbett Park – Uttarakhand
(c) Sundarbans – Paschim Bangal
(d) Bandipur – Karnataka

61 Brown-antlered deer is one of the rarest mammal found in India. It is found in
(a) Nanda Devi – Himachal Pradesh
(b) Keibul Lamjao National Park – Manipur
(c) Dudhwa National Park – Uttar Pradesh
(d) Periyar Wildlife Sanctuary – Kerala

62 Choose the incorrect match pair.
(a) BRP – Biosphere Reserve Programme
(b) CITES – Convention of International Trade in Endangered Species
(c) UNEP – United Nations Environment Programme
(d) IBWL – International Board of Wildlife

63 Choose the incorrect match pair.
(a) Biodiversity Bill – 2020
(b) Wildlife Protection Act – 1970
(c) Forest Consevation Act – 1980
(d) All of the above

64 The convention on biological diversity consists of
(a) 45 articles
(b) 42 articles
(c) 52 articles
(d) 75 articles

65 The country which hosted the first World Earth Summit on conservation of environment is
(a) India (b) Brazil (c) Peru (d) Spain

(B) Cumulative Exercise

(Assorted Questions of the Chapter for Advanced Level Practice)

1 Match the following columns.

Column I	Column II
A. Rare species	1. No species
B. Vulnerable species	2. Facing at high risk of extinction
C. Endangered species	3. Localised species
D. Extinct species	4. Species under threat

Codes

	A	B	C	D		A	B	C	D
(a)	1	2	3	4	(b)	1	2	4	3
(c)	3	4	1	2	(d)	3	4	2	1

2 Choose the incorrect statements.
I. WWF has renamed as World Wonder Fund for Nature (WFN).
II. Hotspots are also known as island of pristine forests.
III. 50% of plants in India are endemic.
IV. Greater the species abundance greater its species diversity.

Codes
(a) I and III (b) II, III and IV
(c) I, III and IV (d) Only I

3 A survey was carried out to investigate the relationship between the human population density and elephant population density in Zimbabwe.

Twenty five sites were sampled, all within a 15000 km^2 area in the North of the country. Elephant populations were estimated by flying over the area and counting elephants seen from the air. The results are shown in the figure. Each point represents the results from one of the sites sampled.

Why elephant populations are very low in areas where human population density is high?

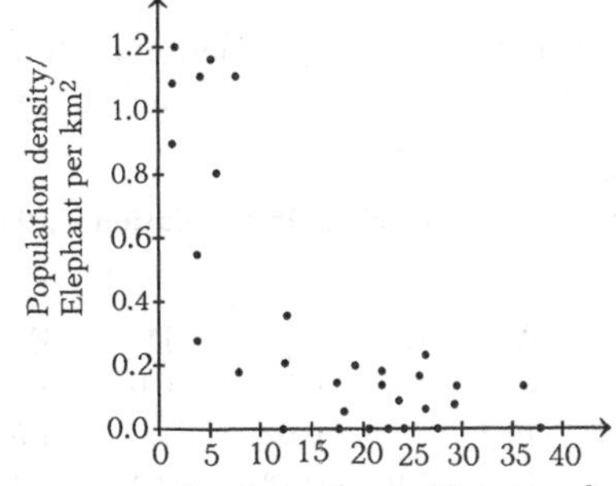

(a) Elephants occupy more grassland areas and this reduces the habitats available to humans
(b) High human population causes decline in elephant populations
(c) More humans are threat to elephants as they compete for land needed for the agriculture and settlement
(d) All of the above

4 In Mexico, coffee is an important crop as coffee trees grow well in areas in which tropical rainforest is found and so, the planting of coffee plantations frequently means that rainforest is destroyed. The given table shows four different coffee-growing systems that are used in Mexico. It also shows the results of a survey of the number of different bird species found in each system.
Which of the following is the reason for the pattern shown by the number of bird species in systems *A*, *B*, *C* and *D*?

Coffee-growing system		Mean total number of bird species per unit area
A. Traditional polyculture of 'coffee garden'	Coffee and many other useful species grown beneath the original forest tree	184
B. Commercial polyculture 'coffee garden'	Original forest trees removed and replaced with a mixture of other tall trees such as rubber, coffee and other crops beneath them	106
C. Light shaded monoculture	Original forest trees removed and replaced with a single species of leguminous trees, only coffee trees grown beneath them	50
D. Unshaded monoculture	Original forest trees removed, coffee trees grown alone	9

Increasing fertiliser and pesticide use and increase in yield of coffee (arrow from A down to D)

(a) Fewer habitats being available in tall trees to protect the bird species from the predators
(b) The number of the bird species reduces as more of the original forest trees are removed in *B*, *C* and *D*
(c) The number reduces drastically in *D* as there are less food resources for the bird species that depend on original forest trees
(d) Both (b) and (c)

5 The table below gives the population (in thousands) of ten species (A-J) in four areas (I-IV) consisting of the number of habitats given within brackets against each. Study the table and answer the question which follows.

Area and number of habitats	**Species and their population** (in thousands) **in the area**									
	A	B	C	D	E	F	G	H	I	J
I (11)	23	1.2	0.52	6.0	—	3.1	1.1	9.0	—	10.3
II (11)	10.2	—	0.62	—	1.5	3.0	—	8.2	1.1	11.2
III (13)	11.3	0.9	0.48	2.4	1.4	4.2	0.8	8.4	2.2	4.1
IV (12)	3.2	10.2	11.1	4.8	0.4	3.3	0.8	7.3	11.3	2.1

Which out of I to IV shows maximum species diversity?
(a) II (b) III (c) IV (d) I

6 Match the following columns and choose the correct option from the codes given below.

	Column I		Column II
A.	Rhinoceros	1.	Bharatpur
B.	Tiger project in Karnataka	2.	Tropical evergreen forest
C.	Assemblage protection	3	Kaziranga
D.	Silent valley	4	National park
		5.	Bandipur

Codes

	A	B	C	D		A	B	C	D
(a)	5	3	1	4	(b)	2	4	3	1
(c)	4	3	1	2	(d)	3	5	1	2

7 Consider the following statements.

I. The average annual production of dry grass or hay in India is about 250 million tonnes.

II. Red list has catalogue of taxa facing risk of extinction.

III. β-diversity is a diversity within a community.

IV. *Rauwolfia vomitaria* shows differences in chemical, is an example of species diversity.

V. Total diversity in an area is Epsilon diversity.

Choose the option containing true statements.

(a) I and II (b) II, III and IV
(c) I, II and V (d) III, IV and V

8 Which of the following statements are incorrect?

I. There is always one type of ecosystem in a region.

II. Genetic diversity comprises of different type of gene in different type species as well as same species.

III. Amphibian species diversity is more in Eastern Ghats than the Western Ghats.

Codes

(a) II and III (b) I and II (c) Only II (d) Only III

9 Match the following columns.

	Column I		Column II
A.	Species diversity	1.	Biogeographical areas where biological diversity along with natural and cultural resources is protected, maintained and managed.
B.	Biosphere reserves	2.	Influence adaptability and distribution of a species in diverse habitats.
C.	Threatened species	3.	Multipurpose protected areas, which are meant for preserving genetic diversity in the ecosystem of various natural biomass and unique biological communities.
D.	Protected areas	4.	Moving towards extinction if not allowed to realise their biotic potential and protection against human exploitation alien species, scarcity of food, etc.

Codes

	A	B	C	D
(a)	2	4	1	3
(b)	1	4	2	3
(c)	3	1	2	4
(d)	2	3	4	1

10 Consider the following statements.

I. Approximately 30% of endemic flowering plants is in India.

II. Biodiversity was coined by G Rosen.

Choose the correct option.

(a) Statement I is true, but II is false
(b) Statement I is false, but II is true
(c) Both statements I and II are true
(d) Both statements I and II are false

11 Extinction is a naturally occurring phenomenon that has occurred on earth, since life began. Scientists are so concerned about extinction now because

(a) human activities are directly responsible for today's mass extinctions
(b) extinction is occurring faster than ever before and faster than rates of respeciation
(c) large numbers of plant species, which form the base of terrestrial food webs are becoming extinct
(d) All of the above

12 Consider the following statements regarding endangered flora.

I. *Coptis teeta* is an endangered plant species of India.

II. The pteridophyte which is endangered in India is *Abies delavayi.*

Choose the correct option.

(a) Statement I is true, but II is false
(b) Statement I is false, but II is true
(c) Both statements I and II are true
(d) Both statements I and II are false

Assertion and Reason

Direction (Q. Nos. 13-21) *In each of the following questions, a statement of Assertion (A) is given followed by the corresponding statement of Reason (R). Of the statements, mark the correct answer as*

(a) Both A and R are true and R is the correct explanation of A
(b) Both A and R are true, but R is not the correct explanation of A
(c) A is true, but R is false
(d) A is false, but R is true
(e) Both A and R are false

13 **Assertion** (A) The term 'species' is given by John Ray.
Reason (R) The species are a distinct unit of diversity.

14 Assertion (A) β-diversity is a community diversity.

Reason (R) It is the diversity of organisms sharing the same habitat.

15 Assertion (A) The biological diversity is unchangeable with the change in latitude.

Reason (R) Environmental conditions are favourable in speciation.

16 Assertion (A) There is a little diversity at the poles.

Reason (R) Environmental conditions are unfavourable for the organisms at the poles.

17 Assertion (A) Red Data Book categorises all the plant species occurring on the earth.

Reason (R) Blue whale, blackbuck and snow leopard are some animals mentioned in Red Data Book.

18 Assertion (A) *In situ* conservation means conservation of organism in their natural habitat, in which they naturally occur.

Reason (R) Zoo is an *in situ* conserved area.

19 Assertion (A) Garden is an example of *ex situ* conservation.

Reason (R) It is an artificial habitat resembling to the natural habitat of organisms.

20 Assertion (A) Great Indian Bustard is a rare species.

Reason (R) Vulnerable species are rare species.

21 Assertion (A) Tropical rainforests are disappearing fast from developing countries such as India.

Reason (R) No value is attached to these forests because these are poor in biodiversity.

(C) Medical Entrances' Gallery

(Collection of Questions Asked in NEET & in Various Medical Entrance Exams)

1 According to Alexander von Humboldt, **[NEET 2020]**

(a) species richness decreases with increasing area of exploration
(b) species richness increases with increase area, but only up to limit
(c) there is no relationship between species richness and area explored
(d) species richness goes on increasing with increasing area of exploration

2 In the following in each set a conservation approach and an example of method of conservation are given

I. *In situ* conservation — Biosphere reserve
II. *Ex situ* conservation — Sacred groves
III. *In situ* conservation — Seed bank
IV. *Ex situ* conservation — Cryopreservation

Select the option with correct match of approach and method. **[NEET 2020]**

(a) I and III (b) I and IV (c) II and IV (d) I and II

3 Which of the following regions of the globe exhibits highest species diversity? **[NEET 2020]**

(a) Madagascar (b) Himalayas
(c) Amazon forest (d) Western Ghats of India

4 According to Robert May, the global species diversity is about **[NEET 2020]**

(a) 20 million (b) 50 million
(c) 7 million (d) 1.5 million

5 Which of the following is the most important cause for animals and plants being driven to extinction? **[NEET 2019, 2016]**

(a) Drought and floods
(b) Economic exploitation
(c) Alien-species invasion
(d) Habitat loss and fragmentation

6 Decline in the population of Indian native fishes due to introduction of *Clarias gariepinus* in river Yamuna can be categoriesd as **[NEET 2019]**

(a) coextinction
(b) habitat fragmentation
(c) overexploitation
(d) alien-species invasion

7 Western Ghats have a large number of plant and animal species that are not found anywhere else. Which of the following terms will you use to notify such species? **[NEET 2019]**

(a) Endemic (b) Vulnerable
(c) Threatened (d) Keystone

8 Read the following statements carefully.

I. Species diversity increases as we move away from the equator towards the poles.
II. Stellar's sea cow and passenger pigeon got extinct due to overexploitation by man.
III. *Lantana* and *Eichhornia* are invasive weed in India.
IV. The historic convention on biological diversity was held in 1992.

Choose the option containing correct statements. **[AIIMS 2019]**

(a) I and II (b) I, II and IV
(c) I, III and IV (d) II, III and IV

9 Which one of the following is not a method of *in situ* conservation of biodiversity? **[NEET 2019]**

(a) Wildlife sanctuary
(b) Botanical garden
(c) Sacred grove
(d) Biosphere reserve

10 The Earth Summit held in Rio de Janeiro in 1992 was called **[NEET 2019]**
(a) for conservation of biodiversity and sustainable utilisation of its benefits
(b) to assess threat posed to native species by invasive weed species
(c) for immediate steps to discontinue the use of CFCs that were damaging the ozone layer
(d) to reduce CO_2 emissions and global warming

11 All of the following are included in *ex situ* conservation except **[NEET 2018]**
(a) botanical gardens (b) sacred groves
(c) wildlife safari parks (d) seed banks

12 Alexander von Humboldt described for the first time
(a) Ecological biodiversity **[NEET 2017]**
(b) Law of limiting factor
(c) Species-area relationship
(d) Population growth equation

13 Refer to the following figures represent global biodiversity. Identify *A-E* and choose the correct option from the codes given below.

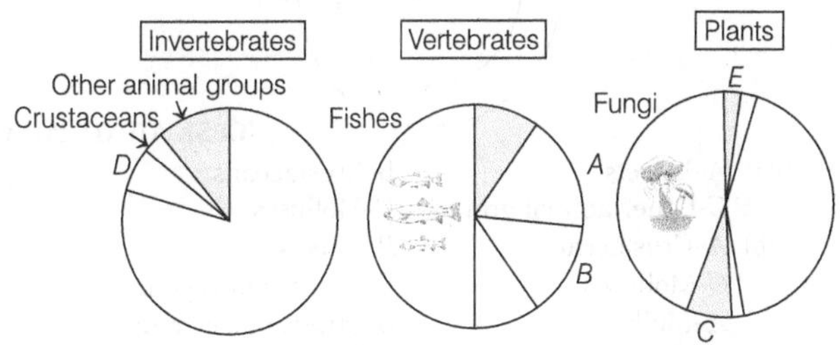

Codes **[NEET 2017]**

	A	B	C	D	E
(a)	Birds	Reptiles	Algae	Molluscs	Mosses
(b)	Mammals	Birds	Lichens	Molluscs	Mosses
(c)	Birds	Amphibians	Mosses	Insects	Algae
(d)	Birds	Reptiles	Algae	Insects	Mosses

14 Which one of the following is related to *ex situ* conservation of threatened animals and plants?
(a) Wildlife Safari parks **[NEET 2017]**
(b) Biodiversity hotspots
(c) Amazon rainforest
(d) Himalayan region

15 The region of biosphere reserve, which is legally protected and where no human activity is allowed, is known as **[NEET 2017]**
(a) core zone (b) buffer zone
(c) transition zone (d) restoration zone

16 **Assertion** (A) Gene bank is a type of *ex situ* conservation of biodiversity.

Reason (R) It involves maintaining stocks of viable seeds, living growing plants, tissue culture, etc. **[AIIMS 2017]**
(a) Both A and R are true and R is the correct explanation of A
(b) Both A and R are true, but R is not the correct explanation of A
(c) A is true, but R is false
(d) Both A and R are false

17 IUCN stands for **[JIPMER 2017]**
(a) Indian Union for Conservation of Nature
(b) International Union for Conservation of Nature
(c) Indian Union for Chemical Nomenclature
(d) International Union for Conservation of Nutrients

18 Red List contains data or information on **[NEET-II 2016]**
(a) all economically important plants
(b) plants whose products are in international trade
(c) threatened species
(d) marine vertebrates only

19 Which of the following National Parks is home to the famous musk deer or hangul? **[NEET-II 2016]**
(a) Keibul Lamjao National Park, Manipur
(b) Bandhavgarh National Park, Madhya Pradesh
(c) Eaglenest Wildlife Sanctuary, Arunachal Pradesh
(d) Dachigam National Park, Jammu and Kashmir

20 How many hotspots of biodiversity in the world have been identified till date by Norman Myers? **[NEET-II 2016]**
(a) 17 (b) 25 (c) 34 (d) 43

21 Which of the following is correctly matched? **[NEET-I 2016]**
(a) Aerenchyma — *Opuntia*
(b) Age pyramid — Biome
(c) *Parthenium hysterophorus* — Threat to biodiversity
(d) Stratification — Population

22 With reference to competitive exclusion, which one of the following became extinct when browsing goats were introduced in Galapagos Islands? **[EAMCET 2016]**
(a) Darwin's finches (b) *Chathamalus*
(c) Abingdon tortoise (d) Warblers

23 Which one of the following methods does not fall under *ex situ* conservation of biodiversity?
[EAMCET 2016, Karnataka CET 2015, Karala CEE 2014]
(a) Cryopreservation (b) *In vitro* culture
(c) Gene Bank (d) Biosphere reserves

24 Which is the National Aquatic Animal of India?
(a) River dolphin (b) Blue whale **[NEET 2016]**
(c) Seahorse (d) Gangetic shark

25 In which of the following both pairs have correct combination? **[CBSE AIPMT 2015]**
(a) *In situ* conservation/National park
Ex situ conservation/Botanical garden
(b) *In situ* conservation/Cryopreservation
Ex situ conservation/Wildlife sanctuary
(c) *In situ* conservation/Seed bank
Ex situ conservation/National park
(d) *In situ* conservation/Tissue culture
Ex situ conservation/Sacred groves

26 Cryopreservation of gametes of threatened species in viable and fertile condition can be referred to as
(a) *in situ* conservation of biodiversity [CBSE AIPMT 2015]
(b) advanced *ex situ* conservation of biodiversity
(c) *in situ* conservation by sacred groves
(d) *in situ* cryoconservation of biodiversity

27 Select the correct combination(s) from the following. [WB JEE 2015]
(a) Gir – Asiatic lion
(b) Sunderbans – Rhinoceros
(c) Periyar – Indian elephant
(d) Corbett National Park – Red panda

28 What is the full form of MAB? [WB JEE 2015]
(a) Man and Biosphere
(b) Man and Biosphere Reserve
(c) Man and Biosphere Reserve Programme
(d) Man and Biosphere Programme

29 Beta (β) diversity refers to diversity [WB JEE 2015]
(a) within a community (b) between communities
(c) between two eco zones (d) within a population

30 Wildlife Protection Act, India was implemented in the year [WB JEE 2015]
(a) 1982 (b) 1988 (c) 1972 (d) 1970

31 Which one of the following is an *in situ* method of biodiversity conservation? [WB JEE 2015]
(a) National park
(b) Botanical garden
(c) Zoological garden
(d) Scientific laboratory

32 An area is declared as hotspot when [WB JEE 2015]
(a) it has 1500 more endemic species and 75% of its original habitat is lost
(b) it has 1500 or more vertebrate species and 75% of its original habitat is lost
(c) it has more than 2000 species of plants
(d) most of the species inhabiting the area is facing the risk of extinction

33 *Antilope cervicapra* is [WB JEE 2015]
(a) a mammal
(b) commonly known as blackbuck
(c) an animal under data deficient category of wildlife
(d) a threatened Indian wildlife

34 The distribution of species diversity on earth may be best described as [AMU 2015]
(a) it is uniformly distributed
(b) it is highest in tropics
(c) it is highest in polar regions
(d) it is highest in Southern hemisphere and lowest in Northern hemisphere

35 Rajaji National Park is situated in [AMU 2015]
(a) Tamil Nadu (b) Uttarakhand
(c) Assam (d) Karnataka

36 The following graph depicts changes in two populations (*A* and *B*) or herbivores in grassy field. *A* possible reason for these changes is that

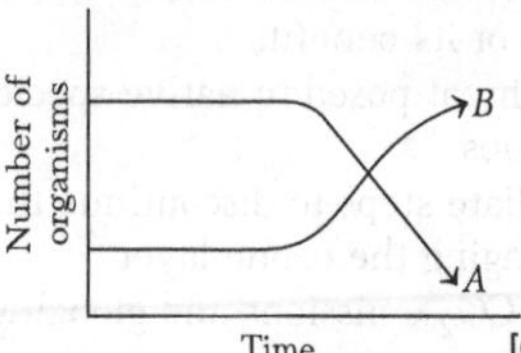

[CBSE AIPMT 2015]
(a) both plant populations in this habitat decreased
(b) population *B* competed more successfully for food than population *A*
(c) population *A* produced more offspring than population *B*
(d) population *A* consumed the members of population *B*

37 Given below is the representation of the extent of global diversity of invertebrates. What groups the four portions (*A*-*D*) represent, respectively?

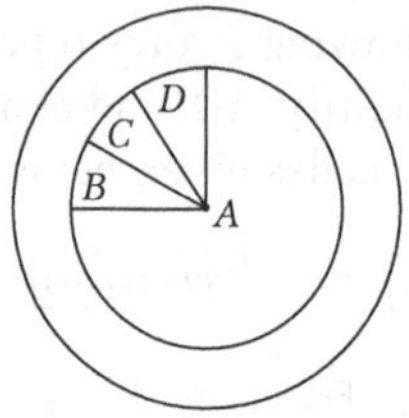

[CBSE AIPMT 2014
(a) *A*-Insects *B*-Crustaceans *C*-Other animal groups *D*-Molluscs
(b) *A*-Crustacean *B*-Insects *C*-Molluscs *D*-Other animal groups
(c) *A*-Molluscs *B*-Other animal groups *C*-Crustaceans *D*-Insects
(d) *A*-Insects *B*-Molluscs *C*-Crustaceans *D*-Other animal groups

38 In IUCN Red List, 2004 documents, the extinction of 784 species, it includes [J&K CET 2014]
(a) 335 vertebrates, 360 invertebrates and 89 plants
(b) 337 vertebrates, 362 invertebrates and 88 plants
(c) 338 vertebrates, 359 invertebrates and 87 plants
(d) 340 vertebrates, 357 invertebrates and 87 plants

39 Maximum biodiversity is found in [UK PMT 2014]
(a) tropical rainforests (b) temperate rainforests
(c) mangrove vegetation (d) tundra

40 One of the following statements is incorrect with reference to biodiversity. Identify it. [Karnataka CET 2014]
(a) Biodiversity increases with higher altitudes to lower altitudes
(b) Depletion in genetic diversity of crop plants is mainly due to the introduction of better varieties with high yield, disease resistance, etc
(c) The richest reservoirs of animal and plant life (species richness) with few or no threatened species are called 'biodiversity hotspots'
(d) Biodiversity decreases from the equator to polar regions

41 One of the chief reason among the following for the depletion in the number of species making it endangered is **[Karnataka CET 2014]**
(a) greenhouse effect
(b) habitat destruction
(c) overhunting and poaching
(d) competition and predation

42 An example of *ex situ* conservation is **[CBSE AIPMT 2014]**
(a) national park (b) seed bank
(c) wildlife sanctuary (d) sacred grove

43 Find the incorrectly matched pair. **[Kerala CEE 2014]**
(a) Endemism – Species confined to one region and not found anywhere else
(b) Hotspots – Regions with species richness
(c) Alien species to India – *Clarias gariepinus*
(d) Lungs of the planet – Amazon rainforest
(e) *In situ* – IVF conservation

44 The concept of hotspot was first introduced by **[WB JEE 2014]**
(a) Mayer (b) Simpson (c) Myers (d) David

45 The objective of 'Ramsar Convention' was **[WB JEE 2014]**
(a) forest conservation (b) wildlife conservation
(c) wetland conservation (d) biodiversity conservation

46 Management of national parks is controlled by **[WB JEE 2014]**
(a) State Government
(b) Central Government
(c) United Nations
(e) Non-government Organisations

47 Match the following columns.

	Column I		Column II
A.	Jim Corbett National Park	1.	Gujarat
B.	Kaziranga National Park	2.	Andhra Pradesh
C.	Mahavir Harina Vanasthali National Park	3.	Rajasthan
D.	Keoladeo Ghana National Park	4.	Uttarakhand
		5.	Assam

Codes **[EAMCET 2014]**

	A	B	C	D		A	B	C	D
(a)	2	5	4	3	(b)	2	1	3	4
(c)	4	1	2	5	(d)	4	5	2	3

48 Breeding ground for migratory flamingo is **[Gujarat CET 2014]**
(a) area of Gulf of Kachchh (Kutch)
(b) area between Khadir and Pachham islands in great Rann of Kachchh (Kutch)
(c) area of great Rann of Kachchh (Kutch) and little Rann of Kachchh (Kutch)
(d) area of Nal Sarovar Bird Sanctuary

49 The organisation which publishes the Red List of species is **[CBSE AIPMT 2014]**
(a) ICFRE (b) IUCN (c) UNEP (d) WWF

50 Which of the following rainforests is home to more than 40,000 species of plants, 3000 of fishes, 1300 of birds, 427 of mammals, 427 of amphibians, 378 of reptiles and more than 1,25,000 invertebrates? **[AIIMS 2013]**
(a) Amazonian (b) Tropical
(c) Arctic tundra (d) Temperate

51 The government of India in 1980s has introduced a concept to work closely with the local communities for protecting and managing forests. The concept is **[AIIMS 2013]**
(a) Forest Research Institutes
(b) Panel of Local Communities for Forest Management
(c) Joint Forest Management
(d) Jhum Cultivation

52 5th June is celebrated as **[Odisha JEE 2013]**
(a) Water Day (b) World Environment Day
(c) Conservation Day (d) World Earth Day

53 Chipko movement is related to **[Odisha JEE 2013]**
(a) Swaminathan (b) Bahuguna
(c) Odum (d) Mishra

54 Which one of the following is not used for *ex situ* plant conservation? **[NEET 2013]**
(a) Seed banks (b) Shifting cultivation
(c) Botanical gardens (d) Field gene banks

55 Biosphere reserve programme started in India, **[Manipal 2013]**
(a) 1986 (b) 1984
(c) 1982 (d) 1988

56 The single-horned rhinoceros is protected at **[BHU 2012, Chandigarh CET 2012. Odisha JEE 2011, Karnataka CET 2013]**
(a) Anshi National Park
(b) Rajiv Gandhi National Park
(c) Kanha National Park
(d) Kaziranga National Park

57 The term 'alpha diversity' refers to **[WB JEE 2013]**
(a) genetic diversity
(b) community and ecosystem diversity
(c) species diversity
(d) diversity among the plants

58 Which one is odd for species diversity? **[UP CPMT 2013]**
(a) α diversity (b) γ diversity
(c) β diversity (d) δ diversity

59 Most of the tree dwellers are found in which of the forests? **[Kerala CEE 2013]**
(a) Northern conifer forest
(b) Deciduous forest
(c) Mediterranean scrub forest
(d) Tropical rainforest

60 Select the correct statement about biodiversity. **[CBSE AIPMT 2012]**
(a) The desert areas of Rajasthan and Gujarat have a very high level of desert animal species as well as numerous rare animals
(b) Large scale planting of *Bt* cotton has no adverse effect on biodiversity
(c) Western Ghats have a very high degree of species richness and endemism
(d) Conservation of biodiversity is just a fad pursued by the developed countries

61 Which one of the following is exotic species? **[Manipal 2012]**
(a) *Parthenium* (b) *Lantana*
(c) *Eichhornia* (d) All of these

62 Silent valley is tropical evergreen forest located in **[Manipal 2012]**
(a) Kerala (b) Karnataka
(c) Maharashtra (d) Odisha

63 India has only 2.4% of the world's land area, its share of the global species diversity is **[AMU 2012]**
(a) 1.8% (b) 3.1% (c) 5.1% (d) 8.1%

64 Kanha National Park is located in .... and is famous for .... **[AMU 2012, Odisha JEE 2011]**
(a) Madhya Pradesh, elephant (b) Madhya Pradesh, tiger
(c) Odisha, tiger (d) Assam, elephant

65 Sacred groves are specially useful in **[CBSE AIPMT 2012]**
(a) year round flow of water in rivers
(b) conserving rare and threatened species
(c) generating environmental awareness
(d) preventing soil erosion

66 Arrange the following in ascending order based on their numbers in India. **[Haryana PMT 2012]**
I. Biosphere reserves
II. Hotspots
III. National parks
IV. Wildlife sanctuaries

Codes
(a) II → I → III → IV
(b) II → III → IV → I
(c) I → II → III → IV
(d) IV → III → II → I

67 Which one of the following expanded forms of the following acronyms is correct? **[CBSE AIPMT 2011]**
(a) UNEP – United Nations Environmental Policy
(b) EPA – Environmental Pollution Agency
(c) IUCN – International Union for Conservation of Nature and Natural Resources
(d) IPCC – International Panel for Climate Change

ANSWERS

Check Point 25.1

1. (b)	2. (b)	3. (c)	4. (b)	5. (c)	6. (c)

Check Point 25.2

1. (b)	2. (b)	3. (c)	4. (c)	5. (c)	6. (b)

Check Point 25.3

1. (c)	2. (c)	3. (d)	4. (b)	5. (b)	6. (a)

(A) Topical Exercise

1. (a)	2. (b)	3. (a)	4. (c)	5. (c)	6. (b)	7. (d)	8. (b)	9. (a)	10. (b)
11. (a)	12. (d)	13. (c)	14. (a)	15. (a)	16. (a)	17. (d)	18. (b)	19. (b)	20. (c)
21. (b)	22. (a)	23. (d)	24. (c)	25. (b)	26. (d)	27. (b)	28. (a)	29. (c)	30. (b)
31. (a)	32. (d)	33. (b)	34. (a)	35. (d)	36. (c)	37. (c)	38. (c)	39. (c)	40. (b)
41. (c)	42. (a)	43. (b)	44. (a)	45. (b)	46. (b)	47. (a)	48. (c)	49. (a)	50. (b)
51. (a)	52. (a)	53. (c)	54. (a)	55. (c)	56. (b)	57. (b)	58. (c)	59. (d)	60. (a)
61. (b)	62. (d)	63. (b)	64. (b)	65. (b)					

(B) Cumulative Exercise

1. (d)	2. (b)	3. (c)	4. (d)	5. (c)	6. (d)	7. (c)	8. (d)	9. (d)	10. (c)
11. (d)	12. (a)	13. (b)	14. (c)	15. (d)	16. (a)	17. (d)	18. (c)	19. (a)	20 (c)
21. (c)									

(C) Medical Entrances' Gallery

1. (b)	2. (b)	3. (c)	4. (c)	5. (d)	6. (d)	7. (a)	8. (d)	9. (b)	10. (a)
11. (b)	12. (c)	13. (a)	14. (a)	15. (a)	16. (a)	17. (b)	18. (c)	19. (d)	20. (c)
21. (c)	22. (c)	23. (d)	24. (a)	25. (a)	26. (b)	27. (a, c)	28. (d)	29. (b)	30. (c)
31. (a)	32. (a)	33. (a,b,d)	34. (b)	35. (b)	36. (b)	37. (d)	38. (c)	39. (a)	40. (c)
41. (b)	42. (b)	43. (e)	44. (c)	45. (c)	46. (b)	47. (d)	48. (b)	49. (b)	50. (a)
51. (c)	52. (b)	53. (b)	54. (b)	55. (a)	56. (d)	57. (c)	58. (d)	59. (d)	60. (c)
61. (d)	62. (a)	63. (d)	64. (b)	65. (b)	66. (a)	67. (c)			

Explanations

(A) Topical Exercise

5 (*c*) Coral reefs are the most productive ecosystem and form the most diverse part of coastal region providing a home to fish molluscs, crustaceans, sponges, etc.

Other options are explained as

Mangroves, found in coastal regions usually have plants growing in swampy and saline water, deserts have mostly xerophytic species and Alpine meadows are related to high altitudes and do not show much tree growth.

16 (*a*) Statement I is true, but II is false. Incorrect statement can be corrected as

The Amazon rainforest possesses the greatest biodiversity on the earth.

20 (*c*) In Amazon rainforests, vegetation continuously rcycles carbon dioxide into oxygen. 20% of the oxygen on the earth is produced by the Amazon rainforests. So, Amazon rainforest is known as the lungs of the earth.

38 (*c*) Option (c) is incorrect match pair and can be corrected as

Great Indian Bustard is a critically endangered species.

54 (*a*) Option (a) is odd combination of the habitat and the particular animal concerned because

Dachigam National Park is famous for Kashmir stags.

57 (*b*) Option (b) is incorrect match pair and can be corrected as

Dudhwa National Park is situated in Uttar Pradesh.

62 (*d*) Option (d) is incorrect match pair and can be corrected as

IBWL stands for Indian Board of Wildlife.

63 (*b*) Option (b) is incorrect match pair and can be corrected as

Wildlife Protection Act was enacted in 1972.

(B) Cumulative Exercise

7 (*c*) Statements I, II and V are true whereas III and IV are false. Incorrect statements can be corrected as

- β-diversity is a diversity between the communities.
- *Rauwolfia vomitaria* shows differences in chemical, is an example of genetic diversity.

8 (*d*) Only statement III is incorrect and can be corrected as

Amphibian species diversity is more in Western Ghat than in the Eastern Ghat.

12 (*a*) Statement I is true, but II is false. Incorrect statement can be corrected as

Abies delavayi is a threatened species.

13 (*b*) Both A and R are true, but R is not the correct explanation of A.

The term species was given by John Ray. These are distinct units of diversity and has a specific role in an ecosystem.

14 (*c*) A is true, but R is false. R can be corrected as

β -diversity refers to the diversity of different organisms occurring in different habitats. It is also called diversity between communities.

15 (*d*) A is false, but R is true. A can be corrected as

The biological diversity is changeable with the change in latitude and altitude due to change in environmental conditions.

16 (*a*) Both A and R are true and R is the correct explanation of A.

There is a little biodiversity at the poles due to unfavourable environmental conditions (decrease in temperature).

17 (*d*) A is false, but R is true. A can be corrected as

Red Data Book categorises those species, which are under high risk of extinction, e.g. blue whale, blackbuck and snow leopard.

18 (*c*) A is true, but R is false because

In situ conservation means conservation of organisms within the natural ecosystem, in which they occur, e.g. national parks, sanctuaries. Zoo is an example of *ex situ* conservation.

19 (*a*) Both A and R are true and R is the correct explanation of A.

Ex situ conservation means conservation of living organisms in an artificial habitat resembling to the natural habitat of these organisms, e.g. zoos, gardens, seed banks, etc.

20 (*c*) A is true, but R is false. R can be corrected as

Rare species are those, which have small population in the world. They are usually confined to limited areas or are thinly scattered over a more wide area. While vulnerable species are present in sufficient number, but becomes endangered due to several reasons.

Great Indian Bustard are the rare species, which are in danger of extinction, hence are endangered species.

21 (*c*) A is true, but R is false because
Tropical rainforests are very rich in biodiversity due to climatic factors. These are disappearing fast from developing countries because of less awareness to the biodiversity conservation.

(C) Medical Entrances' Gallery

1 (*b*) Alexander von Humboldt was a German naturalist and geographer. He proposed that within a region, species richness increases with increasing explored area, but only up to a limit.
Accordingly, the relation between species richness and area for a wide variety of taxa turn out to be rectangular hyperbola. The relationship appears as a straight line on logarithmic scale and described by the equation

$$\log S = \log C = Z \log A$$

Where, S-Species richness,
A-Area
Z-Regression coefficient,
C-Y-Intercept.

2 (*b*) Option (b) is correct. It can be explained as
In situ conservation is on-site conservation technique, i.e. the species are protected in their natural habitats only. In this approach, the important components of biological diversity are protected and managed through protected areas, biosphere reserves and sacred forests or lakes.
On the other hand, *ex situ* conservation involves the conservation of selected rare flora or fauna in places outside their natural habitat. It includes off-site collection and gene banks. In gene banks, germplasm, tissue or embryos are stored in preserved conditions using the technologies like orchards, tissue culture and cryopreservation.

3 (*c*) The Amazonian rainforest in South America has the greatest biodiversity on the earth. Rainforests have high biodiversity because they are abundant in nutrients, energy and have a favourable climalte for the biodiversity to prosper.

4 (*c*) Robert May estimated global species diversity at about 7 million. Although some other scientists estimate its range from 20-50 million. India has only 2.4% of the world 's land area, it shares of the global species diversity of an impressive 8.1%.

5 (*d*) Habitat loss and fragmentation is the most important cause for animals and plants being driven to extinction. Due to habitat loss and fragmentation, a 14% of the earth's land surface, rainforest has shrunk to only 6% in last few years.
Fragmentation and loss of large habitats due to various human activities badly affect mammals and birds requiring large territories. Certain animals with migratory habits are also affected by habitat loss and fragmentation. Thus, their populations are driven towards decline and extinction.
On the other hand, droughts and floods, economic exploitation and alien-species invasion affect only a small part of population at a time.

6 (*d*) Decline in the population of Indian native fishes due to introduction of *Clarias gariepinus* in river Yamuna can be categorised as alien-species invasions. It is posing a threat to the indigenous catfishes in our rivers and causing a loss of biodiversity.

7 (*a*) Endemic species are those species which are confined to a particular region and not found anywhere else. For example, species of Western Ghats. On the other hand, vulnerable and threatened species are the species which are facing high risk of extinction. Keystone species are the species whose presence or absence significantly affects others species in an ecosystem.

8 (*d*) Statements II, III and IV are correct. Only statement I is incorrect and can be corrected as
Species diversity on the earth is not uniformly distributed but shows interesting patterns. It is generally highest in the tropics and decreases as we move towards the poles. Species richness of the tropics is due to relatively constant environment and more solar energy with constitute to greater productivity.

9 (*b*) Botanical garden is not a method of *in situ* conservation of biodiversity. It is a type of *ex situ* or off-site conservation in which rare plants are conserved in places outside their natural habitat.
Rest all are methods of *in situ* conservation of biodiversity.

10 (*a*) The Earth Summit held in Rio de Janeiro in 1992 was called for the conservation of biodiversity and sustainable utilisation of its benefits. In this summit, more than 130 nations signed a convention on Biodiversity and Climate Change. Canada was the key player in the development of this convention.

11 (*b*) Sacred groves is a mode of *in situ* conservation in which forest fragments of varying size are protected by religious communities. It helps to protect the biota of that area on-site.
On the other hand, botanical gardens, seed banks and wildlife safari parks are the examples of *ex situ* conservation in which the biota is protected outside its natural habitat.

12 (*c*) Alexander von Humboldt did extensive exploration in the wilderness of South America. He established species-area relationship. He observed that within a region, species richness increases with increasing explored area, but up to a certain limit. Infact, the relationship between species richness and area for a variety of taxa is a rectangular hyperbola as seen below

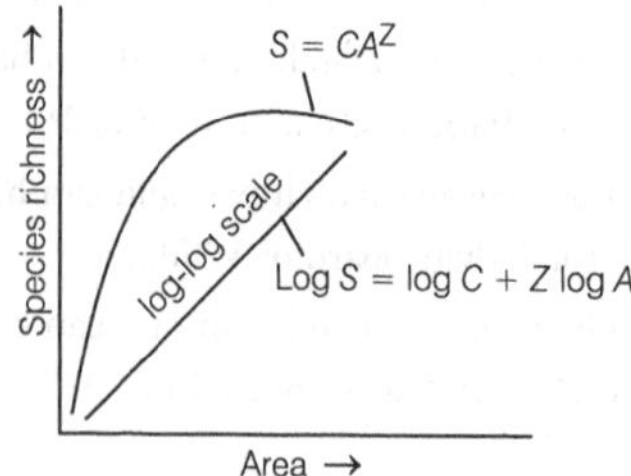

13 (*a*) Option (a) represents the correct matches of global diversity indicating major taxa of plants, vertebrates and invertebrates where,
A - Birds *B* - Reptiles
C - Algae *D* - Molluscs
E - Mosses

14 (*a*) Wildlife Safari parks are used for the *ex situ* conservation of threatened animals and plants. Such organisms are taken out from their natural habitat and placed in special settings (Wildlife Safari Park, zoo).

15 (*a*) Biosphere reserve consists of three zones, i.e. core, buffer and transition zone. Core zone is the region of biosphere reserve which is undisturbed and legally protected ecosystem, where no human activity is allowed.

Buffer zone surrounds the core area and transition zone is the outermost area of the biosphere reserve, where active cooperation between reserve management and the local people occurs.

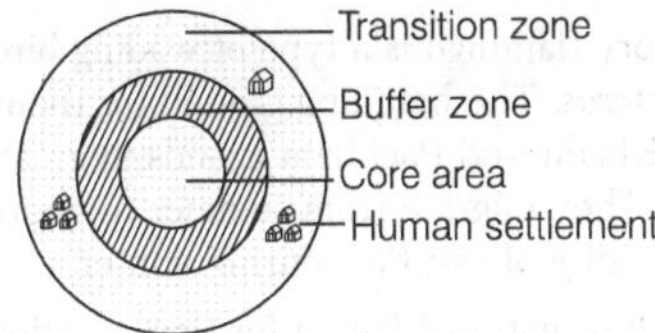

16 (*a*) Both A and R are true and R is the correct explanation of A.

Gene banks are institutes that maintain stocks of viable seeds (seed banks), live growing plants (e.g. orchards), tissue culture and frozen germplasm with the whole range of genetic variability. These are methods of *ex situ* conservation of biodiversity.

17 (*b*) Full form of IUCN is International Union for Conservation of Nature and Natural Resource. It works for the conservation of nature and sustainable use of various natural resources.

18 (*c*) IUCN maintains a Red Data Book which is a catalogue of the taxa facing the risk of extinction. The threatened species are the one which are at more risk of becoming extinct. The list of such species is called Red List.

19 (*d*) Dachigam National Park, situated at Jammu and Kashmir and is famous for conservation of musk deer.

Other options are explained as

- At Keibul Lamjao National Park, Manipur, brown deer (Sangai) is protected.
- At Bandhavgarh National Park, MP, tiger is protected.
- Eaglenest Wildlife Sanctuary, Arunachal Pradesh, protects elephants and red panda.

20 (*c*) The total number of biodiversity hotspots in the world at present are 34. These are the areas of high endemism and high level of species richness.

21 (*c*) Option (c) is correctly matched.

Parthenium hysterophorus (carrot grass) is an alien species introduced inadvertently for some economic use, turned invasive causing decline or extinction of the indigenous species.

22 (*c*) Browsing goats when introduced in Galapagos island, then Abingdon tortoise became extinct, because these goats destroyed their food and territory. Galapagos island is also famous for adaptive radiation phenomenon in Darwin finches.

25 (*a*) Option (a) represents correct combination, i.e.

In situ conservation-National park

Ex situ conservation-Botanical garden

Other options are incorrect and can be corected as

The process of protecting endangered plant and animal species in their natural habitat is *in situ* conservation.

It involves the creation of protected areas such as national parks, biosphere reserves, etc.

Ex situ conservation is the technique of conservation of all levels of biological diversity outside their natural habitat through different techniques like zoo, captive breeding aquarium, cryopreservation, botanical garden and gene bank.

26 (*b*) Cryopreservation at -196°C in liquid nitrogen is an advanced method for *ex situ* conservation of gametes, tissue culture, embryos, etc., for indefinite periods. To prevent extinction of threatened species, cryopreservation is done. *In situ* conservation occurs at ecosystem level of threatened or endangered species.

27 (*a, c*) Options (a) and (c) are correct combinations.

The Gir, the largest compact, dry deciduous forests in the semiarid Western part of India is the last abode of big and regal predator, Asiatic lion (*Panthera leo persica*) an endangered species. It is situated in Gujarat. Periyar National Park is notable as an elephant reserve and a tiger reserve. It is situated in Kerala. Other options are incorrect combinations and can be corrected as

Sunderbans for tigers present in West Bengal. Corbett National Park for tigers, leopards and elephants, situated in Nainital.

28 (*d*) Man and Biosphere Programme (MAB) is an intergovernmental scientific programme that aims to establish a scientific basis for the improvement of relationship between people and their environment. This programme was launched in 1971 by UNESCO.

30 (*c*) Wildlife Protection Act in 1972 is an act of the Parliament of India. It was enacted for protection of plant and animal species. It establishes schedules of protected plant and animal species. Hunting or harvesting these species was largely outlawed.

32 (*a*) Biodiversity hotspots are geographical areas that contain high levels of species diversity, but are threatened with extinction.

To qualify as a hotspot, a region must meet two strict criteria.

(i) It must contain at least 1500 species of vascular plants (> 0.5 per cent of the world total) as endemics.

(ii) It has lost at least 75% of its original habitat.

33 (*a, b, d*) *Antilope cervicapra* (the blackbuck) is an ungulate species of *Antilope*, native to the Indian subcontinent that has been classified as near threatened by IUCN since 2003. It is a mammal belonging to order—Artiodactyla.

34 (*b*) The distribution of species diversity is highest in tropical regions of the earth, while it is lowest in the polar regions due to the optimum conditions prevailing in tropics.

36 (*b*) The individuals of population-*B* have increased because they have adapted better to their environment than population-*A*. Population-*B* had proved to be superiorly adapted for survival and attainment of resources like food, water, shelter, etc., leading to an increase in their number of outgrowing the offsprings, as compared to those of population-*A*.

37 (*d*) In the given diagram, the largest portion is of phylum-Arthropoda, the largest phylum of the animal kingdom with its largest group, i.e. Insecta (*A*). The second largest population is of phylum-Mollusca (*B*). The third one is occupied by crustaceans (*C*). All the other invertebrates combinedly indicate the (*D*) portion of pie chart.

38 (*c*) The IUCN Red List which is issued in 2004 documents, the extinction of 784 species including 338 vertebrates, 359 invertebrates and 87 plants in the last 500 years.

39 (*a*) Maximum biodiversity is found in tropical rainforests. In these forests, rainfall is above 140 cm/yr usually between 200-500 cm/yr. It may also reach upto as 1000 cm. Rain occurs through major parts of the year.

Due to high humidity, plant growth is luxuriant. That is why, it shows maximum biodiversity in terms of flora and fauna.

40 (*c*) Out of all the options, the only incorrect statement with reference to biodiversity is option (c). It can be corrected as Biodiversity hotspots are the biogeographic regions which are both, biologically rich reservoirs and deeply threatened by habitat loss and other human activities destruction.

Rest of the statements are correct with reference to biodiversity.

41 (*b*) One of the chief reason is habit at destruction. Destruction for depletion in number of species making it endangered.

Due to habitat destruction, the rainforest once covering 14% of earth's land surface has gone down to only 6% now.

This is badly affecting the mammals and birds and certain animals with migratory habits leading to decline in their population.

42 (*b*) Among the given options, seed bank is an example of *ex situ* conservation. *Ex situ* or off-site conservation is the process of protecting endangered species of plants and animals outside their natural habitats. It also involves the conservation of genetic resources as well as species.

43 (*e*) Out of all the pairs given in the options, all are correctly matched except option (e) for *in situ* conservation because it is an on-site conservation that provides protection of the whole ecosystem and its biodiversity at all levels in order to protect the threatened species, e.g. sacred groves. The IVF is a technique of assisted reproductive technique to facilitate parenthood in infertile couples.

44 (*c*) The concept of hotspot was first introduced by Norman Myers in 1989. Biodiversity hotspot is an approach for the *in situ* conservation. These are certain regions identified as the maximum protection areas for species conservation.

45 (*c*) Ramsar Convention is an intergovernmental treaty. The objective is the conservation and sustainable utilisation of wetlands and also, for recognising the fundamental ecological functions of wetlands and their economic, cultural, scientific and recreation value.

This convention was named after the city of Ramsar in Iran and the convention was signed in 1971 and was effective from 25th December in 1975. The Ramsar list of wetlands of international importance now includes over 2000 sites known as Ramsar sites.

46 (*b*) The management of National Parks is controlled by Central government. National parks are large areas of native land designed for the conservation purposes of plants and animals.

47 (*d*) A–4, B–5, C–2, D–3

48 (*b*) Migratory flamingo is a type of wading bird in the genus *Phoenicopterus*. The breeding ground for them is the area between Khadir and Pachham islands in great Rann of Kachchh. They migrate from summer to winter due to the extreme aridity of salt flats during winter.

49 (*b*) IUCN (International Union for Conservation of Nature and Natural Resources) which publishes the Red List of threatened species or Red Data List. It possesses the status of all the species. It is an international organisation established in October (1948). Its headquarter is in Switzerland.

53 (*b*) In 1973, the Chipko movement was launched by Chandi Prasad Bhatt and Sundar Lal Bahuguna against large scale cutting of trees (deforestation) by timber contractors in Uttaranchal hills.

54 (*b*) Shifting cultivation results into deforestation (not used for *ex situ* plant conservation). On the other hand, botanical gardens have collection of living plants for reference. Seed banks store seeds as a source for planting in case seed reserves elsewhere are destroyed. Field gene banks are a type of biorepository, which preserve genetic material.

55 (*a*) Biosphere Reserve Programme was launched by UNESCO in 1971 under its 'Man and Biosphere Programme' (MAB). But in India, it was launched in 1986.

56 (*d*) Kaziranga National Park is situated in the Golaghat and Naugaon District of Assam. It is inhabited by the world's largest population of one-horned rhinoceros.

58 (*d*) δ diversity is odd for species diversity. Ecosystem diversity is of three types, i.e. α, β and γ. Alpha diversity is within community diversity, beta diversity is between community diversity and gamma diversity is the diversity present in ranges of communities, as represented by diversity of habitats/ecosystem over a total landscape or geographical area.

59 (*d*) Most of the tree dwellers and insect species are found in tropical rainforest. The warm humid climate of tropical rainforests supports the broad leaves, evergreen plants and trees. Animal life is also highly diverse. Some of the animals of tropical rainforests are monkeys, snakes, tropical birds, bats, carnivorous animals, variety of fishes, etc.

CHAPTER 26

Environmental Issues

Human population has been growing rapidly and in turn, per capita consumption of resources is also increasing. This has strained the life supporting systems on earth and brought about a number of environmental changes. These changes resulted into desertification, irregular rainfall, global warming, increase in quantity of pollutants, etc. Environmental issues include all the aspects which adversely affect our biophysical environment. Pollution, global warming, deforestation, etc., are the topics of major concern in current perspective.

POLLUTION

It is an undesirable change in physical, chemical or biological characteristics of air, water and soil. It is harmful to both nature and man, directly or indirectly. Before discussing the various aspects of pollution, we must know about the pollutants.

Pollutants

It is a chemical or biological substance that deteriorates our natural environment. Pollutants can be categorised on the basis of their chemical nature, degradation, etc.

Based upon chemical nature

On the basis of their chemical nature, pollutants are of following types

- **Organic pollutants**, e.g. DDT (Dichlorodiphenyl Trichloro ethane), Polychlorinatedbiphenyls (PCBs), oils.
- **Inorganic pollutants**, e.g. nitrates, acids found in acid rain, metals.
- **Acid pollutants** Found in run-off from coal mining, HCl formed by a reaction of HCl gas with moisture.
- **Radiological pollutants** Radioactive chemicals found naturally in rocks, soil and water.
- **Biological pollutants** These are pathogenic microorganisms such as infectious bacteria, viruses and protozoans.
- **Multiple pollutants** There are many pollutants that affect the organisms at one time, e.g. xenobiotics (foreign chemicals).
- **Physical pollutants** These may have both inorganic and organic components, e.g. soil carried in rainwater, run-off from agricultural fields, etc.

Inside

Based upon existence in nature

On the basis of their existence in nature, pollutants are of following types

- **Quantitative pollutants** These normally occur in nature. However, they become pollutant when their concentration reaches above a threshold value in nature, e.g. CO_2, nitrogen oxides, etc.
- **Qualitative pollutants** These do not occur in environment naturally, but are added by man, e.g. pesticides, fungicides, etc.

Based upon natural degradation

On the basis of their natural degradations, pollutants are of two types, i.e. biodegradable and non-biodegradable. These are discussed in below table

Table 26.1 Differences between biodegradable and non-biodegradable pollutants

Biodegradable pollutants	Non-biodegradable pollutants
These can be decomposed and degraded by microbes.	These cannot be decomposed by microbes.
Their degradation is rapid.	Their degradation is slow.
Biodegradable pollutants do not accumulate in nature.	They often accumulate in nature.
Used to produce energy, manure, compost and biogas.	Some of the pollutants, if properly separated, can be recycled.
These do not combine with other substances to produce toxins.	These may combine with other substances in nature to produce toxins.
They become a part of rapid turn over in biogeochemical cycles. For example, sewage, livestock wastes.	Most of them do not enter in biogeochemical cycle. Often are very slow and toxic. For example, DDT, BHC, polyethylene bags.

Based upon persistence

On the basis of their form in which it persists after the release, pollutant may be of two types, i.e. primary and secondary.

These are discussed in below table

Table 26.2 Differences between primary and secondary pollutants

Primary pollutants	Secondary pollutants
These are the pollutants, which enter the environment directly from the source.	These develop from the interaction of primary pollutants with atmospheric constituents.
No photochemical reaction.	These are formed through photochemical reactions that release nascent oxygen.
These are found in different states including reduced, oxidised, etc.	They are commonly oxidants.
There is no enhancement of effect of primary pollutants.	Secondary pollutants are more potent than the primary pollutants due to synergism.
For example, DDT, CO_2, SO_2 , flyash.	For example, Ozone (O_3), Peroxyacetyl Nitrate (PAN), nitrogen oxides, olefins, benzpyrene, PBN.

Types of pollution

Based upon different parameters, pollution can be divided into following types

(i) On the basis of its origin

- **Natural** This type of pollution is caused by natural phenomenon. It accounts for 99.95% of atmospheric pollution. For example, volcanic eruptions, release of methane (CH_4) by paddy fields and cattle, release of carbon monoxide (CO) by plants and animals, emission of natural gases, ozone, nitrogen oxides, cosmic rays, UV rays, etc.
- **Anthropogenic** This type of pollution is caused by human activities. It accounts for only 0.05% of atmospheric pollution. For example, burning of fossil fuels, deforestation, mining, sewage, industrial effluent, pesticides, fertilisers, etc.

(ii) On the basis of the most affected component of the environment

- Air pollution
- Water pollution
- Soil pollution

(iii) On the basis of physical nature of pollutants

- Gaseous pollution
- Dust pollution
- Thermal pollution
- Noise pollution
- Radioactive pollution

(iv) On the basis of emission of pollutants

- **Point source pollution** Pollution from a single source, e.g. chimney, municipal sewer.
- **Line source pollution** Pollution is passed along a narrow belt, e.g. roads due to automobile exhaust.
- **Area source pollution** Pollution from a whole area, e.g. mining area, industrial estate.
- **Diffuse source pollution** Pollution emitted from a large area, e.g. sprayed pesticides or fertilisers through run-off.
- **Fixed source pollution** Pollutants are passed from fixed spots, e.g. large factories, small scale industries, mineral smelters and electrical power plants.

AIR POLLUTION

The presence of any material or gas in air in concentration that can be harmful to men and environment is called air pollution.

Sources of air pollution

Various sources of air pollution are as follows

- Combustion of fossil fuels like coal, petroleum, etc., produce carbon monoxide and carbon dioxide along with sulphur oxide.
- Pollutants from automobiles, locomotives, aircrafts and exhausts in cities constitute the major part of the total air pollution.
- Smokestack of thermal power plants, smelters and other industries release particulate and gaseous air pollutants together with harmless gases such as N_2 and O_2.
- Natural sources include pollen, dust and smoke.

Air pollutants

These are of following two types

1. Primary air pollutants

These include the directly emitted pollutants from sources. These are further divided into following types

(i) **Particulate matter** These are added into the air by industries, automobiles and by many operations like drilling, crushing, grinding, etc.

- Various types of particulate matter include either solid or liquid particles.
- Settable particulate matter (diameter $\geq 10\ \mu m$) - settles in less than one day.
- Suspended particulate matter (diameter $\leq 10\ \mu m$) - remains suspended in air for weeks.
- Aerosols (less than 1 mm) - found in the form of fluorocarbons, chlorofluorocarbon, oxides of sulphur and nitrogen.
- It is emitted through jet and supersonic planes, refrigerators and air conditioners and solid plastic foams. Smoke is the visible suspension of carbon. It is released from burning and smouldering of organic matter.
- According to Central Pollution Control Board (CPCB), particulate size 2.5 mm or less in diameter (PM 2.50) are responsible for causing serious health hazards.

(ii) **Carbon monoxide** It is released from incomplete combustion of fossil fuels.

(iii) **Hydrocarbons** or **Volatile organic carbons** These are produced naturally (e.g. CH_4) or due to incomplete combustion.

(iv) **Sulphur dioxide** It is produced during the combustion of sulphur containing fossil fuels and smelting of ore.

(v) **Nitrogen oxides** These are mainly produced during the combustion of fossil fuels at high temperature in automobile engine.

2. Secondary air pollutants

- These are formed through reaction between primary pollutants, e.g. smog.
- Smog is opaque or dark fog having condensed water vapours, dust, smoke and gases. It was first described by **Des Voeux** in 1905.
- It is of two types, namely classical (London) smog and photochemical (Los Angeles) smog.

Table 26.3 Differences between classical smog and photochemical smog

Classical smog	Photochemical smog
It was first reported in London in 1952.	It was first reported in Los Angeles in 1946.
It occurs at low temperature.	It occurs at high temperature.
It has reducing effect on environment.	It has oxidising effect on environment.
It is dark brown in colour.	It is grey in colour.
It does not contain secondary pollutants.	It contains secondary pollutants (O_3, PAN).
It is formed by condensation of water vapours with H_2S and SO_2 over dust or smoke particles.	It is formed due to still air, emission of nitrogen oxides and hydrocarbons from automobile exhaust.

Effects of air pollution

Air pollution not only affects human health, but also plants and climate in many ways.

1. Effects on humans

Effects of air pollution on humans are as follows

- It causes many acute and chronic diseases in humans. The leakage of Methylisocyanate (MIC) gas killed over 2500 people in Bhopal, Madhya Pradesh in 1980.
- Carbon monoxide combines with haemoglobin in the blood to form Carboxyhaemoglobin (COHb). Affinity of CO for haemoglobin is 200 times more as compared to O_2.

  It reduces the oxygen carrying capacity of the blood, impair vision and psychomotor activity.
- Smoke causes respiratory problems like asthma, bronchitis. It also decreases visibility.
- Hay fever is very common form of pollen allergy.

- Besides these, a table describing the effects of different air pollutants is given below

Table 26.4 Common air pollutants and their effects on human body

Pollutants	Effects on human body
Aldehydes	Irritate nasal and respiratory tract.
Ammonia	Inflame upper respiratory passages.
Arsenic	Breakdown red blood cell, damage kidneys, causes jaundice, lung and skin cancer.
Carbon monoxide	Reduce O_2 carrying capacity of blood.
Chlorine	Attack entire respiratory tract and mucous membrane of eyes, cause pulmonary oedema.
Cyanides	Interfere with nerve cells, produce dry throat, indistinct vision, headache.
Fluorides	Irritate and corrode all body passages, causes osteoporosis.
Sulphides	Cause nausea, irritate eyes and throat.
Nitrogen oxides	Inhibit ciliary action of nose, causes bronchitis.
Phosgenes (carbonyl chloride $COCl_2$)	Induce coughing, irritation and sometimes fatal pulmonary oedema.
Sulphur	Causes chest constriction, headache, vomiting and death from respiratory elements.
Suspended particles (ash, soot, smoke)	Cause emphysema, eye irritations and possibly cancer.

2. Effects on plants

Air pollution affects plants in many ways. It causes damage to the crops and trees. Estimated crop losses from ozone pollution are 5-10%.

The effects of various pollutants on plants are tabulated below

Table 26.5 Injury thresholds and effects of air pollutants on plants

Pollutants	Effects on plants	ppm	Sustained exposure time
Ozone (O_3)	Fleck, bleaching, bleached spotting, growth suppression. Tips of conifer needles become brown and necrotic.	0.03	4 hrs
Sulphur dioxide (SO_2)	Bleached spots, bleached areas between veins, chlorosis, growth suppression, reduction in yield, leaf curling, inhibits ETS in plants, phaeophytisation in lichens.	0.03	8 hrs
Peroxyacetyl Nitrate (PAN)	Glazing silvering or bronzing on the lower surface of leaves.	0.01	6 hrs
Hydrogen Fluoride (HF)	Chlorosis, dwarfing leaf abscission, lower yield.	0.00 01	5 weeks
Chloride (Cl_2)	Bleaching between veins, tips and leaf abscission.	0.01	2 hrs
Ethylene (C_2H_4)	Withering, leaf abnormalities, flower dropping and failure of flower to open.	0.05	6 hrs

3. Effects on climate

- Air pollution have highly adverse effects on climate and one such effect is **acid rain**. This term was coined by **Robert August** in 1872.
- It refers to the rainfall having pH less than 5.65, due to the presence of acids such as H_2SO_4 and HNO_3.
- Acid rain is caused when oxides of nitrogen and sulphur react with water in the atmosphere.
- The concerned reactions are given below

$$2SO_2 + O_2 \longrightarrow 2SO_3$$
$$SO_3 + H_2O \longrightarrow H_2SO_4$$
$$2NO + O_2 \longrightarrow 2NO_2$$
$$N_2O_5 + H_2O \longrightarrow 2HNO_3$$

- These acids from atmosphere are deposited over earth in two forms *viz.*,
  (i) **Wet deposition** It includes rain, snow and fog.
  (ii) **Dry deposition** It includes wind blow, acidic gases and particles over trees.
- **Effect of acid rain** Acid rain damages plants by direct effect on foliage. It causes leaching of essential minerals of soil. It also affects freshwater reservoirs.
- The H_2SO_4 present in acid rain can corrode metals, marble, painted surfaces, slate, stone, etc. This phenomenon is called **stone leprosy**.
- The Taj Mahal at Agra is threatened by the corrosive action of acid deposition.
- It is believed that Taj Mahal is degrading due to air pollutants released from the oil refinery of Mathura. The H_2SO_4 present in acid rain combines with $CaCO_3$ of marble of Taj to form unstable $CaSO_4$.

$$CaCO_3 + H_2SO_4 \longrightarrow CaSO_4 + H_2O$$

Control of air pollution

Some of the methods to control air pollution are as follows

(i) **Use of high chimneys** Industrial plants should be advised to use high chimneys for the emission of smoke, fumes or heated air.

(ii) **Use of Compressed Natural Gas** (CNG) This has reduced vehicular pollution in Indian cities with a substantial fall in carbon monoxide, nitrogen oxides, sulphur dioxides, etc.

(iii) **Use of unleaded petrol** Tetraethyl lead is an antiknocking agent. It is added to unleaded petrol to control pollution.

Other control measures to control air pollution

I. Methods to control particulate pollutants are as follows

(i) **Arresters** These are the devices to separate particulate pollutants. These are of various types

- Cyclonic separators centrifugal force causes the settling of particulate matter and clean air is allowed to pass out.
- **Trajectory separators** Heavier particles settle down when dirty air is passed from a chamber as an oblique jet.
- **Filters** These are large-sized porous bags of polyester, polyprolene, polyamide, etc. Through these bags, dry emissions are passed under pressure to filter out particulate matter.
- **Electrostatic precipitators** Particulate matters present in dirty air are charged electrically. These are then passed through a chamber where they loose the charge and settle down.
  Electrostatic precipitators are the most efficient devices to remove over 99% of particulate matter present in the exhaust. They consist of high voltage electrode wires which produce a corona that release electrons.

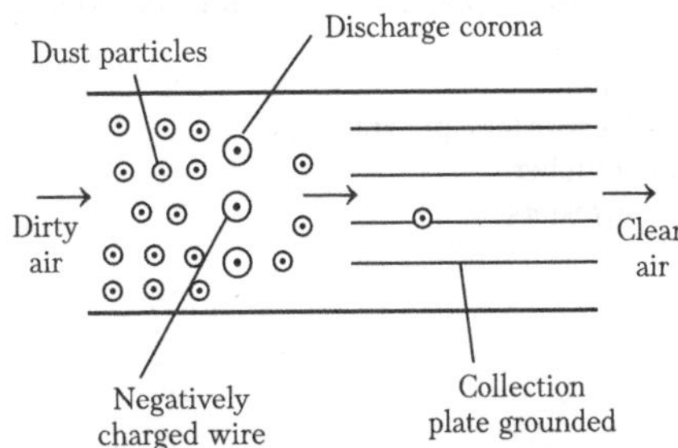

Fig. 26.1 Electrostatic precipitator

These electrons attach to dust particles and give them a net negative charge.
The collecting plates attract the charged dust particles. The velocity of air between the plates must be low enough to allow the dust to fall.

(ii) **Scrubber** It can remove gases like sulphur dioxide. In a scrubber, the effluent containing sulphur dioxide is passed through a slurry of water and crushed limestone ($CaCO_3$). The calcium in limestone combines with the sulphur to produce calcium sulphate ($CaSO_4$) which is collected separately.

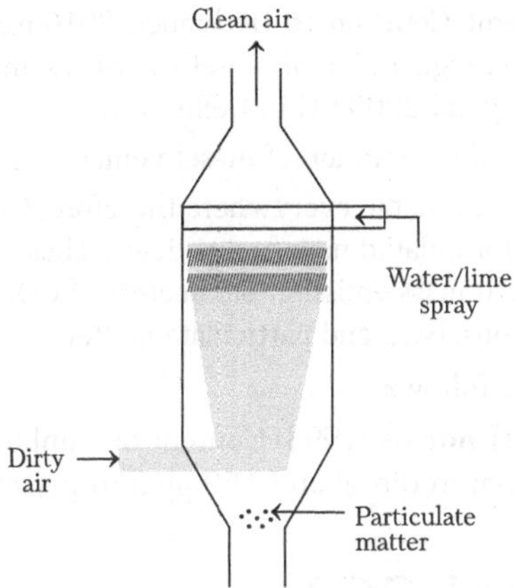

Fig 26.2 Scrubber

II. Methods to control gaseous pollutants are as follows

(i) **Adsorption technique** Very fine solid particles (e.g. charcoal) are used to remove toxic gases from dirty air.

(ii) **Combustion technique** The emission are burnt at high temperature to remove gaseous pollutants. It is applicable to oxidisable pollutants.

(iii) **Absorption technique** Gaseous pollutants are absorbed by scrubber having packing materials. The gaseous pollutants are absorbed here.

(iv) **Catalytic convertors** They contains expensive metals like platinum-palladium and rhodium as the catalysts. These catalysts are fitted into automobiles for reducing poisonous gaseous emissions.
As the exhaust passes through the catalytic converter, unburnt hydrocarbons are converted into carbon dioxide and water.
Carbon monoxide and nitric oxide are also changed into carbon dioxide and nitrogen gas, respectively.

Case study on air pollution

- In 2000, the Supreme Court directed the government to take appropriate measure for reducing air pollution.
- The government was asked to take appropriate measures within a specified time period. These measure include
  - Switch over of public transport from diesel/petrol to CNG.
  - Phasing out of old vehicles.
  - Compulsory use of unleaded petrol.
  - Fitting the vehicles with catalytic converter.
- Delhi became the first city of the world to use CNG in public transport and autorikshaw by the end of 2002.
- The Supreme Court on 16 December, 2016 passed an order and banned registration of diesel-run SUVs and cars having engines beyond 2000 CC in Delhi-NCR.
- NGT banned registration of diesel vehicles in Delhi.
- CNG is not available everywhere therefore, Government of India has formulated new fuel policies. These are related to the standard mass emission parameters of CO, hydrocarbons, NO_x and particulate matter.

These are as follows

(a) **Euro II norms** (1993) Content of sulphur at 350 ppm in diesel and 150 ppm in petrol.

(b) **Bharat stage II norm** It is equivalent to Euro II norms. It was first applicable in 11 cities of India and latter got applicable to all automobiles throughout the country from 1st April, in 2005.

(c) **Euro III norms** All automobiles (fuel-petrol and diesel) had to met the Euro III emission specifications in 11 cities of India from 1st April, in 2005.

(d) **Euro IV norms** They have to meet in 11 cities of India by 1st April in 2010.

(e) **Other European emission standards** That are applied to vehicles are Euro II (1993), Euro III (2000), Euro IV (2005), Euro V (2008) and Euro VI (2014).

Mass emission parameters in India

Types of vehicles	Norms	Cities of implementation
4 Wheelers	Bharat stage IV	Throughout the country since April 2017
3 Wheelers	Bharat stage IV	Throughout the country since 1st April 2017
2 Wheelers	Bharat stage IV	Throughout the country since April 2017

CHECK POINT 26.1

1. In pollution, the term synergism is used for
   (a) biomagnification of non-degradable pollutants
   (b) dangerous effect when two pollutants are present together
   (c) decreasing effect to a degradable pollutant
   (d) formation of more potent secondary pollutant from primary pollutants
2. Choose the correct statement.
   (a) Primary pollutants are more harmful than secondary pollutants
   (b) DDT is a secondary pollutant
   (c) Secondary pollutants are more harmful than primary pollutants
   (d) Both (b) and (c)
3. Select the correct match of air pollution source with the type of pollutant and the effect it produce.
   (a) Chemical factory $\rightarrow NO_2 \rightarrow$ Ozone hole
   (b) Automobile exhaust $\rightarrow N_2O \rightarrow$ Asphyxia effect
   (c) Heavy industry $\rightarrow CO_2 \rightarrow$ Acid rain
   (d) Incinerators $\rightarrow NO_x$ gases $\rightarrow$ Photochemical smog
4. Photochemical smog formed in congested metropolitan cities mainly consists of
   (a) ozone, peroxyacetyl nitrate and NO_x
   (b) smoke, peroxyacetyl nitrate and SO_2
   (c) hydrocarbons, SO_2 and CO_2
   (d) hydrocarbons, O_3 and SO_x
5. According to Central Pollution Control Board (CPCB), which particulate size in diameter (in micrometre) of the air pollutants is responsible for greatest harm to human health?
   (a) 2.5 or less (b) 1.5 or less
   (c) 1.0 or less (d) 5.2 or 2.5
6. A device 'X' used to control air pollution, remove gases which are involved in acid rain formation. Identify the device 'X'.
   (a) Filters
   (b) Electrostatic precipitators
   (c) Scrubber
   (d) Arresters

WATER POLLUTION

Water is said to be polluted when its quality gets degraded. It is caused due to the addition of various inorganic, organic, biological and radiological substances in water. It make water unfit and poses health hazard for human and all aquatic organisms.

Water pollutants may be of three types. These are as follows

(i) **Physical** These include floating debris, cans, paper, leaves, etc. These affect general appearance, turbidity, colour, taste and odour of water.

(ii) **Chemical** These include all the possible inorganic and organic substances, such as chlorides, sulphates, nitrates, nitrites, boron, heavy metals, pesticides, phenol, cyanide, oil, etc. They affect pH, acidity, alkalinity, hardness, conductivity, etc., of water.

(iii) **Biological** These include various pathogens. These may affect the quality of water and makes it unfit for use.

Sources of water pollution

Various sources of water pollution are as follows

- **Fertilisers and farm wastes** Run-off from agricultural fields.
- **Synthetic detergents** Washing clothes near water bodies.
- **Household wastage and sewage** Include carbohydrates, proteins, sugars, starch, cellulose, dextrin, glycogen, alginic acid, etc.
- **Pesticides** Include DDT, 2, 4-D, TEPP, aldrin, BHC, parathion.
- **Toxic metal** Pb, Zn, Ar, Cu, Cd, Hg, Ni from electroplating, chemical and copper pickling industries.
- **Oils** Tanks, machines, lubricants, factories and refineries waste.
- **Gaseous pollutants** NH_3, Cl, H_2S, O_2, phosphine, etc.
- **Fats, soaps and waxes** Food and household industries.
- **Dyes** Chemical industries.
- **Acids** HNO_3, H_2SO_4, etc.
- **Industrial agents**
  - **Paper and pulp** Free chlorine
  - **Textile** Minor acids, fats, oils and grease
  - **Food processing** Starch
  - **Chemical** Mineral acids, NH3, tartaric acid and nitrocompounds
  - **Metal** Fluorides, cyanogen and nuisance dust containing limestone and titanium dioxide.
  - **Petroleum** Hydrocarbons, phenols and fats.
  - **Tanneries** Sulphide, chromium, phenol and tannic acid.
  - **Acid and grease** Bad taste and odour to H_2O.
  - **Battery** Lead mineral acids.
  - **Wool scouring** Alkalis, fats, oils and grease.

Effects of water pollution

The various effects of water pollution are as follows

(i) Increase in BOD

- Water pollution may decrease the percentage of dissolved oxygen (DO) content of water bodies.
- Polluted water usually have higher **Biochemical Oxygen Demand** (BOD). It is the amount of O_2 (in mg) required to decompose organic matter present in one litre of water which is heavily polluted.
- Domestic sewage is rich in biodegradable organic matter. It stimulates the activity of several decomposers and thus, increases the BOD.
- This increase in BOD causes a sharp decline in dissolved oxygen in polluted water. It leads to mortality of fish and other aquatic creatures.

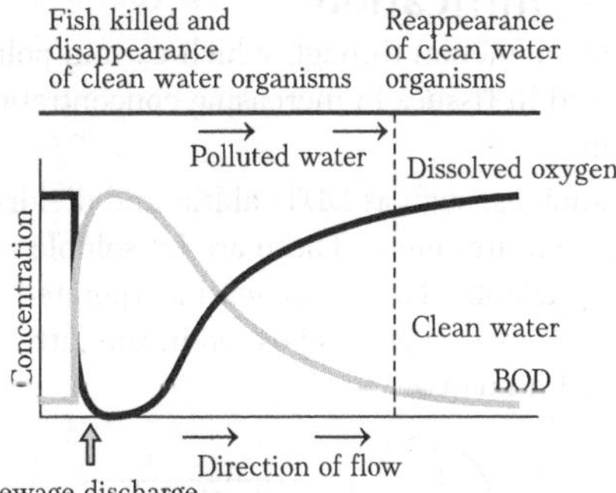

Fig. 26.4 Effect of sewage discharge and its recovery in a river

Note
- *Chemical Oxygen Demand (COD) is a measure of the capacity of water to consume oxygen during decomposition of organic matter and the oxidation of inorganic chemicals such as ammonia and nitrite.*
- *BOD below 1500 mg/L is regarded as low polluted, BOD 1500-4000 mg/L is regarded as medium polluted and above 4000 mg/L is regarded as highly polluted water.*

(ii) Eutrophication

- Due to the continuous addition of sewage waste, phosphates, nitrates, etc., in water bodies, these may become nutrient enriched. This is known as eutrophication.
- Such water bodies are highly productive and they support a dense growth of plants and algae.
- This extensive increase of algae growth in water bodies is called **algal bloom** (water bloom).

The impacts of algal bloom growth in water bodies are as follows

- It imparts a distinct colour to the water bodies due to their pigments.
- The blooms are generally not utilised by zooplanktons and they cause deterioration of the water quality and lead to fish mortality.
- Some bloom forming algae (e.g. *Microcystis*) are extremely toxic to animals.
- *Eichhorina crassipes* (water hyacinth) grows abundantly in eutrophic lakes and causes imbalance in ecosystem. For this reason, this weed is also known as **'Terror of Bengal'**.

The process of eutrophication occur *via* two modes as follows

(a) **Natural eutrophication** is natural ageing of lake due to nutrient enrichment of water body. It is a slow process.

(b) **Accelerated eutrophication** is caused by human activities like effluents from the industries and homes, etc. It shows a rapid growth of organisms.

Note *Tubifex and Chironomus can survive in a eutrophic lake therefore, they are considered to be pollution indicators.*

(iii) Biomagnification

- It is the phenomenon through which certain pollutants get accumulated in tissues in increasing concentrations along the food chain.
- Many pesticides, such as DDT, aldrin and dieldrin, sustain for long in the environment. These are fat soluble and generally non-biodegradable. Thus, they get incorporated into the food chain and ultimately gets deposited in the fatty tissues of animals and humans.

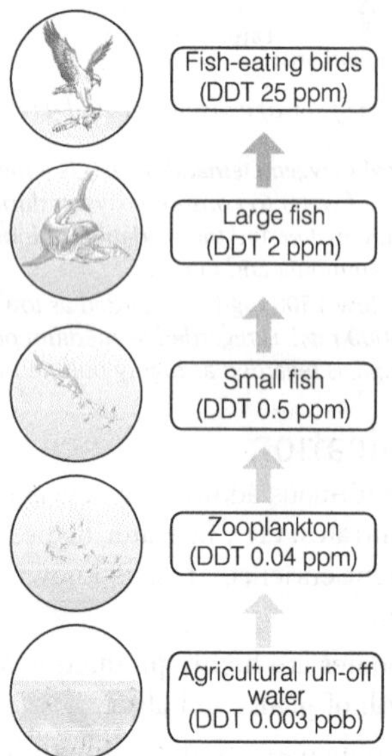

***Fig. 26.5** Biological magnification : The amount of DDT in an organism increases as we go up the food chain. This illustration depicts an eight million-fold amplification of the DDT*

- In the food chain, these pollutants get magnified in the higher trophic levels.
- The phenomenon of biological magnification has also been reported for certain other pollutants, such as heavy metals like lead, mercury and copper and radioactive substances such as strontium-90.
- It can be destructive for organisms at higher trophic levels.
- For example, high concentration of DDT disturb calcium metabolism in birds. It causes thinning of egg shell and their premature breaking. It eventually cause decline in bird population.

Note *Recently microorganisms capable of metabolising chlorinated hydrocarbons have been discovered. They possess enzyme **dehalogenase**.*

Table 26.6 Some water pollutants and their toxic effects in humans

Pollutant elements	Toxic effects
Aluminium	Interferes with phosphate metabolism, inhibit absorption of fluorides, Ca and iron compounds.
Arsenic	Loss of appetite, copious secretion of mucus in respiratory tract, black foot disease.
Cadmium	Itai-itai disease (Japan), kidney damage.
Fluorine	Fluorosis, about 5-12 ppm is toxic, enamel becomes brittle, bones lose their elasticity and are prone to fractures, impairs glycolysis, knock-knee disease.
Lead	Anaemia and mental retardation due to degenerative changes in motor nerves.
Mercury	Minamata disease, main site of injury is CNS leading to tremors, inability to coordinate, impairment of vision and loss of hearing. Two major episodes of mercury poisoning have occurred in Japan, in Minamata bay and Niigata. Mercury was absorbed, bioaccumulated and biomagnified to higher levels. Fish collected from this bay had 10-12 mg of Hg per kg of their flesh and bones. The largest mercury epidemic occurred in 1971-72 in Iraq, when 6000 people were affected and 500 died; infertility in human.
Nitrate	Fatal for infants, reacts with haemoglobin and forms methaemoglobin that impairs oxygen transport. This causes methaemoglobinemia or blue-baby syndrome in infants.
DDT	Causes cancer, affects sex hormones in mammals, hormonal disturbances, delayed ovulation and inhibition of gonad development.

Control of water pollution

Water pollution of natural resources can be reduced and controlled by following methods

- Biomagnification of toxic chemicals can be controlled by limited use of fertilisers and pesticides.
- Effect of acid rain can be reduced by the use of less sulphur, tall chimneys, etc.
- Sewage contains a large quantity of human excreta, organic matter and microbes. It should be first treated in sewage treatment plant before discharging into the water bodies.
- **Ecosanitation** is a sustainable system for handling human excreta using dry composting toilets. This composting method recycles human excreta into a natural fertiliser, which reduces the need of chemical fertilisers.
- **NEERI** (National Environmental Engineering Research Institute) have devised a very cheap and unconventional process of sewage treatment in especially constructed large shallow ponds.

Integrated wastewater treatment

Waste or Polluted water can be treated in an integrated manner by utilising a mix of artificial and natural process. These are as follows

- **Conventional method** Filtering, sedimentation and chlorine treatment for removing organic remains and microbes.
- **Innovative approach** A series of six connected marshes in 60 hectares of marshland is developed which is seeded with bacteria, algae, fungi and plants. This biota neutralises, assimilates and absorbs the pollutants. As the water flows through the marshes, it gets purified naturally. These marshes also constitute a sanctuary with a high level of biodiversity. A citizen group called **Friends Of Arcata Marsh** (FOAM) looks after the project.

Note
- *Stoneflies are very sensitive to pollution and only live in the very cleanest streams.*
- *In a polluted lake, Daphnia acts as index of pollution.*
- *E. coli grows rapidly in water containing faecal organic matter.*

THERMAL POLLUTION

It can be defined as 'warming up of an aquatic ecosystem to the point, where desirable organisms are adversely affected' (Owen; 1985).

Cause of thermal pollution

- A large number of industrial plants use cold water from the rivers and discharge hot water into it. The electric power, steel and chemical industries are the most important users of cold water.
- A single 1000 MW power plant may use one-half million gallons of cold water per minute.
- In many countries, atomic energy plants have become a major source of thermal pollution, which is harmful to the fishes and aquatic invertebrates.

Sources of thermal pollution

Major sources of thermal pollution are large scale industries, thermal power plants, oil refineries, etc.

Effects of thermal pollution

Harmful effects of thermal pollution on aquatic ecosystem are as follows

- Reduction in dissolved oxygen.
- Interference with reproduction of aquatic animals.
- Increased vulnerability of diseases.
- Direct mortality of aquatic organisms.
- Invasion of destructive organisms.
- Undesirable changes in algal population.
- Elimination of flora and fauna of cold water.

Control of thermal pollution

Thermal pollution can be controlled by the following ways

(i) **Cooling ponds** are used to store hot water from condensers. Evaporation cools the water and after cooling, water is discharged into the nearby water bodies.

(ii) **Spray ponds** are used to receive hot water from condensers. Water is sprayed through the nozzles and heat is dissipated in the air through droplets.

(iii) **Cooling towers** These are of following two types

- **Wet cooling tower** It contains baffles in which cool air enters from sides, takes away the heat and cools the water.
- **Dry cooling tower** It contains a system of pipes, which contains hot water. Air is allowed to flow through these pipes with fans. It is a costly method.

SOIL POLLUTION

It is the unfavourable alteration of soil caused by the removal or addition of substances, which decreases its productivity, quality of plants and ground water, etc.

It can be of following two types

(i) **Negative soil pollution** It is the reduction in soil productivity due to erosion, overuse, deforestation, desertification, etc.

(ii) **Positive soil pollution** It is the reduction in soil productivity due to the addition of undesirable substances, e.g. agrochemicals, industrial wastes, etc.

Sources of soil pollution

- Pesticides and fertilisers are the major factors that cause soil pollution.
- Landscape or third pollution also contributes to soil pollution by converting the fertile land into barren land.
- Major sources are discussed below

(i) **Biological agents** These include excreta of human, animals and birds, digested sewage sludge.

(ii) **Industrial and urban waste** These include

(a) Coal and mineral mines, metal processing industries and engineering industries.

(b) Domestic wastes, i.e. sludge.

(c) Garbage, rubbish materials such as paper, residues from home, fuels, street sweepings, glasses and abandoned vehicles, etc.

(iii) **Agricultural practices** These include the use of fertilisers, pesticides, fumigant, chemical agents, phosphates, nitrates, DDT, BHC, endrin, aldrin, dieldrin, organosulphurous compounds, organic compounds with Pb, Hg, Ar. Lindane has been reported to taint carrots.

(iv) **Radiological agents** These are derived from nuclear explosion and radioactive wastes (nuclear testing and laboratories) like, ruthenium 106, rhodium 106, iodine 131, barium 140, lanthanium 140, cerium 144, promethium 144, carbon 14, caesium 137.

Effects of soil pollution

- Crops and plants grown on polluted soil absorb much of the pollution and then pass these into the food chain.
- Plants are unable to adapt when the chemistry of the soil changes.
- The toxic chemicals present in the soil can decrease soil fertility and therefore, decrease the crop yield.

Control of soil pollution

These are as follows

- It may be done by safer land use, planned urbanisation, controlled developmental activities, safe disposal and the management of solid wastes.
- Soil pollution can be controlled by recovering and recycling waste items like plastics, tincans, other metals, glass, polyethylenes, rags, papers, etc. These are picked up by rag pickers and recycled in recycling units to make new items.
- To reduce soil pollution, solid waste is sometimes disposed off by burning.

  The methods of burning are

  (i) **Incineration** Carried out at very high temperature, i.e. 900-1300°C.

  (ii) **Pyrolysis** It is combustion at temperature of 1650°C, in the absence of oxygen.
- **Integrated organic farming** It is a cyclic zero waste procedure of farming where waste of one process are cycled as nutrients for the other processes.
  In this procedure, instead of chemical fertilisers cattle excreta is used as manure. **Ramesh Chandra Dagar**, a farmer in Sonipat, Haryana is doing organic farming. He includes bee-keeping, dairy management, water harvesting, composting and agriculture in a chain of processes that allow a sustainable venture.
- **Reforestation** is the process of restoring a forest that once existed, but was removed at some point of time in the past.

CHECK POINT 26.2

1. A lake near a village suffered heavy mortality of fishes within a few days. Which of the following statements could be the incorrect explanation?
   (a) Phosphate fertilises when used in the crops near by fields
   (b) Phytoplankton populations in the lake declined initially which reduces photosynthesis
   (c) The lake water tuns green and stinky
   (d) Due to growth of *Eichhornia crassipes* in lake
2. *E. coli* is used as an indicator organism to determine the pollution of water with
   (a) industrial effluents (b) heavy metals
   (c) pollen of aquatic plants (d) faecal matter
3. A dental disease characterised by molting of teeth due to the presence of 'X' in drinking water. Which of the following is that 'X' element?
   (a) Chlorine (b) Boron (c) Fluorine (d) Arsenic
4. Formation of non-functional methaemoglobin causes blue-baby syndrome. This is due to
   (a) excess of arsenic concentration in drinking water
   (b) excess of nitrates in drinking water
   (c) deficiency of iron in food
   (d) increased methane content in the atmosphere
5. In which one of the following options, the BOD (Biological Oxygen Demand) of Sewage (S), Distillery Effluent (DE), Paper Mill Effluent (PE) and Sugar Mill Effluent (SE) have been arranged in ascending order?
   (a) SE < S < PE < DE
   (b) SE < PE < S < DE
   (c) PE < S < SE < DE
   (d) S < DE < PE < SE
6. Which of the following is not a bioindicator of water pollution?
   (a) Sludge worms
   (b) Blood worms
   (c) Stone flies
   (d) Sewage fungus
7. In an area where DDT has been used extensively, the population of birds declined significantly. What can be the reason?
   (a) Birds stopped laying eggs, they become sterile
   (b) Cobras were feeding on their eggs
   (c) The egg shells are weak
   (d) Both (a) and (c)

NOISE POLLUTION

Noise is defined as any loud disturbing sound dumped into the ambient atmosphere. It is measured by a sound meter and is expressed in a unit called **decibel** (dB). Any value more than 80 dB causes noise pollution. The intensity of sound in normal conversation is 30-60 dB. Noise becomes unhearable at 140 dB.

Sources of noise pollution

The various sources of noise pollution are as follows

- Sounds from industries such as textile mills, construction site, etc.
- Agricultural machines like tractors, tubewells, etc.
- Defence equipment such as tanks, artillery, explosion.
- Public address system like loudspeakers.
- Dynamite blasting.
- Crackers used during marriages and festivals.
- Bull dozing, stone crushings, etc.
- Transport automobiles and other vehicles such as trucks, buses, etc.

Effects of noise pollution

The various effects of noise pollution are as follows

- Prolonged and continuous high intensity noise may cause a partial or even permanent loss of hearing. A sudden loud noise such as an explosion can damage the tympanic membrane.

Table 26.7 High intensity noise and human health hazards

Noise intensity (dB)	Health hazards
80 (scooter, radio)	Annoying
90 (truck, bus)	Hearing damage (8 hrs)
95	Very annoying
110 (train)	Stimulation of reception in skin
120	Pain threshold
130-135	Nausea, vomiting and dizziness
140	Pain in ear, prolong exposure causing insanity
150 (jet aeroplane)	Significant change in pulse rate
160	Other minor permanent damage if prolonged
180 (rocket)	Eardrum ruptures and major permanent damage
194	Lung damage

- Noise can cause anxiety and stress. However, it can lead to fright. It causes headache by dilating blood vessels of the brain, eye strain by dilating the pupil, etc.
- It can increase the rate of heartbeat, constriction of blood vessels, decreased heart output and sleeplessness.
- It can impair the development of nervous system of unborn babies.
- Functioning of many internal organs, including endocrine glands gets disturbed.
- Reproductive cycle gets disturbed.
- Hatching of birds is disturbed.

Control of noise pollution

The following measures can be used to control noise pollution

(i) **By enforcing concerned laws** The laws should be strictly enforced as per the provisions. The permissible sound level in different areas are given in the following table

Table 26.8 The permissible sound levels in different areas

Zones	Day	Night
Industrial	75 dB	70 dB
Commercial	65 dB	55 dB
Residential	55 dB	45 dB
Silent	50 dB	40 dB

(ii) **Machines** All machines should be designed to produce lesser noise. These should be maintained properly and lubricated from time to time.

(iii) **Loudspeakers** The volume should be kept low.

(iv) **Green belt vegetation** Green muffler or green belt vegetation is rows of trees and shrubs grown and maintained to serve as noise absorbers. Neem and Ashoka trees absorb sound vibrations to a great extent.

(v) **Ear plugs and ear muffs** Traffic police personal and factory workers exposed to high noise pollution should be provided with the ear plugs or ear muffs.

(vi) **Sound diversion** These devices should be used to deflect the sound.

RADIOACTIVE POLLUTION

It is physical pollution of air, water and soil caused due to the presence of radioactive materials. These materials have the ability to emit ionizing radiations containing α-particles, β-particles and γ-rays spontaneously by the disintegration of their atomic nuclei.

Sources of radioactive pollution

Various sources of radioactive pollution are given below

- Elements such as radium 224, uranium 235, uranium 238, thorium 232, radon 222 and carbon 14 naturally emit radiations.
- Man-made sources of radioactive pollution include mining and refining of plutonium and thorium, atomic explosions, atomic reactors and nuclear fuel.
- Accidental leakage may also be a source of radioactive pollution. It had occurred in the three mile Island incident of USA in 1979 and chernobyl incident.
- Some radioactive materials found in tobacco smoke, e.g. polonium 210, also contributes to radioactive pollution.
- Radioactive Iodine (RAI) is a therapy used in the treatment of some thyroid cancers, especially papillary and follicular thyroid cancer.

  A certain form of radioactive iodine is used : I-131. It is found to be the most effective in eliminating thyroid cells, but it may also cause radioactive pollution.

Effects of radioactive pollution

Radioactive pollution adversely affect living forms in following ways

- Bioaccumulation of radioisotopes takes place in the aquatic food chains. As a result, river insects have many times more radioactivity than the water they inhabit. Fishes also take up radioactive materials by the ingestion and assimilation with food and by absorption. The most abundant nuclides found in river animals are P 32, Cu 64, Cr 51, Zn 65 and Na 24.
- Embryo is particularly susceptible to damage by radiation due to mutations.
- At high doses, nuclear radiations are lethal. At lower dose, it may cause several disorders. For example, Strontium 90 (Sr 90) is a dangerous radioactive pollutant that causes bone cancer, leukaemia and degradation of body tissues.

Control of radioactive pollution

- Leakage of radioactive elements from nuclear reactors, laboratories and industries should be checked.
- Radioactive wastes should be transformed into harmless form or stored in safe place.

SOLID WASTES

These are discarded or left over solid materials produced due to human activities. These wastes refer to everything that goes out in trash.

Types of solid wastes

Depeneding upon source, solid waste is of three types

(i) **Municipal solid wastes** These wastes are from homes, offices, schools, hospitals, etc. The municipal wastes generally comprise paper, food wastes, plastic, glass, metals, rubber, leather, textile, etc.

(ii) **Hospital wastes** Hospitals generate hazardous wastes that contain disinfectants and harmful chemicals and also pathogenic microorganisms.

(iii) **Electronic wastes** (e-wastes) These include irreparable computers, mobiles and other electronic goods. Recycling is the only solution for the treatment of e-wastes.

Control of solid wastes

These are as follows

- Solid wastes can be recovered or recycled. These articles are tins, cans and other metal wastes, etc.
  For example, polyblend is a fine powder of recycled modified plastic developed by **Ahmed Khan**. He also proved that when polyblend and bitumen were mixed together and used to lay roads, the water repellant property of bitumen gets increased.
- Dumping or landfilling is pilling of waste on selected low lying land. Open landfilling is dumping of waste material on uncovered low lying area. The waste is burnt periodically or compressed at intervals. In sanitary landfilling, wastes are dumped in a depression or trench after compactions.
- A scientific method of treating e-wastes in an environment friendly manner is called **evencs**. e-wastes are buried in landfill.
- Other methods of disposing wastes are source reduction, composting, incineration, etc.

CHECK POINT 26.3

1. The intensity level of whispering noise (daytime) is
(a) 10-15 dB (b) 20-30 dB (c) 45 50 dB (d) 55-60 dB

2. The effect of today's radioactive fall out will probably be more harmful to children of future generation than the present day children because
(a) as infants are more susceptible to radiations
(b) susceptibility to radiations increases with age
(c) mutated genes are usually recessive
(d) All of the above

3. Choose the incorrectly matched pair.
(a) Polonium 210 – Tobacco smoke
(b) Strontium 90 – Least harmful to humans
(c) Zinc 65 – Abundant in aquatic animals
(d) None of the above

4. Which of the following is correct regarding the remedy for plastic waste?
(a) Polyblend is a fine mixture of recycled modified plastic
(b) It is a zero waste procedure
(c) The blend of polyblend and bitumen helps to increase road life
(d) Both (a) and (c)

5. For which of the following, incineration is crucial or necessary?
(a) Agriculture waste
(b) Industrial waste
(c) Radioactive waste
(d) Hospital waste

CONSEQUENCES OF POLLUTION

Pollution causes major problems, which affect organisms globally. Some of these problems are discussed below

Ozone layer depletion

- Ozone (O_3) is a triatomic gas lying 17-26 km above the earth's surface in the stratosphere. It absorbs about 99% of the harmful incoming Ultraviolet (UV) radiations from the sun and prevents them from reaching the earth's surface.
- Ozone layer is continuously being formed and degraded by the action of UV rays in the stratosphere.
- The mechanism of formation of ozone is depicted in the figure given below

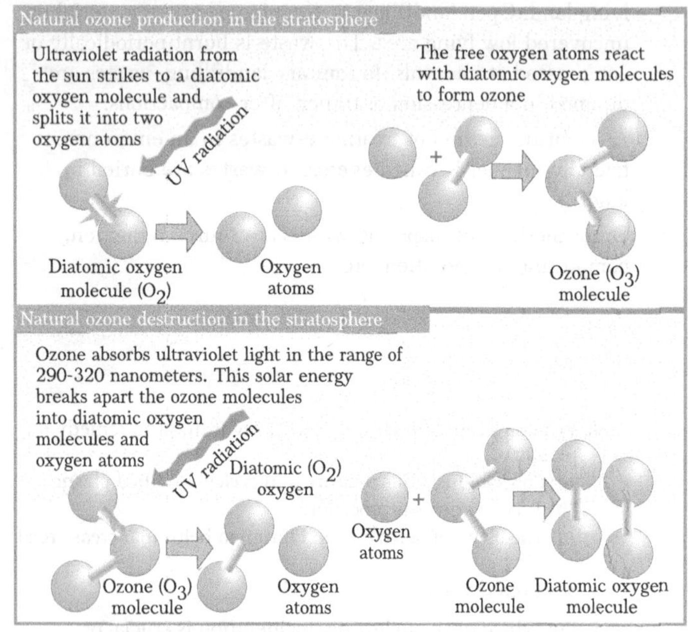

Fig. 26.6 Ozone production and destruction in nature

Various features of ozone layer are as follows

- Ozone layer found in stratosphere protects the earth from harmful UV rays. Hence, it is also known as **'good ozone'**.
- Apart from stratosphere, ozone is found in lower atmosphere. This ozone is harmful for food plants and animals. It is also known as the **'bad ozone'**.
- **Dobson Unit** (DU) is a measurement of column ozone levels (the ozone between the earth's surface and outer space).
- In the tropics, ozone levels are typically between 250 and 300 DU year-round.
- In temperate regions, seasonal variations can produce large swings in ozone levels. These variations occur even in the absence of ozone depletion.
The problem of ozone depletion was first detected in 1985 by **Farman *et al.*** Researchers discovered that the ozone in the upper stratosphere over Antarctica is being constantly destroyed during the Antarctic spring (September - December).
- **American Nimbus** seven satellite recorded a substantial depletion of ozone layer over Antarctica. This has resulted in the formation of a large area of thinned ozone layer known as **ozone hole**. These holes are usually thinner in tropics and denser towards poles.

Mechanism of ozone depletion

- Ozone is being depleted by the excessive use of certain chemicals known as **Ozone Depleting Compounds** (ODCs).
- For example, chlorofluorocarbon, CH_4, CCl_4, halons, N_2O, etc. Among these, CFCs are the major ozone depleting compounds used in refrigerators.
- These are extremely stable and are able to stay in atmosphere for long time. These also act as hungry 'ozone eaters'.
- The CFCs discharged in the lower part of the atomosphere move upward and reach to the stratosphere.
- There, CFC destroy ozone in following steps
  (i) In the stratosphere, UV rays act on CFC and release Cl atoms.

$$CFCl_3 \xrightarrow{UV-C} CFCl_2 + Cl$$

$$CFCl_2 \xrightarrow{UV-C} CFCl + Cl$$

  (ii) Chlorine reacts with ozone in chainomatic method and convert it into oxygen.

$$Cl + O_3 \longrightarrow ClO + O_2$$

$$ClO + O_3 \longrightarrow Cl + 2O_2$$

- One active chlorine can destroy 5000 molecules of ozone in one month and about 1 lac ozone molecuels during its stay in stratosphere.
- Cl atoms merely act as catalyst and are not consumed in the reaction. Thus, CFCs have permanent and continuing affects on ozone layer.

Harmful effects of ozone layer depletion

Depletion of ozone layer has some direct as well as indirect harmful effects. Some of them are given below

(i) **Rain failure** Due to the depletion of ozone layer in stratosphere, the temperature of earth increases and cause failure of rainfall.

(ii) **Increase in radiation** Reduction of O_3 in stratosphere would allow UV rays to reach the earth.

(iii) **Cancer** Due to thinning of ozone layer, threat of skin cancer (melanoma) may increase. A 5% decrease in stratospheric ozone is likely to increase 10-20% cases of skin cancer globally.

(iv) **High dose of UV-B** causes inflammation of cornea, thus leading to **snow blindness**, cataract, etc. UV-B affects the human skin maximally whereas UV-A has least effects.

(v) **Other effects** Destruction of aquatic flora and fauna, loss of immunity are some other effects of O_3 depletion.

Table 26.9 Effects of ozone on human health

Concentrations (ppm)	Effects observed
0.2	No ill effects
0.3	Nose and throat irritation
3.0	Extreme fatigue after two hours
9.0	Severe pulmonary oedema

Since 1987, nations and their leaders have cut their consumption of ozone depleting substances by 70%. Although, the phase out is still not complete and there is a significant black market in CFCs. Ozone loss is projected to diminish gradually untill around 2050, so that the polar ozone holes would return to 1975 levels.

Note *Ozone Day is observed on **16th September** every year.*

Greenhouse effect

It is a naturally occurring phenomenon responsible for heating of earth's surface and atomosphere.

It was first described by **Fourier** in 1827. Without greenhouse effect, the average temperature at surface of earth would have been chilly (–18°) rather than the present average temperature of 15°C.

Concept of greenhouse

- The term greenhouse effect has been derived from a phenomenon that occurs in a greenhouse.
- A **greenhouse** looks like a small glass house and is used for growing plants, especially during winters.
- In a greenhouse, the glass panel lets the light come in, but does not allow the heat to escape. Therefore, the greenhouse gets warm up and allow the growth of plants.
- Similarly, some gases called **greenhouse gases** absorb the irradiatied waves, but prevent the long wave (infrared) radiations from escaping the earth. IPCC (Intergovernmental Panel on Climate Change) periodically monitors the atmospheric concentration of Greenhouse Gases (GHGs).

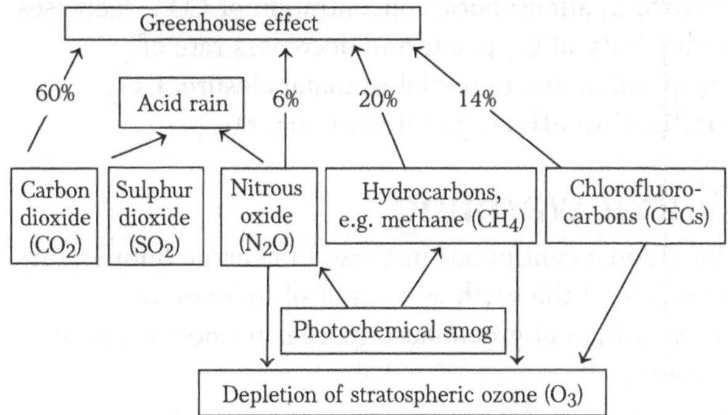

Fig. 26.7 Differential greenhouse effect

Mechanism of greenhouse effect

- Clouds and gases reflect about one-fourth of the incoming solar radiation and absorb some of it. Almost half of incoming solar radiation falls on earth's surface and heat it.
- A small portion of these radiation is reflected back in the form of infrared (IR) radiation.
- In greenhouse effect, these IR radiations does not escape into space as greenhouse gases (CO_2, CH_4) absorb a major fraction of it.
- The molecules of these gases radiate heat energy and a major part of it again comes to earth's surface. This downward flux of radiation is called **greenhouse flux**. This cycle is repeated many a times.
- Various sources of greenhouse gases are as follows

(i) **Carbon dioxide** (CO_2) Present level in atmosphere is 380 ppm (parts per million) and its atmospheric lifetime is 5-200 yrs. It is increasing due to fossil fuel's burning, deforestation and change in land use.

(ii) **Nitrous oxide** (N_2O) Present atmospheric concentration is 316 ppb (parts per billion). Major sources are agriculture, biomass burning, nylon industries, nitrogen rich fertilisers and fuels.

(iii) **Methane** (CH_4) Present level in atmosphere is 1750 ppb (parts per billion). Methanogen bacteria increase greenhouse effect by producing methane. The major sources are freshwater wetlands, enteric fermentation in cattle, flooded rice fields along with biomass burning.

(iv) **Chlorofluorocarbons** (CFCs) Present atmospheric concentration is 282 ppt (part per trillion). Atmospheric lifetime is 45-260 yrs. Major sources include leaking from air conditioners, refrigeration units, evaporation of industrial solvents, production of plastic foams and propellants in aerosol and spraycans.

Effects

Increase in atmospheric concentration of CO_2, increases productivity of C_3 plants and decreases rate of transpiration due to partial stomatal closure, **CO_2 fertilisation effect**, global warming, etc.

Global warming

The gradual continuous increase in average temperature of surface of the earth as a result of increase in concentration of greenhouse gases is termed as global warming.

The carbon dioxide in our atmosphere acts like a light filtre. It allows certain wavelengths of visible light to pass through, but absorbs others, especially infrared light.

Effects of global warming

Various effects of global warming are as follows

- The temperature of the earth has increased by 0.6°C in last three decads. It has lead to changes in precipitation patterns.
- Rise in temperature leads to deleterious changes in environment, resulting in odd climatic changes called **El Nino effect.**
- The rise in temperature has lead to increased melting of polar ice caps. It can cause rise in sea level and thus, many coastal areas are at the risk of getting submerged.
- Increased temperature causes increased weed growth, eruption of disease and pests. Thus, crop productivity also decreases.

International initiative for mitigating global changes

(i) Kyoto protocol

- Kyoto protocol hosted an international conference 1997 of G-77 (a group of 140 developing countries) from December 1-10 to discuss global warming.
- The detailed rules for the implementation of the protocol were adopted at COP-7 in Marrakesh, Morocco, in 2001 and these are referred to as the **Marrakesh Accords**. Its first commitment period started in 2008 and ended in 2012 .
- This protocol requires countries to take appropriate measures to reduce their overall GHGs emission to a level at least 5% below 1990 level by the commitment 2008-2012.
- To assess the role of human activities in climate change, the World Meteorological Organisation (WMO) and United Nations Environmental Programme (UNEP) setup an Intergovernmental Panel on Climate Change (IPCC) in 1988.
- The IPCC and United Nations Framework on Climate Change (UNFCC) that had reviewed the situation in October 1997, submitted their report in Kyoto in Kyoto Protocol.
- **Doha amendment** In Doha, Qatar on 8th December 2012, Kyoto protocol was given second commitment period from 1st January 2013 to 31st December 2020.

(ii) Montreal protocol

It aimed at protecting stratospheric ozone. It was proposed in 1987, but became effective in 1989.

(iii) Earth summit

United Nations Conference on Environment and Development, 1992 was held in Rio de Janeiro (Brazil) and adopted the recommendations of Convention on Climate Change (CCC) for reducing greenhouse gases.

Laws for controlling pollution

There are some laws for controlling the pollution. These are as follows

- **Environment** (protection) **Act, 1986** This act is implemented for air, water, soil and noise pollution.
- **Water** (prevention and control of pollution) **Act, 1974** This rule ensures quality of water, ways and means to control water pollution, prevention of detrimental effects on human health, etc.
- **Insecticide Act, 1968** It controls manufacture, import, sale, distribution and use of insecticides to reduce the risk to human health and pollution of natural resources.
- **Air** (prevention and control of pollution) **Act, 1981** It is applied to prevent quality degradation of air by controlling air pollution. The act was amended in 1987 to include noise in it as an air pollutant.
- Other laws are as follows
  - Management and Handling of Hazardous Toxic Waste Rules, 1989.
  - Biomedical Waste Management and Handling Rules, 1998.
  - Recycled Plastic Manufacture and Usage Rules, 1999.

- Noise Pollution Rules, 2000.
- Ozone Depleting Substances Rules, 2000.
- Municipal Solid Wastes Rules, 2000.
- Hazardous Wastes Management, Handling and Transboundary Rules, 2008.

Note
- *World Environment Day is observed on **5th June** every year.*
- *National Pollution Prevention Day is observed on 2nd December.*

Deforestation

- It is the conversion of forested areas to non-forested areas. It is estimated that about 40% forests have been lost in the tropics, compared to only 1% in the temperate regions.
- In India, at the beginning of the 20th century, forests covered was about 30% of the total land. By the end of the century, was shrunk to 19.4%.
- The National Forest Policy (1988) of India has recommended 33% forest cover for the plains and 67% for the hills.

Causes of deforestation

Various causes of deforestation are listed below

- Deforestation is contributed by a number of human activities. For example, trees are axed for timber, firewood, cattle ranching, human establishment, etc.
- Jhum cultivation or slash and burn agriculture is one of the major source of deforestation. It is the farming practice in North-Eastern states of India. In Jhum cultivation, the farmers cut down the trees of the forest and burn the plant remains. The ash is used as a fertiliser and the land is then used for farming or cattle grazing. After cultivation, the area is left for several years so as to allow its recovery. The farmers then move on to other areas and repeat this process.

Effect of deforestation

The effects of deforestation includes

- Increase in carbon dioxide (CO_2) concentration in the atmosphere because trees that could hold a lot of carbon in their biomass are lost with deforestation.
- It also causes loss of biodiversity due to habitat destruction.
- Soil erosion that may lead to desertification.

Forest conservation

Various case studies in forest conservation are as follows

(i) Amrita devi movement

- A Bishnoi woman, Amrita Devi in 1731, showed exemplary courage by hugging a tree and daring King's people to cut her first before cutting the tree.
- The king's men did not consider her pleas and cut down trees along with Amrita Devi.
- Her three daughters and hundreds of villagers followed her and lost their life while saving trees.
- On her honour and memory, Government of India instituted, the **Amrita Devi Bishnoi Wildlife Protection Award** for individuals or communities from rural areas that have shown extraordinary courage and dedication to save forests and wildlife.

(ii) Chipko movement

- The Chipko Movement (Chipko means to hug or stick to) was launched in 1974 by **Chandi Prasad Bhatt** and **Sunder Lal Bahuguna** against large scale falling of trees by timber contractors in the Uttarakhand hills.
- The starting of movement occurred from Chamoli district of Garhwal region in Uttarakhand.
- The unique feature of Chipko Movement was that local hill women from villages, were organised and made aware of the ecological threat in the hills.
- They took active part in the campaign.
- They embraced trees, when the timber contractors reached and compelled them to leave.
- This novel campaign of saving hill forests and greenery soon spread all along the hill region.
- Later in Karnataka in the South, by Panduranga hedge, in 1983, it was named **Appiko**.

(iii) Joint Forest Management (JFM)

- This concept started by government in 1980s for protecting and managing forests with the help of local people.
- In return, the local communities can obtain forest products like fruits, gum, rubber, medicine, etc., to earn their livelihood. Thus, forests can be conserved in sustainable ways.

CHECK POINT 26.4

1. Which one of the following is the correct percentage of the two (out of the total of four) greenhouse gases that contribute to the global warming?
   (a) CFCs 14%, CH_4 20%
   (b) CO_2 40%, CFCs 30%
   (c) N_2O 6%, CO_2 86%
   (d) CH_4 20%, N_2O 18%
2. Find the odd statement about global warming.
   (a) Increased CO_2 concentration has led to global warming
   (b) Industrialisation and deforestation are the major factors responsible for global warming
   (c) Global warming has helped in generation of greenhouse effect
   (d) Global warming has caused melting of glaciers and flooding of low lying costal areas
3. Among the following greenhouse gases, whose atmospheric concentration is least?
   (a) CH_4
   (b) CFC
   (c) N_2O
   (d) CO_2
4. Select the correct arrangement of the types of UV radiation according to the intensity of their effect on human skin.
   (a) UV-A > UV-B > UV-C
   (b) UV-B > UV-C > UV-A
   (c) UV-C > UV-B > UV-A
   (d) UV-A > UV-C > UV-B
5. Which of the following is the correct approaches to reduce global warming?
   I. Use of fossil fuel
   II. Improving efficiency of energy usage
   III. Afforestation
   IV. Increasing growth of human population
   Codes
   (a) I and III
   (b) II and III
   (c) III and IV
   (d) I, II and III
6. An international initiative of year ...*A*... to mitigate climatic changes to reduce greenhouse emission is called ...*B*... .

	A	B
(a)	1987	Montreal protocol
(b)	1997	Kyoto protocol
(c)	1992	Earth summit
(d)	1985	Vienna convention

EXAM POINTS

- O_3 is a secondary pollutant, SO_2 is primary pollutant, while CO_2 is a quantitative as well as primary pollutant. **[NEET 2018]**
- Particulate matter is any matter suspended in the atmosphere which causes various breathing and respiratory problems. These matters are controlled by electrostatic precipitators. **[NEET 2019]**
- According to Central Pollution Control Board (CPCB), particulate of size 2.5 micrometers is responsible for causing greater harm to human health. **[NEET 2020]**
- Lichens are the most suitable indicators of SO_2 pollution in the environment. **[CBSE AIPMT 2015]**
- The Air Prevention and Control of Pollution Act came into force in 1981. **[NEET 2013]**
- Secondary air pollutants include smog, O_3 and PAN. **[J&K CET 2015]**
- A location with luxuriant growth of lichens on the trees indicates that the location is not polluted. **[CBSE AIPMT 2014]**
- Biological Oxygen Demand (BOD) is the presence of organic matter, present in 1 L of water. Higher BOD indicates decrease the amount of dissolved O_2 in water, hence indicating that the water is polluted. **[NEET 2018]**
- Increase in BOD in water leads to higher mortality rate of fishes in water due to lack of O_2. **[NEET-I, NEET-II 2016]**
- Eutrophication is caused due to the accumulation of minerals in water bodies, it is the process of natural ageing of lake by the biological enrichment in lake. **[NEET 2019]**
- The species which was introduced for ornamentation, but has become a trouble for some breed in India is *Eichhornia crassipes*. **[NEET 2020]**
- Biomagnification is the phenomenon through which certain pollutants get accumulated in tissues in increasing concentration along the food chain. Higher the trophic level, higher is the concentration of pollutant, e.g. DDT in an aquatic food chain.

  $$\underset{(0.003\text{ ppm})}{\text{Water}} \rightarrow \underset{(0.04\text{ ppm})}{\text{Zooplankton}} \rightarrow \underset{(0.5\text{ ppm})}{\text{Small fish}} \rightarrow \underset{(2\text{ ppm})}{\text{Large fish}}$$

  [NEET 2017, 16]
- Now-a-days, use of DDT as insecticide is banned because it has long residual effect. **[Chhattisgarh PMT 2015]**
- Natural insecticide which is obtained form neem is azadirachtin. **[Chhattisgarh PMT 2015]**
- The polluting strength of sewage is usually characterised by its BOD. **[J&K CET 2015]**
- The term biomagnification refers to increase in concentration of non-degradable pollutant through a food chain. **[J&K CET 2014]**
- Salinity of soil is a problem faced by farmers if they liberally irrigate for a prolonged period of time. **[NEET 2019]**
- Air (prevention and control of pollution) Act was amended in 1987 to include noise pollutants. **[NEET 2020]**
- The anxiety and stress reactions are caused by noise pollution. **[Chhattisgarh PMT 2015]**
- Nuclear waste is usually disposed by burying it within rocks deep below the earth surface. Before burying them, they all sealed in large container to reduce its radiation effects because it is hazardous. **[NEET 2019]**
- Ahmed Khan proved that blends of polyblend (plastic waste) and bitumen, when used to lay roads, enhanced the bitumen's water repellant properties and helped to increase road life. **[Kerala CEE 2015]**
- Polyblend is an innovative remedy for plastic waste. It is a fine powder of recycled modified plastic which is mixed with bitumen and used to construct roads. **[NEET 2019]**
- World Ozone Day is celebrated on 16th September to control O_3 depletion. Depletion of O_3 leads to disease like skin cancer. **[NEET 2018, NEET-I 2016]**
- Chlorofluorocarbons (CFCs) are widely used in refrigerator. These when reached in atmosphere, react with UV rays and release Cl atoms. These work as catalyst in the degradation of O_3 and release oxygen molecule. **[NEET 2018]**
- Stratosphere forms ozone which protects us from UV radiation, it is 'good ozone' whereas bad ozone' is formed troposphere. **[NEET 2019]**
- Gases responsible for greenhouse effect are carbon dioxide (60%), methane (20%) along with nitrous oxides (6%) and chlorofluorocarbons (14%). **[AIIMS 2016, NEET 2019]**
- Snow blindness in Antarctic region is caused due to inflammation of cornea due to high dose of UV-B radiation. **[NEET 2020]**
- Montreal protocol was signed in 1987 for the control of emission of ozone depleting substances like chlorofluorocarbon. **[NEET 2020, 2019]**
- The UN conference on climate change in the year 2012 was held at Doha. **[CBSSE AIPMT 2015]**
- The UN conference on climate change in the year 2011 was held in South Africa. **[CBSE AIPMT 2015]**
- Rachel Carson's famous book, *Silent Spring*, is related to pesticide pollution. **[CBSE AIPMT 2015]**
- Increase skin cancer, reduced immune system and damage to eyes are some of the prime health risks associated with greater UV radiation through the atmosphere due to the depletion of stratospheric zone. **[CBSE AIPMT 2015]**
- Greenhouse effect is caused due to the accumulation of O_3 and depletion of O_2. **[Chhattisgarh PMT 2015]**
- Redesigning landfill dumps to allow methane to be collected would most likely help to slow down the greenhouse effect. **[Karnataka CET 2015]**
- If there was no carbon dioxide on the earth's atmosphere, the temperature of the earth's surface would be less than the present level. **[Karnataka CET 2014]**
- The ozone hole over Antarctica develops each year between late August and early October. **[Kerala CEE 2014]**
- Kyoto protocol is a multinational international treaty for phasing out greenhouse gases. **[WB JEE 2014]**
- Kyoto protocol was endorsed at COP-3. **[NEET 2013]**
- Global warming can be controlled by reducing deforestation and cutting down use of fossil fuel. **[NEET 2013]**
- Ozone hole is measured in Dobson Unit (DU). **[J&K CET 2014]**

Chapter Exercises

(A) Topical Exercise

Air Pollution

1 Xenobiotics can be categorised into which of the following category of pollutants?
(a) Multiple pollutant (b) Biological pollutant
(c) Acid pollutant (d) None of these

2 The most harmful types of environmental pollutants are
(a) human organic wastes
(b) wastes from faecal
(c) non-biodegradable chemicals
(d) natural nutrients present in excess

3 Which of the following is normally not an atmospheric classified pollutant?
(a) CO (b) CO_2
(c) NO_2 (d) Sulphur

4 Primary constituents of photochemical smog are
(a) SO_2 and CO (b) O_3 and PAN
(c) NO_2 and hydrocarbons (d) CO_2

5 Which of the following materials takes the longest time for biodegradation? **[NCERT Exemplar]**
(a) Cotton (b) Paper (c) Bone (d) Jute

6 Consider the following statements.
I. Secondary pollutants are more harmful than primary pollutant.
II. Peroxyacyl Nitrates (PAN) are formed by photochemical reaction.
Choose the correct option.
(a) Statement I is true, but II is false
(b) Statement I is false, but II is true
(c) Both statements I and II are true
(d) Both statements I and II are false

7 Decomposition of domestic wastes under natural process is included in
(a) industrial pollution
(b) thermal pollution
(c) non-biodegradable pollution
(d) biodegradable pollution

8 Photochemical reaction of nitrogen oxides with unsaturated hydrocarbons produces
(a) methyl isocyanate (b) phosgene
(c) benzypyrene (d) peroxyacyl nitrates

9 Photochemical smog brings about
(a) defoliation
(b) bleaching and blazing of foliage
(c) floral bud shedding
(d) discolouration and curling of petals

10 Suspended particles such as ash, soot, smoke may affect human body as they cause ....
(a) eye irritation (b) emphysema
(c) possibly cancer (d) All of these

11 Which kind of power station produces sulphur dioxide, causing air pollution and acid rain?
(a) Coal-fired (b) Nuclear
(c) Hydroelectric (d) Wind-powered

12 The Taj Mahal may be destroyed due to
(a) flood in Yamuna river
(b) high temperature
(c) acid rain
(d) All of the above

13 Choose the incorrect statement.
(a) Mosses are indicators of SO_2 pollution
(b) PCB is released when plastic is burned
(c) Etching of marble, limestone, jewellery, etc., is caused by SO_2 pollution
(d) Pollutants of jet planes are NH_3

14 Consider the following statements.
I. CNG burn most efficiently without leaving any unburnt remnant behind.
II. CNG cannot be siphoned off by thieves and adultered like petrol or diesel.
Choose the correct option.
(a) Statement I is true, but II is false
(b) Statement I is false, but II is true
(c) Both statements I and II are true
(d) Both statements I and II are false

15 Which air pollutant could cause rains to be acidic?
(a) Dust particles from cement factories
(b) Insecticides from crop sprays
(c) Smoke from wood fires
(d) Sulphur dioxide from coal-fired power stations

16 Consider the following statements for acid rain.
I. The phenomenon called stone leprosy is due to acid rain.
II. Rain is acidic when its pH is below 6.5 due to the presence of H_2SO_4 and HNO_3.

Choose the correct option.
(a) Statement I is true, but II is false
(b) Statement I is false, but II is true
(c) Both statements I and II are true
(d) Both statements I and II are false

17 Which of the following health problems originate due to inhalation of fine particulate matter?
(a) Irritation
(b) Inflammation of respiratory tract
(c) Damage of lungs
(d) All of the above

18 Identify the incorrectly matched pair.
(a) Particulate matter – Breathing and respiratory symptoms
(b) Photochemical smog – Secondary pollutants
(c) Leaf curling – Hydrogen Fluoride (HF)
(d) Both (b) and (c)

19 The gas which was released in Bhopal gas tragedy was
(a) ethylene
(b) methyl isocyanate
(c) mustard gas
(d) potassium isocyanate

20 Which one of the following statements regarding CO gas is incorrect?
(a) It is produced by the incomplete combustion of fossil fuels
(b) It combines with haemoglobin to form carbamino haemoglobin
(c) It impairs oxygen transport resulting in giddiness, headache, asphyxia and even death
(d) Affinity of CO for haemoglobin as compared to O_2 is 200 times more

21 Select the correct match of air pollution source with the type of pollutant and the effect it produces.
(a) Chemical factory $\rightarrow NO_2 \rightarrow$ Ozone hole
(b) Automobile exhaust $\rightarrow N_2O \rightarrow$ Asphyxia effect
(c) Heavy industry $\rightarrow CO_2 \rightarrow$ Acid rain
(d) Incinerators $\rightarrow NO_x$ gases $\rightarrow$ Photochemical smog

22 Catalytic converters are fitted into automobiles to reduce emission of harmful gases. They change unburnt hydrocarbons into **[NCERT Exemplar]**
(a) carbon dioxide and water
(b) carbon monoxide
(c) methane
(d) carbon dioxide and methane

23 The antiknock agent added to unleaded petrol is
(a) tetraethyl lead
(b) tetramethyl lead
(c) dibromo ethane
(d) methyl tertiary butyl ether

24 Why is it necessary to remove sulphur from petroleum products? **[NCERT Exemplar]**
(a) To reduce the emission of sulphur dioxide in exhaust fumes
(b) To increase efficiency of automobiles engines
(c) To use sulphur removed from petroleum for commercial purposes
(d) To increase the lifespan of engine silencers

25 In a coal-fired power plant, electrostatic precipitators are installed to control emission
(a) SO_2 (b) NO_x (c) SPM (d) CO

26 Which of the following statements is incorrect regarding the Euro II norms?
(a) It stipulates that sulphur be controlled at 350 ppm in diesel
(b) It stipulates that sulphur be controlled at 150 ppm in petrol
(c) Aromatic hydrocarbons are to be contained at 42% of the concerned fuel
(d) None of the above

27 In cyclonic separators, which of the following act as major factor for separating particulate matter?
(a) Electricity (b) Centrifugal force
(c) Polyester bags (d) All of these

Water, Thermal and Soil Pollution

28 Choose the correct statement.
(a) Physical variables of water pollution include pale colour and bad taste
(b) Bad taste and odour of the water bodies of tanks, ponds, etc., is due to acids and grease
(c) Aluminium in drinking water may influence phosphate metabolism
(d) All of the above

29 World's most problematic aquatic weed is
(a) *Azolla* (b) *Wolffia* **[NCERT Exemplar]**
(c) *Eichhornia* (d) *Trapa*

30 By what method, the quality of organic pollutant in water can be determined?
(a) pH (b) Change of colour
(c) Measuring BOD (d) Transparency measurement

31 Algal bloom in a lake
(a) leads to O_2 depletion
(b) increases CO_2 level
(c) kills fishes and other organisms
(d) All of the above

32 Algal blooms impart a distinct colour to water due to
(a) their pigments **[NCERT Exemplar]**
(b) excretion of coloured substances
(c) formation of coloured chemicals in water facilitated by physiological degradation of algae
(d) absorption of light by algal cell wall

33 Eutrophication in lakes is the direct result of
(a) a diminished supply of nitrates and phosphates
(b) industrial poisons
(c) nutrient enrichment such as nitrate and phosphate run-offs from the land
(d) an increase in predators

34 Population explosion of small organisms due to nutrient enrichment of a lake causes a visual aspect, called
(a) primary production (b) algal bloom
(c) climax state (d) dominance

35 Often in water bodies subjected to sewage pollution, fishes die due to
(a) pathogens related to sewage
(b) reduction of dissolved O_2 caused by microbial activity
(c) clogging of their gills by solid substance
(d) foul smell

36 If water pollution continues at its present rate, it will eventually
(a) stop the water cycle
(b) make O_2 molecule unavailable to water plants
(c) make nitrate molecules unavailable to water plants
(d) prevent precipitate

37 The expanded form of DDT is **[NCERT Exemplar]**
(a) Dichloro Diphenyl Trichloroethane
(b) Dichloro Diethyl Trichloroethane
(c) Dichloro Dipyridyl Trichloroethane
(d) Dichloro Diphenyl Tetrachloroacetate

38 Increasing concentration of DDT in organisms of a food chain in higher trophic levels is known as
(a) biological chain (b) biological value
(c) biological magnification (d) biotic potential

39 The major drawback of DDT as a pesticide is that
(a) it is not degraded in nature
(b) its cost of production is high
(c) it is significantly less effective than other pesticides
(d) the organisms at once develop resistance to it

40 Which of the following is responsible for kidney damage?
(a) Cadmium (b) Fluorine
(c) Arsenic (d) Calcium

41 Environment planning organisation is
(a) CSIR (b) NEERI
(c) ICAR (d) CEPHERI

42 Choose the incorrect matched pair.
(a) Water bloom – *Hydrilla*
(b) DDT – Organochloride
(c) BOD – Microbes and organic matter
(d) Both (b) and (c)

43 Ecosanitation is a sustainable system for handling
(a) soil pollution (b) human excreta
(c) water (d) radioactive material

44 Blue-baby syndrome occurs by the pollution of
(a) CO (b) fluorine
(c) nitrate (d) mercury

45 Minamata disease was caused due to the consumption of
(a) sea food containing lot of cadmium
(b) fish contaminated with mercury
(c) oysters with lots of pesticides
(d) sea food contaminated with selenium

46 Which of the following statements is correct?
(a) There are working 'EcoSan' toilets in many areas of Kerala and Sri Lanka
(b) Municipal solid wastes are wastes from homes, offices, stores, schools, hospitals, etc., that are collected and disposed by the municipality
(c) In a sanitary landfill, wastes are dumped in a depression or trench after compaction and covered with dirt everyday
(d) All of the above

47 The chemicals released due to unsustainable agricultural practices and causing soil pollution are
(a) pathogens (b) chemical fertilisers
(c) strontium-90 (d) None of these

48 Slash and burn agriculture is known as
(a) striping farming (b) intercrop farming
(c) jhum cultivation (d) None of these

49 Result of deforestation is
(a) increase in CO_2 concentration
(b) decrease in CO_2 concentration
(c) water pollution
(d) All of the above

50 Which of the following is carried out at 900-1300°C?
(a) Pyrolysis (b) Incineration
(c) Both (a) and (b) (d) All of these

51 Who initiated organic farming in Sonipat, Haryana?
(a) Ramesh Dagar (b) Amrita Devi
(c) Ahmed Khan (d) None of these

52 Which of the following statements is not correct regarding jhum cultivation?
(a) It is also called as shifting cultivation and has resulted in deforestation
(b) It helps in increasing crop yield to a considerable extent
(c) A time-gap of several years is required for the recovery of the land after cultivation
(d) It involves cutting down of trees of the forest, burning of the plant remains and then using the land for farming

53 Consider the following statements.

I. Reforestation is the process of restoring a forest that once existed, but was removed at some point of time in the past.

II. Reforestation may occur naturally in a deforested area, however it can be speeded up by planting trees with due consideration to biodiversity that earlier existed in that area.

Choose the correct option.

(a) Statement I is true, but II is false
(b) Statement I is false, but II is true
(c) Both statements I and II are true
(d) Both statements I and II are false

54 Amrita Devi Bishnoi Wildlife Protection Award is for the individuals or communities form rural areas that have shown extraordinary courage in

(a) reducing environmental pollution
(b) reducing global warming
(c) protecting wildlife
(d) reforestation in deforested area

Noise Pollution, Radioactive Pollution and Solid Waste

55 Noise pollution is measured in

(a) fathoms (b) decibels
(c) tonne (d) kilogram

56 Choose the correct statement.

(a) Most dangerous radioactive pollutant is strontium-90
(b) Radioactive isotope used in the detection of thyroid cancer is I-131
(c) Chemical causing bone cancer and degeneration of tissues is Sr-90
(d) All of the above

57 A brief exposure to 150 dB sound may

(a) damage ear drums
(b) cause permanent impairing hearing ability
(c) cause temporary impairing hearing ability
(d) Both (a) and (b)

58 A prolonged exposure to noise at 65 dB can produce

(a) respiratory trouble
(b) skin cancer
(c) nervous tension and increased blood pressure
(d) digestive spasm

59 Which of the following actions can be taken to control noise pollution?

(a) Delimitation of horn free zone around hospitals nad schools
(b) Permissible sound levels of crackers and of loudspeakers
(c) Set the timing after which loudspeakers cannot be played
(d) All of the above

60 Consider the following statements.

I. The range of normal human hearing lies between 20-2000 Hzs.

II. The threshold of pain of human ears is 120-140 dB.

Choose the correct option.

(a) Statement I is true, but II is false
(b) Statement I is false, but II is true
(c) Both statements I and II are true
(d) Both statements I and II are false

61 The material generally used for sound proofing of rooms like a recording studio and auditorium, etc., is **[NCERT Exemplar]**

(a) cotton (b) coir
(c) wood (d) styro foam

62 The loudness of a sound that a person can withstand without discomfort is about **[NCERT Exemplar]**

(a) 150 dB (b) 215 dB
(c) 30 dB (d) 80 dB

63 Consider the following statements.

I. Noise intensity of jet aeroplane is 150 dB.

II. Maximum noise permissible during daytime is residential area is 65 dB.

Choose the correct option.

(a) Statement I is true, but II is false
(b) Statement I is false, but II is true
(c) Both statements I and II are true
(d) Both statements I and II are false

64 Noise was recognised as air pollutant through amendment of

(a) Environment (Protection) Act
(b) Air (Prevention and Control of Pollution) Act
(c) Noise (Control and Pollution) Act
(d) All of the above

65 Green muffler scheme helps to reduce

(a) air pollution (b) noise pollution
(c) e-wastes (d) Both (a) and (b)

66 Radioactive element found in tobacco smoke is

(a) iodine-131 (b) polonium-210
(c) caesium-137 (d) strontium-90

67 Among the following which one causes more indoor chemical pollution? **[NCERT Exemplar]**

(a) burning coal (b) burning cooking gas
(c) burning mosquito coil (d) room spray

68 Radioactive pollution is caused by

(a) α-particles (b) β-particles
(c) γ-particles (d) All of these

69 The most abundant nucleides found in river insects are

(a) P-32 (b) S
(c) Zn-65 (d) Both (a) and (c)

70 Thyroid cancer is treated by radiation therapy is known as
(a) endoscopy (b) chemotherapy
(c) radioiodine (d) None of these

71 Contamination of radioactive materials are dangerous because it causes
(a) biological magnification
(b) gene mutation
(c) photochemical smog
(d) ozone destruction

72 The most outstanding danger at present for the survival of living beings on earth is
(a) glaciation (b) deforestation
(c) radiation hazards (d) desertification

73 The term 'Nuclear war' is associated with
(a) soil pollution (b) water pollution
(c) radioactive pollution (d) All of these

74 Sources of solid wastes are
(a) municipal wastes
(b) electronic wastes
(c) hospital wastes
(d) All of the above

75 A fine powder of recycled modified plastic developed by Ahmed Khan is known as
(a) polycarbon (b) polynol
(c) polyblend (d) polycol

Ozone Depletion and Greenhouse Effect

76 Ozone gas is formed by the action of ....
(a) UV rays (b) microorganisms
(c) low temperature (d) All of these

77 Ozone hole is present above
(a) Antarctica (b) India (c) USA (d) USSR

78 Chlorofluorocarbons are not recommended to be used in refrigerators because they
(a) increase temperature (b) deplete ozone
(c) affect environment (d) affect human body

79 Ozone hole result is
(a) rainfailure (b) cataract
(c) increase in skin cancer (d) All of these

80 ODS means
(a) Ozone Developing Substance
(b) Ozone Depleting Substance
(c) Ozone Data Source
(d) Office Data Secrecy

81 Ozone hole over Antarctica was firsty detected by
(a) Molina and Rowland
(b) Farman *et. al.*
(c) Augus
(d) Molina and Molina

82 Ozone is
(a) harmful in the upper atmosphere
(b) beneficial in the upper atmosphere
(c) beneficial in the lower atmosphere
(d) harmful in the upper atmosphere and beneficial in the lower atmosphere

83 Ozone hole is the
(a) absence of O_3 in troposphere
(b) absence of O_3 in stratosphere
(c) deficiency of O_3 in stratosphere
(d) deficiency of O_3 in troposphere

84 Ozone depletion in stratosphere would result in
(a) forest fires (b) glaciation
(c) skin cancer incidence (d) None of these

85 Ultraviolet radiations from sunlight causes a reaction that produces
(a) fluorides (b) carbon monoxide
(c) sulphur dioxide (d) ozone

86 Greenhouse effect refers to
(a) cooling of earth (b) trapping of UV rays
(c) production of cereals (d) warming of earth

87 Who described greenhouse effect?
(a) Fourier (b) Ahmed Khan
(c) Both (a) and (b) (d) None of these

88 Gases referred to as 'greenhouse gases' are
(a) CO_2, O_2, NO_2, NH_3 (b) CFCs, CO_2, NH_3, N_2
(c) CH_4, N_2, CO_2, NH_3 (d) CFCs, CO_2, CH_4, N_2O

89 Which of these gases is not involved in global warming?
(a) Methane (b) Chlorofluorocarbon
(c) Nitrogen (d) Carbon dioxide

90 Loss of forests, urbanisation and increasing pollution are all due to
(a) greenhouse effect (b) global warming
(c) ozone depletion (d) population explosion

91 The Montreal protocol aimed at
(a) persistent organic pollutants
(b) global warming and climate change
(c) protecting stratospheric ozone
(d) biosafety of genetically modified organisms

92 Consider the following statements with respect to greenhouse effect.
I. Global warming will result in an increase in the number of tropical storms.
II. Global warming will result in rising sea level.
Choose the correct option.
(a) Statement I is true, but II is false
(b) Statement I is false, but II is true
(c) Both statements I and II are true
(d) Both statements I and II are false

93 Given pie-diagram represents the relative contribution of various GHGs to total global warming. Select the correct statement(s) regarding *A*, *B* and *C*.

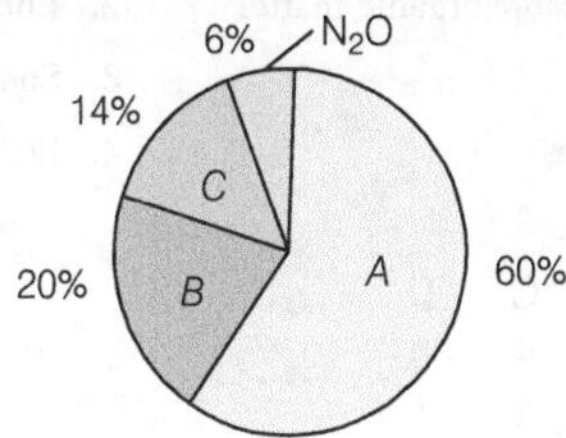

(a) *A* is the gas which is produced during the combustion of fossil fuels
(b) *B* are the chemicals which are used as coolants in refrigerators
(c) *C* is the gas which is the major constituent of biogas
(d) All of the above

94 Consider the following statements.

I. Average temperature of earth has increased by 0.6°C during the past century.

II. There has been a progressive increase in the use of the fossil fuels generating more greenhouse gases.

Choose the correct option.
(a) Statement I is true, but II is false
(b) Statement I is false, but II is true
(c) Both statements I and II are true
(d) Both statements I and II are false

95 Select the correct arrangement of the types of ultraviolet radiations according to the intensity of their effect on human skin.
(a) UV-A > UV-B > UV-C
(b) UV-B > UV-C > UV-A
(c) UV-C > UV-B > UV-A
(d) UV-A > UV-C > UV-B

96 Which of the following is correct regarding 'El Nino' effect?
(a) Temperature rise leads to odd climatic changes
(b) Cutting down the use of fossil fuels
(c) Planting more trees
(d) Slowing down the growth of human population

(B) Cumulative Exercise

(Assorted Questions of the Chapter for Advanced Level Practice)

1 A lake near a village suffered heavy mortality of fishes within a few days. Consider the following reasons for this.

I. Lots of urea and phosphate fertiliser were used in the crops in the vicinity.
II. The area was sprayed with DDT by an aircraft.
III. The lake water turned green and stinky.
IV. Phytoplankton populations in the lake declined initially thereby greatly reducing photosynthesis.

Which of the above were the main causes of fish mortality in the lake?
(a) II and III (b) III and IV
(c) I and III (d) I and II

2 Match the following columns.

Column I	Column II
A. DDT	1. CO, CO_2
B. PAN	2. Smog
C. Acid rain	3. Biological magnification
D. Global warming	4. SO_2

Codes

	A	B	C	D
(a)	4	3	2	1
(b)	1	2	3	4
(c)	2	3	4	1
(d)	3	2	4	1

3 The diagram shows changes in the concentrations of two substances *X* and *Y* in the sewage river polluted.

Concentration
Substance *Y*
Substance *X*
Sewage added
Distance downstream

What are the substances *X* and *Y*?

	X	*Y*
(a)	Carbon dioxide	Oxygen
(b)	Oxygen	Nitrogen compound
(c)	Carbon dioxide	Nitrogen compound
(d)	Nitrogen compound	Carbon dioxide

4 Match the following columns.

Column I	Column II
A. El Nino effect	1. Rio de Janeiro
B. Earth summit	2. 1974
C. Amrita Devi	3. Global warming
D. Sunder Lal	4. 1731

Codes

	A	B	C	D		A	B	C	D
(a)	1	2	4	3	(b)	3	1	4	2
(c)	3	4	1	2	(d)	1	4	3	2

5 Lichens are organisms, which are very sensitive to air pollution. The graph shows how the distance from a coal-fired power station affects the number of different types of growing lichen.

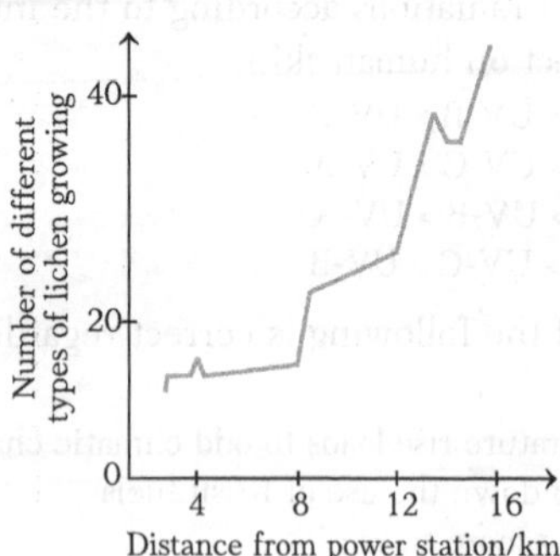

What conclusion can be drawn from this information?

(a) Lichens grow faster near the power station
(b) Lichens grow more fast near the power station
(c) There are fewer different types of lichens growing near the power station
(d) There are more different types of lichens growing near the power station

6 Which of the following statements is correct?

I. Montreal Protocol was signed in 1987.
II. Earth Summit 1992 was held at Rio de Janeiro.
III. World Environment Day is 5th June.
IV. World Environment Day coincides with commemoration of First United Nations Conference on Human Environment.
V. At DO below 4 mg/L water at normal temperature is heavily polluted.

Choose the correct option from the codes given below.

(a) I, II, III, IV and V (b) All except IV
(c) All except II and III (d) None of these

7 Which of the following statements is correct?

I. Global warming will result is an increase in the number of tropical storms.
II. Eutrophication is commonly associated with high level of nitrates and sulphates.
III. Global warming will result in rising sea level.
IV. Eutrophication is the result of pteridophytes.

Codes

(a) I, II and III (b) II and III
(c) II, III and IV (d) I, III and IV

8 Match the following columns.

Column I	Column II
A. UV	1. Biomagnification
B. Biodegradable organic matter	2. Eutrophication
C. DDT	3. Snow blindness
D. Phosphates	4. BOD

Codes **[NCERT Exemplar]**

	A	B	C	D
(a)	2	1	4	3
(b)	3	2	4	1
(c)	3	4	1	2
(d)	3	1	4	2

9 Match the following columns.

Column I	Column II
A. World Environment Day	1. 2nd December
B. World Ozone Day	2. 29th December
C. National Pollution Prevention Day	3. 16th September
D. Biological Diversity Day	4. 5th June

Codes

	A	B	C	D
(a)	1	2	3	4
(b)	4	2	1	3
(c)	1	2	3	4
(d)	4	3	1	2

10 Fill up the blanks.

I ...*A*... used as refrigerants which react with UV in ...*B*... to release ...*C*... atoms.
II Chlorine atoms act as ...*D*... to degrade ozone and release molecular ...*E*... .
III Bad ozone is formed in ...*F*... and is harmful to plant and animals.
IV Good ozone is formed in ...*G*... and absorbs harmful ...*H*... from the sun.

Complete the given set of statements by filling appropriate options in the blanks *A*-*H*.

(a) *A*-NO_2, *B*-troposphere, *C*-fluoride, *D*-catalyst, *E*-CO_2, *F*-stratosphere, *G*-atmosphere, *H*-infrared radiation
(b) *A*-CFCs, *B*-stratosphere, *C*-chlorine, *D*-catalyst, *E*-oxygen, *F*-troposphere, *G*-stratosphere, *H*-UV radiations
(c) *A*-CO_2, *B*-ionosphere, *C*-calcium, *D*-catalyst, *E*-chlorine, *F*-ionosphere, *G*-troposphere, *H*-infrared radiation
(d) *A*-CH_4, *B*-stratosphere, *C*-sodium, *D*-catalyst, *E*-oxygen, *F*-atmosphere, *G*-ionosphere, *H*-UV radiation

11 Match the following columns.

Column I	Column II
A. Environment Protection Act	1. 1974
B. Air prevention and Control of Pollution Act	2. 1987
C. Water Act	3. 1986
D. Amendment of Air act to include noise	4. 1981

Codes **[NCERT Exemplar]**

	A	B	C	D		A	B	C	D
(a)	3	4	1	2	(b)	1	3	2	4
(c)	4	1	2	3	(d)	3	4	2	1

12 Given diagram represents the greenhouse effect.

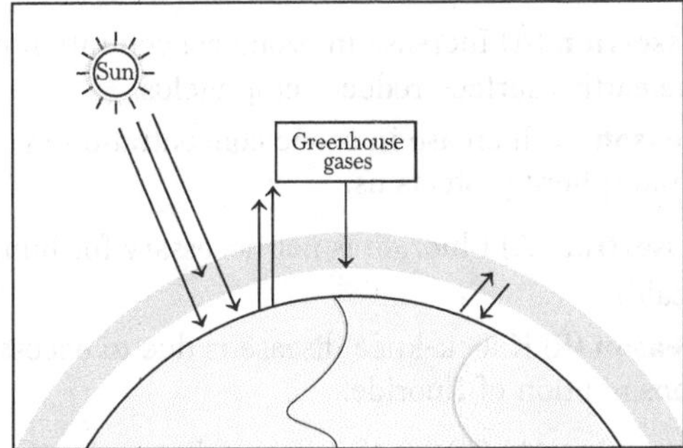

I. Greenhouse gases absorb infrared radiation from the earth. The absorbed radiations again come to earth's surface and heat it up.
II. CO_2, CH_4, CFCs and N_2O are the gases responsible for greenhouse effect.
III. Increase in the level of greenhouse gases results in the reduction of global warming.

Which of the statements given above are correct?
(a) I and II (b) II and III (c) I and III (d) I, II and III

13 Fill up the blanks.

I ...*A*...in soil results from irrigation without proper drainage of water. This affects the plants and draws salts to the soil surface. The salt is either deposited as a layer on land surface or collects at ...*B*... of plants.
II *A* water logged soil has poor ...*C*... .
III Removal of forest areas to fulfil the need of growing human population is called ...*D*... .
IV ...*E*... of India has recommended 33% forest cover for the plains and 67% for the hills.

Here *A-E* refer to
(a) *A*-Soil erosion, *B*-stems, *C*-structure, *D*-reforestation, *E*-The National Forest Policy (1987)
(b) *A*-Water logging, *B*-roots, *C*-aeration, *D*-deforestation, *E*-The National Forest Policy (1988)
(c) *A*-Soil succession, *B*-leaves, *C*-nutrients, *D*-afforestation, *E*-The National Forest Policy (1989)
(d) *A*-Desertification, *B*-fruits, *C*-minerals, *D*-deforestation, *E*-The National Forest Policy (1986)

14 Choose the correct statement regarding the process of biomagnification of DDT in an aquatic food chain as described by the figure given below.

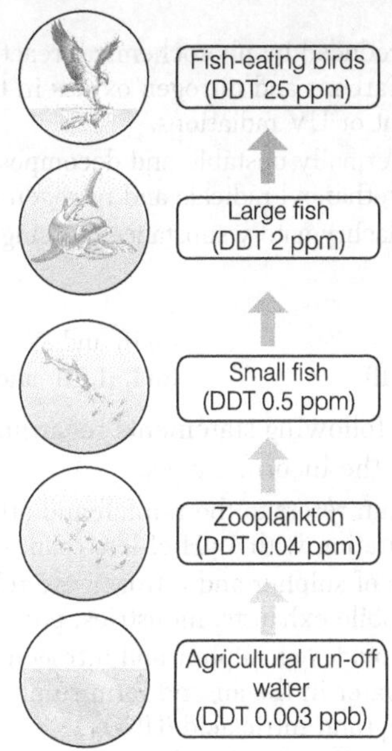

I. Biomagnification refers to increase in concentration of the toxicant at successive trophic levels.
II. High concentrations of DDT disturb calcium metabolism in birds, which cause thinning of eggshell and their premature breaking.
III. River water may have a very low concentration of DDT, but the carnivorous fish in that river may contain high concentration of DDT, which is still suitable for consumption by human beings.

Which of the statements given above are correct?
(a) I and II (b) I and III (c) II and III (d) I, II and III

15 Read the following statements regarding particulate matter and select the incorrect ones.

I. Particulate Matter (PM) consists of shoot, flyash, dust, spores, pollen grains, etc.
II. Particulate matter is differentiated into settleable (larger than 10 μm, remaining in air for less than one day) and suspended (less than 10 μm remaining in air for more than one day to several weeks) particulate matter.
III. SPM (Suspended Particulate Matter) consists of aerosol, dust and mist.
IV. Particulate matter causes respiratory diseases such as tuberculosis, allergy and many more diseases in animals and plants.
V. According to Central Pollution Control Board (CPCB), particulate size of 2.5 μm or less in diameter are responsible for causing the greatest harm to human health.

(a) I and II (b) III and IV
(c) Only II (d) None of these

16 Read the following statements regarding the PAN (Peroxyacyl Nitrate) and select the correct ones.

I. It is a secondary pollutant present in photochemical smog.
II. It is produced by photochemical reactions between hydrocarbons and nitrogen oxides in the presence of sunlight or UV radiations.
III. It is thermally unstable and decomposes into peroxyethanoyl radicals and nitrogen dioxide gas.
IV. It is a lachrymatory substance, causing irritation of eyes.

Codes

(a) I and II (b) III and IV
(c) I II and III (d) I, II, III and IV

17 Study the following statements regarding acid rain and select the incorrect ones.

I. Acid rain refers to the rainfall and other forms of precipitation with a pH of less than 5.
II. Oxides of sulphur and nitrogen are released from automobile exhausts, industries, power plants, etc.
III. These oxides of sulphur and nitrogen may react with water in the air and form sulphuric acid (H_2SO_4) and nitric acid (HNO_3).
IV. Acid rain has harmful effects on animals and human beings but no characteristic impact on plants.

Codes

(a) I and III (b) III and IV
(c) Only IV (d) Only II

18 Match the following columns.

Column I	Column II
A. Mercury	1. Methaemoglobinemia or Blue baby syndrome
B. Nitrate	2. Black foot disease
C. Arsenic	3. Itai-itai disease
D. Cadmium	4. Minamata disease

Codes **[NCERT Exemplar]**

	A	B	C	D
(a)	4	1	2	3
(b)	4	1	3	2
(c)	2	3	1	4
(d)	2	4	1	3

Assertion and Reason

Direction (Q. Nos. 19-30) *In each of the following questions, a statement of Assertion (A) is given followed by the corresponding statement of Reason (R). Of the statements, mark the correct answer as*

(a) Both A and R are true, but R is the correct explanation of A
(b) Both A and R are true, but R is not the correct explanation of A
(c) A is true, but R is false
(d) A is false, but R is true
(e) Both A and R are false

19 **Assertion** (A) Greenhouse effect is due to thick layer of CO_2.
Reason (R) CO_2 acts as the glass panels of a greenhouse allowing the sunlight to filter through, but preventing the heat from being re-radiated in outer space.

20 **Assertion** (A) The problem of acid rain has dramatically increased due to industrialisation.
Reason (R) Industries are responsible for most of the emission of oxides of sulphur and nitrogen.

21 **Assertion** (A) Acid rain disrupts ecological balance.
Reason (R) It affects flora and fauna.

22 **Assertion** (A) Increase in ozone concentration near the earth's surface reduces crop yields.
Reason (R) Increase in ozone concentration in stratosphere protects us.

23 **Assertion** (A) Fluoride is not necessary for human health.
Reason (R) Knock-knee disease is due to excess consumption of fluoride.

24 **Assertion** (A) CO_2 is the main pollutant causing greenhouse effect.
Reason (R) Incomplete combustion of fossil fuels in automobiles releases 80% of CO_2.

25 **Assertion** (A) Liquid waste products from industrial processes and domestic activity are termed as effluents.
Reason (R) Fertiliser factories, steel and textile sugar mills are some industries, which release effluents.

26 **Assertion** (A) Phosphorus and nitrogen compounds in a lake, favour the luxuriant growth of algae.
Reason (R) Water bloom condition occurs in eutrophic ponds.

27 **Assertion** (A) Inhabitants close to very busy airports are likely to experience health hazards.
Reason (R) Sound level of jet aeroplanes usually exceeds 160 dB.

28 **Assertion** (A) Noise is considered as a pollutant.
Reason (R) It adversely affects our health.

29 **Assertion** (A) Jhuming practice causes soil erosion.
Reason (R) It involves deforestation.

30 **Assertion** (A) Use of weedicides affects photosynthetic ability of plants.
Reason (R) Weedicides are metabolic inhibitors.

(C) Medical Entrances' Gallery

(Collection of Questions Asked in NEET & in Various Medical Entrance Exams)

1 A species which was introduced for ornamentation, but has become a trouble some weed in India? [NEET 2020]

(a) *Parthenium hysterophorus* (b) *Eichhornia crassipes*
(c) *Prosopis juliflora* (d) *Trapa spinosa*

2 Air Prevention and Control of Pollution Act was amended in 1987 to include among pollutants, [NEET 2020]

(a) vehicular exhaust
(b) allergy causing pollen
(c) noise
(d) particulates of size 2.5 micrometer or below

3 According to Central Pollution Control Board (CPCB), what size (in diameter) of particulate is responsible for causing greater harm to human health? [NEET 2020]

(a) 3.5 micrometers (b) 2.5 micrometers
(c) 4.0 micrometers (d) 3.0 micrometers

4 Montreal protocol was signed in 1987 for control of [NEET 2020]

(a) emission of ozone depleting substances
(b) release of greenhouse gases
(c) disposal of e-wastes
(d) transport of genetically modified organisms from one country to another

5 Snow blindness in Antarctic region is due to [NEET 2020]

(a) inflammation of cornea due to high dose of UV-B radiation
(b) high reflection of light from snow
(c) damage to retina caused by infrared rays
(d) freezing of fluids in the eye by low temperatures

6 Identify the correctly matched pair. [JIPMER 2019]

(a) Particulate matter - Breathing and respiratory symptoms
(b) Particulate mattter - Electrostatic precipitator
(c) SO_2- Catalytic converter
(d) Both (a) and (b)

7 Eutrophication is caused due to [JIPMER 2019]

(a) accumulation of minerals
(b) effect of UV- C
(c) accumulation of metals only
(d) accumulation of zooplankton

8 Which of these following methods is the most suitable for disposal of nuclear waste? [NEET 2019]

(a) Bury the waste under Antarctic ice-cover
(b) Dump the waste within rocks under deep ocean
(c) Bury the waste within rocks deep below the earth's surface
(d) Shoot the waste into space

9 If an agricultural field is liberally irrigated for a prolonged period of time, it is likely to face problem of [NEET 2019]

(a) metal toxicity (b) alkalinity
(c) acidity (d) salinity

10 Which of the following pairs of gases is mainly responsible for greenhouse effect? [NEET 2019]

(a) Oxygen and nitrogen
(b) Nitrogen and sulphur dioxide
(c) Carbon dioxide and methane
(d) Ozone and ammonia

11 Which of the following statements about ozone is correct? [NEET 2019]

(a) Tropospheric ozone protects us from UV radiations
(b) Stratospheric ozone is 'bad'
(c) Tropospheric ozone is 'good'
(d) Stratospheric ozone protects us from UV radiations

12 Which of the following protocols did aim for reducing emission of chlorofluorocarbons into the atmosphere? [NEET 2019]

(a) Kyoto Protocol (b) Gothenburg Protocol
(c) Geneva Protocol (d) Montreal Protocol

13 Which of the following is an innovative remedy for plastic waste? [NEET 2019]

(a) Burning in the absence of oxygen
(b) Burying 500 m deep below soil surface
(c) Polyblend
(d) Electrostatic precipitator

14 Polyblend, a fine powder of recycled modified plastic, has proved to be a good material for [NEET 2019]

(a) use as a fertiliser (b) construction of roads
(c) making tubes and pipes (d) making plastic sacks

15 Which of the following is a secondary pollutant? [NEET 2018]

(a) SO_2 (b) CO_2
(c) CO (d) O_2

16 **Assertion** (A) BOD is an indicator of pollution in water.

Reason (R) High BOD is observed in highly polluted water. [AIIMS 2018]

(a) Both A and R are true and R is the correct explanation of A
(b) Both A and R are true, but R is not the correct explanation of A
(c) A is true, but R is false
(d) Both A and R are false

17 World Ozone Day is celebrated on **[NEET 2018]**
(a) 16th September (b) 21st April
(c) 5th June (d) 22nd April

18 In stratosphere, which one of the following elements acts as a catalyst in degradation of ozone and release of molecular oxygen? **[NEET 2018]**
(a) Fe (b) Cl
(c) Carbon (d) Oxygen

19 Which one option is incorrectly matched regarding biological magnification of DDT in aquatic ecosystem? **[AIIMS 2017]**
(a) Small fish - 0.5 ppm
(b) Large fish - 2 ppm
(c) Fish-eating birds - 25 ppm
(d) Zooplankton - 0.003 ppm

20 Biochemical Oxygen Demand (BOD) may not be a good index for pollution in water bodies receiving effluents from **[NEET-II 2016]**
(a) domestic sewage
(b) dairy industry
(c) petroleum industry
(d) sugar industry

21 A lake which is rich in organic waste may result in **[NEET-II 2016]**
(a) increased population of aquatic organisms due to minerals
(b) drying of the lake due to algal bloom
(c) increased population of fish due to lots of nutrients
(d) mortality of fish due to lack of oxygen

22 The highest DDT concentration in aquatic food chain shall occur in **[NEET-II 2016]**
(a) phytoplankton (b) seagull
(c) crab (d) eel

23 Joint forest management concept was introduced in India during **[NEET-I2016]**
(a) 1970s (b) 1980s
(c) 1990s (d) 1960s

24 A river with an inflow of domestic sewage rich in organic waste may result in **[NEET-I 2016]**
(a) increased population of aquatic food web organisms
(b) an increased production of fish due to biodegradable nutrients
(c) death of fish due to lack of oxygen
(d) drying of the river very soon due to algal bloom

25 Depletion of which gas in the atmosphere can lead to an increased incidence of skin cancer? **[NEET-I 2016]**
(a) Ozone (b) Ammonia
(c) Methane (d) Nitrous oxide

26 Identify the wrong statement with reference to UV rays. **[EAMCET 2016]**
(a) UV radiation is classified into 3 categories
(b) UV radiation kills microorganisms
(c) UV-A is more harmful to animals than UV-B
(d) UV radiation falls in the range between 100 mm-380 nm (wavelength)

27 Match the environmental activists in Column I with the environmental issues in Column II and choose the right option.

Column I	Column II
A. Ramesh Chandra Dagar	1. Conservation of forests
B. Ahmed Khan	2. Organic farming
C. Amrita Devi	3. Plastic waste recycling

Codes **[Kerala CEE 2016]**

	A	B	C		A	B	C
(a)	2	3	1	(b)	3	1	2
(c)	1	2	3	(d)	2	1	3
(e)	1	3	2				

28 A scrubber in the exhaust of a chemical industry removes **[Karnataka CET 2016, 14, CBSE AIPMT 2014]**
(a) nitrous oxide (b) hydrogen sulphide
(c) carbon dioxide (d) sulphur dioxide

29 One greenhouse gas contributes 14% to total global warming and another contributes 6%. These are respectively, identified as **[AIIMS 2016]**
(a) N_2O and CO_2
(b) CFCs and N_2O
(c) CH_4 and CO_2
(d) methane and CFCs

30 The figure given below is the diagrammatic representation of relative contribution of various greenhouse gases to total global warming what do *A*, *B*, *C* and *D* represent, respectively ?

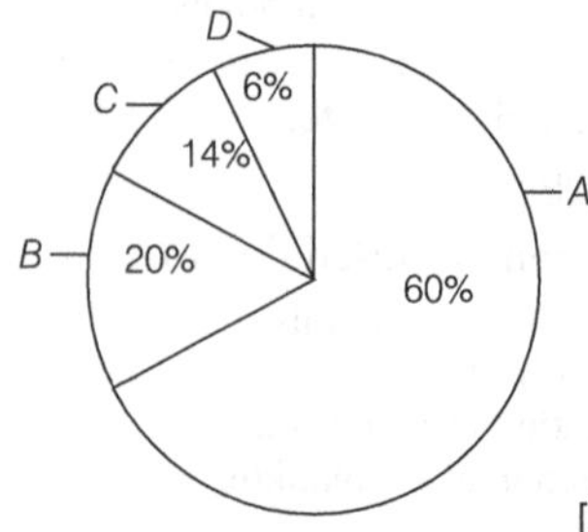

[Kerala CEE 2016]
(a) *A*-Carbon dioxide, *B*-Methane, *C*-CFCs, *D*-N_2O
(b) *A*-Carbon dioxide, *B*-CFCs, *C*-Methane, *D*-N_2O
(c) *A*-Carbon dioxide, *B*-N_2O, *C*-CFCs, *D*-Methane
(d) *A*-Carbon dioxide, *B*-Methane, *C*-N_2O, *D*-CFCs
(e) *A*-CFCs, *B*-Carbon dioxide, *C*-Methane, *D*-N_2O

31 Which of the following are most suitable indications of SO_2 pollution in the environment? **[CBSE AIPMT 2015]**

(a) Lichens (b) Conifers
(c) Algae (d) Fungi

32 The UN conference of parties on climate change in the year 2012 was held at **[CBSE AIPMT 2015]**

(a) Hurban (b) Doha
(c) Lima (d) Warsaw

33 Increase in concentration of the toxicant at successive trophic levels is known as **[CBSE AIPMT 2015]**

(a) biomagnification (b) biodeterioration
(c) biotransformation (d) biogeochemical cycling

34 Acid rain is caused by increase in the atmospheric concentration of **[CBSE AIPMT 2015; Odisha JEE 2011]**

(a) SO_2 and NO_2 (b) SO_2 and CO
(c) CO_2 and CO (d) O_3 and dust

35 The UN conference of parties on climate change in the year 2011 was held in **[CBSE AIPMT 2015]**

(a) Poland (b) South Africa
(c) Peru (d) Qatar

36 Rachel Carson's famous book '*Silent Spring*' is related to **[CBSE AIPMT 2015]**

(a) pesticide pollution (b) noise pollution
(c) population explosion (d) ecosystem management

37 Which of the following is not one of prime health risks associated with greater UV radiation through the atmosphere due to depletion of stratospheric zone? **[CBSE AIPMT 2015]**

(a) Increased skin cancer
(b) Reduced immune system
(c) Damage to eyes
(d) Increase liver cancer

38 Match the following columns.

	Column I		Column II
A.	Mercury	1.	Plumbism
B.	Lead	2.	Minamata
C.	Cadmium	3.	Itai-itai
D.	Hydrocarbon	4.	Cancer

Codes **[Chhattisgarh PMT 2015]**

	A	B	C	D
(a)	2	1	3	4
(b)	1	2	3	4
(c)	2	3	1	4
(c)	2	1	4	3

39 The anxiety and stress reactions are caused by **[Chhattisgarh PMT 2015]**

(a) water pollution (b) nuclear pollution
(c) noise pollution (d) air pollution

40 Now-a-days, use of DDT as insecticide is banned because **[Chhattisgarh PMT 2015]**

(a) it is less effective than other pesticides
(b) organisms develop resistance to it
(c) production cost is very high
(d) it has long residual effect

41 Match the following columns.

	Column I		Column II
A.	Photochemical smog	1.	Itai-itai disease
B.	Arsenic pollution	2.	Parkinson's disease
C.	Manganese pollution	3.	Black foot disease
D.	Cadmium pollution	4.	Burning of petrol and diesel with oxides of nitrogen

Codes **[Chhattisgarh PMT 2015]**

	A	B	C	D
(a)	4	2	3	1
(b)	4	3	2	1
(c)	4	3	1	2
(c)	4	1	2	3

42 Natural insecticide which is obtained from neem is **[Chhattisgarh PMT 2015]**

(a) azadirachtin (b) nicotine
(c) DDT (d) Both (a) and (b)

43 Greenhouse effect is due to the **[Chhattisgarh PMT 2015]**

(a) accumulation of O_3 and depletion of O_2
(b) accumulation of O_3 and CO_2
(c) depletion of CO_2 and O_3
(d) accumulation of green plants

44 Examples of secondary air pollutants is/are **[J&K CET 2015]**

(a) smog (b) O_3
(c) PAN (d) All of these

45 The polluting strength of sewage is usually characterised by its **[J&K CET 2015]**

(a) BOD (b) nitrogen content
(c) ozone content (d) eutrophication

46 Match the following Column I with Column II.

Column I	Column II
A. Pollen grains	1. Photochemical smog
B. PAN	2. Particulate pollution
C. CO_2	3. Global warming
D. Cadmium	4. Itai-itai disease

Codes **[WB JEE 2015]**

	A	B	C	D
(a)	2	1	3	4
(b)	4	2	1	3
(c)	1	2	3	4
(d)	3	1	2	4

47 Which one of the following combinations is incorrect? **[WB JEE 2015]**
(a) Rio convention – Air pollution
(b) Kyoto protocol – Climate change
(c) Montreal protocol – Ozone depletion
(d) Ramsar convention – Wetland conservation

48 Match the following columns.

Column I	Column II
A. Eutrophication	1. Rise in sea level
B. Biomagnification	2. Water hyacinth
C. Terror of Bengal	3. Increase of quantity of pollutant at successive trophic levels
D. Greenhouse effect	4. Enrichment with nutrients

Codes **[EAMCET 2015]**

	A	B	C	D
(a)	2	1	3	4
(b)	4	2	1	3
(c)	1	2	3	4
(d)	4	3	2	1

49 High value of BOD (Biochemical Oxygen Demand) indicates that **[CBSE AIPMT 2015]**
(a) water is pure
(b) water is highly polluted
(c) water is less polluted
(d) consumption of organic matter in the water is higher by the microbes

50 Which of the following would most likely help to slow down the greenhouse effect? **[Karnataka CET 2015]**
(a) Converting tropical forests into grazing land for cattle
(b) Ensuring that all excess paper packaging is burned to ashes
(c) Redesigning landfill dumps to allow methane to be collected
(d) Promoting the use of private rather than public transport

51 Who proved that blends of polyblend (plastic waste) and bitumen, when used to lay roads, enhanced the bitumen's water repellant properties and helped to increase road life ? **[Kerala CEE 2015]**
(a) Amrita Devi (b) Ramdeo Misra
(c) WH Pearsall (d) Ramesh Chandra Dagar
(e) Ahmed Khan

52 Match the following Column I with Column II.

Column I	Column II
A. Zooplankton	1. 0.003 ppm
B. Small fishes	2. 2 ppm
C. Water	3. 25 ppm
D. Fish eating birds	4. 0.04 ppm
E. Big fishes	5. 0.5 ppm

[Gujarat CET 2015]

Codes

	A	B	C	D	E
(a)	2	1	4	5	3
(b)	4	5	1	2	3
(c)	4	5	3	2	1
(d)	4	5	1	3	2

53 If there was no carbon dioxide on the earth's atmosphere, the temperature of the earth's surface would be **[Karnataka CET 2014]**
(a) same as the present level
(b) more than the present level
(c) less than the present level
(d) dependent on the oxygen content in the atmosphere

54 Which of the option shows following examples in ascending order in terms of BOD? **[Gujarat CET 2014]**
I. Distilled water
II. Tap water
III. Sewage wastes drained in river
Codes
(a) II, I and III (b) I, II and III
(c) III, I and II (d) III, II and I

55 The zone of atmosphere in which the ozone layer is present is called **[CBSE AIPMT 2014]**
(a) ionosphere (b) mesosphere
(c) stratosphere (d) troposphere

56 A location with luxuriant growth of lichens on the trees indicates that the **[CBSE AIPMT 2014]**
(a) trees are very healthy (b) trees are heavily infested
(c) location is highly polluted (d) location is not polluted

57 Afforestation is **[MHT CET 2014]**
(a) restoring a forest
(b) plantation in barren lands
(c) cultivation under agriculture
(d) Jhum cultivation

58 The ozone hole over Antarctica develops each year between **[Kerala CEE 2014]**
(a) late December and early February
(b) late February and early April
(c) late April and early June
(d) late August and early October
(e) late October and early December

59 Which of the following statements does not apply to eutrophication? **[Kerala CEE 2014]**
(a) It is the natural ageing of a lake by nutrient enrichment of its water
(b) In a young lake, the water is cold and clear and supports less life
(c) The nutrients such as sulphur and phosphorus encourage the growth of aquatic organisms in the lake
(d) Pollutants released by man radically accelerate the ageing process of a lake
(e) Overgrowth of algae leads to scum that depletes the level of dissolved oxygen in water

60 With the rise of water temperature, dissolved oxygen **[WB JEE 2014]**
(a) remains unchanged
(b) increases in amount
(c) decreases in amount
(d) is more available to the aquatic organisms

61 'Kyoto protocol' is a multinational international treaty for **[WB JEE 2014]**
(a) phasing out greenhouse gases
(b) controlling ozone destroying substances
(c) management of hazardous wastes
(d) conservation of biodiversity

62 Main cause of eutrophication is **[WB JEE 2014]**
(a) fluctuation of temperature
(b) unusual growth of aquatic vegetations
(c) enrichment of nutrients
(d) abundance of microorganisms

63 Carbon dioxide, methane, nitrogen oxide and chlorofluorocarbons are called greenhouse gases because they can absorb **[J&K CET 2014]**
(a) ultraviolet radiations
(b) visible light radiations
(c) γ-rays radiations
(d) long wave infrared radiations

64 Hyacinth is termed as the terror of Bengal how it causes death of fishes? **[J&K CET 2014]**
(a) Covers the surface of the water that inhibits sunlight to pass through
(b) Drains oxygen from the water that causes oxygen deficiency
(c) Absorbs nutrients from the water that causes malnutrition
(d) Releases carbon dioxide in a huge amount which is lethal to fishes

65 Ozone hole is measured in **[J&K CET 2014]**
(a) Decibel (b) Dobson Units (DU)
(c) Parts Per Million (PPM) (d) Cubic Centimeter

66 The term 'biomagnification' refers to **[J&K CET 2014]**
(a) increase in concentration of non-degradable pollutant through a food chain
(b) growth of organisms due to food consumption
(c) decrease in population size
(d) increase in population size

67 Which of the following is true for eutrophicated water body? **[Karnataka CET 2014]**
(a) High mineral content (b) High oxygen content
(c) Rich species diversity (d) Low organic content

68 The Air Prevention and Control of Pollution Act came into force in **[NEET 2013]**
(a) 1981 (b) 1985
(c) 1990 (d) 1975

69 Global warming can be controlled by **[NEET 2013]**
(a) reducing reforestation, increasing the use of fossil fuels
(b) increasing deforestation, slowing down the growth of human population
(c) increasing deforestation, reducing efficiency of energy usage
(d) reducing deforestation, cutting down use of fossil fuel

70 Kyoto protocol was endorsed at **[NEET 2013]**
(a) CoP-5 (b) CoP-6 (c) CoP-4 (d) CoP-3

71 Measuring Biochemical Oxygen Demand (BOD) is a method used for **[CBSE AIPMT 2012]**
(a) working out the efficiency of oil driven automobile engines
(b) measuring the activity of *Saccharomyces cerevisae* in producing curd on a commercial scale
(c) working out the efficiency of RBCs about their capacity to carry oxygen
(d) estimating the amount of organic matter in sewage water

72 Which one of the following is a wrong statement? **[CBSE AIPMT 2012]**
(a) Ozone in upper part of atmosphere is harmful to animal
(b) Greenhouse effect is a natural phenomenon
(c) Eutrophication is a natural phenomenon in freshwater bodies
(d) Most of the forests have been lost in tropical areas

73 High amount of *Escherichia coli* in water indicates **[Chandigarh CET 2012]**
(a) hardness of water
(b) industrial pollution
(c) sewage pollution
(d) pollution due to electromagnetic radiations

74 The range of biomagnification of DDT in an aquatic food chain, if starting from 0.003 ppm level in water, may go at fish eating bird level upto **[AMU 2012]**
(a) 0.5 ppm (b) 5.0 ppm
(c) 15.0 ppm (d) 25.0 ppm

75 Environment Protection Act, to protect and improve the quality of our environment (air, water and soil) was passed in the year **[AMU 2012]**
(a) 1971 (b) 1974
(c) 1981 (d) 1986

76 In an area where DDT had been used extensively, the population of birds declined significantly because **[CBSE AIPMT 2012]**
(a) birds stopped laying eggs
(b) earthworms in the area got eradicated
(c) cobras were feeding exclusively on birds
(d) many of the eggs laid, did not hatch

77 If a water body is contaminated with a toxicant, its biomagnification will be more marked in **[AMU 2012]**
(a) water (b) planktons
(c) small fishes (d) birds

78 Which one of the following pair of gases are the major cause of 'greenhouse effect'? **[CBSE AIPMT 2011]**
(a) CO_2 and CO (b) CFCs and SO_2
(c) CO_2 and N_2O (d) CO_2 and O_3

79 Which one of the following statements is wrong in case of Bhopal gas tragedy? **[CBSE AIPMT 2011]**
(a) Thousands of human being died
(b) Radioactive fall out engulfed Bhopal
(c) It took place in the night of December 2/3, 1984
(d) Methyl isocyanate gas leakage took place

80 Eutrophication is often seen in **[CBSE AIPMT 2011]**
(a) freshwater lakes (b) ocean
(c) mountains (d) deserts

81 At present, the concentration of CO_2 in the atmosphere is about **[DUMET 2011]**
(a) 100 ppm (b) 240 ppm
(c) 380 ppm (d) 520 ppm

82 The main cause of pollution in metrocities is **[UP CPMT 2011]**
(a) burning of fossil fuels (b) water plants
(c) domestic products (d) None of these

83 Minamata disease first occurred in **[Odisha JEE 2011]**
(a) Japan (b) Australia (c) India (d) China

84 Which one of the following is mainly responsible for greenhouses effect? **[WB JEE 2011]**
(a) SO_2 (b) CO_2 (c) CO (d) O_2

85 Match the following columns.

Column I	Column II
A. Electrostatic precipitator	1. Removes gases like SO_2
B. Scrubber	2. Reduces automobile emission
C. Catalytic converter	3. Removes particulate matter

Codes **[Kerala CEE 2011]**

	A	B	C		A	B	C
(a)	3	2	1	(b)	1	2	3
(c)	3	1	2	(d)	1	3	2
(e)	2	3	1				

86 Which one of the following is a correct option with reference to pathogenic bacteria and DDT? **[Gujarat CET 2011]**
(a) Bacteria can undergo multiplication and DDT is degraded by living cells
(b) Bacteria can be degraded by living cells and DDT cannot be degraded by living cells
(c) Bacteria can undergo biological magnification and DDT can be degraded by living cells
(d) Bacteria can undergo biological magnification and DDT cannot be degreded by living cells

ANSWERS

Check Point 26.1

1. (d)	2. (c)	3. (d)	4. (a)	5. (a)	6. (c)

Check Point 26.2

1. (b)	2. (d)	3. (c)	4. (b)	5. (d)	6. (b)	7. (c)

Check Point 26.3

1. (b)	2. (c)	3. (b)	4. (d)	5. (d)

Check Point 26.4

1. (a)	2. (c)	3. (c)	4. (b)	5. (d)	6. (c)

(A) Topical Exercise

1. (a)	2. (c)	3. (b)	4. (b)	5. (c)	6. (c)	7. (d)	8. (d)	9. (b)	10. (d)
11. (a)	12. (c)	13. (d)	14. (c)	15. (d)	16. (a)	17. (d)	18. (c)	19. (b)	20. (b)
21. (d)	22. (a)	23. (a)	24. (a)	25. (c)	26. (d)	27. (b)	28. (d)	29. (c)	30. (c)
31. (d)	32. (a)	33. (c)	34. (b)	35. (b)	36. (b)	37. (a)	38. (c)	39. (a)	40. (c)
41. (b)	42. (a)	43. (b)	44. (c)	45. (b)	46. (d)	47. (b)	48. (c)	49. (a)	50. (b)
51. (a)	52. (b)	53. (c)	54. (c)	55. (b)	56. (d)	57. (d)	58. (c)	59. (d)	60. (c)
61. (b)	62. (d)	63. (a)	64. (b)	65. (d)	66. (b)	67. (c)	68. (d)	69. (d)	70. (c)
71. (b)	72. (c)	73. (c)	74. (d)	75. (c)	76. (a)	77. (a)	78. (b)	79. (d)	80. (b)
81. (b)	82. (b)	83. (c)	84. (c)	85. (d)	86. (d)	87. (a)	88. (d)	89. (c)	90. (d)
91. (c)	92. (c)	93. (a)	94. (c)	95. (b)	96. (a)				

(B) Cumulative Exercise

1. (c)	2. (d)	3. (b)	4. (b)	5. (c)	6. (a)	7. (a)	8. (d)	9. (d)	10. (b)
11. (a)	12. (a)	13. (b)	14. (a)	15. (d)	16. (d)	17. (c)	18. (a)	19. (a)	20. (a)
21. (a)	22. (b)	23. (d)	24. (c)	25. (b)	26. (b)	27. (b)	28. (a).	29. (a)	30. (a)

(C) Medical Entrances' Gallery

1. (b)	2. (c)	3. (b)	4. (a)	5. (a)	6. (d)	7. (a)	8. (c)	9. (d)	10. (c)
11. (d)	12. (d)	13. (c)	14. (b)	15. (d)	16. (a)	17. (a)	18. (b)	19. (d)	20. (c)
21. (d)	22. (b)	23. (b)	24. (c)	25. (a)	26. (d)	27. (a)	28. (d)	29. (b)	30. (a)
31. (a)	32. (b)	33. (a)	34. (a)	35. (b)	36. (a)	37. (d)	38. (a)	39. (c)	40. (d)
41. (b)	42. (a)	43. (a)	44. (d)	45. (a)	46. (a)	47. (a)	48. (d)	49. (b)	50. (c)
51. (e)	52. (d)	53. (c)	54. (b)	55. (c)	56. (d)	57. (b)	58. (d)	59. (d)	60. (c)
61. (a)	62. (c)	63. (d)	64. (b)	65. (b)	66. (a)	67. (a)	68. (a)	69. (d)	70. (d)
71. (d)	72. (a)	73. (c)	74. (d)	75. (d)	76. (d)	77. (d)	78. (c)	79. (b)	80. (a)
81. (c)	82. (a)	83. (a)	84. (a)	85. (c)	86. (b)				

Explanations

(A) Topical Exercise

16 (*a*) Statement I is true, but II is false because
Sulphuric acid present in acid rain can cause corrosion of metals, marbles, stone, etc. This process is termed as stone leprosy.
Rain is acidic when its pH is below 5.65 due to the presence of H_2SO_4 and HNO_3.

13 (*d*) Statement in opiton (d) is incorrect and can be corrected as
Pollutants in jet planes are fluorocarbons.

20 (*b*) Statement in option (b) is incorrect and can be corrected as
CO gas combines with haemoglobin to form carboxyhaemoglobin.

40 (*c*) Arsenic is responsible for kidney damage.
Other options are explained as
Fluorine causes osteoporosis.
Cadmium leads to cancer.
Calcium helps in building and protecting bones.

52 (*b*) Statement in option (b) is not correct and can be corrected as
Jhum cultivation has no role in increasing crop yield. However, it is supposed to increase the soil fertility to some extent.

93 (*a*) In given pie chart, *A* is CO_2, *B* – Methane (CH_4), *C* = Chlorofluorocarbon (CFC).
Statement in option (a) is correct, while other statements are incorrect regarding *A*, *B* and *C*. Incorrect statements can be corrected as
B is the constituent of biogas and *C* is used as coolant.

(B) Cumulative Exercise

7 (*a*) Statements I, II and III are correct while IV is incorrect.
Incorrect statment can be corrected as
Eutrophication is the result of abundant growth of algae in water bodies.

12 (*a*) Statements I and II are correct for greenhouse effect.
Statement III is incorrect and can be corrected as
Increase in the level of greenhouse gases results in the considerable heating of the earth, leading to global warming.

14 (*a*) Statements I and II are correct, while III is incorrect.
Incorrect statement can be corrected as
River water may have a very low concentration of DDT, but the carnivorous fish in that river may contain high concentration of DDT, which is not suitable for consumption by human beings.

17 (*c*) Statement IV is incorrect and can be corrected as
Acid rain is harmful for all living organisms including plants and animals.

19 (*a*) Both A and R are true and R is the correct explanation of A.
CO_2 is confined exclusively to the troposphere. The thick layer of CO_2 in the troposphere behaves like the glass panels of a greenhouse and allows the sunlight to filter through, but prevents the heat from being re-radiated in the outer space. This is called greenhouse effect. CO_2 and water vapours absorb most of the heat present in the atmosphere and add it to the heat, which is already present on earth. Thus, the net result is the warming up of the earth's atmosphere.

20 (*a*) Both A and R are true and R is the correct explanation of A.

Oxides of sulphur and nitrogen are mainly responsible for the acid rain. These combine with the water vapour and form harmful H_2SO_4 and HNO_3, which then fall to the ground as acid rain. The problem of acid rain dramatically increased due to industrialisation, because the burning of fossil fuels in industries for power generation contributes oxides of sulphur and nitrogen to the atmosphere.

21 (*a*) Both A and R are true and R is the correct explanation of A.

Acid rain disrupts ecological balance, because it increases soil acidity, thus affecting the land flora (plants) and fauna (animals). It also causes acidification of lakes and streams thus, affecting aquatic life, crop productivity and finally, human health. Acidification kills many bacteria and blue-green algae (microorganisms) also.

22 (*b*) Both A and R are true, but R is not the correct explanation of A.

An increase in the concentration of ozone near earth's surface reduces crop yields because it enters in the plants through the stomata and produces visible damage to the leaves and other parts. It may decrease yield and quality of crop production, while higher concentration of O_3 in stratosphere protects us from the harmful UV rays coming from the sun.

23 (*d*) A is false, but R is true. A can be corrected as

Fluoride is necessary for the proper growth of human teeth. But excess consumption of fluoride causes knock-knee disease, in which pain in bones and joints and outward bending of legs from the knees takes place.

24 (*c*) A is true, but R is false because

Carbon dioxide forms a blanket around the earth and functions like a glass panel of a greenhouse. This allows the sunlight to pass out through it, but does not allow the heat from being re-radiated back into the outer space. This phenomenon is called greenhouse effect. Incomplete combustion of fossil fuels in automobiles releases 80% of carbon monoxide (CO).

25 (*b*) Both A and R are true, but R is not the correct explanation of A.

Effluents are industrial wastes released from steel, textile mills and fertiliser factories as waste products.

26 (*b*) Both A and R are true, but R is not the correct explanation of A.

In polluted water, the concentration of phosphorus and nitrogen compounds increases. These compounds favour the luxuriant growth of algae which generate an overproduction of these algae called water bloom.

27 (*b*) Both A and R are true, but R is not the correct explanation of A.

Prolonged exposure to noise level to 80 dB or more leads to the loss of hearing ability fatigue, nervousness, fever, hypertension, gastric disorder, increase in cholesterol level and dilation of pupil of the eye. As the jet aeroplanes have the noise upto 150-160bB, the inhabitants in the vicinity of busy airports are likely to experience the health hazards. Maximum noise level is recorded in rocket are 180 dB.

28 (*a*) Both A and R are true and R is the correct explanation of A.

Noise has been well-defined as 'unwanted sounds' which is being 'dumped' into the atmosphere to disturb the unwilling ears. It adversely affects our physiological and mental health. Prolonged and continued high intensity noise may cause permanent loss of hearing.

29 (*a*) Both A and R are true and R is the correct explanation of A.

Jhuming practice consists of cutting down of trees and burning the fallow trees and raising crops on the ash formed. It destroys forest and causes soil erosion.

30 (*a*) Both A and R are true and R is the correct explanation of A.

The weedicides or herbicides are usually metabolic inhibitors, which stop photosynthesis and other metabolic activities and hence kill the plants. Some weedicides cause death due to proliferation of phloem cells, so as to block the transport of organic food.

(C) Medical Entrances' Gallery

1 (*b*) *Eichhornia crassipes* (water hyacinth) was introduced in several tropical countries including India for ornamentation but later this exotic species became a trouble-some aquatic weed.

This free-floating weed clogged rivers and lakes and threatened the survival of many native species to the point of extinction. This species was called 'Terror of Bengal' in India.

2 (*c*) Air Prevention and Control of Pollution Act was amended in 1987 to include noise among pollutants. This act is meant for preserving quality of air, controlling air and noise pollution and prevent their detrimental effects on human health and health of other biological entities.

3 (*b*) According to Central Pollution Control Board (CPCB), particulate size 2.5 micrometers or less in diameter (PM 2.5) are responsible for causing the greatest harm to human health. These fine particulates can be inhaled deep into the lungs and can cause breathing and respiratory symptoms, irritation, inflammation and damage to the lungs and premature deaths.

5 (*a*) Snow blindness in Antarctic region is caused due to inflammation of cornea due to high dose of UV-B radiation. It is a painful temporary loss of vision due to overexposure to the sun's UV rays. It also called photo keratitis (photo—light, keratitis—inflammation of the cornea).

6 (*d*) Both options (a) and (b) represent the correctly matched pairs.

Particulate matter is any matter suspended in the atmosphere and causes various breathing and respiratory problems. Particulate matter parsent in atmosphere is controlled by electrostatic precipitator.

Option (c) is incorrectly matched pair and can be corrected as SO_2 is removed from industrial exhaust by scrubber and catalytic converter converts unburnt hydrocarbons into CO_2 and water.

7 (*a*) Eutrophication is caused due to accumulation of minerals in water body. It is the process of natural ageing of lakes by the biological enrichment of its water.

In a young lake, the water is clear, supporting little life. With time, due to the introduction of nutrients such as nitrogen and phosphorus, microorganisms which deteriorate the water quality grow and deplete the dissolved O_2 in water.

8 (*c*) Method in option (c) is the most suitable for disposal of nuclear waste.

Nuclear waste is usually disposed by burying it within rocks deep below the earth's surface.

Nuclear waste disposal is extremely hazardous. Before burying the waste, it is sealed in large containers so as to reduce its radiation effects.

9 (*d*) Salinity of soil is a problem faced by farmers if they liberally irrigate agricultural field for a prolonged period of time.

Irrigation salinity is the accumulation of salts in the top soil under irrigation. It is caused by over irrigation of agricultural land, inefficient water use, poor drainage and the irrigation of unsuitable and leaky soils.

10 (*c*) Greenhouse effect is mainly contributed by carbon dioxide (60%) and methane (20%) along with nitrous oxide, nitrogen dioxide and chlorofluorocarbons. It results in the rise in temperature of earth because greenhouse gases have the ability to trap the heat of solar radiations.

11 (*d*) Statement in option (d) is correct.

Stratospheric ozone protects us from UV radiations of the sun.

Rest of the statements about ozone are incorrect and can be corrected as

Good ozone is found in the upper part of the atmosphere, i.e. stratosphere. Bad ozone is formed in the lower atmosphere (troposphere) that harms plants and animals.

12 (*d*) Montreal protocol aimed to reduce the emission of chlorofluorocarbons into atmosphere because of their deleterious effects on stratospheric ozone. This protocol was signed in Montreal, Canada in 1987. Other options are explained as

- Kyoto protocol aimed to reduce the emission of CO_2, NO_2 and methane.
- It was signed by 160 countries in a convention held in Kyoto, Japan in 1997.
- Geneva protocol is a treaty to prohibit the use of chemical or biological weapons in international armed conflicts.
- Gothenberg protocol is a multipollutant protocol which focuses to reduce eutrophication, acidification, emission standards for SO_2, etc.

14 (*b*) Polyblend has proved to be a good material for the construction of roads. It is a fine powder of recycled plastic and it is mixed with bitumen to lay roads. The first polyblend road was laid in Bengaluru by the effort of Ahmed Khan.

15 (*d*) Ozone (O_3) is a secondary pollutant as it is formed by the reaction amongst the primary pollutants in the atmosphere and are not directly released. On the other hand, SO_2 is a primary pollutant. These pollutants persist in the environment in their actual form. CO is quantitative pollutant. It is considered as a pollutant only when its concentration reaches beyond a threshold value in the environment.

CO_2 is a quantitative as well as a primary pollutant.

16 (*a*) Both A and R are true and R is the correct explanation of A.

Biological Oxygen Demand (BOD) is the amount of O_2 (in miligrams), required to decompose organic matter present in one litre of water which is heavily polluted. Increase in BOD value causes sharp decline in dissolved oxygen in water hence, indicating that the water is polluted.

17 (*a*) 'World Ozone Day' is celebrated on 16th September to control O_3 depletion. Ozone layer is a fragile shield of gas that protects earth from harmful UV-rays.

Other options are explained as

On 21st April, the Civil Service Day and National Yellow Bat Day is celebrated. 5th June of every year is celebrated on World Environment Day. Earth Day is an annual event, celebrated on 22nd April of every year.

18 (*b*) In stratosphere, Cl acts as a catalyst in the degradation of ozone and release of molecular oxygen. It is released by action of UV-rays on chlorofluorocarbons.

Chlorine reacts with ozone in a series of chain reaction, converting it into oxygen.

19 (*d*) The zooplankton is incorrectly matched regarding biological magnification of DDT in aquatic ecosystem. It can be corrected as

Zooplankton- 0.04 ppm whereas water has 0.003 ppm of DDT.

Rest options are correctly matched pairs.

20 (*c*) BOD may not be a good index for pollution in water bodies receiving effluents from petroleum industry. This is because petroleum effluents contain waste which is non-biodegradable.

21 (*d*) When much of organic matter is present in lake, lots of microbial activity takes place in its decomposition process. So, demand for oxygen increases. This increased O_2 demand depletes the dissolved oxygen in water at faster rates. This adversely affects the living conditions for other organisms like fishes, etc., ultimately causing their death.

22 (*b*) DDT is a toxic substance which gets concentrated subsequently in a food chain of an aquatic ecosystem in the following manner

Phytoplanktons → Eel → Crab → Seagull
(0.04 ppm) (0.5 ppm) (2 ppm) (25 ppm)

Thus, the animal or organism acquiring the highest position in a food chain would have the highest DDT concentration (here seagull).

28 (*d*) Scrubber is used to remove gases, e.g. SO_2 from industrial exhausts.

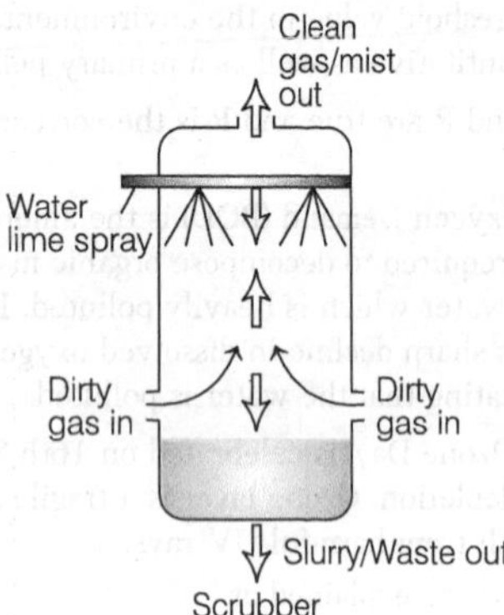

Scrubber

The dirty air is cleaned by capturing gases like SO_2 and other oxides in water/lime spray.

29 (*b*) One greenhouse gas CFCs contributes 14% to total global warming and another, N_2O contributes 6%. The total contribution of greenhouse gases is as follows

Greenhouse gases		Percentage
CO_2	–	60
CH_4	–	20
CFCs	–	14
N_2O	–	6

32 (*b*) The UN conference of parties (CoP-18), the UN Framework Convention on Climate Change (UNFCCC) was held in Doha, Qatar from 26th Nov-8th Dec 2012.

35 (*b*) The UN conference of parties on climate change in the year 2011 from 28th November to 1st December was held at Durban, South Africa.

36 (*a*) *Silent Spring* documents the detrimental effects of indiscriminated use of pesticides on the environment and both its components. The book spured the authorities and caused a reversal in pesticide usage policies also, ensuring a nationwide ban on DDT use in agricultural fields.

Environmental protection agencies and acts were created as the result of jarring awareness caused by the book.

37 (*d*) Depletion of stratospheric ozone UV radiation is able to reach earth's surface. The exposure to these radiations has increased the occurrence of skin cancer, snow blindness (damage to eyes), herpes and deficient functioning of immune system, etc. Liver cancer is not a consequence of UV exposure.

39 (*c*) High noise levels cause cardiovascular, neurological effects on the human body. If one person is exposed to such condition for a longer period of time, he will suffer from stress and anxiety disorders.

40 (*d*) DDT is banned because, it shows deleterious effects on organisms and is found in considerably high toxic amount in all trophic level organisms. It is degraded biologically and has long residual effects on almost all living organisms due to the high concentration of accumulation in higher trophic levels, i.e. biomagnification.

42 (*a*) The natural insecticide in neem (*Azadirachta indica*) is azadirachtin. It provides the indigenous way to kill wide variety of insects and pests and serves as broad spectrum pesticide for fruit, vegetables and other agricultural crops. The best part in insects cannot develop resistance against it and remains completely safe for non-targeted insects and human beings.

44 (*d*) The secondary pollutants are not emitted directly, but are formed in the air when primary pollutants react or interact photochemically to form photochemical oxidants. These include smog, O_3, PAN, etc.

Thus, option (d) is correct.

45 (*a*) There will be more microbial activity in the sewage if more dead organic matter is present. More microbial activity will require more oxygen which, we call technically as biological oxygen demand. So, the pollution strength of any sewage can be determined by its Biological Oxygen Demand (BOD).

47 (*a*) Option (a) is incorrect combination and can be corrected as

The historic convention on biological diverstiy, the earth summit held in Rio de Janeiro in 1992 called upon all nations to take appropriate measures for sustainable utilisation of its benefits.

Rest options are correct combinations.

49 (*b*) BOD is the measure of oxygen required for chemical breakdown of organic pollutants or wastes. High value of BOD in a water source indicates high level of pollutants.

50 (*c*) Methane is a greenhouse gas which contributes about 20% to total global warming. Redesigning the landfill dumps in a way which will permit the collection of methane, will most likely help in slowing down the greenhouse effect.

51 (*e*) Ahmed Khan developed the method of plastic waste recycling.

Polyblend is a recycled modified plastic, which on mixing with bitumen increases its water repellant properties.

This mixture was used to lay many roads in Bengaluru and helped to increase road life.

53. (*c*) If there was no CO_2 in the earth's atmosphere, the temperature of the earth's surface would be less than the present level because CO_2 has the property of trapping heat on earth surface.

Hence, CO_2 as a greenhouse gas has made the earth habitable by maintaining the adequate amount of temperature on earth's surface.

54 (*b*) The correct order (ascending) of BOD is I, II and III.
BOD (Biochemical Oxygen Demand) is the amount of dissolved oxygen needed by aerobic organisms in a water body to breakdown organic material present in it, at certain temperature, over a specific period of time.

56 (*d*) The situation suggests that the site is not polluted as lichens are the bioindicators for air pollution. These respond to change in the environment. The lichens are useful indicators of especially SO_2 pollution because they derive their water and essential nutrients mainly from the atmosphere rather than from the soil.

60 (*c*) If temperature of water rises, the amount of dissolved oxygen decreases. Dissolved Oxygen (DO) is a relative measure of the amount of oxygen dissolved or carried in a given medium. Water contains very limited amount of dissolved oxygen. It comes from the atmosphere and from photosynthesis by aquatic plants. The aquatic organisms in turn, uses this oxygen for respiration and to survive.

63 (*d*) Greenhouse gases absorb long wave infrared radiation from the earth and emit it again towards the earth. The cycle continues till the earth's surface has no long wave radiation to emit.

68 (*a*) The Air Prevention and Control of Pollution Act, came into force in 1981. The act is meant for preserving quality of air, controlling air pollution and preventing detrimental effects of air pollutants on human health and health of other biological entities.

69 (*d*) Global warming is the term that describes the average rise of temperature on earth. Thus to reduce global warming, deforestation must be reduced and fossil fuel usage should be decreased.

73 (*c*) High amount of *Escherichia coli* in water indicates sewage pollution. *E. coli* bacteria are good indicator of faecal contamination because they generally live longer than pathogens and are found in greater number.

79 (*b*) Statement in option (b) is wrong in case of Bhopal gas tragedy and can be corrected as
Bhopal gas tragedy (Bhopal disaster) is the world's worst industrial catastrophes. It occurred on the night of December 2/3, 1984 at the Union Carbide India Limited (UCIL) pesticide plant in Bhopal, Madhya Pradesh. A leak of methyl isocyanate gas and other chemicals from the plant resulted the exposure of hundreds to thousands of people. The official immediate death toll was 2259 and the government of Madhya Pradesh has confirmed a total of 3787 deaths related to the gas releases.

80 (*a*) Eutrophication is nutrient enrichment of water body resulting in increased growth of algae, other plants and animals. It is often seen in freshwater lakes. Actually, it is the natural ageing of a lake by biological enrichment of its water.

82 (*a*) Main causes of pollution in metrocities is burning of fossil fuels. It releases CO_2, CO, SO_2, H_2S and H_2SO_4. All these form strong air pollutants.

85 (*c*) A-3, B-1, C-2
Electrostatic precipitators are used in thermal power plants to remove particulate matter upto 99% by electrically changing the particles.
A scrubber can remove gases like SO_2. In a scrubber, the exhaust is passed through a spray of water of lime.

Catalytic converter has expensive metals namely platinum, palladium, rhodium that can convert NO_x to nitrogen and CO to CO_2. In this way, it reduces automobile emission.
Thus, option (c) is correct.

86 (*b*) Option (b) is correct with reference to pathogenic bacteria and DDT.

Bacteria is a prokaryotic organism that can be degraded by living cells and DDT is a non-biodegradable pollutant and undergoes biological magnification.

Appendix

Emergence of contemporary biology

Some historical events in biology

Years	Names	Contributions
460-377 BC	Hippocrates	Known as Father of Medicine, he wrote fifty books. Hippocratic Oath for graduate physicians is being administered even today.
384-322 BC	Aristotle	Father of Biology, Zoology and Embryology.
380-287 BC	Theophrastus	A student of Aristotle, considered as Father of Botany due to contribution in plant morphology.
1690	Leonardo da Vinci	Father of Palaeontology, who stated that fossils are evidences of past.
1707-1778	Carolus Linnaeus	Father of Taxonomy and Nomenclature and introduced system of Binomial nomenclature.
1721-1797	Lazzaro Spallanzani	Rejected the Theory of Abiogenesis in 1765.
1802	Lamarck and Treviranus	Proposed the term 'Biology'.
1809-1882	Charles Darwin	Proposed the Theory of Natural Selection, Theory of Pangenesis and Survival of the Fittest.
1813	AP Candolle	Introduced the term 'Taxonomy'.
1838	TR Malthus	Suggested that human population increases much faster than its food supply.
1840-1935	Hugo de Vries	Proposed Mutation Theory of Evolution. He worked on *Oenothera lamarckiana* (evening primrose).
1861	Louis Pasteur	Proved biogenesis by experiments, Proposed Germ Theory of Disease.
1834-1919	Ernst Haeckel	Proposed Theory of Recapitulation in 1864, Coined the term 'Protista'.
1875	Wallace	Described zoogeographical regions of the world.
1885	August Weismann	Proposed Theory of Germplasm.
1889	Martinus Beijerinck	Concept of virus.
1892	Dimitri Ivanovsky	Discovered virus.
1924	AI Oparin	Chemical origin (synthetic evolution) of organisms.
1926	T Svedberg	Discovered ultracentrifuge.
1927	Hermann J Muller	Proved that the X rays cause mutation, artificial mutation in *Drosophila*.
1929	Haldane	Proposed the Theory of Origin of Life.
1929	A Fleming	Discovered penicillin from *Penicillium notatum*.
1932	Knoll and Ruska	Invented electron microscope.
1935	W M Stanley	Isolated TMV in crystal form.
1942	Mayer	Described species as interbreeding individuals of population.
1946	HJ Muller	Discovered that the mutations are produced by X ray irradiation.
1953	Urey and Stanley Miller	Explained the presence of organic elements in primitive atmosphere by an experiment.

Major branches of botany

Branches	Descriptions
Agriculture	Cultivation of useful plants.
Agronomy	Study of crop cultivation and farm management.
Algology (Phycology)	Study of algae.
Anthology	Study of flowers.
Aphidology	Study of aphids (plant lice).
Carcinology	Study of crustaceans.
Bryology	Study of bryophytes.
Biochemical Taxonomy	Study of taxonomy of related plants based on chemical reactions.
Cnidology	Study of coelenterates (cnidarians).
Conchology	Study of shells secreted by mantle as in molluscs.
Dendrochronology	Counting and analysing annual growth rings of trees.
Economic Zoology	Study of useful and harmful activities of animals.

Branches	Descriptions
Entomology	Study of insects.
Ethology	Study of behaviour of animals in response to the environmental stimuli.
Eugenics	Study of improvement of future human race.
Economic Botany	Study of commercially useful plants.
Edaphology (Pedology)	Study of soil.
Ethnobotany	Study of relationship between the primitive humans and plants.
Floriculture	Cultivation of flower yielding plants.
Forestry (Silviculture)	Study of development and conservation of forests and their products.
Horticulture	Development and management of orchards and gardens.
Helminthology	Study of worms (round and flatworms).
Herpetology	Study of reptiles and amphibians
Ichthyology	Study of fishes.
Lepidoteriology	Study of moths and butterflies.
Lichenology	Study of lichens.
Limnology	Study of freshwater ecology.
Mycology	Study of fungi.
Mammalogy	Study of mammals.
Myremecology	Study of ants.
Palaeobotany	Study of plant life of past based on fossil studies.
Palynology	Study of pollen grains.
Parasitology	Study of parasites.
Protistology	Study of protists (unicellular plants and animals)
Physiology	Study of functions and processes of life.
Phytography	Branch of botany dealing with descriptive features of plant parts.
Pomology(Carpology)	Science dealing with fruits and fruit yielding plants.
Saurology	Study of lizards.
Termitology	Study of termites.
Zootomy	Dissection and anatomy of animals.

Major discoveries in cell biology

Years	Names	Contributions
1632-1723	AV Leeuwenhoek (an amateur lens grinder)	Discovered single lens high power microscope. Observed bacteria, Protozoa, spermatozoa, RBCs, etc. Father of Microbiology/Protozoology.
1665	Robert Hooke	Discovered cell, compound microscope, Father of Cytology.
1781	Fontana	Discovered nucleus although credit goes to Robert Brown.
1773-1858	Robert Brown	Described Brownian movement in 1831. Observed nuclei in flowering plant cell of *Tradescantia* in 1835.
1837	JE Purkinje	Used the term 'protoplasm' for the first time.
1838-39	Schleiden and T Schwann	Proposed cell theory which states that organisms are made up of cells.
1841	Robert Remak	Described the amitotic cell division for the first time.
1843	Claude	First recognised the ribosomes as basophilic granules rich in nucleic acids.
1858	R Virchow	Stated that all cells arise from pre-existing cells, *Omnis cellula e cellula.*
1800-85	Milne Edwards	Explained the division of labour in cells of the body.
1866	GJ Mendel	Father of Genetics, proposed law of inheritance.
1868	Huxley	Proposed that protoplasm is the physical basis of life.
1869-71	Frederick Miescher	Isolated nucleoproteins from pus cells in 1870 and discovered DNA in 1897.
1879	W Flemming	Coined the term 'Chromatin' and described the splitting of chromosomes, described mitosis in 1882.
1884	Christian Gram	Gram staining method.
1887	Waldeyer	Used the term chromosome for the first time.

Years	Names	Contributions
1888	T Boveri	Described the term centrosome.
1897	C Benda	Named mitochondria.
1898	Camillo Golgi	Described and named Golgi complex.
1900	Correns, Hugo de Vries and Tschermak	Rediscovered the Mendel's laws of inheritance.
1902	Sutton and Boveri	Explained the importance of meiotic cell division, propounded chromosome theory of inheritance (genes are part of chromosomes).
1905	Farmer and Moore	Called reduction division as meiosis.
1906	Bateson and Punnett	Applied Mendel's laws on animals and named the science of heredity as Genetics.
1908	Barr Murray	Discovered Barr body in man.
1909	Johannsen	Coined the term gene, genotype and phenotype.
1910	TH Morgan	Discovered sex-linked inheritance in *Drosophila* and laid foundation of gene theory.
1914	Robert Feulgen	Described a stain for DNA and showed that chromosomes contain DNA.
1915	Twort and d'Herelle	Discovered bacteriophage virus.
1928	F Griffith	Discovered transformation in bacteria.
1941	George Beadle and Edward Tatum	One-gene-one enzyme hypothesis.
1949	L Pauling	Demonstrated that the protein structure is controlled by genes.
1950	Barbara McClintock	Discovered jumping genes or transposons in maize.
1950	E Chargaff	Studied that purines and pyrimidines are in equal amounts in DNA.
1952	M Chase and AD Hershey	Suggested that the DNA is a carrier of genetic information in T_2-phase.
1952	Lederberg and Zinder	Bacterial transduction.
1953	JD Watson and FH Crick	Proposed double helix model of DNA.
1954	F Jacob and J Monod	Demonstrated that the genetic expression is controlled by regulatory genes and proposed *lac* operon model of *E. coli*.
1955	Kornberg and S Ochoa	Biologically synthesised nucleic acid of *E. coli* (Nobel Prize in 1959).
1955	Fraenkel Conrat and RC Williams	Studied the nature of TMV virus and showed that it was made up of RNA and protein-A.
1955	M Hoagland	Discovered *t*RNA.
1956	H Fraenkel and Conrat	Showed that RNA is the genetic material in TMV.
1959	S Ochoa	Artificially synthesised RNA (*in vitro*).
1959	Robertson	Proposed unit membrane model of plasma membrane.
1961	Nirenberg and Methaei	Discovered the genetic code and its triplet nature.
1965	H Harris and JF Watkins	Discovered protoplast fusion in cells of different species.
1970	HG Khorana	Discovered DNA ligase enzyme. Synthesised gene (DNA) artificially.
1970	Norman Borlaug	Developed rust resistant wheat varieties.
1975	JW Sanger	Chromosome migration on spindle fibres.

Nobel Prize winners in physiology and medicine

Scientist (s)	Years of Nobel Prize	Contributions
Arvid Carlsson	2000	Proved that dopamine is a neurotransmitter in the brain whose depletion leads to symptoms of Parkinson's disease.
Paul Greengard	2000	Described how neurotransmitters act on the cell and can activate a central molecule known as DARPP-32.
Eric R Kandel	2000	Described how short-term and long-term memory is formed on the molecular level.
Leland H Hartwell, R Timothy Hunt and Sir Paul M Nurse	2001	Discovery of cyclin and cyclin dependent kinase, central molecules in the regulation of the cell cycle.
Paul Lauterbur and Sir Peter Mansfield	2003	Discoveries concerning magnetic resonance imaging.
Linda B Buck and Richard Axel	2004	Discoveries of odorant receptors and the organisation of the olfactory system.

Scientist (s)	Years of Nobel Prize	Contributions
Barry J Marshall and Robin Warren	2005	Discovery of the bacterium *Helicobacter pylori* and its role in gastritis and peptic ulcer disease.
Andrew Z Fire and Craig C Mello	2006	Discovery of RNA interference-gene silencing by double-stranded RNA.
Mario R Capecchi, Sir Martin and Oliver Smithies	2007	Discoveries of principles for introducing specific gene modifications in mice by the use of embryonic stem cells.
Harald zur Hausen	2008	Discovery of human papilloma viruses causing cervical cancer.
Francoise Barre Sinoussi and Luc Montagnier	2008	Discovery of human immunodeficiency virus.
Elizabeth H Blackburn, Carol W Greider and Jack W Szostak	2009	Discovery of how chromosomes are protected by telomeres and the enzyme telomerase.
Robert G Edward	2010	Development of *in vitro* fertilisation.
Bruce A Beutler, Jules A Hoffmann	2011	Discoveries concerning the activation of innate immunity.
Ralph M Steinman	2011	Discovery of the dendritic cells and its role in adaptive immunity.
Sir John B Gurdon, Shinya Yamanaka	2012	Discovery that mature cells can be reprogrammed to become pluripotent.
James E Rothman, Randy W Schekman and Thomas C Siidhof	2013	Discoveries of machinery regulating vesicle traffic, a major transport system in our cells.
JohnO' keefe, May-britt Moser Edward I. Moser	2014	Discovery of cells that constitute a positioning system in the brain.
William C, Campbell, Satoshi Omura, Youyou Tu	2015	Discovery concerning a novel therapies against malaria and roundworm infections.
Yoshinori oh sumi	2016	Discovery of mechanism for autophagy.

Major discoveries in genetics and biotechnology

7000 BC.	Chinese discovered fermentation through beer making
1862	Louis Pasteur discovered the bacterial origin of fermentation
1864	Antonin Prandtl invents first centrifuge to separate cream from curd
1881	Louis Pasteur developed vaccines against cholera and Anthrax in chickens.
1919	Karoly Ereky, a Hungarian agriculture engineer first used the word biotechnology
1928	Alexander Fleming discovered penicillin
1953	James D Watson and Francis Crick described the structrue of DNA
1972	DNA composition of chimpanzees and gorillas was discovered to be 99% similar to humans
1973	Stanley Norman Cohen and Herbert Boyer performed the first successful recombinant DNA experiment using bacterial genes.
1975	Methods for monoclonal antibodies developed by Kohler and Cesar Milstein
1980	US Patent gene for gene cloning was awarded to Cohen and Boyer.
1982	Humulin, human insulin drug was produced by genetically engineered bacteria for the treatment of diabetes.
1983	Polymerase chain reaction technique was conceived
1990	Immune disorder in a girl was treated using gene therapy
1994	'*Flavr Savr*' GM tomato were approved for the first time by US food and drug administration
1997	First cloned animal, Dolly sheep was created by Ian Wilmut
2000	Human Genome Project Draft was completed
2002	Rice genome was first decoded
2003	Human Genome Project was completed
2009	Cedars-Sinai Heart Institute used modified SAN Heart genes to create the first pacemaker in guinea pigs now known as is SANs.

Famous Indian biologists and their contributions

Biologists	Contributions
MOP Iyengar	Father of Indian Phycology
Y Bhardwaj	Indian Phycologist
RN Singh	Indian Phycologist
GS Venkataraman	Indian Phycologist
EJ Butler	Father of Indian Mycology and Pathology
Dhanwantri	God of Medicine/Ayurveda
R Misra	Father of Indian Plant Ecology
Birbal Sahni	Father of Indian Palaeobotany
P Maheswari	Father of Indian Plant Embryology
PKK Nair	Father of Indian Palynology
RN Dastur	Father of Indian Physiology
V Puri	Plant Morphologist
KA Chaudhary	Plant Anatomist and Xylotomist
William Roxburgh	Father of Indian Botany and Father of Indian Herbaria
Ram Udar	Bryologist
TS Sadasivan	Mycologist
DD Awasthi	Lichens
JJ Chinoy	Plant Physiologist
PN Mehra	Great Pteridologist
RN Singh	Role of Blue Green Algae (BGA) in nitrogen-fixation and utility of BGA in reclamation of Kallar grass
Susruta	Father of Surgery and Plastic Surgery
Charaka	Father of Ayurveda
MS Swaminathan	Father of Green Revolution in India. He developed wheat triple dwarf variety (Pusa Larma and Sharbati Sonora)
Salim Ali	Ornithologist (Birdman of India)
Indira Hinduja, Subhas Mukherjee	Test tube Baby
Col. Stevenson	Father of Indian Zoology
Lalji Singh	Father of DNA Fingerprinting in India
H Santapu	Father of Indian Systemic Botany (Taxonomy)
V Kurien	Father of White Revolution in India
Sir Ronald Ross	A doctor in Indian Army established that malarial parasite is transmitted by the bite of female *Anopheles* mosquito. In 1972, he got Nobel Prize for this discovery

Books and authors (Years of publishing)

Books	Authors
De Historia Plantarum	Theophrastus (320 BC)
De Causis Plantarum	Theophrastus (320 BC)
Naturalis Historia	Pliny the Elder (77-79 AD)
Anatomical Preparations	Galen (131-200 AD)
On Animals	Albertus Magnus (1249)
De Humani Corporis Fabrica	Andreas Vesalius (1543)
Micrographia	Robert Hooke (1665)
Historia Generalis Plantarum	John Ray (1686)
Systema Naturae	Carolus Linnaeus (1735)
Genera Plantarum	Carolus Linnaeus (1737)
Species Plantarum	Carolus Linnaeus (1753)
Philosophie Zoologique (Inheritance of acquired characters)	Jean Baptiste de Lamarck (1809)
Histology	Albrecht von Kolliker (1852)
On the Origin of Species	Charles Darwin (1859)

Important human disorders

Names of disorder	Related to body systems	Agents/Reasons of disorder
Arthritis	Skeleton system	Inflammation in one or more joints cause pain.
Asthma	Respiratory system	Inflammation in respiratory system due to genetic and environmental factors.
Baldness	Skin and hair	Due to fungal infection, traumatic damage, radio or chemotherapy or genetically.
Cancer	Any body system	Due to loss of control over cell division and cell cycle.
Dandruff	Skin	Due to dry skin, fungal infection (by *Malassezia furfur*), etc.
Diabetes	Digestive /Endocrine system	Due to loss of control over regulatory mechanism of carbohydrate metabolism of pancreatic hormones in insulin and glucagon.
Dyslexia	Nervous system	Due to neurological, genetical and environmental reasons.
Enlarged	Prostate gland	Excessive secretion of androgens.
Epilepsy	Brain	Due to brain injury, brain cancer, genetical, drug, alcohol, etc.

Names of disorder	Related to body systems	Agents/Reasons of disorder
Fracture	Skeleton system	As a result of high pressure/force or impact of stress on bones and also due to osteoporosis.
Gall stone	Digestive system/Gall bladder	Due to deposition of crystalline substances of bile in gall bladder.
Gout	Joints/Skeleton system	Also termed as acute inflammatory arthritis due to elevated level of uric acid.
Heart attack	Heart	Happens when blood stops flowing properly to any part of heart
Hypertension	Blood vascular system	Due to increase in blood pressure in the arteries.

Names of disorder	Related to body systems	Agents/Reasons of disorder
Migraine	Nervous system	Exact mechanism not known. May be due to genetic or environmental reason.
Osteoporosis	Bones	Due to decrease in the mineral content of bones that lead to fracture.
Parkinson's disease	Nervous system	As result of death of dopamine generating cells in the midbrain.
Tennis elbow	Muscles and skeleton system	Caused by changes in the tendons that attache the forearm muscle to the elbow.
Ulcers	Digestive system	Due to excess secretion of acid, pepsin in digestive tract.

Viral infections of human body

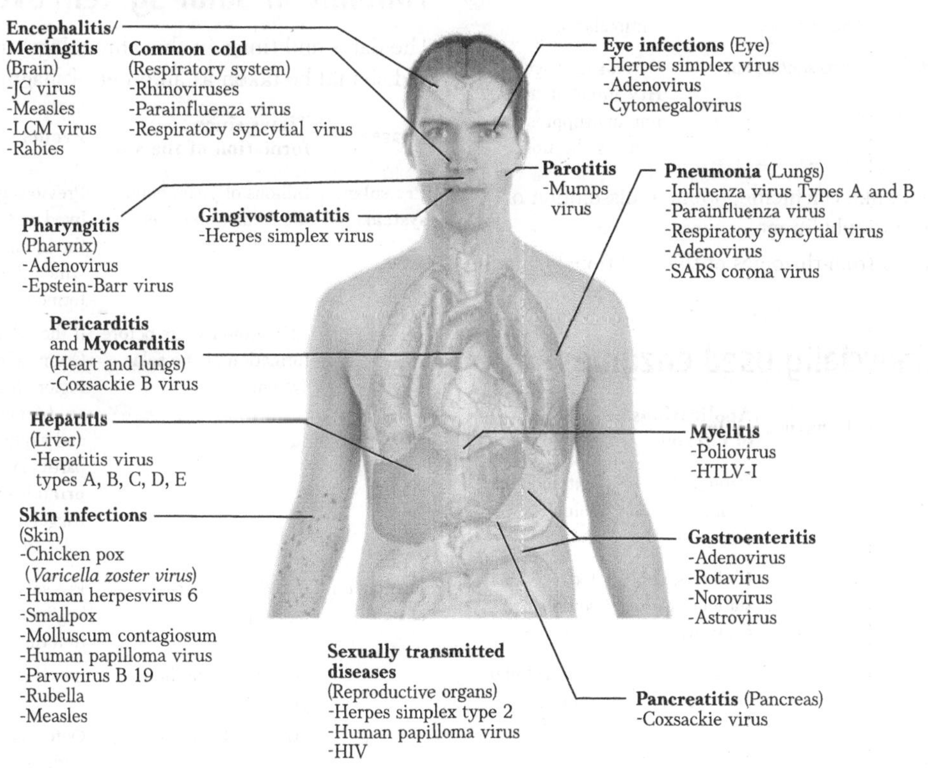

Some important compounds, their medicinal values and source plant

Compounds	Plant species	Medicinal values
Shikonin	*Lithospermum erythrorhizon*	Antiseptic (also used as dye for silk and cosmetics)
Berberine	*Coptis joponica*	Antibacteria, anti-inflammatory
Codeine	*Papaver somniferum*	Analgesic
Diosgenin	*Dioscorea deltoidea*	Antifertility agents
Quinine	*Cinchona*	Antimalarial
Scopolamine	*Datura stramonium*	Antihypertensive
Vincristine	*Catharanthus roseus*	Antileukaemic
Ajamalicine	*C. roseus*	
Taxol*	*Taxus* species	Breast and ovarian cancer treatment
Artemisin	*Artemisia* sp.	Antimalarial
Tirchosanthin and Karasorin**	*Trichosanthes* sp.	Cytotoxicity against HIV infected cells, immunosuppressant, induces abortion

* Acts on spindle like colchicine; promote dissolution of microtubules into tubulin molecules.

** Proteins isolated from rhizomes of the traditional Chinese medicinal plant.

Some commercially used enzymes

Enzymes	Sources of enzyme	Applications of enzyme	Usable forms
Alkaline protease	*B. licheniformis, B. subtilis*	Detergents (protein digestion)	Extracellular, soluble
α-amylase	*Bacillus licheniformis,* *B. amyloliquefaciens*	Hydrolysis of starch to dextrans	Extracellular, soluble
Acid protease, e.g. rennet	*A. niger*	Milk coagulation and cheese flavour enhancement	Extracellular, soluble
Cellulase	*A. niger, Trichoderma reesei*	Cellulose hydrolysis, in fruit juices	Extracellular, soluble
Glucoamylase	*Aspergillus niger*	Dextran hydrolysis to glucose	Extracellular, soluble
Lipase	*Rhizopus* species	Detergents, lipid hydrolysis	Extracellular, soluble
Lactase	*A. niger*	Milk lactose hydrolysis to glucose+galactos e	Immobilised on glass beads
Neutral protease	*B. amyloliqufaciens, B. subtilis*	Protein digestion in brewing substances	Extracellular, soluble
Pectinase	*A. niger, B. subtilis*	Pectin hydrolysis in fruit	Extracellular, soluble
Xylose (glucose) isomerase	*Bacillus coagulans*	Pure glucose to equilibrium mixture of glucose + fructose	Immobilised whole cells

Timeline of solar system evolution

The dates and times in this chronology are approximate and should be taken as an order of magnitude only.

Phases	Times since formation of the sun	Events
Pre-solar system	Billions of years before the formation of the Solar System	Previous generations of stars lived and died, injecting into the interstellar medium of which the solar system is formed.
	~50 million years before formation of the solar system	If the solar system formed in an Orion nebula-like star-forming region, the most massive stars are formed, live their lives, die, and explode in supernova. One particular supernova, called **the primal** supernova, possibly triggers the formation of the solar system.
Formation of sun	0-100,000 years	Pre-solar nebula forms and begins to collapse. Sun begins to form.
	100,000-50 million years	Sun is a T Tauri protostar.
	100,000-10 million years	Outer planets formed. By 10 million years, gas in the protoplanetary disc has been blown away and outer planet formation is likely to complete.
	10 million-100 million years	Terrestrial planets and the moon formed. Giant impacts occurred. Water delivered to earth.

Phases	Times since formation of the sun	Events
Main Sequence	50 million years	Sun became a main sequence star.
	200 million years	Oldest known rocks on the Earth formed.
	500 million-600 million years	Resonance in Jupiter and Saturn's orbits moved Neptune out into the Kuiper belt. Later heavy bombardment occurred in the inner solar system.
	800 million years	Oldest known life on earth. Oort cloud reached maximum mass.
	4.6 billion years	Today, sun remains a main sequence star, continually growing, warmer and brighter by ~10% every 1 billion years.
	6 billion years	Sun's habitable zone moved outside of the Earth's orbit, possibly shifting on to Mars's orbit.
	7 billion years	The Milky Way and Andromeda Galaxy begin to collide. Slight chance the Solar System could be captured by Andromeda before the two galaxies fuse completely.

Relation between some food items and genes

Specific genes	Functions of the gene	Link to the gene	Food	Long-term effects
HER-2	Triggers growth signals in cells	Helps to inhibit genes that fuel breast cancer	**Green Tea**	Slow HER-2 signalling in tumours
GST	Produces the body's master antioxidant - glutathione	Boosts genes that protect against heart disease	**Broccoli**	The additional glutathione helps to keep arteries healthy
p53	Kill mutant cells	Affect 123 genes involved in prostate cancer	**Soyabeans**	Increase activity of the p53 gene to block tumour formation
Cox-2	Makes inflammatory compounds	Suppresses genes that bump up inflammation	**Turmeric (a curry ingredient)**	Helps to ward off heart disease, colon cancer and Alzheimer's disease

A, B, C and D forms of DNA

DNA can exist in A, B, C and D forms depending upon different condition. B form (B-DNA) is the structure proposed by **Watson** and **Crick**. It has metabolically stable configuration and can undergo transformation to A, C and D forms at relative humidity lower than 92% and temperature variation.

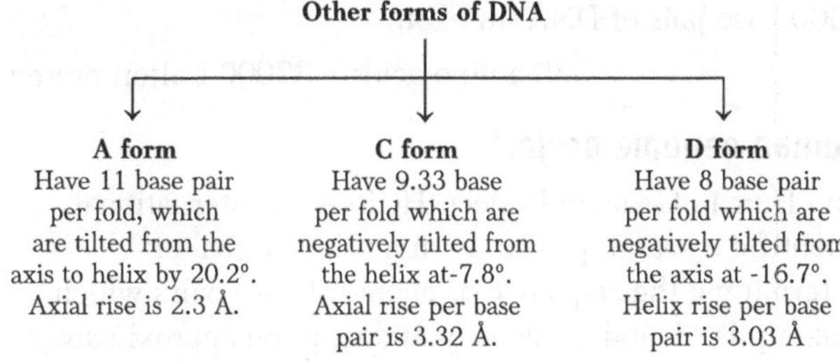

RL and Z forms of DNA

GA Rodley Group of New Zealand and V Sasisekharan Group of India have independently proposed a structure of DNA, which is different from right handed helix model of Watson and Crick. According to this model, DNA duplex is formed by alternating right and left handed helices arranged side by side, thus, called **RL** (Right Handed-Left Handed) **helix** or **side by side helix.** The repeating unit of helix is 10 base pairs thus, the helices aligned 10 base pairs with 5 each in right and left handed helix. The model can more easily explain the supercoiling of DNA in eukaryotic chromosomes. Rich and his group at MIT, USA have studied molecular structure of DNA at atomic resolution. They have proposed a left handed helix model with *ziq-zaq* sugar phosphate backbone in antiparallel organisation. This DNA has been called **Z-DNA.**

Comparison of major forms of DNA

Features	B form	A form	Z form
Major groove	Wide and deep	Narrow and deep	Flat
Minor groove	Narrow and deep	Wide and shallow	Narrow and deep
Helix coiling	Right handed	Right handed	Left handed
Pitch of helix (turn of helix)	33.2 Å	24.6 Å	45.6 Å
Diameter	20 Å	23 Å	18 Å
Repeating unit	1 base pair	1 base pair	2 base pairs
Rotation/Base pair	34.3°	33.6°	60°/2
Mean base pair/turn	10.4 or 10	10.7 or 11	12
Rise/Base pair	3.32 Å	2.3 Å	3.8 Å

Conversion factor of nucleic acid

Average molecular weight of DNA base pair = 650 Dalton
1 piconode of DNA = 1000 base pair = 0.66 microgram
1 A_{260} unit = ~ 33 microgram /mL of single-stranded DNA
1 A_{260} unit = ~ 40 microgram / mL of double-stranded RNA
1 A_{260} unit = ~ 50 microgram / mL of single-stranded DNA
A_{260} unit is the absorbance by nucleic acid at 260 nm
1000 base pair of DNA (in exon)
= 333 amino acids = 37000 Dalton protein

Human genome project

The Human Genome Project (HGP) is an international scientific research project with a primary goal of determining the sequence of chemical base pairs which makeup DNA and to identify and map the approximately 20,000-25,000 genes of the human genome from both physical and functional standpoint. A parallel project was conducted outside of government by the Celera Corporation, which was formally launched in 1998. Most of the government-sponsored sequencing was performed in universities and research centres from the United States, the United Kingdom, Japan, France, Germany and China. The mapping of human genes is an important step in the development of medicines and other aspects of healthcare. Following table gives a brief history of development and completion of human genome project in connection with genomes of other organisms.

Years	Contributors (Person/Organisation)	Contributions
Mid 1980	Watson and Crick, and Sanger	Ideological origin of human genome project based on previous information about DNA, i.e. its structure by Watson and Crick, development of sequencing techniques by Sanger.
1988	National Institute of Health and Department of Energy, USA	These agencies were funded by government for making coordination in the research of human genome.
1988	James Watson	Appointed as Head to lead Human Genome Research at NIH in a separate office of human genome research which was later called as National Centre for Human Genome Research (NCHGR).
1990	–	Initial planning was made by desiging a report 'Understanding Our Genetic Inheritance: The Human Genome Project, The First Five Years, FY 1991-1995.' The aim of this report was to plan out the goals of study on human genome.
1992	Michael Gottesman and Francis S Collins	Watson resigned and Michael Gottesman was appointed as Director of the NCHGR. Francis S Collins was latter appointed as Director of the centre.
1992	NIH and DOE	Second generation human genetic map was developed. Rapid data guidelines established by NIH and DOE.
1993	NCHGR	1990th Five Year Plan updated and Second Five Year Plan introduced. Sanger Centre founded which was later called Welcome Trust Sanger Institute.
1994	–	Human genome project's human genetic mapping goal achieved.
1995	–	HGP's physical mapping goal achieved. First bacterial genome (*H. influenzae*) sequenced.
1996	–	First human gene map established. Pilot project for human genome sequencing began in USA. First archeal genome sequenced. Yeast (*S. cerevisiae*) genome sequenced. HGP's mouse genetic mapping goal achieved.
1997	NCHGR	NCHGR received full status of institute at NIH. It is now called as National Human Genome Research Institute (NHGRI). Department of energy forms joint genome institute. *E. coli* genome was sequenced.
1998	NHGRI	Third Five Year Plan was announced. Incorporation of 30,000 genes into human genome sequenced. Single nucleotide polymorphism initiative begins.

Years	Contributors (Person/Organisation)	Contributions
1999	–	Full scale human sequencing began. Sequence of first human chromosome, i.e. chromosome 22 completed.
2000	Bill Clinton and Tony Blair (President of USA and Prime Minister of UK, respectively)	Majority of human genome had been sequenced. A rough draft announced jointly by Bill Clinton and Tony Blair on June 26, 2000. They supported the free access of the data of human genome. Fruitfly (*D. melanogaster*) genome sequenced. Mustard cress (*A. thaliana*) genome sequenced.
2001	Nature magazine	90% of the genome sequence was published in 'Nature' magazine. Draft version of rice genome sequence completed and published.
2002	–	Draft version of mouse genome sequence completed and published. Draft version of rice genome sequence completed and published.
2003	–	In April 2003, Human Genome Project was completed.
Latest about human genome project		
2003	Nature magazine	Human chromosome 6,7,Y,14 published.
2004	Nature magazine	Human chromosome 16,5,9,10,19,13,18 published.
2005	Nature magazine	Haplotype map of human genome published. Human chromosome 4, 2, X published.
2006	Nature magazine	Human chromosome 1,3,17,15,11,12,8, published.

Ageing symptoms of human body

Organs	Ageing symptoms
Arteries	Cholesterol and calcium buildup, walls thicken, arteries harden, high blood pressure, risk of heart attack.
Bladder	Connective tissue weakens, lower capacity to store urine and reduced efficiency of emptying content.
Blood	White blood cells and red blood cells count decrease.
Body weight	Weight declines between age 55 and 75, due to mostly loss of lean tissue, muscle mass, water and bone.
Bones	Loss of bone cells accelerates at about age 35, bones become porous and brittle in the demineralising process. Osteoporosis is common in women.
Brain	Gradual loss of brain tissue (5-10% by age 90), slow reaction and faltering memory.
Breast	Mammary (milk secreting) glands reduce in size, as does the breast.
Ear	Gradual loss of the ability to hear higher frequencies, starting around age of 30; hair grows in auditory canal.
Eye	More far-sighted problem with focusing, difficulty in adjusting to light intensity, perception of hues alter.
Face	Wrinkles, facial hair, bags under the eyes, double chin, longer ears, thinning cheek.
Fat	Fat content and distribution change, storage increases.
Hair	Greying, thinning, balding.
Heart	Thickening of heart wall, gradual loss of effectiveness as a pumping machine.
Hormones	The level of several hormones, e.g. GH, DHEA, IGF, falls with age, may be a major cause on ageing.
Immunity	Body's power to combat infection declines, autoimmune responses increase.
Joints	Cartilage becomes cracks and frays, cushioning fluid gets thinner, tendons and ligaments are less resilient.
Kidneys	Weight and volume of the kidneys shrink, marked reduction in the cleansing of impurities from the blood.
Liver	The ageing process does not affect the liver adversely. Only colour changes occur.
Lungs	Loses elasticity and capacity (40% between ages 20 and 80), increasing difficulty to oxygenate blood.
Metabolism	Ability to metabolise sugar decreases with age, reduction of food intake may prolong life.
Muscles	Loss of muscular mass, partly due to unuse, other causes include loss of blood flow and energy supply.
Nerve	Demyelination - loss of myelin covering of nerve fibres, which is a characteristic of neurological disorders.
Nose	Ability to smell declines after age 65, amount of reduction varies widely between individuals.
Prostate	Reduction in semen making after 60, enlargement in size may cause difficulty to urinate.
Reaction time	Mental and physical responses to specific stimuli become slower.
Reproductive system	Women go through menopause at the age of 45-50; reduced level of oestrogen affects the whole body. Men's reproductive change with age is more likely to undergo reduction than a cessation.
Skin	Wrinkles (related to decreased mitochondrial function), dryness and dark spots.

Organs	Ageing symptoms
Teeth	Teeth gum recession.
Thermoregu-lation	Response to changes in environmental temperature becomes impaired.
Tongue	Sense of taste loses only gradually with age, with equal reduction of all flavours.
Voice	Voice becomes weak and muffled.

GH - Growth Hormone, DHA - Dehydroandrosterone, IGF - Insulin/Insulin-like Growth Factor (GF).

ELISA test

Enzyme Linked Immunosorbent Assay (ELISA) is a very sensitive immunological and serological (because it uses antibody containing sera) test employed to determine an unknown antigens (bacterium, virus, toxin, etc.) with the help of a known antibody. The test is based on specific antibody interaction involving labelling of known antibody with specific enzyme.

The method of measurement of the amount of antigen (Ag) or antibody (Ab) by the addition of a labelled reagent is referred to as Immuno Assays. When radio isotopic labels are used in the measurement, the technique is known as **Radio Immuno Assay** (RIA).

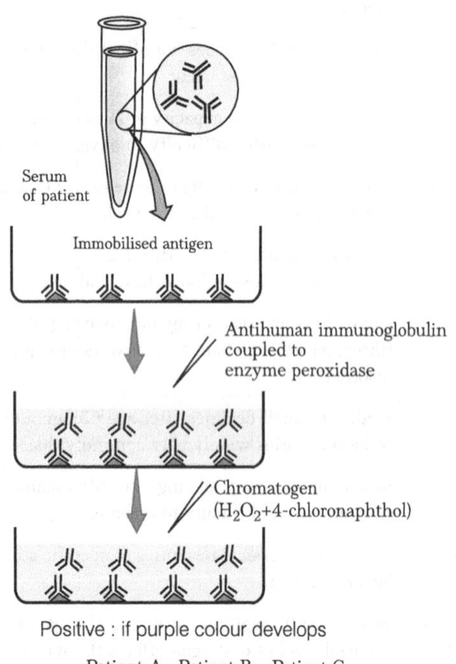

Enzyme Linked Immunosorbent Assay (ELISA)

When enzyme labels are used in the determination, then the technique is known as **Enzyme Linked Immunosorbent Assay** (ELISA). It is a standard test for detecting the presence of antibody directed against HIV. ELISA is the most widely used test in serological diagnosis. It is well used for the detection of viruses, fungi, bacteria, MLOs (Mycoplasma Like Organisms), mycotoxins and hormones. It is a rapid test with high sensitivity and specificity that make it a most important test in the diagnosis of many diseases.

Lipid profile

Blood cholesterol tests measure the levels of lipids (fatty acids), cholesterol and low density lipoprotein, very low density lipoprotein and high density lipoprotein and triglycerides in the blood. Elevated lipid levels indicate heart disease or stroke which may be due to smoking, overweight or diabetes mellitus.

The two important cholesterol types are HDL (High-Density Lipoprotein) and LDL (Low-Density Lipoprotein).
HDL have protective effect against atherosclerosis whereas high blood level of LDL is a risk factor, as increased LDL causes increased plasma fluidity. Total blood cholesterol of more than 200 mg/dL is considered harmful, optimal LDL levels are below 100 mg/dL.

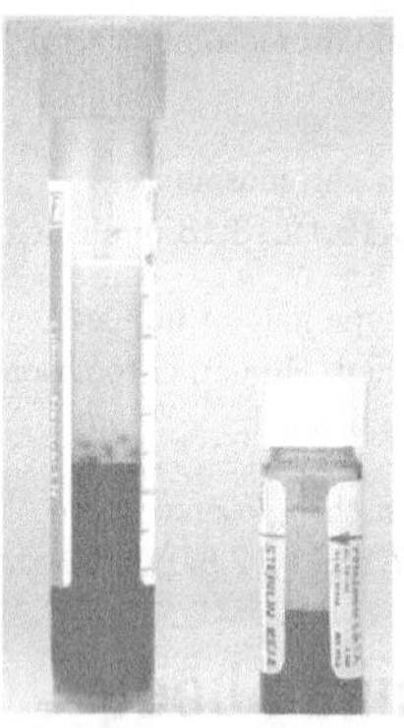
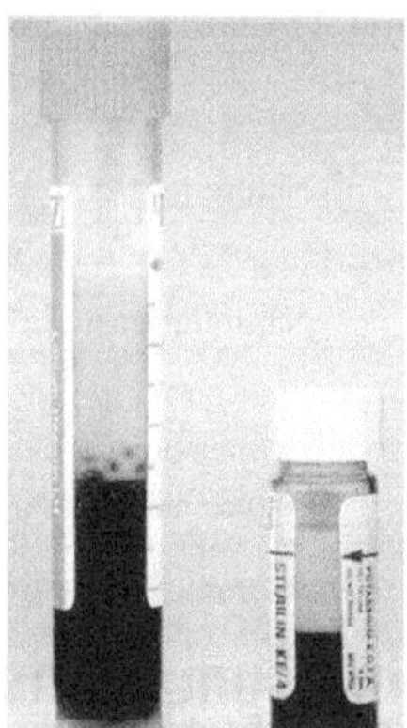

Tubes containing lipids in the upper layers

External prosthetics

In medicine, a prosthesis is an artificial device that replaces a missing body parts which may be lost through trauma, disease or congenital defects. It initially included artificial limbs (hands and legs) and artificial teeth. The modern technology has developed body powered arms, sockets, wrists, foot, knee joints, etc. Besides this, myoelectric arms enables a patient to control the movement of prosthetic wrists and hands.

In India, Dr. PK Sethi from Jaipur has designed Jaipur foot which resembles natural foot. He used rubber and aluminium to make this prosthetic device. Robotic prosthetic is a new energy research area for solving disabled person's problems.

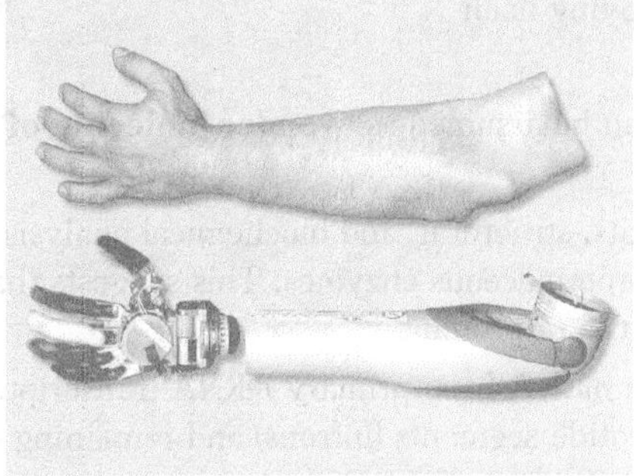

Cloning milestones

Cloning is the creation of an organism that is an exact genetic copy of another. This means that every single bit of DNA is the same between the two. Here are some milestones in the field of cloning of living organisms.

Years	Events
1938	Cloning envisioned. Dr Hans Spemann (Germany) proposed an experiment to remove the nucleus from an unfertilised egg and replace it with the nucleus from a differentiated cell.
1953	Structure of DNA (Deoxyribonucleic Acid) discovered by Francis C Crick (UK) and James D Watson (US).
1970	Dr John B Gurdon (UK) cloned a frog by transplanting the intestinal cell of a tadpole into an enucleated frog egg, which developed into an adult frog.
1973	First successful gene splicing (Recombinant DNA) by Paul Berg and Stanley N Cohen (US). A major breakthrough in genetic engineering.
1978	Birth of first child, conceived by *in vitro* (literally in glass) fertilisation to Leslie Brown (UK).
1980	US Supreme Court rules that a genetically created new bacterium (a non-natural man-made microorganism) may be patented.
1984	Dr Steen M Willesden (Denmark) cloned a lamb from a developing sheep embryo cell. His experiment was repeated by other scientists who cloned a variety of animals.
1994	Dr Ned First (US) cloned calves from the cells of early embryos.
1995	Dr Ian Wilmut and Keith Campbell (UK) created the world's first cloned sheep, Megan and Morag, from embryo cells.
1996	Dr Ian Wilmut and his team cloned the world's first sheep from adult cells. The lamb born in July 1996 was named 'Dolly'.
1997	Scientists at Oregon Regional Primate Research Centre (US) created first primates-two rhesus monkeys named Neti and Ditto-from DNA taken from cells of developing monkey embryos. They ware not genetically identical because two different embryos were used.
1997	A team led by Dr Ian Wilmut and Keith Campbell (UK) created the first sheep with a human gene in every cell of its body. The genetically engineered lamb was named 'Polly'.
1999	Dr Gerald Schatten (US) lead a team of researchers who became the first to create a clone (Tetra, a rhesus monkey) by embryo splitting.
1999	Dr Xiangzhong Yang lead a US experiment to clone calves from frozen cells taken from a Japanese bull. The experiment was successful and proved that cells can be stored for later cloning.
2000	The first patents for cloning were given to the scientists who cloned 'Dolly', giving their company, Geron Bio-med, exclusive right to the technologies they used.
2000	Japanese scientists cloned a baby bull from a bull that was a clone itself, the first recloning case involving a large mammal.
2000	Five piglets were cloned by a company, they eventually wanted to reproduce organs for humans.
2001	Scientists at Advanced Cell Technology in Massachusetts cloned human embryos for the first time.
2001	President Bush limits federally funded human embryonic stem cell research to stem cell lines that have already been created.
2001	A cat, called CC for 'carbon copy' was cloned by a company that wanted to go into business of reproducing pets.
2002	California became the first US state to approve a law legalising the therapeutic cloning of embryos.
2003	Britain became the first country to issue research licences for human embryonic cloning to create stem cells. It specifies therapeutic, not reproductive and cloning.
2004	Britain announces the first embryonic stem cell bank.
2005	South Korea cloned a dog names 'Snuppy'. Dogs are considered particularly difficult to clone because of their complex reproductive biology.

Ribozyme : The only non-proteinaceous enzyme

The key step in the evolution of life was the evolution of RNA molucule. It is because RNA could copy both, carry information and cause chemical reactions to happen. In fact, biologists suggest that RNA occupied centre stage and performed most jobs in the cells like

(i) Storing genetic information (ii) Copying itself

(iii) Performing basic metabolic functions

So, how it is proved that RNA was the first molecule of heredity and can be assumed as **'wonder molecule of early life'**.

Although, the ribosome is made up of both RNA and protein components, structural and biochemical analysis reveals that mechanism central to translation is catalysed by RNA and not by proteinaceous enzymes. This suggests that the use of RNA by early lifeforms to carryout chemical reaction proceeded the use of proteins.

The recent researches have proved that in the maturation of eukaryotic *m*RNA from primary *m*RNA transcript, only about 25% of RNA molecules are converted to *m*RNA by excising nucleotide segments (introns) and remaining sequences (exons) are sliced back together before translation.

This complex process is carried out with the help of a large complex called **spliceosome**. It comprises of 150 proteins and 5 RNA and is 100-300 nucleotides long and is complexed with many proteins. These RNA protein complexes are called **small nuclear RNAs** (*sn* RNAs). These have catalytic functions in the process of splicing.

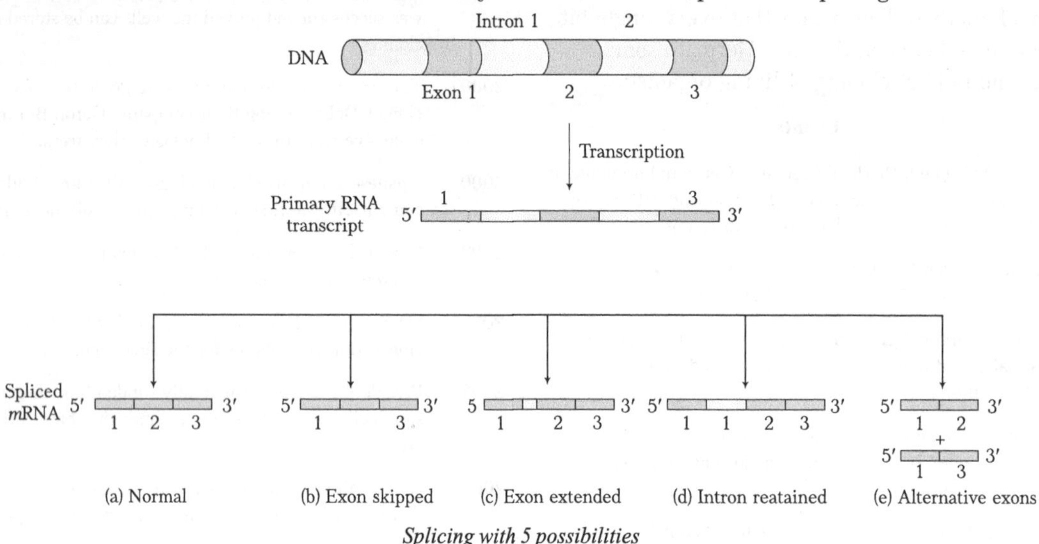

Splicing with 5 possibilities

A remarkable event was noticed in the splicing of a ribosomal RNA precursor in ciliate *Tetrahymena.* Here, the intron is found to work as an enzyme in catalysing the splicing reaction. This self splicing *Tetrahymena* RNA molecule was the first example of a RNA molecule that could function as an enzyme in catalysing a chemical reaction. Such enzymatic RNA molecules are usually called **ribozymes** (Thomas Cech, 1981). For his discovery of ribozymes, Thomas Cech got the Nobel Prize of 1986.

MULTI-COLOURED PICTURES & DIAGRAMS

Biology as a subject always requires visualisation of concept for better understanding. Thus, some diagrams & pictures are given below with coloured visual effects to improve your grafting.

Immune system

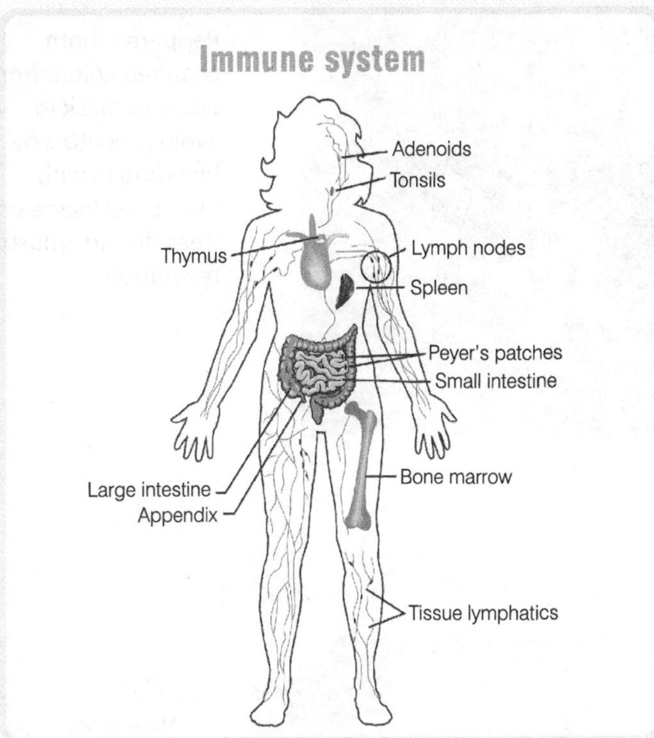

Immune system is a complex system of cellular and molecular components whose primary function is to distinguish self from non-self and defence against foreign organisms or substances. Various organs related to immune system are listed in the diagram.

Antibody structure

1. Fab region
2. Fc region
3. Heavy chain with one variable domain (VH) followed by a constant domain (CH_1), a hinge region, and two more constant domains (CH_2 and CH_3).
4. Light chain with one variable (VL) and one constant (CL) domain
5. Antigen binding site (Paratope)
6. Hinge regions

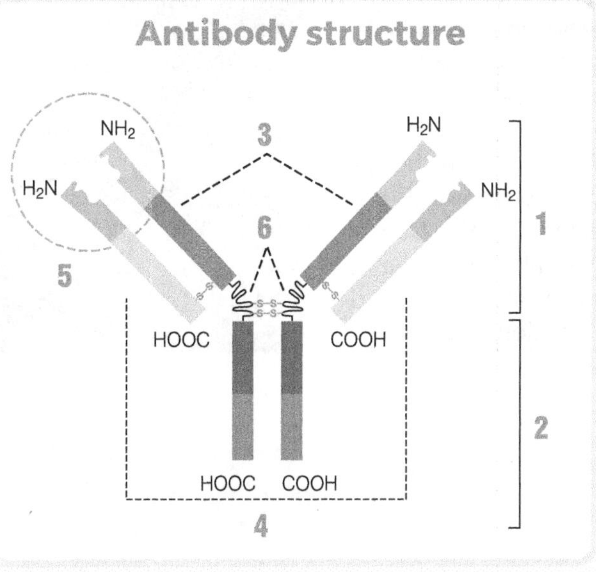

Industrial melanism

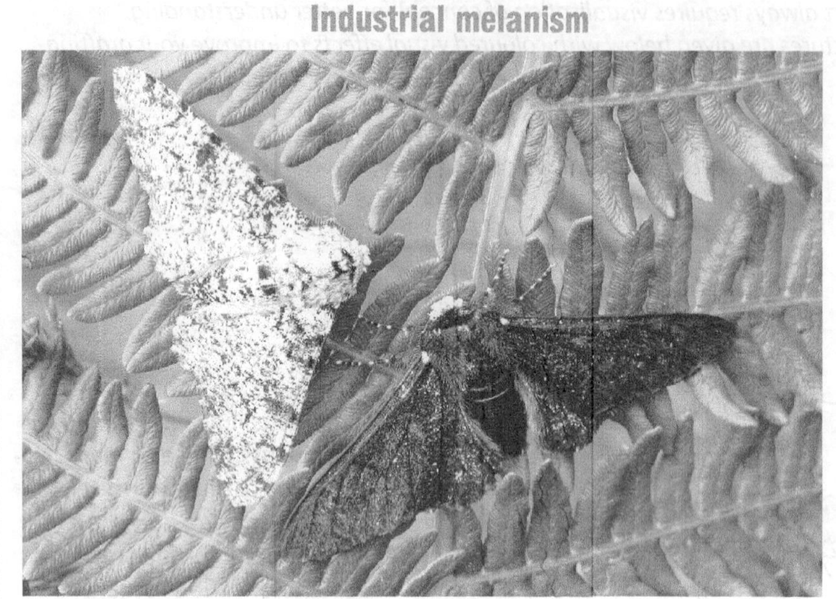

Peppered moth changed colour from white to black to avoid predators by blending in with blackened leaves on trees during industrial revolution.

HIV infecting macrophage

Macrophage

Virus infects macrophage

Macrophage attack

HIV

This illustration depicts white blood cells swarming to attack HIV (AIDS virus). A recent genetic studies showed that the stage of HIV infection in some people does not progress to AIDS. It is related to the presence of certain amino acids in the body that can destroy cells infected with HIV. Due to these amino acids, the stage of HIV infection did not develop into AIDS.

Genetically engineered tomato

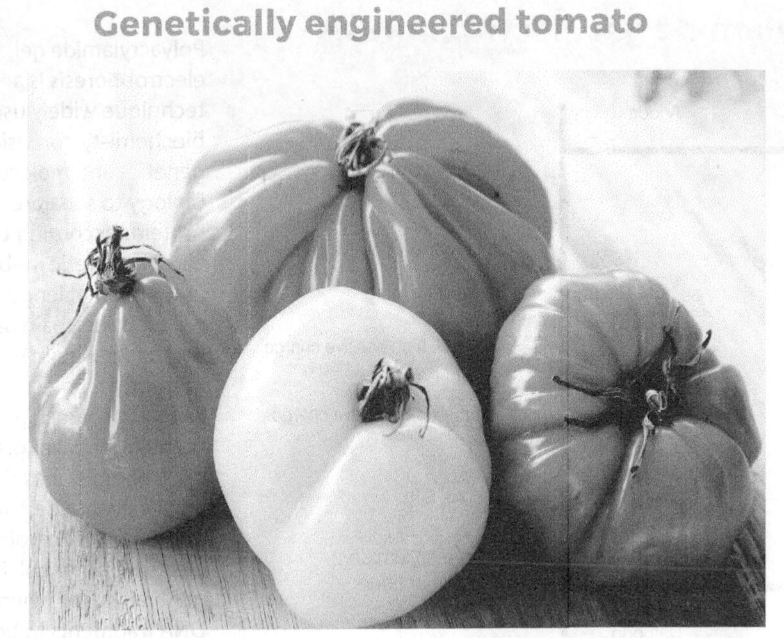

The photograph shows the genetically-engineered redish tomato made by inserting genes of a pigment called anthocyanin. So, these are anthocyanin rich tomato varieties. Anthocyanin is a water-soluble pigment that may appear red, purple, or blue according to pH. These are powerful antioxidant. The increase in antioxidant capacity of blood seen after the consumption of anthocyanin-rich foods may not be caused directly by the anthocyanin in food, but instead by increased uric acid levels derived from metabolising flavonoids in the food.

Infection by *Rhizobium* on the roots of leguminous plants

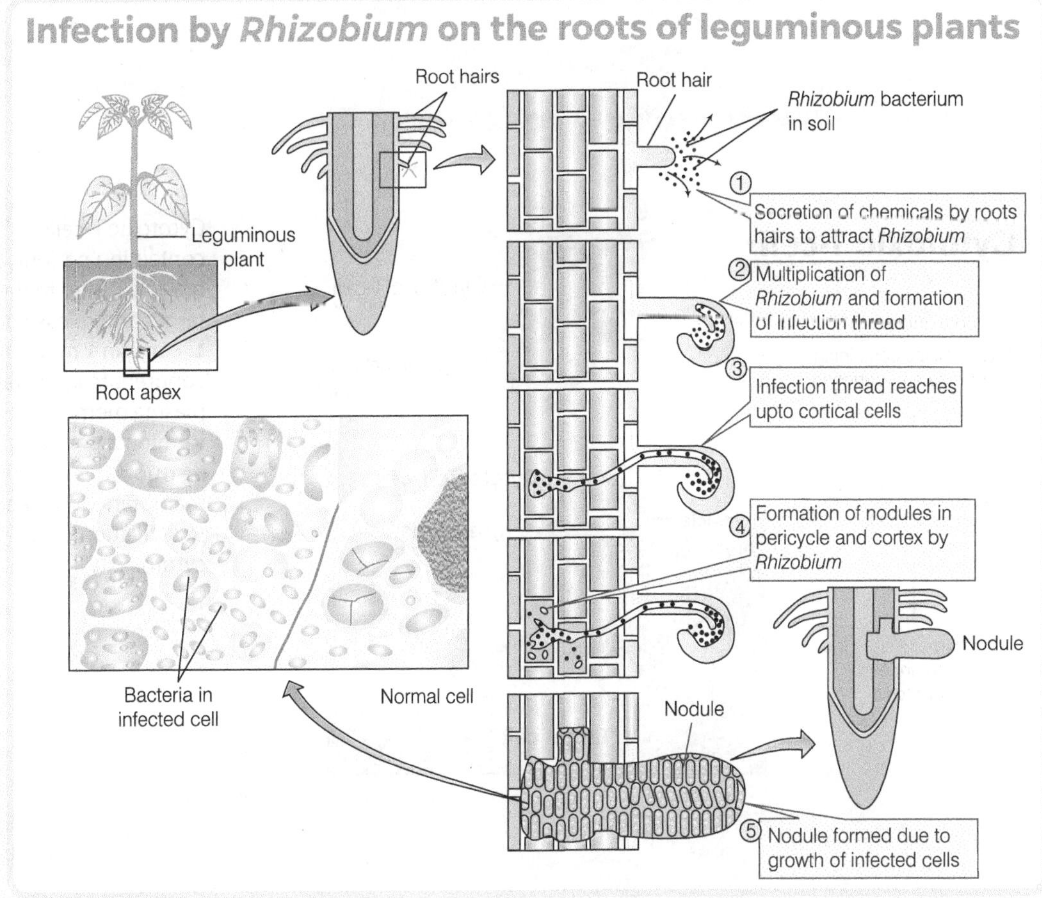

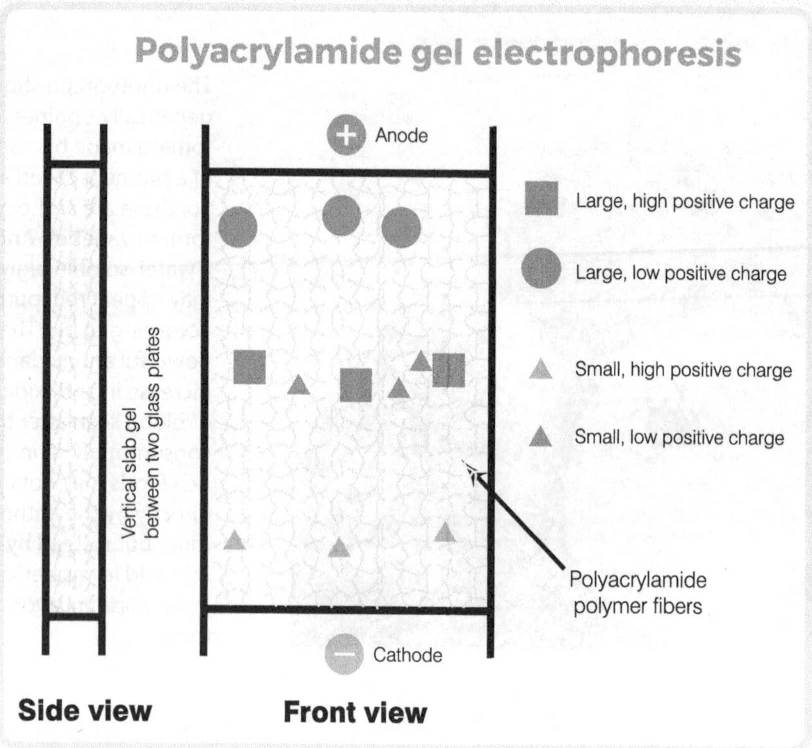

Polyacrylamide gel electrophoresis is a technique widely used in biochemisty, forensics, genetics and molecular biology to separate proteins according to their electrophoretic mobility (a function of length of polypeptide chain or molecular weight). It is a method of molecular separation which relies on the differential migration rates of molecules through a polyacrylamide matrix upon application of an electrical potential. PAGE, is generally used when the DNA fragments to be separated are small.

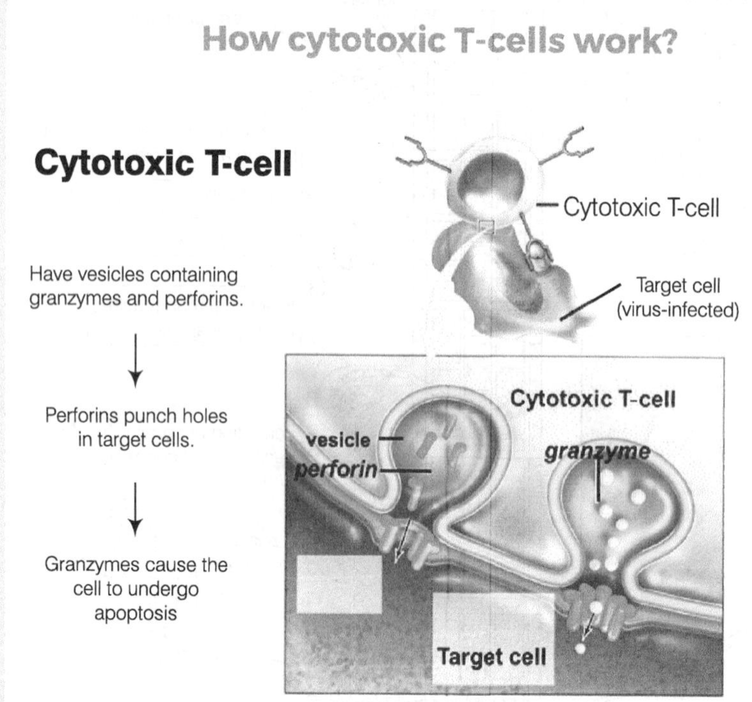

Cytotoxic T-cells containing perforin 1 granules, bind to their target and release perforin 1. Perforin 1 molecules congregate in the target plasma membrane, forming a pore that distrupts the plasma membrane thus, leading to activation of cell cytotoxicity.

Diagrams showing embryonic similarities amongst different vertebrates

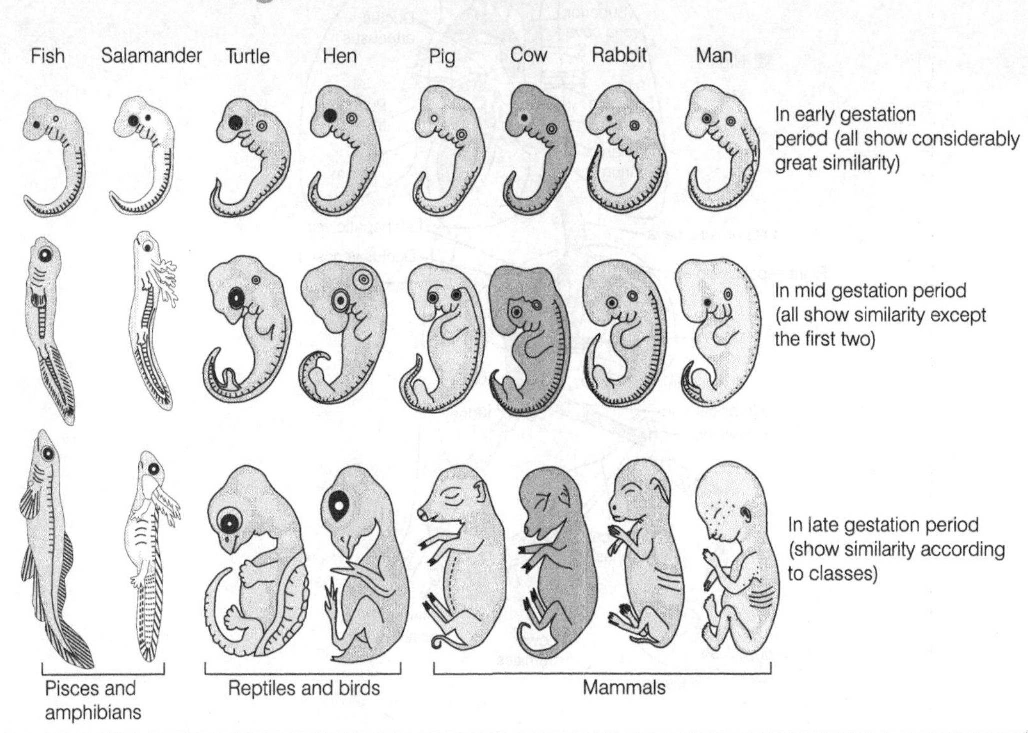

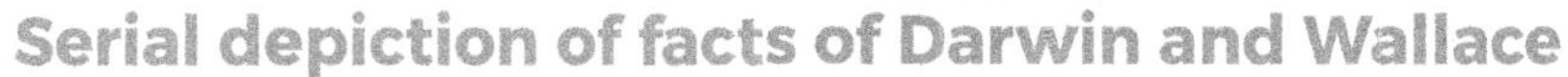

Serial depiction of facts of Darwin and Wallace

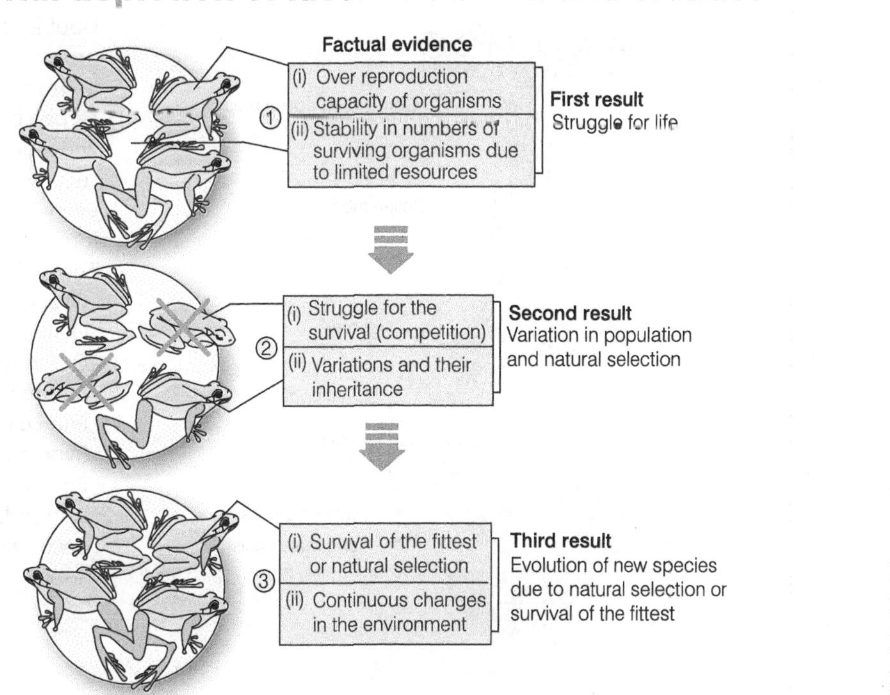

Foetal circulation

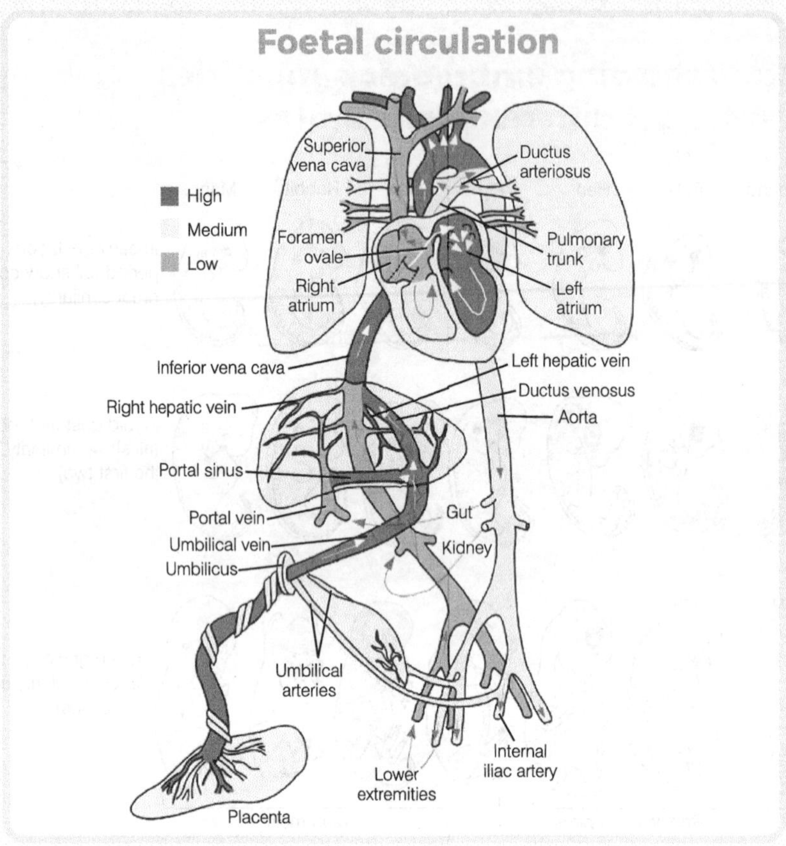

Double fertilisation shown in LS of flower

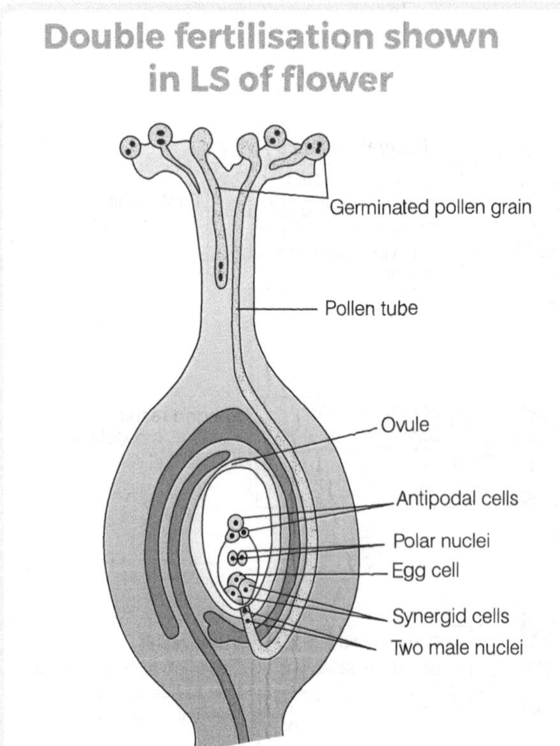

Double fertilisation is unique process found in angiosperms. In this process, two male nuclei are carried by pollen tube, one fuses with egg cell and other with secondary nucleus. After this, every part of the flower changes into the some part of fruit/seed. These changes are as follows :

- Ovary wall – fruit wall
- Ovule – seed
- Outer integument and inner integument – seed coat
- Funiculus – stalk
- Synergids – get destroyed
- Egg cell – embryo
- Antipodal cell – get destroyed
- Secondary nucleus – endosperm.

DNA organisation in eukaryotes

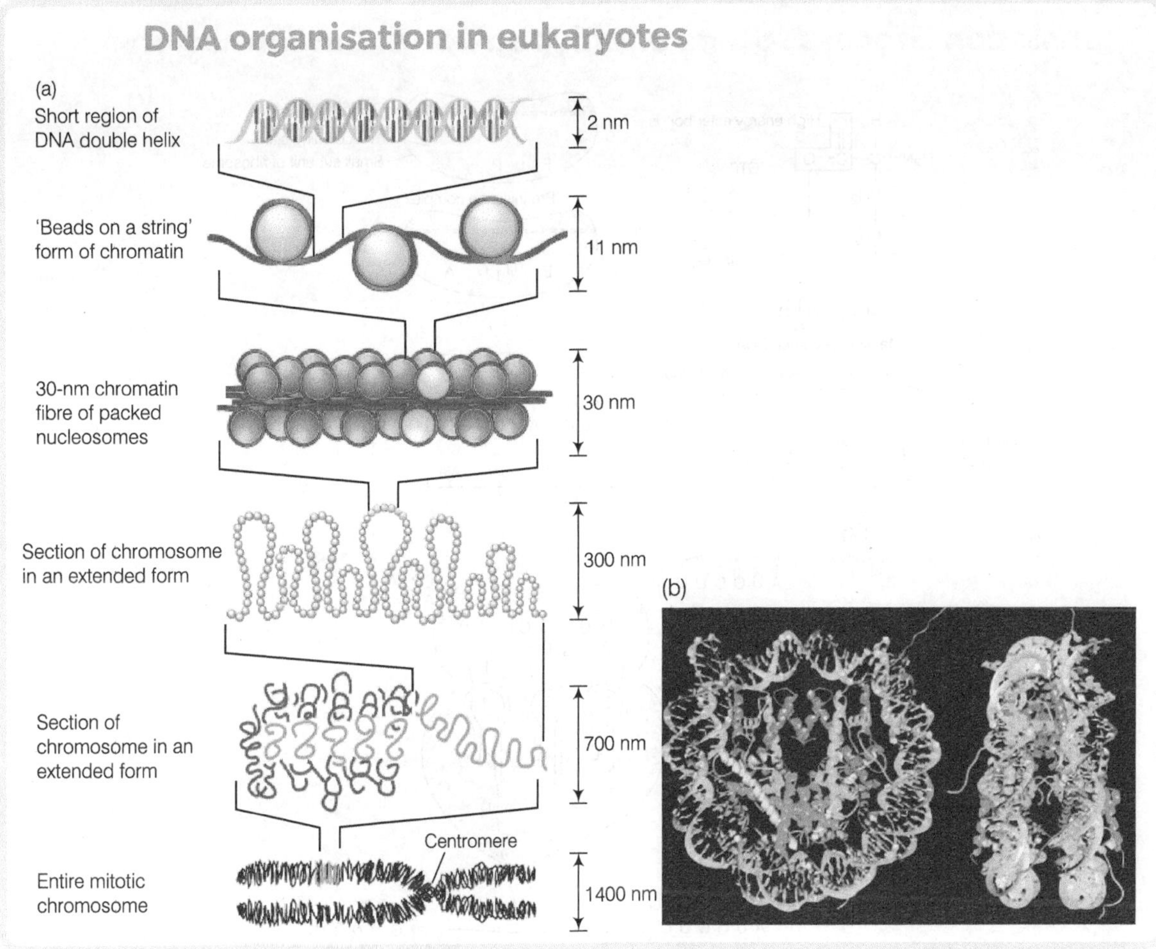

Oogenesis and follicular development

Vitelline layer
Protein receptors
Egg plasma membrane
Egg cytoplasm
Mitochondrial material
Nucleus
Actin
Acrosomal granule
Jelly coat
Perivitelline space
Cortical granule content
Cortical granule
Acrosome reaction
Fused plasma membrane

Plasma membrane of sperm and the outer membrane of acrosome fuse and the membrane breakdown, releasing enzyme that allow the sperm to penetrate the corona radiata. Sperm digest their way through the zona pellucida *via* enzymes associated with the inner acrosomal membrane. Sperms are engulfed by the oocyte plasma membrane. Cortical granules are released when the sperm cell contacts the membrane. These granules cause other sperm in contact with the membrane to detatch from it.

Translation process : Steps of polypeptide chain formation

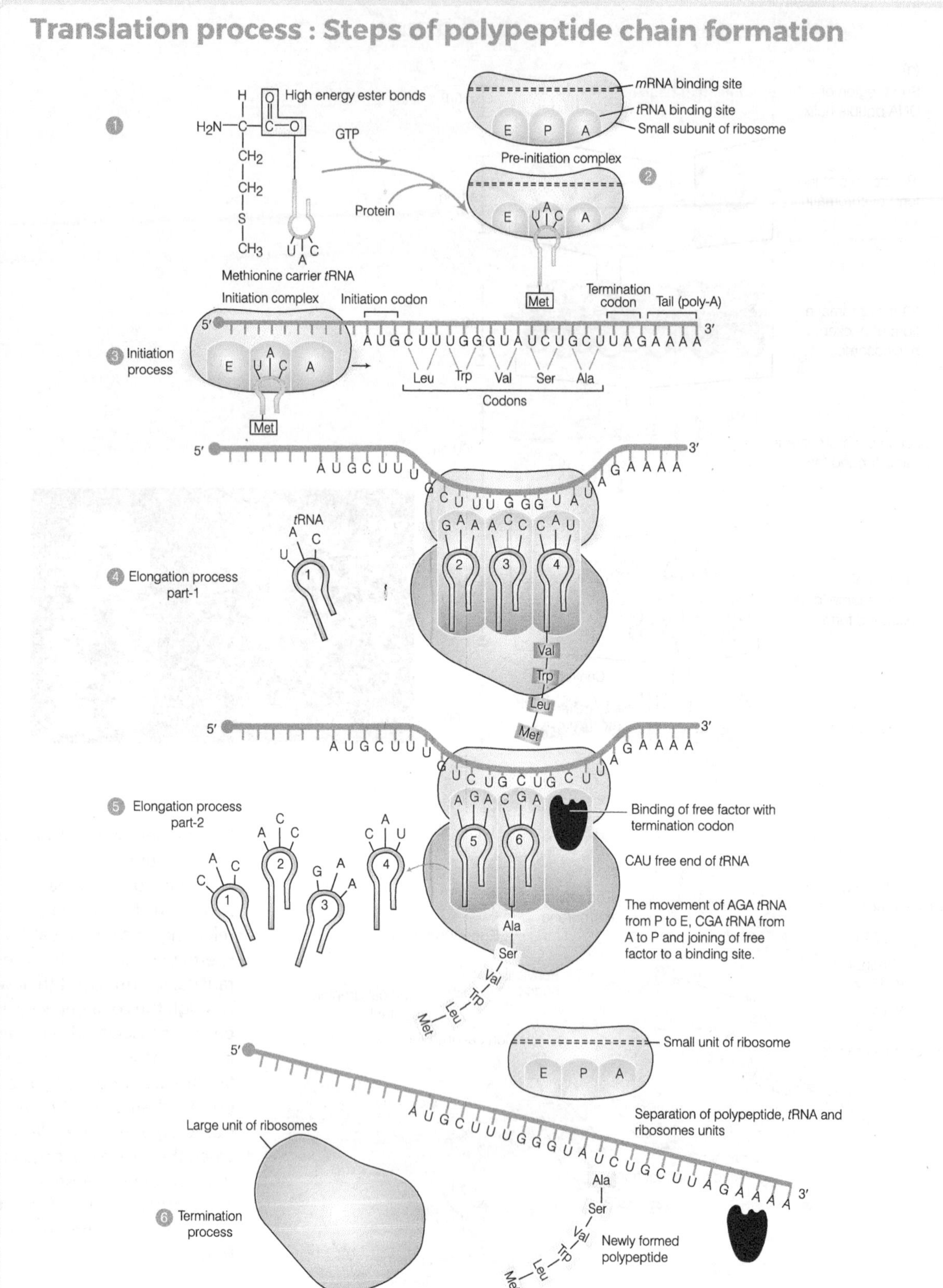